Applied Nutrition, Dietetics and Biochemistry for Basic BSc Nursing

Applied Nutrition, Dietetics and Biochemistry for Basic BSc Nursing

Previously known as Essentials of Nutrition and Biochemistry for Basic BSc Nursing

As per the Revised INC Syllabus for BSc Nursing

I Clement

PhD (Nursing) MSc (Nursing) Medical Surgical Nursing
MBA (Education) MSW (Master of Social Work) MA (Sociology) MSc (Physiology) MA (Child Care and Education)
Postgraduate Diploma in Hospital Administration

Presently
Professor and Head, Department of Research and Development
RV College of Nursing, Bengaluru, Karnataka, India

Former, Professor and Principal
Columbia College of Nursing
VSS College of Nursing, Bengaluru, Karnataka, India

Professional Assignment
PhD (N) Guide
INC PhD (N) Guide
Chief Editor for Nursing Journals
Rajiv Gandhi University of Health Sciences
Bengaluru, Karnataka, India

Professional Life Member
PhD Society of India, Chennai, Tamil Nadu, India
Nursing Research Society of India, New Delhi, India
Trained Nurses Association of India, New Delhi
Christian Medical Association of India, New Delhi
Indian Society of Psychiatric Nursing, Bengaluru
Medical Surgical Nursing Society of India, Chennai
Indian Society of Neuroscience Nursing, New Delhi
Asian Association of Cardiac Nurses, Kolkata, West Bengal, India

Health Organization Member
Indian Red Cross Society, Bengaluru
St Johns Ambulance Association, Bengaluru
General Secretary, Indian Society of Medical Surgical Nurses

Assignments and Examiner
Faculty of Nursing, RGUHS, Bengaluru, Karnataka, India
LIC Inspector, Chief Squad, Observer
PhD Research Guide, RGUHS, Bengaluru
UG and PG Examiner, Paper-setter, Valuator other Universities in India

Professional Activity and Editorial
MAT Nursing Journal Chief Editor and PUB Journals
Indian Journal of Practical Nursing
National Editorial Advisory Board, New Delhi
Nurses of India (Former) Bengaluru
Chairman-Souvenir Committee, Florence Nightingale Awards-2012

Winner
Florence Nightingale Awards-2013
Rajiv Gandhi Education Excellence Award

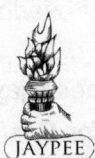

JAYPEE BROTHERS MEDICAL PUBLISHERS
The Health Sciences Publisher
New Delhi | London

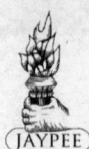 **Jaypee Brothers Medical Publishers (P) Ltd**

Headquarter
EMCA House
23/23-B, Ansari Road, Daryaganj
New Delhi 110 002, India
Landline: +91-11-23272143, +91-11-23272703
+91-11-23282021, +91-11-23245672
E-mail: jaypee@jaypeebrothers.com

Corporate Office
Jaypee Brothers Medical Publishers (P) Ltd.
4838/24, Ansari Road, Daryaganj
New Delhi 110 002, India
Phone: +91-11-43574357
Fax: +91-11-43574314
E-mail: jaypee@jaypeebrothers.com

Website: www.jaypeebrothers.com
Website: www.jaypeedigital.com

Overseas Office
JP Medical Ltd.
83, Victoria Street, London
SW1H 0HW (UK)
Phone: +44-20 3170 8910
Fax: +44(0)20 3008 6180
E-mail: info@jpmedpub.com

© 2022, Jaypee Brothers Medical Publishers

The views and opinions expressed in this book are solely those of the original contributor(s)/author(s) and do not necessarily represent those of editor(s) and publisher of the book.

All rights reserved. No part of this publication may be reproduced, stored or transmitted in any form or by any means, electronic, mechanical, photocopying, recording or otherwise, without the prior permission in writing of the publishers.

All brand names and product names used in this book are trade names, service marks, trademarks or registered trademarks of their respective owners. The publisher is not associated with any product or vendor mentioned in this book.

Medical knowledge and practice change constantly. This book is designed to provide accurate, authoritative information about the subject matter in question. However, readers are advised to check the most current information available on procedures included and check information from the manufacturer of each product to be administered, to verify the recommended dose, formula, method and duration of administration, adverse effects and contraindications. It is the responsibility of the practitioner to take all appropriate safety precautions. Neither the publisher nor the author(s)/editor(s) assume any liability for any injury and/or damage to persons or property arising from or related to use of material in this book.

This book is sold on the understanding that the publisher is not engaged in providing professional medical services. If such advice or services are required, the services of a competent medical professional should be sought.

Every effort has been made where necessary to contact holders of copyright to obtain permission to reproduce copyright material. If any have been inadvertently overlooked, the publisher will be pleased to make the necessary arrangements at the first opportunity.

Inquiries for bulk sales may be solicited at: jaypee@jaypeebrothers.com

Applied Nutrition, Dietetics and Biochemistry for Basic BSc Nursing
First Edition: 2018
Second Edition: **2022**
ISBN: 978-93-5465-796-2
Printed at Rajkamal Electric Press, Kundli, Haryana.

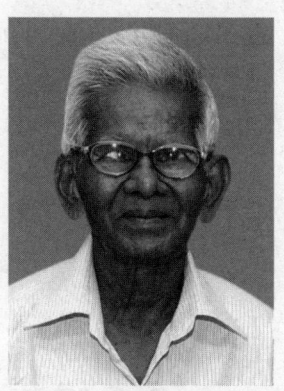

Dedicated to
My Beloved Father
Mr Irudayanathan (Late)

Preface to the Second Edition

Nursing as a profession and a discipline utilizes knowledge derived from arts, sciences (physical, biological and behavioral), humanities and human experience. Nursing science incorporates clinical competence, critical thinking, communication, teaching learning, professionalism, and caring and cultural competency. Nurses collaborate with other health disciplines to solve individual and community health problems. Nursing facilitates evidence-based practice, compassionate caring among its practitioners in response to emerging issues in healthcare and new discoveries and technologies in profession. Nursing practice requires personal commitment to professional development and life-long learning.

Textbook on applied nutrition, dietetics and biochemistry for BSc Nursing students [as per New Indian Nursing Council (INC) Syllabus] has 23 chapters, 14 chapters framed for nutrition and dietetics, 9 chapters framed for biochemistry, prepared carefully in simple language with adequate tables, diagrams, chemical structures and clinical aspects for easy understanding of the basic nutrition and biochemistry.

The book has glossary, review questions are given at the end of each chapter for better understanding.

Applied nutrition and dietetics, the subject is designed to assist the students to acquire basic knowledge and understanding of the principles of nutrition and dietetics and apply this knowledge in the practice of nursing. The students will be able to identify the importance of nutrition in health and wellness, apply nutrient and dietary modifications in caring patients, explain the principles and practices of nutrition and dietetics identify nutritional needs of different age groups and plan a balanced diet for them, dietary principles for different diseases. Plan therapeutic diet for patients suffering from various disease conditions and prepare meals using different methods and cookery rules.

Applied biochemistry, the subject is designed to assist the students to acquire knowledge of the normal biochemical composition and functioning of human body, its alterations in disease conditions and to apply this knowledge in the practice of nursing. This book has complete coverage of subjects for the students will be able to—describe the metabolism of carbohydrates and its alterations, the metabolism of lipids and its alterations, metabolism of proteins and amino acids and its alterations, clinical enzymology in various disease conditions, acid base balance, imbalance and its clinical significance, metabolism of hemoglobin and its clinical significance, different function tests and interpret the findings and immunochemistry.

I wish all the best for all nursing students.

I Clement

Preface to the First Edition

Nursing is a noble profession that is integrated with scientific principles and can be practiced well only when the nurses are sound in their knowledge and have good attitude to empathize any patient under their care and provide quality nursing care by updating their knowledge and skill.

Understanding basic requirement of macronutrients and micronutrients demands in human body and its metabolism help every nurse to plan better nursing care since administering the medications and carrying out the doctor's order will never bring a complete health; to attain a complete health, an appropriate healthy diet and its adaptation in daily life is important to lead a healthy life.

In collaboration with dietitian every nurse should know about all different types of therapeutic diet, balanced diet and its importance. Nurse should understand complete perspective of nutrition and biochemistry to give better care for the patients.

This book on *Essentials of Nutrition and Biochemistry for Basic BSc Nursing* in nursing will definitely help every Basic BSc Nursing student to understand the basic nutrition and biochemistry and its application in nursing care. This book has totally 19 chapters, 11 chapters framed for nutrition and 8 chapters for biochemistry framed carefully in simple language with adequate tables and diagrams for easy understanding of the basic nutrition and biochemistry.

The book has glossary and exercises are given at the end of each chapter for better understanding; to attain good clarity on the content and also has previous years' question papers from the 2015 to 2008 which will help the students to understand the subject better and all these topics are designed based on Indian Nursing Council (INC) requirements.

This book will be student-friendly guide for BSc Nursing students and also a refreshing book for teachers.

First of all I would like to thank my God for showering me abundant blessing to complete this book successfully, then my parents for their powerful prayers and my beloved wife, for her constant support and care to finish this book.

I wish all the best for all nursing students.

I Clement

Acknowledgments

I am thankful to the Lord Almighty who strengthens me with his abundant blessing through innumerable means, helping me in all my accomplishment. My heartfelt thanks to Shri Sommana, Minister of Karnataka and Chairman of VSS Group of Institutions, Bengaluru, Karnataka, India, for his constant support and encouragement. My sincere thanks to my Guru Dr BT Basavanthappa, Principal, Rajarajeswari College of Nursing, Bengaluru, Karnataka, India and Professor PV Ramachandran, Chairman, College of Nursing, Sri Ramachandra University, Chennai, Tamil Nadu, India, a great philosopher and internationally renowned teacher of nursing, who helped me in discovering the world of knowledge. I am thankful to Ms Shylaja Sommana, Managing Directors: Dr BS Naveen, Dr BS Arun and Ms Divya from VSS Group of Institutions, Bengaluru, for their support and encouragement. I am also grateful to Dr BC Bhagavan, Syndicate Member of RGUHS, Bengaluru, Professor, Department of Surgery, Kempegowda Institute of Medical Sciences, Bengaluru, Karnataka, India and Dr Aswathnarayanan MLA, Deputy Chief Minister of Karnataka, Chairman, Padmashree Group of Institutions, Bengaluru, Karnataka, India. Special thanks to Dr Gajender Singh Principal, RV College of Nursing, Bengaluru. Special thanks to Dr TV Ramakrishnan, Professor of Anesthesiology and Head, Clinical Services, Department of Accident and Emergency Medicine, Sri Ramachandra University, Chennai, India; Dr Jeyaseelan Manickam Devadassan, Syndicate Member, The Tamil Nadu Dr MGR Medical University, Chennai, Dean, Annai JKK Sampoorani Ammal College of Nursing, Erode, Tamil Nadu, India; Dr Tamilmani, Principal, Annai JKK Sampoorani Ammal College of Nursing, Erode, Tamil Nadu, India, Professor Mrs Jessie Sudarsanum, Head, Department of Medical Surgical Nursing, Annai JKK Sampoorani Ammal College of Nursing, Erode, Tamil Nadu, India and all my teachers and students. I convey my sincere thanks to my beloved parents, brothers and sisters and my wife Nisha Clement for her continuous support and constant encouragement in each step of my life. I take this opportunity to thank my little ones, Cibin, Cynthia and Cavin. I extend thanks to my beloved friend and brother, Mr Regi T Kurien, USA.

I am very grateful to the whole team of M/s Jaypee Brothers Medical Publishers (P) Ltd, New Delhi, India, who helped and guided me, Shri Jitendar P Vij (Group Chairman), Mr Ankit Vij (Managing Director), Mr MS Mani (Group President), Dr Madhu Choudhary (Publishing Head-Education), Ms Pooja Bhandari (Production Head), Ms Sunita Katla (Executive Assistant to Group Chairman and Publishing Manager), Ms Samina Khan (Executive Assistant to Publishing Head-Education), Mr Rajesh Sharma (Production Coordinator), Ms Seema Dogra (Cover Visualizer), Mr Vakil Khan (Proofreader), Mr Ajeet Rathor (Typesetter), Mr Pappu Kumar (Graphic Designer) and their team members, for all their support to work in this project and make it a success. Without their cooperation, I could not have completed this project. I would also like to thank Mr Venugopal V (Associate Director-South), Mr Santhosh Kumar (Author Coordinator, Bengaluru), and other staff members of M/s Jaypee Brothers Medical Publisher (P) Ltd, Bengaluru branch.

Contents

Section 1: Applied Nutrition and Dietetics

1. **Introduction to Nutrition** 3
   - Definition 4
   - Nutrition: History and Concepts 4
   - History of Nutrition 5
   - Role of Nutrition in Maintaining Health 10
   - Facts About Basic Nutrition and Health 10
   - Importance of Nutrition in Health 11
   - Factors Affecting Food and Nutrition 13
   - Nutrients 14
   - Macro- and Micronutrients 15
   - Energy Yielding and Non-energy Yielding 16
   - Elements of Nutrients: Macro and Micro 16
   - Mineral Elements 20
   - Food 22
   - Five Food Group Plans 23
   - Basic Seven Food Groups 24
   - Functions of Food 24
   - Nutrition Problems in India 26
   - National Nutritional Policy 27
   - Role of Food and Medicinal Values 28
   - Nurses Role in Food and Nutrition 30

2. **Carbohydrates and Energy** 32
   - Definition and Meaning of Carbohydrate 33
   - Classifications of Carbohydrate 33
   - Calorie 34
   - Recommended Dietary Allowances 35
   - Sources of Carbohydrate 37
   - Functions of Carbohydrate 38
   - Digestion and Absorption of Carbohydrate 38
   - Regulation of Blood Sugar 39
   - Units of Energy 42
   - Components of Energy Requirements 44
   - Measurement of Energy 45
   - Body Mass Index and Basic Metabolism 45
   - Basal Metabolic Rate 46
   - Determinants and Factors Affecting 46
   - Nurses Role in Carbohydrate 47

3. **Proteins** 49
   - Definitions 49
   - Chemical Composition 50
   - Structure of Protein 50
   - Properties of Protein 50
   - Classifications of Protein 51
   - Sources of Protein 53
   - Examples of Protein in Biology and Diet 55
   - Amino Acids 56
   - Biological Value of Protein 57
   - Functions of Protein 57
   - Digestion of Protein 59
   - Deficiencies of Proteins 61

4. **Fats** 64
   - Classifications of Fats 65
   - Saturated and Unsaturated Fats 66
   - Calorie Value 66
   - Properties of Fats 66
   - Recommended Dietary Allowances 67
   - Dietary Sources of Fats 68
   - Functions of Fat in the Diet 68
   - Digestion and Absorption of Fats 70
   - Essential Fatty Acids 73
   - Lipids in Blood 73
   - Deficiency of Fats 73
   - LDL 74
   - HDL 74
   - VLDL 75
   - Over Consumption of Fat 75
   - Obesity 75
   - Dietary Management of Atherosclerosis 77
   - Role of Nurse in Fats 78

5. **Vitamins** 79
   - Classifications of Vitamins 80
   - Fat-soluble Vitamins 82
   - Water-soluble Vitamins 93
   - Vitamin Deficiencies and Hypervitaminosis 103

6. **Minerals** 106
   - Definition and Meaning 107
   - Classifications of Minerals 107
   - Calcium 108
   - Phosphorus 111
   - Iron 112
   - Zinc 115
   - Iodine 115
   - Fluoride 117
   - Sodium 118
   - Potassium 120
   - Magnesium 121
   - Chlorine 124
   - Trace Elements 124

7. Water and Electrolytes — 127
- Water Requirement and Regulation — 128
- Water Metabolism and Distribution — 130
- Electrolytes: Type, Sources and Consumption of Body Fluids — 131
- Maintenance of Fluid and Electrolyte Balance — 134
- Dehydration, Over Hydration and Water Intoxication — 139
- Electrolyte Imbalance — 143

8. Balanced Diet — 155
- Definition — 156
- Meaning of Balanced Diet — 156
- Elements of Balanced Diet — 156
- RDA—Definition, Limitations, Uses — 157
- Components of Healthy Balanced Diet — 158
- Factors Influencing Balanced Diet — 159
- Importance of Balanced Diet — 160
- Calculation of Balanced Diet — 161
- Effects of Unbalanced Diets — 162
- Specific Nutritional Deficiencies — 162
- Conditions with Specific Dietary Requirement — 163
- Food Exchange System — 164
- Dietary Fiber — 166
- Meal Planning — 170
- Meal Planning for Different Meals in a Day — 174
- Budget for Food — 176
- Infant and Young Child Feeding Guidelines—Breastfeeding, Infant Foods — 177
- Diet Plan for Different Age Groups—Children, Adolescents and Elderly — 180
- Diet in Pregnancy—Nutritional Requirements and Balanced Diet Plan — 185
- Anemia in Pregnancy—Diagnosis, Diet for Anemic Pregnant Women, Iron and Folic Acid Supplementation and Counseling — 186
- Nutrition in Lactation—Nutritional Requirements, Diet for Lactating Mothers, Complementary Feeding/Weaning — 188
- Weaning — 189
- Complementary Feeding — 190

9. Nutritional Deficiency Disorders — 193
- Protein-energy Malnutrition — 193
- Severe Acute Malnutrition — 196
- Childhood Obesity — 199
- Vitamin Deficiency Disorders — 202
- Vitamin A Deficiency — 202
- Vitamin D Deficiency — 203
- Vitamin C Deficiency — 206
- Vitamin B1 Deficiencies — 208
- Riboflavin — 211
- Niacin — 212
- Pyridoxine — 213
- Pantothenic Acid — 214
- Folic Acid — 215
- Cyanocobalamin — 216
- Mineral Deficiency Diseases — 217
- Iron Deficiency — 219
- Iodine Deficiencies — 222
- Calcium Deficiencies — 223

10. Therapeutic Diets — 226
- Concept and Meaning of Diet Therapy — 227
- Definition — 227
- Diet as a Therapeutic Agent — 228
- Principles of Diet Therapy — 228
- Factors to Consider in Planning Therapeutic Diets — 229
- Modification of Nutrients in Therapeutic Diets — 229
- Team Approach — 229
- Diet in Sickness — 230
- Therapeutic Diet — 231
- Regular Diet — 231
- Types of Diet Used in Hospitals — 233
- Special Feeding Methods (Management of Special Diets) — 235
- Tube Feeding — 236
- Parenteral Feeding — 236
- Dietary Modifications — 236
- High-Calorie and High-protein Diets — 237
- Kilocalorie-controlled and Low-kilocalorie Diets — 237
- Very Low-calorie Diet — 238
- Carbohydrate Modified Diets — 238
- Dumping Syndrome — 240
- Lactose Intolerance — 240
- Fat-modified Diets — 240
- Protein, Electrolyte and Fluid-modified Diets — 241
- Nurses Responsibilities in Food Serving — 243
- Diet Therapy for Perioperative Conditions — 244
- Diet Therapy in Fevers — 247
- Diet Therapy for Gastrointestinal Disorders — 249
- Diarrhea — 249
- Constipation — 249
- Peptic Ulcer — 250
- Modification of Diet in Bleeding Ulcer — 251
- Diet Therapy for Liver Diseases — 251
- Infective Hepatitis (Jaundice) — 252

- Cirrhosis of Liver — 253
- Hepatic Coma — 254
- Cholelithiasis — 255
- Dietary Restriction for Liver Diseases — 256
- Diet for Metabolic Disorders — 257
- Gout — 257
- Diet Therapy for Urinary Disorders — 259
- Nephrosis (Degenerative Bright's Disease) — 259
- Acute Renal Failure — 259
- Chronic Renal Failure — 260
- Urolithiasis or Urinary Calculi — 261
- Diet Therapy for Cardiovascular Disorders — 262
- Hypertension — 262
- Diet Therapy for Respiratory Disorder — 263
- Role of Nurse in Therapeutic Diet — 263

11. Cookery Rules and Preservation of Nutrients — 265

- Objectives of Cooking — 266
- Cooking Methods — 266
- Combination of Cooking Methods — 272
- Preservation of Nutrients — 273
- Food Preservation — 274
- Food Spoilage — 275
- Uses of Temperatures — 278
- Canning Procedure — 279
- Drying Method of Preservation — 280
- Preservation by High Concentration of Sugar and Salt — 281
- Food Additives — 283
- Food Adulteration — 286
- Packaging Materials and Hazards — 288
- Food Laws — 291
- Consumer Protection — 292
- Prevention of Food Adulteration, Act 1954 — 292
- Sale of Certain Admixtures Prohibited — 292
- Procedure for Sampling and Analysis — 293
- Penalties — 293
- Important Miscellaneous Provisions — 293
- Food Standards — 293
- Bureau of Indian Standards — 293
- Food and Nutrition Board — 294
- Nutrition Society of India — 294
- Food and Agricultural Organization — 294

12. Nutrition Assessment and Nutrition Education — 298

- Definition — 299
- Meaning of Nutrition Assessment — 299
- Purpose — 299
- Objectives — 299
- Goals — 299
- Systems of Nutritional Assessment — 299
- Methods of Nutritional Assessment — 300
- Types of Assessment — 300
- Clinical Assessment (Signs and Symptoms) — 304
- Dietary History — 306
- Nutritional Education — 307
- Meaning — 307
- Aims — 308

13. National Nutritional Programmes and Role of Nurse — 311

- National Nutritional Programmes — 311
- History of Nutritional Programs — 312
- Guiding Principles — 313
- Current Nutritional Deficiency Status — 313
- Five Year Plans on Nutritional Aspects — 313
- Nutrition Interventions — 314
- Nutritional Problems in India — 314
- National Nutritional Policy — 315
- Special Nutritional Programme — 316
- Integrated Child Development Services Scheme — 317
- Mid-day Meal Programme — 318
- National Nutritional Anemia Program — 319
- Special Nutrition Programme — 319
- National Goitre Control Programme — 320
- National Programme for Prophylaxis Against Blindness Due to Vitamin-D Deficiency — 320
- Balwadi Nutrition Programme — 321
- World Food Programme — 321
- Applied Nutrition Programme — 322
- Integrated Child Development Services — 322
- Minimum Need Programme — 323
- 20-Points Programme — 323
- Child Survival and Safe Motherhood Programmes — 324
- Reproductive and Child Health Programme — 324
- National Nutritional Programs and Role of Nurse — 324

14. Food Safety — 327

- Concept of Food Safety — 328
- Four Steps to Food Safety — 329
- Major Foodborne Illnesses and Causes — 329
- The Evolving World and Food Safety — 330
- Food Safety: A Public Health Priority — 331
- Food Safety Considerations and Measures — 331
- Tips for Maintaining Food Safety — 332
- Food Hygiene/Sanitation — 332
- Food Poisoning — 333
- Hygiene Control — 335

- Effects of Unsafe Practices 336
- Role of Food Handlers in Foodborne Diseases 337
- Essential Steps in Safe Cooking Practices 338
- Consumer Control Points for Food Safety 339

Section 2: Applied Biochemistry

15. Introduction to Biochemistry 343
- Definition and Significance in Nursing 343
- Meaning and Concept of Biochemistry 344
- History of Biochemistry 344
- Need of Studying Biochemistry 345
- Review of Structure, Composition and Functions of Cell 345
- Structure and Composition of Cell 346
- Structure of the Unit Membrane 347

16. Carbohydrates 362
- Glycolysis 370
- Glycogenesis 371
- Cori Cycle or Lactic Acid Cycle 372
- Pentose Phosphate Pathway 373
- Citric Acid Cycle 375
- Glycogenolysis 377
- Regulation of Blood Sugar Level 378
- Hereditary Fructose Intolerance 386

17. Lipids 388
- Fatty Acids 389
- Essential Fatty Acids 389
- Properties of Lipids 390
- Lipid Metabolism 391
- Cholesterol 395
- Steroid Hormones 396
- Atherosclerosis 397
- Lipoproteins 397

18. Proteins 400
- Structural Organization of Protein 401
- Importance of Protein 402
- Classifications of Protein 402

19. Clinical Enzymology 415
- Mechanism of Enzyme Activity 417

20. Acid Base Maintenance 424
- Concept and Meaning of Acid Base Maintenance 424
- Definition 425
- Blood Gases 425
- Organ Systems Involved in pH Balance 426
- Respiratory Acidosis 429
- Metabolic Alkalosis 432
- Acid-base Balance: Ketoacidosis 433

21. Heme Catabolism 436
- Function of Heme 437
- Mechanism 437
- Pathophysiology 438
- Iron Absorption and Transport 438
- Heme Degradation 440
- Heme Catabolism 440
- Heme Degradation Pathway 441
- Jaundice 443

22. Organ Function Tests 450
- Kidney Function Test 450
- Liver Function Test 452
- Thyroid Function Test 455

23. Immunochemistry 459
- Historical Perspectives 459
- Macrophages 461
- Major Histocompatibility 461
- Immunity 463
- Antigen 464
- Antibodies 465
- Enzyme-linked Immunosorbent Assay 467
- Human Leukocyte Antigens 469
- Specialized Proteins 469

Biochemistry Glossary 471
Index 491

INC Syllabus

APPLIED NUTRITION AND DIETETICS

Placement: II Semester
Theory: 3 Credits (60 hours)
Theory: 45 hours
Lab: 15 hours
Description: The course is designed to assist the students to acquire basic knowledge and understanding of the principles of nutrition and dietetics and apply this knowledge in the practice of nursing.
Competencies: On completion of the course, the students will be able to—
1. Identify the importance of nutrition in health and wellness.
2. Apply nutrient and dietary modifications in caring patients.
3. Explain the principles and practices of nutrition and dietetics.
4. Identify nutritional needs of different age groups and plan a balanced diet for them.
5. Identify the dietary principles for different diseases.
6. Plan therapeutic diet for patients suffering from various disease conditions.
7. Prepare meals using different methods and cookery rules.

Course Outline

T: Theory

Unit	Time (Hrs)	Learning outcomes	Content	Teaching/Learning activities	Assessment methods
I.	2 (T)	Define nutrition and its relationship to health	**Introduction to nutrition** *Concepts:* • Definition of nutrition and health • Malnutrition—undernutrition and overnutrition • Role of nutrition in maintaining health • Factors affecting food and nutrition *Nutrients:* • Classification • Macro- and micronutrients • Organic and inorganic • Energy yielding and non-energy yielding *Food:* • Classification—food groups • Origin	• Lecture-cum-discussion • Charts/slides	• Essay • Short answer • Very short answer
II.	3 (T)	Describe the classification, functions, sources and recommended daily allowances (RDA) of carbohydrates Explain BMR and factors affecting BMR	**Carbohydrates** • Composition—starches, sugar and cellulose • Recommended daily allowance (RDA) • Dietary sources • Functions **Energy** • Unit of energy—Kcal • Basal metabolic rate (BMR) • Factors affecting BMR	• Lecture-cum-discussion • Charts/slides • Models • Display of food items	• Essay • Short answer • Very short answer
III.	3 (T)	Describe the classification, functions, sources and RDA of proteins	**Proteins** • Composition • Eight essential amino acids • Functions • Dietary sources • Protein requirements—RDA	• Lecture-cum-discussion • Charts/slides • Models • Display of food items	• Essay • Short answer • Very short answer

Contd...

Contd...

Unit	Time (Hrs)	Learning outcomes	Content	Teaching/Learning activities	Assessment methods
IV.	2 (T)	Describe the classification, functions, sources and RDA of fats	**Fats** • Classification—saturated and unsaturated • Calorie value • Functions • Dietary sources of fats and fatty acids • Fat requirements—RDA	• Lecture-cum-discussion • Charts/slides • Models • Display of food items	• Essay • Short answer • Very short answer
V.	3 (T)	Describe the classification, functions, sources and RDA of vitamins	**Vitamins** • Classification—fat soluble and water soluble • Fat soluble—vitamins A, D, E, and K • Water soluble—thiamine (vitamin B1), riboflavin (vitamin B2), nicotinic acid, pyridoxine (vitamin B6), pantothenic acid, folic acid, vitamin B12, ascorbic acid (vitamin C) • Functions, dietary sources and requirements—RDA of every vitamin	• Lecture-cum-discussion • Charts/slides • Models • Display of food items	• Essay • Short answer • Very short answer
VI.	3 (T)	Describe the classification, functions, sources and RDA of minerals	**Minerals** • Classification—major minerals (calcium, phosphorus, sodium, potassium and magnesium) and trace elements • Functions • Dietary sources • Requirements—RDA	• Lecture-cum-discussion • Charts/slides • Models • Display of food items	• Short answer • Very short answer

VII.	7 (T)
	8 (L)
		Describe and plan balanced diet for different age groups, pregnancy, and lactation	**Balanced diet**
			• Definition, principles, steps
			• Food guides—basic four food groups
			• RDA—definition, limitations, uses
			• Food exchange system
			• Calculation of nutritive value of foods
			• Dietary fiber
			Nutrition across life cycle
			• Meal planning/menu planning—definition, principles, steps
			• Infant and young child feeding (IYCF) guidelines—breastfeeding, infant foods
			• Diet plan for different age groups—children, adolescents and elderly
			• Diet in pregnancy—nutritional requirements and balanced diet plan
			• Anemia in pregnancy—diagnosis, diet for anemic pregnant women, iron and folic acid supplementation and counseling
			• Nutrition in lactation—nutritional requirements, diet for lactating mothers, complementary feeding/weaning
				• Lecture-cum-discussion
				• Meal planning
				• Lab session on:
				  ▪ Preparation of balanced diet for different categories
				  ▪ Low cost nutritious dishes
					• Short answer
					• Very short answer

VIII.	6 (T)	Classify and describe the common nutritional deficiency disorders and identify nurses' role in assessment, management and prevention	**Nutritional deficiency disorders** • Protein energy malnutrition—magnitude of the problem, causes, classification, signs and symptoms, severe acute malnutrition (SAM), management and prevention and nurses' role • Childhood obesity—signs and symptoms, assessment, management and prevention and nurses' role • Vitamin deficiency disorders—vitamin A, B, C and D deficiency disorders—causes, signs and symptoms, management and prevention and nurses' role • Mineral deficiency diseases—iron, iodine and calcium deficiencies—causes, signs and symptoms, management and prevention and nurses' role	• Lecture-cum-discussion • Charts/slides • Models	• Essay • Short answer • Very short answer

Contd...

Contd...

Unit	Time (Hrs)	Learning outcomes	Content	Teaching/Learning activities	Assessment methods
IX	4 (T) 7 (L)	Principles of diets in various diseases	**Therapeutic diets** • Definition, objectives, principles • Modifications—consistency, nutrients • Feeding techniques • Diet in diseases—obesity, diabetes mellitus, CVD, underweight, renal diseases, hepatic disorders constipation, diarrhea, pre- and postoperative period	• Lecture-cum-discussion • Meal planning • Lab session on preparation of therapeutic diets	• Essay • Short answer • Very short answer
X	3 (T)	Describe the rules and preservation of nutrients	**Cookery rules and preservation of nutrients** • Cooking—methods, advantages and disadvantages • Preservation of nutrients • Measures to prevent loss of nutrients during preparation • Safe food handling and storage of foods • Food preservation • Food additives and food adulteration • Prevention of food adulteration act (PFA) • Food standards	• Lecture-cum-discussion • Charts/slides	• Essay • Short answer • Very short answer
XI	4 (T)	Explain the methods of nutritional assessment and nutrition education	**Nutrition assessment and nutrition education** • Objectives of nutritional assessment • Methods of assessment—clinical examination, anthropometry, laboratory and biochemical assessment, assessment of dietary intake including food frequency questionnaire (FFQ) method • Nutrition education—purposes, principles and methods	• Lecture-cum-discussion • Demonstration • Writing nutritional assessment report	• Essay • Short answer • Evaluation of Nutritional assessment report
XII	3 (T)	Describe nutritional problems in India and nutritional programs	**National Nutritional Programs and role of nurse** • Nutritional problems in India • National nutritional policy • National nutritional programs—vitamin A supplementation, Anemia Mukt Bharat Programme, Integrated Child Development Services (ICDS), Midday Meal Scheme (MDMS), National Iodine Deficiency Disorders Control Programme (NIDDCP), Weekly Iron and Folic Acid Supplementation (WIFS) and others as introduced • Role of nurse in every program	• Lecture-cum-discussion	• Essay • Short answer • Very short answer
XIII	2 (T)	Discuss the importance of food hygiene and food safety Explain the Acts related to food safety	**Food safety** • Definition, food safety considerations and measures • Food safety regulatory measures in India—relevant acts • Five keys to safer food • Food storage, food handling and cooking • General principles of food storage of food items (e.g., milk, meat) • Role of food handlers in foodborne diseases • Essential steps in safe cooking practices	• Guided reading on related acts	• Quiz • Short answer

Foodborne diseases and food poisoning are dealt in Community Health Nursing I.

APPLIED BIOCHEMISTRY

Placement: II Semester

Theory: 2 credits (40 hours) (includes lab hours also)

Description: The course is designed to assist the students to acquire knowledge of the normal biochemical composition and functioning of human body, its alterations in disease conditions and to apply this knowledge in the practice of nursing.

Competencies: On completion of the course, the students will be able to—
1. Describe the metabolism of carbohydrates and its alterations.
2. Explain the metabolism of lipids and its alterations.
3. Explain the metabolism of proteins and amino acids and its alterations.
4. Explain clinical enzymology in various disease conditions.
5. Explain acid base balance, imbalance and its clinical significance.
6. Describe the metabolism of hemoglobin and its clinical significance.
7. Explain different function tests and interpret the findings.
8. Illustrate the immunochemistry.

Course Outline

T: Theory

Unit	Time (Hrs)	Learning outcomes	Content	Teaching/Learning activities	Assessment methods

I.	8 (T)	Describe the metabolism of carbohydrates and its alterations	**Carbohydrates**
			• Digestion, absorption and metabolism of carbohydrates and related disorders
			• Regulation of blood glucose
			• Diabetes mellitus—type 1 and type 2, symptoms, complications and management in brief
			• Investigations of diabetes mellitus
			   ▪ OGTT—Indications, procedure, interpretation and types of GTT curve
			   ▪ Mini GTT, extended GTT, GCT, IV GTT
			   ▪ HbA1c (only definition)
			• Hypoglycemia—definition and causes
				• Lecture-cum-discussion
				• Explain using charts and slides
				• Demonstration of laboratory tests
					• Essay
					• Short answer
					• Very short answer

II.	8 (T)	Explain the metabolism of lipids and its alterations	**Lipids** • Fatty acids—definition, classification • Definition and clinical significance of MUFA and PUFA, essential fatty acids, trans fatty acids • Digestion, absorption and metabolism of lipids and related disorders • Compounds formed from cholesterol • Ketone bodies (name, types and significance only) • Lipoproteins—types and functions (metabolism not required) • Lipid profile • Atherosclerosis (in brief)	• Lecture-cum-discussion • Explain using charts and slides • Demonstration of laboratory tests	• Essay • Short answer • Very short answer
III.	9 (T)	Explain the metabolism of amino acids and proteins Identify alterations in disease conditions	**Proteins** • Classification of amino acids based on nutrition, metabolic rate with examples • Digestion, absorption and metabolism of protein and related disorders • Biologically important compounds synthesized from various amino acids (only names) • In born errors of amino acid metabolism—only aromatic amino acids (in brief) • Plasma protein—types, function and normal values • Causes of proteinuria, hypoproteinemia, hypergammaglobulinemia • Principle of electrophoresis, normal and abnormal electrophoretic patterns (in brief)	• Lecture-cum-discussion • Explain using charts, models and slides	• Essay • Short answer • Very short answer

Contd...

Contd...

Unit	Time (Hrs)	Learning outcomes	Content	Teaching/Learning activities	Assessment methods

IV	4 (T)	Explain clinical enzymology in various disease conditions	**Clinical Enzymology**
			• Isoenzymes—definition and properties
			• Enzymes of diagnostic importance in
			   ▪ Liver diseases—ALT, AST, ALP, GGT
			   ▪ Myocardial infarction—CK, cardiac troponins, AST, LDH
			   ▪ Muscle diseases—CK, Aldolase
			   ▪ Bone diseases—ALP
			   ▪ Prostate cancer—PSA, ACP
				• Lecture-cum-discussion
				• Explain using charts and slides
					• Essay
					• Short answer
					• Very short answer

V	3 (T)	Explain acid base balance, imbalance and its clinical significance	**Acid base maintenance** • pH—definition, normal value • Regulation of blood pH—blood buffer, respiratory and renal • ABG—normal values • Acid base disorders—types, definition and causes	• Lecture-cum-discussion • Explain using charts and slides	• Short answer • Very short answer
VI	2 (T)	Describe the metabolism of hemoglobin and its clinical significance	**Heme catabolism** • Heme degradation pathway • Jaundice—type, causes, urine and blood investigations (Van den Bergh test)	• Lecture-cum-discussion • Explain using charts and slides	• Short answer • Very short answer
VII	3 (T)	Explain different function tests and interpret the findings	**Organ function tests (biochemical parameters and normal values only)** • Renal • Liver • Thyroid	• Lecture-cum-discussion • Visit to lab • Explain using charts and slides	• Short answer • Very short answer
VIII	3 (T)	Illustrate the immunochemistry	**Immunochemistry** • Structure and functions of immunoglobulin • Investigations and interpretation—ELISA	• Lecture-cum-discussion • Explain using charts and slides • Demonstration of laboratory tests	• Short answer • Very short answer

Note: Few lab hours can be planned for observation and visits (less than 1 credit, lab hours are not specified separately).

SECTION 1

Applied Nutrition and Dietetics

SECTION OUTLINE

1. Introduction to Nutrition
2. Carbohydrates and Energy
3. Proteins
4. Fats
5. Vitamins
6. Minerals
7. Water and Electrolytes
8. Balanced Diet
9. Nutritional Deficiency Disorders
10. Therapeutic Diets
11. Cookery Rules and Preservation of Nutrients
12. Nutrition Assessment and Nutrition Education
13. National Nutritional Programmes and Role of Nurse
14. Food Safety

CHAPTER 1

Introduction to Nutrition

CHAPTER OUTLINE

- ❖ Concepts
  - Definition of Nutrition and Health
  - Malnutrition–Under Nutrition and Over Nutrition
  - Role of Nutrition in Maintaining Health
  - Factors Affecting Food and Nutrition
- ❖ Nutrients
  - Classification
- Macro- and Micronutrients
- Organic and Inorganic
- Energy Yielding and Non-energy Yielding
- ❖ Food
  - Classification—Food Groups
  - Origin

TERMINOLOGY

- **Allergic reaction:** Immunologically-induced tissue response to a foreign substance (allergen).
- **Alpha-linolenic acid:** 18 carbon fatty acid with three double bonds; the first double bond is on the third carbon atom from the methyl end and therefore, it is called n-3 fatty acid. It is abbreviated as 18:3 n-3.
- **Amino acid:** The fundamental building block of proteins.
- **Anabolism:** Process by which complex materials in tissues and organs are built up from simple substances.
- **Antioxidants:** A group of substances that prevent the damage caused by the oxidation of fatty acids and proteins by oxygen free radicals.
- **Balanced diet:** A diet containing all essential (macro and micro) nutrients in optimum quantities and in appropriate proportions that meet the requirements.
- **Beta-Carotene:** A yellow-orange plant pigment which yields vitamin A by oxidation in the body.
- **Bifidus factor:** A substance in human milk which stimulates the growth of a microorganism (*Lactobacillus bifidus*) in the infants' intestine.
- **Body mass index:** Body weight in relation to height. Body weight in kilograms divided by 2 heights in meters.
- **Calorie:** Unit used to indicate the energy value of foods. Quantitative requirements are expressed in terms of energy, i.e., kilocalories (kcals). Newer unit for energy is kjoules.
- **Catabolism:** Process of breakdown of complex organic constituents in the body.
- **Cholesterol:** A lipid constituent of blood and tissues derived from diet as well as from synthesis within the body.
- **Colostrum:** The milk produced by mammals during the first few days after delivery.
- **Consumption unit (CU):** One unit represents recommended dietary allowance of energy for a sedentary man.
- **Empty calories:** Term used for foods that provide only energy without any other nutrient, e.g., white sugar and alcohol.
- **Enzymes:** Biological catalysts which enhance the rate of chemical reactions in the body.
- **Essential fatty acids (EFA):** Fatty acids, such as linoleic acid and alpha linolenic acid which are not made in the human body and must be supplied through the diet.
- **Fatty acids:** Fundamental constituents of many lipids.
- **Fiber:** Collective term for the structural parts of plant tissues which are resistant to the human digestive enzymes.
- **Flavonoids:** Pigments widely distributed in nature in flowers, fruits and vegetables.
- **Food exchange:** Foods are classified into different groups for exchange. Each "exchange list" includes a number of measured foods of similar nutritive value that can be substituted interchangeably in meal plans.
- **Free radicals:** Highly reactive oxygen-derived species formed in the body during normal metabolic processes. They have the capacity to damage cellular components by oxidation.
- **High-density lipoproteins (HDL):** These transport cholesterol from the extra-hepatic tissues to the liver. They are antiatherogenic.
- **Hormones:** Substances produced by a gland (endocrine) which are secreted directly into the blood stream to produce a specific effect on another organ.
- **Hyperlipidemia:** An increase in the concentration of blood lipids (triglycerides and cholesterol).
- **Invisible fats:** Fat present as an integral component of plant and animal foods such as in cereals, legumes and spices.

- **Lactoferrin:** Minor protein of milk containing iron. Lactose intolerance: Disorder resulting from improper digestion of milk sugar called lactose, due to lack of an enzyme, lactase, in the intestinal mucosa.
- **Linoleic acid:** Fatty acid containing 18 carbon atoms and two double bonds. The first double bond is on the sixth carbon atom from the methyl end. Therefore, it is called n-6 fatty acid and is abbreviated as 18:2 n-6.
- **Lipids:** A technical term for fats. They are important dietary constituents. The group includes triglycerides, steroids, cholesterol and other complex lipids.
- **Lipoproteins:** Lipids are not soluble in blood; they are therefore transported as lipid and protein complexes.
- **Low-density lipoproteins (LDL):** These transport cholesterol from the liver to tissues. High blood levels indicate that more cholesterol is being transported to tissues.
- **Macrocytic anemia:** Anemia characterized by red blood cells which are larger than normal.
- **Macronutrients:** Nutrients, such as carbohydrates, proteins and fats which are required in large quantities.
- **Metabolism:** Includes catabolism and anabolism.
- **Microcytic anemia:** Anemia characterized by red blood cells which are smaller than normal.
- **Micronutrients:** Nutrients which are required in small quantities, such as vitamins and trace elements.
- **Monounsaturated fatty acids:** Unsaturated fatty acids with one double bond. n-6 PUFA—linoleic acid and its longer chain polyunsaturated fatty acids are collectively called n-6 PUFA. n-3 PUFA—alpha-linolenic acid and its longer-chain polyunsaturated fatty acids are collectively called n-3 PUFA.
- **Phytochemicals:** General name for chemicals present in plants.
- **Polyunsaturated fatty acids (PUFA):** Unsaturated fatty acids with two or more double bonds.
- **Processed foods:** Foods that are produced by converting raw food materials into a form suitable for eating.
- **Protein energy malnutrition (PEM):** A marked dietary deficiency of both energy and protein resulting in under nutrition.
- **Recommended dietary allowances (RDA):** The amounts of dietary energy and nutrients considered sufficient for maintaining good health by the people of a country.
- **Refined foods:** Foods which have been processed to improve their appearance, color, taste, odor or keeping quality.
- **Saturated fatty acids:** Fatty acids containing maximum number of hydrogen atoms that each carbon atom can carry. They do not have double bonds.
- **Satiety:** Feeling of satisfaction after food intake.
- **Trans-fatty acids:** Are mainly produced during hydrogenation of oils; a few also occur naturally in very small quantities.
- **Triglycerides (Neutral fat):** The major type of dietary fat and the principal form in which energy is stored in the body. A complex of fatty acids and glycerol.
- **Unsaturated fatty acids:** Fatty acids in which there is a shortage of hydrogen atoms. The carbon atoms then become linked by double bonds. Unsaturated fatty acids are less stable than saturated fatty acids.
- **Visible fats:** Fats and oils that can be used directly or in cooking.
- **Weaning foods:** Foods which are used during gradual transition of the infant from breastfeeding to a normal diet.

INTRODUCTION

Food is prime necessity of life. The food we eat is digested and assimilated in the body and used for its maintenance and growth. Food also provides energy for doing work. Man has exhibited much thought and foresight in cultivating a variety of grains, fruits, vegetables, nuts and oil seeds and in rearing birds and animals for use as food. Nutrition deals with the way in which the human body receives and uses all the substance or materials necessary for its growth and development and for keeping it in good condition. This begins in eating food. The food swallowed then digested as it is passed through the stomach and small intestines. During digestion, the food is broken up into simple substances. These are absorbed into bloodstream and carried to the liver, where they are either stored or changed further or sent out to other parts of the body for use as required.

DEFINITION

- **Food:** Food is defined as anything solid, liquid or semi-solid, which when ingested putting into the mouth, digested and assimilated, nourishes the body.
- **Nutrients:** Nutrients are defined as those chemicals substances, which are supplied by food and are needed as a source of energy and as a structural material for every cell of the body.
- **Food:** The edible stuff that provides us with nutrients is termed as food. Food is broadly classified as cereals, pulses, vegetable, fruits, milk, eggs, flesh food, fats and sugar.
- **Nutrients:** These are the constituents in food that must be supplied to the body in suitable amounts. They include proteins, fats, carbohydrates, minerals, water and vitamins.
- **Nutrition status:** It is defined as the extent to which a customary diet meets the body's requirement. In other words, it signifies the condition of the body after the consumption of food. The condition of health of individuals as influenced by the utilization of nutrients. It can be assessed by dietary survey, anthropometry, clinical and laboratory investigations

NUTRITION: HISTORY AND CONCEPTS

Nutrition is the combination of processes by which the living organism receives and utilizes the materials necessary for

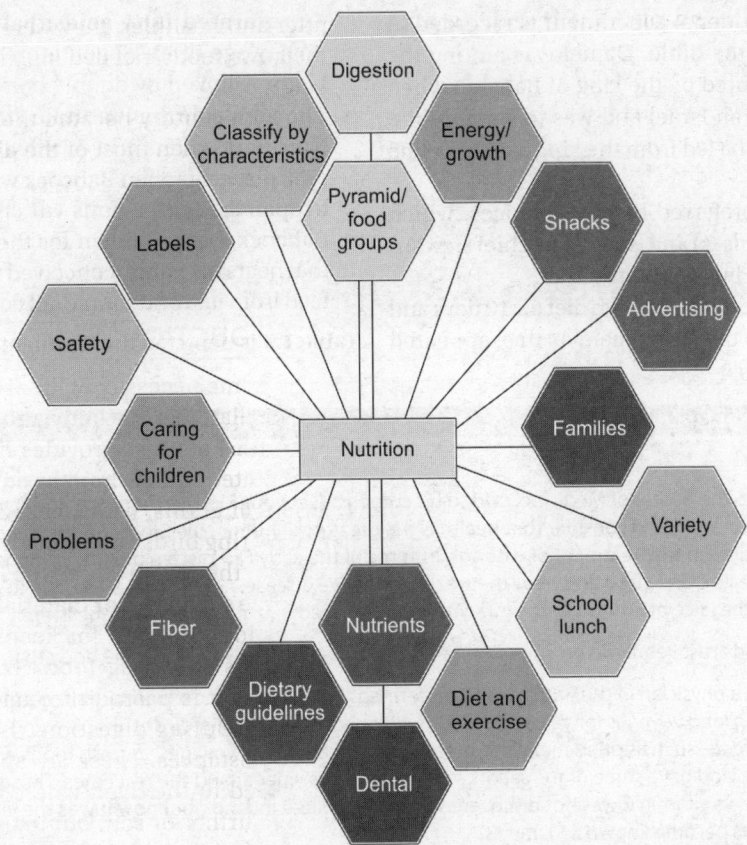

Fig. 1.1: Nutrition and related concepts.

the maintenance of its function and for the growth and renewal of its components. Nutrition is that condition, which permits the development and maintenance of the highest state of fitness is processes or activities by which the human body receives and uses all the food necessary for its growth, development, regulation and repair. It is the science of food, the nutrients and other substances therein, their action, interaction and balance in relationship to health and disease.

Figure 1.1 is depicted the nutrition and related concepts.

Box 1.1 is depicted the history of nutrition I.

HISTORY OF NUTRITION

- Nutritional discoveries from the earliest days of history have had a positive effect on our health and well-being. The word nutrition itself means "the process of nourishing or being nourished, especially the process by which a living organism assimilates food and uses it for growth and replacement of tissues."

> **Box 1.1:** History of nutrition I.
> - **Lavoisier** is generally credited as being the "father" of nutrition
> - Until the first quarter of 19th Century, we thought the nutritive value of food resided only in one component
> - Near the end of the 19th Century research started to focus primarily on the need for protein, lipids and carbohydrates
> - Minerals were considered important, but their essentiality was unknown

- Nutrients are substances that are essential to life, which must be supplied by food. Today more than ever, obtaining nutritional knowledge can make a big difference in lives. Air, soil and water pollution in addition to modern farming techniques, have depleted soils of vital minerals.
- The widespread use of food additives, chemicals, sugar and unhealthy fats in the diets contributes too many of the degenerative diseases of our day such as cancer, heart disease, arthritis and osteoporosis. Here is a brief history of the science that offers the hope of improving health naturally.

Box 1.2 is depicted the historical milestones in nutrition.

> **Box 1.2:** Historical milestones in nutrition.
> - In pre-agricultural era, entire mankind consumed meat as early man was hunter. Possibly he ate from plants sources which grew in the wilderness.
> - With the advent of agriculture as an outcome of civilization, man acquired the ability to cultivate what he wanted, as by now he was influenced to some extent by the selection of the food that he wanted to eat.
> - **The Bible, Book of Daniel:** Daniel was captured by the king of Babylon and had to serve in the King's court. Daniel objected to being fed fine foods and wine, saying he preferred vegetables, pulses and water. The chief steward reluctantly agreed to a trial, comparing Daniel's dietary preference to those of the court of the King of Babylon. For then days Daniel and his man had their vegetarian diet, while the King's men had theirs. The trial revealed that Daniel and his men were healthier and fitter, so they were allowed to carry on with their diet.

- The first recorded nutritional experiment is recorded in the book of Daniel in the Bible. Daniel was among the finest young men captured by the king of Babylon when the Babylonians over ran Israel and was to serve in the king's court. He was to be fed from the king's table of fine foods and wine.
- Daniel objected and preferred his own choices, which included vegetables (pulses) and water. The chief steward was afraid for his head, but agreed to a trial.
- Daniel and his friends received his own diet for 10 days and then were compared to the king's men. As they appeared fitter and healthier, they were allowed to continue with their own foods, not defiling themselves with those of the king.
- The 20th century became the era of the Golden Age of Nutrition, when most of the discoveries of the nutrients took place. Stephen Babcock was instrumental in helping to open the age.
- Babcock, better known for the Babcock test for milk fat that bears his name, conceived the idea to feed dairy cattle feed from just one source, all corn plant or all wheat plant.

Table 1.1 is depicted the highlights of history of nutrition.

Table 1.1: Highlights of history of nutrition

Sl. No.	Year	Description
1.	400 BC	Hippocrates, the 'Father of Medicine', said to his students, 'Let your food be medicine and thy medicine be food'. He also said "A wise man should consider that health is the greatest of human blessings." Foods were often used as cosmetics or as medicines in the treatment of wounds. In some of the early Far-Eastern biblical writings, there were references to food and health. One story describes the treatment of eye disease, now known to be due to a vitamin A deficiency, by squeezing the juice of liver on to the eye. Vitamin A is stored in large amounts in the liver.
2.	1500	Scientist and artist Leonardo da Vinci compared the process of metabolism in the body to the burning of a candle.
3.	1447	James Lind, a physician in the British Navy, performed the first scientific experiment in nutrition. At that time, sailors were sent on long voyages for years and they developed scurvy (a painful, deadly, bleeding disorder). Only non-perishable foods such as dried meat and breads were taken on the voyages, as fresh foods would not last. In his experiment, Lind gave some of the sailors sea water, others vinegar and the rest limes. Those given the limes were saved from scurvy. As vitamin C was not discovered until the 1930s, Lind did not know it was the vital nutrient. As a note, British sailors became known as 'Limey's'.
4.	1770	Antoine Lavoisier, the 'Father of Nutrition and Chemistry' discovered the actual process by which food is metabolized. He also demonstrated where animal heat comes from. In his equation, he describes the combination of food and oxygen in the body and the resulting giving off of heat and water.
5.	1800	It was discovered that foods are composed primarily of four elements carbon, nitrogen, hydrogen and oxygen, and methods were developed for determining the amounts of these elements.
6.	1840	Justus Liebig of Germany, a pioneer in early plant growth studies, was the first to point out the chemical makeup of carbohydrates, fats and proteins. Carbohydrates were made up of sugars, fats were fatty acids and proteins were made up of amino acids.
7.	1897	Christian Eijkman, a Dutchman working with natives in Java, observed that some of the natives developed a disease called beriberi, which caused heart problems and paralysis. He observed that when chickens were fed the native diet of white rice, they developed the symptoms of beriberi. When he fed the chickens, unprocessed brown rice (with the outer bran intact), they did not develop the disease. Eijkman then fed brown rice to his patients and they were cured. He discovered that food could cure disease. Nutritionists later learned that the outer rice bran contains vitamin B1, also known as thiamine.
8.	1912	McCollum EV, while working for the US Department of Agriculture at the University of Wisconsin, developed an approach that opened the way to the widespread discovery of nutrients. He decided to work with rats rather than large farm animals, such as cows and sheep. Using this procedure, he discovered the first fat soluble vitamin, vitamin A. He found that rats fed butter were healthier than those fed lard, as butter contains more vitamin A.
9.	1912	Casimir Funk was the first to coin the term 'vitamins' as vital factors in the diet. He wrote about these unidentified substances present in food, which could prevent the diseases of scurvy, beriberi and pellagra (a disease caused by a deficiency of niacin, vitamin B3). The term vitamin is derived from the words vital and amine, because vitamins are required for life and they were originally thought to be amines—compounds derived from ammonia.
10.	1930	William Rose discovered the essential amino acids, the building blocks of protein.
11.	1940	1. The water soluble B and C vitamins were identified. 2. Russell Marker perfected a method of synthesizing the female hormone progesterone from a component of wild yams called diosgenin.
12.	1950	The roles of essential nutrients as a part of bodily processes have been brought to light. For example, more came to known about the role of vitamins and minerals as components of enzymes and hormones that work within the body.

Contd...

Contd...

Sl. No.	Year	Description
13.	1968	Linus Pauling, a Nobel prize winner in chemistry, created the term 'Orthomolecular Nutrition'. Orthomolecular is, literally, 'pertaining to the right molecule'. Pauling proposed that by giving the body the right molecules in the right concentration (optimum nutrition), nutrients could be used by people to achieve better health and prolong life. Studies in the 1970s and 1980s conducted by Pauling and colleagues suggested that very large doses of vitamin C given intravenously could be helpful in increasing the survival time and improving the quality of life of terminal cancer patients.
14.	1994–2000	Have you ever wondered why vitamin bottle labels and nutritional websites include a phrase saying that their products and information are not intended to diagnose, cure or prevent any disease? These also usually state that their health claims have not been evaluated by the food and drug administration (FDA). Here is why: the Dietary and Supplement Health and Education Act was approved by congress in October of 1994 and updated in January 2000. It sets forth, what can and cannot be said about nutritional supplements without prior FDA review.

Concept of Nutrition

Nutrition is also known as nourishment or aliment in the form of food in order to support life. The diet of an organism refers to what they eat. Many common health problems can be prevented by having a healthy diet. Dietitians are professionals who specializes human nutrition, meal planning, preparation and so on. They are trained people to provide dietary advice for every individual in health and disease. **Box 1.3** is depicted the basic nutrition concepts.

- There are seven major classifications of nutrients, they are, carbohydrates, fiber, fats, protein, minerals, water and vitamins. These classes of nutrients are categorized as macronutrients are needed in relatively large amounts.
- Micronutrients are needed in smaller quantities. Macronutrients' are carbohydrates, fats, fibers, water and protein, while micronutrients are vitamins and minerals.
- The macronutrients provide energy, which is measured in Joules or kilocalories and written with a capital 'C' to distinguish them from gram calories. Carbohydrates and proteins provide 17 kJ (4 kcal) of energy per gram, while fats provide 37 kJ (9 kcal) of energy per gram.
- Vitamins, minerals, fiber and water do not provide energy, but are necessary for other reasons. Other nutrients include antioxidants and phytochemicals.
- These substances were recently discovered, which have not have been yet recognized as vitamins or contribute to health, but they are necessary in our bodies. Photochemical may act as antioxidant, but not all of them are antioxidants.

Box 1.3: Basic nutrition concepts.

- There is a popular statement that says "Man is what he eats" "whatever a man eats turn into him" which means it is what a man eats that is digested, absorbed and utilized in his body to ensure that growth and maintenance of the body cells, and the proper functions of the organs and tissues.
- Good feeding is intrinsically linked to the body components and good health. A man in good health can work more efficiently towards the achievement of his goals and also live a comfortable and happy life.
- No single food item can supply all the necessary nutrients.
- All the nutrients needed by the body can be obtained from combinations of adequate quantities/proportions of different food items.

Nutrition: A Basic Human Need

Nutrition is a basic human need that changes throughout the life cycle and along the health-illness continuum. The body requires food to provide energy for organ functions, body movement and work, maintain body temperature and to provide raw materials for enzymes function, growth replacement of cells and repair. Food provides nutrition for both the body and mind. Eating has evolved from being simply a necessity; is an integral component of medical treatment **(Fig. 1.2)**.

- The science of nutrition encompasses the study of nutrients and how they are handled by the body, as well as the impact of human behavior and environment on the process of nourishment.
- Nutrients alter specific substances used by the body for growth and development, activity, reproduction, lactation, heath maintenance and recovery from illness or injury.

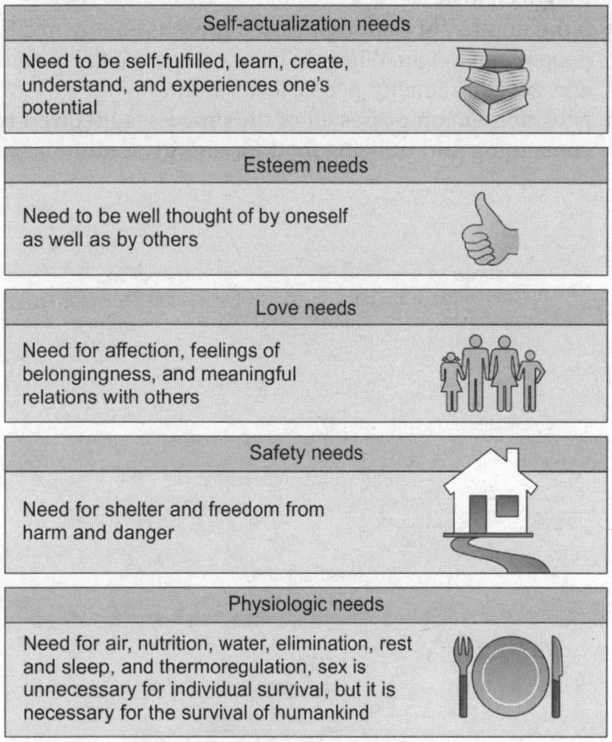

Self-actualization needs
Need to be self-fulfilled, learn, create, understand, and experiences one's potential

Esteem needs
Need to be well thought of by oneself as well as by others

Love needs
Need for affection, feelings of belongingness, and meaningful relations with others

Safety needs
Need for shelter and freedom from harm and danger

Physiologic needs
Need for air, nutrition, water, elimination, rest and sleep, and thermoregulation, sex is unnecessary for individual survival, but it is necessary for the survival of humankind

Fig. 1.2: Nutrition: A basic human need.

- Good nutrition is a basic component of health, growth and development for maintaining health throughout the life. Proper nutrition of the nation is necessary for the nation's growth and economic development.
- Nurses must understand the functions of the basic nutrients and metabolism. An understanding of the guidelines for adequate diet is essential so that, nurses can teach about nutrients and answer for the questions related to diet.
- Nurses must be able to assist the nutrients of the diet. They must also recognize that many divergent factors influence food intake and considering the factors when attempting to modify food intake.
- The factors that influence nutrient requirements are developmental consideration, i.e., age, sex, health status, culture and religion, socioeconomic status, personal preference, medications, alcohol and drugs, etc.
- Nurse also must be able to identify clients at risk for nutritional problems and be aware of common nutritional conditions.
- Metabolism refers to all the biochemical reactions within the body. It consists of anabolic reactions that build substances, body tissues and catabolic reactions those breakdown substances.
- Food is ingested, digested and absorbed to produce the energy needed for these reactions. The energy requirement of an awake person at rest is called the 'basal metabolic rate' (BMR).
- BMR is the energy needed at a person's lowest level of cellular functions. Age, body size, temperature, growth, sex, nutritional status, emotional status and good intake affect individual energy requirements beyond the BMR.
- When energy requirements are completely met by caloric intake in food, people maintain that activity levels without weight change.
- If the number of calories ingested exceeds energy needs, people gain weight. When the calories ingested fail to meet energy requirements, people lose weight.
- Nutrition encompasses all of the processes involved in consuming and utilizing food for energy, maintenance and growth. The processes include ingestion, digestion, absorption, metabolism and excretion.

Figure 1.3 is depicted the classifications of nutrition.

Physiology of Nutrition

Five processes are involved in the body's use of nutrients:
1. Ingestion
2. Digestion
3. Absorption
4. Metabolism
5. Excretion

> There are 5 steps involved in the process of nutrition of human beings:
> 1. **Ingestion:** The process of taking in food into the body is called ingestion
> 2. **Digestion:** It involves the break down of nutrients such as proteins into amino acids, carbohydrates into starch and fats into fatty acids and glycerol
> 3. **Absorption:** It involves the absorption of nutrients from the food by blood
> 4. **Assimilation:** It involves the process of transporting nutrients and water to all parts of the body by blood
> 5. **Egestion:** It involves the disposal of waste food out form the body

Ingestion
- Nutrition begins with ingestion, taking food into the digestive tract, generally through the mouth.
- In special circumstances, ingestion occurs directly into the stomach, through a feeding tube.

Digestion
- Digestion refers to the mechanical and chemical processes that convert nutrients into a physically absorbable state.
- Mechanical digestion includes mastication (chewing), breaking food into fine particles and mixing it with enzymes in saliva and deglutition (swallowing food), the peristaltic waves and mucus secretions that move the food down the esophagus.
- Chemical digestion includes the digestive juices changes food into the individual nutrients that can be used by the body.
- Digestion begins in the stomach (except in the case of some starches for which digestion begins in the mouth) and is completed in the intestines.
- Peristalsis (rhythmic, coordinated, serial contractions of the smooth muscles of the gastrointestinal tract (GIT) forces, chyme (an acidic, semi-fluid paste) through the small and large intestines.
- Only carbohydrates, proteins and fats require chemical digestion to make the nutrients available or absorption.

Figure 1.4 is depicted the food digestion in digestive system.

Absorption
- Absorption is the process, whereby the end products of digestion (i.e., individual nutrients) pass through the epithelial membranes in the small and large intestines and into the blood or lymph systems.

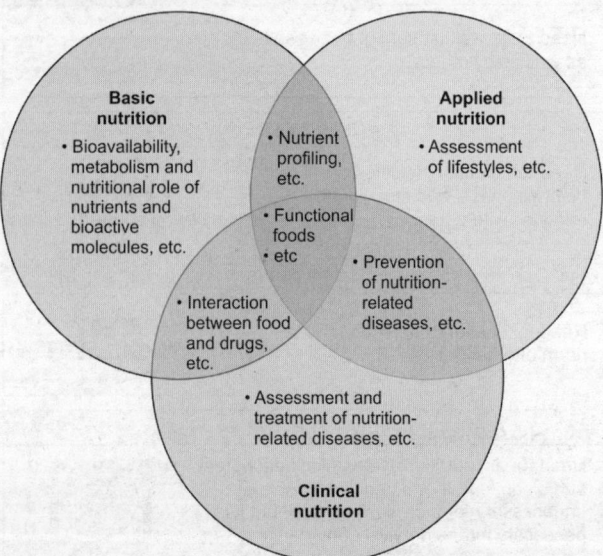

Fig. 1.3: Classifications of nutrition.

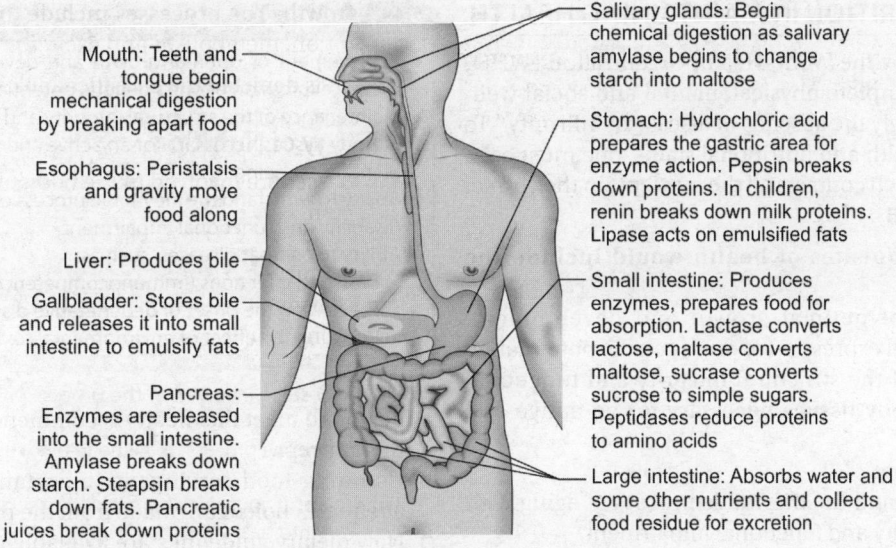

Fig. 1.4: Food digestion in digestive system.

- The nutrients are absorbed and taken to the parts of the body that need them.
- Most nutrients are water soluble and can be absorbed directly through the villi (finger-like projections that line the small intestine) and into the blood.
- Fats, which are not water soluble are absorbed first into the lymph system and eventually enter the circulatory system.

Metabolism

The conversion of nutrients into energy by the body is called metabolism. This process is the sum total of all the biological and chemical processes in the body as they relate to the use of nutrients in everybody cell. Metabolism involves two processes:
1. Anabolism
2. Catabolism

Anabolism

Anabolism is the constructive process of metabolism, wherein new molecules are synthesized and new tissues are formed, as in growth and repair. This process requires energy.

Catabolism

- Catabolism is the destructive process of metabolism, wherein tissues or substances are broken into their component parts. This process releases energy.
- During metabolism, energy is also produced by the process of oxidation, which is the chemical process of combining nutrients with oxygen.
- The energy produced by the body is used in a number of ways such as electrical energy for brain and nerve activities, chemical energy for metabolism, mechanical energy for muscle contractions and thermal energy to keep the body warm.
- Metabolic rate is the rate of energy utilization in the body; it is expressed in units called calories.
- One calorie is the amount of heat required to raise the temperature of 1 g of water by (1°C). Because of the large quantity of energy released during metabolism, the energy is expressed in kilocalories (kcal), each of which is equal to 1,000 calories.
- Basal metabolism is the amount of energy needed to maintain essential physiologic functions, when a person is at complete; rest that is, the lowest level of energy expenditure.
- The major factor affecting basal metabolism is body composition. Lean muscle tissue has a higher metabolic rate and thus produces more energy than fat tissue.
- Generally, women have a lower metabolism than men, because they have a higher percentage of fat tissue; however, metabolism increases during menstruation, pregnancy and lactation.
- Age has also an influence, because growth periods increase metabolism. Glandular activity, especially of the thyroid gland, affects metabolism.
- The rate of metabolism is governed primarily by the hormones triiodothyronine (T3) and thyroxine (T4).
- Hypothyroid activity, a decrease in the secretion of thyroid hormones, causes a lower rate of metabolism, whereas hyperthyroid activity, an increase in the secretion of thyroid hormones, causes a higher rate of metabolism.

Excretion

- Excretion is the process of eliminating or removing waste products from the body.
- Dietary fiber and indigestible materials, salts and other products such as bile and water are converted into feces and excreted from the body as solid waste.
- Other excretory organs that aid the digestive system in the elimination of wastes include the kidneys, bladder, sweat glands, skin and lungs.
- Most liquid waste is sent through the kidneys and bladder to be excreted as urine.
- Some liquid waste is removed through the sweat glands of the skin as perspiration. Gaseous waste is eliminated through the lungs.

ROLE OF NUTRITION IN MAINTAINING HEALTH

Health is defined by the World Health Organization (WHO) as the "state of complete physical, mental and social well-being and not merely the absence of disease or infirmity." To maintain good health and nutritional status, one must eat a balanced food, which contains all the nutrients in the correct proportion **(Fig. 1.5)**.

The essential requisites of health would include the following:
- Achievement of optimal growth and development, reflecting the full expression of one's genetic potential.
- Maintenance of the structural integrity and functional efficiency of body tissues necessary for an active and productive use.
- Mental well-being
- Ability to withstand the inevitable process of aging with minimal disability and functional impairment.
- Ability to combat diseases, such as:
  - Resisting infections (immunocompetence).
  - Preventing the onset of degenerative diseases.
  - Resisting the effect of environmental toxins/pollutants.

Till 3 decades, the role of nutrition in growth and development and tissue integrity alone was clear, but now the persuasive role nutrition plays in the other dimensions of health is implicit. Hence an optimal nutritional status is an indication of good health. This recent advance has brought about a large-scale change in dietary habits and practices of the population.

FACTS ABOUT BASIC NUTRITION AND HEALTH

- The amount and kinds of food eaten affect his/her health and wellbeing.
- Eating the recommended servings of food 'from the food guide pyramid' will provide key nutrients and enable a person to meet the dietary recommendations outlined in this concept.
- Counting food servings is important to assuring that adequate choices are made from the pyramid.
- New dietary guidelines are available to help a person to plan for sound nutrition.
  The number of calories needed per day depends upon the body's metabolic rate (BMR), which in turn, depends upon factors, such as age, sex, size, muscle mass, glandular function, emotional state, climate and exercise.
- Eating well can reduce risk of various health problems and increase quality of life.

Box 1.4 is depicted the relation between nutrition and health.

> **Box 1.4:** Relation between nutrition and health.
> - Achievement of optimal growth and development, reflecting the full expression of one's genetic potential
> - Maintenance of the structural integrity and functional efficiency of body tissues necessary for an active and productive use
> - Mental well-being
> - Ability to withstand the inevitable process of aging with minimal disability and functional impairment
> - Ability to combat diseases, such as:
>   - Resisting infections (immunocompetence)
>   - Preventing the onset of degenerative diseases
>   - Resisting the effect of environmental toxins/pollutants

Dietary Recommendations

- **For facts:**
  - Excess fat in the diet, particularly saturated fat, is associated with an increased risk of disease and is inversely related to optimal health.
  - Modified fats and fat substitutes in the diet can have varying health consequences.
  - There are some recommendations that can be followed to assure healthy amounts of fat in the diet.

  Figure 1.6 is depicted the relationship between nutrition and health.

- **For carbohydrates:**
  - For optimal health, carbohydrates, especially complex carbohydrates, should be the principal source of calories in the diet.
  - There are some recommendations that can be followed to assure healthy amounts of carbohydrate in the diet.

- **For proteins:**
  - Protein is the basic building block for the body, but dietary protein constitutes a relatively small amount of daily calorie intake.
  - There are some recommendations that can be followed to assure healthy amounts of protein in the diet.

- **For vitamins:**
  - Adequate vitamin intake is necessary to good health and wellness, but excessive vitamin intake is not necessary and can be harmful.
  - There are some recommendations that can be followed to assure healthy amounts of vitamins in the diet.

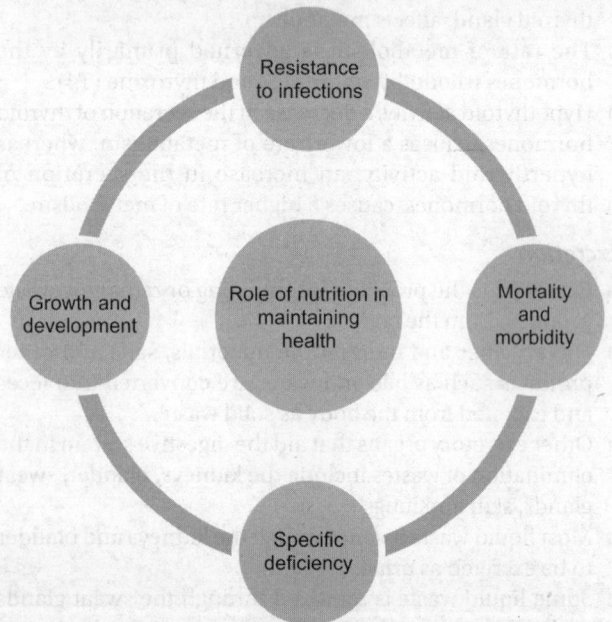

Fig. 1.5: Role of nutrition in maintaining health.

Chapter 1: Introduction to Nutrition

Nutritional situation	Health consequences, outcomes
Optimum nutrition Food—secure individuals with adequate, balanced and prudent diets	Health, well-being, normal development, high quality of life
Undernutrition: Hunger Food-insecure individuals living in poverty, ignorance, politically unstable environments, disrupted societies, war	• Decreased physical and development • Compromised immune systems • Increased infectious diseases • Vicious circle of undernutrition, underdevelopment, poverty
Overnutrition Overconsumption of food, especially macronutrients, plus: • Low physical activity • Smoking, stress, alcohol abuse	Obesity, metabolic syndrome, cardiovascular disease, type 2 diabetes mellitus, certain cancers: chronic NCDs, often characterized by overnutrition of macronutrients and undernutrition of micronutrients
Malnutrition Nutrition transition: Individuals and communities previously food insecure → confronted with abundance of palatable foods → some undernourished, others too many macronutrients and too few micronutrients	Double burden of infectious diseases plus NCDs, often characterized by overnutrition of macronutrients and undernutrition of micronutrients

Fig. 1.6: Relationship between nutrition and health.
(NCD: noncommunicable disease)

- **For minerals:**
  - Adequate mineral intake is necessary for good health and wellness, but excessive mineral intake is not necessary and can be harmful.
  - There are some recommendations that can be followed to assure healthy amounts of minerals in the diet.
- **For water and other fluids:**
  - Water is a critical component in the healthy diet. Beverages other than water are a part of many diets. Some beverages can have an adverse effect on good health.
  - There are some recommendations that can be followed to assure healthy amounts of water and fluids in the diet.

Social factors	Physical factors	Psychological factors
• Poverty • Isolation (living alone or living in a remote area) • Poor nutrition, difficulty with food preparation, poor knowledge of food safety • Elder abuse and neglect • Institutional environment (hospital or old-age home)	• Dental problems and/or dysphagia (difficulty swallowing) • Diminished sense of smell or taste and/or xerostomia (dry mouth) • Effects of medications • Impaired absorption of nutrients • Increased metabolism (as in Parkinson's disease) • Chronic disease or chronic infection • Severe problems with vision • Physical disabilities and/or impaired performance of basic daily activities (including food shopping, cooking, and eating)	• Widowed or bereaved • Depression • Loneliness • Dementia • Alcoholism • Fear of choking and other food-related anxieties • Anorexia (loss of appetite)

Source: Adapted from Damton-Hill et al., 2002.

Facts about Sound Eating Practices
- Healthy snacks can be an important part of good nutrition.
- Consistency (with variety) is a good general rule of nutrition.
- Moderation is a good general rule of nutrition.
- Careful selection of food choices is important for those who rely on fast foods as a significant part of their diet.
- There are some recommendations that can be followed concerning fast foods.

Facts about Nutrition and Physical Performance
- Carbohydrate loading and carbohydrate replacement during exercise can enhance sustained aerobic performances exceeding 1 hour in length.
- The timing may be more important than the makeup of the pre-event meal.
- High protein diets advocated for active people and athletes have been questioned by leading organizations in the areas of health, physical activity and nutrition.
- People who are interested in enhancing physical performance are especially subject to nutrition quackery.

IMPORTANCE OF NUTRITION IN HEALTH

Nutrition may be defined as the science of food and its relationship to health. It is concerned primarily with the part played by nutrients in body growth, development and maintenance. The word nutrient or 'food factor' is used for specific dietary constituents, such as proteins, vitamins and minerals. Dietetics is the practical application of the principles of nutrition; it includes the planning of meals for the well and the sick.

- Good nutrition means 'maintaining a nutritional status that enables us to grow well and enjoy good health'.
- Nutrition deals with the way in which the human body receives and uses all the substance or materials necessary for its growth and development and for keeping it in good condition.
- This begins in eating food. The food swallowed and then digested as it is passed through the stomach and small intestines.
- During digestion, the food is broken up into simple substances. These are absorbed into bloodstream and carried to the liver, where they are either stored or changed further or sent out to other parts of the body for use as required.
- Some are used to supply the body with heat and energy and others for the building and repair of the tissues and yet others are used to control the chemical changes taking place in the body or to protect the body from diseases, finally the waste products, which cannot be used are excreted.

Relation of Nutrition to Health
- Good nutrition is a basic component of health.
- The relation of nutrition to health may be seen from the following view points:

Growth and Development

- Good nutrition is essential for the attainment of normal growth and development. Not only physical growth and development, but also the intellectual development, learning and behavior are affected by malnutrition.
- Malnutrition during pregnancy may affect the fetus resulting in stillbirth, premature birth and 'small-for-dates' babies.
- Malnutrition during early childhood delays physical and mental growth; such children are slow in passing their milestones and are slow learners in school.
- Good nutrition is also essential in adult life for the maintenance of optimum health and efficiency. In short, nutrition affects human health from birth till death.

Specific Deficiency

- Malnutrition is directly responsible for certain specific nutritional deficiency diseases.
- The commonly reported ones in India are kwashiorkor, marasmus, blindness due to vitamin A deficiency, anemia, beriberi, goiter, etc.
- Good nutrition therefore is essential for the prevention of specific nutritional deficiency diseases and promotion of health.

Resistance to Infection

- Malnutrition predisposes to infections, such as tuberculosis. It also influences the course and outcome of many of the clinical disorders.
- Infection, in turn, may aggravate malnutrition by affecting the food intake, absorption and metabolism.

Mortality and Morbidity

- The indirect effects of malnutrition on the community are even more striking; a high general death rate, high-infant mortality rate, high-sickness rate and a lower expectation of life.
- Over-nutrition, which is another form of malnutrition, is responsible for obesity.
- Diabetes, hypertension, cardiovascular and renal disease, disorders of the liver and gallbladder. More recent reports suggest that diet perhaps plays an important role in certain types of gastrointestinal cancers. It is now quite well-accepted that diet and certain diseases are inter-related.

Figure 1.7 is depicted the factors affecting on diet and nutrition and **Figure 1.8** is depicted the role of various parts of body on digestion and absorption.

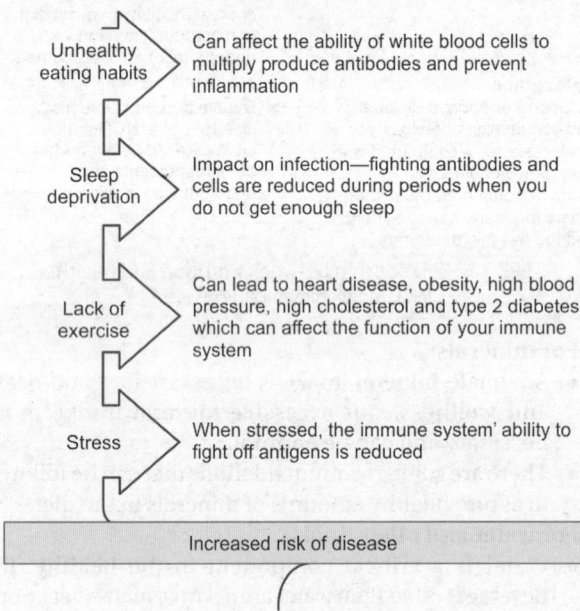

Fig. 1.7: Factors affecting on diet and nutrition.

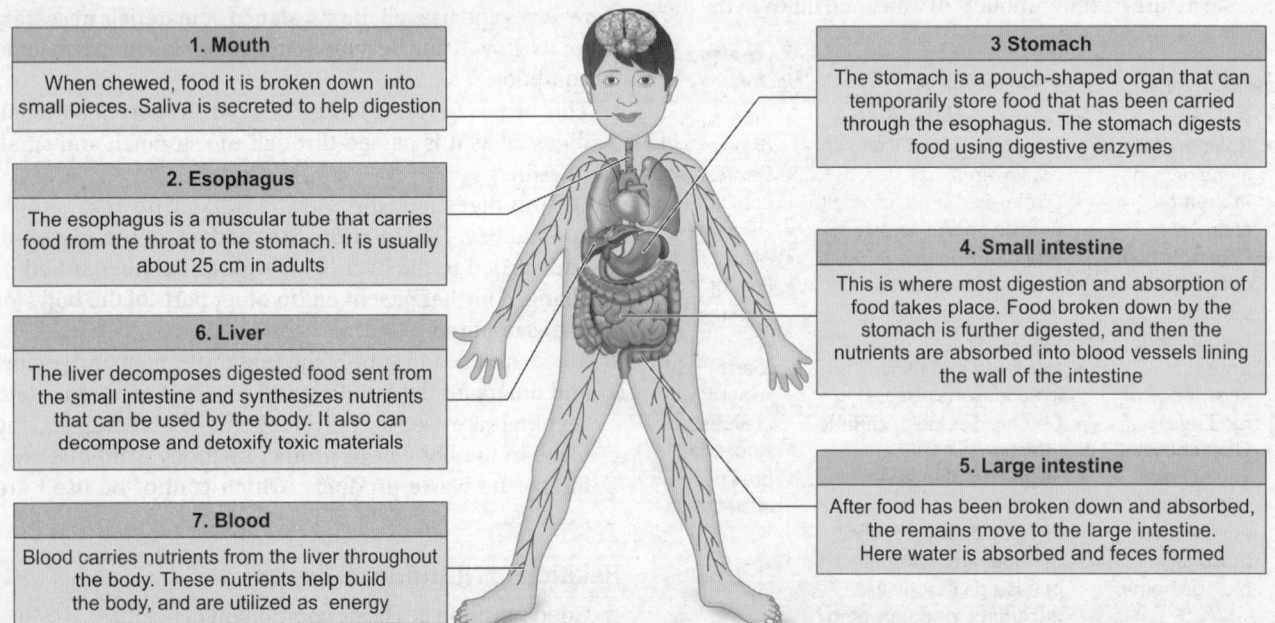

Fig. 1.8: Role of various parts of body on digestion and absorption.

FACTORS AFFECTING FOOD AND NUTRITION

Habits about eating are influenced by developmental considerations, gender, ethnicity and culture, beliefs about food, personal preferences, religious practices, lifestyle, economics, medication and therapy, health, alcohol consumption, advertising, and psychological factors. Although the nutritional content of food is an important consideration when planning a diet, an individual's food preferences and habits are often a major factor affecting actual food intake. Habits about eating are influenced by developmental considerations, gender, ethnicity and culture, beliefs about food, personal preferences, religious practices, lifestyle, economics, medication and therapy, health, alcohol consumption, advertising, and psychological factors.

Sl. No.	Factors	Description
1.	Development	People in rapid periods of growth (i.e., infancy and adolescence) have increased needs for nutrients. Elders, on the other hand, need fewer calories and dietary changes in view of the risk of coronary heart disease, osteoporosis, and hypertension.
2.	Gender	Nutrient requirements are different for men and women because of body composition and reproductive functions. The larger muscle mass of men translates into a greater need for calories and proteins. Because of menstruation, women require more iron than men do prior to menopause. Pregnant and lactating women have increased caloric and fluid needs.
3.	Ethnicity and culture	Ethnicity often determines food preferences. Traditional food (e.g., rice for Asians, pasta for Italians, and curry for Indians) are eaten long after other customs are abandoned. Nurses should not use a "good food, bad food" approach, but rather should realize that variations of intake are acceptable under different circumstances. The only "universally" accepted guidelines are to eat moderately to maintain correct body weight. Food preference probably differs as much among individuals of the same cultural background as it does generally between cultures. Not all Italians like pizza, for example, and many undoubtedly enjoy Mexican food.
4.	Social factors	Food habits are handed over from generation to generation in the society particularly in the developing countries. Though these factors have very little or no scientific basis, people rigidly adhere to them in many parts of India; pregnant women are not allowed to consume papayas as it is believed that papayas produce a lot of heat in the body, which in turn induce abortion.
5.	Religious factors	Many Hindus are vegetarians; Janis do not eat curd and do not eat after sunset. To eat meat is to destroy the seed of compassion. Islamic food laws prohibit the consumption of unclean foods such as swine and animals killed in a manner that prevents their blood from being fully drained from their bodies. Jews do not eat pork and shellfish.
6.	Cultural factors	It is a custom in most of the communities in India that women and girls eat only after men and boys finish their eating. Curd and citrus fruit should not be taken by a person suffering from cold or cough.
7.	Traditional factors	The traditional cooking practices also act as a barrier to achieving a balanced diet, e.g., using polished rice, draining away the rice water and prolonged boiling of vegetables add to the great loss of nutrients. Women should take only bread and coffee for 2 days after the delivery of a child and a very small quantity of water should be given.
8.	Economical factors	Financial resources determine the type of food, depending on the availability one selects the food. People in lower income groups in India consume a combination of cereals and cheaply available green leafy vegetables, roots and tubers.
9.	Beliefs about food	Beliefs about effects of foods on health and well-being can affect food choices. Many people acquire their beliefs about food from television, magazines, and other media. For example, some people are reducing their intake of animal fats in response to evidence that excessive consumption of animal fats is a major risk factor in vascular disease, including heart attack and stroke. Food fads that involve nontraditional food practices are relatively common. A fad is a widespread but short-lived interest or a practice followed with considerable zeal. It may be based either on the belief that certain foods have special powers or on the notion that certain foods are harmful. Food fads appeal to the individual seeking a miracle cure for a disease, the person who desires superior heath, or one who wants to delay aging. Some fad diets are harmless, but others are potentially dangerous. Determining the needs a fad diet fills for the client enables the nurse both to support these needs and to suggest a more nutritious diet.
10.	Personal performance	People develop likes and dislikes based on associations with a typical food. A child who loves to visit his grandparents may love pickled crabapples because they are served in the grandparent's home. Another child who dislikes a very strict aunt grows up to dislike the chicken casserole she often prepares. People often carry such preferences into adulthood. Individual likes and dislikes can also be related to familiarity. Children often say they dislike a food before they sample it. Some adults are very adventurous and eager to try new foods. Others prefer to eat the same foods repeatedly. Preferences in the tastes, smells, flavors (blends of taste and smell), temperatures, colors, shapes, and sizes of food influence a person's food choices. For example, some people may prefer sweet and sour tastes to bitter or salty tastes. Texture plays a great role in food preferences. Some people prefer crisp food to limp food, firm to soft, tender to tough, smooth to lumpy, or dry to soggy.

NUTRIENTS (FIG. 1.9)

A nutrient is a substance used by an organism to survive, grow, and reproduce. The requirement for dietary nutrient intake applies to animals, plants, fungi, and protists. Nutrients can be incorporated into cells for metabolic purposes or excreted by cells to create non-cellular structures, such as hair, scales, feathers, or exoskeletons. Some nutrients can be metabolically converted to smaller molecules in the process of releasing energy, such as for carbohydrates, lipids, proteins and fermentation products (ethanol or vinegar), leading to end-products of water and carbon dioxide. All organisms require water.

Essential nutrients for animals are the energy sources, some of the amino acids that are combined to create proteins, a subset of fatty acids, vitamins and certain minerals. Plants require more diverse minerals absorbed through roots, plus carbon dioxide and oxygen absorbed through leaves. Fungi live on dead or living organic matter and meet nutrient needs from their host.

Definition

Nutrients are chemical compounds in food that are used by the body to function properly and maintain health. Examples include proteins, fats, carbohydrates, vitamins, and minerals.

Classification of Nutrients

The 7 major groups of nutrients performs different and unique functions in our body, they are all essential because they work together and contribute to our good health. The main functions of these major nutrients can be summarized as below:

1. **Carbohydrates:** Carbohydrates are a major source of energy of our body, and they come mainly from grains, such as rice and noodles. Besides, fruit, root vegetables, dry beans and dairy products also contain carbohydrates.
2. **Proteins:** Meat, fish, seafood, eggs, dairy products, dry beans and bean products are good sources of protein. Its major functions include building, repairing and maintaining healthy body tissues.
3. **Fats:** Fats can be found in foods, such as meat, fish, seafood, dairy products, nuts, seeds and oils. Fats serve as an energy source. They prevent heat loss in extreme cold weather and protect organs against shock. They are responsible for making up part of our body cells and transporting fat-soluble vitamins such as vitamin A, D, E and K.

Organic nutrients	Inorganic nutrients
Carbohydrates Proteins Lipids/fats, and vitamins	Minerals Water
The chemical compounds of living things are known as organic compounds because of their association with organisms and because they are carbon-containing compounds	Inorganic nutrients do not contain carbon elements. These nutrients lost in the urine represent that must be consumed in the diet to maintain nutrient balance

4. **Vitamins:** There are many kinds of vitamins from various food groups and they participate in different body metabolism, such as maintaining healthy skin and hair, building bones and releasing and utilizing energy from foods. Vitamins can be classified into water-soluble and fat-soluble vitamins.
5. **Minerals:** Minerals are a group of essential nutrients which regulate many body functions, such as fluid balance, muscle contraction and transmission of nerve impulses. Some minerals also contribute to body structure and build strong and healthy bones, such as calcium

Organic	Inorganic
• Large non-nutrient content • Bulky • Little direct cost • Imprecise content analysis • No direct energy use in manufacture • Readily available • Provides disposal of wastes	• High concentration of nutrients • Ease of transport • Increasing cost • Made from finite resources • Large direct energy use in manufacture • Availability depends on production, cost and region • Creates wastes in processing, but can also utilize wastes from other manufacturing processes

Source: Stout, 1984.

6. **Dietary fiber:** Dietary fiber is the indigestible part found in plant. It helps stabiles blood sugar, promote gastrointestinal health and prevent constipation. Dietary fiber can be classified into soluble and insoluble fibre.
7. **Water:** Water is the most abundant substance in human body and is also an essential nutrient to maintain our health. The major functions of water include regulation of body temperature, production of body fluids, transportation of nutrients and removal of waste products.

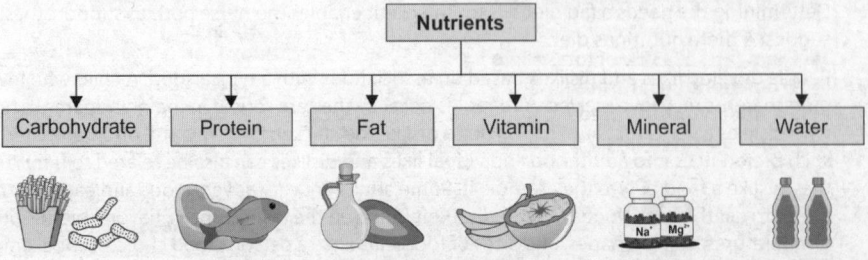

Fig. 1.9: Nutrients.

MACRO- AND MICRONUTRIENTS

Sl. No.	Difference on the basis of	Macro-nutrients	Micro-nutrients
1.	Requirement	Macro-nutrients are required in larger amount/quantity on a daily basis	Micro-nutrients are required in small or tiny amount/quantity on a daily basis
2.	Function	• Macro-nutrients is essential for growth, repair and develop new tissues (carbohydrates), maintain body temperature (fats), conduct nerve impulses, and regulate life process	• Micro-nutrients support macro-nutrients to carry out bodily functions. They are also an essential component for building healthy brain, body and bones.
3.	Benefits/advantages	• Macro-nutrients contribute to the bulk energy needed for the metabolic system • Macro-nutrients provide calories that gives energy to the body	• Micro-nutrients contribute to body growth and disease prevention. • Micro-nutrients comprises of high volume of antioxidants which protects the body against various diseases
4.	Role	Macro-nutrients plays a vital role in the construction of body composition.	Micro-nutrients do not have any role in the construction of body composition.
5.	Concentration	Macro-nutrients are available in high concentration inside the body.	Micro-nutrients are present in minute concentration inside the body.
6.	Composition/known as	Macro-nutrients are also called as major elements.	Micro-nutrients are also called trace elements.
7.	Food composition	Cereals, legumes, meat, fish, yams, potatoes, nuts, oilseeds are rich in macro-nutrients.	Mainly vegetables, fruits, eggs, green leafy vegetables, fermented foods are rich in micro-nutrients.
8.	Types and examples	There are mainly three macro-nutrients required by the body; carbohydrate, protein and fats	Different types of micro-nutrients required by the body include vitamins, minerals and trace elements. Examples: iron, magnesium, calcium, phosphorus, zinc, etc.
9.	Quantity	Macro-nutrients are divided into two classes—primary and secondary, as they are required in large quantities.	Micro-nutrients are not classified in different types, as it is required in trace amount.
10.	Composition	Primary macro-nutrients include nitrogen, phosphorus, and potassium in larger quantities. Secondary macro-nutrients include calcium, magnesium, and sulfur in lesser quantity.	Micro-nutrients include zinc, iron, manganese, copper, boron, molybdenum and chlorine in trace quantities.
11.	Toxicity	Macro-nutrients are normally not toxic to the cell if they are present in comparatively higher concentration than in the normal level.	Micro-nutrients are toxic if present exorbitantly in the cell than the required amount.
12.	Excessive ingestion	Excessive intake of micro-nutrients leads to obesity and diabetes.	Excessive consumption of micro-nutrients leads to suppressing immune function.
13.	Consequences of deficiency	Deficiency of macro-nutrients causes protein–energy malnutrition (PEM), kwashiorkor, marasmus, etc.	Deficiency of micro-nutrients causes different diseases, such as night blindness, beriberi, scurvy, goiter, etc.
14.	Consequences of overdose	Overdose of macro-nutrients causes obesity, heart diseases, diabetes and other metabolic syndromes	Overdose of micro-nutrients may harm specific organs of the body. For example, overdose of vitamins affect liver
15.	Daily recommended requirements	• **From carbohydrates**: 55–75% of total energy • **From protein**: 15–20% of total energy or 1 g/kg body weight per day • **From fats**: 20–35% of total energy • **From monounsaturated fats**: 20% of total energy • **From polyunsaturated fats**: 10% of total energy • **From saturated fats**: 7% of total energy	• Vitamin A—700 µg • Vitamin B12—2.4 mg • Vitamin E—15 mg • Vitamin C—75 mg • Thiamine—1 mg • Riboflavin—1.1 mg • Niacin—14 mg • Folate—400 mg • Iron—18 mg • Selenium—55 mg • Calcium—1000 mg

ENERGY YIELDING AND NON-ENERGY YIELDING

- Carbohydrates, fats, and proteins are also referred to as energy-yielding macro-nutrients because they supply the body with energy. Vitamins and minerals are micro-nutrients, which are required in the body in smaller amounts in comparison to macro-nutrients.
- A common misconception is that vitamins and minerals are energy nutrients. These do not contain energy, though they play essential roles in the production of energy.
- Deficiencies of certain vitamins and minerals can lead to fatigue. Macro- and micro-nutrients work together for optimal physiological function.
- The unit of energy in food is called a kilocalorie, commonly referred to as a calorie or kcal.
- A kilocalorie is the amount of heat it takes to raise the temperature of one kilogram of water by one degree Celsius. A person's energy requirements refer to the number of kilocalories needed each day.
- Food labels list calories per serving of the item. Both carbohydrate and protein contain 4 calories per gram, while lipids provide 9 calories per gram, making lipids more energy dense—i.e., they contain more calories per mass or volume than do carbohydrate or protein.

ELEMENTS OF NUTRIENTS: MACRO AND MICRO

Review of Nutrients: Macro- and Micro-nutrients

- Nutrients which are needed by the body for good nutritional status are provided by food.
- An individual nutritional status is dependent on the provision of sufficient nutrients and the good utilization of these nutrients.
- Power status of nutrition may be caused by eating that is inadequate in amount and kind, or it may be caused by failure in digestion and utilization of these nutrients.
- The nutrients present in foods fall into three major categories—proximate, vitamins and minerals.
- The proximate usually referred to as proximate principles include only those nutrients that yield energy on oxidation, i.e., carbohydrates, proteins and fats.
- Nutrients are organic and inorganic complexes contained in food.

Figure 1.10 is depicted the essential elements.

Macro- and micro-nutrients: Macro-nutrients are carbohydrate, protein and fats which are often called "proximate principles" because they form a main bulk of the food.

- Carbohydrate: 65 to 80%
- Protein: 7 to 15%
- Fats: 10 to 30%

Figure 1.11 is depicted the classification of nutrients.

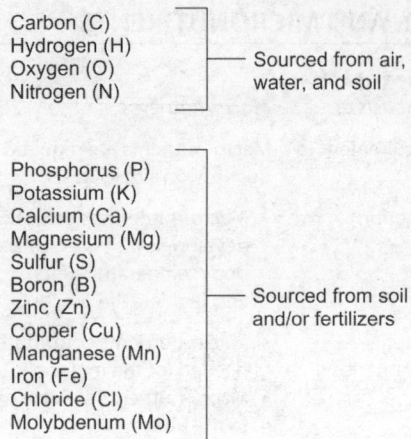

Fig. 1.10: Essential elements.

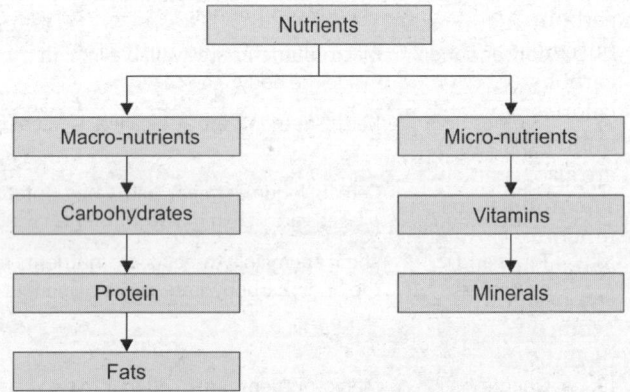

Fig. 1.11: Classification of nutrients.

Micro nutrients:
- These are vitamins and minerals. They are called micro-nutrients because they are required in small amounts.
- A vitamin is an organic compound that cannot be manufactured by the body and is needed in small quantities to catalyze metabolic process. When this vitamins are lacking in the diet, metabolic deficits results.
- Minerals are found in organic compounds, and inorganic compounds as free ions. On oxidation, minerals leave an ash, which can be acid or alkaline.

Macro-nutrients (Fig. 1.12)

Carbohydrates

Carbohydrates are the chief, cheapest and main source of energy. Carbohydrate normally should provide 50–60% of total caloric requirements. All the carbohydrates contain carbon, hydrogen ad oxygen. All the carbohydrates are changed in the body to simple form called glucose.

Carbohydrate can be classified into three categories:
1. Monosaccharide: Glucose, fructose, galactose
2. Disaccharides: Maltose, lactose, sucrose
3. Polysaccharides: Starch, glycogen
- **Food sources of carbohydrates** are the sugars, cereal grains, legumes and dried fruits are the richest sources of

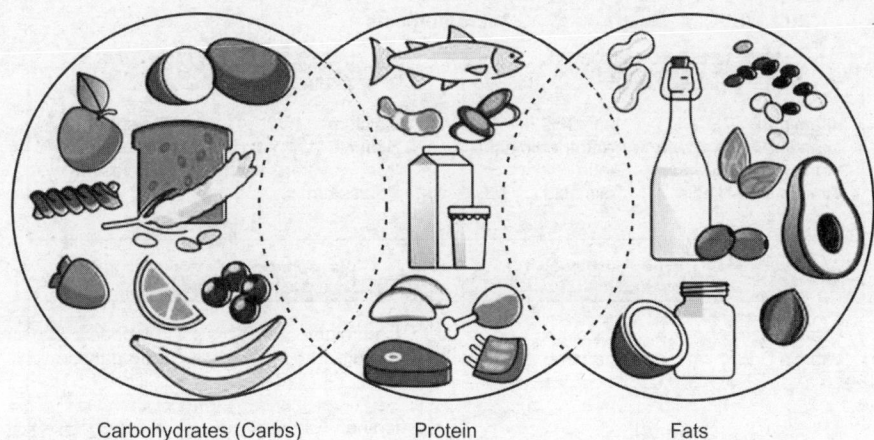

Fig. 1.12: Macro-nutrients.

carbohydrates. White sugar is almost pure carbohydrate but cereal grains, legumes and dried fruits may vary in their carbohydrates content. One gram of carbohydrate gives 4 calories of energy on burning. Intake of carbohydrate is ordinarily greater than that of fat for energy. Carbohydrates are also useful in the detoxication of ammonia.

- **The main functions of carbohydrate** have a variety of functions in the animal and human body. They supply energy for body functions and for doing work. They are essential for the oxidation of fats. They exert a sparing action on proteins and they add flavor to the diet. Diabetes mellitus is a chronic disease in which blood glucose level is raised above 180 mg per 100 mL blood and glucose is excreted in urine. This disease is primarily due to the insufficient production of hormone—insulin by the beta cells of the islets of langerhans of the pancreas.

Proteins

The name "**protein**" was suggested by Mulder in 1838 to the complex organic nitrogenous substances found in animal and plant tissues. Protein constitute about one fifth (20%) of animal body on the fresh weight basis. They are essential for life processes. They plan an important role in many biochemicals, biophysical processes in the body.

Classification of proteins:
1. **Simple proteins:** These include albumins, globulins, glutelins, prolamins, fibrous proteins, histones and protamins.
2. **Conjugated proteins:** These include nucleoprotein glycoprotein, phosphoproteins, hemoglobin and lecithoproteins.
3. **Derived proteins:** These include proteins, metaproteins, coagulated proteins, peptones and peptides.

The main functions of proteins are to replace the daily loss of body protein, to provide amino acids for the formation of tissue proteins during growth and to provide the amino acids necessary for the formation of enzymes, blood, proteins and certain hormones of protein nature and to provide amino acids for growth of fetus in pregnancy and for the production of milk proteins during lactation. Disease due to the deficiencies of protein and calories occur commonly among weaned infants and preschool children in India and other developing countries. They may be classified into three groups—kwashiorkor, nutritional marasmus and marasmic-kwashiorkor.

Lipids

The term "lipids" is applied to a group of naturally occurring substances characterized by their insolubility in water, greasy feel and solubility in some organic solvents. Fats are solid at 20°C they are called "oils" if they are liquid at that temperature. They are classified as—(1) simple lipids, e.g., triglycerides, (2) compound lipids, e.g., phospholipids, (3) derived lipids, e.g., cholesterol.

Sources of fats may be classified as:
1. Animal fats (fat of meat and fish, ghee, butter, milk and eggs.
2. Vegetable fats (some of the plants store fat in the seeds (e.g., ground nut, mustard, sesame, coconut, etc.)
3. Other sources from cereals, pulses nuts and vegetables.

The fats are high energy foods, providing so much as 9 kcal for every gram. Fat in the body support viscera, such as heart, kidney and intestine and fat beneath the skin provides insulation against cold. Cholesterol is essential as a component of membranes and nervous tissue and is a precursor for the synthesis of steroid hormones and bile acid **a diet, rich fat** can pose a threat to human health encouraging obesity, phrynoderma, coronary heart disease, and cancer and skin lesions of kwashiorkor. When the cholesterol level is over 250 mg/100 mL, the incidence of atherosclerosis and coronary heart disease is high.

Micro-nutrients (Fig. 1.13)

Vitamins

Vitamins may be defined as organic compounds occurring in small quantities in the different natural foods and necessary for the growth and maintenance of good health in human being and certain experimental animals. Vitamins may be classified into two groups (a) fat soluble vitamins, (b) water soluble vitamins, fat soluble vitamins, e.g., vitamin A, D, E, and K.

Water soluble vitamins viz vitamins of the B group and vitamin C.

Micro-nutrients

Water soluble vitamins
- Vitamin B6
- Vitamin B2-Riboflavin
- Vitamin B1-Thiamin
- Vitamin B12-Niacin
- Vitamin C
- Pantothenic acid
- Biotin
- Folic acid

Essential minerals
- Calcium
- Sulfur
- Iron
- Potassium
- Phosphorus
- Sodium
- Magnesium

Fat soluble vitamins
- Vitamin A
- Vitamin D
- Vitamin K
- Vitamin E

Trace elements
- Chromium
- Cobalt
- Zinc
- Selenium
- Iodine
- Fluoride
- Manganese
- Silicon
- Boron
- Copper

Fig. 1.13: Types of micronutrients.

Figure 1.14 is depicted the food substances contain micro-nutrients.

Vitamin A:
- Vitamin A occurs only in foods of animal origin. Vitamin A activity is also possessed by carotenoids found in plants. Hence carotenoids are called provitamin A vitamin A is not synthesized in the body and must by supplied by food supplements.
- One of the best defined roles of vitamin A is its requirements for normal vision. Vitamin A is necessary for the health of the epithelial cells.
- Vitamin A deficiency is one of the main causes of blindness in India. The signs of vitamin A deficiency are predominantly ocular. They include night blindness, conjunctival xerosis, Bitot's spots corned xerosis and keratomalacia.
- The term "xerophthalmia" (dry eye) comprises all the ocular manifestations of vitamin A deficiency ranging from night blindness to keratomalacia.

Vitamin D:
- Although do formed bone conditions had been known for countries, it was not until 1922 that the cause of rickets was discovered. Many investigations noted that a poor environment, consisting of poor hygiene, lack of sunshine and exercise and often city dwelling was associated with the incidence of rickets.
- In 1824 cod liver oil was recommended as a remedy for rickets vitamin D helps in absorption of calcium and phosphorous and makes them more available for the development of bones.
- Rickets is the disease caused due to deficiency of vitamin D. The disease is characterized by deformities of the bones, such as knock knees and bow legs which may last throughout fish liver oils provides the most potent sources of this vitamins.
- Also ultraviolet rays of sunlight help in the synthesis of vitamin D in skin.

Vitamin E:
- Vitamin E is the generic name for a group of closely related and naturally occurring fat soluble compounds, the tocopherols of these alpha-tocopherol is biologically the most potent.
- Vitamin E is widely distributed in foods. The usual plasma level of vitamin E in adult is between 0.8 and 1.4 mg per 100 mL.
- A deficiency of vitamin E in various species of animals results in reproductive failure, macrocytic anemia and shorter lifespan of red blood cells.
- Recently the cytotoxic effect of vitamin E on human lymphocytes vitro at high concentrations has been reported.

Vitamin K:
- Vitamin K is necessary for the synthesis of prothrombin and enzyme synthesized by the liver; prothrombin is required for normal clotting of blood.
- Vitamin K is found in plants. Good sources are cauliflower spinach and soyabean.
- In contrast fruits, cereals and animal products contain little vitamin 'K'. It is also synthesized in the intestinal tract by the bacteria.
- In the newborn babies, intestinal bacteria are not sufficiently developed for the synthesis for vitamin 'K'. Thus some infants, especially those who are immature, show susceptibility to hemorrhage.
- Vitamin K is given to infants immediately after birth especially to those who show hemorrhage tendency.

Micro-nutrients

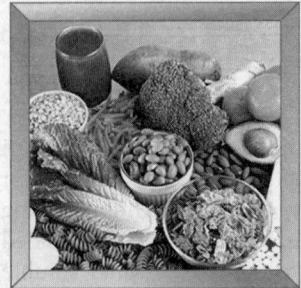
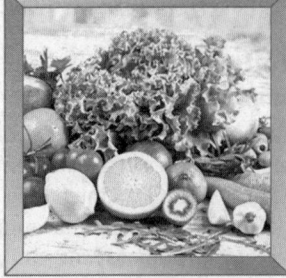

Minerals   Vitamins

Fig. 1.14: Food substances contain micro-nutrients.

Thiamine

- Thiamine (vitamin B1) is a water soluble vitamin. It is essential for the utilization of carbohydrates. In thiamine deficiency there is accumulation of pyruvic and lactic acids in the tissues and body fluids.
- Thiamine occurs in all natural foods, although small amounts. Important sources are whole grain cereals, wheat gram, yeast, pulses, oilseeds and nuts especially groundnut, meat, fish eggs, vegetables and fruits contain smaller amounts.
- Thiamine functions in the release of energy from the metabolism of carbohydrate. As a result thiamine is related to the maintenance of a normal appetite, normal muscle tone in the gastrointestinal tract and healthy nervous system.
- More advanced deficiencies result in the disease beriberi. There are two types of beriberi. The dry form is characterized by sever muscular wasting loss of sensation in the skin, loss of weight and paralysis of lower limbs.
- The wet form produces marked edema which usually starts from lower limbs and develops upward. When it reaches the trunk, involves heart and the result is heart failure.

Riboflavin

- Riboflavin (Vitamin B2) is a member of B group vitamins. It has fundamental role in cellular oxidation. It is a co-factor in a number of enzymes involves with energy metabolism.
- Its richest natural sources are milk, eggs, liver, kidney and green leafy vegetables. Meat and fish contain small amounts.
- There are no real body stores of riboflavin. Low dietary intake of riboflavin may result in fissures at the angle of the mouth, accompanied by the yellow cast.
- The tongue may exhibit glossitis, turning to purplish red in color, accompanied by a painful burning sensation.

Nicotinic Acid (NIACIN)

- Nicotinic acid contains a pyrodine nucleus. It is essential for the metabolism of carbohydrate, fat and protein.
- Nicotinic acid is essential for the normal functioning of the skin, intestinal tract and the nervous system.
- Foods rich in niacin or tryptophan are liver, kidney, meat, poultry, fish, legumes and groundnut. Milk is a poor source of niacin.
- Nicotinic acid deficiency causes the disease "pellagra" in human being.
- This disease is characterized by three D's—dermatitis, diarrhea and dementia. The dermatitis and diarrhea are two distributions and occurs in the hands, feet and neck.

Pyridoxine (B6)

- Pyridoxine (vitamin B6) exists in three forms, pyridoxine, pyridoxal and pyridoxamine.
- It plays an important role in the metabolism of amino acids, fats and carbohydrates. Rice dietary; sources are dried yeast rice polishing, wheat gram and liver.
- Pyridoxine is essential for maintaining the nerves in normal condition. Pyridoxal phosphate acts as coenzyme in the metabolism of amino acids.
- Effects of deficiency in human adults are seborrhea, such as lesion developed around the eyes, nose and mouth within 2-3 weeks.
- In infants deficiency seen as nervous irritability and convulsive seizures.

Pantothenic Acid

- Pantothenic acid is one of the vitamins of the vitamins B2 complex, which can prevent or cure a specific type of dermatitis (chick pellagra) in chicks fed on vitamin B2 deficient.
- Pantothenic acid in the form of coenzyme A takes part in the metabolism of carbohydrates and fats.
- It is essential for the oxidation of pyruvic acid. Burning feet syndrome was observed in prisoners of war during World War II in Japan, and Burma.
- This syndrome was associated with neurological and mental disturbances. Gopalan (1946) found that burning feet syndrome observed in Indian subjects responded to treatment with calcium pantothenate (20–40 mg)

Folic Acid

- Folic acid was known under different names from 1933 by its curative effects in deficiency states in man and in different experimental animals.
- It is essential for the maturation of red blood cells. It acts as a coenzyme in the synthesis of methionine and of purine and pyrimidine rings.
- Foods, such as liver, meat, dairy products, eggs, milk, fruits and cereals are as good dietary sources as leafy vegetables.
- Overcooking destroys much o folic acid and thus contributes of folate deficiency in man.
- Nutritional megaloblastic anemia in adults, the classical studies of wills (1931) in India showed that the megaloblastic anemia prevalent in pregnant women of the low income groups substituting on poor vegetarian diets.
- Megaloblastic anemia has been reported to occur among malnourished children in the developing countries.

Vitamin B12 (Cyanocobalamine)

- Cyanocobalamine was found effective in curing pernicious anemia when administered intramuscularly in small quantities (5-10 mg) for the absorption of vitamin B12 from the intestines, a factor called "Intrinsic factor" (IF) secreted by the stomach is essential vitamin B12 is stored in fair amount in the liver.
- Vitamin B12 promotes the maturation of red blood cells. It acts on the narrow elements and is involved in the formation of white blood cells and blood platelets.
- It cures the neurological symptoms of pernicious anemia. It acts as a coenzyme in the synthesis of methionine.
- Vitamin B12 deficiency causes the disease "pernicious anemia".

Ascorbic Acid

- Ascorbic acid is essential for the production and collagenous or intracellular material which holds the cell in proper relation to each other.
- It also important for healthy development of teeth, bones and cartilage and connective tissues.
- It is an important factor in the healing of wounds and in the ability to withstand stresses of injury and infection.
- A well balanced diet for school children and adults should contain some 30–50 mg of vitamin 'C' per day.
- The major functions of vitamin C is oxidation of tyrosine, reduction of ferric iron to ferrous iron in gastrointestinal tract so that iron is more readily absorbed, and conversion of folic acid into its active form folinic acid.
- Scurvy is the drastic consequence of vitamin 'C' deficiency. The principal symptoms of scurvy are restlessness, loss of appetite generally soreness to touch, sore mouth, bleeding gums and loosening of the health.

■ MINERAL ELEMENTS

There are a number of minerals or inorganic elements that play an important role in nutrition. Mineral elements are present in organic compounds, such as hemoglobin, phospholipids, thyroxin as inorganic compounds in sodium chloride and calcium phosphate and as free ions. They enter the structure of every cell of the body. Hard skeletal structures contain the greater proportions of some elements, such as calcium, phosphorous, and magnesium while soft tissues contain relatively higher proportions of potassium.

Mineral elements enter into numerous regulatory activities of the body. The contraction of muscles, the normal response of nerves to stimulation, the control of water balance, the maintenance of acid base equilibrium and the water balance of the food-stuffs are functions. Sodium, potassium, calcium, phosphorus and chloride are the essential constituents of body fluids. Calcium, magnesium, phosphorus and others are bone constituents. Iron, copper and cobalt function in together with protein, vitamin B12 and other nutrients for the synthesis of hemoglobin and red blood cells.

Element	Plant sources	Animal sources
Ca	Collards, mustard greens, broccoli	Dairy products, fortified juices, sardines, oysters, clams, canned salmon, kale
P	Nuts, beans, peas, lentils, grains	Meats, fish, eggs, dairy products
Mg	Seeds, nuts, beans, peas, lentils, whole grains, dark green vegetables	
Na	Common table salt, seafood	Dairy products, meats, eggs
K	Fruits, dairy products, meats, cereals, vegetables, beans, peas, lentils	

Contd...

Element	Plant sources	Animal sources
Cl	Common table salt	Seafood, dairy products, meats, eggs
Fe		Meats (especially red meats), seafood
Cu	Beans, peas, lentils, whole grains, nuts, organ meats, peanut products, mushrooms	Seafood (e.g., oysters, crab), chocolate
Zn	Nuts, whole grains, beans, peas, lentils, fortified breakfast cereals	Meats, organ meats, shellfish
Se	Grain products, nuts, garlic, broccoli grown on high-sea sales	Meats from Sea-fed livestock, sea fish
I	Iodized salt	Sea fish, kelp
Mn	Whole grains, beans, peas, lentils, nuts, tea	
Mo	Beans, peas, lentils, dark green leafy vegetables	Organ meats

Adapted from Combs (2005).

Calcium

- Body contains calcium in greater amount than other minerals.
- About 2% of the body weight of an adult is due to calcium, out of which about 99% is contained in bones and teeth.
- Calcium is the most important factor in building skeleton and teeth is more important during growing years.
- Normal behavior of heart, nervous system and blood clotting process, etc., depend on the presence of calcium.
- Human body at different levels of intake has suggested the desirability of a daily intake of about 0.4 to 0.6 g of calcium by an adult, the case of growing children and pregnant and lactating mothers, and the requirement is 1.0 g per day.
- Milk and milk products are the richest sources of calcium. Green leafy vegetables, such as spinach, amaranth are rich in calcium but at the same time they are oxalate-rich foods.

Phosphorus

- Phosphorus takes a second place in regard to the total amount of minerals present in the body and constitutes about one fourth of all body minerals.
- About 80% of the phosphorus is found in bones combined with calcium and the rest is found in bones combined with calcium and the rest is found in soft tissues and body fluids.
- Phosphorus plays an important role in the formation of teeth and bones, maintenance of acid base balance of the blood, and supplying energy to the muscles for contraction.
- Phosphorus is found in good amount in the foods which are rich in protein and calcium. Thus milk, cheese, egg yolk, meat, fish are good source of phosphorus.

- Deficiency of calcium and phosphorous cause's rickets in children is generally contributed to lack of vitamin D. Osteomalacia, the adult rickets, may also be due to a calcium deficiency, but usually, the situation is complicated by deficiency phosphorus and vitamin D as well as other factors.

Iron

- Amount of iron in the adult body is about 3 to 5 g of which 70% is in circulating hemoglobin, 4% in the myoglobin of the muscles and 25% in the stores held in liver, bone marrow, spleen and kidneys.
- Iron is essential for the oxidation I the body. Hemoglobin combines with oxygen in the lungs to form oxyhemoglobin and is carried to the tissues by blood circulation.
- Iron containing oxygen in the muscles makes the oxidation of carbohydrate, fat and protein possible within the intact cell.
- Iron is stored chiefly in the liver, spleen and bone-marrow. The amount is variable, ranging from 1 to 2 g.
- Recommended allowances based on the availability and utilization of iron, it is recommended that 20–30 mg of iron per day is sufficient for an adult. The requirements increases in special conditions, such as pregnancy.
- Nutritional anemia's are due to the deficiency of iron, folic acid.
- Liver is an excellent source of iron. Other meat products and egg yolk also have generous amount of this mineral.

Iodine

- Iodine is considered to be an important dietary nutrient because normal functioning of thyroid gland depends upon adequate supply of it in the body. It is an essential component of thyroxine and other iodine containing compounds of thyroid glands.
- Primary function of thyroxine is to influence the rate of oxidation in the cells of the body. Thyroxine also helps in normal growth and development in the Young's all the species.
- Sources of iodine vary widely under different soil and fertilizer conditions. Marine or deep sea fish and shell fish are high in iodine content. The leaves and flowers of plants have higher concentration of iodine than roots.
- The recommended daily allowances of Iodine have been reported to be about 100 to 150 mg.
- Prolonged deficiency of iodine not only develops goiter but also causes sterility in many cases. Development of goiter enlargement of thyroid gland, during pregnant indicates special requirement of iodine.

Fluorine

- Fluorine is found primarily is the bones and teeth. Small amount fluorine brings about striking reduction in teeth decay because this mineral makes tooth enamel more resistant to the action of acid.
- Dental caries is reduced more resistant to the action of acid, water at the rate of 1 part per million.
- Source of fluorine—food as well as water by fluorination of the water at the rate of 1 part per million.
- The recommended level of fluorides in drinking water in this country is accepted as 0.5 to 0.8 mg per liter.
- Fluorine is often called a two-edged sword. Prolonged ingestion of fluorides through drinking water in excess of the daily requirement is associated with dental and skeletal fluorosis and inadequate intake with dental caries.

Sodium

- The adult human body contains about 100 g of sodium ion. It is distributed entirely in the extracellular fluid (plasma, tissue fluid and lymph) of the body.
- The main functions of sodium is regulation of acid base balance of the body, regulation of the osmotic pressure of the plasma or tissue fluids and sodium play a special role in originating and maintaining heartbeat.
- Low sodium diets are prescribed for patients suffering from high blood pressure.

Potassium

- The adult human body contains about 250 g potassium which is present almost in the cells of different tissues, muscle, etc.
- The functions of potassium is regulation of Ph of cell contents, regulation of the osmotic pressure of cell contents and potassium ion increases the relaxation of heart muscle which is antagonized be ca ion.
- Potassium deficiency causes weakness and muscular paralysis. In animals, hypertrophy of the heart has been observed.
- In consumption of excessive amounts of potassium causes muscular weakness and apathy—symptoms similar to those of potassium deficiency.

Magnesium

- Magnesium is a constituent of bones and is present in all body cells.
- Human adult body contains about 25 g of magnesium of which about half is found in the skeleton.
- It appears that magnesium is essential for the normal metabolism of calcium and potassium
- Magnesium deficiency may occur in chronic alcoholic, cirrhosis of liver, toxemias of pregnancy, protein-energy malnutrition and malabsorption syndrome.
- The principal clinical features attributed to magnesium deficiency are irritability, tetancy, hyperreflexia and occasionally hyporeflexia.
- The requirements are estimated to be about 200–300 mg/day for adults.

Trace Elements

Copper

- The healthy human adult body contains about 100–150 mg of copper. Copper present in the blood in the form of copper protein complex hemocuprein in red blood cells ad ceruloplasmin in plasma.

Element	Functions	Element	Functions
Cu	• Superoxide dismutase • Hydrogenase (facultative anaerobes) • Nitrite reductase • Acetyl–CoA synthase	Ni	• CO–dehydrogenase • Acetyl–CoA synthase • Methyl–CoM reductase (F_{430}) • Urease • Stabilizes DNA, RNA • Hydrogenase
Co	• B_{12}–enzymes • Co–dehydrogenase • Methyltransferase	Se	• Hydrogenase • Formate dehydrogenase • Glycin reductase
Fe	• Hydrogenase • CO-dehydrogenase • Methane monooxygenase • NO-reductase • Superoxide dismutase • Nitrite and nitrate reductase • Ntrogenase	W	• Formate dehydrogenase • Formylmethanofuran–dehydrogenase • Aldehyde–oxidoreductase • Antagonist of Mo
Mn	• Stabilizes methyltransferase in methane-producing bacteria • Redox reactions	Zn	• Hydrogenase • Formate dehydrogenase • Superoxide dismutase
Mo	• Formate dehydrogenase • Nitrate reductase • Nitrogenase	V	• Nitrogenase • Chloroperoxidase • Bromoperoxidase

- Anemia produced in infants fed exclusively on milk can be cured only by giving copper salts along with iron. The estimated of average daily intakes in adult diets range from 2-3 mg.
- The high intake in e Indian diets may due to contamination of copper from brass vessels used in cooking.

Zinc

- Zinc is active in the metabolism of glucides and proteins and is required for the synthesis of insulin by the pancreas and for the immunity function.
- Zinc is present is small amount sin all tissues. Zinc plasma level is about 96 mg per 100 mL for healthy adults and 89 mg per 100 mL for healthy children.
- The average adult body contains 1.4 to 2.3 g of zinc. Zinc deficiency in the diet has been reported to the cause of anemia, growth retardation and delayed genital maturation. (Dwarfism) in children.
- Zinc is a constituent of Insulin-the hormone present in the Islets of Langerhans of pancreas.

Cobalt

- Cobalt occurs in small amounts in all tissues, highest concentration occurring in liver and kidneys. Most of the cobalt is present I vitamin B12.
- It is suggested that cobalt may be necessary for the first stage of hormone production. Cobalt may interact with iodine and affect its utilization.

Chromium

- The chromium content of an adult human body is estimated to be 6 mg. Most adult tissues contain 0.02 to 0.4 ppm of chromium on dry basis. The blood contains about 0.009 to 0.055 ppm
- Chromium plays an important role in carbohydrate, lipid and protein metabolism.
- Chromium deficiency is characterized by impaired growth and disturbances in glucose, Lipid and protein metabolism.

Selenium

- Selenium administration to children with kwashiorkor resulted in significant weight increase.
- Studied indicate that human selenium deficiency may occur in protein-energy malnutrition.
- Selenium deficiency especially when combined with vitamin E deficiency reduces production.

FOOD

The term 'food' refers to anything, which nourishes the body. It would obviously include solids, semi-solids and liquids, which can be consumed and which help to sustain the body to keep it healthy. The terms 'food' and 'nutrition' are sometimes used synonymously, but it is not strictly correct.

Definition

- Food is defined as "what one feeds on and is a composite mixture of many nutrient substances ranging from a fraction of a gram in some cases to hundred of gram in others.
- The foodstuff is defined as anything, which can be used as food. Therefore, the word 'nutrition' is derived from the word 'nutricus', which means 'to suckle at the breast'.
- Nutrition is defined as combination of dynamic process by which the consumed food is utilized for nourishment, structural and functional efficiency of every cell of the body.

Classifications of Food (Fig. 1.15)

Food does much more that satisfy your appetite. It provides nutrients that the body uses for growth and health. There are five types of nutrients that fall into two broad categories—macro-nutrients and micro-nutrients. Macro-nutrients, which are required in large amounts, include carbohydrates, proteins and fats. In contrast, micro-nutrients are required in small amounts and include vitamins and minerals. A sixth category includes water, which is essential to life.

Classification by Origin
1. Foods of animal origin
2. Foods of vegetable origin

Classification by Chemical Composition
1. Carbohydrates
2. Proteins
3. Fats
4. Vitamins
5. Minerals

Classification by Predominant Function
1. Body building foods, e.g., milk, meat, poultry, fish, eggs, pulses, ground nuts, etc.
2. Energy giving foods, e.g., cereals, sugars, roots and tubers, fats and oil.
3. Protective foods, e.g., vegetables, fruits, milk.

Figure 1.16 is depicted the food groups.

Classification by Nutritive Value
1. Cereals and millets
2. Pulses (legumes)
3. Vegetables
4. Nuts and oil seeds
5. Fruits
6. Animal foods

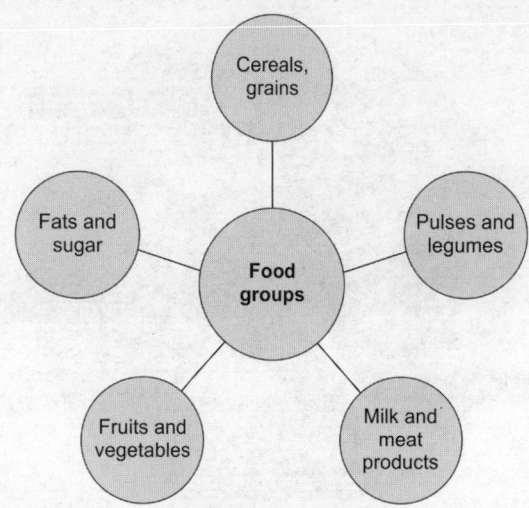

Fig. 1.16: Food groups.

7. Fats and oil
8. Sugar and jaggery
9. Condiments and spices
10. Miscellaneous foods

Since the food is varying in their contents of various nutrients, they have been broadly grouped under three categories from the nutritional point of view.
1. Energy yielding foods
2. Body building foods
3. Protective foods

These are briefly discussed below:

1. **Energy yielding foods:** Food rich in carbohydrates and fats are called energy yielding foods. Cereals, roots and tubers, dried fruits, sugars and fats are included in this group. Cereals contain, in addition, fair amounts of proteins, minerals and certain vitamins and form the important sources of the above nutrients.
2. **Body building foods:** Food rich in proteins are called body building foods. Milk, meat, fish, eggs, pulses, oil seeds and nuts and low-fat oil seed flours are included in the group of body building foods.
3. **Protective foods:** Food rich in protein, vitamins and minerals are termed protective foods. Milk, eggs, liver, green leafy vegetables and fruits are included in this group. Protective foods are broadly classified into two groups:
   a. Food rich in vitamins, minerals and proteins of high biological value, e.g., milk, eggs and liver.
   b. Foods rich in certain vitamins and minerals only, e.g., green leafy vegetables and fruits.

Figure 1.17 is depicted the five food groups.

FIVE FOOD GROUP PLANS

The nutritional expert group of Indian Council of Medical Research, India suggested a five food group plan and the nutrients supplied by each food group are given in **Table 1.2**.

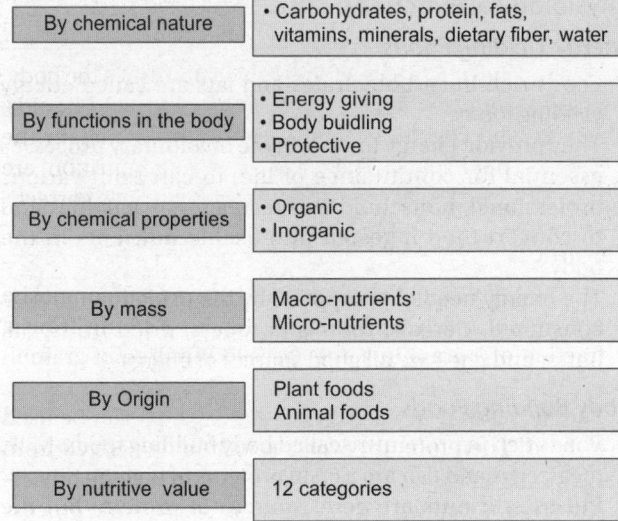

Fig. 1.15: Classification of foods.

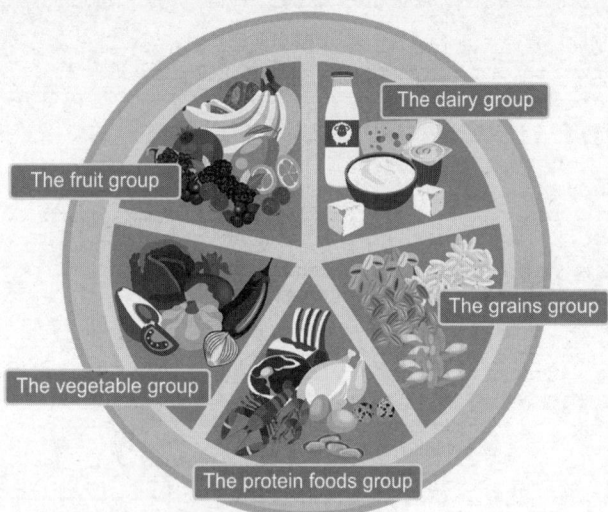

Fig. 1.17: Five food groups.

Table 1.2: Five food group plans.

Sl. No.	Groups	Description
1.	Group-I	**Cereals, roots and tubers:** These entire nutrients primarily supply energy. This group includes foods, such as wheat, jowar, bajra, ragi and other cereals. Tapioca, potato, sweet potato, arbi and yam come under roots and tubers. This group provides calories, protein, iron and vitamins. These foods are cheap and are taken in large amounts by the low-income groups. This also provides thiamine and niacin
2.	Group-II	**Protein-giving foods:** The food stuffs in this group are primary sources of protein; though cereals also furnish protein. Dals, grains, peas, beans, groundnuts, cashew nuts, almonds, coconut, milk, curd, buttermilk, paneer (cottage cheese) khoya, eggs, fish, mutton, chicken, pork and other flesh foods come under this group. It provides protein both from the vegetables and animal kingdom. Milk and dairy products also provide calcium and riboflavin. Meat, fish and eggs are good sources of protein, iron and niacin
3.	Group-III	**Fats/oils, sugar/jaggery:** All these food stuffs supply energy. These include—vegetable oils, vanaspati oil, ghee, butter, cream, sugar and jaggery. This group constitutes about one sixth of the energy value of the diet, but does not add appreciably to the protein, mineral or vitamin levels. Butter is a good source of vitamin A
4.	Group-IV	**Protective vegetables and fruits:** These are rich sources of minerals and vitamins. These include green leafy vegetables, yellow or orange fruits and vegetables and citrus fruits
5.	Group-V	**Other vegetables:** They provide variety in taste and texture and furnish roughage in the diet. These include fruits stems, leaves and flowers of plants, lady's finger, brinjals, bitter gourds and other cauliflower, etc. They are fair sources of certain vitamins and minerals

Table 1.3: Basic seven food groups.

Sl. No.	Groups	Description
1.	Group-I	Green and yellow vegetables—provide carotene, ascorbic acid and iron
2.	Group-II	Oranges, grape fruits, tomatoes or raw cabbage or salad greens. These give ascorbic acid (vitamin C)
3.	Group-III	Potatoes, other vegetables and fruits. There are good sources of vitamin and minerals in general and fiber
4.	Group-IV	Milk and milk products are sources of calcium, phosphorus proteins and vitamins
5.	Group-V	Meat, poultry, fish and eggs provide proteins, phosphorus, iron and vitamin B
6.	Group-VI	Bread flour and cereals provide thiamine, niacin, riboflavin, iron, carbohydrates and fiber
7.	Group-VII	Butter or fortified margarine these are rich sources of fat and vitamin A

BASIC SEVEN FOOD GROUPS

The seven food group plan was developed by US department of agriculture in 1943. The seven groups with their nutrient contribution are given in **Table 1.3**.

FUNCTIONS OF FOOD

Food is the basic necessity of man. It is a mixture of different nutrients, such as carbohydrate, protein, fat, vitamins and minerals. These nutrients are essential for growth, development and maintenance of good health throughout the life. They also play a vital role in meeting the special needs of pregnant and lactating women and patients recovering from illness.

Figures 1.18A and B are depicted the functions of food.

Physiological Functions

Energy Yielding Foods

- Foods rich in carbohydrates and fats are called energy yielding foods.
- They provide energy to sustain the involuntary processes essential for continuance of life, to carry out various professional, household and recreational activities and to convert food ingested into usable nutrients in the body.
- The energy needed is supplied by the oxidation of foods consumed. Cereals, roots and tubers, dried fruits, oil, butter and ghee are all good sources of energy.

Body Building Foods

- Foods rich in protein are called body building foods. Milk, meat, eggs and fish are rich in proteins of high quality.
- Pulses and nuts are good sources of protein, but the protein is not of high quality. These foods help to maintain life and promote growth and also supply energy.

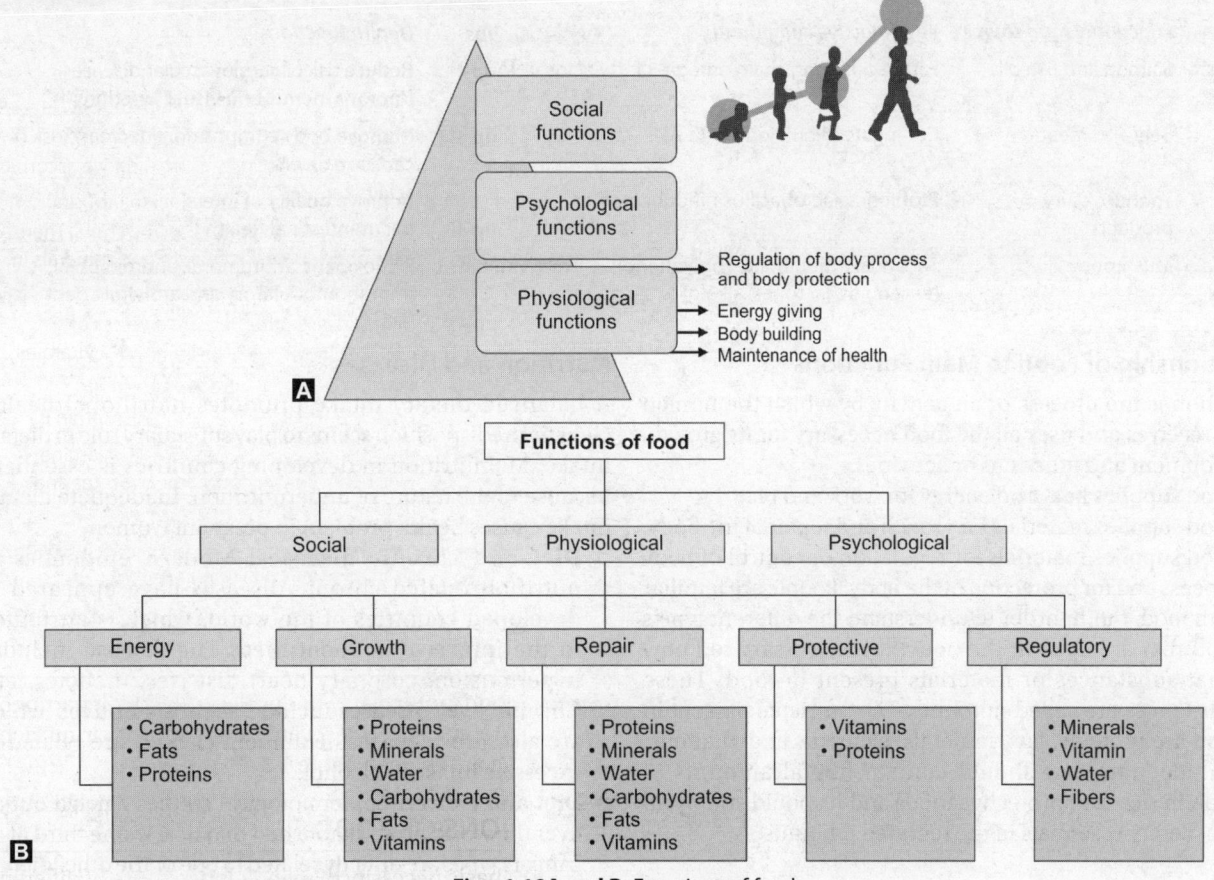

Figs. 1.18A and B: Functions of food.

Protective and Regulatory Food
- Food rich in protein, minerals and vitamins are known as protective and regulatory foods.
- They are essential for health and regulate activities, such as maintenance of body temperature, muscle contraction, control of water balance, clotting of blood, removal of waste products from the body and maintaining heartbeat.
- Milk, egg, liver, fruits and vegetables are protective foods.

Social Function
- Food has always been the central part of our community, social, cultural and religious life.
- It has been an expression of get-togethers. Food is served at many social events, such as teas, breakfasts, banquets, athletic award dinners, dances and meeting of all sorts.
- On all these occasions, food indirectly serves as an instrument to develop social support.

Psychological Function
- Besides other functions, food satisfies certain emotional needs also. People often find it difficult to get adjusted to unfamiliar food, although it may be nutritionally sound.
- Traditional habits are characterized by certain foods, which are pleasing to people of one culture and distasteful for those of another.
- In addition to satisfying physical and social needs, foods also satisfy certain emotional needs of human beings.
- These include a sense of security, love and acceptance. For example, preparation of delicious foods for family members is a token of love and affection.

	Functional food source	Key bioactive compound	Health functions
Plant foods	Tomato	Lycopene	Antioxidant; reduce the risk of prostate cancer
	Carrots, fruits, vegetables	Carotenoids, alpha carotene/beta-carotene anthocyanidins, flavonones, flavones, phenolics	Neutralize free radicals which may cause damage to cells; reduce risk of cancer
	Onion	Prebiotics and probiotics, fructo-oligosaccharides (FOS)	Improve quality of intestinal microflora; gastrointestinal health
	Flaxseed	Lignans	Prevention of cancer; renal failure
	Green vegetables	Lutein	Reduce the risk of muscular degeneration

Contd...

Contd...

	Functional food source	Key bioactive compound	Health functions
Animal foods	Salmon and fish oil	Fatty acids, long chain omega-3 fatty acids-DHA/EPA	Reduce risk of cardiovascular disease; improve mental and visual functions
	Beef and meat	Conjugated linoleic acid (CLA)	Improve body composition; decrease risk of certain cancers
	Yoghurt, dairy products	Probiotics, lactobacillus bifidobacterium	Improve quality of intestinal microflora; gastrointestinal health
Fungal foods	Mushrooms	Secondary metabolite (polyphenols, sterols, vitamins, terpenoids, lactones, alkaloids, sesquiterpenes)	Antioxidant, antitumoral, antimicrobial, immunomodularory and antiviral agent

Relationship of Food to Main Functions

Nutrition is the process or an activity by which the human body receives and uses all the food necessary for its growth, development and functions or activities.
- Food supplies heat and energy for work and play.
- Food supplies materials for growth and repair of the body.
- Food supplies materials for regulation or control of body process and for protection of the body. People are familiar with food, but in order to understand the different type's food that are used in the body, it is necessary to know what substances or materials present in food. These substances are called nutrients. The nutrients present in food are proteins, fats, minerals, elements and vitamins. An adequate diet should contain liberal amounts of protein rich and protective foods and it should supply all the dietary essentials in the required amounts.

■ NUTRITION PROBLEMS IN INDIA

Malnutrition is widely prevalent in India. The specific nutritional problems are:
- **Protein-calorie malnutrition:** This is due to deficiency of calories and proteins in the diet. A large number of children are victims of kwashiorkor and marasmus in India.
- **Endemic goiter:** About 71 million people are estimated to be affected by endemic goiter (i.e., swelling of the thyroid gland in the neck) and other iodine deficiency disorders. This condition is due to iodine deficiency.
- **Vitamin deficiencies:** Deficiency of vitamin A is an important public health problem in India especially in the age group, 3 to 5 years.

Figure 1.19 is depicted the types of malnutrition.

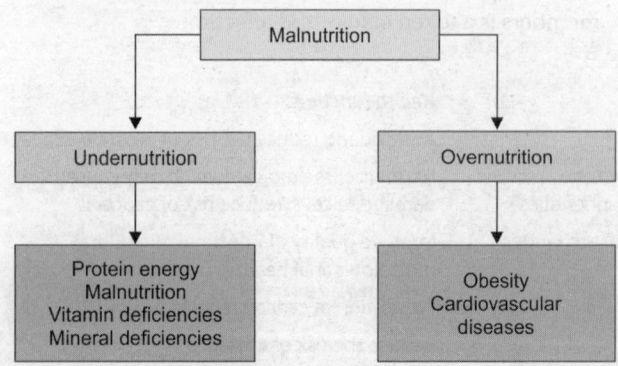

Fig. 1.19: Types of malnutrition.

Nutrition and Diseases

A balanced dietary intake promotes nutritional health. Genetic predisposition seems to play subsidiary role in dietary intake. Malnutrition in developing countries is essentially because of the nature of undernutrition. Inadequate dietary intake causes health problem in pregnant women.
- **Diet and chronic diseases:** Modern epidemics of nutrition-related chronic diseases have appeared in developed countries of the world, which is attributed to the intake of 'affluent diet'. The disease includes hypertension, coronary heart diseases, diabetes, etc. Chronic liver diseases include cirrhosis of liver, which are also prevalent in the affluent classes, are related to excessive intake of alcohol.
- **Diet and cancer:** Epidemiological studies carried out all over the world have established that nearly one third of all cancers types are directly related to one or the other dietary component. Diet rich in saturated fats is particularly linked to colon cancer and prostate cancer. Breast cancer and rectum cancer are also related to high-fat intake. Epidemiological studies have revealed that regular intake of fruits and vegetables, high in fiber content, low in saturated fats and rich in several antioxidants, vitamins namely, retinol, carotene, vitamin C and vitamin E act are potential carcinogenic agents.
- **Diet and dental diseases:** Diet rich in sugar content predispose to dental caries. Sugar has casual association with dental caries; the association is particularly strong during childhood years with sugars that are consumed in between meals rather than with meals. High-starch diet is not cacogenic obviously because it contains complex sugars.
- **Diet and skeletal disease:** Consumption of diet, poor in calcium may predispose to osteoporosis. Alcohol intake and smoking habit are also related to osteoporosis. Osteoporosis predisposes to fracture especially in elderly people.
- **Diet and mental health:** Inadequate dietary intake deficient in nutrients likes iodine, nicotinic acid and iron can retard mental development or impair mental performance. Iodine deficiency can cause an extreme degree of mental impairment as seen in cretinism. Nicotinic acid deficiency can lead to dementias in extreme cases of pellagra.
- **Diet and diet therapy:** Dietetics is the word used to describe the practical application of the principles of

nutrition to the human body in health and disease. Diet therapy is the science dealing with prescription of appropriate diet to patients, which constitutes an important component of their treatment.

NATIONAL NUTRITIONAL POLICY

The Government of India, Ministry of Health & Family Welfare developed and published the "National Health Policy" in 1983. The document gave a general exposition of the policies. The biggest omission in the draft is the lack of any discussion on comprehensive and universal health care. In contrast the NHP 1983 had said: "India is committed to attaining the goal of 'Health for All by the Year 2000 AD'. through the universal provision of comprehensive primary healthcare services". The National Health Policy was endorsed by the Parliament of India in 1983 and updated in 2002. In brief, the draft constitutes a return to the concept of centrally-directed, institution-based health care. If allowed to be enshrined in its present form, the NHP can be used as a tool to legitimize privatization of the health sector.

A further perusal of the document throws up many fundamental concerns, such as the creation of an infrastructure for primary healthcare; close coordination with health-related services and activities (such as, nutrition, drinking water supply and sanitation); active involvement and participation of voluntary organizations; provision of essential drugs and vaccines; qualitative improvement in health and family planning services; provision of adequate training; and medical research aimed at the common health problems of the people. The draft recommends an increase in public health expenditure from the present 0.9% of GDP to 2.0% in 2010.

General Objective

The general objective of the national nutrition policy is to improve the nutritional status of the people.

Specific Objectives

- Promote practices favorable to the improvement of the nutritional status
- Reduce the prevalence of diseases linked to nutritional deficiencies and excesses
- Prevent mother-to-child transmission of HIV through appropriate breastfeeding and infant and young child feeding practice
- Assure adequate treatment of malnutrition due to nutritional deficiencies and excesses
- Provide nutritional care and support for people living with HIV/AIDS

Expected Outcomes and the Link to the Millennium Development Goals

Goal 1: Reduce Poverty and Hungry

The prevalence rate of protein-energy malnutrition in under five of age children is reduced from 45% to 30% for stunting, 22% to 15% for underweight, 4% to 2% for wasting.

Goal 2: Ensure Primary Education

- The prevalence rate of anemia is reduced by from 56% to 37% in children and from 33% to 22% in women.
- Iodine deficiency disorders are eliminated from 26% to less than 5% of total goiter.

Goal 3: Reduce Infant Mortality

- Increase the proportion of women exclusively breast-feeding for the first 6 months with optimal complementary feeding up to 24 months from 17.4% to 60%.
- Reduce vitamin A deficiency in children under five from 25% to 5% in children under five years.

Goal 4: Reduce Maternal Mortality

- Reduce vitamin A deficiency (night blindness) in pregnant women from 7% to less than 1%.
- Reduce the prevalence of anemia in pregnant women from 33% to 22%.

Goal 5

Combat HIV/AIDS and other diseases:
- Nutritional support is provided to PLWA and other vulnerable people.
- Nutrition-related chronic diseases are prevented.

Strategies for Nutrition Improvement:

- Reinforcement of the political commitment
- Promotion of optimal infant and young child feeding
- Scaling up of community-based nutrition programs
- Food fortification
- Promotion of household food security
- Prevention and management of malnutrition and related diseases
- Nutritional support to PLWHA and their families
- Communication for behavior change

Monitoring and Evaluation

- To ensure effective implementation of planned activities, monitoring and evaluation is essential in all development programs.
- In addition, periodic evaluations are necessary for establishing level of objective achievement. In order to follow-up implementation of nutrition programs, data will be collected regularly at the health center and community level.
- In addition, other opportunities for nationwide surveys will be identified and utilized.
- Nutritional surveys and epidemiologic surveillance will be conducted regularly, with appropriate indicators, to evaluate the progress and impact of nutritional interventions.
- Operational research will also be carried out to address specific problems identified during the implementation of nutritional activities.
- To prevent nutritional emergencies, nutrition unit will reinforce collaboration with all existing structures that collect and analyze bioclimatic, environmental, demographic and agricultural data for early warning and timely intervention measures against disasters that can negatively affect the nutrition.

ROLE OF FOOD AND MEDICINAL VALUES

The longer that fruits or vegetables sit around waiting to be sold or eaten, the more nutrients they lose. But fruits and vegetables grown for freezing are usually frozen right after they are picked. Therefore, they have less time to lose their nutrients.

A	Apple	As basic as it may sound, an apple provides you with 13 minerals which our body require daily. A sample mix of apple, walnuts and yoghurt makes for a great breakfast to start the day.
B	Broccoli	The vilayati version of cauliflower is now readily available all over our city. Make good use of it, in a recent survey of greens, broccoli was found to be healthiest, since, it is a powerful anti-carcinogen.
C	Cucumber	As chilly as winter is.
D	Dudhi (melon)	Melon is known to reduce blood pressure. In cooperative dudhi as part of your cuisine to lower your blood pressure, for a healthier heart in general, to lower cholesterol, and many other benefits.
E	Egg (egg white)	Make it a habit to remove the yolk, since egg whites are a great source of protein.
F	Fish	Omega-3 in some fish prevents cardiovascular disease. Also, good source of protein. However, avoid canned varied and over-salted, smoked dishes. Also shell fish, crab and all forms of mussels need to be strictly eaten in moderation.
G	Garlic	There are way too many health benefits.
H	Home grown sprouts	Sprouts while available in the local grocery are a much healthier option to grow at home. It is easy to make these at home (soak them overnight), and they makes for a quiet tasty snack either in chaats, or raitas, or salads of your choice.
I	Iceberg lettuce	Another designer food item that is becoming readily available. This one is great to make salads with at home. Mix with tofu, spoors, tomatoes, chicken and fat free yoghurt to get you through the day.
J	Juice blender	Choose a juice of choice for the year. It could be anything you want. But make sure you make it home. Most bottled juice come with lots of sugar and preservatives.
K	Karela	As bitter and unappetizing as it may sound. The health benefits of this desi veggie far outweigh its sharp taste. It regularizes blood sugar. Aside from a range of other ailments.
L	Lemon	Sprinkle your food with lots of lemon. It is got lots of vitamin C that you need to boost your immune system. Besides, by replacing lemon with salt as it condiment for your meals, you are helping your heart in more ways than one.
M	Milk (skimmed)	Milk (but skimmed), there is no way we have been able to escape milk; it is too ingrained in our culture. So go for it, enjoy your milk, but get a bottle of skimmed milk.
N	Nuts	Nuts reduce coronary heart disease. Almonds and walnuts lower serum LDL cholesterol levels. Dieticians frequently recommended nuts to diabetes patients with insulin resistance. And those who eat nuts live two to three years longer than those who do not.
O	Olive oil	It is clearly the healthiest option to the necessary evil that is oil. Its high content of monounsaturated fatty acids and its high content of anti-oxidants make it the best alternative.
P	Peas	Green peas provide good amount of eight vitamins, seven minerals, dietary fiber and protein. In addition, they are a good source of vitamin K1, which activates osteocalcin, the major non-collagen protein in bone.
Q	Quality fruit	The price of fruits has gone over the top. However, fruits are known to be some of the best anti-oxidants, are a great source of fiber and nutrients. Up to your fridge with quality fruits. Berries, apples, bananas, even the tomato.
R	Red cabbage	Your kids may cringe at sight of regular cabbage. But the flamboyant red cabbage might convince them. Also a source of indole-3-carbinol (13C), which reducing the risk of breast cancer by 50%.
S	Strawberries	It helps to prevent cancer. They also bring out flavor in champagne.
T	Tea	Another desi habit we cannot give up. So why not substitute chai with green tea or black tea. Regular use is known to strengthen bone and cure osteoporosis.
U	Ud-ruck	Sorry but G was taken by garlic. But ginger (adrak) is essential to health.
V	Varan-bhat (dal rice)	Simplicity is a virtue. Amidst your hectic socializing and gourmet fantasies, normal ghar ka khana once a day will do wonders for health.
W	Walnuts	Walnuts reduce the risk of prostate cancer in men.
Y	Yoghurt	Again is a great source of calcium, aid in digestion and can be merged with a range of salads, health food items, marinades. Always keep a bowl of fresh, homemade yoghurt handy in your fridge.
Z	Zucchini	This Italian kakadi ids low in calories and contains a high amount of folate, potassium, vitamin A and manganese. Z though is also for zinc. So do not forget to stack up on your spinach, lentils and salmon.

Nutritive Values of Common Foods

Food contains nutrients in different proposition and different organoleptic properties. Hormonal substance enzymatic substance and antioxidants are present in various propositions in addition, micro- and macro-nutrients.

Cereals
- They are rich in carbohydrate, low protein (6%–12%) low fat, poor in iron and calcium. Rice, barely, ragi, millets and wheat are some of the examples of cereals.
- Insulin stimulants are present in ragi and millets, former is rich in calcium, latter is a source of fiber.
- Except yellow maize and sorghum, cereals are free vitamin A ascorbic acid.
- Wheat has acarbose, a chemical helpful to maintain normal blood sugar level.
- Richest source of iron are bajra and samai (panicum miliare). 100 g of staple food, cereals yield 346 kcal of energy.

Pulses and Legumes
- They are generally called protein foods. They contain 22% protein-soluble and insoluble fiber. They are rich in potassium and vitamin B, deficit in methionine, but rich in lysine.
- More than 40% of protein is present in soybean. It is richest source of protein among plant foods.
- Calorific value of pulses and legumes are ranging from 315 to 372 kcal for every 100 g. But green peas and soybean provide 93–432 kcal respectively.
- Source of pulses and legumes are Bengal gram, black gram, red gram, lentil, rajmah, horse gram, cowpea and field bean.

Green Leafy Vegetables
- They are low-calorie foods, having 90% moisture, high-fiber, low-protein, rich vitamins and minerals particularly beta-carotene and calcium.
- In general greens do not have protein in sufficient amount, but agathi greens contain 8% protein.
- Low-cost nutritous food, such as curry leaves have 800 mg calcium for every 100 g.
- Araikeerai is richest source of iron. Familiar greens, such as Amaranthus gangeticus are good for normal cardiac function, as it provides potassium.
- Amaranthus tristis and *A. viridis* green are excellent source of iron and ascorbic acid respectively.
- Commonly used green leafy vegetables are coriander leaves, drumstick leaves, mint, amaranth, celery, spinach and curry leaves.

Other Vegetables
- They are known as low-caloric foods, which contain potassium, soluble fiber, vitamin B and ascorbic acid. Some types of vegetable are good source of calcium, e.g., sundakkai and field beans.
- Folic acid present in lady's finger and chow chow helps in malnutrition of red blood cell (RBC).
- Choline of pumpkin and cauliflower is vital and regulates fat metabolism.

Roots and Tubers
- They are poor source of protein, but good source of carbohydrate.
- Beta-carotene in carrot and yam, ascorbic acid in potato, magnesium in pink radish, and phosphorus in Colocasia are particularly helpful to meet normal requirements of recommended dietary allowances for an individual.

Healthy Substances of Food
- **Tomato:** It has lycopene, which is anticancer carotenoid.
- **Bitter gourd:** It is an insulin stimulant.
- **Cruciferous vegetables:** Brussels sprouts broccoli and which has indole, which resists cancer of womb.
- **Cucumber:** It is diuretic and has arginine.
- **Green tea:** It contains catechins-an antioxidant.

Fruits
- Fruits are roughage, provide bulk to the stools. Most of the fruits are good sources of vitamins and minerals.
- Ascorbic acid in alma is richer than fruits, such as orange, lime and grapes. 100 g of Indian gooseberry yields 600 mg vitamin C.
- Beta-carotene a precursor of vitamin A, found in mango and papaya helps to maintain good vision because of an action similar to pepsin.
- Papain relieves the symptoms of episiotomy (surgical incision of vulva during delivery).
- Watermelon is very meager energy yielder, whereas dried fruits provide high calories.
- A report by national academy of sciences found that resveratrol, a chemical known to be highly concentrated in grapes skin, acts, such as estrogen, a hormone known to protect against heart diseases.

Nuts and Oil Seeds
- They are rich saturated fat; contain tocopherol thiamine and niacin. Almond, cashew nut, groundnut, walnut, sesame seed, linseed are some sources of nuts and oil seeds.
- Groundnuts contain monounsaturated fatty acid, 25% protein and 40% fat. Nutritious ball made from groundnut and jaggery in healthy food for children.
- Coconut meals raises hemoglobin content, as it provides approximately 70 mg iron.
- Most of the nuts and oil seeds are energy yielder and rich in phosphorus. Short- and medium-chain fatty acid of coconut oil is good for infant-intestine.

Eggs
- They are good mixture of all nutrients except carbohydrate and fiber; supplies essential amino acids and termed as good quality proteins.
- Raw egg white contains antinutritional factor avidin, which is binding with biotin and makes it unavailable.
- Ovalbumin, ovomucoid, flavoprotein are egg white proteins. One egg yolk contains 200 g cholesterol and

proteins, such as lipovitellin and phosvitin. 13% fat, 170 kcal energy, 2 mg iron, 60 mg calcium, 220 mg phosphorus can be obtained from 100 g of egg. Cooked egg is better than raw egg.

Meat Poultry and Fish

- Beef meal is richest source of iron among meat products. Protein in the meat and meat products are superior compared to vegetable proteins.
- Essential amino acids and biological value are responsible to upgrade the quality.
- Protein value of mutton is less than that of chicken, but fat percentage is higher than fish and chicken. They all are moderate source of phosphorus.
- Common fish varieties rohu and katla have 1.4% and 2.4% of fat respectively. Cat fish is free from fat.
- Fatty fish are hilsa, tapsee and dried chela. Omega fatty acid content of fish is helpful in preventing cardiac diseases. Consumption of cod-liver oil protects eyes from night blindness.

Milk and Milk Products

- Milk is ideal food since infant to aged. Skimmed milk, cheese, tinned milk powder, khoya and supplementary foods are made from milk.
- Cow milk, buffalo milk and processed milk are widely consumed. Protein content of cow milk is higher than human milk, but buffalo milk is rich in fat.
- High protein and calcium content among milk products is in skimmed milk powder. This group of foods have sufficient phosphorus, thiamine, niacin, but deficit in iron and vitamins.
- Energy value of 100 g cow milk, buffalo milk, goat milk, human milk is 67, 117, 72 and 65 calories respectively.

NURSES ROLE IN FOOD AND NUTRITION (BOX 1.5)

Why is nutrition so important and what is the nurse's role in nutrition? Nutrition is essential because it is required for growth, healing and all body functions. The nurse's role in nutrition is to educate patients about good nutrition to promote health. In this research paper, we will be discussing the nurse's role in nutrition and strategies that can be implemented in the hospital, nursing home and community.

Box 1.5: Role of nurse in nutrition.

- Assess nutritional health needs
- Nutritional surveillance
- Health education
- Nutritional supplementation
- National nutrition programs
- In-service education, training
- Special care for vulnerable groups
- Community participation
- Referrals
- Records and reports
- Participate in research
- Evaluation

Hospital

- In a hospital setting, physicians will issue orders for a diet type just as they write orders for medications or treatments.
- Knowledge of nutrition plays a role for the nurse because she must be aware of the significance of each diet.
- A nurse must know the component of each diet because if a patient asks for a carton of milk on a clear-liquid diet, this is not permitted. A full-liquid diet permits dairy products, however.
- Knowing low-sodium and low-sugar choices for cardiac and diabetic patients, respectively, also is important for ensuring that the patient does not eat foods that would adversely affect his nutrition is believed to be a key issue for healthcare professionals in hospital settings, yet the management of nutritional problems is often poor.
- According to O'Regan (2009) "nutrition should be viewed as an integral and central component of patient care irrespective of the patient's physical diagnosis, condition, age or psychological status".
- A failure to address the issue of malnutrition is a failure of the duty of nurses to protect the health of patients. In hospital environments, nurses are obliged to make observations about physical status, food intake, weight changes and response to therapy.

Nursing Home

- The nurse's role in nutrition can affect the nutritional status of residents of a nursing home. Many nutritional issues arise in residents of a nursing home (**Box 1.6**).
- Nurses play a major role in ensuring that the resident's nutritional needs are met.
- Documenting changes in weight loss, decreased appetite, oral health, and physical activity are examples of the important role that we play in our evaluation of the nutritional status of our patient.
- Morley and Silver (1995) raise the important fact that "Without input from staff, the physician is not likely to be successful in evaluation and treatment".
- It is important that we include nutrition as we evaluate our patients and plan their care. Authors, Morley and Silver (1995), stressed "Careful attention to the nutritional of nursing home residents is both a clinical and a quality-of-life issue".

Preventive Care

- Nurses are constantly engaged in teaching moments, particularly for preventive care.

Box 1.6: Role of the nurse in promoting nutrition.

The nurse can promote good nutrition by:
- Helping the patient understand the importance of the diet and encouraging dietary compliance
- Serving meal trays to patients in a prompt and positive manner
- Assisting some patients with the eating process
- Taking and recording patient weight
- Recording patient intake
- Observing clinical signs of poor nutrition and reporting them
- Serving as a communication link

- For example, if a patient has a family history of high blood pressure, a nurse may wish to teach her about healthy choices, such as a low-sodium diet, that can slow the onset of high blood pressure.
- Nurses also can help to review a patient's current diet to pinpoint areas where she can make healthier food selections.

Nutrition Knowledge and Medications

- Nutrition plays a further role in nursing when it comes to reviewing a patient's medication list.
- For example, patients who are on therapies to prevent blood clotting may need to avoid leafy, green vegetables and other vitamin K-containing foods. This is because vitamin K can decrease the beneficial effects of blood thinners.
- Some foods, such as grapefruits and foods containing tyramine, an amino acid or building block of protein responsible for regulating blood pressure, can interfere with medication therapies.
- Examples of tyramine-containing foods include aged cheeses, soy sauce and draft beer. When educating a patient on a new medication, nutrition must be a key component discussed to ensure safe drug administration.

Community

- People in the community that was studied show their lack of knowledge when they make poor food choices.
- The nurse's role in nutrition is to educate patients on how to improve eating habits to promote good health.
- To effectively manage and prevent malnutrition in either setting, it is important to recognize the barriers to nutritional care for patients.
- According to Dupertuis as cited by O'Regan (2009) inadequate nutrition can lead to an increase in hospitalization and mortality.
- As nurses provide nutritional care for patients in each of these settings, they should be educated on the importance of nutrition and the healing process to assist patients in avoiding a failure to thrive diagnosis.

CONCLUSION

The importance of food in the care and treatment of hospital patients has been championed by the nursing profession for many years. Nonetheless, it is still a neglected branch of nursing. As nurses and nurse practitioners become more involved with nutritional interventions, the health of patients will improve. Starting in the community, with meaningful nutrition interventions, patient outcomes and health can be changed. Much of the result depends on nursing's focus. In the busy lives of nurses, patients often get looked at as a disease; while that is not a nursing concept, it is often a fact of life. If instead we see clients as the complex individuals that they are, the advantage of early nutrition intervention becomes obvious.

Proper nutrition is important for staying healthy and is particularly vital for the elderly. The nutritional state of a patient often affects patient outcomes during illness and recovery. The nurse is the logical person to provide nutritional information because nurses are the primary interface between the patient and the healthcare system. Nursing plays a key role in nutrition education because nutrition is a part of patient outcomes. The healing of the body can take place only when the nutrients that provide the building blocks for repair are present. The nurse as a nutrition educator is a vital role in the overall healthcare system. Prehospital nursing has the opportunity to provide nutrition education that can help to preserve the health of all populations and particularly of older adults.

BIBLIOGRAPHY

1. Antia FP. Clinical Dietetics and Nutrition, 3rd edition. Oxford University Press, Bombay, 1986.
2. Briggs GM, Doris H. Calloway: Nutrition and Physical Fitness, 11th Ed. Harcourt College Publishers, New York, USA, 1984.
3. Cataldo CB, Whitney EN, DeBruyne LK: Nutrition and Diet Therapy—Principles and Practice, West Publishing Co. St. Paul, 2003.
4. Chaney MS, Margaret LR, Jelia CW. Nutrition, 9th edition. Houghton. Mifflin, Boston 1979 (Indian reprint, Surjeet Publications, New Delhi, 1979).
5. Davidson SR, Passmore, Brock JF. Human Nutrition & Dietetics, 8th edition. Churchill Livingstone, London, UK, 1986.
6. Mahan K, Escott-Stump S. Krause's Food, Nutrition, and Diet Therapy, 11th edition. Philadelphia: Saunders; 2004.
7. Schmidl MK, Labuza TP (Eds). Essentials of Functional Foods. Gaithersburg, MD: Aspen Publishers; 2000.

REVIEW QUESTIONS

Long Essays

1. Discuss the highlights of history of nutrition.
2. Explain in detail about physiology of nutrition.
3. Enumerate the factors affecting food and nutrition.
4. Define nutrition, explain the types of nutrients.
5. Define food, explain the classifications of food.
6. Enumerate the functions of food.
7. Discuss in detail about nurses role in food and nutrition.

Short Essays

1. **Nutrition:** History and concepts.
2. **Nutrition:** A basic human need.
3. Role of nutrition in maintaining health.
4. Importance of nutrition in health
5. Discuss the difference between macro and micro-nutrients.
6. Energy yielding and non-energy yielding.
7. Five food group plans.
8. Nutrition problems in India.
9. National nutritional policy.
10. Role of food and medicinal values.

Short Answers

1. Digestion.
2. Metabolism.
3. Relation between nutrition and health.
4. Food sources of carbohydrates.
5. Classification of proteins.
6. Sources of fats.
7. Inorganic elements.
8. Body building foods.

CHAPTER 2

Carbohydrates and Energy

CHAPTER OUTLINE

- ❖ Carbohydrates
  - Composition—Starches, Sugar and Cellulose
  - Recommended Daily Allowance (RDA)
  - Dietary Sources
  - Functions
- ❖ Energy
  - Unit of Energy—Kcal
  - Basal Metabolic Rate (BMR)
  - Factors Affecting BMR

TERMINOLOGY

- **Sugars:** The term "sugars" describes all mono- and disaccharides. Sugars are found naturally in fruits, vegetables, and milk products, or added to foods and beverages.
- **Basal metabolic rate (BMR):** BMR is a measurement of the level of energy required to maintain the body's vital life functions. Measured when the body is at complete rest.
- **Bioavailability:** Bioavailability is the ease at which a substance can be absorbed from the digestive tract and into the bloodstream. The higher the bioavailability, the greater the absorption.
- **Body mass index (BMI):** BMI is a measure of a person's body size by calculating their weight in relation to their height. BMI = kg/m_2
- **Antioxidant:** Antioxidants are chemical substances that help protect against cell damage from free radicals. Well-known antioxidants include vitamin A, vitamin C, vitamin E, carotenoids, and flavonoids.
- **Dietary fiber:** Dietary fiber comes from the thick cell walls of plants. It is an indigestible complex carbohydrate. Fiber is divided into two general categories—water-soluble and water-insoluble
- **Dietary supplements:** A dietary supplement is a product you take to supplement your diet. It contains one or more dietary ingredients (including vitamins; minerals; herbs or other botanicals; amino acids; and other substances). Supplements do not have to go through the testing that drugs do for effectiveness and safety.
- **Nutrient:** Nutrients are chemical compounds in food that are used by the body to function properly and maintain health. Examples include proteins, fats, carbohydrates, vitamins, and minerals.
- **Electrolytes:** Electrolytes are minerals in body fluids. They include sodium, potassium, magnesium, and chloride. When you are dehydrated, your body does not have enough fluid and electrolytes.
- **Digestion:** Digestion is the process the body uses to break down food into nutrients. The body uses the nutrients for energy, growth, and cell repair.
- **Calories:** Calories are a measurement of energy. One calorie is equivalent to 4.18 kJ.
- **Carbohydrate**
- Carbohydrates are the most readily converted energy source. Good sources include rice, bread, cereal, legumes, fruits and vegetables which also provide important nutrients. Additional carbohydrate sources include refined sugars, which do provide instant energy but unfortunately do not offer the nutrients that the more complex sources of carbohydrates do.
- **Catabolism:** Catabolism is the breaking down of a larger molecule into a smaller molecule. For example, the breakdown of carbohydrates to release energy.
- **Cellulose:** Cellulose is an insoluble fiber that makes up the framework of plant cell walls.
- **Energy:** Energy is the fuel we need from food to function and be active. Energy requirements vary depending on your age, body size and physical activity. It is important to monitor your energy consumption as too much energy can lead to weight gain. Fat, protein and carbohydrates all provide energy (known as kilojoules or calories) in the foods we eat. Fats provide more energy per gram than protein or carbohydrates.
- **Energy balance:** Endosperm is the inner part of the grain. It contains carbohydrate, protein and B vitamins.
- **Soluble fiber:** Soluble fiber is beneficial to help lower blood cholesterol levels and, in people with diabetes, helps to control blood sugar. Soluble fiber is found in fruits, vegetables, dried peas, soybeans, lentils, oats, rice and barley.

- **Insoluble fiber:** Because of its 'bulking properties', insoluble fiber helps keep us 'regular'. Foods containing insoluble fiber include whole grain and whole meal wheat-based breads, cereals and pasta.
- **Resistant starch:** Resistant starch is a type of starch found in plant foods that escapes digestion in the small intestine. Resistant starch may provide similar benefits to other types of fiber, such as helping to prevent constipation. Foods containing resistant starch include firm bananas, roasted chickpeas, boiled long grain white rice, baked beans, cooked and cooled potato, as well as cornflakes.
- **Flavonoids:** Flavonoids are water soluble plant pigments and are a subgroup of the polyphenol group of plant compounds. Flavonoids are believed to function as antioxidants, and are produced by plants to assist in photosynthesis.
- **Fructose:** Fructose is a type of sugar that is found naturally in fruit and honey.
- **Functional foods:** Functional foods are foods that have been manufactured to contain a specific compound to provide a particular health benefit. Also called nutraceuticals or designer foods.
- **Lactase:** Lactase is the enzyme produced in the small intestine that is required to breakdown lactose.
- **Lactose:** Lactose is the sugar found in milk. The body breaks it down to glucose and galactose.
- **Dietary fiber:** A type of carbohydrate that the body cannot easily digest. It occurs naturally in fruits, vegetables, nuts, seeds, beans, and whole grains.
- **Total sugars:** Which include sugars that occur naturally in foods, such as dairy products, as well as added sugars, which are common in baked goods, sweets, and desserts. The body very easily digests and absorbs sugars.
- **Sugar alcohols:** A type of carbohydrate that the body does not fully absorb. They have a sweet taste and fewer calories than sugar. Sugar alcohols are added to foods as reduced-calorie sweeteners, such as in chewing gum, baked goods, and sweets.

INTRODUCTION

Carbohydrates are macro-nutrient, containing carbon, hydrogen and oxygen. They are primary energy yielder, present in plant foods as well as animal foods. Polyhydroxy aldehyde or ketones group occurs in some sugar units. Glucose is physiologically significant among carbohydrate. Carbohydrates are the chief, cheapest and main source of energy. Carbohydrate normally should provide 50-60% of total caloric requirements.

Figure 2.1 is depicted the health benefits of carbohydrates.

All the carbohydrates contain carbon, hydrogen and oxygen. All the carbohydrates are changed in the body to simple form called glucose. Carbohydrates are organic compounds composed of carbon, hydrogen and oxygen with the later elements in the ratio of 2:1. The general formula is $C_nH_{2n}O_n$. They are viewed as hydrated carbon atoms.

Carbohydrates, all coming from the process of photosynthesis, represent the major part of organic substance on earth, are the most abundant organic components in the major part of fruits, vegetables, legumes and cereal grains, carry out many functions in all living organisms and are the major energy source for humans in Western diet of Mediterranean type. Finally, they provide flavor and texture in many processed foods.

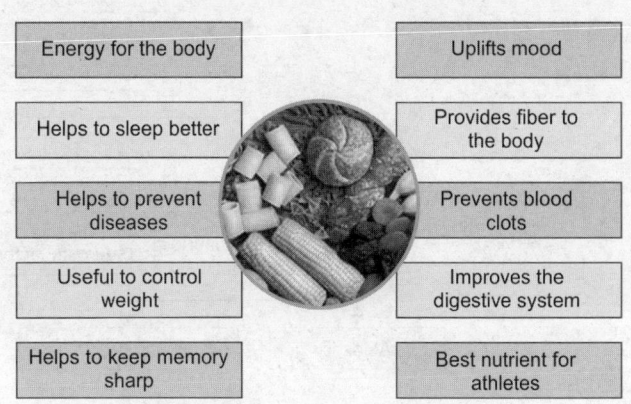

Fig. 2.1: Health benefits of carbohydrates.

DEFINITION AND MEANING OF CARBOHYDRATE

Carbohydrates-fiber, starches and sugars—are essential food nutrients that your body turns into glucose to give you the energy to function. Complex carbs in fruits, vegetables and whole-grain products are less likely to spike blood sugar than simple carbs (sugars). Low-carb diets, such as keto can be high in fats.

CLASSIFICATIONS OF CARBOHYDRATE (FIG. 2.2)

Chemical classification of carbohydrates: Carbohydrates, also called Carbs, are defined as aldehydic or ketonic compounds with some number of oxydrilic groups (so polyhydroxy aldehydes or ketones as well). Many of them, but not all, have general formula $(CH_2O)_n$ (only molecules with are considered carbohydrates); some, in addition to carbon (C), oxygen (O) and hydrogen (H), include nitrogen or sulfur. On the basis of the number of forming units, three major classes of carbohydrates can be defined—monosaccharides, oligosaccharides and polysaccharides. The term "saccharide" derives from the Greek word "sakcharon", which means sugar. Carbohydrates are chemically known as saccharides, they are classified according to number of sugar units present in the molecular structure.

Oligosaccharides

- Oligosaccharides yield 2–10 molecules of monosaccharide on hydrolysis, e.g., disaccharides (maltose, lactose and, sucrose), trisaccharides (raffinose) and tetrasaccharides (stachyose).
- Oligosaccharides are formed by short chains of monosaccharidic units (from 2 to 20) linked one to the next by chemical bounds, called glycosidic bounds.

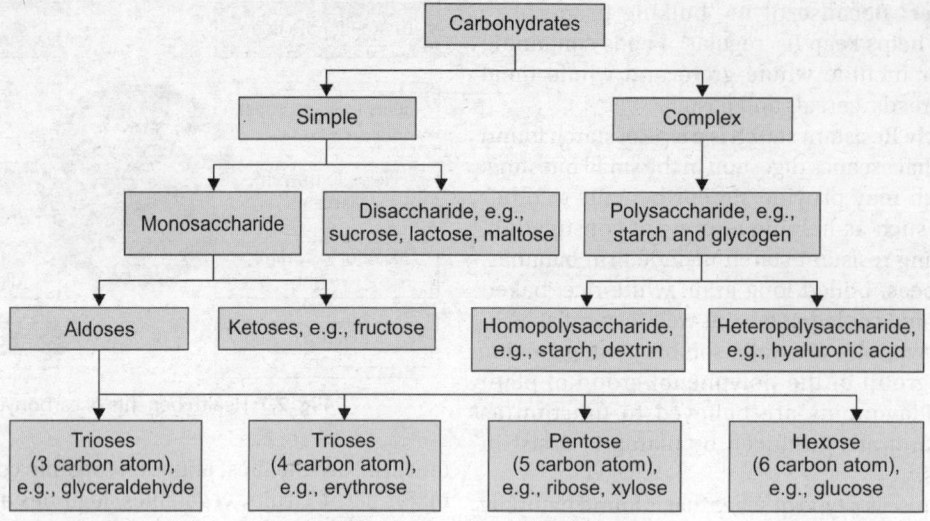

Fig. 2.2: Classification of carbohydrates.

- The most abundant oligosaccharides are disaccharides, formed by two monosaccharides, and especially in the human diet the most important are sucrrose (common table sugar), lactose and maltose.
- Within cells many oligosaccharides formed by three or more units do not find themselves as free molecules but linked to other ones, lipids or proteins, to form glycoconjugates.

Table 2.1 is depicted the classification of oligosaccharides.

Polysaccharides

- Polysaccharides are polymers consisting of 20 to 10^7 monosaccharidic units; they differ each other for the monosaccharides recurring in the structure, for the length and the degree of branching of chains or for the type of links between units.
- Whereas in the plant kingdom several types of polysaccharides are present, in vertebrates there are only a small number.
- Polysaccharides are defined homopolysaccharides if they contain only one type of monosaccharide as starch, glycogen and chitin; heteropolysaccharides, instead, contain two or more different kinds (e.g., hyaluronic acid).
- Polysaccharides yield many molecules of monosaccharide on hydrolysis.

Table 2.1: Classification of oligosaccharides.

	No 'C'	Example	Type of monosaccharide
Disaccharides	2	Maltose	Glucose + Glucose
		Lactose	Glucose + Galactose
		Lactose	Glucose + Fructose
Trisaccharides	3	Raffinose	Glu + Fruc + Galactose
Tetrasaccharides	4	Stachyose	2 Galactose + Glucose + Fructose
Pentasaccharides			3 Galactose + Glucose + Fructose

1. **Pentosans:** For example, araban, xylan
2. **Hexosans:**
   - Starch, dextrin and glycogen
   - Cellulose, inulin, man

Complex polysaccharides: They are not digested by human enzymes, e.g., hemicelluloses, gums, mucilages and pectins.

CALORIE

The scientific definition of a calorie is a unit of energy, for heat in particular. One calorie is the amount of heat that increases the temperature of 1 kg of water by 1°C. Any food may contain one or more nutrients, but carbohydrates, fats and protein are the nutrients, which gives calories to the body. The caloric value of these nutrients and of any common foods has been determined by burning a known weight of the nutrient or food in an atmosphere of oxygen in what is known as a bomb calorimeter. The caloric values of the nutrients are given in **Table 2.2**.

The following examples of calorie intake are based on US Department of Agriculture (USDA) guidelines: A person's daily calorie intake should be based on age, gender and physical activity level. Men generally need more calories than women and active people need more calories than sedentary (inactive) people.

- Children aged 2 and 8: 1,000–1,400
- Active women aged 14 and 30: 2,400
- Sedentary women aged 14 and 30: 1,800–2,000
- Active men aged 14 and 30: 2,800–3,000
- Sedentary men aged 14 and 30: 2,000–2,600
- Active men and women above 30: 2,200–3,000
- Sedentary men and women 30: 1,800–2,200

Table 2.2: Caloric values of the nutrients.

Sl. No.	Caloric value	Kcal/g
1.	Carbohydrate	4
2.	Protein	4
3.	Fat	9

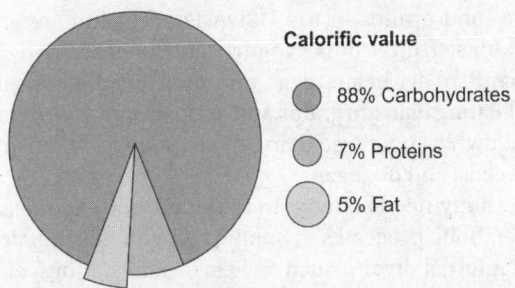

Fig. 2.3: Proportion of nutrients.

Caloric Value

Calories are needed to provide energy so the body functions properly. The number of calories in a food depends on the amount of energy the food provides. The number of calories a person needs depends on age, height, weight, gender, and activity level. People who consume more calories than they burn off in normal daily activity or during exercise are more likely to be overweight. The energy value of a food indicates how much energy the human body can gain through metabolism. The energy value is specified in kilojoules (kJ) per 100 g or 100 mL. In addition, the specification is often in kilocalories (kcal). The total energy value of a food product results from the addition of the energy content of each nutrient components. These are defined as follows:

1 g fat	37 kJ (9 kcal)
1 g carbohydrates	17 kJ (4 kcal)
1 g protein	17 kJ (4 kcal)
1 g alcohol (ethanol)	29 kJ (7 kcal)
1 g polyhydric alcohols (polyols)	10 kJ (2.4 kcal)
1 g dietary fiber	8 kJ (2 kcal)

For example, fat has a higher calorific value than the same amount of carbohydrates. Calorific value details **Figure 2.3** shows the proportion of nutrients on the calorific value in a small graphic.

▎RECOMMENDED DIETARY ALLOWANCES

The RDA for carbohydrates is set at 130 g per day. That is the minimum amount of glucose (the breakdown product of carbohydrate) needed by the brain. Carbohydrate intake is typically higher to meet calorie needs. In a healthy diet, the acceptable range for carbohydrates is set at 45 to 65% of total calories. Carbohydrate from of sugar added to processed foods should not exceed 10% of total calories. Carbohydrate in the form of dietary fiber should measure at least 25 g a day. As carbohydrate is utilized as main source of energy, at least 40% of the total energy in the food should come from carbohydrates. In our country, 60–80% of a day's energy needs are met from carbohydrates in the form of starch furnished by cereals and pulses. In developed countries, only 30–40% of days energy needs are met from carbohydrates.

❑ The body has a specific need for carbohydrates as a source of energy for the brain and other tissue cells, for synthesis of lactose of milk (lactating women) and galactose and other sugars present in the cerebrosides, mucopolysaccharides, etc.
❑ Carbohydrate is essential for the oxidation of fat and for the synthesis of certain non-essential amino acids.
❑ The carbohydrate calories should be at least 40% in well-balanced diets. The level of carbohydrates calories in the diet will also depend on the availability of fat and the economic conditions of the people as fat is about twice as costly as cereals on equicalorie basis in the developing countries and per caput production of fat per day is low (10–15 g).
❑ The optimal levels of carbohydrates in the diet, taking into physiological needs for proteins and fats.

Sl. No.	Age group	Optimal level calories as per cent of total calories
1.	Adults	50–70
2.	Expectant and nursing mothers	40–60
3.	Infants (1–12 months)	40–50
4.	Pre-school children (1–5 years)	40–60
5.	Older children and adolescents	50–70

The RDA daily value percentage listed on food labels can give you a general idea of what percentage the carbohydrates in a single serving of the food will contribute to your overall daily intake. This information is based on a 2,000-calorie diet, which is average for adult males. Women may need slightly less, and as you age, caloric needs continue to decrease. The Recommended Daily Allowances, or RDA, are a part of a larger nutrition system called the Dietary Reference Intake, or DRI, determined by the Institute of Medicine. Because the exact number of carbohydrates needed each day varies from person to person, the DRI is given as a percentage of total daily caloric intakes. Carbohydrates contribute four calories per gram; the USDA recommends that between 45 and 65% of your total caloric intake should come from carbohydrates. Based on a 2,000-calorie diet, this would equate to between 225 and 325 g of carbohydrates daily.

DRIs actually include four different reference values:
1. The **RDA**, which is the daily intake of a nutrient sufficient to meet the needs of almost all healthy people in an age and gender group.
2. The **AI**, or **Adequate Intake**, which is used if the RDA cannot be established. This is based on looking at how much of a nutrient healthy people actually eat.
3. The **UL** is the **Tolerable Upper Intake Level**, or the amount of a nutrient that a healthy person can eat without any risk of toxicity.
4. The **EAR**, or **Estimated Average Requirement**, is the amount of a nutrient that is estimated to meet the requirement of half of all healthy individuals in the population.

Of these four reference values, the **RDA, AI** and **UL** are of most use to individuals who want to know a safe and healthy level of nutrient intake. The **EAR** is mainly of use to people who are planning diets for large population groups, or developing new foods.

Estimated amounts of calories needed to maintain energy balance for various gender and age groups at three different levels of physical activity. The estimates are rounded to the nearest 200 calories and were determined using the Institute of Medicine equation.

Gender	Age (years)	Activity level		
		Sedentary	Moderately active	Active
Child	2–3	1,000	1,000–1,400	1,000–1,400
Female	4–8	1,200	1,400–1,600	1,400–1,800
	9–13	1,600	1,600–2,000	1,800–2,200
	14–18	1,800	2,000	2,400
	19–30	2,000	2,000–2,200	2,400
	31–50	1,800	2,000	2,200
	51+	1,600	1,800	2,000–2,200
Male	4–8	1,400	1,400–1,600	1,600–2,000
	9–13	1,800	1,800–2,200	2,000–2,600
	14–18	2,200	2,400–2,800	2,800–3,200
	19–30	2,400	2,600–2,800	3,000
	31–50	2,200	2,400–2,600	2,800–3,000
	51+	2,000	2,200–2,400	2,400–2,800

1. These levels are based on Estimated Energy Requirements (EER) from the Institute of Medicine Dietary Reference Intakes macronutrients report, 2002, calculated by gender, age, and activity level for reference-sized individuals. "Reference size," as determined by IOM, is based on median height and weight for ages up to age 18 years of age and median height and weight for that height to give a BMI of 21.5 for adult females and 22.5 for adult males.
   Table 2.3 is depicted the sources of carbohydrate.
2. Sedentary means a lifestyle that includes only the light physical activity associated with typical day-to-day life.
3. Moderately active means a lifestyle that includes physical activity equivalent to walking about 1.5 to 3 miles per day at 3 to 4 miles per hour, in addition to the light physical activity associated with typical day-to-day life
4. Active means a lifestyle that includes physical activity equivalent to walking more than 3 miles per day at 3 to 4 miles per hour, in addition to the light physical activity associated with typical day-to-day life.
5. The calorie ranges shown are to accommodate needs of different ages within the group. For children and adolescents, more calories are needed at older ages. For adults, fewer calories are needed at older ages.

Table 2.3: Sources of carbohydrate.

Sl. No.	Age group	Optimal level of carbohydrate calories as % of total calories
1.	Adults	50–70%
2.	Expectant and nursing mothers	40–60%
3.	Infants (1–12 month)	40–50%
4.	Preschool children (1–5 years)	40–60%
5.	Older children and adolescents	50–70%

The food groups in the USDA Food Guide are grains; vegetables; fruits; milk, yogurt, and cheese; and meat, poultry, fish, dry beans, eggs, and nuts. Food groups in the DASH Eating Plan are grains and grain products; vegetables; fruits; low-fat or fat-free dairy; meat, poultry, and fish; and nuts, seeds, and dry beans.

The body needs energy to maintain body temperature for metabolic processes to support growth, for functioning of the internal organs, such as heart, kidney, lungs, etc and for physical activity. Energy needs are influenced by factors such as body size, age, climate, extent of physical activity and altered physiological status such as pregnancy and lactation.

Energy allowance for infants:

Age	Kcal/Kg
3 months	120
3–5 months	115
6–8 months	110
9–11 months	105
Average during 1st year	112

Recommendation of energy intake of infants is based on breast milk intake. These allowances would form guidelines in feeding children who do not get sufficient breast milk. Usually the breast milk would be sufficient to meet the calorie recommendation up to 5–6 months and later require supplementation with other food stuffs besides milk in order to fulfill not calories but also other nutritional requirements.

Age group	Body weight (kg)	Energy allowance (kcal)
1–3 years	12.03	1220
4–6 years	18.87	1720

The allowances for calories are based on ideal body weight and not on actual body weights.

Energy allowances for adults: Recommendation for adults is made on a "Reference man" and "Reference women" who belong to the age group 20–39 years and weighing 55 kg and 45 kg respectively.

Energy allowances for women performing moderate activity:

Category	Energy allowance (kcal)
Women (Normal)	2200
Pregnancy	2500
Lactation (1st 6 months)	2750
6–12 months	2600

During pregnancy additional energy is needed to support the growth of the fetus, placenta and maternal tissues as well as to meet the increased metabolic rate. 300 extra calories is provided during pregnancy. Extra energy is provided during lactation for encouraging optimum secretion of milk. During the 1st 6 months, the quantity of milk produced by the mother is more and an extra allowance of 550 kcal is made during this period. Since women continue to lactate beyond 6 months, with reduced milk output up to one year, an extra allowance of 400 kcal/day recommended for periods from 6–12 months.

SOURCES OF CARBOHYDRATE (FIG. 2.4 AND TABLE 2.4)

Carbohydrates are broken down into three main categories—starches and starchy vegetables, fruits and dairy products. The USDA recommends that at least half of the starches and grains included in your diet be whole grains, such as bran, whole-wheat breads and pastas, brown rice and oatmeal. Other complex carbohydrates recommended include fruits and vegetables and low-fat or fat-free dairy products. On average, each serving provides between 12 and 15 g of carbohydrate, and a serving may be made up of a slice of bread, 1/3 cup of rice or pasta, a cup of milk or a small piece of fresh fruit.

Carbohydrates are classified as simple or complex. The classification depends on the chemical structure of the food, and how quickly the sugar is digested and absorbed. Simple carbohydrates have one (single) or two (double) sugars. Complex carbohydrates have three or more sugars. Examples of single sugars from foods include: Fructose (found in fruits), Galactose (found in milk products).

Double sugars include: Lactose (found in dairy), maltose (found in certain vegetables and in beer), sucrose (table sugar), honey is also a double sugar. But unlike table sugar, it contains a small amount of vitamins and minerals. (Note: Honey should not be given to children younger than 1 year old.) Complex carbohydrates often referred to as "starchy" foods, include—legumes, starchy vegetables, whole-grain breads and cereals. Simple carbohydrates that contain vitamins and minerals occur naturally in—fruits, milk and milk products, vegetables.

Simple carbohydrates are also found in processed and refined sugars, such as—candy, regular (nondiet) carbonated beverages, such as soda, syrups, table sugar. Refined sugars provide calories, but lack vitamins, minerals, and fiber. Such simple sugars are often called "empty calories" and can lead to weight gain. Also, many refined foods, such as white flour, sugar, and white rice, lack B vitamins and other important nutrients unless they are marked "enriched." It is healthiest to get carbohydrates, vitamins, and other nutrients in as natural a form as possible—for example, from fruit instead of table sugar.

Table 2.5 is depicted the food groups suggested by ICMR (2011).

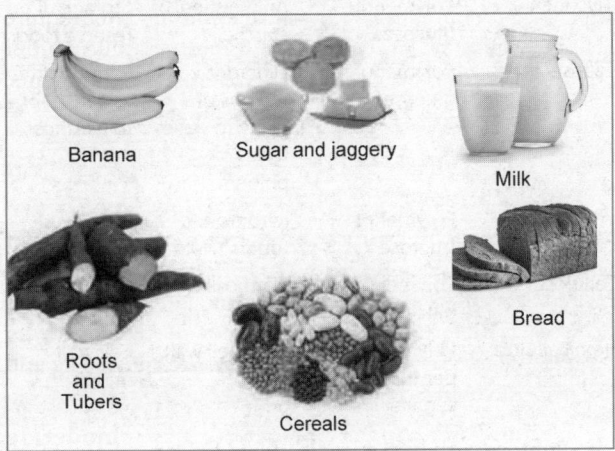

Fig. 2.4: Food sources of carbohydrates.

Table 2.4: Sources of carbohydrate.

Sl. No.	Source	Percentage
1.	Arrowroot powder	83%
2.	Sago	87%
3.	Syrup, jelly, jam	65–85%
4.	Rice	79%
5.	Barley, dates dried	75%
6.	Mango powder	64%
7.	Ragi	72%
8.	Tapioca	38%
9.	Jaggery	90%
10.	Bread	55%
11.	Honey	79%

Table 2.5: Food Groups Suggested by ICMR (2011).

Nutrient content of food groups	Nutrients
Cereals, millets and pulses:	
Rice, wheat, ragi, bajra, maize, jowar, barley, rice flakes, wheat flour, breakfast cereals	Energy, protein, invisible fat, vitamin B1, vitamin B2, folic acid, iron, fiber
Pulses and Legumes: Bengal gram, black gram, green gram, red gram, lentil (whole as well as dhal), cowpea, peas, rajmah, soya bean, beans	Energy, protein, invisible fat, vitamin B1, vitamin B2, folic acid, calcium, iron, fiber
Milk and animal products:	
Milk, curd, skimmed milk, cheese, chicken, liver, fish, egg, meat	Protein, fat, vitamin B1, vitamin B2, calcium, iron
Vegetables and fruits:	
Fruits: mango, guava, tomato, papaya, orange, sweet lime, water melon	Carotenoids, vitamin C, fiber, invisible fat, vitamin B2, folic acid, Iron
Green leafy vegetables: Amaranth, spinach, gogu, drumstick leaves, coriander leaves, fenugreek leaves	Carotenoids, vitamin B2, folic acid, calcium, iron, fiber
Other vegetables: Carrots, brinjal, ladies finger, beans, capsicum, onion, drumstick, cauliflower	Carotenoids, folic acid, calcium, fiber
Oils, fats and nuts:	
Fats: Butter ghee, hydrogenated fat, cooking oils, such as groundnut, mustard, sunflower	Energy, fat, essential fatty acids
Sugar: Jaggery and cane-sugar	Energy
Almonds, walnuts and gingelly seeds	Protein, ω-3 fatty acids

FUNCTIONS OF CARBOHYDRATE

Carbohydrates perform the following functions (Box 2.1).

- **Yield energy:** Yield energy—principle function of carbohydrates is to serve as a major source of energy for the body. Each gram of carbohydrate yields 4 kcal of energy regardless of its source. In Indian diets, 60–80% of energy is derived from carbohydrate.
- **Glucose maintenance:** Glucose maintenance is indispensable for the maintenance of the functional integrity of the nervous tissue and is the sole source of energy for the proper functioning of the brain. Prolonged lack of glucose may cause irreversible damage to the brain.
- **Protein sparing action:** Carbohydrates exert a protein sparing action. If sufficient amounts of carbohydrates are not available in the diet, the body will convert protein to glucose in order to supply energy. Hence to spare proteins for tissue building, carbohydrates must be supplied in optimum amounts in the diet. This is called the protein sparing action of carbohydrates.
- **Fat metabolism:** Carbohydrates are essential to maintain normal fat metabolism. Insufficient carbohydrates in the diet results in larger amounts of fat being used for energy than the body are equipped to handle. This leads to accumulation of acidic intermediate products called ketone bodies.
- **Synthesis of body substances:** Carbohydrates aid in the synthesis of non-essential amino acids, glycoproteins (which function as antibodies) and glycolipids (which form a part of cell membrane in body tissues especially brain and nervous system). Lactose remains in the intestine longer than other disaccharides and thus encourages growth of beneficial bacteria.
- **Precursors of nucleic acid:** Carbohydrates and products derived from them, serve as precursors of compounds, such as nucleic acids, connective tissue matrix and galactosides of nervous tissue.
- **Detoxification function:** Glucuronic acid, a metabolite of glucose serves as a detoxifying agent. It combines with harmful substances containing alcohol or phenolic group converting them to harmless compounds, which are later excreted.
- **Roughage of the diet:** Insoluble fibers known as composite carbohydrates can absorb water and give bulk to the intestinal contents, which aids in the elimination of waste products by stimulating peristaltic movements of the gastrointestinal tract.
- **Other roles:** Carbohydrate has a variety of functions in the animal and human body. It plays crucial role in biological system they are:
  - 1 g of carbohydrate provides 4 kcal on oxidation.
  - Protein sparing action helps to regulate protein metabolism. When carbohydrate and fat is adequate amount in the diet, major protein is used for tissues building.
  - Ketone body from fat metabolism is prevented when carbohydrate is sufficient.

> **Box 2.1:** Functions of carbohydrates in the human body.
> - Carbohydrate oxidation provides energy
> - Carbohydrate storage, in the form of glycogen, provides a short-term energy reserve
> - Carbohydrates supply carbon atoms for the synthesis of other biochemical substances (proteins, lipids, and nucleic acids)
> - Carbohydrates form part of the structural framework of DNA and RNA molecules
> - Carbohydrates linked to lipids are structural components of cell membranes
> - Carbohydrates linked to proteins function in a variety of cell-cell and cell-molecule recognition processes

Name of the polysaccharide	Composition	Occurrence	Function
Starch	Polymer of glucose containing a straight chain of glucose molecules and a branched chain of glucose molecules	In several plant species as main storage carbohydrate	Storage of reserve food
Glycogen	Polymer of glucose	Animals (eq. of starch)	Storage of reserve food
Callose	Polymer of glucose	Different regions of plant, in sieve tubes of phloem	Formed often as a response to wounds
Insulin	Polymer of fructose	In roots and tubers	Storage of reserve food
Cellulose	Polymer of glucose	Plant cell wall	Cell wall matrix
Hemicellulose	Polymer of pentoses and sugar acids	Plant cell wall	Cell wall matrix

- Pentose carbon-5 sugar is utilized in formation of DNA and RNA.
- It supplies fuel to brain tissues, otherwise irreversible damage occurs.
- If carbohydrate exceeds the normal requirement, fat synthesis in adipose tissue.
- Lactose in gastrointestinal tract promotes the growth of bacteria, which is responsible for the synthesis of B-complex vitamins.
- Complex polysaccharides cellulose and hemicellulose contribute bulk to the stool.
- Carbohydrate in well-balanced diet keeps the blood sugar level within normal limits

DIGESTION AND ABSORPTION OF CARBOHYDRATE

Digestion:
- The first stage of digestion of carbohydrate takes place in the mouth. Chewing breaks up food and exposes starch

Chapter 2: Carbohydrates and Energy

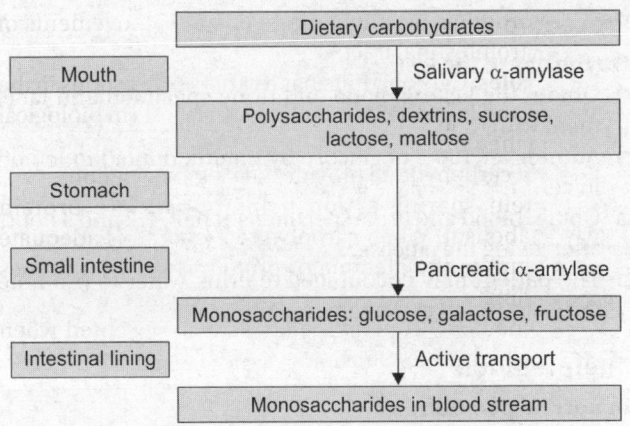

Fig. 2.5: Digestion of carbohydrate.

and sugars to the action of enzymes. Saliva contains salivary amylase (ptyalin).
- It converts starch to maltose, but time limits the action of salivary amylase, because as food enters the stomach, the acid present in the stomach blocks the action of salivary amylase.
- In the stomach, the acid causes hydrolysis of sucrose. In the small intestine, pancreatic amylase and intestinal amylase digest starch up to the stage of maltose.
- Starch salivary, pancreatic maltose + Isomaltose and intestinal amylase
- Glycogen is also broken by these enzymes to disaccharides. Enzymes maltase, sucrase and lactase present in the brush borders of the columnar cells of small intestine convert disaccharides to monosaccharides.
  Maltase: Maltose glucose + Glucose
  Lactase: Lactose glucose + Galactose
  Sucrase: Sucrose glucose + Fructose
- Cellulose and other polysaccharides are not digested by enzymes, so undigested material passes to large intestine forming bulk, which contributes to feces.
- The end products of carbohydrate digestion are monosaccharides—glucose, galactose and fructose. They are absorbed by process of active absorption by the mucosa of the small intestine.

Figure 2.5 is depicted the digestion of carbohydrate.

Metabolism

Metabolism occurs inside the various cells of the body. There are two types of metabolism—anabolism (building up) and catabolism (breaking down).
1. The major carbohydrate anabolic pathways are conversion of glucose into glycogen (glycogenesis) is tale place in the liver and muscles.
2. The conversion of glucose into fat (lipogenesis) in the liver and adipose tissue.
3. Carbohydrates follow two major catabolic pathways:
   a. The breakdown of glucose releasing energy (glycolysis) and converting it into usable energy (ATP) and the converting into of glycogen glucose (glycogenolysis).
   b. After digestion and absorption of glucose into the blood stream it is utilized directly by the tissues for energy.

When the absorbed glucose exceeds the body's need for energy, it is stored as glycogen in the liver and muscle and excess glucose is converted to triglycerides and stored as fat in adipose tissue.

Glucose Formation from Non-carbohydrate Sources

- Glucose can be formed the metabolism of protein and from the glycerol of fat. It has been estimated that the glycerol present in 100 g of fat can give rise to 50-60 g glucose.
- Lactate which is formed from glucose can be reconverted into glucose in the liver.

REGULATION OF BLOOD SUGAR

- Blood circulates glucose continuously to each and every cell of the body as a source of energy and for the synthesis of a number of substances.
- In fasting state blood sugar level is 60-85 mg/100 mL of blood. Soon after a meal it raises to 140-150 mg/100 mL.
- If the body is in a good carbohydrate metabolic pathway this concentration will fall down to a normal blood sugar level of 60-85 mg/100 mL.
- The liver very efficiently maintains the normal blood sugar level. The liver is the only organ in our body, which can either supply glucose to the circulation or to remove the excess sugar from blood.
- If the blood sugar concentration is high this condition is known as hyperglycemia. Hypoglycemia occurs when the blood sugar level is below normal level. This occurs in certain abnormalities of liver function or when insulin is produced in excessive amount by the pancreas.

Glucose Tolerance Test (Fig. 2.6)

Glucose tolerance test (GTT) is done to detect the abnormalities of carbohydrate metabolism.

Indications: 1. Hypoglycemia, 2. Diabetes mellitus, 3. Adrenocortical diseases.

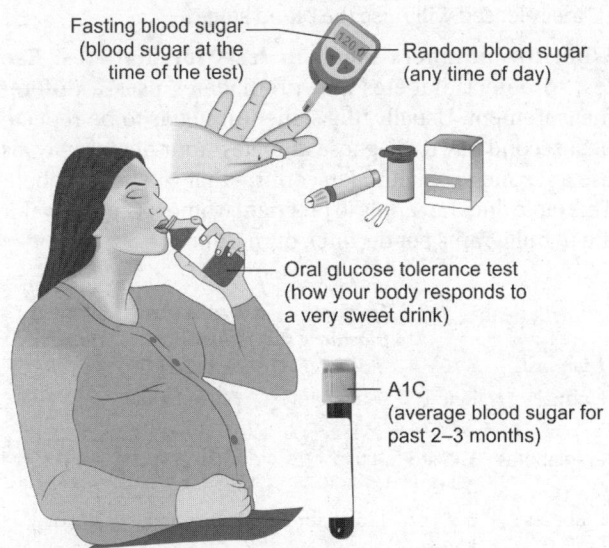

Fig. 2.6: Glucose tolerance test.

Preparation of the patient

- At least 2 weeks of good health is desirable in the patient prior to the test. Patient with inadequate dietary intake may show high curve than normal.
- They should receive a high carbohydrate diet for at least 3 days prior to the test and then the patient should fast 8 to 12 hours.
- On the previous day of the test, approximately 12 hours prior to the test, the patient is given evening meal. Thereafter no food is allowed until the test is over.
- On the day of test, the patient should not have even black coffee or tea and should not smoke.
- Undue exercise and mental stress should be avoided and the patient should relax for 30 minutes before the test is started.

General Instructions

- The GTT test curve shows abnormal in thyroid diseases, adrenal insufficiency, hyper functioning of the adrenal cortex, excess insulin due to pancreatic tumors, physical and mental stress.
- The abnormal GTT curve also seen in patients receiving diuretics, glucocorticoids, estrogens, oral-contraceptives, etc.
- Patient should be monitored for hypoglycemic reactions, such as profuse. Sweating and dizziness, a drop in blood sugar much below normal and must be watched.
- The glucose (dextrose) could be given intravenously at the dose of 0.2 g/kg body weight, as 50% glucose solution. intravenous administration of glucose given for patients with decreased absorption of sugar from the intestine.
- The GTT test should not be performed on patients with intital fasting blood sugar of over 200 mg/dL.
- The delayed return (beyond 2 hours) of blood glucose to a fasting (if normal) level indicates abnormal glucose tolerance.

Factors affecting GTT test:

- **Coffee and tea:** These substances alter the body's response to carbohydrate.
- **Stress control:** Because epinephrine and cortisone that are released will raise the blood sugar.

What the numbers mean in tests for diabetes: Each test to detect diabetes and prediabetes uses a different measurement. Usually, the same test needs to be repeated on a second day to diagnose diabetes. Your doctor may also use a second test method to confirm that you have diabetes. This table does not apply to pregnant women. Glucose values are in milligrams per deciliter, or mg/dL.

Diagnosis	A1C	Fasting plasma glucose (FPG)	Oral glucose tolerance test (OGTT)	Random plasma glucose test (RPG)
Normal	Below 5.7%	99 or below	139 or below	
Prediabetes	5.7% to 6.4%	100 to 125	140 to 199	
Diabetes	6.5% or above	126 or above	200 or above	200 or above

Soruce: American Diabetes Association.

Procedure

On the day of the test:

- Obtain the fasting blood and urine specimen and label them with time.
- Administer 100 g of glucose by mouth, diluted in lemon juice.
- Obtain blood and urine specimens at half, 1, 2 and 3 hours after giving the glucose.
- The patient may encouraged to drink water to promote urine excretion at the required times.

Interpretation

In normal person:

- In a normal individual the fasting blood sugar will be 55 to 110 mg/dL.
- In first hour, the maximum blood sugar level reached after the oral glucose intake. It blood sugar level will be 140 to 180 mg/dL (usually not more than 160 mg/dL).
- The blood sugar level returns to normal fasting limits after I hour or at least by 2 hours.
- There is usually no sugar in any of the urine specimens in normal persons.

In diabetic mellitus:

- In the post-oral glucose period, the blood sugar level is rises to a peak much higher than 160 mg/dL.
- Sometimes it may reach high as 400 mg/dL and does not return to normal by the second or third hour.
- All the specimens of urine will contain glucose.

Deficienies of Carbohydrate

Low level of glucose (40 mg% or below) in the blood is called hypoglycemia. This is not common in healthy individual. Diabetic people may get this condition on poor or irregular treatment. The signs and symptoms of diabetes are tiredness, convulsions, dizziness, tingling, faintness, headache, firmness, tachycardia, palpation, confusion, slurred speech, staggering gait, lack of coordination and coma.

Figure 2.7 is depicted the main symptoms of diabetes.

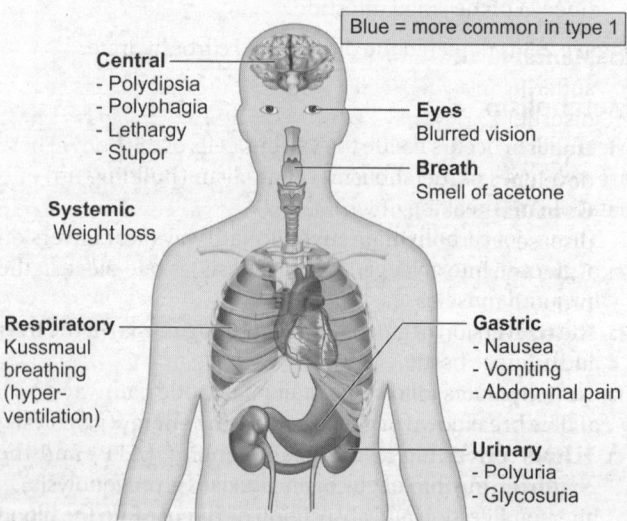

Fig. 2.7: Main symptoms of diabetes.

Diabetes mellitus:
- Diabetes mellitus is a chronic disease in which blood glucose level is raised above 180 mg/dL of blood and glucose is excreted in urine.
- The disease is primarily due to the insufficient production of the hormone, insulin by the beta-cells of the islets of langerhans of the pancreas.
- The two types of diabetes are referred to as type 1 and type 2. Former names for these conditions were insulin-dependent and non-insulin-dependent diabetes, or juvenile onset and adult onset diabetes.
- Symptoms of diabetes include increased urine output, thirst, hunger, and fatigue.
- Diabetes is diagnosed by blood sugar (glucose) testing. The major complications of diabetes are both acute and chronic.

Acute complications: Dangerously elevated blood sugar (hyperglycemia) or abnormally low blood sugar (hypoglycemia) due to diabetes medications

Chronic complications: Disease of the blood vessels (both small and large) that can damage the feet, eyes, kidneys, nerves, and heart. Diabetes treatment depends on the type and severity of the diabetes. Type 1 diabetes is treated with insulin, exercise, and a diabetic diet. Type 2 diabetes is first treated with weight reduction, a diabetic diet, and exercise. When these measures fail to control the elevated blood sugars, oral medications are used. If oral medications are still insufficient, insulin and other injectable medications are considered.

Complications linked to badly controlled diabetes:
- **Eye complications**—glaucoma, cataracts, diabetic retinopathy, and some others.
- **Foot complications**—neuropathy, ulcers, and sometimes gangrene which may require that the foot be amputated
- **Skin complications**—people with diabetes are more susceptible to skin infections and skin disorders
- **Heart problems**—such as ischemic heart disease, when the blood supply to the heart muscle is diminished
- **Hypertension**—common in people with diabetes, which can raise the risk of kidney disease, eye problems, heart attack and stroke
- **Mental health**—uncontrolled diabetes raises the risk of suffering from depression, anxiety and some other mental disorders
- **Hearing loss**—diabetes patients have a higher risk of developing hearing problems
- **Gum disease**—there is a much higher prevalence of gum disease among diabetes patients
- **Gastroparesis**—the muscles of the stomach stop working properly
- **Ketoacidosis**—a combination of ketosis and acidosis; accumulation of ketone bodies and acidity in the blood.
- **Neuropathy**—diabetic neuropathy is a type of nerve damage which can lead to several different problems.
- **HHNS (Hyperosmolar Hyperglycemic Nonketotic Syndrome)**—blood glucose levels shoot up too high, and there are no ketones present in the blood or urine. It is an emergency condition.
- **Nephropathy**—uncontrolled blood pressure can lead to kidney disease
- **PAD (peripheral arterial disease)**—symptoms may include pain in the leg, tingling and sometimes problems walking properly
- **Stroke**—if blood pressure, cholesterol levels, and blood glucose levels are not controlled, the risk of stroke increases significantly
- **Erectile dysfunction**—male impotence
- **Infections**—people with badly controlled diabetes are much more susceptible to infections
- **Healing of wounds**—cuts and lesions take much longer to heal

Figure 2.8 is depicted the complications of diabetes and **Figure 2.9** is depicted the major complications of diabetes.

Energy

Energy is defined as the capacity for doing work. It is the heat produced in the body, which is utilized for performing the involuntary and voluntary activities, to maintain body temperature to synthesize new body constituents.

Definitions
- **Unit:** The standard quantity (constant quality), used for comparison is called unit.
- **Measurement:** Measurement is the comparison of an unknown quantity with a known standard quantity (constant quantity) or unit.
- **GCS system:** This system is generally adopted for smaller measurement of mass, length and time. In this system, C stands for centimeter (length), G-stands for gram (mass), and S-stands for seconds (time).
- **MKS system:** In this system, M-stands for meter (length); K-stands for kilogram (mass) and S-stands for second (time). This system is generally adopted for longer measurements.

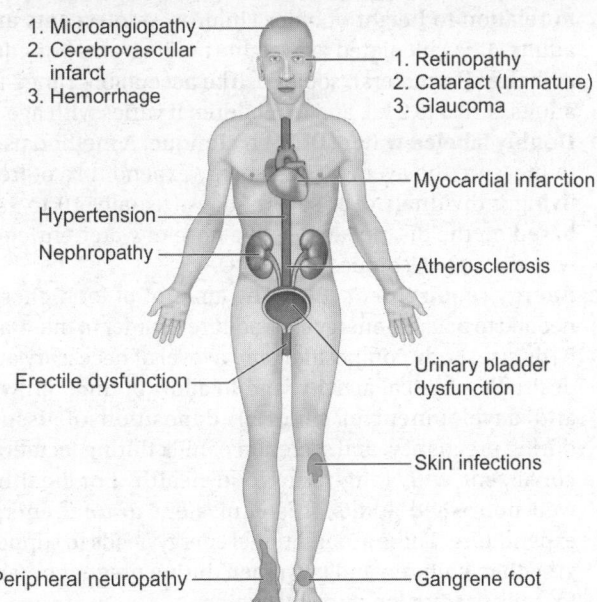

Fig. 2.8: Complications of diabetes.

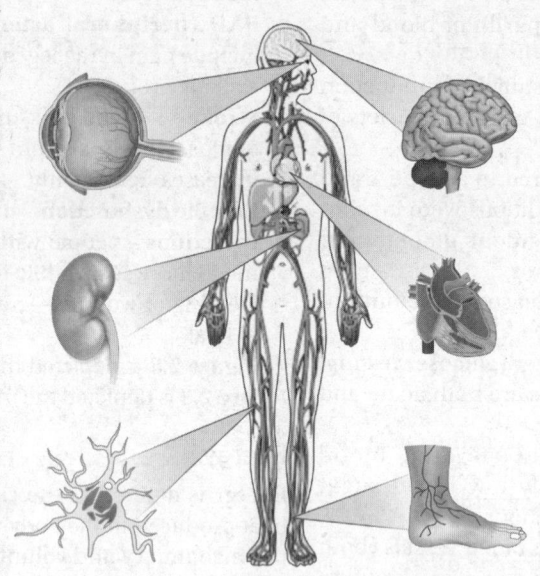

Fig. 2.9: Major complications of diabetes.

- **SI system:** It is standard international system, in this system the units of mass, length and time are same, as that of MKS system.
- **Fundamental unit:** A unit which is indepentable of any other unit, or which can neither be changed nor related to any other fundamental unit, is a fundamental unit.
- **Basal metabolic rate (BMR):** The minimal rate of energy expenditure compatible with life. It is measured in the supine position under standard conditions of rest, fasting, immobility, thermoneutrality and mental relaxation. Depending on its use, the rate is usually expressed per minute, per hour or per 24 hours.
- **Body mass index (BMI):** The indicator of weight adequacy in relation to height of older children, adolescents and adults. It is calculated as weight (in kilograms) divided by height (in meters), squared. The acceptable range for adults is 18.5 to 24.9, and for children it varies with age.
- **Doubly labeled water (DLW) technique:** A method used to measure the average total energy expenditure of free-living individuals over several days (usually 10 to 14), based on the disappearance of a dose of water enriched with the stable isotopes ^2H and ^{18}O.
- **Energy requirement (ER):** The amount of food energy needed to balance energy expenditure in order to maintain body size, body composition and a level of necessary and desirable physical activity, and to allow optimal growth and development of children, deposition of tissues during pregnancy, and secretion of milk during lactation, consistent with long-term good health. For healthy, well-nourished adults, it is equivalent to total energy expenditure. There are additional energy needs to support growth in children and in women during pregnancy, and for milk production during lactation.
- **Heart rate monitoring (HRM):** A method to measure the daily energy expenditure of free-living individuals, based on the relationship of heart rate and oxygen consumption and on minute-by-minute monitoring of heart rate.
- **Total energy expenditure (TEE):** The energy spent, on average, in a 24-hour period by an individual or a group of individuals. By definition, it reflects the average amount of energy spent in a typical day, but it is not the exact amount of energy spent each and every day.
- **Physical activity level (PAL):** TEE for 24 hours expressed as a multiple of BMR, and calculated as TEE/BMR for 24 hours. In adult men and non-pregnant, non-lactating women, BMR times PAL is equal to TEE or the daily energy requirement.
- **Physical activity ratio (PAR):** The energy cost of an activity per unit of time (usually a minute or an hour) expressed as a multiple of BMR. It is calculated as energy spent in an activity/BMR, for the selected time unit.

UNITS OF ENERGY

The words "power" and "energy" are often used interchangeably. While energy in the ability to do work, power is the rate at which energy is transferred, used, or transformed. Energy is defined as the capacity of a system to perform work. Suppose a body having mass M kg moving with a linear velocity of v meter/sec so its energy is in the form of kinetic energy which is equal to $KE = 21\ mv^2$. SI unit of energy is Joule. CGS unit of energy is erg.

Example of a unit of energy: A related unit is the Watt, which is a unit of power (energy per unit time). Power units can be converted to energy units through multiplication by seconds [s], hours, [h], or years [yr]. For example, 1 kWh [kilowatt hour]

= 3.6 MJ [mega Joule]. The energy value of food is expressed in terms of kilocalories (kcal or C). A kilocalorie is defined as the amount of heat required to raise the temperature of 1 kg of water by 10°C. In the metric system, the international unit, which is kilojoules, is used instead of kilocalories. Kilojoules energy is expended when 1 kg of mass is moved by 1 meter using a force of a Newton.

- 1 Calorie = 4.184 Joule
- 1 kcal or C = 4.184 kjoule
- 1,000 kcal or C = 4.184 MJoule
- 1 MJoule = 239 kcal

Joule (J): This is the basic energy unit of the metric system, or in a later more comprehensive formulation, the International System of Units (SI). It is ultimately defined in terms of the meter, kilogram, and second.

Calorie (cal): Historically the calorie was defined in terms of the heating of water. Thus, in a traditional definition, one calorie is the amount of heat required to raise the temperature of 1 gram of water by 1°C, from 14.5°C to 15.5°C. (This is sometimes referred to as the 15°C calorie, and differs slightly from the "calorie" measured for other temperature intervals.) More recently the calorie has been defined in terms of the joule; the equivalence between the calorie and joule is historically known as the mechanical equivalent of heat.

Energy Requirements of Different Categories of People

An adequate, healthy diet must satisfy human needs for energy and all essential nutrients. Furthermore, dietary energy needs and recommendations cannot be considered in isolation of other nutrients in the diet, as the lack of one will influence the others. Thus, the following definitions are based on the assumption that requirements for energy will be fulfilled through the consumption of a diet that satisfies all nutrient needs.

Energy requirement is the amount of food energy needed to balance energy expenditure in order to maintain body size, body composition and a level of necessary and desirable physical activity consistent with long-term good health. This includes the energy needed for the optimal growth and development of children, for the deposition of tissues during pregnancy, and for the secretion of milk during lactation consistent with the good health of mother and child.

Scenario	Physical activity level
Sedentary	Light physical activity associated with daily living, 1976–2003
Moderately active	Walking 2.4 to 4.8 km/d in addition to light physical activity associated with daily living, 1976–2003
Active	Walking >3.8 km/d in addition to light physical activity associated with daily living, 1976–2003
Moderate → sedentary	Progressing from moderate physical activity level in 1976 to sedentary physical activity level in 2003

The recommended level of dietary energy intake for a population group is the mean energy requirement of the healthy, well-nourished individuals who constitute that group. Based on these definitions, a main objective for the assessment of energy requirements is the prescription of dietary energy intakes that are compatible with long-term good health. Therefore, the levels of energy intake recommended by this expert consultation are based on estimates of the requirements of healthy, well-nourished individuals. It is recognized that some populations have particular public health characteristics that are part of their usual, "normal" life. Foremost among these are population groups in many developing countries where there are numerous infants and children who suffer from mild to moderate degrees of malnutrition and who experience frequent episodes of infectious diseases, mostly diarrhoeal and respiratory infections. Special considerations are made in this report for such sub-populations.

Daily energy requirements and daily energy intakes: Energy requirements and recommended levels of intake are often referred to as daily requirements or recommended daily intakes. These terms are used as a matter of convention and convenience, indicating that the requirement represents an average of energy needs over a certain number of days, and that the recommended energy intake is the amount of energy that should be ingested as a daily average over a certain period of time. There is no implication that exactly this amount of energy must be consumed every day, nor that the requirement and recommended intake are constant, day after day. Neither is there any biological basis for defining the number of days over which the requirement or intake must be averaged. As a matter of convenience, taking into account that physical activity and eating habits may vary on some days of the week, periods of seven days are often used when estimating the average daily energy expenditure and recommended daily intake.

Energy requirements of children: Although children of all ages grow rapidly, their energy needs vary. For example, the amount of energy needed—on a per kilogram (pound) basis—by an 18-year-old teenager is much lower than that of an 18-month-old toddler. Babies double their body weight over a few months, whereas older children and adolescents may double their weight over five to ten years.

Age	Boys per day	Girls per day
0–3 months	545 calories	515 calories
4–6 months	690 calories	645 calories
7–9 months	825 calories	765 calories
10–12 months	920 calories	865 calories
1–3 years	1230 calories	1165 calories
4–6 years	1715 calories	1545 calories
7–10 years	1970 calories	1740 calories
11–14 years	2220 calories	1845 calories
15–18 years	2755 calories	2110 calories

Energy requirements will vary in special cases. For example, children who use up a lot of energy in sport or those who are very physically active will need more calories every day than children who are less active. In addition, children who are ill or recovering from an injury need almost double their normal amount of calories to aid the healing process and continue growing normally.

		Activity level		
Gender	Age	Sedentary	Moderately active	Active
Child	2–3	1,000	1,000–1,400	1,000–1,400
Female	4–8	1,200	1,400–1,600	1,000–1,800
	9–13	1,600	1,600–2,000	1,800–2,200
	14–18	1,800	2,000	2,400
	19–30	2,000	2,000–2,200	2,400
	31–50	1,800	2,000	2,200
	51+	1,600	1,800	2,000–2,200
Male	4–8	1,400	1,400–1,600	1,600–2,000
	9–13	1,800	1,800–2,000	2,000–2,600
	14–18	2,200	2,400–2,800	2,800–3,200
	19–30	2,400	2,600–2,800	3,000
	31–50	2,200	2,400–2,600	2,800–3,000
	51+	2,000	2,200–2,400	2,400–2,800

COMPONENTS OF ENERGY REQUIREMENTS

Human beings need energy for the following:

Basal Metabolism

- This comprises a series of functions that are essential for life, such as cell function and replacement; the synthesis, secretion and metabolism of enzymes and hormones to transport proteins and other substances and molecules; the maintenance of body temperature; uninterrupted work of cardiac and respiratory muscles; and brain function.
- The amount of energy used for basal metabolism in a period of time is called the basal metabolic rate (BMR), and is measured under standard conditions that include being awake in the supine position after ten to 12 hours of fasting and eight hours of physical rest, and being in a state of mental relaxation in an ambient environmental temperature that does not elicit heat-generating or heat-dissipating processes.
- Depending on age and lifestyle, BMR represents 45 to 70% of daily total energy expenditure, and it is determined mainly by the individual's age, gender and body size and body composition.

Metabolic Response to Food

- Eating requires energy for the ingestion and digestion of food, and for the absorption, transport, interconversion, oxidation and deposition of nutrients.
- These metabolic processes increase heat production and oxygen consumption, and are known by terms such as dietary-induced thermogenesis, specific dynamic action of food and thermic effect of feeding.
- The metabolic response to food increases total energy expenditure by about 10% of the BMR over a 24-hour period in individuals eating a mixed diet.

Physical Activity

- This is the most variable and, after BMR, the second largest component of daily energy expenditure.
- Humans perform obligatory and discretionary physical activities. Obligatory activities can seldom be avoided within a given setting, and they are imposed on the individual by economic, cultural or societal demands.
- The term "obligatory" is more comprehensive than the term "occupational" that was used in the 1985 report (WHO, 1985) because, in addition to occupational work, obligatory activities include daily activities, such as going to school, tending to the home and family and other demands made on children and adults by their economic, social and cultural environment.

Discretionary Activities

Discretionary activities: Although not socially or economically essential, are important for health, well-being and a good quality of life in general. They include the regular practice of physical activity for fitness and health; the performance of optional household tasks that may contribute to family comfort and well-being; and the engagement in individually and socially desirable activities for personal enjoyment, social interaction and community development.

Growth

The energy cost of growth has following components:
1. The energy needed to synthesize growing tissues; and
2. The energy deposited in those tissues.
3. The energy cost of growth is about 35% of total energy requirement during the first three months of age, falls rapidly to about 5% at 12 months and about 3 percent in the second year, remains at 1 to 2% until mid-adolescence, and is negligible in the late teens.

Pregnancy

During pregnancy, extra energy is needed for the growth of the fetus, placenta and various maternal tissues, such as in the uterus, breasts and fat stores, as well as for changes in maternal metabolism and the increase in maternal effort at rest and during physical activity.

Lactation

The energy cost of lactation has two components:
1. The energy content of the milk secreted; and
2. The energy required producing that milk. Well-nourished lactating women can derive part of this additional requirement from body fat stores accumulated during pregnancy.

MEASUREMENT OF ENERGY

Energy or work

The SI unit of energy or work is the **joule**. To change any of these other units of energy or work into their **equivalent values ID joules** use the operation and conversion factor given.

Calories–cal	x 4.1868
Calorie (food)	x 4186 (approx.)
Ergs	Divide by 10000000
Gigajoules [GJ]	x 1000000000
Horsepower hours	x 2684520 (approx.)
Joules (J)	1
Kilocalories	x 4186.8
Kilogram-force meters	x 9.80665
Kilojoules (kJ)	x 1000
Kilowatt hours (kWh)	x 3600000
Megajoules (MJ)	x 100000
Newton meters [Nm]	x 1
Therms	x 105500000 (approx.)
Watt seconds (Ws)	1
Watt hours (Wh)	x 3600

BODY MASS INDEX AND BASIC METABOLISM

Body Mass Index (BMI) is a simple index of weight-for-height that is commonly used to classify underweight, overweight and obesity in adults. It is defined as the weight in kilograms divided by the square of the height in meters (kg/m^2). For example, an adult who weighs 70 kg and whose height is 1.75 m will have a BMI of 22.9. BMI = 70 kg/(1.75 m^2) = 70/3.06 = 22.9.

BMI	Weight status
Below 18.5	Underweight
18.5–24.9	Normal weight
25.0–29.9	Overweight
30.0–34.9	Obesity class I
35.0–39.9	Obesity class II
Above 40	Obesity class III

Body Mass Index (Quetelet's Index): The body mass index is used as a reference standard for assessing the prevalence of obesity in the community.

Body mass index = weight in kg/height in meters. Ideal body mass index:
- Ideal body mass index for Indian women: 19–24.
- Ideal body mass index for Indian man: 20–26.

Once the body mass index exceeds the normal limit; the person can be termed as overweight or obese.

Classification	BMI (kg/m^2)	
	Principal cut-off points	*Additional cut-off points*
Underweight	<18.50	<18.50
Severe thinness	<16.00	<16.00
Moderate thinness	16.00–16.99	16.00–16.99
Mild thinness	17.00–18.49	17.00–18.49
Normal range	18.50–24.99	18.50–22.99
		23.00–24.99
Overweight	≥25.00	≥25.00
Pre-obese	25.00–29.99	25.00–27.49
		27.50–29.99
Obese	≥30.00	≥30.00
Obese class I	30.00–34.99	30.00–32.49
		32.50–34.99
Obese class II	35.00–39.99	35.00–37.49
		37.50–39.99
Obese class III	≥40.00	≥40.00

The basal metabolic rate is the minimum number of calories needed to maintain vital functions, such as breathing and keeping the heart beating. It is the energy expenditure necessary to maintain basic physiologic conditions, such as; respiration, cardiac contraction, conduction of nerve impulses, metabolic activity, such as synthesis of macromolecules under standard conditions, reabsorption of kidney, iron transport across impulse. This function occurs continuously with one's own conscious or awareness. Basal metabolic needs are surprisingly large person whose total energy expenditure amounts to 2,000 calories/day, spends as much as 1,200–1,400 calories to support usual metabolism.

BMI Classifications: The International Classification of adult underweight, overweight and obesity according to BMI.

Definition
- Basal metabolism is the minimum amount of energy needed by the body for maintenance of life when the person is at post-absorptive state, physical and emotional rest.
- Basal metabolic rate is a measure of the energy required by the activities of resting tissue can be measured directly from the heat produced (using a respiration calorimeter and metabolic chamber) or indirectly from O$_2$ intake and CO$_2$ expenditure when the subject is at rest.

Normal Values
- Basal metabolic rate values are expressed as kcal or kJ square meter of body surface per hour.
- In adults, basal metabolic rate for healthy males 40 kcal/h (168 KJ) per hour and in healthy females is 37 kcal/h (155 KJ).

BASAL METABOLIC RATE

The basal metabolic rate is the minimum number of calories needed to maintain vital functions, such as breathing and keeping the heart beating. It is the energy expenditure necessary to maintain basic physiologic conditions, such as; respiration, cardiac contraction, conduction of nerve impulses, metabolic activity, such as synthesis of macromolecules under standard conditions, reabsorption of kidney, iron transport across impulse. This function occurs continuously with one's own conscious or awareness. Basal metabolic needs are surprisingly large person whose total energy expenditure amounts to 2,000 calories/day, spends as much as 1,200–1,400 calories to support usual metabolism.

Basal Metabolic Rate Formulas in Metric

The original Harris-Benedict equations published in 1918 and 1919	Men	BMR = 66.5 + (13.75 × weight in kg) + (5.003 × height in cm) – (6.755 × age in years)
	Women	BMR = 655.1 + (9.563 × weight in kg) + (1.850 × height in cm) – (4.676 × age in years)
The Harris-Benedict equations revised by Roza and Shizgal in 1984	Men	BMR = 88.362 + (13.397 × weight in kg) + (4.799 × height in cm) – (5.677 × age in years)
	Women	BMR = 447.593 + (9.247 × weight in kg) + (3.098 × height in cm) – (4.330 × age in years)
The Harris-Benedict equations revised by Mifflin and St Jeor in 1990	Men	BMR = (10 × weight in kg) + (6.25 × height in cm) – (5 × age in years) + 5
	Women	BMR = (10 × weight in kg) + (6.25 × height in cm) – (5 × age in years) – 161

Definitions
- Basal metabolism is the minimum amount of energy needed by the body for maintenance of life when the person is at post absorptive state, physical and emotional rest.
- Basal metabolic rate is a measure of the energy required by the activities of resting tissue can be measured directly from the heat produced (using a respiration calorimeter and metabolic chamber) or indirectly from O_2 intake and CO_2 expenditure when the subject is at rest.

Normal Values
- Basal metabolic rate values are expressed as kcal or kJ square meter of body surface per hour.
- In adults, basal metabolic rate for healthy males 40 kcal/h (168 KJ) per hour and in healthy females is 37 kcal/h (155 KJ).

Meaning of BMR
Basal metabolic rate is a number of processes go on in the body without any conscious effort, even when subject is at complete rest and no physical work is done. These include involuntary processes, such as the beating of heart, the circulation of blood, etc. These activities are called basal metabolic processes. The energy used for carrying out these activities is known as the basal metabolic rate. The basal energy need constitute more than half of the total energy need, for most of the people.

Factors Affecting basal Metabolic Rate
There are many factors, which affect the basal metabolic rate; the most common factors are:

Sl. No.	Caloric value	Kcal/g
1.	Surface area of the body	The larger the surface area of the body in relation to its bulk, the greater is the heat lost by radiation
2.	Sex	The basal metabolic rate is higher per square meter of body surface area in men than in women. According to Western standards the requirements are: • 40 cal/m^2/h men • 37 cal/m^2/h for women
3.	Age	Growing children and adolescent have high-basal metabolic rates in relation to their weight than adults
4.	Diseases	Some diseases, especially of thyroid gland, may raise or lower the basal metabolic rates. A rise of body temperature of 1°F is found to increase basal metabolic rate by about 7%
5.	Nutritional status	Basal metabolic rate is lower in starvation and under nourishment as compared to well-fed state. Under-prolonged or chronic under nutrition, the basal metabolic rate is decreased
6.	Stress	Psychological stress and tension caused by worry or stress will increase the basal metabolic rate
7.	Environmental factors	In cold climate, the basal metabolic rate is increased and in tropical climate, the basal metabolic rate is proportionally low
8.	Drugs	Smoking (nicotine), coffee (caffeine) increases the basal metabolic rate, whereas β-blockers tend to decrease energy expenditure

DETERMINANTS AND FACTORS AFFECTING

Among factors, which influences energy needs are age, sex, body size, climate,

Secretion of endocrine glands, status of health, altered physiological activity.

Age
- During the growth period, the BMR is high, therefore during infancy; the energy need per kilogram of body weight is higher than during adulthood.
- Energy requirement also decline progressively after early adulthood due to steady decline in BMR thereafter.
- The basal metabolism during rapid growth is at a high level. The younger the individuals the higher, the basal metabolism since, much energy are stored for growth.

- The period at which the basal metabolism reaches its highest level is between the ages of 1 and 2 years. A gradual decline occurs between the age of 2 and 5 years, with a more rapid decline until adult age is reached.

Table 2.6 is depicted the factors affecting basal metabolic rate (BMR).

Sex

- The BMR is higher in adolescent boys and adult males as compared to adolescent girls and adult females though it is not due to direct influence of sex differences, but are due to the differences in body composition.
- Males have a greater amount of muscles and glandular tissues, which is metabolically more active whereas, females have greater adipose tissues, which is metabolically less active. Hence, energy requirement of males is higher than of females.

Body Size

- It will have an important effect on energy needs, because a larger body has a greater amount of muscles and glandular tissue to maintain, thus requiring higher energy allowances.
- Heat is continuously lost through the skin by radiation. Since, the heat loss is proportional to the skin surface; the basal heat production is directly proportional to the surface area.
- A tall thin individual has a greater surface area than an individual of the same weight who is short and fat and the former will therefore, have a higher basal metabolic rate.

Climate

It is known that the BMR is lower in tropics then in temperate zones. Hence, the energy cost of work is slightly higher when the temperature falls below 140°C. However, it is felt that there is no need to make any adjustment for temperature in India.

Secretion of Endocrine Glands

- The thyroid gland in particular exerts a marked influence on the energy requirement.

Table 2.6: Factors affecting basal metabolic rate (BMR).

Increasing age	BMR falls with age
Growth in childhood and pregnancy	Raises BMR
Body muscle: Fat ratio	Muscle has higher BMR than fat tissue
Fever and physical injury	Raises BMR
Extreme heat or cold	Both raise BMR
Reduced food and energy consumption	Body automatically adjusts to lower BMR
Thyroid hormone levels in the body	Thyroid hormones drive BMR up
Nicotine and caffeine	Increase BMR slightly

- If it is overactive (hyperthyroidism), the BMR will increase; if the activity of the gland decreases (hypothyroidism), the BMR will be reduced. Thereby, increasing or decreasing energy requirement accordingly.

Status of Health

- During the periods of fever as well as malnutrition, the BMR of an individual is affected.
- Illness involving an elevation of body temperature markedly increases the basal heat production thus increasing the BMR, hence increased energy requirement.

Altered Physiological States

- During pregnancy and lactation, the energy needs are increased because of an elevated BMR.
- In pregnancy, this additional energy is needed to support the growth of fetus and maternal tissues. During lactation, energy is required for synthesis of milk.

Effect of Food

- A certain amount of work is expended in the digestion of food, its absorption, transfer to the tissues and utilization.
- The increased heat production as a result of the ingestion of food is known as the specific dynamic action of the food.
- Protein, when eaten alone has been shown to increase the metabolic rate by 30%.
- On the basis of the mixed diets, which are usually consumed, the specific dynamic action of food is approximately 10% of the energy requirement.

Extent of Physical Activity

- Any kind of physical activity increases the energy expenditure above the basal energy need.
- Energy for the performance of all types of physical activities ranks next to basal metabolism in amount of energy expended.
- Sleep causes a reduction of about 10% in the BMR depending on the number of hours spent in sleeping and its manner, i.e., restless/peaceful.
- The energy need is determined by the nature and duration of physical activity.
- Sedentary work, which includes office work, book keeping, typing, teaching, etc., calls for lesser energy than moderate work (more active and strenuous occupations) such as nursing, homemaking or gardening.
- A still greater amount of energy is required by those individuals who are involved in heavy work (hard manual laborer), such as ditch digging, shifting freight, etc. Energy needs vary with age, occupation and physiological state.

NURSES ROLE IN CARBOHYDRATE

Carbohydrates not only serve nutritional functions, but are also thought to play important roles in cellular recognition processes. For example, many immunoglobulins (antibodies) and peptide hormones contain glycoprotein sequences. These sequences are composed of amino acids linked to carbohydrates. During the course of many hours or days, the carbohydrate polymer linked to the rest of the protein may be cleared by circulating enzymes or be degraded spontaneously. The liver can recognize differences in length and may internalize the protein in order to begin its own degradation. In this way, carbohydrates may mark the passage of time for proteins. Nurses have an important role to play in improving patients' diets.

CONCLUSION

Carbohydrates are either simple or complex, and are major sources of energy in all human diets. They provide energy of 4 Kcal/g. The simple carbohydrates, glucose and fructose, are found in fruits, vegetables and honey, sucrose in sugar and lactose in milk, while the complex polysaccharides are starches in cereals, millets, pulses and root vegetables and glycogen in animal foods. The other complex carbohydrates which are resistant to digestion in the human digestive tract are cellulose in vegetables and whole grains, and gums and pectins in vegetables, fruits and cereals, which constitute the dietary fibre component.

Energy is the capacity of a physical system to perform work. Energy exists in several forms such as heat, kinetic or mechanical energy, light, potential energy, electrical, or other forms. Energy is the ability to do work. Energy sources could be classified as Renewable and non-renewable.

BIBLIOGRAPHY

1. Garrow JSS, James WPT, Ralph A. Human Nutrition & Dietetics, 10th edition. WB Saunders, Philadelphia, USA, 1999.
2. Henrietta F. Introduction to Nutrition, 4th edition. Macmillan, New York, 1981.
3. Joshi SA. Nutrition and Dietetics, Tata McGraw Hill, New Delhi, India, 1992.
4. Leverton RM. Food Becomes You: Better Health through Better Nutrition, Doubleday Publishing, Boston, USA, 1980.
5. Lutz CA. Karen RP. Nutrition and Diet Therapy, 4th edition. In: Davis FA (Ed). Philadelphia, USA, 1995.
6. Martin EA, Ardath A. Coolidge: Nutrition in Action, 4th edition. Holt Rinehart and Winston, New York, 1978.
7. McDivitt ME, Sumati RM. Human Nutrition—Principles and Applications in India, Revised Edition, Prentice Hall, New Delhi, 1973.
8. Patwardhan VN. Nutrition in India, 2nd edition. Indian Journal of Medical Sciences, New Delhi, 1961.

REVIEW QUESTIONS

Long Essays

1. Define carbohydrate, explain the classifications in detail.
2. Explain the function of carbohydrate in detail.
3. Define basal metabolic rate, describe the factors affecting basal metabolic rate.

Short Essays

1. Health benefits of carbohydrates.
2. Define calorie, explain the calorie requirements of nutrients.
3. Enumerate the sources of carbohydrate.
4. Describe digestion and absorption of carbohydrate.
5. Explain regulation of blood sugar.
6. Discuss glucose tolerance test.
7. Explain deficiencies of carbohydrate.
8. Explain various units of energy.
9. Components of energy requirements.
10. Body mass index and basic metabolism.
11. Nurses role in carbohydrate.

Short Answers

1. Dietary supplements.
2. Dietary fiber.
3. Flavonoids.
4. Antioxidant.
5. Basal metabolic rate.
6. Oligosaccharides.
7. Recommended dietary allowances.
8. Food groups suggested by ICMR.
9. Factors affecting GTT test.
10. MKS system.
11. GCS system.
12. Quetelet's index.

CHAPTER 3

Proteins

CHAPTER OUTLINE

- ❖ Proteins
  - Composition: Eight Essential Amino Acids
  - Functions
- Dietary Sources
- Protein Requirements–RDA

TERMINOLOGY

- **Amino acid:** Any of 20 naturally occurring α-amino acids (having the amino, and carboxylic acid groups on the same carbon atom), and a variety of side chains, that combine, via peptide bonds, to form proteins.
- **Polypeptide:** Any polymer of (same or different) amino acids joined via peptide bonds.
- **Catalyze:** To accelerate a process.
- **Simple proteins:** On hydrolysis they yield only the amino acids and occasional small carbohydrate compounds. Examples are—albumins, globulins, glutelins, albuminoids, histones and protamines.
- **Conjugated proteins:** These are simple proteins combined with some non-protein material in the body. Examples are—nucleoproteins, glycoproteins, phosphoproteins, hemoglobins.
- **Derived proteins:** These are proteins derived from simple or conjugated proteins by physical or chemical means. Examples are: denatured proteins and peptides.

INTRODUCTION

In Greek proteins means the first importance, they are nitrogenous constituents made up of chain of amino acids present in both plant and animal foods. The name protein was suggested by mulder in 1838 to the complex organic nitrogenous substances found in animal and plant tissues. They are essential for life processes; they play an important role in many biochemical, biophysical and physiological processes in the body.

Proteins are important molecules in cells. Proteins are the major component of the dry weight of cells. The name protein is derived from a Greek word Proteios which means pre-eminent or first. This name was fist suggested in 1838 by a Swedish chemist Berzelius. He suggested it to a Dutch chemist Mulder and he referred it to the complex organic substances found in the cells of living beings. Proteins are the most abundant intracellular macromolecules. Proteins are connected intimately with all chemical and physical activity, which constitutes the life of the cell.

DEFINITIONS

- A large molecule composed of one or more chains of amino acids in a specific order, formed according to genetic information. More—each protein has a unique structure and plays a specific role in the function, structure, or regulation of cells, tissues and organs.
- Proteins are an important class of molecules found in all living cells. A protein is composed of one or more long chains of amino acids, the sequence of which corresponds to the DNA sequence of the gene that encodes it. Proteins play a variety of roles in the cell, including structural (cytoskeleton), mechanical (muscle), biochemical (enzymes), and cell signaling (hormones). Proteins are also an essential part of diet.

Figure 3.1 is depicted the levels of protein organization.

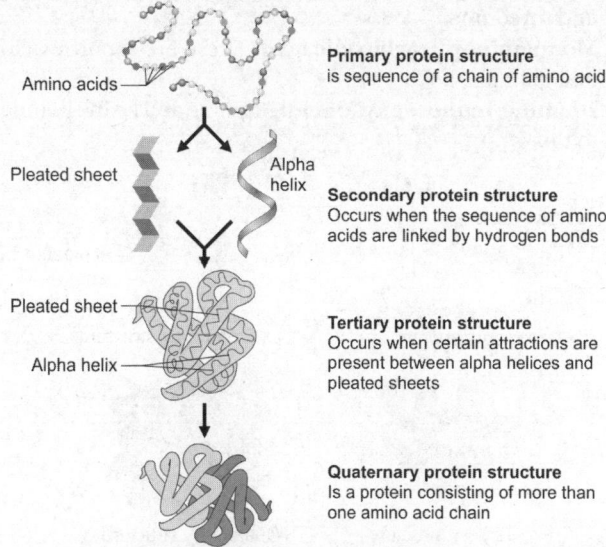

Fig. 3.1: Levels of protein organization.

CHEMICAL COMPOSITION

- Proteins contain carbon, hydrogen, nitrogen and sulphur and some contain also phosphorus.
- Proteins are large molecules formed from the combination of a number of simpler substances known as amino acids.
- Proteins are larger than carbohydrates and fat molecules; its molecular weight is 13,000.
- They are colloids which is large particles and do not pass through semi-permeable membrane.
- The nitrogen content of proteins varies from about 14 to 20% and in most of the proteins; the value is near about 16%.
- This average figure of 16% is used commonly for converting nitrogen content of food stuffs or tissues into proteins by multiplying by the factor 6.25 (100/16).

STRUCTURE OF PROTEIN

Proteins differ from carbohydrates and fats in that they contain nitrogen in addition to carbon, hydrogen and oxygen and with few contain sulphur. Most of the proteins also contain phosphorus, and some specialized proteins contain iron, iodine, copper and other organic elements. Contribution made by proteins to the energy value of most well-balanced diets is usually between 10 and 15% of the total. But they are most important because every cell in the body is composed of proteins which are subjected to continuous wear and replacement.

Figure 3.2 is depicted the types of protein structure.

Proteins are present in and vital to all living cells. They provide structure, protection to the body of multicellular organism in the form of skin, hair, callus, cartilage, ligaments, muscles, tendons. Proteins regulate and catalyze the body chemistry in the form of hormones, enzymes, immunoglobulins, etc. Proteins are large molecules formed by the combination of a number of amino acids. About 23 amino acids have been found to occur in proteins.

- **Monoamine-monocarboxylic acids:** These include glycine, alanine, valine, isoleucine, norleucine, serine, and threonine.
- **Monoamino-dicarboxylic acid:** These are aspartic acid and glutamic acid.
- **Diamino-monocaoxylic acid:** Arginine and lysine belong to this group.
- **Sulfur containing amino acids:** These are cystine, cysteine and methionine.
- **Aromatic and heterocyclic amino acids:** These include phenylalanine, tyrosine, histidine, tryptophan, proline and hydroxyproline.

PROPERTIES OF PROTEIN

The common property of all proteins is that they consist of long chains of α-amino (alpha amino) acids. The general structure of α-amino acids is shown in. The α-amino acids are so called because the α-carbon atom in the molecule carries an amino group ($-NH_2$); the α-carbon atom also carries a carboxyl group (–COOH).

General Characteristics of Proteins

- Proteins are organic substances; they are made up of nitrogen and also, oxygen, carbon and hydrogen.
- Proteins are the most important biomolecules; they are the fundamental constituent of the cytoplasm of the cell.
- Proteins are the structural elements of body tissues.
- Proteins are made up of amino acids.
- Proteins give heat and energy to the body and also aid in building and repair.
- Only small amounts of proteins are stored in the body as they can be used up quickly on demand.
- Proteins are considered as the bricks, they make up bones, muscles, hair and other parts of the body.
- Proteins, such as enzymes are functional elements that take part in metabolic reactions.
- Antibodies, blood hemoglobin are also made of proteins.
- Proteins have a molecular weight of 5 to 300 kilo-daltons.

Physical Properties of Proteins

- Proteins are colorless and tasteless.
- They are homogeneous and crystalline.
- Proteins vary in shape; they may be simple crystalloid structure to long fibrilar structures.
- Protein structures are of two distinct patterns—globular proteins and fibrilar proteins.
- Globular proteins are spherical in shape and occur in plants. Fibrilar proteins are thread-like, they occur generally in animals.
- In general proteins have large molecular weights ranging between 5×10^3 and 1×10^6.
- Due to the huge size, proteins exhibit many colloidal properties.
- The diffusion rates of proteins is extremely slow.
- Proteins exhibit Tyndall effect.
- Proteins tend to change their properties, such as denaturation. Many a times, the process of denaturation is followed by coagulation.
- Denaturation may be a result of either physical or chemical agents. The physical agents include, shaking, freezing, heating, etc. Chemical agents are, such as X-rays, radioactive and ultrasonic radiations.
- Proteins, such as the amino acids exhibit amphoteric property, i.e., they can act as acids and alkalies.

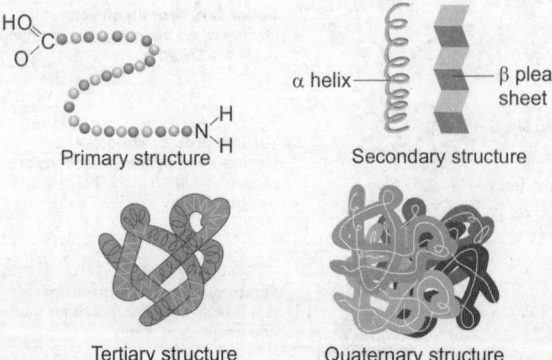

Fig. 3.2: Types of protein structure.

- As the proteins are amphoteric in nature, they can form salts with both cations and anions based on the net charge.
- The solubility of proteins depends upon the pH. Lowest solubility is seen at isoelectric point, the solubility increases with increase in acidity or alkalinity.
- All the proteins show the plane of polarized light to the left, i.e., laevorotatory.

Box 3.1 is depicted the chemical properties of proteins.

Chemical Properties of Proteins

- Proteins when hydrolyzed by acidic agents, such as conc. HCl yield amino acids in the form of their hydrochlorides.
- Proteins when are hydrolyzed with alkaline agents leads to hydrolysis of certain amino acids, such as arginine, cysteine, serine, etc., also the optical activity of the amino acids is lost.
- Proteins with reaction with alcohols give its corresponding esters. This process is known as esterification.
- Amino acids react with amines to form amides.
- When free amino acids or proteins are said to react with mineral acids, such as HCl, the acid salts are formed.
- When amino acids in alkaline medium react with many acid chlorides, acylation reaction takes place.
- **Sanger's reaction:** Proteins react with FDNB reagent to produce yellow colored derivative, DNB amino acid.

> **Box 3.1:** Chemical properties of proteins
> - **Heat:** The weak side-chain attractions in globular proteins are easily disrupted by heating
> - **Mechanical agitation:** The most familiar example of denaturation by agitation is the foam produced by beating egg whites. Denaturation of proteins at the surface of the air bubbles stiffens the protein and causes the bubbles to be held in place
> - **Detergents:** Even very low concentrations of detergents can disrupt the association of hydrophobic side chains
> - **Organic compounds:** Polar solvents interfere with hydrogen bonding by competing for bonding sites
> - **pH change:** Excess H^+ or OH^- ions react with basic or acidic side chains in amino acid residues and disrupt salt bridges
> - **Inorganic salts:** High concentrations of ions can disturb salt bridges

- **Xanthoproteic test:** On boiling proteins with conc. HNO_3, yellow color develops due to presence of benzene ring.
- **Folin's test:** This is a specific test for tyrosine amino acid, where blue color develops with phosphomolybdotungstic acid in alkaline solution due to presence of phenol group.

CLASSIFICATIONS OF PROTEIN

1. **Simple proteins:** These include albumins, globulins, glutelins, prolamines, fibrous proteins, histones and protamins.
2. **Conjugated proteins:** These include neucleoproteins, glycoproteins, phosphoproteins, hemoglobins and lecithoproteins.
3. **Derived proteins:** Include proteans, metaproteins, coagulated proteins, peptones and peptides.

Figure 3.3 is depicted the classification of proteins and Figure 3.4 is depicted the classification of proteins based on structure.

Classification of proteins based on content of amino acids:
1. **Complete proteins:** It contains enough essential amino acids to maintain the growth and the development of cells and it has high biological valve. For example, milk and meat. These foods are referred to be having a high biological valve.
2. **Partially complete proteins:** It will maintain life, but they lack some of the amino acids which are necessary for growth and development. For example, Gliadin of wheat.
3. **Incomplete proteins:** They are incapable of replacing or building new tissues and hence cannot support life. For example, Zein in corn.

Classification of Proteins Based on Composition and Solubility

These proteins are made of only one type of amino acid, as structural component, on decomposition with acids, they liberate constituent amino acids. They are mostly globular type of proteins except for scleroproteins, which are fibrous in nature.

Simple proteins are further classified based on their solubility.
1. **Protamines and histones:** These proteins occur only in animals and are basic proteins. The possess simple

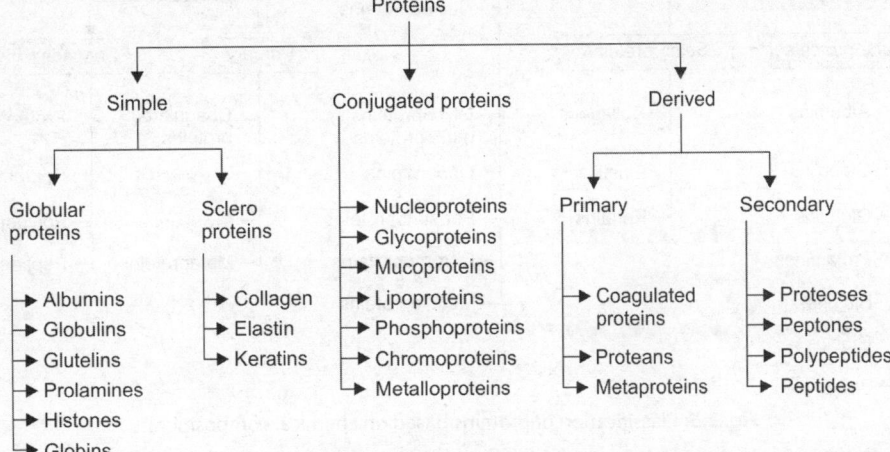

Fig. 3.3: Classifications of protein.

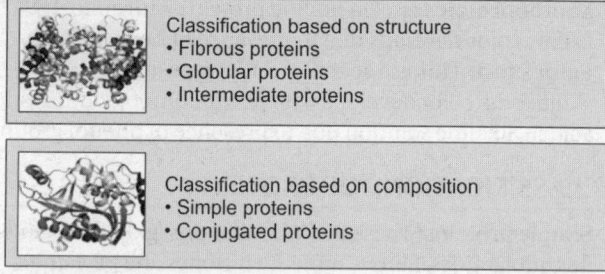

Fig. 3.4: Classification of proteins based on structure.

structure and low molecular, are water soluble and are not coagulated by heat. They are strongly basic in character due to the high content of lysine, arginine. For example, protamines—salmine, clupine, cyprinine; Histones—nucleoshistones, globin.

2. **Albumins:** Albumin is the most abundant plasma protein. It is essential role is to regulate passage of water and solutes through the capillaries by maintaining colloidal oncotic pressure within the vasculature. Plasma proteins have long been considered integral to assessment of nutritional status.
3. **Globulins:** They are of two types, pseudoglobulins which are soluble in water; other is euglobulins which are insoluble in water. They are coagulated by heat. For example, pseudo-globulin, serum globulin, glycinine, etc.
4. **Scleroproteins or albuminoids:** These occur mostly in animals and are commonly known as animal skeleton proteins, they are insoluble in water, and in dilute solution of acids, based and salts.

Complex proteins are further classified based on the type of prosthetic group present:
1. **Metalloproteins:** These are proteins linked with various metals. For example, casein, collagen, ceruloplasmin, etc.
2. **Chromoproteins:** These are proteins that are coupled with a colored pigment. For example, myoglubin, hemocyanin, cytochromes, flavoproteins, etc.
3. **Glycoproteins and mucoproteins:** These proteins contain carbohydrates as the prosthetic group. For example, glycoproteins—egg albumin, serum globulins, serum albumins; mucoproteins—ovomucoid, mucin, etc.
4. **Phosphoproteins:** These proteins are linked with phosphoric acid. For example, casein.
5. **Lipoproteins:** Proteins forming complexes with lipids are lipoproteins. For example, lipovitellin, lipoproteins of blood.
6. **Nucleoproteins:** These are compounds containing nucleic acids and proteins. For example, nucleoproteins, nucleohistones, nuclein.
7. **Derived proteins:** These are proteins that are derived from the action of heat, enzyme or chemical reagents. Derived proteins are of two types, primarily derived proteins and secondary derived proteins. Primary derived proteins are derivatives of proteins, in which the size of the protein molecule is not altered materially, while in secondary derived proteins, hydrolysis occurs, as a result the molecules are smaller than the original proteins.
    a. Primary derived proteins are classified into three types—proteans, infraproteins and coagulated proteins. For example, edestan, coagulated egg white.
    b. Secondary derived proteins are further classified into three types—proteoses, peptones and polypeptides.

Figure 3.5 is depicted the classification of proteins based on chemical composition.

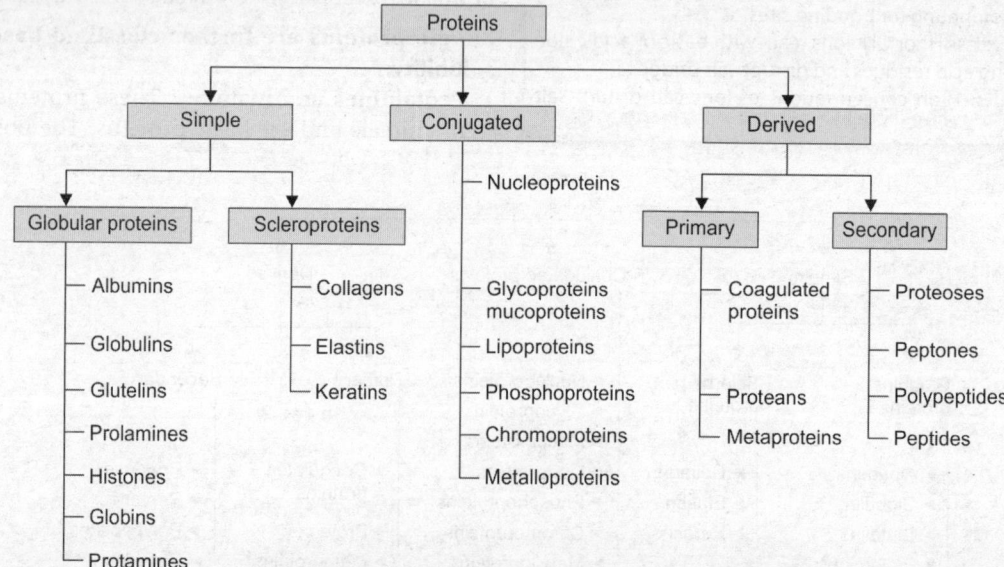

Fig. 3.5: Classification of proteins based on chemical composition.

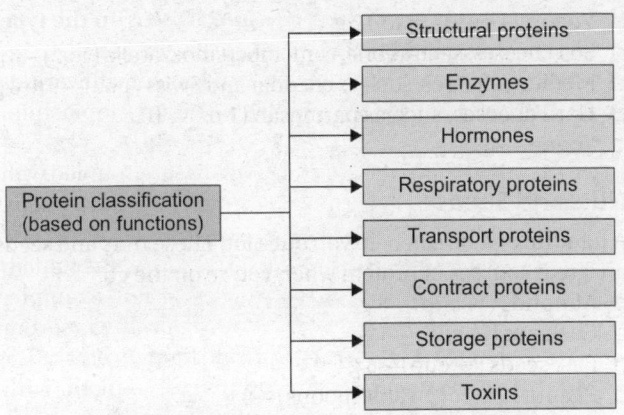

Fig. 3.6: Protein classification based on functions.

Classification of Proteins on Biological Function

Proteins depending upon their physical and chemical structure and location inside the cell, they perform various functions. Proteins are grouped as follows, based on their metabolic function they perform.

- **Enzymic proteins:** They are the most varied and highly specialized proteins with catalytic activity. Enzymes catalyze a variety of reactions. For example, urease, catalase, cytochrome C, etc.
- **Structural proteins:** These proteins aid in strengthening or protecting biological structures. For example, collagen, elastin, keratin, etc.
- **Transport or carrier proteins:** These proteins help in transport of ions or molecules in the body. For example, myoglobin, hemoglobin, etc.
- **Nutrient and storage proteins:** These proteins provide nutrition to growing embryos and store ions.
- **Contractile or motile proteins:** These proteins function in the contractile system. For example, actin, myosin, tubulin, etc.
- **Defense proteins:** These proteins defend against other organisms. For example, antibodies, fibrinogen, thrombin.
- **Regulatory proteins:** They regulate cellular or metabolic activities. For example, insulin, G proteins, etc.
- **Toxic proteins:** These proteins hydrolyze or degrade enzymes. For example, snake venom, ricin.

Figure 3.6 is depicted the protein classification based on functions.

SOURCES OF PROTEIN

Excellent sources of protein include turkey, tuna, shrimp and cod.

Very good sources of protein include halibut, salmon, scallops, sardines, pasture-raised chicken, lamb, grass-fed beef, calf's liver, spinach, tofu, mustard greens, asparagus, soybeans, salmon, and cheese.

Good Sources of Protein

- Good sources of protein include crimini mushrooms, eggs, summer squash, collard greens, cauliflower and many legumes including lentils, split peas, kidney beans, black beans, pinto beans and garbanzo beans.

- When discussing food sources of protein, nutritionists often speak in terms of "complete" and "incomplete" proteins.
- Foods that provide complete protein are those that include all of the essential amino acid, while foods that provide some or none of the essential amino acids are said to be incomplete.
- Eggs, dairy foods, meat, fish and poultry are typically considered to be complete proteins.
- Vegetarians, and especially vegans, often do not have a source of complete protein in their diets, but can easily obtain all of the essential amino acids by eating a variety of beans, grains, nuts, seeds, and vegetables.

	Source	*Percentage*
Plant sources	Soybean	43%
	Roseted groundnut	26%
	Skimmed milk	38%
	Field bean	25%
	Black gram dal	24%
	Green gram dal	24%
	Peas (dried)	24%
	Cow pea	24%
	Moth beans	23%
	Almond	20%
	Bengal gram	20%
	Wheat	12%
	Agathi greens	8%
	Sundakkai (dried)	8%
	Wood apple	7%
Animal source	Chicken	25%
	Cheese	24%
	Fish (seer-vanjaram)	22%
	Prawn	19%
	Mutton	18%
	Pork	18%
	Egg	13%
	Cow milk	3.2%

High-Protein Foods

Here are examples of proteins in food with the number of grams of protein per 100 grams:
- Soybeans—35.9 g
- Cheese—30.9 g
- Venison—30.21
- Pumpkin seeds—28.8 g
- Lobster—26.41
- Canned tuna fish—26.3 g
- Tuna fish—25.6 g
- Monkfish—24 g
- Crunchy peanut butter—24.9 g
- Tilapia—24 g
- Skinless chicken breast—23.5 g
- Sunflower seeds—23.4 g
- Orange roughy—22.64 g
- Skinless turkey breast—22.3 g

- Boneless salmon fillets—21.6 g
- Sardines—21.5 g
- Almonds—21.1 g
- Beef fillet—20.9
- Lamb steak—19.9 g
- Pork chops—19.3 g
- Crab meat—18.1 g
- Cod—17.9 g
- Shrimp—17.0 g
- Haddock—16.4 g
- Bacon—15.9 g
- Couscous—15.1 g
- Anchovies—14.5 g
- Pork sausages—13.9 g
- Eggs—12.5 g
- Pasta—12.5 g
- Goji berries—12.3 g
- Cottage cheese—12.2 g
- Tofu—12.1 g
- Pepperoni pizza—11.4 g
- Whole grain bread—11.0 g
- Porridge oats—11.0 g
- Baked beans—9.5 g
- Hummus—7.4 g
- Brown rice—6.9 g
- Peas—5.9 g
- Spaghetti—5.1 g
- Yogurt—4.5 g
- Broccoli—4.2 g
- Coconut—3.33 g
- Whole milk—3.3 g
- Asparagus—2.9 g
- Spinach—2.8 g
- Potatoes—2.1 g
- Avocado—1.9 g
- Bananas—1.2 g
- Orange—1.1 g

Beans and Legumes

Whether you eat meat or you are a strict vegan, beans and legumes are an excellent place to find protein. Check out these simple ways to add protein to your diet.

- Tofu (½ cup)—20 g
- Soy milk (1 cup)—6 to 10 g
- Soybeans (½ cup cooked)—14 g
- Split peas (½ cup cooked)—8 g
- Other beans, such as black, pinto, lentils (1/2 cup)—7 to 10 g

Eggs and Dairy

You may know that dairy products are good sources of calcium, but protein too? Both eggs and dairy are helpful ways to boost your protein intake.

- Egg (1 large)—6 g
- Cottage cheese (½ cup)—15 g
- Milk (1 cup)—8 g
- Yogurt (1 cup)—8 to 12 g
- Soft cheeses, such as brie, camembert mozzarella (1 oz)—6 g
- Medium cheeses, such as cheddar and Swiss (1 oz)—7 to 8 g
- Hard cheeses, such as parmesan (1 oz)—10 g
- Yogurt—4.5 g

Nuts and Seeds

A handful of nuts can help you out a lot! These nuts and seeds are great sources of protein when you're on the go.

- Almonds (¼ cup)—8 g
- Cashews (¼ cup)—5 g
- Flax seeds (¼ cup)—8 g
- Peanut butter (2 Tablespoons)—8 g
- Peanuts (¼ cup)—9 g
- Pecans (¼ cup)—2.5 g
- Pumpkin seeds (¼ cup)—8 g
- Sunflower seeds (¼ cup)—6 g

Meat and Poultry

Every grill master can tell you that meat is an important source of protein in your diet. If you are forming a diet without meat, you will need to replace the large amount of protein found in a small serving of meat and poultry.

- Hamburger patty (4 oz)—28 g
- Steak (6 oz)—42 g
- Venison (6 oz)—30.21 g
- Chicken breast (3.5 oz)—30 g
- Chicken thigh—10 g
- Drumstick—11 g
- Wing—6 g
- Chicken meat (4 oz cooked)—35 g
- Pork chop (average size)—22 g
- Pork loin or tenderloin (4 oz)—9 g
- Ham (3 oz)—19 g
- Ground pork (3 oz cooked)—22 g
- Bacon, 1 slice—3 g
- Canadian-style bacon (slice)—5 to 6 g

Fish and Seafood

Seafood is an excellent source of lean fats and protein. Most cuts of fish have over 20 g of protein in just a few ounces.

- Most cuts of fish (3.5 oz) - around 22 g
- Tuna (6 oz)—48 g
- Canned tuna fish—26.3 g
- Cod (6 oz)—30 g
- Salmon (6 oz)—34 g
- Shrimp (6 oz)—41 g
- Lobster (6 oz)—28 g

Recommended Dietary Allowances

Proteins are needed for building and repairing of body tissues, muscles and vital fluids, such as blood to help enzymes and antibodies to fight infections. Protein requirements are based upon actual estimation of the lowest amount of nitrogen intake necessary to maintain nitrogen equilibrium and have been evolved by N balance studies.

Sl. No.	Age group	Requirements
1.	0–3 months	2.3 g/kg
2.	3–9 months	1.8 g/kg
3.	9–12 months	1.5 g/kg
4.	1–3 years	22 g/day
5.	4–6 years	29 g/kg
6.	7–9 years	36 g/day
7.	10–12 years	43 g/day
8.	13–15 years	47.5 g/day
9.	16–18 years	48.5 g/day
10.	Adult	One gram/kg body weight
11.	Pregnancy	+ 14 g/day
12.	Lactation	+ 25 g/day

Protein requirements are expressed in terms of body weight. In a diet with energy deficiency, some of the protein would be burnt or wasted in providing energy and will not be available for the synthesis of body protein. The efficiency with which protein is utilized, also decreases.

Energy allowance for infants:

Age	Protein allowance per day g/kg
0–3 months	1.3
3–6 months	1.8
6–9 months	1.8
9–12 months	1.5

Allowances for infants should be made for the rapid growth. The allowances for the first 6 months are met by milk proteins. Later the child has to be supplemented with other sources of protein.

Age group	Body weight	Protein allowances g/kg/day	g/day
1–3 years	12	1.8	22
4–6 years	19	1.6	29

Protein allowances during pregnancy and lactation: Allowance for pregnant women must cover the additional needs for the development of the fetus, placenta and material tissues, while those of lactating women must cover what is secreted in milk. During the 2nd and 3rd trimester, an extra allowance of 14 g/day have been made. During the first 6 months of lactation, an extra allowance of 25 g/day have been made. This is over and above the normal protein requirement of 45 g/day.

EXAMPLES OF PROTEIN IN BIOLOGY AND DIET

Proteins are the basic component of living cells. They are made of carbon, hydrogen, oxygen, nitrogen, and one or more chains of amino acids. The three structures of proteins are **fibrous, globular** and **membrane**, which can also be broken down by each protein's function. Keep reading for examples of proteins in each category and in which foods you can find them.

Fibrous Proteins

Also called scleroproteins, fibrous proteins form muscle fiber, tendons, connective tissue and bone. They have an elongated shape and play many structural roles in the body. The main types of fibrous proteins include structural proteins and storage proteins.

Structural Proteins

These can be found in the fibers of both smooth muscles and skeletal muscles, as well as in cardiac muscle around the heart. Collagen, for example, is the most abundant protein in human and animal bodies. Some structural proteins also have contractile functions, which aid in the movement of muscles.

Examples of the proteins in this category include:
- Actin—found in muscle cells and used during cellular processes
- Collagen—found in connective tissue and cartilage throughout the body
- Dystrophin—links actin to other proteins in muscle fibers
- Elastin—makes tissues and organs elastic
- Fibrin—works with platelets to clot blood
- Keratin—protein found in human hair, skin and nails, as well as animal hooves, wool, horns, claws, and feathers
- Myosin—found in muscle cells; involved with contracting movements
- Nebulin—large protein found in muscle filament
- Pikachurin—binds different proteins in the retina of the eye
- Titin—large protein that aids in contractions
- Tropomyosin—found throughout the body and used for movement
- Tubulin—present in the cytoskeletal structure of a cell

Storage Proteins

Some fibrous proteins store amino acids and metal ions for later use. Both plants and animals alike have storage proteins in their cells, though many are distinctive to various organisms.

Examples of storage proteins are:
- Casein—stores amino acids in animal and human milk
- Ferritin—stores iron in plants and animals
- Gliadin—storage protein in wheat; component of gluten
- Kafirin—found in sorghum and millet
- Oryzin—found in rice
- Ovalbumin—stores amino acids in egg whites
- Zein—found in corn

Globular Proteins

The other main protein structure is globular. Globular proteins are spherical and more water soluble than the other classes of proteins. They have several functions including transporting, catalyzing and regulating within the body. Antibodies, enzymes, transport proteins, and many kinds of hormones are examples of globular proteins.

Antibody Proteins

Antibodies, which are called immunoglobulins, are proteins created by your immune system to fight off harmful invaders. There are five main types of antibodies; however, their binding site is made to fight a specific pathogen, including viruses and bacteria.

Examples of antibody proteins include:
1. Immunoglobulin A (IgA)—found in saliva and tears from mucosal tissues
2. Immunoglobulin D (IgD)—low-quantity protein that signals the immune system to work
3. Immunoglobulin E (IgE)—begins an allergic reaction when exposed to an allergen
4. Immunoglobulin G (IgG)—high-quantity protein that tags pathogens and releases toxins to destroy them
5. Immunoglobulin M (IgM)—triggers the pathogen "memory" in your immune system

Enzyme Proteins

Proteins that carry out biochemical reactions are called enzymes. They are a type of biological catalyst that keeps the body going. Other enzymes, called inhibitors, slow down reactions.

Some protein examples that carry out enzymatic functions include:
- C1-inhibitor—anti-inflammatory protein
- Carboxypeptidase—created in the pancreas for digestive aid
- Hydrolase enzymes—catalyze hydrolysis in chemical bonds
- Helicase—unzips DNA for decoding
- Lactase—breaks down lactose from dairy products
- Lipase—breaks down fats in the pancreas
- Maltase—found in the saliva; breaks down sugars into glucose
- Oxidoreductases—catalyze the transfer of electrons between molecules
- Thrombin—converts proteins in the blood to clot blood
- Trypsin—breaks down proteins during digestion

Messenger Proteins

Proteins that send messages throughout the body are known as messenger proteins. These proteins include different types of hormones, which can transmit signals to coordinate processes between parts of the body. They are different from steroid hormones, which come from lipids, not proteins.

Some examples of messenger proteins include:
- Angiotensin—maintains blood pressure
- Antidiuretic hormone (ADH)—carries messages to the kidneys to balance water levels in the blood
- Epinephrine—controls respiration and other involuntary functions
- Follicle-stimulating hormone (FSH)—controls the stimulation of eggs and sperm in female and male reproductive system
- Insulin—regulates glucose levels in the blood
- Norepinephrine—controls the body's response to stress
- Oxytocin—regulates emotions related to the reproductive system
- Somatotropin—hormone that controls growth rates in the body
- Tryptophan—regulates the sleep-wake cycle in the body

Transport Proteins

When atoms need to be taken across a cell membrane, a transport membrane can do it. These types of proteins, also known as escort proteins, aid in cellular transport. They include:
- Albumin—transports hormones and vitamins in the bloodstream
- Alpha globulin—found in blood plasma
- Beta globulin—functions as a transport and an enzyme
- Hemoglobin—carries oxygen from the lungs to body tissue
- Hemopexin—transports heme in blood plasma
- Myoglobin—transports and stores oxygen from hemoglobin
- Transferring—delivers iron to different organs in the body

Membrane Proteins

Membrane proteins are found within the membranes of cells. They aid with many cellular functions, including transporting substances across the membrane and adhering cells to other structures.

Membrane protein examples include:
- Cystic fibrosis transmembrane conductance regulator (CFTR)—regulates sodium levels in the lungs
- Estrogen receptor—activated by the hormone estrogen
- Forkhead box P2 (FOXP2)—found in the major organs, including brain and heart
- Forkhead box P3 (FOXP3)—regulates T cell activation
- Glucose transporter—carries glucose across the membrane
- Histones—pack DNA into cells and chromosomes
- Integrin—adheres cells to other cells
- Selectin—adheres white blood cells to other cells in the bloodstream

AMINO ACIDS

Amino acids are simplest molecule derived from large molecule of protein. Animal foods have good quality amino acids compare to plant containing amino acid. There are 23 amino acids.

1. **Essential amino acids (EAA):** 8, it can be defined as, body cannot synthesis certain amino acids which must be supplied by the diet. For example, methionine, tryptophan, valine, isoleucine, lysine and phenylalanine.
2. **Semi-essential amino acids (SEAA):** 2, Methionine essential amino acids can be converted to cystine, but cystine cannot be converted to methionine. Likewise phenylalanine is converted to tyrosine, but tyrosine cannot

be converted to phenylalanine. When cystine and tyrosine are present in the diet the requirement for methionine and phenylalanine.
3. **Non-essential amino acids (NEAA):** 13, they are synthesized in the body, i.e., they are derived from other amino acids, e.g., alanine, aspartic acid, cystine, glutamine, glutamic acid, glycine, hydroxylysine, praline, serine, tyrosine and cysteine

Types	Amino acids
Essential amino acids	
1.	Leucine
2.	Isoleucine
3.	Lysine
4.	Methionine
5.	Phenylalanine
6.	Threonine
7.	Valine
8.	Tryptophan and histidine
Non-essential amino acids	
1.	Arginine
2.	Aspartic acid
3.	Serine
4.	Glutamic acid
5.	Praline
6.	Glycine

Sources of Amino Acid

Amino acid	Source
Valine	Rice, jackfruit, agathi, cheese, brewer's yeast, egg, apple, sweet potato, cauliflower, pumpkin, radish, horsegram, potato, bitter gourd.
Leucine	Thinai (millet), cholam (jower), kambu (bajra), rice, Bengal gram, dal, black gram dhal, whole green gram, agathi, potato, yam, brinjal, cashew net, apple, beef, pork, curd, buffalo milk, wheat, egg.
Isoleucine	Ragi, rice, kesari dal, black gram dhal, agathi, radish, potato, tomato, pork, cheese, banana, egg.
Methionine	Ragi, celery, leaves, yam, ladies finger, dried, coconut, grapes, egg.
Phenylalanine	Dairy products, egg, pork, banana, almond, groundnut, yam, colocasia, spinach, agathi, rice, barley, red gram dal, horse gram, Bengal gram dal
Tryptophan	Kambu (bajra), rice, potato, cauliflower, egg, papaya, mango, milk, radish, carrot, beetroot.

■ BIOLOGICAL VALUE OF PROTEIN

Biological value of protein is the percentage of protein nitrogen that is absorbed and available for use by the body for growth and maintenance.
- **Proteins are functionally divided into:** Complete, partially complete and incomplete proteins.
- **A complete protein:** Contains all essential amino acids in relatively the same amounts as human beings require promoting and maintaining normal growth, e.g., protein derived from animal foods.
- **A partially complete protein:** Contains sufficient amounts of amino acids to maintain life, but fail to promote growth, e.g., gliadin in wheat.
- **Incomplete proteins:** Are incapable of replacing or building new tissue and cannot support life or growth, e.g., protein in wheat germ.
- **The quality of a protein is determined** by the kind and proportion of amino acid it contains. Proteins that contain all essential amino acids in proportions capable of promoting growth are described as complete protein, good quality protein or proteins of high biological value.
- **A good quality protein is digested and utilized well:** Egg protein is a complete protein and is considered as a reference protein with the highest biological value. The quality of other proteins is determined based on their comparison with egg protein.
- **The protein of animal foods like milk, meat and fish** generally compare well with egg in the essential amino acid composition and are categorized as good quality proteins. Plant proteins are of poor quality, since the essential amino acid composition is not well balanced. The amino acid, which is not present in sufficient amount in food protein, is called the limiting amino acid of that food. For, e.g., lysine in cereal protein, tryptophan in wheat germ.

■ FUNCTIONS OF PROTEIN (FIG. 3.7)

Protein, providing 4 calories per gram, is an important source of energy for the body, when carbohydrates and fats are not available. In addition to using protein to generate energy for cellular function whenever necessary, the body uses the amino acids contained in the protein we eat to manufacture its own proteins. The proteins synthesized by the body perform a variety of important physiological functions:
- **Growth and maintenance:** Each body cell contains proteins. All growth depends on a sufficient supply of amino acids. The amino acids are needed to make the proteins required to support muscle, tissue, bone formation, and the cells themselves.

Maintaining our bodies also requires a constant supply of amino acids. There is a continual turnover of body cells, which are composed of protein. The cells break down and must immediately be replaced. Each replacement cell requires the formation of additional protein.

Also needed for growth and maintenance is the protein collagen, found throughout the body. Collagen forms connective tissues such as ligaments and tendons and acts as a glue to keep the walls of the arteries intact. In addition, collagen has a role in bone and tooth formation by forming the framework structure that is then filled with minerals, such as calcium and phosphorus. Synthesis of scar tissue also depends on collagen. Other structures, such as hair, nails, and skin are composed of similar protein substances.

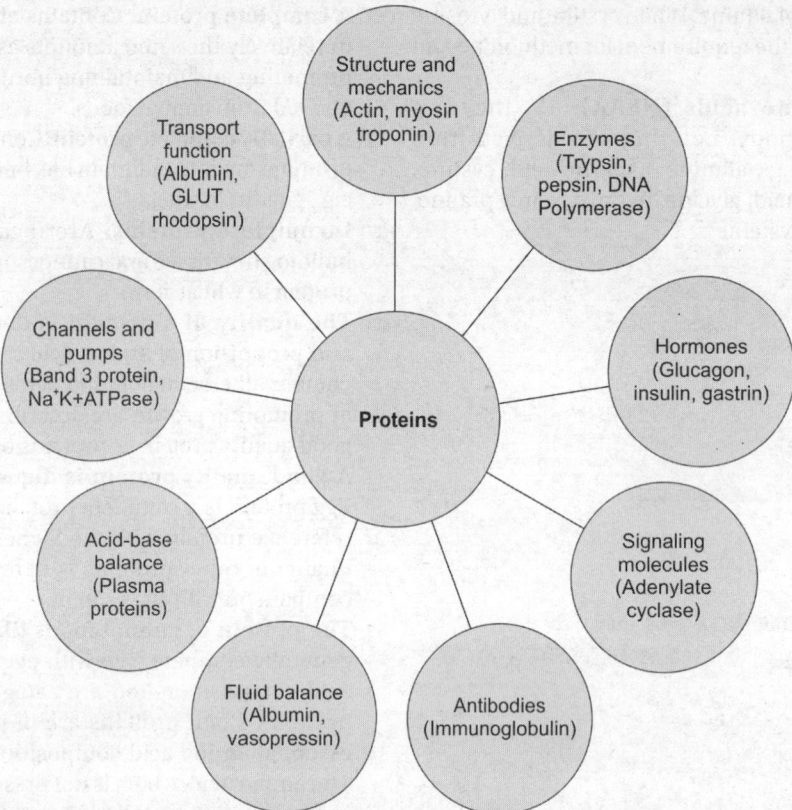

Fig. 3.7: Functions of protein.

- **Production and maintenance of structural proteins:** The body manufactures several structural proteins, such as myosin, actin, collagen, elastin, and keratin that maintain the strength and integrity of muscles, connective tissues (ligaments and tendons), hair, skin, and nails.
- **Production of enzymes and hormones:** All of the enzymes, which are compounds that catalyze chemical reactions in the body, are made from protein. In addition, the hormones involved in blood sugar regulation (insulin and glucagon) as well as the thyroid hormones are synthesized from proteins.
- **Production of transport proteins and lipoproteins:** Certain proteins are used by the body to carry various substances to body tissues. These transport proteins include hemoglobin (carries oxygen), transferrin (carries iron), ceruloplasmin (carries copper), retinol-binding protein (carries vitamin A), albumin and transthyretin (both carry other proteins). Lipoproteins participate in the transportation of fat and cholesterol.
- **Production of antibodies:** Antibodies, which are proteins, play an important role in the immune system by attaching to antigens (viruses, bacteria, or other foreign invaders), thereby inactivating the antigens and making them more visible to the immune cells (called macrophages) that destroy antigens.
- **Maintenance of proper fluid balance:** Proteins participate in the maintenance of osmotic pressure, which controls the amount of water that is found inside of cells. Water is balanced among three compartments in the body: intravascular (within veins and arteries), intracellular (inside cells), and interstitial (between cells). Proteins and minerals attract water, creating osmotic pressure. As proteins circulate through our bodies, they maintain body fluid and electrolyte balance by keeping water appropriately divided among the three compartments.
- **Maintenance of proper acid-base balance:** Due to their ability to combine with both acidic and basic substances, proteins help to maintain the normal acid-base balance in the body. Some reactions occurring within the body lead to the release of acidic substances; others cause basic matter to enter the fluids of the body. Blood proteins can buffer the effects of fluids to maintain a safe acidic level in body fluids. The ability of protein to regulate the balance between the acidic and base characteristics of fluids is called the buffering effect of protein. Because the chemical structure of amino acids combines an acid [the carboxyl group (COOH)] and base (amine), an amino acid can function either as an acid or a base depending on the pH of its medium. This is why the buffering effect of blood proteins is possible. This function is crucial to protect all proteins in the body. If fluids become either too acidic or too basic, the shape of proteins is altered or denatured. Denatured proteins are not able to perform their usual functions.
- **Creation of communicators and catalysts:** Many vital substances produced by our bodies are formed of protein. Some hormones are proteins. Hormones act as communicators to alert different parts of the body

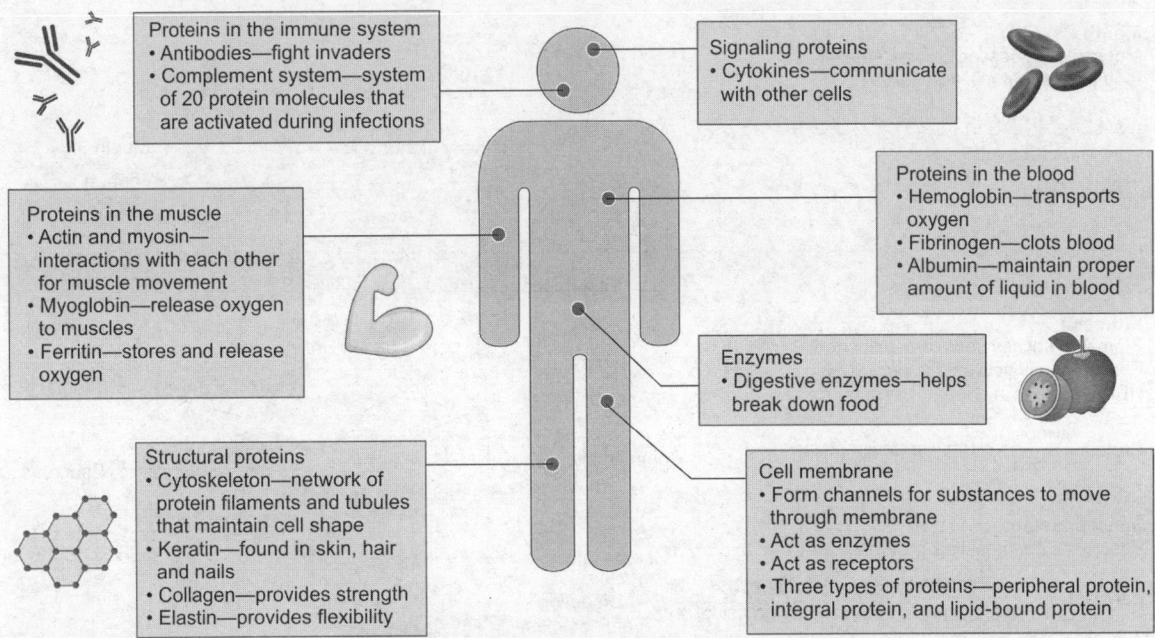

Fig. 3.8: Proteins in the human body.

to changes or to regulate functions of organs. Insulin, a hormone that directs cells to take in glucose, is a protein. Enzymes are also proteins. Enzymes are catalysts that enable chemical reactions or biologic changes to occur within the body. Each enzyme has a specific target; consequently, numerous enzymes are continually formed.

Blood clotting depends on protein substances as well. Twelve blood clotting factors must be in place for blood to clot when injury has occurred; several of the factors, such as fibrogen, are composed of protein.

- **Immune system response:** The defense system of our bodies depends on proteins produced in response to foreign viruses and bacteria that invade our bodies. The proteins, or antibodies, are specific to each intruder. If sufficient levels of amino acids are not available to form these antibodies, we may have difficulties maintaining our health. Our overall immunologic response—our resistance to disease—depends on proteins formed within our bodies.

Figure 3.8 is depicted the proteins in the human body.

DIGESTION OF PROTEIN

Because of the complex structure of proteins, a number of protein enzymes, or proteases, produced by the stomach and pancreas are required to hydrolyze proteins into smaller and smaller peptides until individual amino acids are ready for absorption.

Mouth: Only mechanical digestion of protein occurs in the mouth. Mastication breaks protein-containing food into smaller pieces that mix with saliva passing through to the stomach.

Stomach: Pepsinogen, an inactive form of the gastric protease pepsin, is secreted by the stomach mucosa. Pepsin becomes activated when it mixes with hydrochloric acid (HCl), also produced by stomach secretions. Pepsin then begins the process of protein hydrolysis, breaking the bonds linking the amino acids of the protein peptide bonds. The result is smaller-sized polypeptides rather than single amino acids or dipeptides. The polypeptides pass through to the small intestine for further hydrolysis.

Figure 3.9 is depicted the digestion and absorption of protein.

Small intestine
- In the small intestine, pancreatic and intestinal proteases continue the hydrolysis of polypeptides. As these smaller peptides touch the intestinal walls, peptidases are released that complete the hydrolysis of protein into absorbable units of individual amino acids and dipeptides.
- The primary pancreatic enzyme is trypsin. It is first secreted as trypsinogen, an inactive form. The intestinal hormone enteropeptidase activates trypsinogen into trypsin, which continues the hydrolysis of polypeptides.
- Two other pancreatic enzymes assist in the hydrolysis process: chymotrypsin hydrolyzes polypeptides into dipeptides, and carboxypeptidase breaks polypeptides and dipeptides into amino acids.
- Two intestinal peptidases are aminopeptidase, which releases free amino acids from the amino end of short-chain peptides, and dipeptidase, which completes the hydrolysis of proteins to amino acids.
- Absorption of amino acids occurs through the intestinal walls by means of competitive active transport that requires vitamin B_6 (pyridoxine) as a carrier. Because amino acids are water soluble, they easily pass into the bloodstream.

Intestinal digestion: The digestion of proteins is further carried on in the intestines by the action of proteolytic enzymes (trypsin, chymotrypsin, and peptidases) present in the pancreatic and intestinal juices. The polypeptides

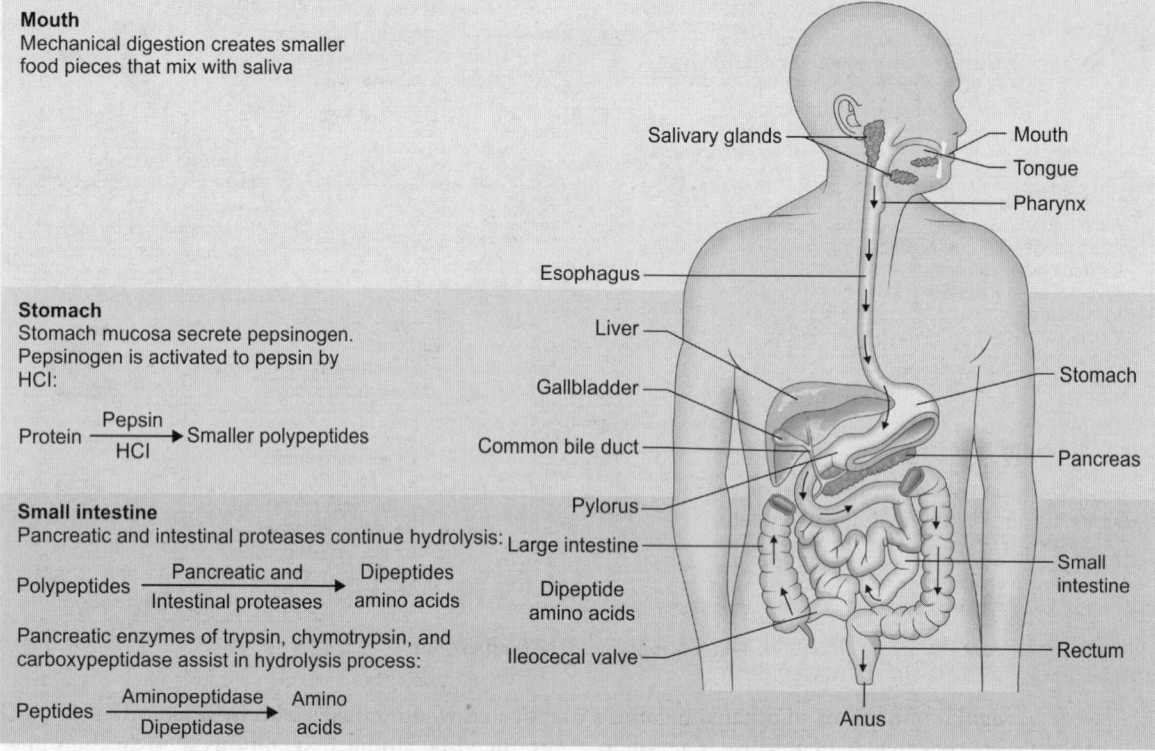

Fig. 3.9: Digestion and absorption of protein.

produced by gastric digestion are hydrolyzed to free amino acids by the above enzymes. The amioacids are absorbed in the small intestines and enter the blood circulation through the portal vein.

- There are no proteins-splitting enzymes in saliva and so in salivary digestion protein is not affected.
- Hydrolysis of protein begins in the stomach, protein, the enzymes secreted by gastric glands in the stomach, breaks down proteins into proteoses and peptones.
- Milk proteins are first converted to casein by a special enzyme called rennin. Casein combines with calcium to form calcium caseinate, pepsin converts this into peptones. All the peptide linkages are not broken by gastric digestion.
- A stronger enzyme of pancreatic and intestinal juice contains trypsin and chymotrypsins. They hydrolyses peptones and proteoses into polypeptides.
- The final breakdown of all protein fractions to amino acids is brought about by erepsin secreted by intestinal mucosa.
- Amino acids are absorbed by the small intestine and they are carried to the tissues or to the liver.

Figure 3.10 is depicted the protein digestion in small intestine.

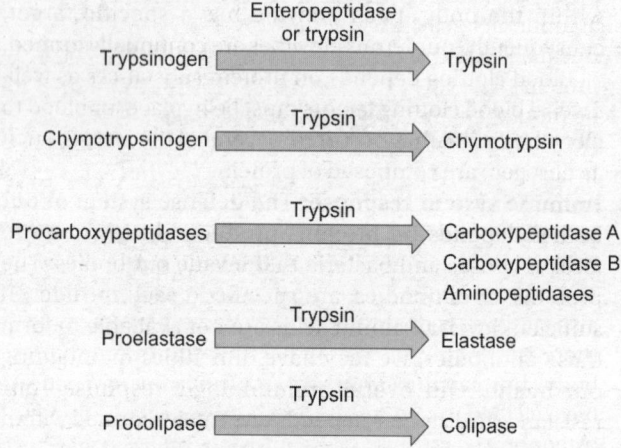

Fig. 3.10: Protein digestion in small intestine.

growth hormone (from the pituitary gland) and the male hormone testosterone.
- Hormones affecting the catabolism (break down) of proteins are the glucocorticoids that are enhanced by adrenocorticotropic hormone (ACTH); these hormones are secreted from the adrenal cortex.
- This process releases proteins in the cells to break down to amino acids, and then the amino acids travel in the bloodstream, contributing to an available pool of amino acids.
- The liver cells begin the process of catabolism through deamination. Deamination results in an amino acid (NH_2) group breaking off from an amino acid molecule, resulting in one molecule each of ammonia (NH_3) and a keto acid.

Metabolism

- To understand the importance of protein metabolism in the growth and maintenance of the body, consider that most protein functions are a result of protein anabolism (synthesis) in cells.
- Hormones have a major role in the regulation of protein metabolism. Anabolism is enhanced by the effect of

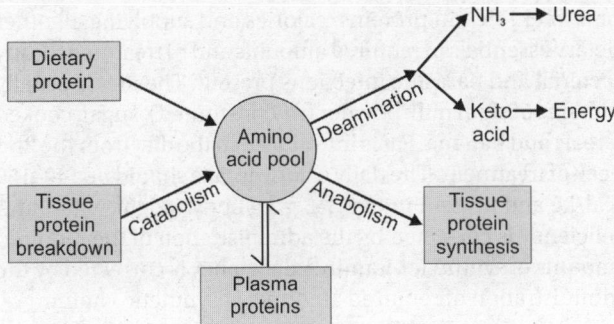

Fig. 3.11: Protein metabolism.

- Liver cells convert most of the ammonia to urea, which is later excreted in urine.
- The keto acid may enter the tricarboxylic acid (TCA) cycle to be used for energy or, through gluconeogenesis and lipogenesis, be converted to glucose and fat.

Figure 3.11 is depicted the protein metabolism.

Protein Excess

- An excessive intake of protein results in increased deamination by the liver. The increased deamination may result in high levels of keto acids, possibly putting the body into a state of ketosis.
- The increased urea is excreted by the kidneys. Because the liver and kidneys are involved with the deamination process, the increased stress on the organs could initiate an underlying disorder of these organs.
- Because there are no definitive benefits of excessive protein intake, the general recommendation is to consume no more than twice the Recommended Dietary Allowance (RDA) for protein.
- In fact, the source of excess protein may be a health concern. Animal-derived protein sources, such as meats may also be high in saturated fat and cholesterol. This may increase the risk of coronary artery disease (CAD) and some cancers.
- The relationship between protein intake and osteoporosis also has been considered. When protein intake is high, there is a slight increase of calcium excretion from the body, but calcium absorption is not affected. Studies have yielded mixed results about this effect on the risk of osteoporosis. Because osteoporosis is multifactorial, this specific relationship is difficult to determine.
- Recommendations to consume moderate amounts of protein and to meet the new Dietary Reference Intake (DRI) levels for calcium are the best dietary approaches to decrease the risk of CAD and cancer.

■ DEFICIENCIES OF PROTEINS

Protein energy leads to kwashiorkor. In Greek word, it means the displaced child when the next baby is born. This is widely prevalent among weaned infants and preschool children due of lack of protein, calories, vitamins and minerals. It is usually occurs in the age group of 1–4 years. The following symptoms are observed. They are muscles wasting, mental change, edema, moon face, grey hair, necrosis, vitamin A deficiencies, anemia, fatty liver, nervous irritability, diarrhea, low serum level, disturbances of gastrointestinal tract.

Symptoms of protein deficiency and excess:

Protein deficiency	Protein excess
• Loss of muscle tone	• Acidosis and dehydration
• Confusion	• Constipation
• Slow wound healing	• Putrefaction in the gut if stomach acid is low
• Irritability	• Loss of bone (if vitamin D and calcium are low)
• Fluid retention	
• Food cravings	
• Too acid or alkaline	• Musculoskeletal issues
• Low libido	• Kidney dysfunction

Treatment: High quality protein and adequate amount of calories are requirement. Protein in the form of milk protein 3–5 g per day is required.
- **Calories:** 140–150 kcal/kg body weight
- **Vitamin A:** 50,000 international units
- **Iron:** iron salts and tablets of folic acid are prescribed.
- **Electrolytes:** potassium chloride 3–4 g, magnesium chloride 5 g to be given daily.

Marasmus

In Greek word, it means withering. It is usually occurring in earlier age than kwashiorkor. Marasmus is caused by both protein and calories, widely prevalent among infants in the age group of 0–12 months. Signs and symptoms are, growth failure—more severe than kwashiorkor, edema is absent, acid stool, dehydration, lack of subcutaneous fat and apathy (lack of interest in surrounding).

Marasmic kwashiorkor: In this condition, both kwashiorkor and marasmus symptoms are noticed. So, calories and protein allowances are required in adequate amounts.

Clinical features of kwashiorkor and marasmus:

Sl. No.	Clinical features	Kwashiorkor	Marasmus
1.	Weight (growth for age)	Below normal, may be marked by edema	Very much below normal
2.	Muscles	Thin upper arms can be marked by edema	Very thin upper arms
3.	Edema of feet and legs	Present	Not present
4.	Hair color and texture	Bright than in others or reddish and brittle	Lighter but softer than others
5.	Skin	Stretched and taut, flaking off of skin, pale patches	Shriveled and wrinkled
6.	Appetite and behavior	Poor appetite looks miserable or irritated weak cry	Usually accepts food offered, alter but looks anxious
7.	Stools	Often loose	Sometimes loose, Motion may also be constipated
8.	Diarrhea	Often	Sometimes
9.	Anemia	Sometimes	Sometimes
10.	Vitamin deficiencies	Usually found	Sometimes found

Protein Energy Malnutrition

Protein energy malnutrition is a disease due to the deficiencies of protein and calories occur commonly among weaned infants and preschool children in India and other developing countries. These may be classified into three groups
1. Kwashiorkor
2. Nutritional marasmus
3. Marasmic-Kwashiorkor

Kwashiorkor: It is caused by deficiency of proteins in the diet. The important symptoms of the disease by; deficiency of proteins in the diet muscle wasting, fatty liver, loss of appetite and diarrhea, changes in the color of the skin and hair and anemia.

Nutritional marasmus: This is caused by severe deficiency of proteins and calories in the diet. The important features of growth retardation and sever wasting of muscle and loss of subcutaneous fat. The skin is dry and a atrophic. Eye lesions due to vitamin A deficiency and anemia may also be present.

Maraaasmic kwashiorkor: Children suffering from this disease show the signs of both kwashiorkor and marasmus described above.

Assessment: The anthrometeric measurements which are monitored to recognize PEM include weight, height and arm circumference. Weight for age is an easy method of assessing nutritional status. But it does not differentiate between acute and chronic malnutrition. Chronic malnutrition is defined when there is decrease in height but the weight is normal in relation to height. The PEM ranges from retardation of growth to occurrence of kwashiorkor. It can be graded as under.

Classification of malnutrition based on weight for age:

Nutritional status	% of reference weight for age (%RWA)
Normal	80–100%
Grade I	70–79%
Grade II	60–69%
Grade III	50–59%
Grade IV	<50

The classification of malnutrition is based on weight for age of the child. It is recommended by the Indian Academy of pediatrics and is used by integrated child Development scheme. The expected body weight is in this system is 50th percentile of hardware standards. The interpretation of nutritional anthropometric data is made simple and easy by Kapil and Gupta by developing slide in and out Assessment Table (KGAT).

The measurement of mid arm circumference (MAC) is another measure which is a sensitive and reliable index of malnutrition in children in age group of 1 to 5 years. The MAC does not change during this period.
- MAC 13.5 cm normal
- MAC 12.5-13.5 mild to moderate malnutrition (Gread I and II)
- MAC <12.5 severe (Grade III) malnutrition

Treatment: The main principles of treatment are to ensure an acceptable and readily digestible diet (liquid diet initially for a week) rich in proteins, calories and supplying all other dietary essentials in required amounts and b) treatment of any bacterial and parasitic infections present. The diet is usually contains of skim milk powder (re-constituted), sugar, cooked cereals and banana. Fat is introduced in the diet from the 2nd week of treatment. The daily calorie intake should be 140–150 kcal/kg and protein intake 3–5 g/kg body weight. Vitamin A deficiency is corrected by the administration of the required amounts of synthetic vitamin A deficiency is corrected by the administration of required amounts of synthetic vitamin A.

Prevention and control: The PEM, such as any other disease can be prevented and controlled by comprehensive approach involving primary level secondary level and tertiary level preventive measures. Primary preventive measures include health promotion and specific protection. The secondary and tertiary level preventive measures include early diagnosis treatment and rehabilitation.

Over consumption of proteins: Eating too much protein can worsen kidney problems, and over time can cause symptoms, such as bad breath, indigestion and dehydration. Certain sources of protein, such as meat, dairy, and processed foods can increase the risk of chronic illnesses, such as heart disease and cancer.

Total Serum Protein: Nursing Implications

Total serum protein test can be indicated to assess a patient's overall nutritional status, especially if the patient has a history of unexplained, significant weight loss. The other indications of this test are to assess liver disorders as part of liver function tests, to assess renal disorders and bone marrow disorders, and to investigate the cause of edema. This test finds a place in comprehensive metabolic panel test. The normal range for total protein in serum is 6–8 g/dL, and in albumin is 3.5–5 g/dL. The normal ratio of albumin to globulin is from 0.8 to 2.

The following are the interpretations of the total serum protein test:
- A decrease in total protein level may indicate severe malnutrition, disorders associated with mal-absorption, such as celiac or hepatic disease, or renal disorder which interferes with protein metabolism.
- An increased total protein level can occur in chronic inflammation or infections. It can also occur in bone marrow disorders, such as multiple myeloma.
- A decrease in the albumin to globulin (A/G) ratio reflects low albumin or elevated globulin levels. Elevated total globulins can occur in multiple myeloma, collagen disorders, rheumatoid arthritis, and some chronic inflammatory diseases, such as tuberculosis and syphilis. Low albumin levels can occur due to underproduction as in cirrhosis, or due to selective loss of albumin as in nephrotic syndrome.
- A high A/G ratio occurs due to underproduction of immunoglobulins as seen in leukemias and certain genetic deficiencies.
- A low total protein with normal A/G ratio typically occurs due to expansion of plasma volume where both albumin and globulin are diluted to the same extent.

CONCLUSION

Protein is an essential macro-nutrient, but not all food sources of protein are created equal, and you may not need as much as you think. Protein is found throughout the body—in muscle, bone, skin, hair, and virtually every other body part or tissue. It makes up the enzymes that power many chemical reactions and the hemoglobin that carries oxygen in your blood. Protein is made from twenty-plus basic building blocks called amino acids. Because we do not store amino acids, our bodies make them in two different ways—either from scratch, or by modifying others. Nine amino acids—histidine, isoleucine, leucine, lysine, methionine, phenylalanine, threonine, tryptophan, and valine—known as the essential amino acids, must come from food. In conclusion providing good nutrition is important in the prevention of malnutrition, degenerative diseases and overall well being of patients. It is vital for nurses to develop good nutritional knowledge and interpersonal skills to be able to provide holistic quality care towards the recovery of patients.

BIBLIOGRAPHY

1. Joshi SA. Nutrition and Dietetics, Tata McGraw Hill, New Delhi, India, 1992.
2. Lutz CA, Karen R. Przytuski: Nutrition and Diet Therapy, 4th edition. Davis FA, Philadelphia, USA, 1995.
3. Patwardhan VN. Nutrition in India 2nd edition. Indian Journal of Medical Sciences, New Delhi, 1961.
4. Robinson CH, Marilyn RL, Wanda LC, Anne EG. Normal and Therapeutic Nutrition, 17th edition. Macmillan Publishing Co., New York, USA, 1996.
5. Shils MS, Benjamin CA, Catherine R, Robert J. Cousins: Modern Nutrition in Health and Disease, 10th edition. Lippincott, Williams & Wilkins, Baltimore, USA, 2005.
6. Swaminathan M. Essentials of Food and Nutrition, Volume I and II, 2nd edition. Ganesh, Madras, India, 1985.

REVIEW QUESTIONS

Long Essays
1. Define protein, explain the chemical composition of protein.
2. Describe the classifications of proteins.
3. Define amino acid, explain types of amino acids.

Short Essays
1. Structure of protein.
2. Chemical properties of proteins.
3. Good sources of protein.
4. Describe enzyme proteins.
5. Biological value of protein.
6. Digestion of protein.
7. Protein energy malnutrition.
8. Clinical features of kwashiorkor and marasmus.

Short Answers
1. Conjugated proteins.
2. Derived proteins.
3. Xanthoproteic test.
4. Folin's test.
5. High-protein foods.
6. Recommended dietary allowances of protein for various age groups.
7. Globular proteins.
8. Antibody proteins.
9. Protein excess.
10. Non-essential amino acids.
11. Messenger proteins.
12. Sources of amino acid.
13. Classification of malnutrition.

CHAPTER 4

Fats

CHAPTER OUTLINE

- Classification—Saturated and Unsaturated
- Calorie Value
- Functions
- Dietary Sources of Fats and Fatty Acids
- Fat Requirements—RDA

TERMINOLOGY

- **Polyunsaturated fat:** A fat found in foods, such as walnuts, salmon, and, soybean oil. Polyunsaturated fats provide essential fatty acids, such as omega-3s and omega-6s to your diet. Most of the fat you eat should be mono- and polyunsaturated.
- **Monounsaturated fat:** A healthy fat found in foods, such as nuts, olive oil, and avocados. When used to replace saturated fats, a diet high in monounsaturated fats can help lower bad cholesterol. Most of the fat in your diet should be mono- and polyunsaturated. All fats have 9 calories per gram.
- **Saturated fat:** Usually solid at room temperature, saturated fats are found in animal products, such as meat and milk, as well as in coconut and palm oil. Saturated fat is often used in foods to prevent rancidity and off flavors. No more than 5% to 10% of your total daily calories should come from saturated fat.
- **Total fat:** This number on a food label indicates how much fat is in a single serving of a food. Limit total fat to less than 25% to 35% of the calories you consume each day. All fats have 9 calories per gram.
- **Trans fat:** Trans fats are created when liquid fats, such as vegetable oil are hydrogenated into more solid fats, such as margarine and shortening. Trans fats are linked with high LDL cholesterol, which can increase your risk of heart disease. Keep intake of trans fats as low as possible.
- **Omega-3 fatty acids:** From marine sources are considered heart healthy, because they lower the level of triglycerides (or fats) and cholesterol circulating in your bloodstream. They also discourage unwanted blood clotting.
- **Cholesterol:** A substance in animal tissue that is an essential component of cell membranes and nerve fiber insulation. Cholesterol is important for the metabolism and transport of fatty acids and in the production of hormones and vitamin D. Cholesterol is manufactured by the liver, and is also present in certain foods (e.g., eggs, shellfish). There are 2 types of cholesterol in the blood, high-density (HDL) and low-density (LDL) lipoproteins. Very low cholesterol levels may indicate malnutrition. Low-density lipoprotein (LDL) cholesterol provides cholesterol for necessary body functions, but in excessive amounts it tends to accumulate in artery walls; known as "bad" cholesterol. High-density lipoprotein (HDL) cholesterol, known as the "good" cholesterol; a high level in the blood is thought to lower the risk of coronary artery disease
- **Total blood cholesterol:** This includes your HDL, LDL, and 20% of your total triglycerides.
- **Triglycerides:** This number should be below 150 mg/dL. Triglycerides are a common type of fat. If your triglycerides are high and your LDL is also high or your HDL is low, you are at risk of developing atherosclerosis.
- **HDL:** The higher this number, the better. It should be at least higher than 55 mg/dL for females and 45 mg/dL for males.
- **LDL:** The lower this number, the better. It should be no more than 130 mg/dL if you do not have heart disease, blood vessel disease, or diabetes. It should be no more than 100 mg/dL if you have any of those conditions or high total cholesterol.

INTRODUCTION

The term lipids are applied to a group of naturally occurring substances characterized by the insolubility in water, greasy feel and solubility in some organic solvents. They occur in the plant and animal kingdoms. Lipids more commonly known as fats and oil are integral part of our food. They are insoluble in water, but soluble in organic solvents. They occur in both plant and animals. Lipids are a concentrated source of energy. Fats are solid at 20°C they are called 'oils' if they are liquid at that temperature. They are classified as—1. Simple lipids, e.g., triglycerides, 2. Compound lipids, e.g., phospholipids, 3. Derived lipids, e.g., cholesterol. Fat does a complex molecule constitute a mixture of fatty acids and an alcohol, generally glycerol. It contains carbon, hydrogen and oxygen, but differs from carbohydrates in that it contains more carbon and hydrogen and less oxygen. When one gram of fat is oxidized it yields 9 kcal.

CLASSIFICATIONS OF FATS

1. **Simple lipids (Oils and fats):** These are esters of fatty acids and glycerol. Oils are liquids at 2°C.
2. **Compound lipids:** The compound lipids contain, in addition to fatty acids and glycerol, some other organic compounds.
   a. *Phospholipids (Phosphatides):* These contain phosphoric acid and a nitrogenous base in addition to fatty acids and glycerol.(e.g., lecithin and cephalin).
   b. *Glycolipids:* Complex lipids containing carbohydrates in combination with fatty acids and glycerol (e.g., cerebrosides).
3. **Waxes:** These are esters of fatty acids and long chain aliphatic alcohols.
4. **Derived lipids:** These include sterols, fatty acids and alcohols.

Lipids are classified into simple, compound and derived lipids, which are further subdivided as follows:
- **Simple lipids:** Fats and oils are included in this type. At room temperature, oils are liquids and fats are solids. Fats and oils contain esters of fatty acid and glycerol, a form in which lipids are present in food.
- **Compound lipids:** They are esters of fatty acids containing phosphorus carbohydrate or protein. Phospholipids contain a phosphoric acid in addition to the alcohol and fatty acids. Glycolipids contain a fatty acid, carbohydrate and a nitrogenous base. Phospholipids and glycolipids form part of the cell membrane and the nervous system. Lipoproteins are macromolecular complex of lipids with proteins.
- **Derived lipids:** These are substances liberated during hydrolysis of simple and compound lipids, which still retain the properties of lipids. The important members of this group are sterols, fatty acids and alcohol.
- **Sterols:** Sterols are solid alcohols and form esters with fatty acids. In nature, they occur in the Free State in the form of esters. Based on their origin sterols are classified as cholesterol (animal origin) and phytosterol (in plants). Cholesterol is a complex type of lipid that is regularly synthesized by and stored in the liver. It is present in all animal products.
- **Fatty acids:** Fatty acids are the main building blocks of fat. They have a methyl group (CH3) at one end and a carboxyl group (COOH) at the other end with a chain of carbon and hydrogen atom in the middle. They have a general formula $CH_3(CH_2)_n COOH$. Where, 'n' denotes the number of carbon atoms, which may vary from 2 to 2l. Fatty acids can be classified into **(Fig. 4.1)**:
   a. *Saturated fatty acids (SFA):* Saturated fatty acids are those that are unable to absorb more hydrogen. They are usually stiff and hard fats, e.g., ghee, butter.
   b. *Unsaturated fatty acids (UFA):* Unsaturated fatty acids have one or more double bond in their molecule and are thus not saturated with hydrogen. They are liquid at room temperature, e.g., sunflower oil. Unsaturated fatty acids may be monounsaturated or polyunsaturated depending on the number of double bonds.
     - Monounsaturated fatty acids (MUFA): MUFA have only one double bond in their molecule, e.g., oleic acid found in olive oil, peanut oil.
     - Polyunsaturated fatty acids (PUFA): PUFA have 2 or more double bonds in their molecule, e.g., linoleic acid, linolenic acid. They are present in corn, safflower, soybean, sunflower oils and fishily. Monounsaturated and polyunsaturated fats are usually soft or liquid at room temperature.

Triglycerides: Fatty acids combine with glycerol to form a glyceride, When only one fatty acid combines with glycerol, it forms a monoglyceride, diglycerides have two fatty acids and triglycerides have three fatty acids attached to glycerol.

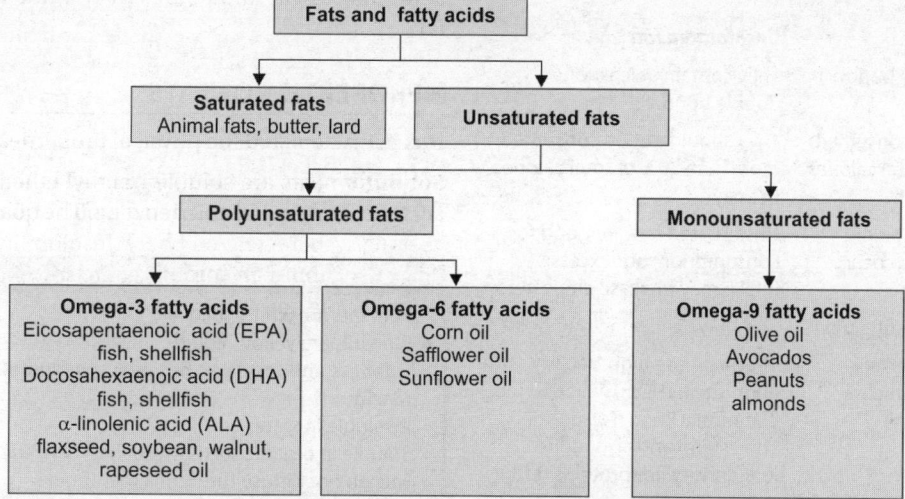

Fig. 4.1: Classification of fat and fatty acids.

Most of the fatty acids present in the body and absorbed from foods occur in the form of triglycerides. During digestion triglycerides are hydrolyzed to form free fatty acid, monoglycerides and glycerol, which are absorbed by the intestinal wall and the majority of these are rebuilt as triglycerides.

- **Long- and short-chain fatty acid:** The number of carbon atom in fatty acids decides the chain length. Thus short chain fatty acids contain 4–6 carbon atoms, medium chain 8–12 carbon atoms and long chain fatty acid have 14–18 carbon atom.
- **Essential and non-essential fatty acid:** Essential fatty acid (EFA) is those, which cannot be synthesized by the body and need to be supplied through diet. Linolenic acid, linoleic acid and arachidonic acid are essential fatty acids.
- **Non-essential fatty acids:** Non-essential fatty acids are those, which can be synthesized by the body and which need not be supplied through the diet. Palmitic acid, oleic acid and butyric acid are examples of non-essential fatty acids.

SATURATED AND UNSATURATED FATS

Our metabolic system provides us with the energy to sustain the proper functioning of the body. This energy comes from the food we consume. Three major macronutrients contribute to the energy in the body—carbohydrates, proteins, and fats. Fat is a vital nutrient that keeps us healthy and protects our tissues. Our daily diet consists of two types of fats—saturated fats and unsaturated fats.

1. **Saturated fats:** Saturated fats have a chemical nature in which the carbon atoms are saturated with hydrogen atoms and do not contain double bonds between carbon atoms. Saturated fats are classically solid at room temperature.
2. **Unsaturated fats:** Unsaturated fats have a chemical nature that contains one or more double or triple bonds between the carbon atoms. These fats are liquid at room temperature in oil form. They also occur in solid foods. These are further divided into monounsaturated fats and polyunsaturated fats.

Differences between saturated and unsaturated fats

Saturated fats	Unsaturated fats
They contain a single bond	They contain at least one double bond
They should not be consumed more than 10% of total calories per day	They should not be consumed more than 30% of total calories per day
Excessive consumption of saturated fats leads to heart diseases	Unsaturated fats are good for consumption, but excessive intake may increase cholesterol
They have a high melting point	They have a low melting point
They increase low-density lipoproteins (LDL), which is called bad cholesterol	They increase high-density lipoprotein (HDL), which is commonly known as good cholesterol and also reduce low-density lipoproteins (LDL)

Contd...

Contd...

Saturated fats	Unsaturated fats
Food sources of saturated fats are whole milk, butter, cheese, margarine, coconut oil, vegetable oil, meat, peanut, fried foods, etc.	Food sources of unsaturated fats are walnuts, flax, avocado, sunflower oil, soybean oil, fish oil, canola oil, red meat, etc.
These are usually found in the solid state in room temperature	These are usually found in the liquid state at room temperature
They do not spoil quickly	They spoil quickly

Saturated and Unsaturated Fats Examples

Saturated fats can be found in a variety of foods, including:
- Animal meat including beef, poultry, pork
- Certain plant oils, such as palm kernel or coconut oil
- Dairy products including cheese, butter, and milk
- Processed meats including bologna, sausages, hot dogs, and bacon
- Pre-packaged snacks including crackers, chips, cookies, and pastries

Foods Containing Unsaturated Fats Include

- Nuts
- Plant oils, such as canola, vegetable, or plant oil
- Certain fish, such as salmon, tuna, and anchovy, which contain omega-3 unsaturated fatty acids
- Olives
- Avocados

CALORIE VALUE

When our body runs out of glucose, it turns to fat for energy, which has 9 calories in every gram. This is a little more than double the amount in carbohydrates. Converting fat into energy takes longer than it does to convert glucose into energy, because fat must be first be broken down into its two component parts: fatty acid and glycerol. Each part follows a separate pathway to ultimately become available as energy. One common saturated fat, palmitic acid, makes 130 molecules of ATP for each molecule of fat.

PROPERTIES OF FATS

Box 4.1 is depicted the physical properties of fats and oils.

Solubility: Fats are soluble in ethyl ether, petroleum ether, acetone, hot alcohol and benzene. The quantity of fat present

> **Box 4.1:** Physical properties of fats and oils.
> - Pure fats are white, solid
> - Pure oils are yellow, liquid
> - Odorless and tasteless, but over a period of time they become rancid
> - Insoluble in water
> - Soluble in organic solvents, such as benzene, acetone, ether
> - Fats do not diffuse through a membrane
> - Fats have a greasy feeling

in food materials is usually determined by extraction with ether or petroleum ether.

Iodine value: This is a measure of the extent of unsaturated fatty acids present in fats and oils. It is defined as the number of grams of iodine absorbed by 100 g of fat. Two atoms of iodine are added to each unsaturated linkage.

Compound lipids: The important compound lipids present in animal and human tissues are:

Phospholipids

- **Lecithin:** This contains glycerol, phosphoric acid, choline and fatty acids.
- **Cephalin:** They contain glycerol, phosphoric acid, ethanolamine and fatty acids.
- **Glycolipids (Cerebrosides):** They contain hexoses (galactose or glucose) fatty acid and amino alcohol, but no phosphoric acid or glycerol.
- **Sterols:** The sterols comprise one of the important groups of lipids. They possess a cyclic structure, i.e., cyclopentanophenanthrene ring with one secondary alcoholic group. In nature, they occur in the Free State and as esters with fatty acids. Sterols are classified as follows: (i) Animal sterols, e.g., cholesterol. (ii) Plant sterols, e.g., phytosterol; and (iii) Mycosterols, e.g., ergosterol.
- **Cholesterol:** The white matter of the brain contains about 4.5% and gray matter 1.0% of cholesterol on the fresh weight basis. Large amounts of cholesterol are also present in sebum secreted by the sebaceous glands. The blood of normal human beings contains 150–250 mg/100 mL.
- **Refined and hydrogenated oils:** The process of refining and hydrogenation is given below
- **Refined oil:** The process of preparation of refined oil consists of the following steps—(i) Alkali refining to remove free fatty acids; (ii) Bleaching with Fuller's earth or activated carbons to remove coloring matter; and (iii) Deodorization with super-heated steam. The refined oils thus obtained are free from odor and color.
- **Hydrogenated oil:** The refined oil obtained as described above is hydrogenated under optimal temperature and pressure in the presence of Nickel catalyst. During the process of hydrogenation, hydrogen is added to the unsaturated linkages. The liquid fat becomes a solid fat and the unsaturated fatty acid contents decrease as a result of hydrogenation. Vanaspathi sold in India consists mostly of hydrogenated refined groundnut oil to which sesame oil (5%) is added. Since it is used as a substitute for ghee, vanaspathi has been fortified with vitamin A.
- **Rancidity in fats:** The development of off-flavors in fats is known as rancidity. There are two main types of rancidity (a) Hydrolytic and (b) Oxidative.
- **Hydrolytic rancidity:** When fat is hydrolyzed by lipase, free fatty acids are formed. The odors of low molecular weight fatty acids contribute to the rancidity.
- **Oxidative rancidity:** The oxidation takes place at the unsaturated linkage (double bond). The addition of oxygen to the unsaturated linkage results in the formation of peroxides which. On decomposition, yields aldehydes and ketones having pronounced off-odor.

RECOMMENDED DIETARY ALLOWANCES

Fat requirements in men: The dietary reference intake (DRI) for fat in adults is 20% to 35% of total calories from fat. That is about 44 grams to 77 grams of fat per day if you eat 2,000 calories a day. It is recommended to eat more of some types of fats because they provide health benefits.

Fat requirements in women: Adults should get 20 to 35 percent of their total daily calories from fat. For those who eat the standard 2,000 calories a day, this ranges from 44 to 77 grams of fat. Each gram of fat contains 9 calories, so this amount ranges from 396 calories to 693 calories of fat per day.

For normal healthy persons:

Age group	Energy (kcal)	Protein (g)	Total fat (g)	SFA (g)	Carbo-hydrates (g)	Dietary fiber (g)	Choles-terol (mg)	Ca (g)	Na (mg)	Fe (mg)	Vit A (µg)	Folic acid (µg)	Vit C (mg)
Men													
18–29 years	2550	68	71	23.6	351	26	300	0.4–0.5	1700	6	750	200	30
30–59 years	2500	68	69	23.0	344	25	300	0.4–0.5	1650	6	750	200	30
60 years and above	2100	68	58	19.3	289	21	300	0.4–0.5	1400	6	750	200	30
Women													
18–29 years	2000	58	56	18.6	275	20	300	0.4–0.5	1350	19	750	200	30
30–59 years	2000	58	57	19.0	275	20	300	0.4–0.5	1350	19	750	200	30
60 years and above	1800	58	50	16.7	248	18	300	0.4–0.5	1200	6	750	200	30
Pregnant women													
Full activity	+285	+9	+8	+6	+39	+3	300	1.0–1.2	+200	19	750	400	50
Reduced activity	+200	+9	+6	+2	+28	+2	300	1.0–1.2	+150	19	750	400	50
Lactating women													
First 6 months	+500	+25	+14	+4.6	+69	+5	300	1.0–1.2	+350	19	1200	400	50
After 6 months	+500	+19	+14	+4.6	+69	+5	300	1.0–1.2	+350	19	1200	400	50

Fat Requirements

The dietary fat should be a good source of essential fatty acids At least 50% of the fat should consist of vegetable oils rich in essential fatty acids.

DIETARY SOURCES OF FATS

Fat is found in meat, poultry, nuts, milk products, butters and margarines, oils, lard, fish, grain products and salad dressings. There are three main types of fat, saturated fat, unsaturated fat, and trans fat. Saturated fat (found in foods like meat, butter, lard, and cream) and trans fat (found in baked goods, snack foods, fried foods, and margarines) have been shown to increase your risk for heart disease. Replacing saturated and trans fat in your diet with unsaturated fat (found in foods, such as olive oil, avocados, nuts, and canola oil) has been shown decrease the risk of developing heart disease.

- **Saturated fats:** Saturated fat is a type of dietary fat. It is one of the unhealthy fats, along with trans fat. These fats are most often solid at room temperature. Foods, such as butter, palm and coconut oils, cheese, and red meat have high amounts of saturated fat. Saturated fats occur naturally in many foods. Most come from animal sources, including meat and dairy products, as well as tropical fats, such as coconut, palm and palm kernel. Saturated fats are found in animal-based foods, such as beef, pork, poultry, full-fat dairy products and eggs and tropical oils, such as coconut, and palm. Because they are typically solid at room temperature, they are sometimes called "solid fats."
- **Unsaturated fats:** Fats that help to lower blood cholesterol if used in place of saturated fats. However, unsaturated fats have a lot of calories, so you still need to limit them. Most (but not all) liquid vegetable oils are unsaturated. (The exceptions include coconut, palm, and palm kernel oils.) There are two types of unsaturated fats— (1) Monounsaturated fats—examples include olive and canola oils, (2) Polyunsaturated fats—examples include fish, safflower, sunflower, corn, and soybean oils.
- **Trans fatty acids:** These fats form when vegetable oil hardens (a process called hydrogenation) and can raise LDL levels. They can also lower HDL levels "good cholesterol".Trans fatty acids are found in fried foods, commercial baked goods (donuts, cookies, crackers), processed foods, and margarines.

Type of fat	Dietary source	State at room temperature	Effects
Mono-unsaturated	Mustard oil, canola oil, groundnut oil, almond oil, walnut oil, avocado oil	Liquid	Lowers the level of bad cholesterol and increases the level of good cholesterol
Poly-unsaturated	Corn oil, soybean oil, safflower, cottonseed oil, fish oil, flax oil	Liquid	Lowers the level of bad cholesterol and increases the level of good cholesterol

Contd...

Contd...

Type of fat	Dietary source	State at room temperature	Effects
Saturated	Whole milk, butter, cheese, desi ghee, coconut oil, chocolate	Solid	Increases the level of bad cholesterol and decreases the level of good cholesterol

- **Hydrogenated and partially hydrogenated fats:** This refers to oils that have become hardened (such as hard butter and margarine). Partially hydrogenated means the oils are only partly hardened. Foods made with hydrogenated oils should be avoided because they contain high levels of trans fatty acids, which are linked to heart disease. (Look at the ingredients in the food label.)

FUNCTIONS OF FAT IN THE DIET

Fat is one of the 3 nutrients that supply calories to the body. Fat provides 9 calories per gram, more than twice the number provided by carbohydrates or protein. Fat is essential for the proper functioning of the body. Fats provide essential fatty acids, which are not made by the body and must be obtained from food.

- The essential fatty acids are linoleic and linolenic acid. They are important for controlling inflammation, blood clotting, and brain development.
- Fat serves as the storage substance for the body's extra calories. It fills the fat cells (adipose tissue) that help insulate the body.
- Fats are also an important energy source. When the body has used up the calories from carbohydrates, which occurs after the first 20 minutes of exercise, it begins to depend on the calories from fat.
- Healthy skin and hair are maintained by fat. Fat helps the body absorb and move the vitamins A, D, E, and K through the bloodstream.

Box 4.2 is depicted the functions of fats.

Fat has several important functions
- It is a concentrated source of energy, yielding more than twice the energy supplied by carbohydrate per unit weight.
- Fats are essential for the absorption of vitamins A, D, E, K, and especially carotenoids (provitamin-A) present in foods of vegetable origin.
- Some animal fats, e.g., fish liver oils, butter and ghee contain vitamin A and many vegetable fats contain vitamin E and red palm oil is a good source of carotene (Provitamin A).

Box 4.2: Functions of fats.
- Provides **energy**
- Keep the **body** warm
- Protect internal organs
- Helps **body** absorb vitamins A, D, E and K through bloodstream
- Produces hormones that help **body** to work properly
- Serves as the storage substances for the body's extra calories

- Fats contain essential fatty acids, viz., linoleic, linolenic and arachidonic acids which are essential for maintaining tissues in normal health.
- Fats help to reduce the bulk of the diet as starchy foods absorb lot of water during cooking.
- Fats improve the palatability of the diet and give satiety value, i.e., a feeling of fullness in the stomach.
- Phosphatides and other complex lipids are essential constituents of nervous tissue.
- Fats are deposited in the adipose tissue and this deposit serves as a reserve source of energy during starvation. Further, adipose tissue functions, such as an insulating material against cold and physical injury.

General Functions of Fats

The functions of lipids may be divided into two categories—(1) Specific characteristics of foods caused by lipids and (2) Maintenance of the physiologic health of our bodies.

Food Functions

- **Source of energy:** Fat is the densest form of stored energy in food and our bodies. This means that gram for gram, food fat—in the form of triglycerides—can produce more than twice the energy in kcal as carbohydrate or protein. For example, a gram of nearly pure fat (9 kcal), such as butter, provides more than twice the kcal as a gram of nearly pure carbohydrate (4 kcal), such as sugar, or a gram of nearly pure protein (4 kcal) such as dried, lean fish.
- **Palatability:** Fat makes food smell and taste good. Deep-fat fried potatoes outrank all other vegetable choices among North Americans. Whether it is bread with butter (or margarine), salad with dressing, or desserts with cream, fat makes these foods taste pleasant for many people. For patients who are anorectic because of illness, strategically adding small amounts of fats to meals may increase their nutrient intake.
- **Satiety and satiation:** Fat helps prevent hunger between meals. Fat slows down digestion because of the hormones released in response to its presence in the gastrointestinal (GI) tract, causing us to feel full and satisfied; we call this feeling satiety. Satiation is another, different aspect of fat consumption that occurs during, not after, eating. In contrast to satiety, satiation tends to increase our desire to eat additional fatty foods, not less. The effect of fat on satiation is likely to be more important than its effect on satiety and may lead to overeating. A situation that often occurs with the last slice of pizza provides a good example—you want it, you eat it, and half an hour later, you feel too full.
- **Food processing:** Certain qualities of lipids, besides their nutritional purposes, make them a valuable resource for the processing of foods. The use of processed hydrogenated fats helps keep the fat in food products from turning rancid. Lecithin, a phospholipid, has an extensive role as an emulsifier. An emulsifier is a substance that works by being soluble in water and fat at the same time. These functions, which will be described in more detail, also increase our overall intake of lipids by allowing their use in numerous processed foods.
- **Nutrient source:** Some fats contain or transport the fat-soluble nutrients of vitamins A, D, E, and K and the essential fatty acids of linoleic and linolenic fatty acids.

Physiologic Functions

- **Stored energy:** Body fat cells contain nearly pure fat, also in the form of triglycerides. This means a pound of adipose tissue, the storage depot of body fat, could produce about 3500 kcal as energy. Because glucose stored in our bodies as glycogen is stored with water, carbohydrate is a bulkier form of stored energy than body fat. Adipose tissue provides important fuel during illness or times of food restriction and is a major energy source for muscle work.
- **Organ protection:** Stored fat safely cushions and protects body organs during bumpy activities, such as participating in impact aerobics or snowboarding.
- **Temperature regulation:** The fat layer just under our skin serves as insulation to regulate body temperature by minimizing the loss of heat.
- **Insulation:** A substance composed largely of fatty tissue, called myelin, covers nerve cells. This covering provides electrical insulation that allows for transmission of nerve impulses.

Functions of Phospholipids and Sterols

- Phospholipids are also important as a part of all cell membrane structure and serve as emulsifiers to keep fats dispersed in body fluids.
- Lecithins are the main phospholipids. Lecithin is a constituent of lipoproteins—carriers or transporters of lipids—including fats and cholesterol in the body.
- This characteristic has earned lecithin a reputation for carrying fat and cholesterol away from plaque deposits in the arteries.
- Although lecithin does play a role in transporting fat and cholesterol, supplementary lecithin from sources outside the body does not help make the body's transportation system more efficient. Instead, dietary lecithin is simply digested and used by the body as any other lipid.
- As a lipid group, sterols are critical components of complex regulatory compounds in our bodies and provide basic material to make bile, vitamin D, sex hormones, and cells in brain and nerve tissue.
- Cholesterol in particular is a vital part of all cell membranes and nerve tissues and serves as a building block for hormones. When exposed to ultraviolet light, a cholesterol substance in our skin can be converted to vitamin D by the kidneys and liver.
- The liver synthesizes cholesterol to make bile, the emulsifying substance necessary to absorb dietary lipids.

Functions of Triglycerides

Triglycerides are used in the body because they provide energy to cells that need it. They are a naturally occurring component of the blood and are deposited in fat deposits.

Excess triglycerides, on the other hand, can cause difficulties in the body and lead to serious ailments. In the human bloodstream, triglycerides play an important role in metabolism as energy sources and transporters of dietary fat. They contain more than twice as much energy as carbohydrates, the other major source of energy in the diet. High triglyceride levels are linked to metabolic syndrome, a collection of illnesses that raises the risk of diabetes, stroke, and cardiovascular disease. A blood level of more than 200 mg/dL is linked to an increased risk of heart attack, stroke, and death.

Function of Lipoproteins

- The function of lipoprotein particles is to transport lipids (fats) (such as cholesterol) around the body in the blood.
- All cells use and rely on fats and cholesterol as building blocks to create the multiple membrane which cells use to both control internal water content, internal water soluble elements and to organize their internal structure and protein enzymatic systems.

Particle	Chol	Trig	Function
Chylomicrons	+	++++	Transport of dietary (exogenous) triglycerides from gut to peripheral tissues
VLDL	+	++++	Transport of triglycerides synthesized in the liver (endogenous) to peripheral tissues
Chylomicron Remnant (CR)	+++	+++	Derived from chylomicrons. Usually rapidly cleared by the liver
IDL	+++	+++	Derived from VLDL. Usually rapidly cleared by the liver or converted to LDL
LDL	+++++	+	Derived from TDL. Transport of cholesterol and fat soluble vitamins to peripheral tisues
HDL	++++	+	Reverse transport of cholesterol from peripheral tissues to the liver; antioxidant

- The lipoprotein particles have hydrophilic groups of phospholipids, cholesterol and apoproteins directed outward. Such characteristics make them soluble in the salt water-based blood pool.
- Triglyceride-fats and cholesterol esters are carried internally, shielded from the water by the phospholipid monolayer and the apoproteins.
- The interaction of the proteins forming the surface of the particles with (a) enzymes in the blood, (b) with each other, and (c) with specific proteins on the surfaces of cells determine whether triglycerides and cholesterol will be added to or removed from the lipoprotein transport particles.
- Regarding atheroma development and progression as opposed to regression, the key issue has always been cholesterol transport patterns, not cholesterol concentration itself.

> **Box 4.3:** Biological significance of cholesterol.
> - In humans and animals, cholesterol is a major constituent of the cell membranes. Cholesterol modulates physical properties of these membranes that in turn affect the function of membrane proteins, such as receptors and transporters
> - Cholesterol is the biosynthetic precursor of bile acids, which are essential for fat digestion
> - Cholesterol is the precursor of all steroid hormones, namely—androgens, estrogens, progestins, glucocorticoids, mineralo-corticoids, and calciferol (vitamin D)
> - Cholesterol also plays a major role in the pathogenesis of atherosclerosis

Functions of Cholesterol

Cholesterol can both be produced by the body itself and obtained from food sources. Cholesterol plays an important part in the human body. Its functions are as follows:

- **Hormone production:** Cholesterol plays a part in producing hormones, such as estrogen, testosterone, progesterone, aldosterone and cortisone.
- **Vitamin D production:** Vitamin D is produced when the sun's ultraviolet rays reach the human skin surface.
- **Bile production:** Cholesterol produces bile acids which aid in digestion and vitamin absorption.
- **Cell membrane support:** Cholesterol plays a very important part in both the creation and maintenance of human cell membrane.

Box 4.3 is depicted the biological significance of cholesterol.

DIGESTION AND ABSORPTION OF FATS

Fat is not digested in the stomach. The presence of fat in the diet delays the emptying of the food from the stomach. Fats are hydrolyzed by the pancreatic and intestinal lipases in the intestines into a mixture of diglycerides, monoglycerides and fatty acids.

- Bile is essential for the digestion and absorption a it helps to emulsify fats before digestion.
- The products of digestion pass into the cells of the intestinal wall, where synthesis of new glycerides characteristic of the animal species takes place.
- The resynthesized lipids pass through the lacteals of the small intestines to the thoracic duct and then to the blood stream in the form of fine particles known as chylomicrons.
- A greater part of the cholesterol present in the diet is absorbed while phytosterols present, in vegetable fats and oils are not absorbed.

Digestion

- **Mouth:** The mouth's primary fat digestive process is mechanical, as teeth masticate fatty foods. The glands of the tongue produce a fat-splitting enzyme (lingual lipase) released with saliva that begins digestion of long-chain fatty acids, such as those found in milk.

- **Stomach:** Mechanical digestion continues through the strong actions of peristalsis. Fat-splitting enzymes, such as gastric lipase hydrolyze some fatty acids from triglycerides.

Small Intestine

- Fats entering the duodenum initiate the release of cholecystokinin (CCK) hormone from the duodenum walls.
- The bile emulsifies fats to facilitate digestion. Mechanical digestion through muscular action allows for increased exposure of the emulsified fat globules to pancreatic lipase.
- This enzyme is the primary digestive enzyme that breaks triglycerides into fatty acids, monoglycerides, and glycerol molecules. Note that fats may not be completely broken down. Some may also pass through without being digested or absorbed.

Use of medium-chain triglycerides: Triglycerides are composed of long chains of fatty acids. To aid fat digestion in those patients with malabsorption, synthetically manufactured medium-chain triglycerides (MCTs) may be incorporated into a patient's dietary intake. MCTs should not be used to completely replace dietary fats because they do not contain EFAs.

Figure 4.2 is depicted the digestion and absorption of fats.

Absorption

- Fatty acids, monoglycerides, and cholesterol are assisted by bile salts in moving from the lumen to the villi for absorption.
- Micelles, created by bile salts encircling lipids, aid diffusion through the membrane wall. When through the membrane wall, fatty acids and glycerol combine back into triglycerides.
- These triglycerides are incorporated into chylomicrons, which are the first lipoproteins formed after absorption of lipids from food. They contain fats and cholesterol and are coated with protein.
- The protein coating allows travel through the lymph system to the blood circulatory system toward the hepatic

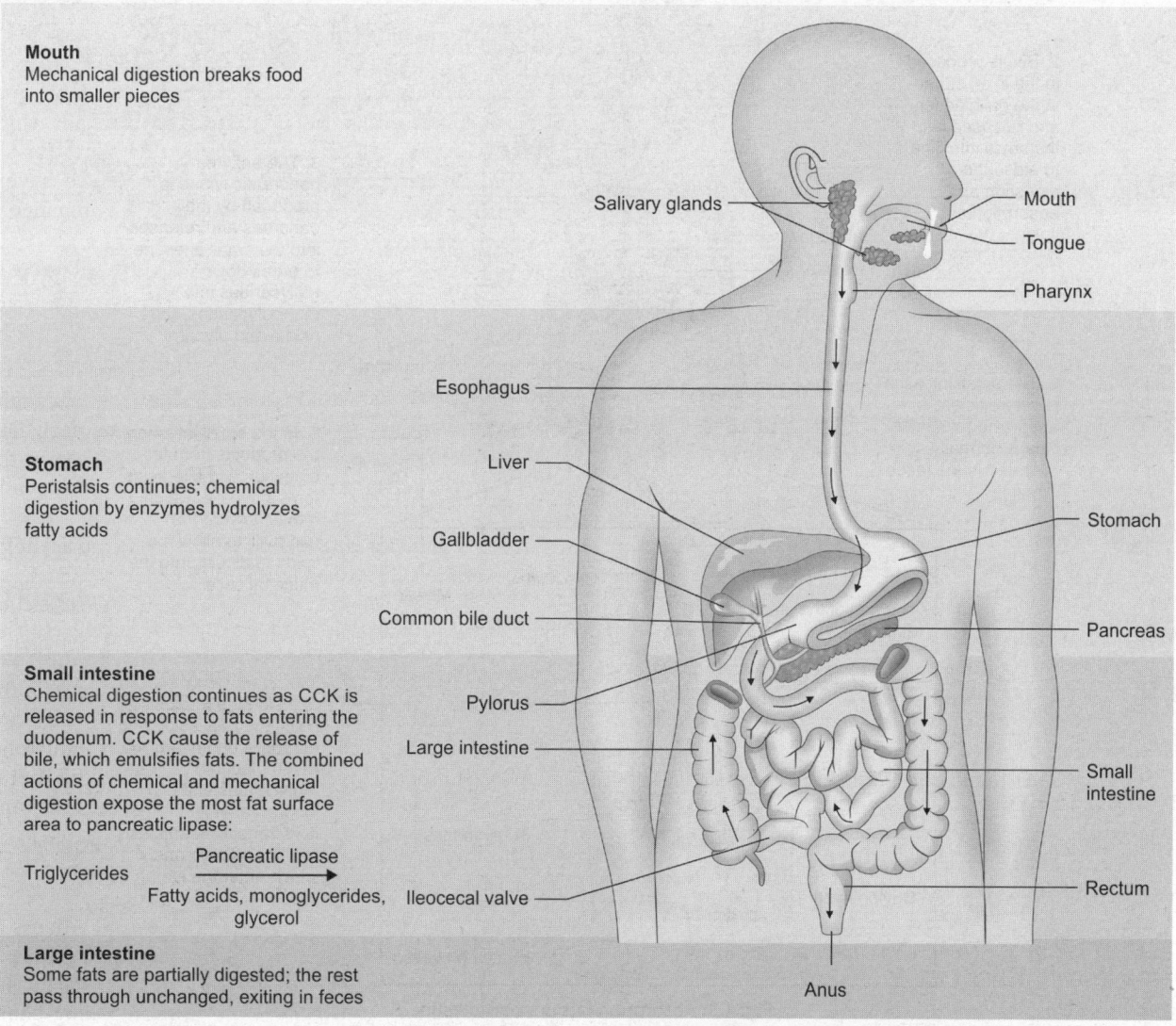

Fig. 4.2: Digestion and absorption of fats.

portal system and the liver. Some glycerol and any short- and medium-chain fatty acids are absorbed directly into the blood capillaries leading to the portal vein and liver.
- At the cell membranes, the triglycerides in the chylomicrons are broken down into fatty acids and glycerol with assistance from an enzyme called lipoprotein lipase.
- Muscle cells, adipose cells, and other cells in the vicinity take up most of the fatty acids released by the breakdown of chylomicrons.
- Cells can use the absorbed fatty acids immediately as fuel, or they can reform them into triglycerides to be stored as reserve energy supplies.

Figure 4.3 is depicted the absorption fats in small intestine.

Metabolism
- Lipid metabolism consists of several processes. Catabolism (breakdown) of lipids for energy involves the hydrolysis of triglycerides into two-carbon units that become part of acetyl coenzyme A (acetyl CoA).
- Acetyl CoA is an important intermediate byproduct in metabolism formed from the breakdown of glucose, fatty acids, and certain amino acids.
- The acetyl CoA then enters the series of reactions called the TCA cycle, eventually leading to the oxidation of the carbon and hydrogen atoms derived from fatty acids (or carbohydrates or amino acids) to carbon dioxide and water with the release of energy as adenosine triphosphate (ATP).

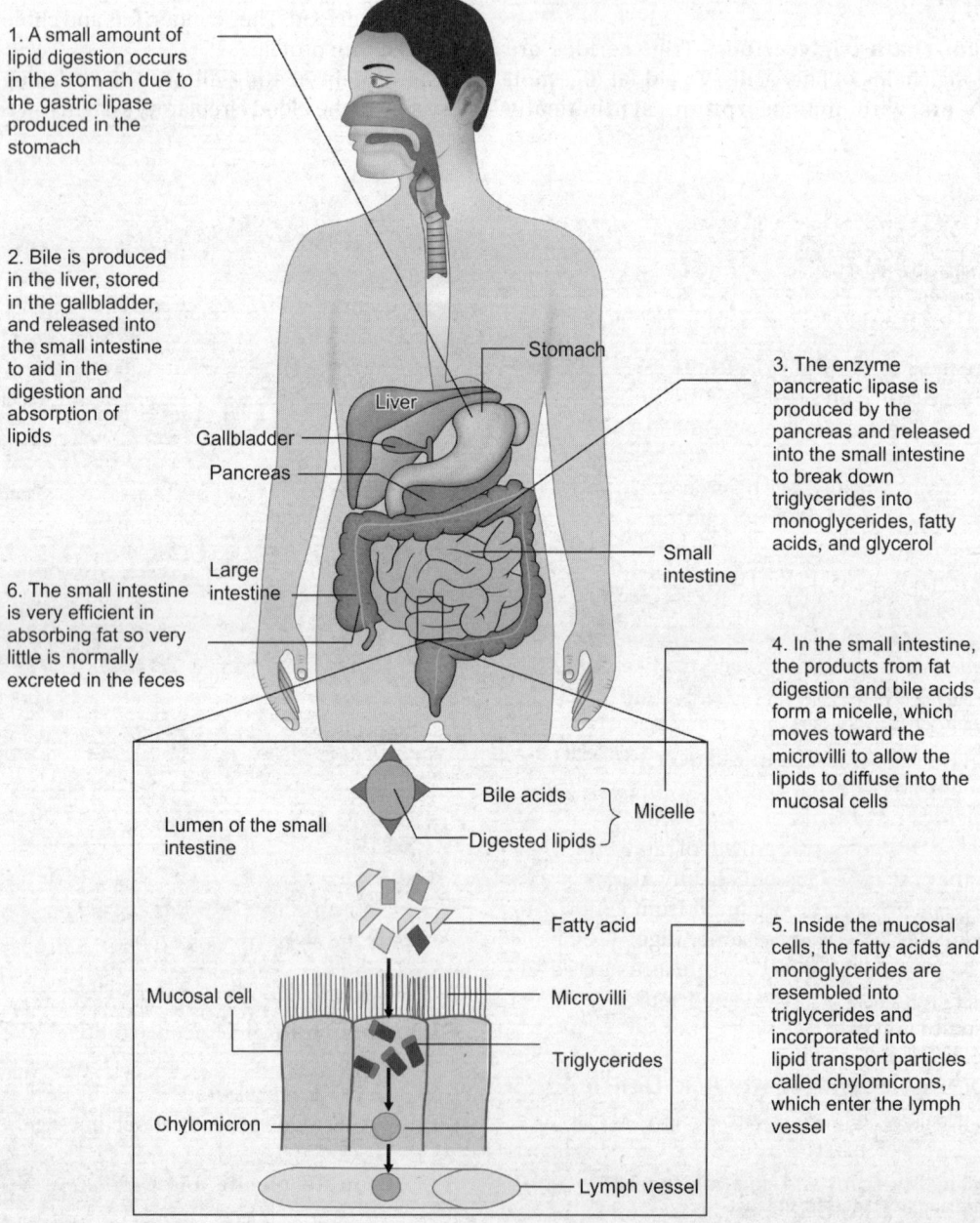

Fig. 4.3: Absorption fats in small intestine.

- If fat catabolizes quickly because of a lack of carbohydrate (glucose) for energy, the liver cells form intermediate products from the partial oxidation of fatty acids called ketone bodies. These ketone bodies may excessively accumulate in the blood, causing a condition called ketosis.
- Anabolism (synthesis) of lipids, or lipogenesis, results in the formation of triglycerides, phospholipids, cholesterol, and prostaglandins for use throughout the body.
- Triglycerides and phosphates form from fatty acids and glycerol or from excess glucose or amino acids. Extra carbon, hydrogen, and oxygen from any source can be converted to and stored as triglycerides in adipose tissues, so we can gain fat from foods other than fat.
- Lipid metabolism is regulated mainly by insulin, growth hormone, and the adrenal cortex hormones; adrenocorticotropic hormone (ACTH), which stimulates secretion of more hormones; and glucocorticoids, which affect food metabolism.

Storage of fats: Fat is stored in the adipose tissues. In normal human subjects, adipose tissue constitutes about 10 to 15 percent of the body weight. In increases up to 30 per cent in obese persons.

ESSENTIAL FATTY ACIDS (EFAs)

Essential fatty acids: Our body is capable of synthesizing maximum fatty acids, apart from these three essential fatty acids Linoleic, linolenic, and arachidonic acids. These designated essential fatty acids must be supplied through the diet. The deficiency symptoms of these fatty acids include poor growth, skin irritation, and have been seen in infants fed with the formula lacking these essential nutrients.

- The term essential fatty acids (EFA) refers to those polyunsaturated fatty acids (PUFA) that must be provided by foods because these cannot be synthesized in the body yet are necessary for health. There are two families of EFA, omega-3 (ω-3) and omega-6 (ω-6).
- Essential fatty acids are fatty acids the body cannot produce on its own. They play a key role in various bodily functions, including heart health, cancer prevention, cognitive function, skin health, and obesity prevention.
- Linoleic, linolenic and arachidonic acids are found to be highly effective in promoting the growth of rats fed fat-free diets. Hence, they are called 'Essential Fatty Acids".
- EFA content of oils: It will be obtained from sunflower seed, safflower seed, soybean, sesame, niger seed and cottonseed oils are rich source, while mustard and groundnut oils and egg yolk fat are good sources of EFA. Butter, vanaspathi and coconut oil are poor sources.

Signs/Symptoms of Essential Fatty Acid Deficiency

- Dry skin (e.g., feet/face/general)
- Scaly or flaky skin (e.g., legs)
- Cracking/peeling fingertips and skin (e.g., heels)
- Lackluster skin
- Small bumps on back of upper arms
- Patchy dullness and/or color variation of skin
- Mixed oily and dry skin ('combination' skin)
- Irregular quilted appearance of skin (e.g., legs
- Thick or cracked calluses
- Dandruff or cradle cap
- Dry, lackluster, brittle or unruly hair
- Soft, fraying, splitting or brittle fingernails
- Dull nails-lack of surface shine
- Slow growing fingernails
- Dry eyes
- Dry mouth/throat
- Inadequate vaginal lubrication
- Menstrual cramps
- Premenstrual breast pain/tenderness
- Excessive ear wax
- Excessive thirst
- Allergic (e.g., eczema/asthma/hay fever/hives)
- Crave fats/fatty foods
- Stiff or painful joints

LIPIDS IN BLOOD

Normal human plasma in the post-absorptive state contains about 500 mg of total lipids (per 100 mL) of which about 120 mg are triglycerides, 160 mg phospholipids, 180 mg cholesterol and about 10–15 mg free fatty acids. Plasma contains two lipoproteins which are involved in the transport of fat.

Fasting Triglyceride Levels

- Optimal triglycerides = <1.5 mmol/L
- Normal triglycerides = <2.0 mmol/L
- Borderline high triglycerides = 2–4 mmol/L
- High triglycerides = 4–11 mmol/L
- Very high triglycerides = >11 mmol/L

High levels of triglyceride are associated with the occurrence of coronary artery disease in some people. However, when triglyceride levels are exceedingly high, the risk is not to the heart but to the pancreas gland which may become inflamed. This condition is called pancreatitis and is very serious often resulting in death.

Table 4.1 is depicted the lipid blood test.

DEFICIENCY OF FATS

- **Infants:** Hansen and co-workers have reported that infants fed on a EFA deficient diet developed perianal irritation and skin changes, such as dryness, etc. within a few weeks. Supplementation of the diet with linoleic acid cured the condition.
- **Adults and children:** Recent studies by Gopalan and associates in India have shown that phrynoderma in adults and children is cured rapidly by the administration of linseed or safflower seed oil rich in essential fatty acids along with vitamins of B2 complex and not by vitamin A.
- **Hypercholesterolemia and coronary heart diseases:** The following factors influence the serum cholesterol level (i) Calorie intake; (2) Cholesterol intake; (3) Fat intake and (4) Essential fatty acid content of the fat. Low

Table 4.1: Lipid blood test.

	Unit	Optimal	Intermediate	High
Total cholesterol	mg/dL	<200	200–239	>239
	mmol/dL	<5.2	5.2–6.2	>6.2
LDL cholesterol (calculated)	mg/dL	<130	130–159	>159
	mmol/dL	<3.36	3.36–4.11	>4.11
HDL cholesterol	mg/dL	>60	60–40	<40
	mmol/dL	>1.55	1.55–1.03	<1.03
Triglycerides	mg/dL	<150	150–199	>199
	mmol/dL	<1.69	1.69–2.25	>2.25
Non-HDL-C (calculated)	mg/dL	<130	130–159	>159
	mmol/dL	<3.3	3.3–4.1	>4.1
TG to HDL ratio (calculated)	mg/dL	<3	3–3.8	>3.8
	mmol/dL	<1.33	1.33–1.68	>1.68

calorie intakes tend to reduce, while calorie excess tends to increase serum cholesterol levels. The dietary intake of cholesterol may vary from 500 to 1200 mg depending on the quantity of milk, butter, eggs, meat and fish in the diet. The adult human body synthesizes daily about 2000 mg cholesterol. Saturated fats viz., animal body fats, butter, coconut oil and hydrogenated fats tend to increase markedly the serum cholesterol level, while fats rich in essential fatty acids viz., sunflower seed, safflower seed, sesame, soybean, niger seed and cottonseed oils and fish oils tend to reduce the serum cholesterol level. When the blood cholesterol level is over 250 mg/100 mL, the incidence of atherosclerosis and coronary heart disease is high. Consumption of fats rich in essential fatty acids has been reported to reduce blood cholesterol level in the above subjects.

Treatment of high triglyceride levels: Lifestyle changes are the most important aspect of treating high triglyceride levels and often the changes alone are sufficient to bring triglyceride levels back to normal.
- Reduce weight. Ideally keep the body mass index between 20–25. The body mass index is the ratio of your weight in kilograms (1 kg = 2.2 pounds) to your height in meters squared (1 inch = 0.0254 meters). Weight in kg/(height in meters)
- Do not take excess quantities of carbohydrates
- Reduce the saturated fat and cholesterol content of in the diet.
- Cut down alcohol intake considerably. If you suffer from very high triglyceride levels, it is best to avoid alcohol entirely.
- Regular exercise helps clear triglyceride levels.
- Some medicines also increase triglyceride levels and you should check this with doctor so as to avoid the problem.
Since high triglycerides are often associated with other risk factors for heart disease, it is important to also treat high blood pressure, high cholesterol levels and diabetes.

LDL

LDL cholesterol, or low-density lipoprotein cholesterol, is a fat that circulates in the blood, moving cholesterol around the body to where it is needed for cell repair and depositing it inside of artery walls. Because cholesterol and triglycerides are insoluble in water, they must be associated with proteins to flow through the hydrophilic blood.

Fundamentals: The LDL particle is made of a monolayer of phospholipid, unesterified cholesterol forms the surface membrane, and fatty acid esters of cholesterol make up the hydrophobic core. One copy of the hydrophobic apo-B protein is embedded in the membrane, mediating the binding of LDL particles to specific cell-surface receptors.

Functions
- Apolipoproteins serve a structural role in phospholipid membranes, act as ligands for lipoprotein receptors, guide the formation of lipoproteins, and serve as activators and inhibitors of enzymes involved in the metabolism of lipoproteins.
- Lipoproteins are critical for absorbing and transporting dietary lipids by the small intestine and moving lipids from the liver to peripheral tissues and back from peripheral tissues to the liver and intestine.
- They are also crucial for transporting toxic foreign hydrophobic and amphipathic compounds, including bacterial endotoxin from areas of invasion and infection.

Testing
- A fasting lipid panel should be ordered in testing for hypercholesterolemia, along with labs to rule out secondary causes.
- In the fasting lipid panel, total cholesterol greater than 200 mg/dL and LDL cholesterol greater than 130 mg/dL are considered abnormal.
- Secondary causes of hyperlipidemia should be ruled out through testing fasting blood glucose, hemoglobin A1c, thyroid-stimulating hormone, alkaline phosphatase, and urinalysis to assess for proteinuria.

Pathophysiology: Hypercholesterolemia occurs from excess cholesterol from diet, bile, or intestines. The liver releases triglycerides into the plasma in the form of VLDL. The intestines release triglycerides into the plasma in the form of chylomicrons. Once in the plasma, the VLDL is converted into LDL. LDL in the plasma then interacts with the LDL receptor on cells in various tissues.

HDL

High-density lipoprotein (HDL) is one of the five major groups of lipoproteins. Lipoproteins are complex particles composed of multiple proteins which transport all fat molecules (lipids) around the body within the water outside cells. They are typically composed of 80–100 proteins per particle (organized by one, two or three ApoA. HDL particles enlarge while circulating in the blood, aggregating more fat molecules) and transporting up to hundreds of fat molecules per particle

HDL is composed of cholesterol, triglycerides, and various apolipoproteins. In particular, the composition of HDL is apolipoproteins Apo-AI, Apo-AII, Apo-AIV, Apo-AV, Apo-C1, Apo-CII, Apo-CIII, and Apo-E.[1]

- Apo-AI is the primary structural apolipoprotein of HDL and activates lecithin cholesterol acyltransferase (LCAT).
- Apo-AII is also a structural protein in HDL and acts as an activator of hepatic lipase.
- Apo-IV has an unknown function.
- Apo-AV activates lipoprotein lipase (LPL), which is responsible for triglyceride lipolysis.
- Apo-CI is responsible for activating LCAT.
- Apo-CII is responsible for activating LPL
- Apo-CIII is responsible for inhibiting LPL.
- Apo-E is a ligand for the LDL receptor.

Function: The primary function of HDL is the transport of cholesterol from the peripheral tissues to the liver, playing a role in the biodistribution of lipids. HDL is known for are anti-atherogenic and anti-inflammatory properties, thanks to its uptake and return of the cholesterol stored in the foam cells of atherosclerotic plaques to the liver. Thus, reducing the size of the plaque and its associated inflammation.

VLDL

Very-low-density lipoprotein (VLDL) cholesterol is produced in the liver and released into the bloodstream to supply body tissues with a type of fat (triglycerides).

- There are several types of cholesterol, each made up of lipoproteins and fats. Each type of lipoprotein contains a mixture of cholesterol, protein and triglycerides, but in varying amounts. About half of a VLDL particle is made up of triglycerides.
- High levels of VLDL cholesterol have been associated with the development of plaque deposits on artery walls, which narrow the passage and restrict blood flow.
- There is no simple, direct way to measure VLDL cholesterol, which is why it is normally not mentioned during a routine cholesterol screening. VLDL cholesterol is usually estimated as a percentage of your triglyceride value. An elevated VLDL cholesterol level is more than 30 milligrams per deciliter (0.77 millimole/Liter).
- VLDL is a type of bad cholesterol that can contribute to the risk of heart attack and stroke. Adopting a heart healthy diet, doing more physical activity, refraining from smoking, and maintaining a moderate weight is the best ways to manage cholesterol levels.
- High cholesterol does not have any symptoms. The only way that people can be sure of their cholesterol levels is to ask a doctor for a lipid profile test. Most adults should ideally have this test every 4–6 years.

OVER CONSUMPTION OF FAT (FIG. 4.4)

Saturated fat is a type of dietary fat. It is one of the unhealthy fats, along with trans fat. These fats are most often solid at

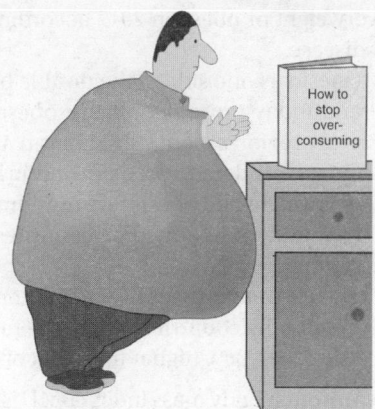

- Eating too much saturated fat has become a problem in our society
- There are many health problems linked with too much saturated fat in the diet, e.g., coronary heart disease, and strokes

Fig. 4.4: Over consumption of fat.

room temperature. Foods, such as butter, palm and coconut oils, cheese, and red meat have high amounts of saturated fat.

- Risks associated with consuming excess fat include heart disease, stroke, and cancer. Although no firm dietary standards exist when it comes to fat consumption, the American.
- Heart Association encourages people to focus on replacing high-fat foods with vegetables, fruit, poultry, lean meat, unrefined whole grains, and fat-free or low-fat dairy products.
- The American Heart Association and other organizations also recommend a ceiling of no more than 300 milligrams of cholesterol per day.
- Vegetarians tend to have lower blood cholesterol because they generally have a higher dietary quality and do not consume as many animal sources that are rich in saturated fats.

OBESITY (FIG. 4.5)

Overweight and obesity are defined as abnormal or excessive fat accumulation that presents a risk to health. A body mass index (BMI) over 25 is considered overweight, and over 30 is obese. The issue has grown to epidemic proportions, with over 4 million people dying each year as a result of being

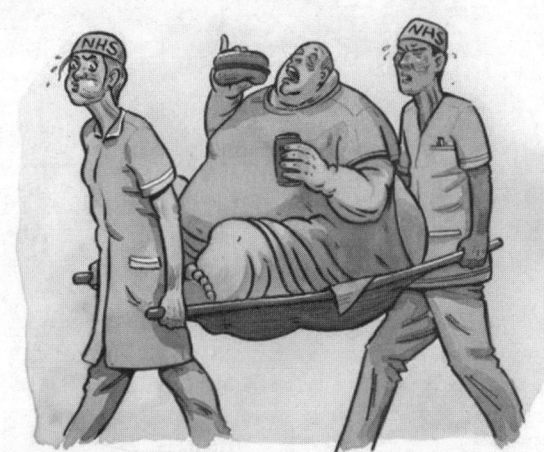

Fig. 4.5: Obesity.

overweight or obese in 2017 according to the global burden of disease.
- Obesity is one side of the double burden of malnutrition, and today more people are obese than underweight in every region except sub-Saharan Africa and Asia.
- Once considered a problem only in high-income countries, overweight and obesity are now dramatically on the rise in low- and middle-income countries, particularly in urban settings.
- The vast majority of overweight or obese children live in developing countries, where the rate of increase has been more than 30% higher than that of developed countries.

Symptoms: Body mass index (BMI) is often used to diagnose obesity. To calculate BMI, multiply weight in pounds by 703, divide by height in inches and then divide again by height in inches. Or divide weight in kilograms by height in meters squared.

BMI	Weight status
Below 18.5	Underweight
18.5–24.9	Normal
25.0–29.9	Overweight
30.0 and higher	Obesity

Asians with BMI of 23 or higher may have an increased risk of health problems. For most people, BMI provides a reasonable estimate of body fat. However, BMI does not directly measure body fat, so some people, such as muscular athletes, may have a BMI in the obesity category even though they do not have excess body fat.

Complications: People with obesity are more likely to develop a number of potentially serious health problems, including (Fig. 4.6):
- **Heart disease and strokes:** Obesity makes you more likely to have high blood pressure and abnormal cholesterol levels, which are risk factors for heart disease and strokes.
- **Type 2 diabetes:** Obesity can affect the way the body uses insulin to control blood sugar levels. This raises the risk of insulin resistance and diabetes.
- **Certain cancers:** Obesity may increase the risk of cancer of the uterus, cervix, endometrium, ovary, breast, colon, rectum, esophagus, liver, gallbladder, pancreas, kidney and prostate.
- **Digestive problems:** Obesity increases the likelihood of developing heartburn, gallbladder disease and liver problems.
- **Sleep apnea:** People with obesity are more likely to have sleep apnea, a potentially serious disorder in which breathing repeatedly stops and starts during sleep.
- **Osteoarthritis:** Obesity increases the stress placed on weight-bearing joints, in addition to promoting inflammation within the body. These factors may lead to complications, such as osteoarthritis.
- **Severe Covid-19 symptoms:** Obesity increases the risk of developing severe symptoms if you become infected with the virus that causes coronavirus disease 2019 (Covid-19). People who have severe cases of Covid-19 may require treatment in intensive care units or even mechanical assistance to breathe.

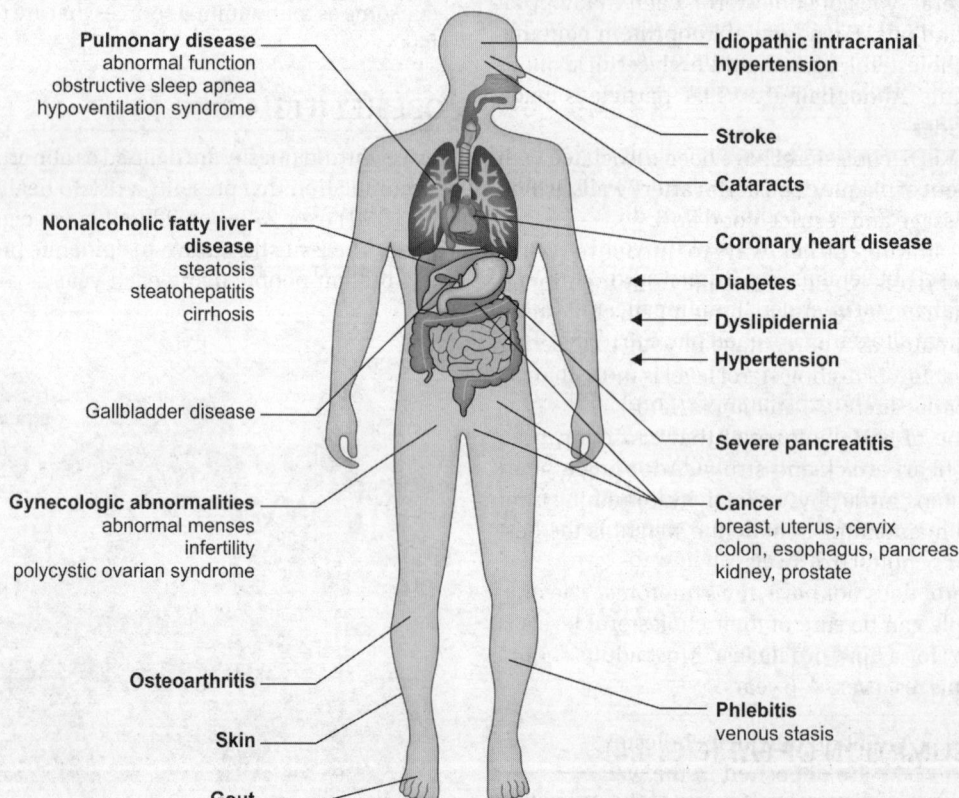

Fig. 4.6: Medical complications of obesity.

Dietary Changes

Reducing calories and practicing healthier eating habits are vital to overcoming obesity. Although you may lose weight quickly at first, steady weight loss over the long-term is considered the safest way to lose weight and the best way to keep it off permanently.

Dietary Management

There is no best weight-loss diet. Dietary changes to treat obesity include:

- **Cutting calories:** The key to weight loss is reducing how many calories you take in. The first step is to review your typical eating and drinking habits to see how many calories you normally consume and where you can cut back. You and your doctor can decide how many calories you need to take in each day to lose weight, but a typical amount is 1,200 to 1,500 calories for women and 1,500 to 1,800 for men.
- **Feeling full on less:** Some foods—such as desserts, candies, fats and processed foods-contain a lot of calories for a small portion. In contrast, fruits and vegetables provide a larger portion size with fewer calories. By eating larger portions of foods that have fewer calories, you reduce hunger pangs, take in fewer calories and feel better about your meal, which contributes to how satisfied you feel overall.
- **Making healthier choices:** To make your overall diet healthier, eat more plant-based foods, such as fruits, vegetables and whole grains. Also emphasize lean sources of protein—such as beans, lentils and soy- and lean-meats. If you like fish, try to include fish twice a week. Limit salt and added sugar. Eat small amounts of fats, and make sure they come from heart-healthy sources, such as olive, canola and nut oils.
- **Restricting certain foods:** Certain diets limit the amount of a particular food group, such as high-carbohydrate or full-fat foods. Ask your doctor which diet plans are effective and which might be helpful for you. Drinking sugar-sweetened beverages is a sure way to consume more calories than you intended. Limiting these drinks or eliminating them altogether is a good place to start cutting calories.
- **Meal replacements:** These plans suggest replacing one or two meals with their products—such as low-calorie shakes or meal bars—and eat healthy snacks and a healthy, balanced third meal that is low in fat and calories. In the short-term, this type of diet can help you lose weight. But these diets likely would not teach you how to change your overall lifestyle.

DIETARY MANAGEMENT OF ATHEROSCLEROSIS

Atherosclerosis is a condition in which cholesterol calcium and biochemical waste are deposited in the walls of blood vessels. It is an underlying cause of most heart attacks and strokes.

Dietary Management for Atherosclerosis

Atherosclerosis is a condition in which cholesterol calcium and biochemical waste are deposited in the walls of blood vessels. It is an underlying cause of most heart attacks and strokes.

Principle of Diet

- A low calorie, complex carbohydrates, normal protein, restricted fat, low sodium and potassium, high fiber, high vitamins and mineral diet should be provided.
- Whole milk should be avoided.
- HDL (high density lipoprotein) is good cholesterol that helps to prevent atherosclerosis.
- Omega-3 fatty acids should be included which protects the heart from clots and inflammation and reduces the risk of heart strokes.
- Drinks and alcohol will be raising blood pressure and triglyceride level. Hence should be restricted.
- Salt should be taken in low amounts.
- Potassium should be restricted as it results in irregular heart beat and may result to death. Hence, Leached fruits and vegetables should be given.

Foods to be included:

- Deep sea fish, omega-3 fish oil, such as salmon and tuna, soy milk, almonds, oat meal, oat bran (contains high amounts of soluble fiber)
- Brown rice, wheat pasta, legumes, such as kidney beans, lentils and chick pea can also be included.

Foods to be avoided:

- Saturated fats, trans-fat, cholesterol, refined carbohydrates, such as sugar foods, soft drinks, sweet baked foods, and salt were avoided.
- Whole milk dairy products including yogurt, cheese, ice creams, margarine, fried foods, egg yogurt, organ meats are not be included.

Sample diet for atherosclerosis: A healthy diet rich in nutrient-dense foods may help reduce the risk of developing clogged arteries. Research has shown that adding foods, such as cruciferous vegetables, fish, berries, olive oil, oats, onions, greens, and beans to the diet may be an effective way to prevent atherosclerosis.

The atherosclerosis diet is similar to those recommended for other conditions associated with heart disease (e.g., hyperlipidemia and hypertension. The aim is to adopt a healthy diet which will prevent further development of coronary heart disease.

The diet:

- Is similar to a Mediterranean-style diet
- Includes large amounts of fresh fruits (2 servings per day) and vegetables (5 servings per day)
- Limits the intake of meat, particularly red meat (1 serving per day)
- Increases consumption of grains and cereals (4–9 servings per day)
- Includes non-fat or low-fat milk and dairy products (2 servings per day)

- Recommends limiting alcohol intake (a maximum of 2 standard drinks for men and 1 for women per day).

Sample daily diet:

Breakfast
- 1 glass of freshly squeezed orange juice
- 1 bowl of porridge with honey and banana
- 1 slice of whole meal toast topped with tomato

Snack
- 1 tub of low-fat yoghurt
- 1 cup of tea or coffee
- 1 slice of fruit bread with thin spread of jam

Lunch
- Tuna salad
- 1 whole meal roll

Snack
- 2 slices of whole meal toast with low-fat cheese melted on top
- 1 cup of tea or coffee

Dinner
- 2 grilled chicken shashlicks with capsicum and onions served on a bed of couscous
- 1 greek salad
- 1 glass of red wine or dark grape juice

ROLE OF NURSE IN FATS

Proper nutrition plays a big role in disease prevention, recovery from illness and ongoing good health. A healthy diet will help you look and feel good as well. Since nurses are the main point of contact with patients, they must understand the importance of nutrition basics and be able to explain the facts about healthy food choices to their patients. Nutrition classes provide the information necessary to sort the fact from fiction about healthy eating and pass that knowledge on to their patients. Not only must nurses be able to explain the ins and outs of a healthy diet, they must also lead by example.

Fat is valuable and necessary to health. It is important to learn about fat in food, what the fat we eat does in our bodies, and how it can be both helpful and harmful to our health. Individual preference for fat is developed either in infancy or early childhood; innate preferences for sweet taste are observed at birth. Thus children learn to prefer tastes, flavors, and textures that are associated with foods that are rich in fat, sweet, or both. Aging may be associated with increasing acceptance of bitter tastes and consumption of more fruits, vegetables, and whole grains. Nonetheless, decreasing fat consumption takes time and effort, perhaps because of food selection habits, symbolic meaning associated with certain foods, and sensory values of fats in foods.

CONCLUSION

Fat actually refers to the chemical group called lipids. Lipids are divided into three classifications—fats (or triglycerides), and the fat-related substances of phospholipids and sterols. Triglycerides are the largest class of lipids and may be in the form of fats (somewhat solid) or oils (liquids). Approximately 95% of the lipids in foods and in our bodies are in the triglyceride form of fat. The other two lipid classifications are the fat-related substances of phospholipids and sterols. Lecithin is the best-known phospholipid; cholesterol is the best-known sterol. All are organic-composed of carbon, hydrogen, and oxygen—and cannot dissolve in water.

BIBLIOGRAPHY

1. Chaney MS, Margaret LR, Jelia CW. Nutrition, 9th Ed. Houghton. Mifflin, Boston 1979 (Indian reprint, Surjeet Publications, New Delhi, 1979).
2. Garrow JSS, James WPT, Ralph A. Human Nutrition & Dietetics, 10th edition. WB Saunders, Philadelphia, USA, 1999.
3. Joshi SA. Nutrition and Dietetics, Tata McGraw Hill, New Delhi, India, 1992.
4. Larsson K. et al. Lipids: Structure, Physical Properties and Functionality: Volume 19. The Oily Press Lipid Library, 2006.
5. Wardlaw GM, Insel PM. Perspectives in Nutrition, 2nd edition. Mosby Year Book Inc, St Louis, USA, 1996.
6. Wendy MW, Robert WL, Alejandro GM. Lipid Modification Strategies in the Production of Nutritionally Functional Fats and Oils. Critical Reviews in Food Science and Nutrition. 1998;38(8):639-74.
7. Williams SR. Basic Nutrition and Diet Therapy, 1st edition. Elsevier Science, New York, 1999.

REVIEW QUESTIONS

Long Essays
1. Define fat; explain the composition and classifications of fats.
2. Describe the dietary sources and functions of fats in diet.

Short Essays
1. Define fatty acids and explain the classifications of fatty acids.
2. Explain the dietary allowances of fats.
3. Describe the digestion and absorption of fatty acids.
4. List out essential fatty acids and explain the deficiencies of fatty acids.
5. Enumerate the deficiencies of fats.

Short Answers
1. Glycolipids.
2. Sterols.
3. Functions of triglycerides.
4. Calorie value of fatty acids.
5. Phospholipids.
6. Properties of fats.
7. Fasting triglycerides level.

CHAPTER 5

Vitamins

CHAPTER OUTLINE

- ❖ Classification
  - Fat Soluble—Vitamins A, D, E and K
  - Water Soluble—Thiamine (Vitamin B1), Riboflavin (Vitamin B2), Nicotinic Acid, Pyridoxine (Vitamin B6), Pantothenic Acid, Folic Acid, Vitamin B12, Ascorbic Acid (Vitamin C)
- ❖ Functions, Dietary Sources and Requirements
  - RDA of Every Vitamin

TERMINOLOGY

- **Beriberi:** A disease of the peripheral nerves caused by a dietary deficiency of thiamine (vitamin B1). Symptoms include fatigue, diarrhea, weight loss, edema, heart failure, and disturbed nerve function.
- **Coenzyme:** A nonprotein substance that combines with a protein molecule to form an active enzyme.
- **Enzymes:** Specialized proteins that catalyze biochemical reactions.
- **Fat-soluble vitamins:** Vitamins that can be dissolved (i.e., are soluble) in fat.
- **Minerals:** Inorganic substances that are ingested and attach to enzymes or other organic molecules.
- **Pellagra:** A disease resulting from a deficiency of niacin or a metabolic defect that interferes with the conversion of tryptophan to niacin (vitamin B3).
- **Rhodopsin:** The purple pigment in the rods of the retina, formed by a protein, opsin, and a derivative of retinol (vitamin A).
- **Rickets:** A condition caused by a deficiency of vitamin D.
- **Scurvy:** A condition resulting from a deficiency of ascorbic acid (vitamin C).
- **Tocopherols:** Biologically active chemicals that make up vitamin E compounds.
- **Vitamins:** Organic compounds essential in small quantities for normal physiologic and metabolic functioning of the body.
- **Water-soluble vitamins:** Vitamins that can be dissolved (i.e., are soluble) in water.
- **Chelating agents:** Drugs used to treat metal poisoning (e.g., from iron, lead, or mercury) that bind to the toxic metal, decrease binding of the metal within the body, and promote elimination of the metal.
- **Electrolytes:** Electrically charged particles found in body fluids and cells (e.g., sodium or potassium ions).
- **Enteral nutrition:** Provision of fluid and nutrients to a functional gastrointestinal tract via a feeding tube in a patient who is unable to ingest enough fluid and food.
- **Fat-soluble vitamins:** Vitamins that are accumulated and stored in the body when taken in excess.
- **Hyperkalemia:** Greater than normal amount of potassium in the blood.
- **Hypokalemia:** Less than normal amount of potassium in the blood.
- **Malabsorption:** Impaired absorption of nutrients from the gastrointestinal tract.
- **Megaloblastic anemia:** Anemia characterized by the presence in the blood of megaloblasts (large, abnormal blood cells); associated with vitamin B12 deficiency.
- **Megavitamins:** Large dose of vitamins in excess of the recommended dietary allowance.
- **Parenteral nutrition:** Intravenous provision of fluid and nutrients to a patient who is unable to ingest enough fluid and food due to a nonfunctional gastrointestinal tract.

INTRODUCTION

The word "vitamin" was coined in 1911 by the Warsaw-born biochemist Casimir Funk (1884–1967). At the Lister Institute in London, Funk isolated a substance that prevented nerve inflammation (neuritis) in chickens raised on a diet deficient in that substance. He named the substance "vitamine" because he believed it was necessary to life and it was a chemical amine. The "e" at the end was later removed when it was recognized that vitamins need not be amines.

The term 'vitamine' derives from the word 'vital amine', which means essential nitrogenous compounds. The term was coined by Polish scientist, Funk, who gave the name 'vitamine' to antiberiberi substance. Later on 'e' was dropped and thus the term 'vitamin' was coined. However, with the discovery of more vitamins, it was soon realized that all the

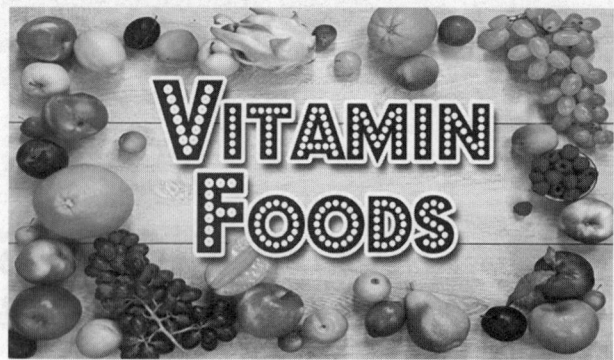

Fig. 5.1: Vitamin foods.

vitamins are not nitrogenous compounds; but all vitamins are essential for health. Vitamins are complex chemical substances, required by the body in very small amounts. They do not yield energy, but act as catalyst in various body processes. Since, vitamins cannot be manufactured in the body (at least in sufficient amounts) they have to be supplied through the diet. Vitamins are organic substances present in small amounts in food; they are required for carrying out vital functions of the body.

Figure 5.1 is depicted the vitamin foods.

CLASSIFICATIONS OF VITAMINS (FIG. 5.2)

Vitamins are involved in the utilization of the major nutrients, such as proteins, fats and carbohydrates. Though, needed in small amounts, they are essential for health and well-being of the body. When these vitamins were discovered on the basis of their function and before their chemical nature were elucidated, they were designated as, B, C and D or in terms of their major functions, such as, antineuritic, antirachitic vitamins.

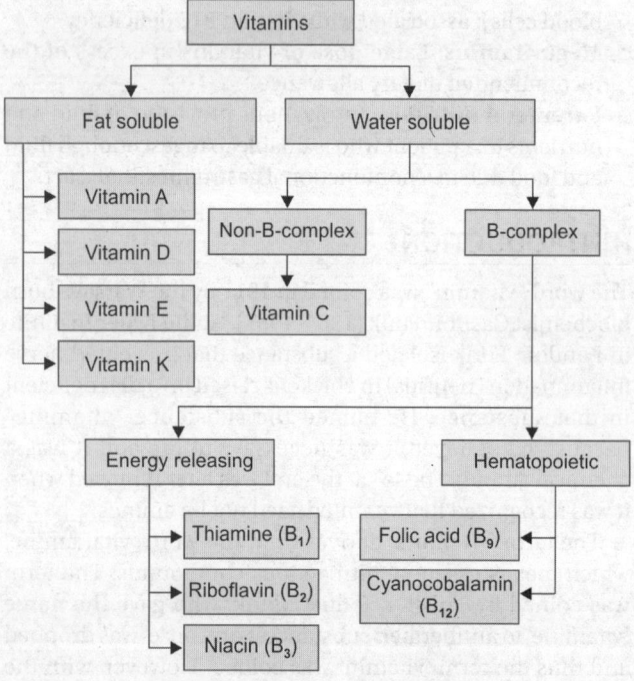

Fig. 5.2: Classifications of vitamins.

Table 5.1 is depicted the types of vitamins and their deficiency diseases.

Vitamins are classified based on their solubility as fat soluble and water-soluble vitamins. Vitamins may be defined as organic compounds occurring in small quantities in the different natural foods and necessary for the growth and maintenance of good health in human being and certain experimental animals. Vitamins may be classified into two group's:
1. Fat-soluble vitamins.
2. Water-soluble vitamins

Fat-soluble vitamins, e.g., vitamin A, D, E and K. Water-soluble vitamins viz vitamins of the B group and vitamin C

- **Vitamin B1:** Thiamin, acts as a coenzyme in body metabolism. Deficiency leads to beriberi, a disease of the heart and nervous system.
- **Vitamin B2:** Riboflavin, essential for the reactions of coenzymes. Deficiency causes inflammation of the lining of the mouth and skin.
- **Vitamin B3:** Niacin, an essential part of coenzymes of body metabolism. Deficiency causes inflammation of the skin, vagina, rectum and mouth, as well as mental slowing.
- **Vitamin B6:** Pyridoxine, a cofactor for enzymes. Deficiency leads to inflammation of the skin and mouth, nausea, vomiting, dizziness, weakness and anemia.

Table 5.1: Types of vitamins and their deficiency diseases.

Sl. No.	Name of vitamins	Sources	Deficiency disease
1.	Vitamin A	Fish liver oil, carrots, butter and milk	Xerophthalmia (hardening of cornea of eye), night blindness
2.	Vitamin B1 (Thiamine)	Yeast, milk, green vegetables and cereals	Beriberi (loss of appe-tite, retarded growth)
3.	Vitamin B2 (Riboflavin)	Milk, egg white, liver, kidney	Cheilosis (fissuring at corners of mouth and lips) digestive disorders and burning sensation of the skin
4.	Vitamin B6	Yeast, milk, egg yolk, cereals and grams	Convulsions
5.	Vitamin B12	Meat, fish, egg and curd	Pernicious anemia (RBC deficient in hemoglobin)
6.	Vitamin C (Ascorbic acid)	Cirtrus fruits, amla and green leafy vegetables	Scurvy (bleeding gums)
7.	Vitamin D	Exposure to sunlight, fish and egg yolk	Rickets (bone deformities in children) and osteomalacia (soft bones and joint pain in adults)
8.	Vitamin E	Vegetable oil, such as wheat germ oil, sunflower oil, etc.	Increased fragility of RBCs and muscular weakness
9.	Vitamin K	Green leafy vegetables	Increased blood clotting time

- **Folate (folic acid):** Folic acid is an important factor in nucleic acid synthesis (the genetic material). Folate deficiency leads to megaloblastic anemia.
- **Vitamin B12:** An essential factor in nucleic acid synthesis (the genetic material of all cells). Deficiency leads to megaloblastic anemia, as can be seen in pernicious anemia.
- **Vitamin C:** Ascorbic acid, important in the synthesis of collagen, the framework protein for tissues of the body. Deficiency leads to scurvy, characterized by fragile capillaries; poor wound healing, and bone deformity in children.
- **Vitamin D:** A steroid vitamin which promotes absorption and metabolism of calcium and phosphorus. Under normal conditions of sunlight exposure, no dietary supplementation is necessary because sunlight promotes adequate vitamin D synthesis in the skin. Deficiency can lead to osteomalacia in adults and bone deformity (rickets) in children.
- **Vitamin E:** Deficiency can lead to anemia.
- **Vitamin K:** An essential factor in the formation of blood clotting factors. Deficiency can lead to abnormal bleeding.

Table 5.2 is depicted the types of vitamin A and their deficiency diseases.

Table 5.2: Types of vitamin A and their deficiency diseases.

Vitamin/Function	Dietary reference intakes	Food sources	Signs and symptoms of deficiency	Signs and symptoms of excess
Fat-soluble vitamin				
Vitamin A (retinol)				
Required for normal vision, growth, bone development, skin and mucous membranes	RDAs **Females** 14 years and older, 700 µg Pregnancy, 750–770 µg Lactation, 1200–1300 µg **Males** 14 years and older, 900 µg **Children** 1–3 year, 300 µg 4–8 years, 400 µg 9–13 years, 600 µg **Infants** 0–6 months, 400 µg 6–12 months, 500 µg	Preformed vitamin A: • Meat, butter, fortified margarine, egg yolk, whole milk, cheese made from whole milk • Carotenoids turnip and collard greens, carrots, sweet potatoes, squash, apricots, peaches, cantaloupe	Night blindness: Xerophthalmia, which may progress to corneal ulceration and blindness; changes in skin and mucous membranes that lead to skin lesions and infections; respiratory tract infections; urinary calculi	• Anorexia, vomiting, irritability, skin changes (itching, desquamation, dermatitis); pain in muscles, bones, and joints; gingivitis; enlargement of spleen and liver; increased intracranial pressure; other neurological sings • Congenital abnormalities in newborns whose mothers took excessive vitamin A during pregnancy • Acute toxicity; with increased intracranial pressure, bulging fontanels, and vomiting, may occur in infants who are given vitamin A
Vitamin D **Vitamin E** Antioxidant Essential in preventing destruction of certain fats, including the lipid portion of cell membranes	RDAs **Females** 14 years and older, 15 mg Pregnancy, 15 mg Lactation, 19 mg **Males** 14 years and older, 15 mg **Children** 1–3 years, 6 mg 4–8 years, 7 mg 9–13 years, 11 mg **Infants** 0–6 months, 4 mg 7–12 months, 5 mg Older adults, 1500 international unit	Cereal, green leafy vegetables, egg yolk, milk fat, butter, meat, vegetable oils	Deficiency is rare	Fatique, headache, blurred vision; nausea, diarrhea

Contd...

Contd...

Vitamin/Function	Dietary reference intakes	Food sources	Signs and symptoms of deficiency	Signs and symptoms of excess
Vitamin K Essential for normal blood clotting. It activates precursor proteins, found in the liver, into clotting factors II, VII, IX and X	RDAs **Females** 19 years and older, 90 μg Pregnancy, 90 μg If 14–18 years, 75 μg Lactation, 90 μg If 14–18 years, 75 μg **Males** 19 years and older, 120 μg **Children** 1–3 y, 30 μg 4–8 y, 55 μg 9–13 y, 60 μg 14–18 y, 55 μg	Green leafy vegetables (spinach, kale, cabbage, lettuce), cauliflower, tomatoes, wheat bran, cheese, egg yolk, liver	Abnormal bleeding (petechiae, ecchymoses, epistaxis, hematemesis, melena, hematuria, hypovolemic shock)	Clinical manifestations rare; however, when vitamin K is given to someone who is receiving warfarin (Coumadin), the patient can be made "warfarin-resistant" for 2–3 week

Table 5.3: Difference between fat-soluble and water-soluble vitamins.

Water-soluble vitamins	Fat-soluble vitamins
Meaning	
As the name states—vitamins that can dissolve in water are called water-soluble vitamins	Similarly, vitamins that dissolve in fat are called fat-soluble vitamins
Example	
Vitamin B, C	Vitamin A, D, E, K
Site of absorption	
Small intestine	Small intestine
Affinity to water	
Hydrophilic	Hydrophobic
How body handles excess	
Excess vitamins are excreted by the kidney	Excess is stored in the body's fatty tissues
Transportation	
Travels freely in the bloodstream	Many vitamins require carriers (proteins) to travel in the blood
Toxicity	
Low toxicity	Comparatively more toxic
Deficiency	
Symptoms appear rather quickly	Symptoms take time to manifest

Difference between Fat-soluble and Water-soluble Vitamins

Vitamin is an organic molecule that the body needs for growth and development. It is a micronutrient and is primarily acquired through food as it cannot be synthesized within an organism. There are many vitamins and they are classified into water-soluble and fat-soluble vitamins. Read on to explore the differences between the two **(Table 5.3)**.

FAT-SOLUBLE VITAMINS (FIG. 5.3)

Fat-soluble vitamins, including vitamins A, D and E, are required for a wide variety of physiological functions. Over the past two decades, deficiencies of these vitamins have been associated with increased risk of cancer, type II diabetes mellitus and a number of immune system disorders. In addition, there is increasing evidence of interactions between these vitamins, especially between vitamins A and D. As a result of this enhanced clinical association with disease, translational clinical research and laboratory requests for vitamin measurements have significantly increased.

These laboratory requests include measurement of 25-OHD (vitamin D), retinol (vitamin A) and α-tocopherol (vitamin E); the most accepted blood indicators for the assessment of body fat-soluble vitamin (FSV) status. There are significant obstacles to precise FSV measurement in blood. These obstacles include their physical and chemical properties, incomplete standardization of measurement and limitations in the techniques that are currently used for quantification.

Vitamin A

Vitamin A occurs only in foods of animal origin. Vitamin A activity is also possessed by carotenoids found in plants. Hence, carotenoids are called provitamin A.
- Vitamin-A combined with vitamin E deficiency reduces production.min A is not synthesized in the body and must by supplied by food supplements.
- One of the best defined roles of vitamin A is its requirements for normal vision.
- Vitamin A is necessary for the health of the epithelial cells. Vitamin A was the first fat-soluble vitamin to be recognized.
- Three forms of vitamin A are active in the body, retinol, retinal and retinoic acid. They are collectively called as retinoids.
- Beta-carotene is the provitamin of vitamin A. Provitamins are substances that are chemically related to a vitamin, but must be changed by the body into the active form of the vitamin.
- Vitamin A in the diet comes in two forms. Retenoids (preformed vitamin A) and carotenoids vitamin A is present in vegetable foods, which contain yellow pigment called carotenes.
- It was isolated from carrots hence called carotenoids, which are provitamins of vitamin A.

Nutrients	What it does to our bodies	In which foods can I find it	How much do I need on a daily basis
Fat-soluble			
Vitamin A	Helps in maintaining good vision. Good for overall growth and development of teeth, skin, white blood cells and the mucous membrane	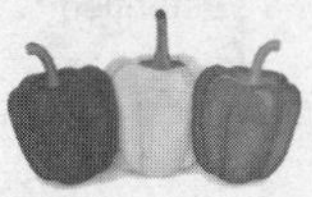 • Sweet potato • Carrots • Sweet peppers • Apricots	At least 350 µg (men) and 350 µg (women) ...less than a teaspoon...
Vitamin D	Essential for the absorption of calcium and phosphorus. Also helps in the maintenance of healthy bones and teeth	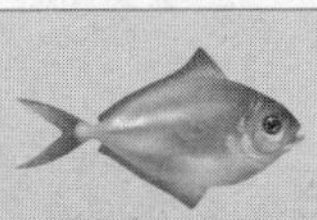 • Tuna • Salmon • Sardines • Mackerel	At least 400 IU or 10 µg (men) and 400 IU or 10 µg (women) ...less than a teaspoon...
Vitamin E	Helps to reduce free radicals in the body and thus prevents the development of diseases as it is a powerful antioxidant. It also helps in balancing hormones and cholesterol levels	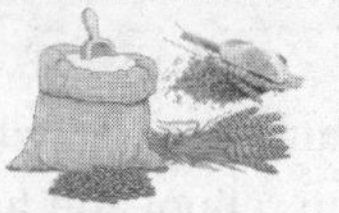 • Wheat germ • Avocado • Spinach • Butternut squash	At least 6 IU or 4 mg (men) and 6 IU or 4 mg (women) ...less than a teaspoon...
Vitamin K	Helps the blood to clot. It is also essential for bone and heart health	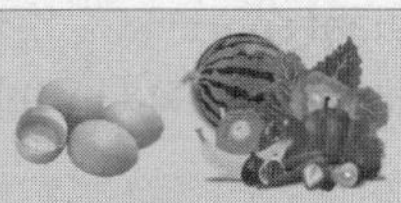 • Collard greens • Parsley • Grapes • Hard boiled eggs	At least 55 µg (men) and 55 µg (women) ...less than a teaspoon..

Fig. 5.3: Fat-soluble vitamins.

Chemistry

- **Vitamin A occurs in several forms:** As retinol, as retinal, as an aldehyde and as retinoic acid. These several forms may be referred to as vitamin A. In its pure form, vitamin A is a pale-yellow crystalline compound and occurs naturally in animals.

  Figure 5.4 is depicted the health benefits of vitamin A.

- It is soluble in fat solvents, but insoluble in water and is relatively stable to heat, acids and alkalies. It is easily oxidized and rapidly destroyed by ultraviolet radiation.
- The ultimate source of all vitamin A is in the carotenes, which are synthesized by plants.

  Figure 5.5 is depicted the vitamin A role in eye.

- Animals, as well as man in turn convert a considerable portion of carotene of the foods they eat into vitamin A.
- Carotenes are dark-red crystalline compounds also known as 'Provitamin A' or 'precursors of vitamin A'.
- Alpha, beta, gamma, molecules of carotene are of significance in nutrition. Each molecule of beta-carotene yields two molecules of vitamin A.

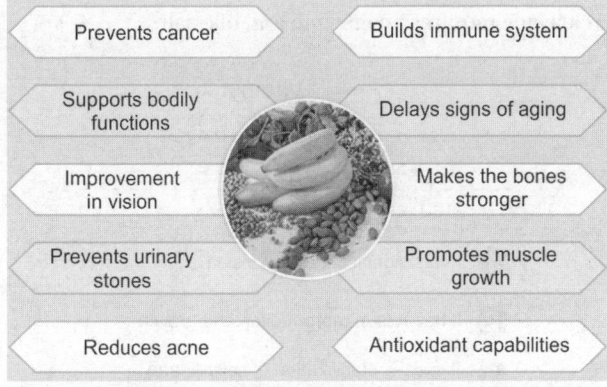

Fig. 5.4: Health benefits of vitamin A.

Absorption, Transport and Storage

Absorption

- Vitamin A is usually complexes with proteins. Before vitamin A can be absorbed, it is hydrolyzed by proteases and pancreatic enzymes to form free retinol.

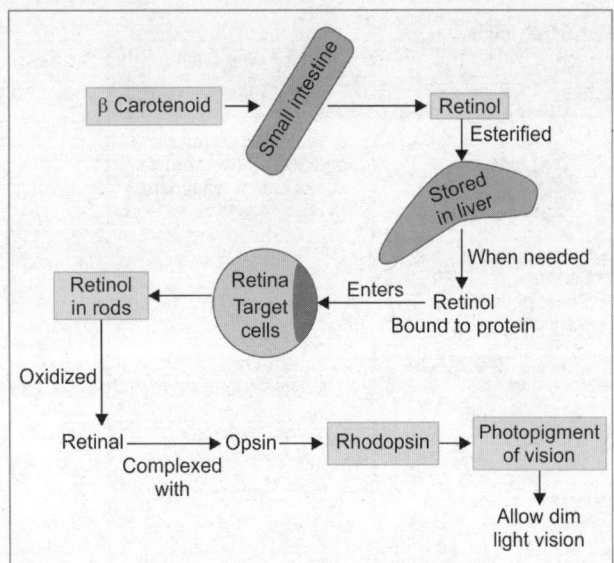

Fig. 5.5: Vitamin A role in eye.

- In addition to this retinyl esters must also be hydrolyzed by lipases in the small intestine to retinol and free fatty acids.
- Vitamin A is absorbed in two forms—as the retinol, which is the preformed vitamin A from animal source and as carotene, which is a precursor from plant sources.
- The absorption of vitamin A and carotene is aided by bile salts, pancreatic lipase and fat.
- After it is absorbed into the mucosal cells, retinol is re-esterified to retinyl esters and these esters are incorporated into chylomicrons for transport through the lymph and eventually the blood stream by way of thoracic duct.
- Carotenes are cleaved in the intestinal mucosa into retinaldehyde, which is then reduced to retinol. This cleavage requires an enzyme and bile salt.

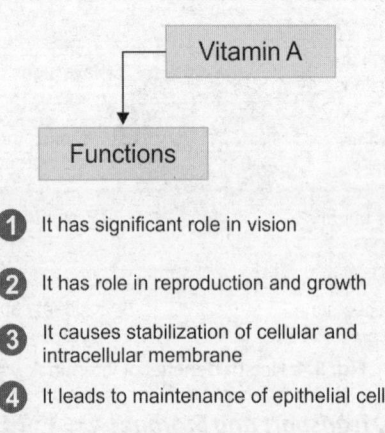

- The conversion of dietary carotene chiefly takes place in the intestine, but some carotene is converted in liver or kidney also. The absorption of vitamin A and carotene follows the same route as that of fat.

Factors affecting vitamin a absorption
- The absorption of vitamin A is seriously affected when the diet contains very low fat or when there is an obstruction of the bile duct.
- The presence of vitamin E in the intestinal tract prevents the excessive oxidation of vitamin A, thus making it available for absorption.
- The presence of mineral oil reduces the absorption because mineral oil itself is not absorbed; it carries vitamin A as well as other fat-soluble vitamins with it. Mineral oil which is used as a laxative should be taken at or around mealtime.
- In premature infants the absorption is poor.
- During protein-energy malnutrition the absorption may be affected due to lack of carrier protein. They have typically low circulating retinol and may not respond to vitamin A supplementation unless protein-energy malnutrition is treated

Transport and storage
- After the absorption of preformed retinol from animal and plant sources, carotene conversion is re-esterified with long-chain fatty acids in the intestinal mucosa.
- Vitamin A is incorporated into the chylomicrons. It enters the bloodstream through the lymphatic system and finally carried to the liver for storage from where it is distributed to the cells as required.
- Liver stores vitamin A (retinol) as retinyl esters in lipid droplets. These retinyl esters are then hydrolyzed and free retinol is bound to a carrier protein, retinol-binding protein (RBP) and is delivered to cells.
- About 90% of vitamin A in the body is found in the liver alone and the remainder is present in the kidney, lungs, adrenal glands and adipose tissue. An average healthy adult stores enough vitamin A for several months to a year.
- These liver stores are reduced during periods of infectious disease. Infants and children do have such reserves; therefore they are more susceptible to develop deficiency symptoms.
- Vitamin A and its products formed on hydrolysis are excreted mainly in the bile. Some amount of vitamin A is reabsorbed, but most of it is excreted in the feces. Some of these products may be excreted in the urine also.

Figure 5.6 is depicted the foods rich in vitamin A and **Figure 5.7** is depicted the importance of vitamin A.

Functions

Vision
- The role of vitamin A in visual process is well-understood, It maintains the normal vision in dim light. There are two types of light receptors in the retina of the eye—the rods for vision in dim light and the cones for vision in bright light and color vision.

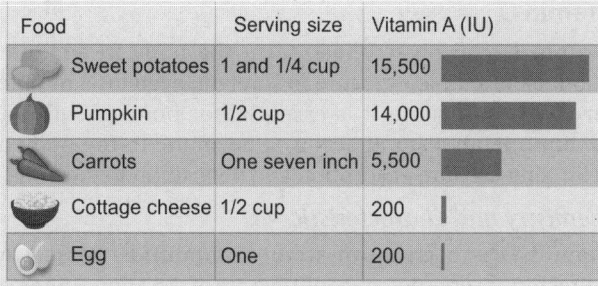

Fig. 5.6: Foods rich in vitamin A.

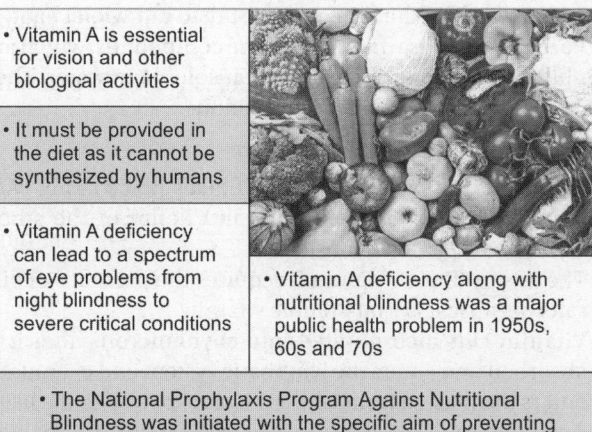

Fig. 5.7: Importance of vitamin A.

- The rods produce rhodopsin or visual purple, a photosensitive pigment and cones produce iodopsin or visual violet. When the light strikes the eye, the rhodopsin is split into its component parts, retinaldehyde (retinal) and protein opsin.
- Due to these changes nerve impulse is initiated, which is then transmitted to the brain by way of optic nerve.
- Rhodopsin is regenerated in the dark, but some retinaldehyde is lost in each cycle, therefore, it becomes necessary to maintain constant supply from the blood.
- Inadequate supply of vitamin A for the synthesis of rhodopsin causes night blindness or nyctalopia.

Maintenance of epithelial tissue
- Vitamin A is associated with the maintenance of healthy tissue covering. It makes the linings of the outside of the body and inside cavities smooth.
- In the presence of adequate amounts of vitamin A, they form columnar, goblet-cells mucus secretion, but in the deficiency of vitamin A, they are keratinized.
- This secret mucus that coats and protects the surface from invasive microorganisms and other harmful particles.
- The mucus lining of the stomach protects itself from digestion by the gastric juices.
- Vitamin A plays a role in maintaining the integrity of cell membranes. It is also essential for healthy skin.

Maintenance of bone growth
- Vitamin A is essential for normal development of skeleton, teeth and soft tissues.
- When vitamin A is deficient, bones do not grow in length and the normal remodeling process does not occur.
- Vitamin A plays an important role of removing old bones and makes way for the new ones.

Reproduction
- Vitamin A is also essential for normal reproduction. It is necessary for spermatogenesis in the males and normal estrous cycle in the females.
- In the absence of vitamin A (retinol and retinal) during fetal development various malformations occur, it also causes sterility and testicular degeneration in males and abortions in females.

Antioxidant
- Beta-carotene (provitamin A) acts as an antioxidant. It has the ability to protect persons from cell damage caused by free radicals.
- These antioxidants neutralize free radicals in the cells thus protecting the persons from oxidative stress.
- These free radicals are the byproducts of normal metabolism in cells or they are created by the exposure to sun light, tobacco smoke, fumes from vehicles or X-rays.
- These free radicals also damage the DNA, cell membranes and cell compounds. Refer to **Table 5.4** for antioxidant rich foods.

Other roles
Some not well-understood roles include helps in the synthesis of corticosterone hormone by the adrenal gland; ensures normal output of thyroid hormone (thyroxin) from the thyroid gland; helps in maintaining nerve cell sheaths; assist in immune reactions; helps in synthesizing red blood cells.

Sources
- Vitamin A in the human diet exists as retinol or as retinal or beta-carotene, which has to be converted to Vitamin A.

Table 5.4: Antioxidant rich foods.

Vitamin	Resources	Deficiency diseases	Symptoms
Vitamin A (retinol)	Leafy vegetables, carrot, tomato, pumpkin, papaya, mango, meat, fish, egg, liver, milk, cod liver oil, shark liver oil	Eye, skin diseases	Night blindness, xerophthalmia, cornea failure, scaly skin
Vitamin D (calciferol)	Liver, egg, better, cod liver oil, shark liver oil, (morning sun rays)	Rickets	Improper formation of bones, knocknees, swollen wrists, delayed dentition, weak bones
Vitamin E (tocopherol)	Fruits, vegetables, sprouts, meat egg, sunflower oil	Fertility disorders	Sterility in males, abortion in females
Vitamin K (Phylloquinone)	Green leafy vegetables, milk	Blood clotting	Delay in blood clotting, over bleeding

- Foods of animal origin contain retinol. Plant sources are rich in beta-carotene. Only one third of the dietary beta-carotene is absorbed.
- Beta-carotene from green leafy vegetables is well-utilized than from carrots and papayas.
- Good sources of vitamin A are sheep liver, butter, ghee, egg, milk, curds, liver oils of shark and halibut.
- Good sources of beta carotene are agathi, amaranth, drumstick leaves, green leafy vegetables, mango, papaya and carrot and jack fruit.

Effects of Deficiency

Deficiency of vitamin A is manifested as nutritional blindness and increased susceptibility to infection. Nutritional blindness is an important public health problem among young children in India.

Night blindness (Fig. 5.8)
- This is an early symptom of vitamin A deficiency. The individual cannot see in dim light. This can be corrected with adequate supply of vitamin A.
- In the absence of adequate vitamin A intake the outer lining of the eye ball loses its usual moist, white appearance and becomes dry and wrinkled called xerosis. This condition is followed by raised muddy dry triangular patches on the conjunctiva called the bitot's spots.
- Redness and inflammation of the eye and gradual loss of vision may follow. The central portion of the eye loses its transparency and becomes opaque and soft, if not treated and leads to total blindness termed xerophthalmia.
- Xerophthalmia encompasses all ocular manifestations of Vitamin A deficiency.
- Increased susceptibility to infection occurs because the mucous membrane lining becomes dry and rough, which is easily invaded by the microorganism.

Hypervitaminosis

Intake of large amount of vitamin A for prolonged periods can lead to toxic symptoms, which include irritability, headache, nausea and vomiting.

Vitamin D

Vitamin D can be synthesized in the body in adequate amounts by simple exposure to sunlight, even for 5 minutes per day is sufficient. It is essential for bone growth and calcium metabolism. It acts as a hormone in the body by facilitating calcium absorption and deposition in the bone.

Chemistry and Characteristic

Vitamin D is a group of sterol compounds possessing antirachitic properties, but only two are of nutritional interest.
1. Vitamin D2 or ergocalciferol found in a plants.
2. Vitamin D3 or cholecalciferol, which occurs in animal cells and activates in the skin on exposure to ultraviolet light.

Pure vitamin D is white, crystalline compounds, which are soluble in fats and fat solvents, but insoluble in water. They are stable to heat, alkalies and oxidation.

Absorption, Transport and Storage

- Absorption of dietary vitamin D takes place along with other lipids into the jejunum and ileum of the small intestine by passive diffusion.
- The absorption of vitamin D requires the presence of bile salts because it is a fat-soluble vitamin.
- Vitamin D is incorporated into chylomicrons after it is absorbed and enters the lymphatic system and eventually enters the plasma from where it is transported to the liver.
- Any conditions, which interfere with fat absorption, will hinder the complete absorption of vitamin D.
- These conditions include pancreatitis, sprue, and colitis and malabsorption syndrome.
- The vitamin D made in the skin from cholesterol enters the blood and is transported by vitamin D binding protein (DBP) to the peripheral tissues.
- Small amount of vitamin D is stored in the liver. The major pathway of vitamin D excretion is through the bile. Daily losses of vitamin D in the urine are very small.

Figure 5.9 is depicted the vitamin D in the body.

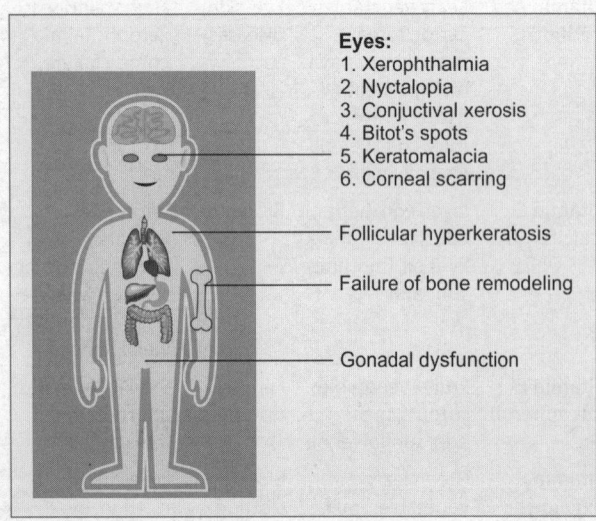

Fig. 5.8: Night blindness.

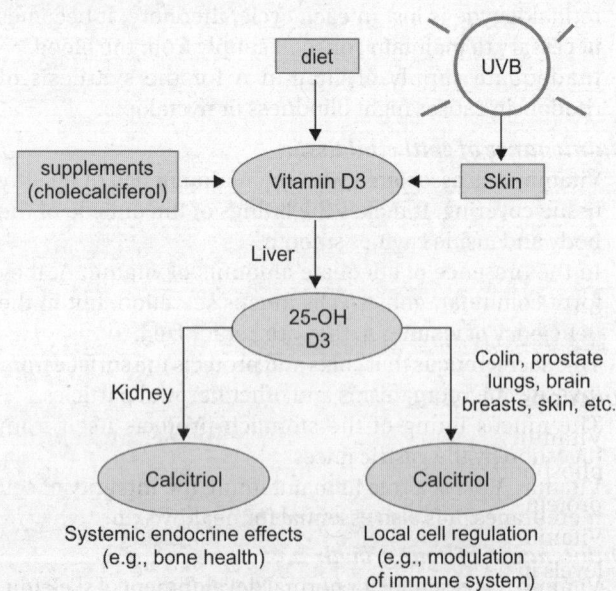

Fig. 5.9: Vitamin D in the body.

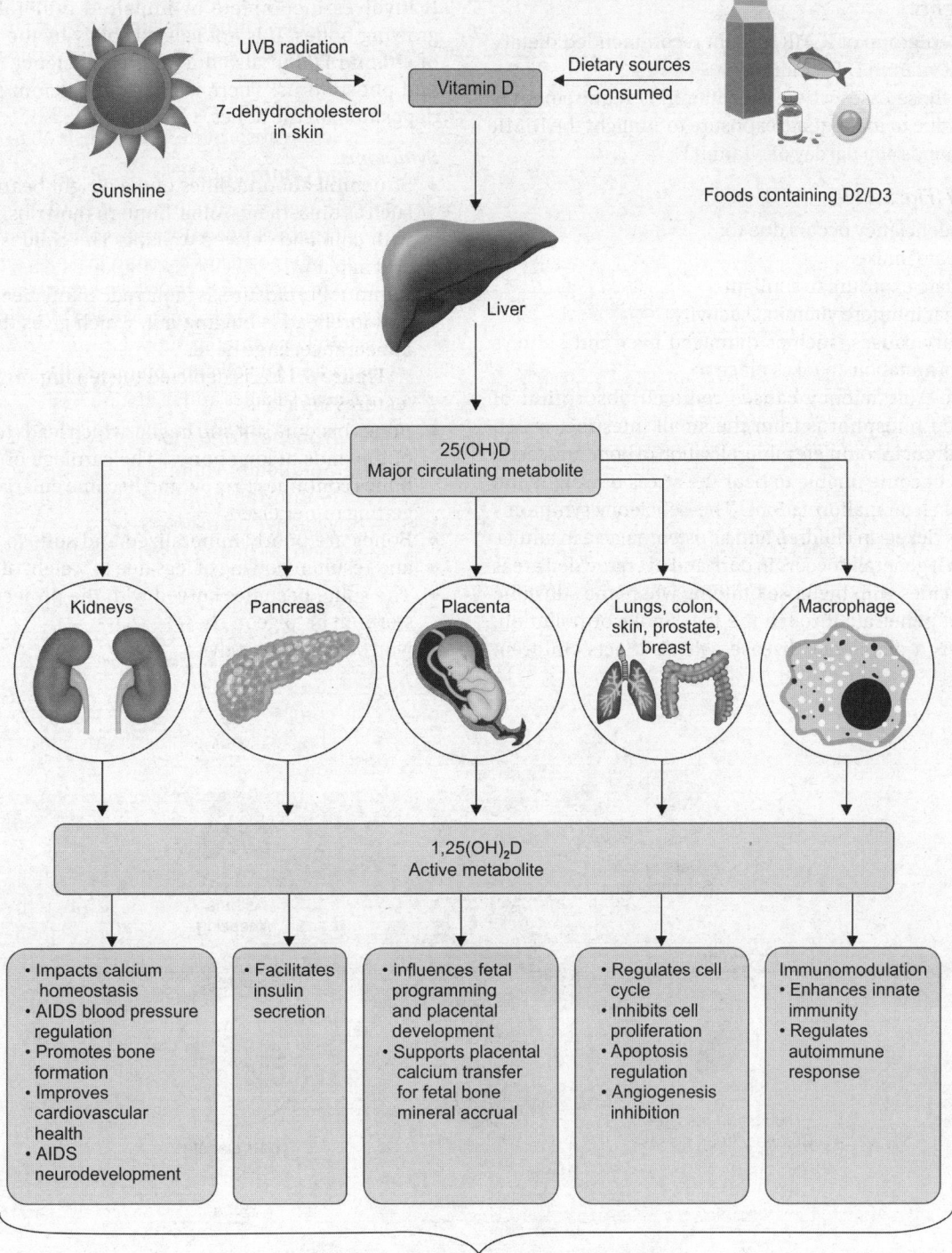

Fig. 5.10: Biological functions of vitamin D.

Functions (Fig. 5.10)

❑ Vitamin D helps in the absorption of calcium and phosphorus by increasing the synthesis of calcium binding protein.
❑ Vitamin D helps to maintain the calcium and phosphorus levels in the body by stimulating.
  ● Absorption in the gastrointestinal tract.
  ● Retention by the kidney.

❑ Vitamin D helps in deposition of calcium in the bones. The bones grow denser and stronger.

Food Sources

❑ The vitamin D content of food sources from animals varies with the diet, breed and exposure to sunlight of the animal.
❑ The good sources of vitamin D are cod liver oil, shrimp, liver, butter, yolk, cheese, milk, spinach and cabbage.

Requirements

- The expert group of ICMR has not recommended dietary intake of vitamin D for Indians.
- Only in those cases where the vitamin D requirement is not met due to inadequate exposure to sunlight the ICMR recommends 400 µg/day of vitamin D.

Deficiency (Fig. 5.11)

Vitamin D deficiency occurs due to:
- Inadequate intake
- Inadequate exposure to sunlight
- Drugs that interfere vitamin D activity
- Secondary causes, such as damaged liver and kidneys where its metabolism takes place

Vitamin D deficiency causes reduced absorption of calcium and phosphorus from the small intestine, which leads to faulty or incomplete mineralization of bone and teeth. Soft bones become unable to bear the stress of weight and results in skeletal malformations. The deficiency symptoms manifest as rickets in children and as osteomalacia in adults.

- **Rickets:** It generally occurs in dark and overcrowded areas of large cities with high rise building where the sunshine does not penetrate through the fog, smoke or pollution. Rickets is a deficiency disease, which affects children. It involves incomplete or impaired mineralization of growing bones. It is not caused solely by the deficiency of vitamin D, but also due to the deficiency of calcium and phosphorus. There is a lack of calcium phosphate deposition on the bones.

Symptoms:
- Structural abnormalities of the weight bearing-bones, such as tibia, radius, ulna, humerus and ribs, associated with pain and delayed walking. The child is miserable and in pain.
- Fontanelle closure is delayed. Skull becomes soft and forehead is bulging out, which gives the box-like appearance; large head.

Figure 5.12 is is depicted the ten important clinical features in rickets.

- Bones become soft and fragile, which leads to widening of the ends of long bones. The cartilage of the end of bones continues to grow and become enlarged without getting mineralized.
- Bones are poorly mineralized and soft, so they bend and result in bowing of legs due to weight of the body.
- The spine becomes curved with the projection of the sternum or 'pigeon chest'.
- Narrowing of the pelvis.

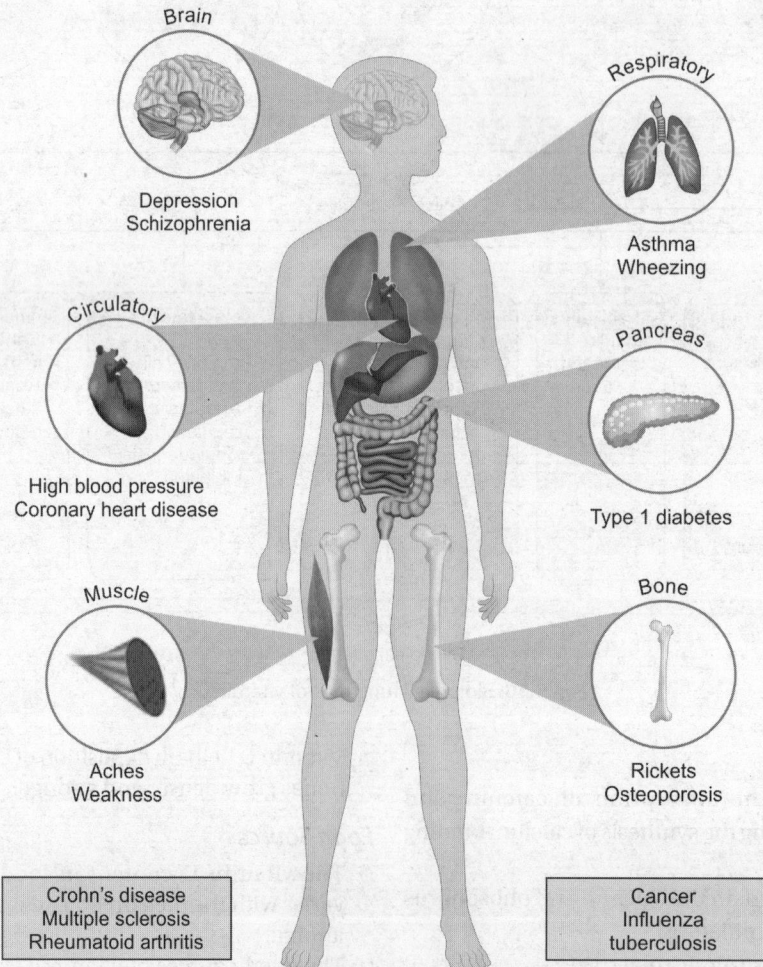

Fig. 5.11: Vitamin D deficiency.

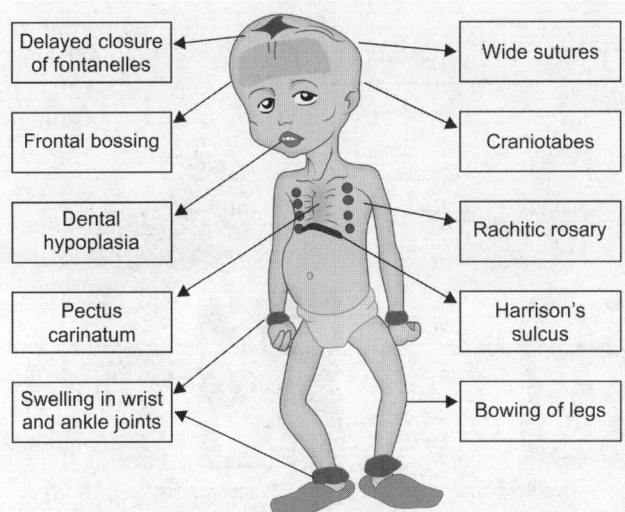

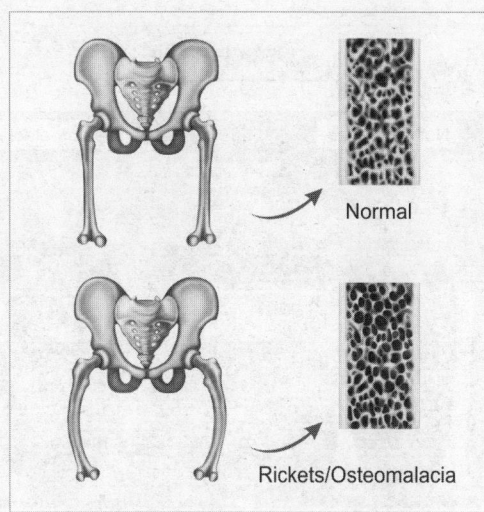

Fig. 5.12: Ten important clinical features in rickets.

Fig. 5.13: Features of osteomalacia.

- Joints of wrist, knees (knock-knees) and ankle are enlarged. The gait becomes waddling due to bowed legs or knock- knees.
- Patients show elevated plasma and serum levels of alkaline phosphatase.
- Restlessness and nervous irritability.
- Neuromuscular irritability. Underdeveloped muscles and lack of muscle tone. Pot belly due to weakness of abdominal muscles.

Causes
- It affects those children who reside in dark and overcrowded areas of large cities where ultraviolet rays of sunshine do not reach due to thick fog, smoke, etc.
- Poverty and failure to obtain required vitamin D concentrates or skin exposure.
- Dark-skinned children are more prone to rickets as compared to white skinned people because the skin pigmentation inhibits the penetration of ultraviolet rays.
- Premature infants are more prone to developing rickets than full-term infants. This is because the growth rate and skeletal calcification impose additional demands for vitamin D.

Treatment:
Rickets can be treated effectively by giving relatively large amounts of vitamin D concentrates orally or by giving vitamin D from natural sources, such as fish-liver oil. Fish-liver oil contains 9 ug (360 IU) of vitamin D.

- **Osteomalacia:** Osteomalacia means bone softening. It is similar to rickets but develops in adults so often refer to as 'adult rickets'. Due to the deficiency of vitamin D and calcium bone mineral density decreases. This deficiency occurs mostly in women who have insufficient calcium intake and little exposure to sunlight. It is also seen in women who have repeated pregnancies in quick succession and periods of lactation and also due to malabsorption of vitamin D. In osteomalacia, lack of calcium phosphate deposition decreases bone mineral content.

Figure 5.13 is depicted the features of osteomalacia.

Symptoms
- Skeletal pain of the rheumatic type especially in bones of the legs and lower back.
- Bone tenderness and spontaneous multiple fractures.
- Muscular weakness with difficulty in walking and climbing.
- Softening of the bones. The bones of the legs, spine, thorax and pelvis may bend and cause deformities.

Causes
- Little exposure to sunlight. Women observing purdah, clothing, which completely shields them from sunlight and dietary calcium is not absorbed properly, ultimately leads to vitamin D deficiency.
- Interference with fat absorption, hence vitamin D absorption also.
- Steatorrhea also reduces the absorption of calcium.
- Chronic renal failure and disease of the parathyroid and liver. Because in the complicated process involved in the metabolism of vitamin D, any liver and kidney disease can lead to bone deterioration. Chronic kidney disease can cause osteomalacia because of the inability of kidneys to convert vitamin D to its active form. Patient on dialysis are frequently prescribed vitamin D supplementation.
- Diet inadequate in calcium.
- Repeated pregnancies and prolonged lactation reduces the body reserves.
- Having dark skin.
- Consumption of cereal grains having high-phytate content hinders calcium absorption.
- Premature infants.
- Elderly people who are housebound.
- Those treated with anticonvulsants

Treatment:
Osteomalacia can be effectively treated with vitamin D3 secondary causes can be treated accordingly.

Prevention
The occurrence of osteomalacia can be prevented with adequate intake of vitamin D, calcium and phosphorus

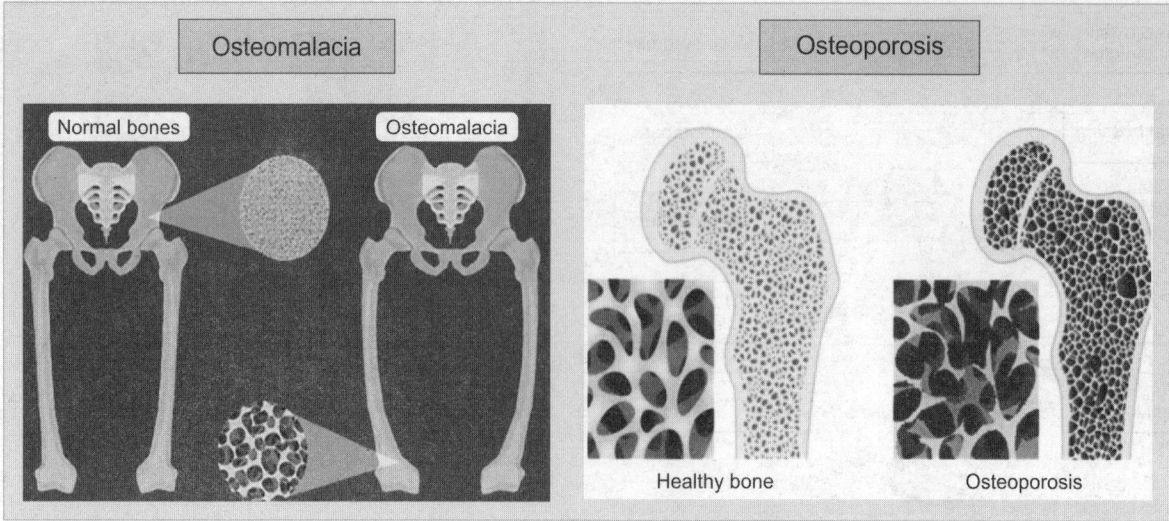

Fig. 5.14: Difference between osteomalacia and osteoporosis.

in the diet. Moderate exposure (10–15 minutes) to sun on a clear sunny day, 2–3 times a week, is enough to prevent osteomalacia.

Figure 5.14 is depicted the difference between osteomalacia and osteoporosis.

- **Osteoporosis:** Osteoporosis is often confused with osteomalacia, but they are very different from each other. In osteoporosis, bone mass is decreased, but the histologic appearance is normal. It is associated with aging.
  - It involves impaired vitamin D metabolism and is associated with low-estrogen levels.
  - This disease is chronic and is most commonly seen in postmenopausal women, but may develop in older men also. It is a decrease in the total bone mass.
  - The onset of the disease is quite gradual and it is asymptomatic in the early stages.
  - The causes of osteoporosis are thought to be multifactorial, but it is also associated with aging.
  - It involves diminished vitamin D metabolism and decreased estrogen levels.
  - It is commonly seen in postmenapausal women and is a major cause of bone fracture.
  - Osteoporosis can be prevented by increase intake of dietary calcium and moderate exercise daily (walking), which improves the calcium status in women.
  - Current approaches include hormonal therapy with estrogen and vitamin D hormone.
  - Prevention must start in youth because it is late when it is diagnosed and the treatment has little effect on reversing the disease, partly because reduced calcium absorption in elderly.
  - Osteoporosis can be treated with hormone replacement therapy in early menopausal women.

Toxicity:
- Massive doses of vitamin D can be dangerous. High intake of vitamin D may cause reabsorption of calcium from the bones resulting in localized osteoporosis.
- Hypervitaminosis D is characterized by hypercalcemia and hyperphosphatemia.
- The common symptoms include headache, nausea, vomiting, diarrhea, excessive thirst, weight loss, polyuria, nocturia (excessive urination at night) and constipation.
- Laboratory tests and history of excessive intake are the basis for diagnosis.
- This can be treated with low-calcium diet, plenty of fluids and stopping vitamin D intake.

Vitamin E

Vitamin E is the generic name for a group of closely related and naturally occurring fat soluble compounds, the tocopherols of these alpha–tocopherol is biologically the most potent. Vitamin E is widely distributed in foods. The usual plasma level of vitamin E in adult is between 0.8 and 1.4 mg per 100 mL. Vitamin E is known as antisterility vitamin because it is required for normal reproduction in animals and men.

Chemistry and Characteristic

- Vitamin E consists of a group of chemical substances called 'tocopherols'.
- Alpha-tocopherol is the compound possessing the greatest vitamin E activity.
- High temperature and acids do not affect the stability of this vitamin, but oxidation takes places in the presence of rancid fats or lead and iron salts.
- Decomposition occurs in ultraviolet light, alkalies and oxygen

Figure. 5.15 is depicted the benefits of vitamin E and **Figure 5.16** is depicted the top ten foods highest in vitamin E.

Absorption, Transport and Storage

- Vitamin E, such as any other fat-soluble vitamin and fat, is absorbed with the help of pancreatic secretions and bile salts.
- The absorption occurs mainly in the upper small intestine by micelle-dependent diffusion. The presence of dietary fat is essential for its absorption.

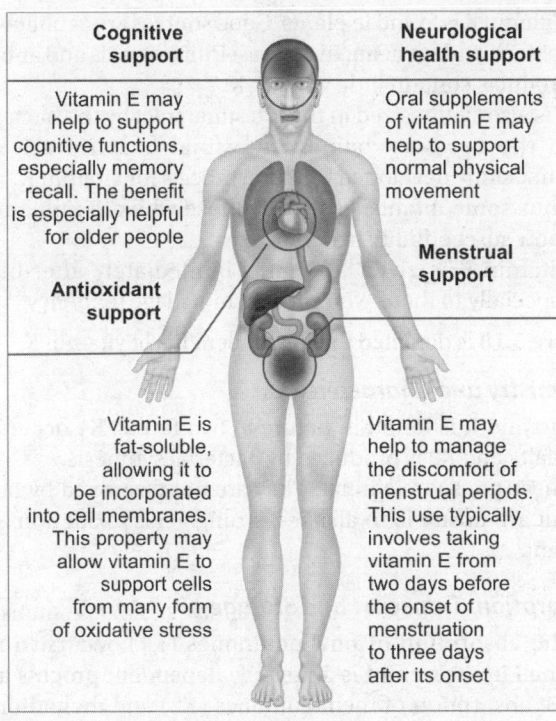

Fig. 5.15: Benefits of vitamin E.

- The absorbed vitamin E are repackaged in the chylomicrons and transported by way of the lymphatic system into the general circulation.
- Vitamin E is incorporated into VLDLs and delivered to the liver and this uses a transport protein specific for vitamin E.
- The absorption of vitamin E is hindered by the presence of fatty diarrhea, celiac disease, intestinal resection and absence of bile.
- Vitamin E is stored in the liver and adipose tissue. A very small amount is excreted in the urine with the normal intake.

Functions

- Vitamin E is the primary antioxidant in the body and serves to protect polyunsaturated fatty acids (PUFA) from oxidation in cells and maintain integrity of the cell membrane. It also prevents the oxidation of beta-carotene and vitamin A. vitamin E helps to maintain cell membrane integrity and protect red blood cells (RBC) against hemolysis.
- Vitamin E reduces platelet aggregation.
- Vitamin E is essential for the iron metabolism and the maintenance of nervous tissues and immune function.
- Vitamin E been promoted as an antiaging vitamin because as cells age they accumulate lipid breakdown products. Vitamin E prevents this accumulation in maintaining cell health.

Box 5.1 is depicted the biochemical functions of vitamin E.

Food Sources

- Vitamin E is widely distributed in foods. It is present in high concentration in vegetable oils and in cereal grains.

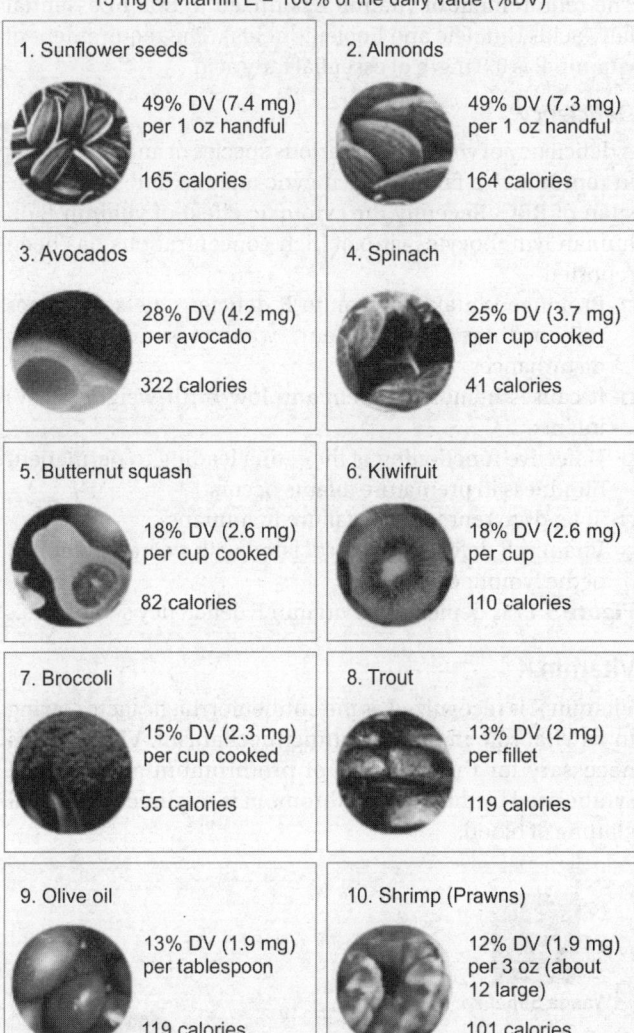

Fig. 5.16: Top ten foods highest in vitamin E.

Box 5.1: Biochemical functions of vitamin E.

Biochemical function of vitamin E are related with its antioxidant property
- Prevents sterility and closely associated with reproductive functions (maintains germinal epithelium of gonads)
- Essential for membrane structure and integrity of cell: a membrane antioxidant (vitamin E-lipophilic in nature) stored in a cell membrane along with lipoproteins and lipids → prevents lipid peroxidation
- Protects RBC from hemolysis by free radicals
- Enhances activity of α aminolevulinic acid (ALA) synthase and ALA dehydratase → enhances heme synthesis
- Required for cellular respiration through electron transport chain (stabilizes coenzyme Q)

- Wheat gum, sunflower seeds, almonds, safflower oil, eggs, butter are good sources.
- Meat, fruits and vegetables contain small amounts. Sesame oil and mustard oil are good sources of vitamin E.

Requirement

The requirement of vitamin E is linked to that of essential fatty acids (linoleic and linolenic acids). The requirement of vitamin E is 0.8 mg/g of essential fatty acid.

Deficiency

A deficiency of vitamin E in various species of animals results in reproductive failure, macrocytic anemia and shorter life span of RBC. Recently the cytotoxic effect of vitamin E on human lymphocytes vitro at high concentrations has been reported.

- Prolonged intake of vitamin E deficient diets produces uncoordinated movement, weakness and sensory disturbances.
- It causes hemolytic anemia in low-birth-weight (LBW) infants.
- Defective functioning of the retina leading to permanent blindness in premature infants occurs.
- It leads to reproductive failure in humans.
- Vitamin E deficiency is associated with decreased ability of the lymphocytes.

Figure 5.17 is depicted the vitamin E deficiency symptoms.

Vitamin K

Vitamin K is recognized as the antihemorrhagic factor owing to its vital role in blood clotting mechanism. Vitamin K is necessary for the synthesis of prothrombin and enzyme synthesized by the liver; prothrombin is required for normal clotting of blood.

- Vitamin K is found in plants. Good sources are cauliflower, spinach and soybean. In contrast fruits, cereals and animal products contain little vitamin K.
- It is also synthesized in the intestinal tract by the bacteria. In the newborn babies, intestinal bacteria are not sufficiently developed for the synthesis for vitamin K.
- Thus some infants, especially those who are immature, show susceptibility to hemorrhage.
- Vitamin K is given to infants immediately after birth especially to those who show hemorrhage tendency.

Figure 5.18 is depicted the health benefits of vitamin K.

Chemistry and Characteristics

- Vitamin K is found in nature in two forms: K1 occurs in alfalfa and K2 is produced by bacterial synthesis.
- These are soluble in fat. They are not destroyed by heat, but are unstable to alkalies, strong acids, oxidation and light.

Absorption, Transport and Storage

- The absorption of phylloquinones (K1) occurs in the small intestine and is an energy dependent process and the absorption of menaquinones (K2) and menadiones (K3) takes place in the small intestine as well as colon by passive diffusion.
- Since, it is a fat-soluble vitamin, it requires bile salts and minimum amounts of dietary fat for its absorption.
- Vitamin K is incorporated in chylomicrons after it is absorbed and travels through the lymphatic system and eventually enters the portal blood from where it is transported to the liver.
- They are incorporated into VLDL and eventually delivered to the tissues where they are needed by LDL.
- Most tissues contain phylloquinones and menaquinones. Vitamin K is apparently stored in the liver in small quantities.
- Vitamin K is excreted in the urine after the administration of therapeutic doses.

Figure 5.19 is depicted the food sources of vitamin E.

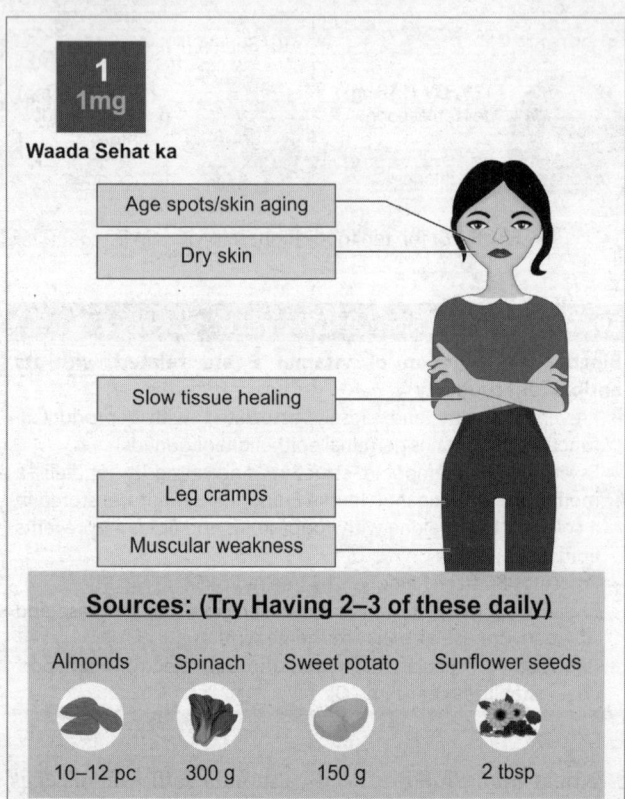

Fig. 5.17: Vitamin E deficiency symptoms.

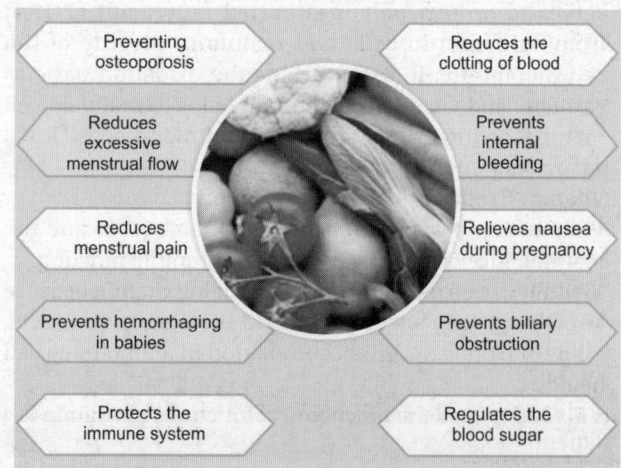

Fig. 5.18: Health benefits of vitamin K.

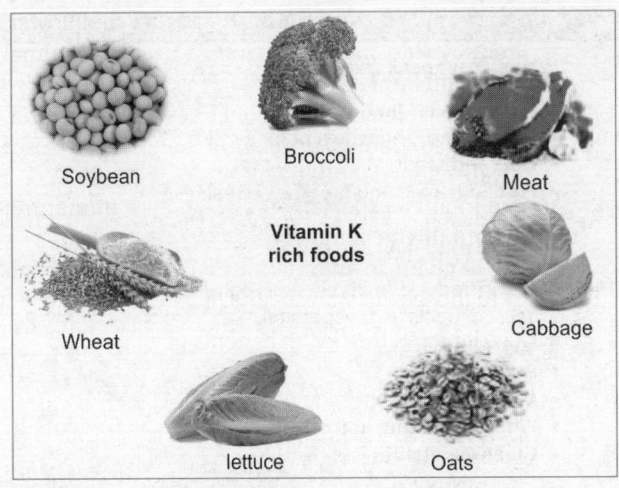

Fig. 5.19: Food sources of vitamin E.

Functions

- Synthesis of blood clotting proteins. Vitamin K is essential for the activation of prothrombin. This gets converted to thrombin, which in turn activates fibrinogen to form fibrin.
- **The process of blood clotting occurs as follows:** Injured tissue releases thromboplastin, which catalyses prothrombin formation.
- Vitamin K catalyses, conversion of prothrombin to thrombin. This in turn causes conversion of fibrinogen to fibrin, which forms the clot.

Food Sources

Dark-green leafy vegetables are good sources of vitamin K. Fruits, tubers, seeds, dairy and meat products contain vitamin K.

Requirements

The ICMR committee considered that no recommendation is needed for this vitamin, as the synthesis of vitamin K occurs in the lower intestine by the colonic bacteria and present widely in foods.

Figure 5.20 is depicted the vitamin K deficiency.

Deficiency

- Deficiency of vitamin K predominantly causes hemorrhage. Newborn infants have sterile intestinal tract, so no intestinal vitamin K is supplied during the first few days of life until intestinal micro flora develops.
- Hemorrhagic disease may occur immediately after birth and it can be prophylactically treated by administering menadione intramuscularly at birth.
- Malabsorption syndrome is the secondary cause of vitamin K deficiency.
- Any obstruction in fat absorption, biliary obstruction will also affect vitamin K absorption because it is a fat-soluble vitamin. Therefore, vitamin K deficiency results in prolonged blood clotting time.
- Patients suffering from this problem are given vitamin K before surgery.
- Normal bile flow is hindered after surgical removal of gallbladder with the result vitamin K is not absorbed properly.

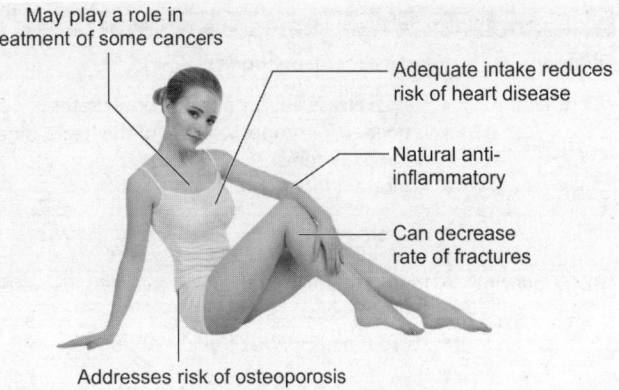

Fig. 5.20: Vitamin K deficiency.

- Vitamin K is involved in several drug-nutrient interactions. An anticlotting drug (dicumerol) inhibits the action of vitamin K.
- Prolonged use of antibiotics kills bacteria and reduces intestinal micro flora, thus reducing the main source of vitamin K

Toxicity

- Both vitamin K1 (phylloquinones) and vitamin K2 (menaquinones) have not shown any toxic effects. However, menadione in large amounts can be toxic.
- Some of the symptoms reported include, liver damage, hypoprothrombinemia, renal tubule degeneration and hemolytic anemia in premature infants.

WATER-SOLUBLE VITAMINS

In 1911, Funk coined the term 'vitamin' for the substance, which he found effective in preventing beriberi. McCullum and Davis applied the term water-soluble B to the concentrates, which cured beriberi. It was soon discovered that vitamin B was not a single substance, but a group of compounds, to which we now designate as the vitamin B complex. Some of these are discussed. The water-soluble vitamins include ascorbic acid (vitamin C), thiamin, riboflavin, niacin, vitamin B6 (pyridoxine, pyridoxal, and pyridoxamine), folacin, vitamin B12, biotin, and pantothenic acid.

Table 5.5 is depicted the water-soluble vitamins.

Thiamine

Thiamine (vitamin B1) is a water-soluble vitamin. It is essential for the utilization of carbohydrates. In thiamine deficiency there is accumulation of pyruvic and lactic acids in the tissues and body fluids.

- Thiamine occurs in all natural foods, although, small amounts. Important sources are whole-grain cereals, wheat gram, yeast, pulses, oil seeds and nuts especially groundnut, meat, fish, eggs, vegetables and fruits contain smaller amounts.
- Thiamine is known as vitamin B1. Deficiency of thiamine leads to beriberi. This condition is widely prevalent among population whose diet contains more of polished cereals.

Table 5.5: Water-soluble vitamins.

Vitamin	What it does for our bodies	Where do we get it from
B1 (thiamin)	• Helps release energy from carbohydrates • Is needed for proper working of the heart, digestive and nervous systems • Important for growth	• Yeast extracts (e.g., vegemite) • Wheat germ and wheat bran • Nuts and seeds • Fortified bread and breakfast cereals • Lean pork • Whole meal flour and cereals
B2 (riboflavin)	• Important for growth and repair of tissues, especially the skin and eyes • Helps release energy from food	• Dairy products (milk, cheese, yoghurt) • Yeast extracts (e.g., vegemite) • Egg whites • Almonds • Mushrooms • Whole meal flour and cereals • Green vegetables
B3 (niacin)	• Helps to release energy from food • Important for growth • Helps control cholesterol levels • Important for nervous system and digestive health	• Lean meat • Yeast • Bran • Peanuts • Tuna and salmon • Legumes • Fortified breakfast cereals • Eggs • Vegetables • Milk
B6 (pyridoxine)	• Helps process protein and carbohydrate • Assists in making red blood cells • Important for brain function and immune system health	• Lean meat and poultry • Fish • Yeast extracts (e.g., vegemite) • Soybeans • Nuts • Wholegrain • Green leafy vegetables
Pantothenic acid	• Helps process carbohydrate, fat and protein for energy • Involved in the formation of fatty acids and cholesterol	• Yeast extracts (e.g., vegemite) • Fish • Lean meat • Legumes • Nuts • Eggs • Green leafy vegetables • Bread and cereals
B12 (cyano-cobalamin)	• Works with folate to produce new blood and nerve cells and DNA • Helps process carbohydrate and fat	• Found only in animal products (lean meat, chicken, fish, seafood, eggs and milk) • Fortified soy products
Biotin	• Helps process fat and protein • Important for growth and nerve cell function	• Egg yolk • Oats • Wholegrain • Legumes • Mushrooms • Nuts
Folate (folic acid)	• Produces red blood cells and DNA • Keeps the nervous system healthy • Important in early pregnancy to prevent neural tube defects	• Yeast extracts (e.g., vegemite) • Green leafy vegetables • Whole grains • Peas • Nuts • Avocado
C (absorbic acid)	• Needed for healthy skin, gums, teeth, bones and cartilage • Assists with absorption of some types of iron • Assists with wound healing and resistance to infection	Fruit and vegetables (citrus fruit and juices, berries, pineapple, mango, pawpaw, capsicum, parsley, broccoli, spinach, cabbage

Chemistry and Characteristics

- Thiamine hydrochloride is a white-crystalline substance. It has a faint yeast-like order and a salty, nut-like taste.
- It is readily soluble in water, but not in fat solvents or fats. It is readily destroyed by heat in neutral or alkaline solution; in acidic medium it is resistant to heat up to 1,200°C.

Absorption, Transport and Storage

- Thiamin taken in food is available either in the free form or in bound form as thiamin pyrophosphate (TPP) or it is also present as protein phosphate complex.
- Before absorption it is split in the digestive tract, and then it is absorbed from the proximal duodenum by active transport and passive diffusion.
- Alcohol consumption interferes with transport of the vitamin and folic acid deficiency interferes with the replication of enterocytes.
- About 90% of thiamin is circulating as TPP and carried by erythrocytes and remaining small amounts exist as free thiamin and thiamin monophosphate (TMP) bound mainly to albumin.
- The bodily stores of thiamin are not so great. About 50% is stored in the skeletal muscles and some amounts are also found in the heart, kidneys, liver and brain.
- Thiamin is excreted in the urine and small amounts are present in the feces, If it is taken in excess, it is excreted in the urine and if small amounts are ingested the amount excreted, falls.

Figure 5.21 is depicted the clinical manifestations of beriberi and **Box 5.2** is depicted the biochemical functions.

Box 5.2: Biochemical functions.

- The coenzyme thiamine pyrophosphate or cocarboxylase is intimately connected with the energy releasing reactions in the carbohydrate metabolism
- Some of the reactions are dependent on TPP, besides the other coenzyme
- α-ketoglutrate dehydrogenase is an enzyme of TCA cycle, this enzyme require TPP
- Transketolase is dependent on TPP. This is an enzyme of hexose monophosphate shunt (HMP)
- The branched chain α-keto acid dehydrogenase (decarboxylase) catalyzes the oxidative decarboxylation of branched chain amino acids (valine, leucine and isoleucine) to the respective keto acids. This enzyme also require TPP.
- TPP plays an important role in the transmission of nerve impulse. It is believed that TPP is required to acetylcholine synthesis and the ion translocation of neural tissue.

Functions

Thiamine functions in the release of energy from the metabolism of carbohydrate. As a result thiamine is related to the maintenance of a normal appetite, normal muscle tone in the gastrointestinal tract and healthy nervous system. More advanced deficiencies result in the disease beriberi. There are two types of beriberi.

- Thiamine is converted to (TPP), which is an important co enzyme in the carbohydrate metabolism.
- It is involved in transmission of nerve impulses across the cells.
- Thiamine as TPP is an essential cofactor for the conversion of amino acid tryptophan to niacin.

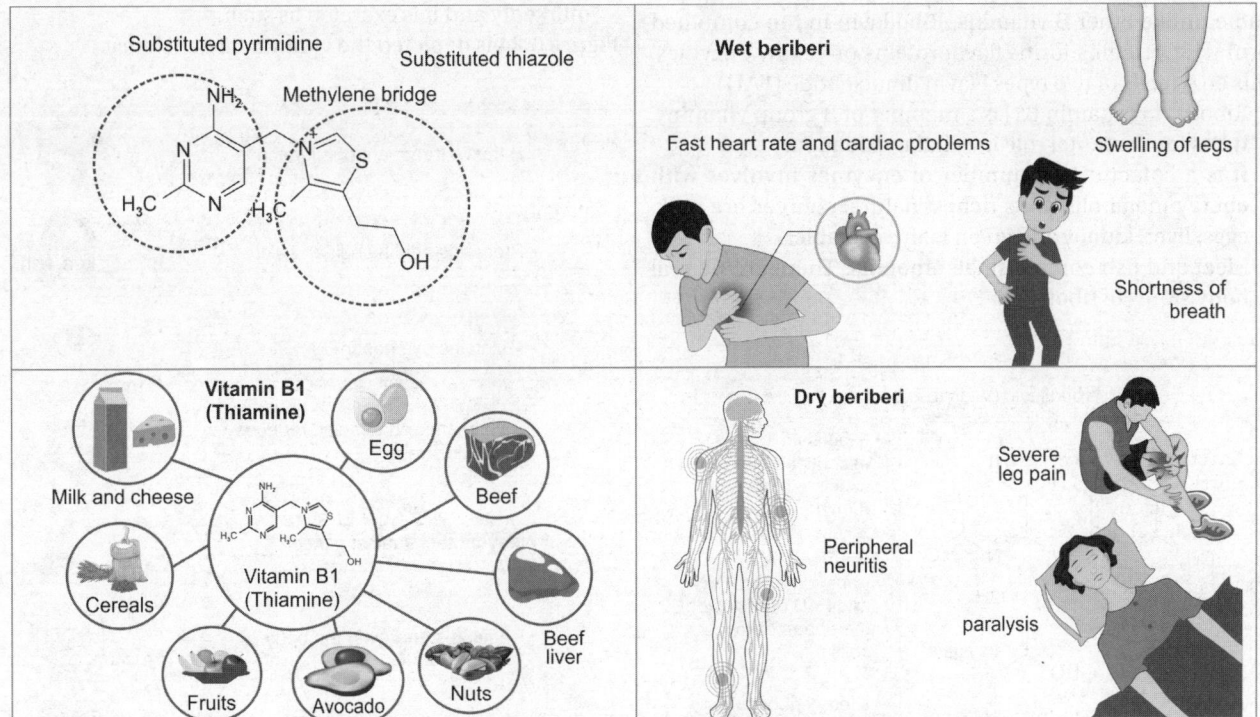

Fig. 5.21: Clinical manifestations of beriberi.

Sources

- Yeast, whole wheat, millets, hand-pounded rice, parboiled rice are good sources of thiamine.
- The bran contains most of the thiamine in the cereals. Gingelly seeds, groundnut, soybean, cashew nuts, organ meats, pork, liver and eggs supply thiamine.

B1 thiamine			
Properties	Sources	Functions	Deficiency
Water soluble	• Whole grain cereals • Meat	Metabolism releases energy from carbs and fat	Fatique Irritability
Unstable in heat	• Spinach • Egg • Milk	Healthy nervous system	Retarded growth
Destroyed by alkalis and milling		Normal growth	Beriberi (build up of pyruvic acid, causing muscle wasting, death)

Requirements

- Thiamine is involved in the carbohydrate metabolism. Its requirement is related to energy derived from carbohydrate.
- The ICMR expert group recommends an allowance of 0.5 mg/1,000 kcal for adults and for infants 0.3 mg/1,000 kcal is suggested.

Riboflavin (Fig. 5.22)

Riboflavin or Vitamin B2 is the yellow enzyme, which is heat stable unlike other B vitamins. Riboflavin in the combined form with proteins forms flavoproteins or yellow enzymes. This enzyme is of two types Flavin dinucleotide (FAD).

- Riboflavin (vitamin B2) is a member of B group vitamins. It has fundamental role in cellular oxidation.
- It is a cofactor in a number of enzymes involves with energy metabolism. Its richest natural sources are milk, eggs, liver, kidney and green leafy vegetables.
- Meat and fish contain small amounts. There are no real body stores of riboflavin.

- Low dietary intake of riboflavin may result in fissures at the angle of the mouth, accompanied by the yellow cast.
- The tongue may exhibit glossitis, turning to purplish red in color, accompanied by a painful burning sensation.

Chemistry and Characteristics

- In its pure form this vitamin is bitter tasting, orange yellow, odorless compound in which crystals are needle-shaped.
- It dissolves sparingly in water to give a typical greenish-yellow fluorescence.
- It is stable to boiling in acids, but in alkaline solutions, it is readily decomposed by heat. It is also destroyed by exposure to light.

Figure 5.23 is depicted the use of riboflavin.

Absorption, Transport and Storage

- Riboflavin is either present in foods in free state or in combination with phosphate or with protein and phosphate together. These compounds are broken down during digestion and free riboflavin is absorbed in the proximal small intestine by a carrier mediated process.
- This process requires adenosine triphosphate (ATP). Riboflavin is present as the coenzyme or as flavoproteins in body tissues.
- The absorption of free riboflavin depends on its phosphorylation in flavin mononucleotide (FMN).
- Riboflavin is transported as free riboflavin and FMN in the plasma and cells by a carrier-mediated process.
- Small amounts are present in the liver, kidney and heart, but it is not stored in appreciable amount, thus it becomes necessary to supply riboflavin in the diet regularly. If intake increases, then the urinary excretion also increases markedly and it is excreted as such.

Figure 5.24 is depicted the vitamin B2 deficiency.

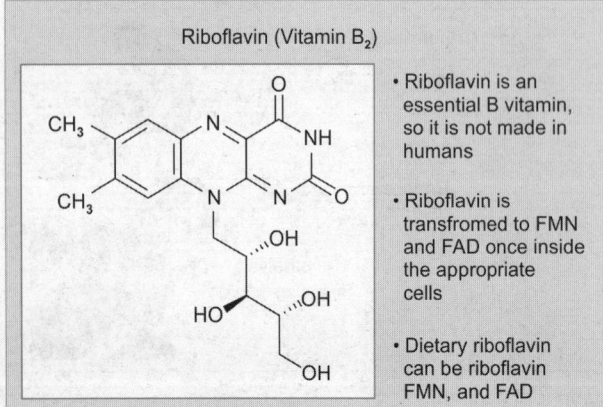

Fig. 5.22: Riboflavin vitamin B2.

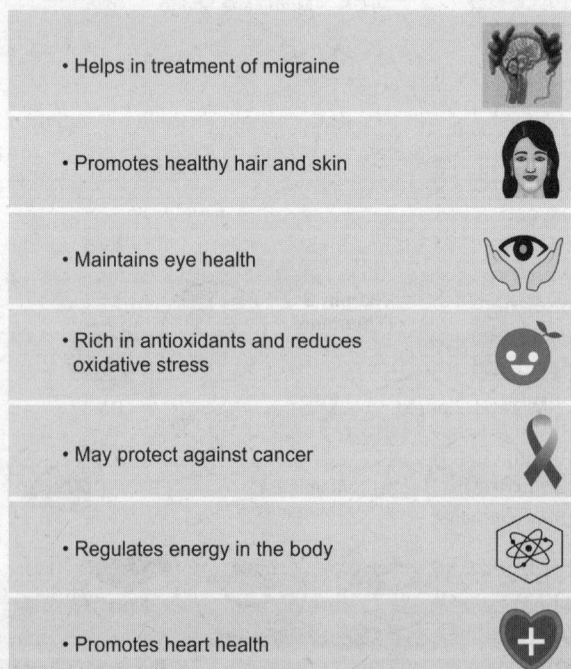

Fig. 5.23: Use of riboflavin.

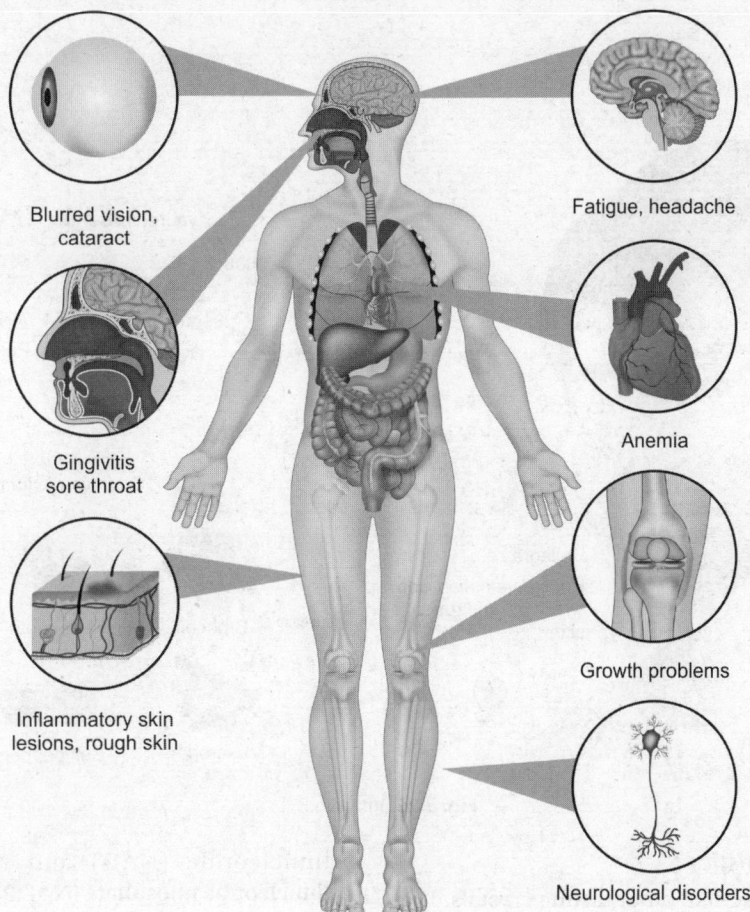

Fig. 5.24: Vitamin B2 deficiency.

Functions

- Riboflavin is part of two coenzymes, FMN and FAD. FMN and FAD are contained in flavoproteins. They are both oxidizing agents and take part in vital reaction points.
- These two act as hydrogen acceptor and form FMNH2 or FADH2. The enzymes are essential for the completion of many reactions in the energy cycle through, which ATP is produced in which hydrogen is transferred from one compound to another and eventually it combines with oxygen to form water.
- FMN and FAD also act as coenzymes of dehydrogenases, which catalyze the initial oxidations of fatty acid and many intermediates in carbohydrate metabolism.
- Pyridoxine (vitamin B6) is converted to active form, pyridoxal phosphate (PLP) in the presence of FMN. Similarly, tryptophan cans biosynthesize vitamin niacin in the presence of FAD.
- Riboflavin is necessary for normal growth and maintenance of tissues. It also plays an important role in the health of the eye.

Recommended Daily Allowances

- The requirement of riboflavin is directly proportional to energy intake. It is 0.6 mg per 1,000 kcals.
- The daily safe intake ranges from 0.7 to 2.2 mg/day, which depends on age, physiological status and level of activity.

Food Sources

- Riboflavin is widely distributed in foods. Dairy products and meats are the best sources. Eggs, liver and green leafy vegetables are also good sources.
- Cereals, such as millets and pulses are fair sources of riboflavin, but vice is specially a poor source as more than half of the vitamin is lost when it is milled. However, the cereals can be enriched with riboflavin to increase its content.

Niacin

Niacin or nicotinamide (amide form) is required by all the cells of our body. Such as thiamine and riboflavin, it plays a vital role in the release of energy from carbohydrates, protein, fat and alcohol.

Nicotinic Acid

- Nicotinic acid contains a pyridine nucleus. It is essential for the metabolism of carbohydrate, fat and protein.
- Nicotinic acid is essential for the normal functioning of the skin, intestinal tract and the nervous system.
- Foods rich in niacin or tryptophan are liver, kidney, meat, poultry, fish, legumes and groundnut. Milk is a poor source of niacin.

Figure 5.25 is depicted the vitamin B3.

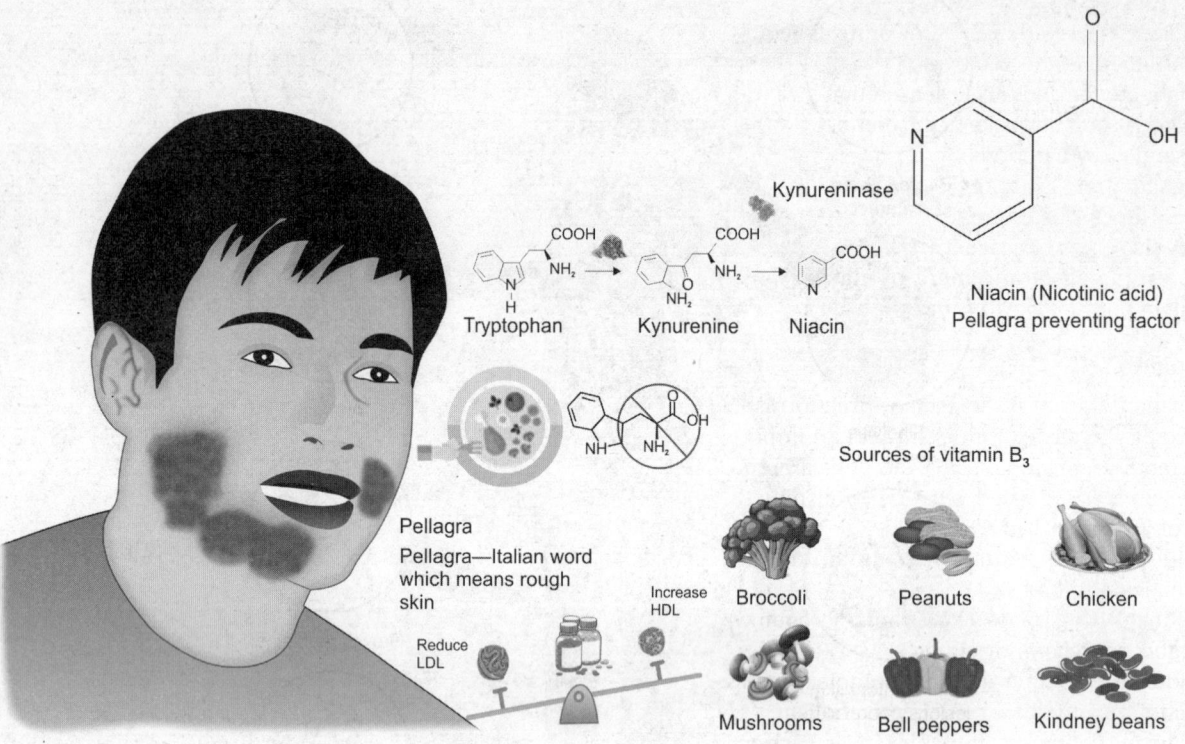

Fig. 5.25: Vitamin B3.

Chemistry and Characteristics
- It occurs in white needle-like bitter tasting crystals. It is moderately soluble in hot water, but only slightly soluble in cold water.
- It is stable to heat, alkalis, acids light and oxidation and unstable to reduction. If fact, it is one of the most stable of the vitamins.
- Niacin occurs in two form: Niacin and proniacin form, i.e., tryptophan.
- Human body can make 1 mg of vitamin from 50 to 60 mg of tryptophan. Thus, if a diet contains large amount of tryptophan, it will provide enough niacin, even thought the diet might be low in its niacin content.

Absorption, Transport and Storage
- Nicotinamide and nicotinic acid are readily absorbed from the small intestine by carrier-mediated facilitated diffusion.
- Body reserves seem to be just enough to meet day-to-day needs. NADH and NADPH, both are transported in the plasma and they are taken up by tissues through passive diffusion.
- Niacin, if taken in excess is excreted in the urine in different forms, N-methylnicotinamide and N-methylpyridine.
- During deficiency state, such as pellagra, the urine content of the metabolites either diminish or are absent altogether.

Functions
- Nicotinamide is essential for tissue metabolism. The active forms of nicotinamide are nicotinamide adenine dinucleotide (NAD) and Nicotinamide adenine dinucleotide phosphate (NADP).

Figure 5.26 is depicted the benefits of vitamin B3 or nicacin.
- NAD and NADP are involved as coenzymes in large number of reversible oxidation reduction reactions.
- Nicotinic acid enhances stomach secretion
- NAD is involved in catabolic reactions and NADP is involved in anabolic reaction in our body.

Food Sources
- Dried yeast, liver, rice polishing, peanut, whole cereals, legumes, meat, fish are good sources.
- Tryptophan present in dietary protein is converted to niacin in humans. 60 mg of tryptophan yields 1 mg of niacin.

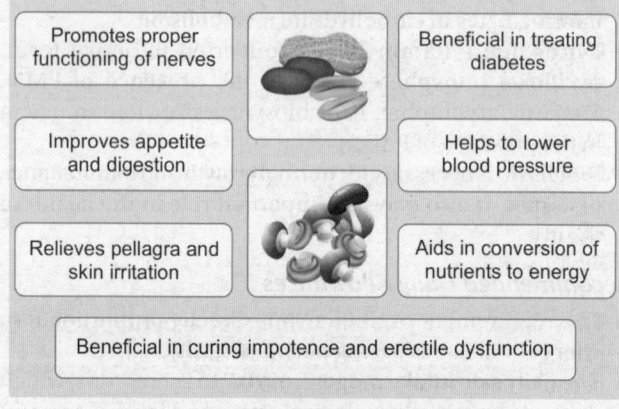

Fig. 5.26: Benefits of vitamin B3 or niacin.

Recommended Daily Allowances

Niacin is expressed in milligrams or niacin equivalent (NE). Its requirement is affected by:
- Metabolic rate and physical excretion
- Daily tryptophan intake in the diet
- Age and growth periods
- Pregnancy and lactation
- Illness and tissue trauma
- Body size and physical activity.

The estimated requirement of niacin is 6.6 mg niacin equivalent per 1,000 kcal.

Pyridoxine

Pyridoxine (vitamin B6) exists in three forms, pyridoxine, pyridoxal and pyridoxamine. It plays an important role in the metabolism of amino acids, fats and carbohydrates. Rice dietary; sources are dried yeast rice polishing, wheat gram and liver.
- Pyridoxine is essential for maintaining the nerves in normal condition.
- Pyridoxal phosphate (PLP) acts as coenzyme in the metabolism of amino acids.
- Pyridoxine is unique among B-complex vitamins in that it functions primarily in protein metabolism.
- Pyridoxine denotes related substances, such as pyridoxine, pyridoxal and pyridoxamine are three forms in which it is present in our body.

> **B6-Pyridoxine**
> **Uses:** Co-factor in >60 enzymes for metabolism (the master vitamin)
> **Deficiency:** Anemia, nervous disorders (especially in almost 50% of NA women, especially those on oral contraceptives)
> **Excess:** Disable nervous system (present in body-building diets)
> **Sources:** Green leafy vegetables, meats, fruit

Chemistry and Characteristics
- Vitamin B6 consists of a group of related pyridines: pyridoxine, pyridoxal and pryridoxamine.
- Vitamin B6 is soluble in water and relatively stable to heat and to acids. It is destroyed in alkaline solutions and is also sensitive to light.

Absorption, Transport and Storage
- Vitamin B6 is absorbed from the small intestine, especially from the jejunum and ileum by passive diffusion of the dephosphorylated forms (pyridoxine, pyridoxal and pyridoxamine).
- Muscle is the major depot and contains 80%–90% of the total body vitamin and stores in the form of PLP bound to glycogen phosphorylase.
- All three vitamins are easily interconverted metabolically by phosphorylation-dephosphorylation, oxidation-reduction and amination-deamination reactions.
- They are excreted in the urine, but 4-pyridoxic is the principal metabolite excreted. Body stores of B6 are small because it is a water-soluble vitamin.

Functions
- **In protein metabolism:** Pyridoxal phosphate is the coenzyme involved in several reactions in amino acid metabolism, for example:
  - **Decarboxylation:** The removal of carboxyl group from amino acid is accomplished in the presence of the coenzyme, PLP. Every amino acid is decarboxylated by a specific enzyme.
  - **Transamination:** The amino group is removed from one amino acid and is transferred to a new carbon skeleton to form a new amino acid. The non-essential amino acids formed by this reaction only.
  - **Deamination:** In this reaction, amino group is removed from amino acid, such as serine and threonine.
  - **Transsulfuration:** In this reaction, sulfur groups are removed from sulfur containing amino acids, such as cysteine in the presence of transulfurases.
  - **Conversion of tryptophan to niacin:** There are several steps that take place in this reaction and one of these reactions requires PLP.
  - **Synthesis of hemoglobin:** This vitamin is essential for the formation of delta-aminolevulinic acid in the synthesis of heme, the chief non-protein core of hemoglobin.
  - **Amino acid transport:** It effectively transports amino acids from the intestine into the circulation. From here it enters the cells.
- **In carbohydrate and fat metabolism:** Through decarboxylation and transamination reactions, PLP supplies metabolites for generating energy in the citric acid cycle. It is also required to convert essential fatty acid, linoleic acid to the fatty acid and arachidonic acid.

Figure 5.27 is depicted the vitamin B6 or pyridoxine functions.

Recommended Daily Allowances
- The need for pyridoxine depends on the amount of protein in the diet. High protein diet increases the requirement, since it is essential for amino acid metabolism.
- The requirement of vitamin B5 has not been established for Indian population. However, a range has been

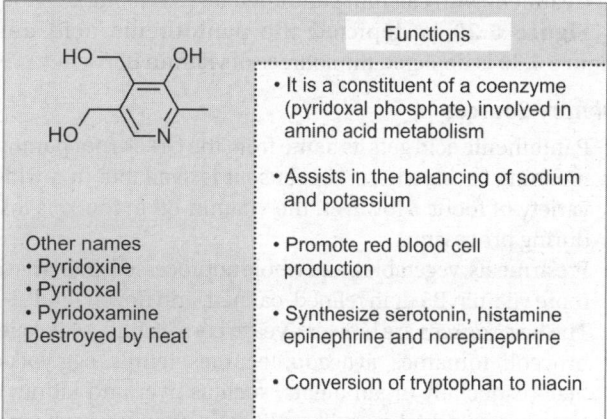

Fig. 5.27: Vitamin B6 or pyridoxine functions.

- Increases stamina and boosts overall health
- Prevents high cholesterol
- Reduce chances of heart attack
- Reduce the impact of radiation exposure
- Effective for sideroblastic anemia
- Decreases chances of lung cancer and kidney stone

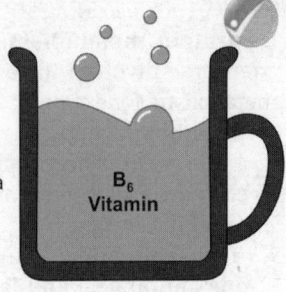

Fig. 5.28: Health benefits of pyridoxine (vitamin B6).

suggested as daily intake, i.e., 0.6–2.5 mg for various age groups, which would meet the requirement.

Figure 5.28 is depicted the health benefits of pyridoxine (vitamin B6).

Food Sources

Meat, pulses and wheat are rich sources. Other cereals are fair sources of this vitamin. Fruits and vegetables are poor sources. Cooking and processing of food causes loss of this vitamin.

Pantothenic Acid

Pantothenic acid is one of the vitamins of the vitamins B2 complex, which can prevent or cure a specific type of dermatitis (chick pellagra) in chicks fed on vitamin B2 deficient. Vitamin B5, also called pantothenic acid, is one of 8 B vitamins. All B vitamins help the body convert food (carbohydrates) into fuel (glucose), which the body uses to produce energy. These B vitamins, often referred to as B complex vitamins, also help the body use fats and protein. B complex vitamins are needed for healthy skin, hair, eyes, and liver. They also help the nervous system function properly.

- Pantothenic acid in the form of coenzyme A takes part in the metabolism of carbohydrates and fats. It is essential for the oxidation of pyruvic acid.
- Burning feet syndrome was observed in prisoners of war during World War II in Japan and Burma.
- This syndrome was associated with neurological and mental disturbances. Gopalan (1946) found that burning feet syndrome observed in Indian subjects responded to treatment with calcium pantothenate (20–40 mg).

Figure 5.29 is depicted the pantothenic acid and **Figure 5.30** is depicted the sources of vitamin B5.

Dietary Sources

- Pantothenic acid gets its name from the Greek root pantos, meaning "everywhere," because it is available in a wide variety of foods. However, the vitamin B5 in foods is lost during processing.
- Fresh meats, vegetables, and whole unprocessed grains have more vitamin B5 than refined, canned, and frozen food.
- The best sources are brewer's yeast, corn, cauliflower, kale, broccoli, tomatoes, avocado, legumes, lentils, egg yolks, beef (especially organ meats, such as liver and kidney), turkey, duck, chicken, milk, split peas, peanuts, soybeans, sweet potatoes, sunflower seeds, whole-grain breads and cereals, lobster, wheat germ, and salmon.

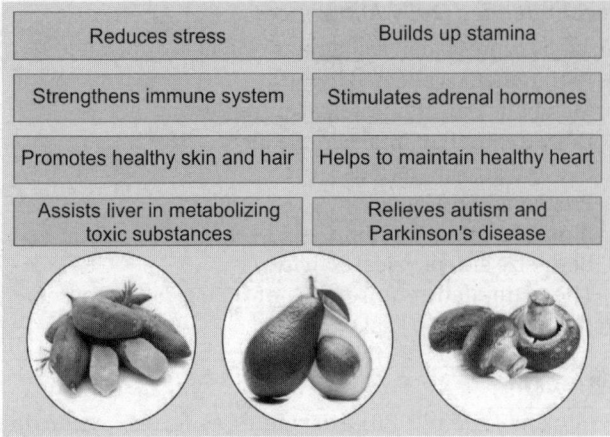

Fig. 5.29: Pantothenic acid.

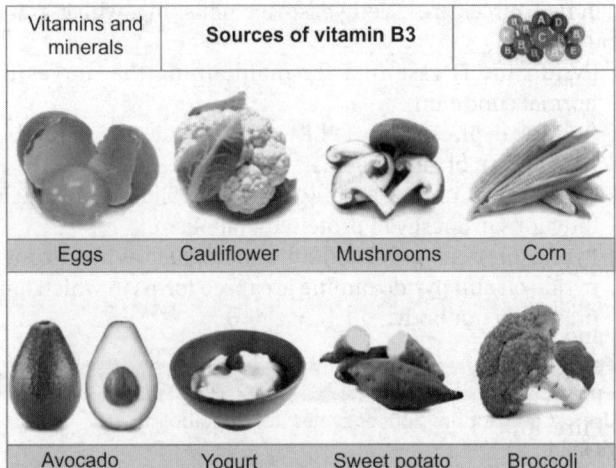

Fig. 5.30: Sources of vitamin B5.

Folic Acid

Folic acid was known under different names from 1933 by its curative effects in deficiency states in man and in different experimental animals. It is essential for the maturation of RBCs. It acts as a coenzyme in the synthesis of methionine and of purine and pyrimidine rings.

- Foods, such as liver, meat, dairy products, eggs, milk, fruits and cereals are as good dietary sources as leafy vegetables.
- Folic acid was first extracted from dark green leafy vegetables.
- It forms yellow crystals and is a conjugated substance made up of three acids namely pteroic, para-aminobenzoic acid (PABA) and glutamic acid.
- Simple folate deficiency results in the bone marrow producing immature cells (megaloblasts cells) and few matured RBCs. These results in reduced oxygen–carrying capacity causing anemia termed megaloblastic anemia.
- Folate deficiency during pregnancy causes neural tube disorders of the fetus.
- Folate deficiency impairs the ability of the immune system to fight infection.

Figure 5.31 is depicted the folic acid benefits and **Figure 5.32** is depicted the funtions of folic acid.

- Helps prevent birth defects
- Promotes heart health
- Natural depression remedy
- Reduces risk of Alzheimer's
- Helps breakdown triglycerides
- Decreases risk of colon cancer
- May lower homocysteine levels

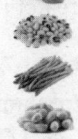

Fig. 5.31: Folic acid benefits.

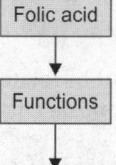

1. Needed for normal function of RBCs
2. Needed for normal function of WBCs
3. For synthesis of purines and pyrimidines (production of DNA)
4. It is more potent growth promoter than vitamin B12
5. With vitamin B12 for normal function of intestinal mucosa
6. Its deficiency leads to megaloblastic anemia
7. Its deficiency leads to short life span of RBCs
8. Its deficiency leads to impaired oxygen carrying capacity

Fig. 5.32: Funtions of folic acid.

Characteristics

- Folate is a generic term for folic acid, pteroylglutamic acid and other compounds having the activity of folic acid. It consists of three linked componets: a pteridine grouping, PABA and glutamic acid, an amino acid.
- Pure folic acid occurs as a bright-yellow crystalline compound, only slightly soluble in water. It is easily oxidized in an acid medium and is sensitive to light.

Absorption, Transport and Storage

- Free folate is generally absorbed throughout the small intestine, but most of it is absorbed mainly in the jejunum by active transport.
- About 75% of dietary folate is in polyglutamyl forms. Before it can be absorbed, these are normally hydrolyzed to free folate by conjugase present in small intestine.
- Alkaline pH of the intestine and intake of sodium bicarbonate collectively decrease the absorption of folic acid.
- The liver is the principal depot for folate. Ascorbic acid maintains an adequate level of the folate for metabolic purposes by preventing the oxidation of tetrahydrofolic acid (active form). Small amounts are lost in the feces and urine.

Functions

- Folic acid coenzyme is essential in bringing about transferring single carbon units for many interconversions. A number of key compounds are formed by these reactions like:
  - Purines, which are essential constituents of living cells.
  - Thymine, which essential compound forms a key part of DNA.
  - The formation of hem group of hemoglobin.
- The conversion of phenylalanine into tyrosin.

Food Sources

Green leafy vegetables, liver, kidney, gingelly seeds, cluster beans are rich sources of folic acid.

Cyanocobalamin

Cyanocobalamin vitamin B12 was found effective in curing pernicious anemia when administered intramuscularly in small quantities (5–10 mg) for the absorption of vitamin B12 from the intestines, a factor called 'Intrinsic factor' (IF) secreted by the stomach is essential vitamin B12 is stored in fair amount in the liver.

- Cyanocobalamin vitamin B12 until 1926, pernicious anemia was a fatal disease of unknown origin with an unknown cure.
- In 1926, Minot and Murphy found that pernicious anemia could be cured by feeding a patient at least 0.3 kg of raw liver per day.
- Also in 1926 Castle noted that patients with pernicious anemia had a low level of gastric secretion. He suggested that the antipernicious anemia factor had two components.
- An 'extrinsic factor' found in food and an 'intrinsic factor' within normal gastric secretions. The extrinsic factor is now known as vitamin B12 or cobalamin.

Figure 5.33 is depicted the benefits of vitamin B12.

Characteristics

- Vitamin B12 is the only cobalt containing substance essential for health. It occurs as dark red needle-like crystals, which are slightly soluble in water.
- This vitamin is absorbed from the ileum only. Its absorption depends on the presence of a muco-protein enzyme produced by the gastric mucosa. The enzyme is called intrinsic factor.

Absorption, Transport and Storage

- Vitamin B12 is absorbed in the ileum in pH of 6.8. However, it must be released from its protein complex by pepsin and by gastric HCl in the stomach before it can be absorbed

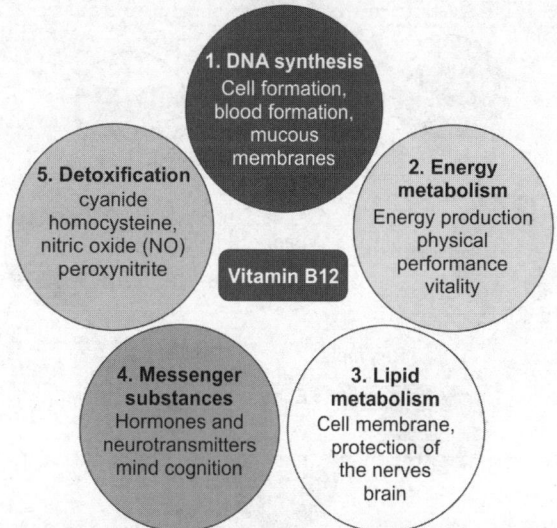

Fig. 5.33: Benefits of vitamin B12.

and then it must be bound to a specific glycoprotein IF secreted by gastric mucosal cells.
- IF is then released and the vitamin is attached to another cobalamin-binding protein carrier and transported to the cells.
- In well-nourished individuals, vitamin B12 is stored in great amounts in the liver, kidney, heart, muscles, pancreas, testes, brain, blood, spleen and bone marrow, but mainly in the liver.
- The liver accumulates a substantial amount enough for 5-7 years. On an average a normal individual excretes about 30 pg of vitamin B12 each day in the urine.

Figure 5.34 is depicted the vitamin B12 rich foods.

Functions
- Vitamin B12 functions as coenzyme in two different forms adenosylcobalamin and methylcobalamin. Adenosylcobalamin is essential for the conversion of homocycine into methionine and for the conversion of L-methylmalonyl-CoA to succinyl-CoA.
- Thus, the deficiency of cobalamin causes two genetic disorders in children—homocystinuria and methylmalonic aciduria. These forms of vitamin play very important roles in metabolism of all cells.
- Cobalamin and folic acid are metabolically interrelated and the deficiency of either causes megaloblastic anemia. Cobalamin provides an activated form of folate for hematopoiesis.

Recommended Dietary Allowances
Vitamin B12 is measured in micrograms. Though the requirement is considerably small, but the suggested intake is sufficient for normal hematopoiesis and good health.

Food Source
- Vitamin B12 is synthesized by the intestinal bacteria in the colon but it is not absorbed.
- The richest sources of dietary cobalamin include liver, kidney, lean meat, milk, egg and cheese.
- Plant foods contain the vitamin through contamination or bacterial synthesis.
- Pure vegetarians who do not include even, milk in their diet are at a greater risk of developing vitamin B12 deficiency.

Vitamin C
The chemical name for vitamin C is ascorbic acid. It was discovered in 1747 by the British physician Lind and demonstrated that citrus fruit juices prevented and cured scurvy.

Figure 5.35 is depicted the health benefits of vitamic C.

Chemistry and Characteristics
- Vitamin C is a white crystalline compound of relatively simple structure and closely related to monosaccharide sugars.
- It can be prepared synthetically at low cost from glucose. Of all the vitamins, vitamin C is the most easily destroyed.
- It highly soluble in water heat, light, alkalis, oxidative, enzymes and trace.

Absorption, Transport and Storage
- Some species, which do not biosynthesize this vitamin, need it from dietary sources. Ascorbic acid is easily absorbed from the small intestine by active transport and passive diffusion.
- Vitamin C is concentrated in the adrenal gland and the retina, but appreciable amounts are present in the spleen, intestine, bone marrow, pancreas, thymus, liver pituitary and kidney also.
- Vitamin C is better absorbed in the oxidized form (dehydroascorbic acid) than in the reduced form (ascorbate or ascorbic acid). It is transported in the plasma in the reduced state.
- Vitamin C is distributed throughout body tissues and if there is any excess, it is slowly excreted in the urine.
- The plasma concentration of vitamin C is usually lower in cigarette smokers and in women on oral contraceptive pills.
- The absorption of vitamin C is hampered by the lack of hypochloric acid or by bleeding from the gastrointestinal tract.
- Normally, kidneys control the excretion of vitamin C. If the tissues have reached the saturation (greater than 0.6 mg per dL), vitamin C taken in excess will be excreted. And if

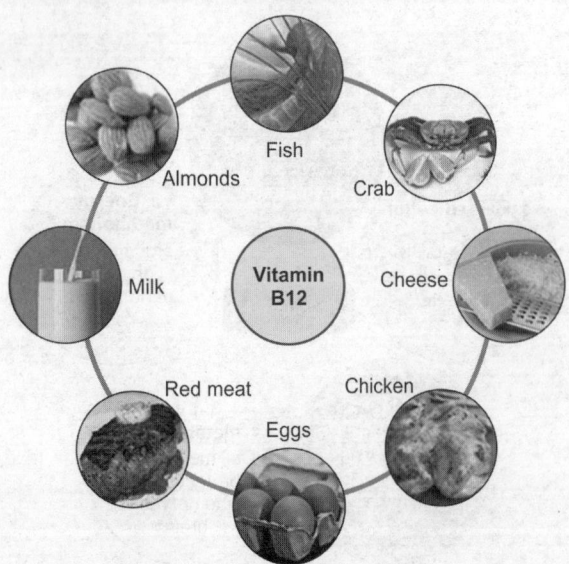

Fig. 5.34: Vitamin B12 rich foods.

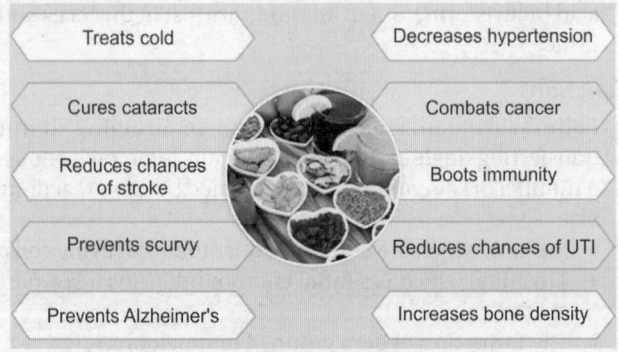

Fig. 5.35: Health benefits of vitamic C.

tissue stores are depleted, very small amount of vitamin C excreted.
- The urinary excretion of ascorbic acid increases during periods of emotional, psychological or physiological stress.

Functions

- Ascorbic acid is essential for formation of cement substances and collagen, which is found in blood vessels teeth and bones.
- It helps in the biosynthesis of non-essential amino acids, e.g., hydroxyproline, tyrosine.
- It is required for absorption of iron as it reduces ferric to ferrous form which is easily absorbed.
- Vitamin C is essential for the formation of collagen a major structural protein of connective tissues.
- It is required for normal wound healing because it helps in the formation of connective tissue.
- Vitamin C is required for carnitine synthesis, which aids in the transport of fatty acids in the cell.
- Vitamin C is essential for the synthesis of norepinephrine a neurotransmitter.
- It activates hormones, e.g., growth hormone, gastrin releasing peptide, calcitonin, gastrin oxytocin.
- Drug detoxifying metabolic systems in the body requires vitamin C for its optimal activity.
- Vitamin C is an excellent antioxidant. It combines with free-radicals oxidizing them to harmless substances that can be excreted.

Figure 5.36 is depicted the functions of vitamic C.

Food Sources (Fig. 5.37)

- Vitamin C is widely distributed in plant foods, especially in fresh fruits and vegetables. But of all the vitamins, it is most easily destroyed by the oxidation.
- Since, it is a powerful reducing agent, it is rapid. Oxidized in the air. Due to this reason, dry and stale vegetables lose considerable amount of vitamin C similarly, if vegetables are cut and left exposed to air, most of the vitamin is destroyed. Therefore, it is advisable that fruits and vegetables should be eaten fresh, whenever possible.

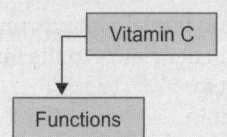

Vitamin C → Functions

1. This is co-factor for the protocollagen hydroxylase, which is important in connective tissue proteins, such as cartilage, dentin and bone.
2. It has function of hydroxylation of Gamma-butyrobetaine to carnitine
3. It is needed for microsomal drugs metabolism
4. It is required for the synthesis of epinephrine, and steroids by the adrenal glands
5. It is required for leukocytes function, anti-inflammatory
6. It takes part in tyrosine metabolism
7. It helps in folic acid metabolism
8. It leads to increased absorption of minerals, e.g., iron

Fig. 5.36: Functions of vitamic C.

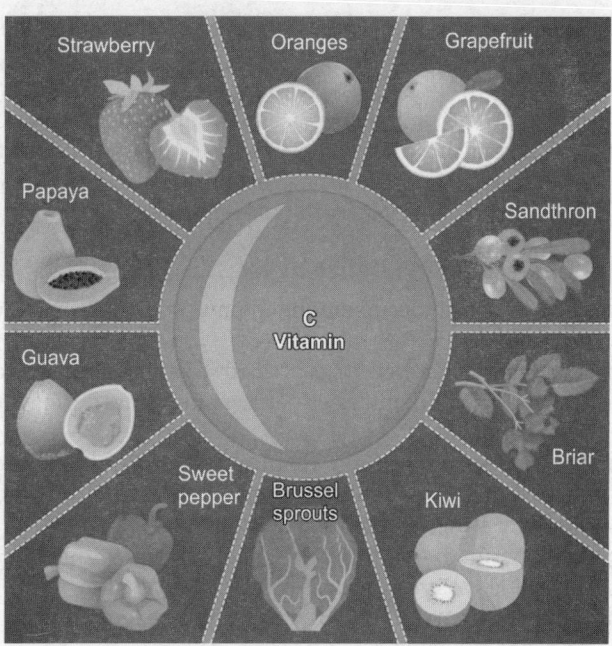

Fig. 5.37: Food sources of Vitamin C.

- Meat, fish, poultry, milk and milk products, and eggs contain very little amounts.
- Dry grains are devoid of vitamin C. Germination of dry pulses considerably increases the vitamin C content.
- Sprouted green gram contains three times more vitamin C as compared to sprouted bengal gram.

Excellent Sources

Amla, guava, citrus fruits, such as oranges, lemon, mausami, kinnu. Fresh strawberries, cantaloupe and pineapple. It is advisable to eat orange sections with thin white peel because it has comparatively more vitamin C than the same amount of strained orange juice.

Excellent-to-good Sources:

Broccoli, Brussels sprouts, capsicum, cabbage and turnips.

Small Amounts

Peaches, pears, apple, bananas.

VITAMIN DEFICIENCIES AND HYPERVITAMINOSIS

Retinol (Vitamin A) Deficiency

- The deficiency of vitamin A is usually manifest clinically as (a) Night blindness, (b) Xerphthalmia, (c) Bitot's spots and Keratomalacia. The commonest cause of blindness among children is vitamin A deficiency.
- The age group most affected is 1–4 years. This condition is closely associated with protein calorie malnutrition.

Xerophthalmia

- It is a disease of the eye in which the cornea and conjunctive become dry. The conjunctive becomes rough and wrinkled.

- Swelling and redness of the lids, pain and aversion to light are also noticed.
- Grayish, silvery or chalky white patches (Bitot's spots) appear on the conjunctive on either side of the cornea.
- The child favors to keep his eyes away from light or closed. If not treat in time the cornea becomes soft and ulcerated (Keratomalacia) resulting in total blindness.

Beriberi (Thiamine Deficiency)

- Beriberi usually occurs among communities that consume over milled rice.
- Two types of Beriberi are described-infantile beriberi and adult beriberi. Infantile beriberi usually occurs during the first year of life.
- Convulsive disorders, respiratory difficulties and gastrointestinal troubles, such as constipation and vomiting are seen among children.
- Adult beriberi occurs among youngsters who experience physiological stress, such as pregnancy, lactation, etc.
- It may be in dry or wet form according to the absence or presence of edema.

Riboflavin Deficiency

- Important clinical manifestations of riboflavin deficiency are: (a) Angular stomatitis, (b) Cheilosis, (c) Scrotal dermatitis, and (d) Corneal vascularization.
- In angular stomatitis, the angles of the mouth are fissured and ulcerated. In cheilosis, the lips get fissured vertically.

Pellagra (Niacin Deficiency)

- Pellagra is caused due to deficiency of niacin. The natural characteristics of pellagra are: (a) Gastrointestinal disturbances, (b) Stomatitis, (c) Dermatitis, and (d) Neurological changes.
- Gastrointestinal disturbances include indigestion, weight loss and diarrhea.
- Stomatitis is swelling and reddening of the tongue. Neurological changes include mental apathy, depression, etc.

Scurvy (Vitamin C Deficiency)

- Scurvy is associated with vitamin C (ascorbic acid) deficiency.
- The condition is not generally seen among breastfed children because they get enough supply of vitamin C from mother's milk. Cow's or buffalo's milk does not contain vitamin C.

Rickets (Vitamin D Deficiency)

- The disease is caused due to deficiency of vitamin D and is directly related to impaired metabolism of calcium and phosphorus.
- The main defect is failure of calcification of the growing portions of the bones. There is enlargement of the long bones at the ends particularly at the wrist and ankles.
- The bone being soft bends under pressure on standing or walking. The knees touch each other.
- The forces legs and assume a bow shape. Adult form of rickets is known as osteomalacia.

Vitamin K Deficiency

- Vitamin K is easily available in nature particularly from various green leaves. It is also synthesized by intestinal bacteria.
- Deficiency of vitamin K causes hemorrhagic disease. Vitamin K is necessary for the synthesis of prothrombin by the liver.
- It this being an important blood clotting mechanism, is not produced hemorrhaging may occur.

Nurses Role and Responsibility in Vitamin Defiencies

The nurse must assess the patient for signs and symptoms of vitamin deficiency before beginning vitamin therapy because vitamin therapy could result in a toxic effect if the patient does not have a vitamin deficiency. In addition, the patient must be assessed for debilitating diseases and GI disorders that may disrupt the absorption, metabolism, and excretion of vitamins used to treat vitamin deficiency. For some patients, vitamin deficiency is caused by inadequate nutrient intake. Therefore, it is critical that the patient's diet be assessed to determine if it is the cause of the deficiency. If so, then the nurse should educate the patient on the importance of maintaining a balanced diet.

In many cases, the nurse may reach one of the following diagnoses:
- Altered nutrition; less than body requirements
- Lack of knowledge related to proper nutrition
- Lack of knowledge related to vitamin use

Based on these diagnoses, the nurse should develop a plan for having the patient eat a well-balanced diet and to take vitamin supplements as prescribed.

The plan should also take into consideration the following interventions:
- Administer vitamins with food to promote absorption.
- Store vitamins in light-resistant container.
- Use a calibrated dropper for administration of liquid vitamins.
- Administer IM if patient is unable to take PO.

Teaching the patient is an important intervention because this gives the patient the knowledge to implement preemptive actions that lower the risk of vitamin deficiency in the future. The nurse should teach the patient to:
- Take prescribed amount of vitamin.
- Read labels carefully.
- Not use megavitamins over a prolonged period of time.
- Check expiration dates on containers before purchasing or taking them (potency is reduced after the expiration date).
- Not take vitamin A with mineral oil because it interferes with the absorption of A.
- Not take mega doses of vitamin C (ascorbic acid) to "cure a cold."
- Not take mega doses of vitamin C with aspirin or sulfonamides.
- Avoid excessive intake of alcoholic beverages. (It can cause vitamin B-complex deficiencies.)

To calculate the desired portions for each food group based on age, sex, and the amount of exercise the patient performs daily. It is important that the patient understands that vitamin supplements are not necessary if he or she is healthy and eats properly.

Alert the patient to the signs and symptoms of hypervitaminosis. Hypervitaminosis A causes nausea, vomiting, headache, loss of hair, and cracked lips. Hypervitaminosis D causes anorexia, nausea, and vomiting.

The nurse should evaluate the patient for proper dietary intake and determine if vitamin therapy is having a therapeutic effect.

CONCLUSION

Vitamin means 'vital for life'. Vitamins and minerals are compounds necessary for the healthy functioning of our bodies. We need vitamins and minerals to help us grow, to see correctly, to form bones, muscles, skin and organs, as well as to help us battle infections. Deficiencies in certain vitamins and minerals can lead to severe problems. The best way to ensure your child receives enough vitamins and minerals for healthy growth and development is to provide a wide variety of fresh foods from the five food groups including whole grain bread and cereals, vegetables, fruit, meat, fish, poultry, eggs, nuts and legumes, and dairy products, such as milk, cheese and yoghurt.

BIBLIOGRAPHY

1. Antia FP. Clinical Dietetics and Nutrition, 3rd edition. Oxford University Press, Mumbai, 1986.
2. Berdanier CD, Berdanier L. Advanced Nutrition: Macronutrients, Micronutrients, and Metabolism, Second Edition. Oakville: CRC Press, 2015.
3. Briggs GM, Doris HC. Nutrition and Physical Fitness, 11th edition. Harcourt College Publishers, New York, USA, 1984.
4. Duyff RL. Academy of Nutrition and Dietetics Complete Food and Nutrition Guide, Fifth edition. Boston: Houghton Mifflin Harcourt, 2017.
5. Gropper SA, Smith JL, Carr TP. Advanced Nutrition and Human Metabolism, Seventh Edition. 2018.

REVIEW QUESTIONS

Long Essays

1. Define vitamins, classify vitamins; explain the dietary sources daily requirements of vitamin A.
2. Define vitamins. Classify vitamins; explain the dietary sources daily requirements, absorption, functions, deficiency of Vitamin D.
3. Define vitamins. Mention fat soluble vitamin. Explain vitamin K in detail.
4. Explain the dietary sources, functions, deficiency manifestations and daily requirements of vitamin C.
5. What are water soluble vitamins? Write a note on functions and deficiency of thiamine.

Short Essays

1. Describe the dietary sources, deficiency manifestations and daily requirements of thiamine.
2. Describe the dietary sources, deficiency manifestations and daily requirements of riboflavin.
3. What is the requirement and functions of vitamin D?
4. What are the sources and functions of vitamin K?
5. What are the sources, function, and deficiencies of vitamin C?
6. Explain functions of vitamin A.
7. Explain deficiency and hypervitaminosis of vitamin A.
8. Explain functions of vitamin D.
9. Mention deficiency and hypervitaminosis of vitamin D.
10. Write a short essay on vitamin E.
11. Write a short essay on vitamin K.
12. Define vitamins. Classify vitamins.
13. What are fat soluble vitamins?
14. What is the role of vitamin A in vision?
15. What are functions of vitamin C.
16. List the deficiencies of vitamin C.
17. Mention the B complex vitamins and sources.
18. Mention deficiency disorders of B complex vitamins.
19. Mention sources, requirements and deficiency of vitamin C.
20. What is vitamin K. Sources, uses and requirements?
21. Explain vitamin A. Deficiency and effects.
22. Mention sources, requirements, deficiency disorders of thiamine.
23. Mention sources, requirements, deficiency disorders of Riboflavin.
24. Mention sources, requirements, deficiency disorders of vitamin B3.
25. Mention sources, requirements, deficiency disorders of vitamin B9.
26. Mention sources, requirements, deficiency disorders of vitamin B12.

Short Answers

1. Define pro-vitamins.
2. What are carotenes?
3. Define night blindness.
4. Define exophthalmia.
5. What is the cause of rickets?
6. Mention the cause of osteomalacia.
7. Vitamin E has selenium sparing action. Give reason.
8. What is caused by tonicity of vitamin A?
9. What are sources of vitamin D?
10. Define beri-beri.
11. What is cheilosis?
12. Define pellagra.
13. Define pernicious anemia.
14. What is vitamin B12?
15. Define megaloblastic anemia.
16. Define scurvy.
17. Define Wernicke's encephalopathy.

CHAPTER 6

Minerals

CHAPTER OUTLINE

- ❖ Classification—Major Minerals (Calcium, Phosphorus, Sodium, Potassium and Magnesium) and Trace Elements
- ❖ Functions
- ❖ Dietary Sources
- ❖ Requirements—RDA

TERMINOLOGY

Calcium: Calcium builds strong bones and teeth and helps in muscle contraction, blood clotting, nerve transmission, cell signaling and regulation of metabolism. The deficiency of calcium makes bone fragile and easy to fracture. Milk and dairy products, cashew, dates, broccoli, parsley and greens are good sources of dietary calcium.

Sodium: Sodium helps in muscle contraction, conducts nerve impulses and controls the fluid balance in the body. The primary source of dietary sodium is table salt. However, salt should be taken in moderation.

Potassium: Potassium plays a crucial role in maintaining fluid balance, muscle contraction and nerve impulse conduction. It supports brain health and reduces the risk of stroke. Low potassium causes irregular heartbeats, edema (swelling), brain damage, etc. Bananas, sweet potatoes, avocados, beets and dates are rich sources of potassium.

Chloride: Chloride in association with sodium maintains the normal fluid balance in the body. It is used in the formation of hydrochloric acid (stomach acid) for digestion and to sustain electrical neutrality in the body. Table salt, tomatoes, celery and lettuce are rich sources of chloride.

Magnesium: Magnesium acts as a cofactor in several enzymatic reactions and is required for the synthesis of deoxyribonucleic acid (DNA) and an antioxidant, glutathione. Green leafy vegetables, legumes, nuts, seeds and whole grains replenish dietary magnesium.

Phosphorous: Phosphorus helps build and repair bones and teeth, helps nerves function and makes muscles contract. Phosphorus deficiency leads to bone diseases and growth restriction in children. Meats, poultry, beans, nuts, seeds and dairy products are rich sources of phosphorus.

Iodine: It is the mineral used to produce thyroid hormones. It is necessary for the body's metabolism and physical and mental development. Phosphorus deficiency leads to impaired growth in children and metabolic disorders such as goiter and mental problems and affects menstrual health and pregnancy-related issues. Iodized table salt is the main source and is easily available.

Iron: It is used in hemoglobin formation, which carries oxygen in the blood. Iron deficiency can lead to cellular hypoxia (decreased oxygen) and cell death. Green leafy vegetables and meats such as beef, chicken and pork are rich sources of iron.

Zinc: This mineral aids in cell division, immunity and wound healing. Low zinc levels impair the immune system. Oysters, red meat, poultry, beans, nuts and whole grains provide major quantities of zinc.

Copper: Copper helps in energy production and facilitates iron uptake from the gut. Chocolate, liver, shellfish and wheat bran cereals are rich sources.

Manganese: Manganese plays an important role in protein, carbohydrate and cholesterol breakdown and cell division. Along with vitamin K, it helps in blood clotting. Whole grains, nuts, soybeans and rice are rich in manganese.

Sulfur: Sulfur has antibacterial properties and helps fight acne-causing bacteria in the skin. It also repairs DNA damage. Seafood and legumes, especially soybeans, black beans and kidney beans are rich sources of sulfur.

Selenium: Selenium helps prevent oxidative damage to the cells. It is also very important for the metabolism of the thyroid hormone. Brazil nuts, seafood and organ meats are good sources of selenium.

Atom: Composed of protons, electrons and neutrons

Crystallization: Liquid to solid phase change

Density: Mass divided by volume

Electron: Negatively charged particles surrounding the nucleus of an atom. Has an atomic mass of nearly zero (0).

Elements: Definable substances composed of atoms

Magma: Liquid rock

Mass: The amount of stuff

Matter: Anything which has mass and occupies space

Minerals: Solid matter composed of elements in specific combinations and arrangements

Neutron: Non-charged particle found in the nucleus of an atom. Has an atomic mass of one (1).
Phase change: Based on temperature (and pressure) all matter can exist in one of 4 separate phases - solid, liquid, vapor, or plasma
Proton: Positively charged particle found in the nucleus of an atom. Has an atomic mass of one (1).
Rocks: Composed of minerals in specific combinations
Sub-atomic particles: Fundamental building block of matter, including quarks and such
Volume: How much space is occupied by a mass.

INTRODUCTION

There are a number of minerals or inorganic elements that play an important role in nutrition. Mineral elements are present in organic compounds, such as hemoglobin, phospholipids, thyroxin as inorganic compounds in sodium chloride and calcium phosphate and as free ions. They enter the structure of every cell of the body. Hard skeletal structures contain the greater proportions of some elements, such as calcium, phosphorus and magnesium, while soft tissues contain relatively higher proportions of potassium.

Figure 6.1 is depicted the nutrient in food.

Mineral elements enter into numerous regulatory activities of the body. The contraction of muscles, the normal response of nerves to stimulation, the control of water balance, the maintenance of acid base equilibrium and the water balance of the foodstuffs are few functions. Sodium, potassium, calcium, phosphorus and chloride are the essential constituents of body fluids. Calcium, magnesium, phosphorus and others are bone constituents. Iron, copper and cobalt function in an intendated manner together with protein, vitamin B_{12} and other nutrients for the synthesis of hemoglobin and RBCs.

DEFINITION AND MEANING

Minerals may be defined as those elements, which remain largely as ash when plant and animal tissues are burnt. The human body contains more than 19 minerals, all of which must be derived from foods. A total of 4% of the body weight is made up of minerals.

- Some of the important minerals found in our body include calcium, phosphorus, iron, iodine, sodium, potassium, zinc and chloride. All these minerals are derived from the food we eat. Of these, calcium, phosphorus, sodium, potassium, chloride and magnesium are the minerals required in larger amounts by the body.
- Calcium and phosphorus account for 3–4 of the minerals present in the body and five other elements account for most of the rest.
- Many of these elements are present in such minute amounts that they are referred to as a trace elements or micronutrients.
- Minerals are important for the body in various ways. They are required to form such organic compounds-like phosphoproteins, hemoglobin and thyroxin.
- Hard skeletal structures are formed with the help of elements, such as calcium, phosphorus and magnesium, whereas soft tissues contain a relatively high proportion of potassium.
- Mineral elements are also required in the constitution of enzymes; for maintaining osmotic pressure and water balance between intracellular and extracellular compartments; for proper functioning of the nervous system; for muscular contraction and so on.

Major minerals		
Minerals	Major roles	Natural sources
Calcium	Bone and tooth formation; muscle and nerve function	Dairy products, leafy greens, dry beans
Iron	Used to make hemoglobin and myoglobin	Red meats, eggs, nuts, whole grains, leafy greens
Zinc	Component of certain enzymes, required for growth	Meats, whole grains, nuts, legumes
Phosphorous	Bone and tooth formation; pH of body fluids, phospholipids	Dairy products, grains
Potassium	Maintains pH of body fluids; used in action potentials	Many fruits and vegetables, meats, milk
Sodium	Maintains pH of body fluids; used in action potentials	Table salt, meats
Selenium	Used by the immune system	Nuts, especially Brazil nuts; many fruits and vegetables

CLASSIFICATIONS OF MINERALS

Macrominerals are present at larger levels in the animal body or required in larger amounts in the diet. Macrominerals include calcium, chlorine, magnesium, phosphorus, potassium, sodium, and sulfur.

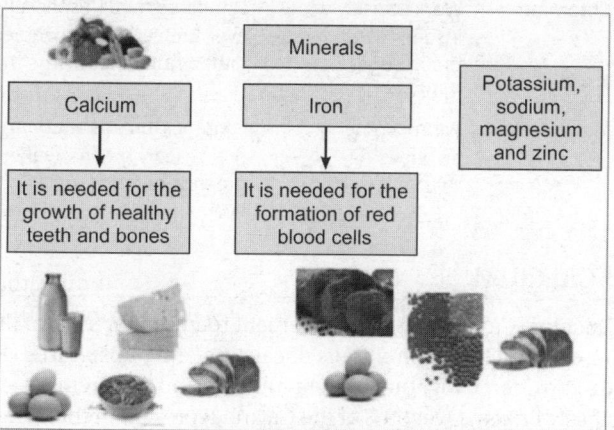

Fig. 6.1: Nutrient in food.

- Microminerals are often referred to as trace minerals, meaning they are present at low levels in the body or required in smaller amounts in the animals diet.
- Microminerals include chromium, cobalt, copper, fluorine, iodine, iron, manganese, molybdenum, selenium, and zinc. Microminerals are also known as trace elements.
- The microminerals are iron, iodine, zinc (Zn), copper (Cu), fluoride (F), selenium (Se), chromium (Cr), manganese (Mn), cobalt (Co) and molybdenum (Mo). However, only the deficiency of few of these elements is observed in humans.
- Iron and iodine deficiencies are widespread, while deficiency of Cu, Zn, Cr and Se has been reported in recent years

Macrominerals

Mineral	Function	Sources
Sodium	Needed for proper fluid balance, nerve transmission, and muscle contraction	Table salt, soy sauce; large amounts in processed foods; small amounts in milk, breads, vegetables, and unprocessed meats
Chloride	Needed for proper fluid balance, stomach acid	Table salt, soy sauce; large amounts in processed foods; small amounts in milk, meats, breads, and vegetables
Potassium	Needed for proper fluid balance, nerve transmission, and muscle contraction	Meats, milk, fresh fruits and vegetables, whole grains, legumes
Calcium	Important for healthy bones and teeth; helps muscles relax and contract; important in nerve functioning, blood clotting, blood pressure regulation, immune system health	Milk and milk products; canned fish with bones (salmon, sardines); fortified tofu and fortified soy milk; greens (broccoli, mustard greens); legumes
Phosphorus	Important for healthy bones and teeth; found in every cell; part of the system that maintains acid-base balance	Meat, fish, poultry, eggs, milk, processed foods (including soda pop)
Magnesium	Found in bones; needed for making protein, muscle contraction, nerve transmission, immune system health	Nuts and seeds; legumes; leafy, green vegetables; seafood; chocolate; artichokes; "hard" drinking water
Sulfur	Found in protein molecules	Occurs in foods as part of protein: meats, poultry, fish, eggs, milk, legumes, nuts

Microminerals

Trace minerals (microminerals): The body needs trace minerals in very small amounts. Note that **iron** is considered to be a trace mineral, although the amount needed is somewhat more than for other micro minerals.

Trace minerals

Mineral	Function	Sources
Iron	Part of a molecule (hemoglobin) found in red blood cells that carries oxygen in the body; needed for energy metabolism	Organ meats; red meats; fish; poultry; shellfish (especially clams); egg yolks; legumes; dried fruits; dark, leafy greens; iron-enriched breads and cereals; and fortified cereals
Zinc	Part of many enzymes; needed for making protein and genetic material; has a function in taste perception, wound healing, normal fetal development, production of sperm, normal growth and sexual maturation, immune system health	Meats, fish, poultry, leavened whole grains, vegetables
Iodine	Found in thyroid hormone, which helps regulate growth, development, and metabolism	Seafood, foods grown in iodine-rich soil, iodized salt, bread, dairy products
Selenium	Antioxidant	Meats, seafood, grains
Copper	Part of many enzymes; needed for iron metabolism	Legumes, nuts and seeds, whole grains, organ meats, drinking water
Manganese	Part of many enzymes	Widespread in foods, especially plant foods
fluoride	Involved in formation of bones and teeth; helps prevent tooth decay	Drinking water (either fluoridated or naturally containing fluoride), fish, and most teas
Chromium	Works closely with insulin to regulate blood sugar (glucose) levels	Unrefined foods, especially liver, Brewer's yeast, whole grains, nuts, cheeses
Molybdenum	Part of some enzymes	Legumes; breads and grains; leafy greens; leafy, green vegetables; milk; liver

■ CALCIUM

Calcium (Ca) is an essential element required for several life processes. The requirements of calcium and phosphorus (P) are considered together as their function and requirement are closely linked. Over 99% of the Ca and P present in the bones and the remaining 1% in the body fluids. The Ca and P are present in the ratio of 2:1 in our body. In the skeletal system, Ca and P is present in the form of hydroxyapatite crystals.

Hydroxyapatite is a compound made up of Ca and P that is deposited into the bone matrix to give it strength and rigidity.

Figure 6.2 is depicted the functions of calcium.

Description of Calcium

- Body contains Ca in greater amount than other minerals.
- About 2% of the body weight of an adult is due to Ca, out of which about 99% is contained in bones and teeth.
- Calcium is the most important factor in building skeleton and teeth is more important during growing years.
- Normal behavior of heart, nervous system and blood clotting process, etc., depend on the presence of calcium.
- Human body at different levels of intake has suggested the desirability of a daily intake of about 0.4–0.6 g of Ca by an adult, the case of growing children and pregnant and lactating mothers and the requirement is 1.0 g per day.
- Milk and milk products are the richest sources of calcium. Green leafy vegetables, such as spinach, amaranth are rich in Ca, but at the same time they are oxalate-rich foods.

Absorption and Excretion

Absorption

- The absorption of minerals are not as efficient as of vitamins and the macronutrients. It is not necessary that all the minerals taken as a part of our food are available to the body.
- The extent to which the body utilizes a particular nutrient is called bioavailability of a nutrient. This depends on many factors.
- Ca absorption takes place in all parts of the small intestine but mainly in the duodenum because of its acidic pH (< 7) as compared to the other parts of the intestine-normally, only 10–30% of dietary calcium is absorbed by the adults.

Calcium is absorbed by two mechanisms:

- Active transport, which mainly works when the luminal concentration of calcium ion is low.
- Passive transfer or paracellular movement, which mainly works when the luminal concentration of calcium ion is high.
- The active transport mainly takes place in the duodenum, but jejunum has a limited capacity. Also it is controlled by the action of 1, 25-dihydroxyvitamin D or vitamin D.
- This hormone enhances the uptake of Ca at the brush borders of the intestinal mucosal cell. This mechanism is not well-understood.
- The passive transfer mechanism occurs throughout the small intestine. When a single meal supplies large amount of Ca, much of it is absorbed through passive transfer.
- The active transport mechanism plays an important role when Cal intakes are low due to which the body requirements are not being met.
- Ca is absorbed in ionic form only. The unabsorbed Ca is excreted in the feces as Ca oxalates and Ca soaps.

Figure 6.3 is depicted the health benefits of calcium.

Excretion

- If the intake of dietary Ca exceeds the requirements, it remains unabsorbed in the intestine and is secreted in the feces.
- Normally, approximately 50% of the ingested Ca is excreted in the urine daily.
- Urinary calcium excretion continues to change throughout the life cycle, but during the growth periods it is very low.
- Ca excretion increases markedly during menopause but in postmenopausal stage, if the woman is on estrogen therapy, less Ca is excreted.
- After the age of 65 years, calcium excretion decreases, may be because of diminished intestinal absorption of Ca.
- A diet high in sodium decreases renal resorption of Ca and increased urinary Ca losses.
- Under normal conditions the losses of calcium from the skin are very small.
- Approximately 15 mg of Ca is lost in sweat each day. During increased physical activity, when sweating increases, Ca losses also increase even if the ingested Ca is low.

Figure 6.4 is depicted the common calcium sources.

Factors increasing calcium absorption

- **Body needs:** During the growth periods, such as infancy, childhood, during pregnancy and lactation more Ca is absorbed. In elderly persons especially in postmenopausal women the calcium absorption is reduced.

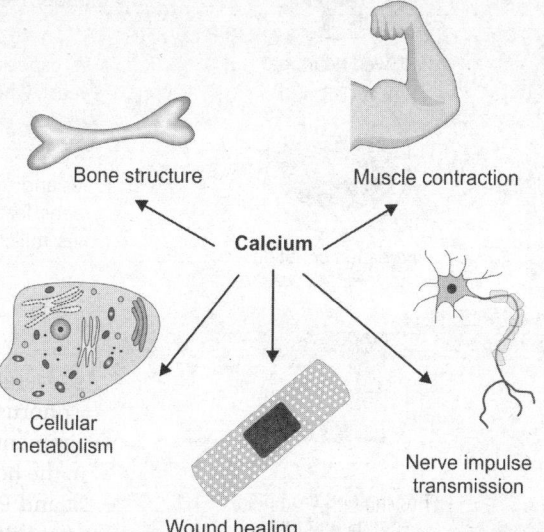

Fig. 6.2: Functions of calcium.

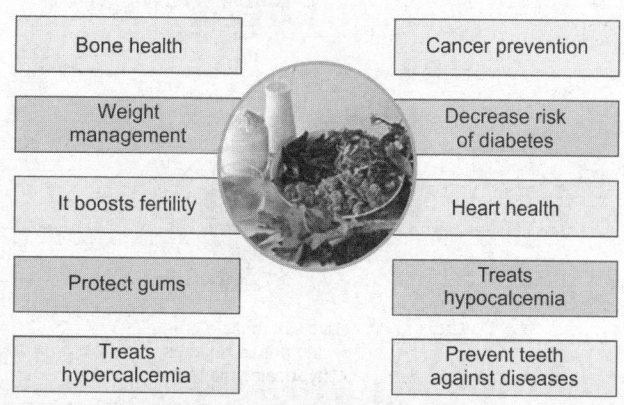

Fig. 6.3: Health benefits of calcium.

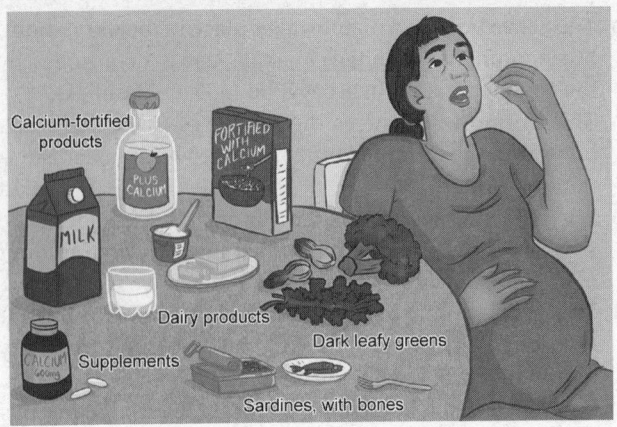

Fig. 6.4: Common calcium sources.

- **Concentration:** The higher concentration of Ca in the intestine the greater the absorption.
- **Dietary protein:** When the diet is high in protein, higher percentage of Ca is adsorbed, but this higher amount of Ca absorbed results in higher renal excretion after which a negative Ca balance follows. This means that high-protein diets increase calcium requirements to maintain Ca balance.
- **Lactose:** It is enhances Ca absorption through the action of lactobacilli, which produces lactic acid and this in turn reduces the pH.
- **Acidity:** The acid medium (lower pH) enhances the absorption of Ca. The HCl secreted in the stomach during a meal, increases Ca absorption, therefore, it is advised to take calcium supplements with a meal especially in older adults.
- **Body mechanisms:** The two most important mechanisms that control the calcium absorption involve vitamin D and the parathyroid hormone (PTH). The low-blood calcium concentration triggers the secretion of PTH. PTH then stimulates the kidneys to synthesize calcitriol, which is the active form of vitamin D. Due to this, metabolite increases the absorption from the intestine and along with PTH it also mobilizes calcium from the bones.

Functions of Calcium

- **Formation and maintenance of bone and teeth:** An adult human body has approximately 1,200 g of Ca, out of which 99% is maintained in the skeletal tissue and used for developing bones out of cartilage. They form salts, which provide structural rigidity to bones and teeth as hydroxyapatite. Small amounts of magnesium, sodium, carbonate, citrate, chloride and fluoride are also present in bone salts. The bones not only provide the rigid structure and framework to the body, but are also a storehouse for Ca which is mobilized to maintain serum levels constant at all times. The remaining 1% of Ca is distributed throughout the extracellular and intracellular fluids of the body.

Figure 6.5 is depicted the calcium deficiency.

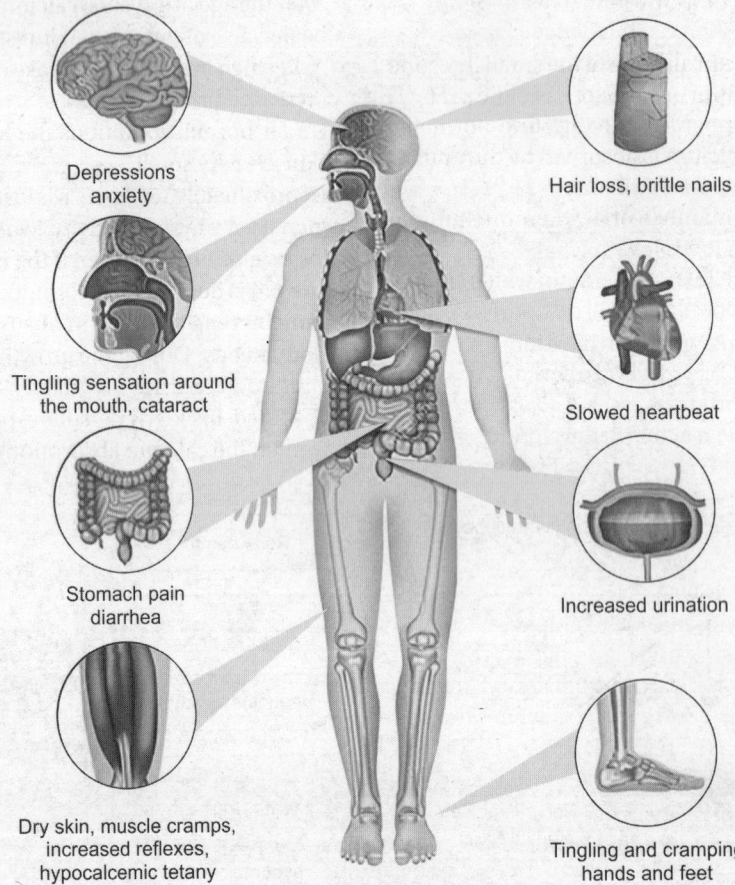

Fig. 6.5: Calcium deficiency.

- **Growth:** Calcium is essential for the growth of children.
- **Enzyme activation:** Calcium activates many enzymes, such as pancreatic lipase, adenosine triphosphatase (ATPase) and some protein splitting enzymes.
- **Nerve impulse transmission:** It is needed for the synthesis of acetylcholine, which is necessary for transmission of nerve impulse.
- **Muscle contraction and relaxation:** Each muscle fiber contains hundreds of myofibrils, which are small contractile units. These myofibrils are composed of muscle protein filaments myosin and actin. Each myofibril has T-tubules and sarcoplasmic reticulam along its sides. Calcium is firmly bound to these reticulams. Whenever the body receives a signal, Ca is suddenly released, ionized and mobilized. This free calcium ion acts as an activator for the chemical reaction between actin and myosin filament and a large amount of energy in the form of adenosine triphosphate (ATP) is released and brings about muscle contraction. The Ca ions again attach themselves back to sarcoplastic reticulam and cause relaxation. Minerals-like magnesium and potassium also play a role in this process. Calcium also regulates the heartbeat and is necessary for the functioning of heart muscle.
- **Cell membrane permeability:** It increases the cell membrane permeability, therefore helps in the process of absorption. Calcium ions control the passage of fluids through cell membranes.
- **Absorption:** It aids in the absorption of vitamin B1
- **Blood clotting:** Calcium ions catalyze several steps in the process of blood clotting. The inactive form of blood coagulation protein (prothrombin) is catalyzed by Ca$^+$ and converted to an active form (thrombin). Thrombin then catalyzes the next protein (fibrinogen) to form fibrin (the clot).

Recommended Dietary Allowances

- The dietary requirement of calcium has been studied extensively universally, but there is no general agreement among the experts.
- Some studies on Western population have indicated much higher requirements of Ca (1 g) whose diet consists of high levels of milk and milk products.
- On the other hand people residing in developing countries take about 500 mg without any symptoms of deficiency.
- The FAQ/WHO committee has recommended 400–500 mg Ca as 'practical allowance' adults.

Deficiency

Calcium related health problems occur due to inadequate intake, improper absorption or utilization of Ca.
- **Osteoporosis:** Osteoporosis is a condition found primarily among middle aged and elderly woman, where the bone mass of the skeleton is diminished. It is a condition of multiple origins. It results due to the following reasons:
  - Prolonged dietary inadequacy
  - Poor absorption and utilization of Ca
  - Immobility
  - Decreased levels of estrogen in postmenopausal women

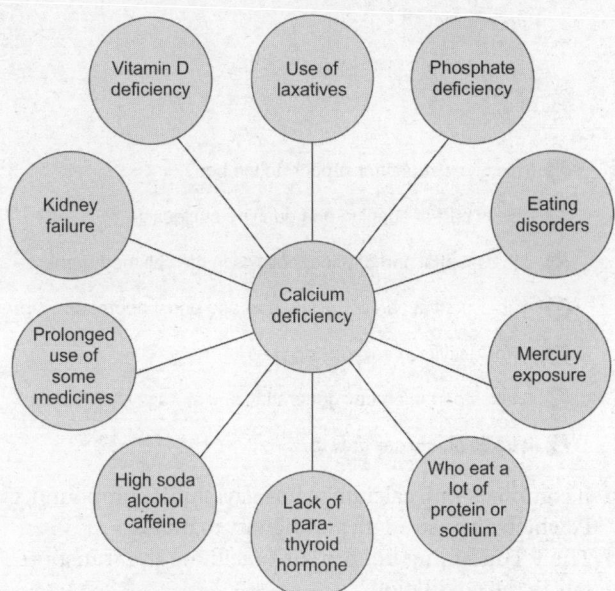

Fig. 6.6: Causes of calcium deficiency.

  - Hyperparathyroidism
  - Vitamin D deficiency
- **Osteomalacia:** Osteomalacia is a condition in which the quality but not the quantity of bone is reduced. This condition is discussed in detail under deficiency of vitamin D.
- **Tetany:** Tetany occurs when Ca in the blood drops below the critical level. There is a change in the stimulation of nerve cells resulting in increased excitability of the nerve and uncontrolled contraction of the muscle tissue. Hence Ca and P ratio in the diet should be maintained at 1:1 for proper utilization of Ca in the body.

Figure 6.6 is depicted the causes of calcium deficiency.

PHOSPHORUS

- Phosphorus (P) takes a second place in regard to the total amount of minerals present in the body and constitutes about one fourth of all body minerals.
- About 80% of the P is found in bones combined with Ca and the rest is found in bones combined with Ca and the rest is found in soft tissues and body fluids.
- Phosphorus plays an important role in the formation of teeth and bones, maintenance of acid base balance of the blood and supplying energy to the muscles for contraction.
- Phosphorus is found in good amount in the foods, which are rich in protein and Ca. Thus milk, cheese, egg yolk, meat, fish are good source of P.
- Deficiency of Ca and P causes rickets in children is generally contributed to lack of vitamin D. Osteomalacia, the adult rickets, may also be due to a Ca deficiency, but usually, the situation is complicated by deficiency P and vitamin D as well as other factors.

Functions

Phosphorus is one mineral which performs widely differing functions. These are:

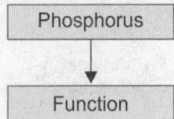

1. This gives structural support to the body
2. This is part of adenine and guanine nucleoside
3. It is essential part of phospholipids in the cell membrane
4. It is essential part of nucleic acid and phosphoprotien
5. It has activity in enzyme sysytem
6. It takes part in energy generation and storage of ATP
7. It takes part in cell growth

- It combines with calcium to form insoluble compound, Ca P, which gives strength and rigidity to bones.
- The P containing lipoproteins facilitate the transport of fats in the circulation.
- Phosphorus is a constituent of nucleoproteins, the basic genetic material.
- Phospholipids are constituents of cell membranes, thus regulating the transport of solutes into and out of the cell.
- Phosphorylation is the key reaction in many metabolic processes.
- Phosphorus captures and store vital energy in the cells of many tissues by forming a high-energy compound. Muscle tissue is a prominent example where P helps in energy store and thus fuel muscle contraction.
- Inorganic P in the body fluids constitutes an important buffer system in the regulation of body neutrality.

Food Sources

Phosphorus is widely distributed in foods; the milk and meat groups being important contributors. Whole grain cereals and flours contain much more P that refined cereals and flours. Vegetables and fruits contain only small amount of P.

Figure 6.7 is depicted the rich sources of calcium.

Deficiency

A deficiency of P is generally not seen in human beings because diets having cereals as major food are seldom inadequate in phosphorus.

■ IRON

The total body iron is 4 g in adults. Iron exists in a complex form in our body. It is present as:
- Iron porphyrin compounds—hemoglobin in RBC, myoglobin in muscle.
- Enzymes: Peroxidases, succinate dehydrogenase and cytochrome oxidase.
- Transport and storage forms—transferrin and ferritin:
  - Amount of iron in the adult body is about 3–5 g of which 70% is in circulating hemoglobin, 4% in the myoglobin of the muscles and 25% in the stores held in liver, bone marrow, spleen and kidneys.

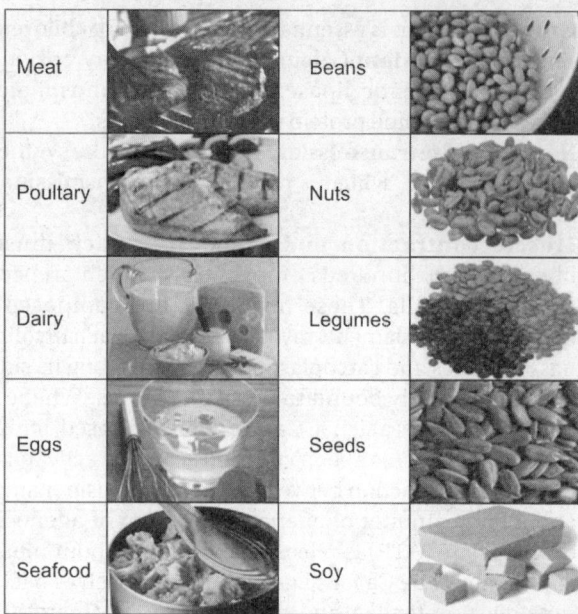

Fig. 6.7: Rich sources of calcium.

- Iron is essential for the oxidation the body. Hemoglobin combines with oxygen in the lungs to form oxyhemoglobin and is carried to the tissues by blood circulation.
- Iron-containing oxygen in the muscles makes the oxidation of carbohydrate, fat and protein possible within the intact cell.
- Iron is stored chiefly in the liver, spleen and bone marrow. The amount is variable, ranging from 1 to 2 g.
- Recommended allowances based on the availability and utilization of iron, it is recommended that 20–30 mg of iron per day is sufficient for an adult. The requirements increase in special conditions-like pregnancy.
- Nutritional anemia's are due to the deficiency of iron, folic acid.
- Liver is an excellent source of iron. Other meat products and egg yolk also have generous amount of this mineral

Figure 6.8 is depicted the iron metabolism and deficiencies and **Figure 6.9** is depicted the health benefits of iron.

Functions (Fig. 6.10)

The chief functions of iron in the body are:
- Iron forms a part of the protein: hemoglobin, which carries oxygen to different parts of the body.
- It forms a part of the myoglobin in muscles, which makes oxygen available for muscle contraction.
- Iron is necessary for the utilization of energy as part of the cells metabolic machinery.
- As part of enzymes iron catalyzes many important reactions in the body.

Examples are:
- Conversion of beta-carotene to active form of vitamin A.
- Synthesis of carnitine, purines, collagen and neurotransmitters.
- Detoxification of drugs in the liver.

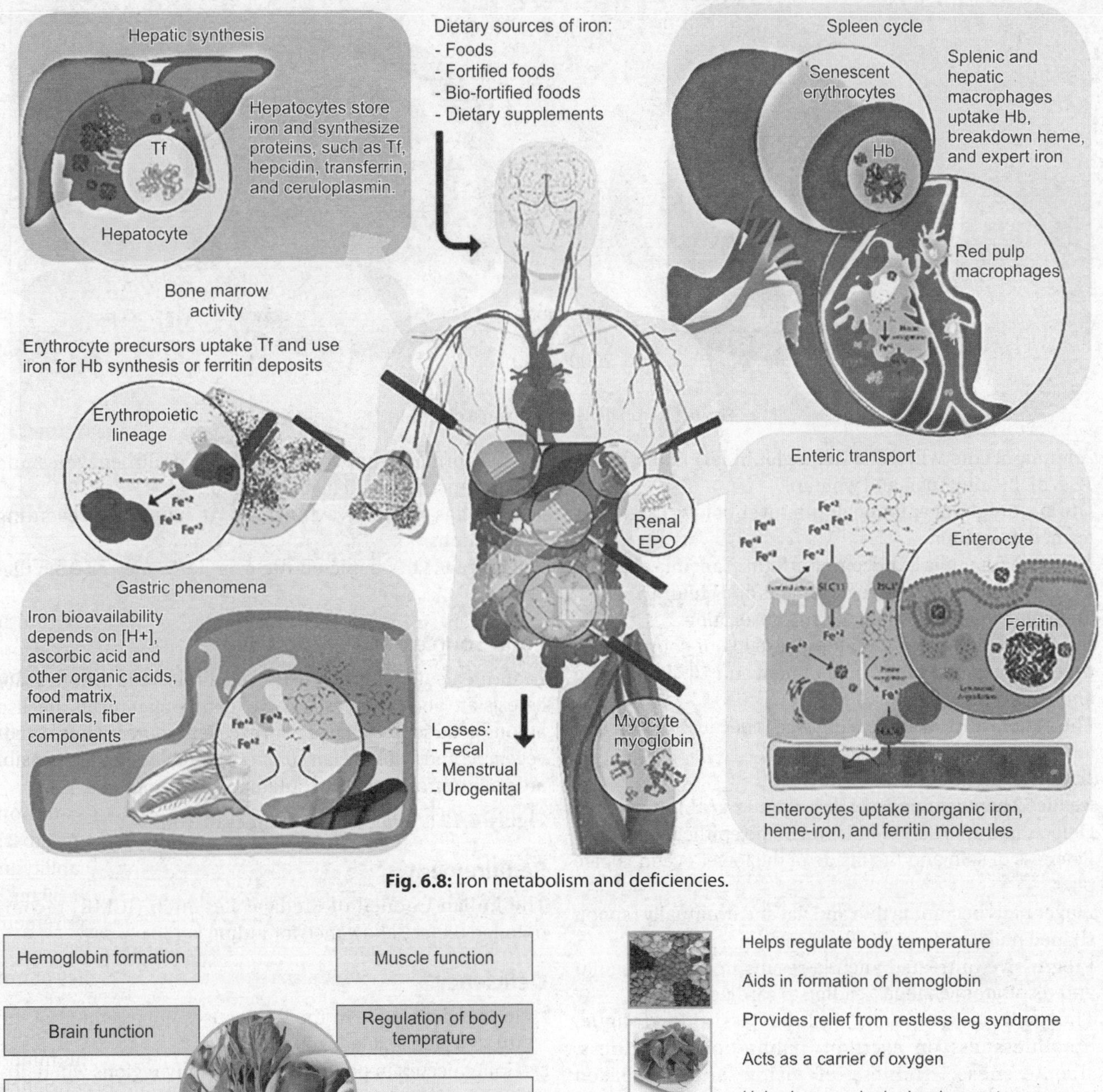

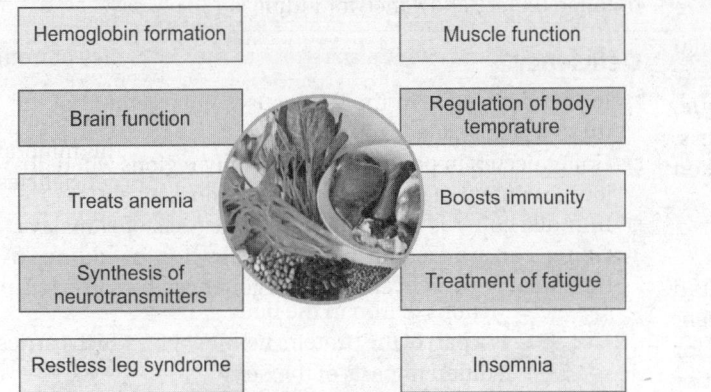

Fig. 6.8: Iron metabolism and deficiencies.

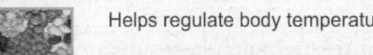
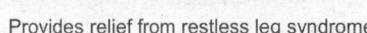
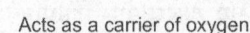
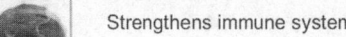

Fig. 6.9: Health benefits of iron.

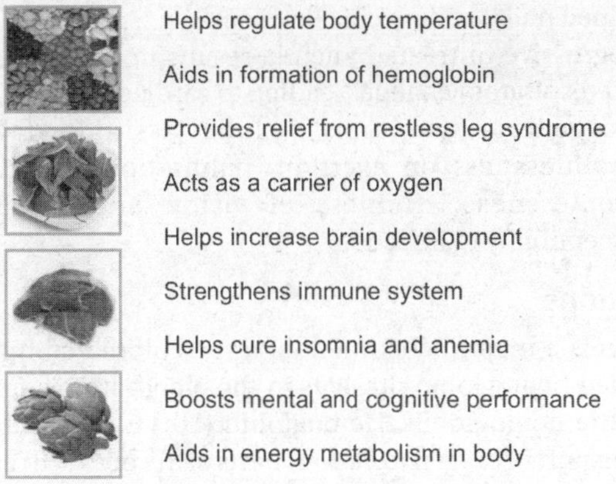

Fig. 6.10: Functions of iron.

Food Sources

- The iron present in food can be as heme and non-heme iron depending upon the source from which it is obtained.
- Heme iron is obtained from animal tissues; non-heme iron is obtained from plant foods. Sources of non-heme iron are ragi, green leafy vegetables, dried fruits and jaggery.
- Liver, fish, poultry, meat, eggs dates are good sources of heme iron. Heme iron is absorbed and utilized better than the non-heme iron. Iron absorption from Indian diets is only 3% as it is mainly cereal-based diet.

Deficiency

- Dietary iron deficiency leads to nutritional anemia. Nutritional anemia is defined as the condition that results from the inability of the erythropoietic tissue to maintain a normal hemoglobin concentration.

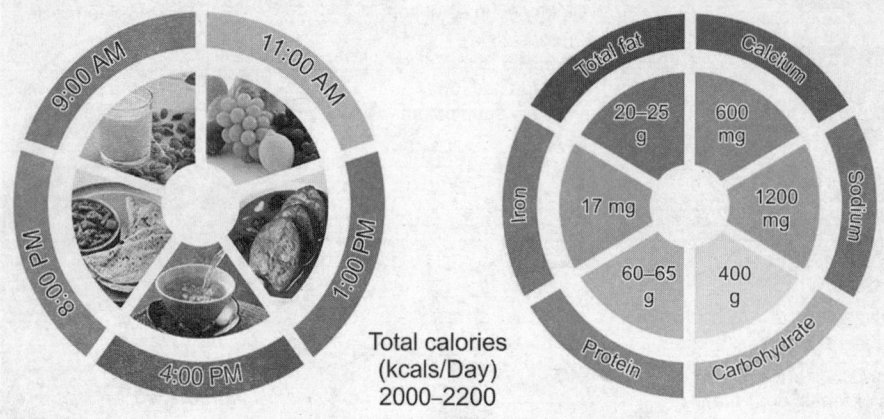

Fig. 6.11: Iron deficiency anemia diet chart.

- Anemia occurs when the hemoglobin level falls below 12 g/dL in adult man and woman.
- During pregnancy, hemoglobin level below 11 g/dL is termed as anemia.
- Nutritional anemia is the common form of anemia affecting women in reproductive years, infants and children, which are mainly due to poor intake and absorption.
- Iron deficiency anemia is widespread in our country. The prevalence varying from 45% in men and 70% in women and children.
- The major cause of anemia in India is because of iron and folic acid deficiency.

Nutritional anemia is manifested as:
- Reduced hemoglobin level (less than 12 g/dL).
- Defects in the structure function of the epithelial tissues.
- Paleness of skin and the inside of the lower eyelid is pale pink.
- Finger nails becoming thin and flat and eventually (spoon shaped nails) koilonychia develops.
- Progressive untreated anemia results in cardiovascular and respiratory changes leading to cardiac failure.
- The general symptoms include lassitude, fatigue, breathlessness on exertion, palpitations, dizziness, sleeplessness, dimness of vision and increased susceptibility to infection.

Functions

- Iron is a major constituent of a red colored compound called hemoglobin presents in the blood. Iron is present in the hemoglobin. Hemoglobin (Hb) is necessary for transport of oxygen to various parts of the body. Hb carries oxygen from the lungs to the tissues and in turn helps in carrying carbon dioxide from the tissue to the lungs. From the lungs carbon dioxide is then exhaled out.
- Iron is also present in the muscle in the form of myoglobin. Myoglobin has the capacity to store oxygen. This oxygen is used for muscle contraction and for other immediate needs of the muscle cells.
- Iron facilitates the complete oxidation of carbohydrate fats and proteins within the cell.
- Iron plays on important role in maintenance of specific brain.
- Iron forms a vital component of certain enzymes and substances that aid in metabolism.
- Iron has protective function. It helps in preventing infections.

Figure 6.11 is depicted the iron deficiency anemia diet chart.

Food Sources

Lean meats, deep green leafy vegetables and whole-grain cereals are good sources. Egg, yolk and organ meats are also among good sources. Liver is an excellent source of iron. Other vegetable and fruits are fair source. Milk, cheese and ice-cream are poor sources. Jaggery contains a good amount of iron.

Figure 6.12 is depicted the sources of iron.

Requirement

The Indian Council of Medical Research (ICMR) recommended dietary allowance for iodine is 150 µg/day.

Deficiency

- Iodine deficiency in the diet causes enlargement of the thyroid gland called 'goiter'.
- Goiter occurs in people staying in hilly regions where the iodine content of water and soil is comparatively less.
- In India, goiter is common in hilly districts of Himalaya. Goiter can be treated by administration of iodine. If treatment is given in early stages goiter can be corrected.

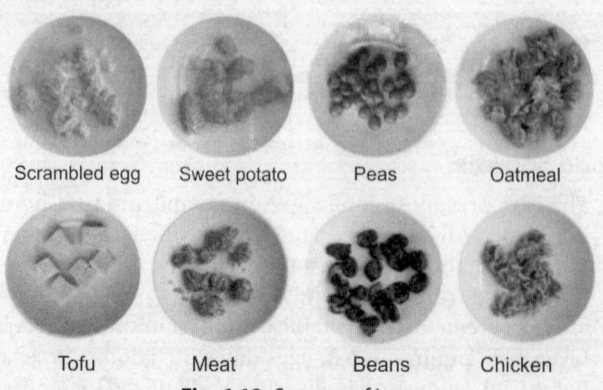

Fig. 6.12: Sources of iron.

- Severe iodine deficiency in children leads to hypothyroidism resulting in retarded physical and mental growth. This condition is known as cretinism.
- Goitrogens are substances present in foods, which cause goiter. These substances react with iodine present in the food making it unavailable for absorption. Foods, such as cabbage, cauliflower, raddish contain goitrogens.

ZINC

Zinc (Zn) is primarily intracellular substance. Its total quantity in the body is 2.3 g. largest stores of Zn are present in the bones. Zinc forms a constituent of the blood. Zinc is an important element performing a range of function in the body as it is a cofactor for a number of enzymes.

Figure 6.13 is depicted the role of zinc in human body.

Functions

Zinc is necessary for carrying out many primary functions in the body, such as:
- Bolstering immunity
- Enhancing nervous system function, brain activity, memory and concentration
- Lowering inflammation in certain conditions in the body like acne
- Accelerating wound healing process, in instances of tissue injury
- Preventing chronic diseases in old age, such as diabetes, heart disease and age-related macular degeneration, by fostering healthy aging process
- Preserving a normal sense of taste and smell
- Promoting optimal cell growth, division as well as DNA and protein synthesis

Sources

Meat, unmilled cereals and legumes are good sources. Fruits and vegetables are poor sources. Some of the food sources that offer profuse amounts of the trace mineral zinc include:

- Legumes such as channa, kidney beans, chickpeas
- Nuts and seeds, such as almonds, cashews, pumpkin seeds
- Dairy products including milk, cheese and yoghurt
- Whole grains, such as quinoa, oats
- Vegetables including mushrooms, peas and greens like spinach, kale

Requirements

- The daily requirement of Zn in adults is 15.5 mg/day as recommended by the ICMR expert group.
- Apart from iron, iodine, zinc, copper, selenium and fluoride are essential trace elements.
- Copper is essential element in iron absorption. Selenium is an essential element along with vitamin E for maintaining integrity of the liver cells.
- Fluoride is required in minimum amounts to prevent dental caries. Excessive consumption leads to mottling of teeth.

Deficiency

A deficiency in the quantity of zinc being consumed as part of diet causes many symptoms of discomfort and hampers the functioning of the immune system. Zinc deficiency invariably results in sudden weight loss, opens sores and wounds that do not heal, decreased appetite, diarrhea and lowered sense of smell and taste.

Figure 6.14 is depicted the zinc deficiency and excess symptoms and **Figure 6.15** is depicted the symptoms and hidden causes of a severe zinc deficiency.

Toxicity

Excessive intake of zinc through food can result in dangerous levels of the metallic substance accumulating in the body. This causes grave complications, such as abdominal cramps, high blood cholesterol levels and severe headaches that affect normal brain functions. Hence, it is advised to consume only the recommended daily intake of zinc and not ingest surplus amounts, in order to steer clear of its toxic effects.

IODINE

About one-third of iodine present in an adult body variously estimated from 25 to 50 mg is found in the thyroid gland. The concentration in thyroid tissue is 2,500 times as great as is any other tissue, all of which contain traces.

- Iodine is considered to be an important dietary nutrient because normal functioning of thyroid gland depends upon adequate supply of it in the body. It is an essential component of thyroxine and other iodine containing compounds of thyroid glands.
- Primary function of thyroxine is to influence the rate of oxidation in the cells of the body. Thyroxine also helps in normal growth and development in the Young's all the species.
- Sources of iodine vary widely under different soil and fertilizer conditions. Marine or deep sea fish and shellfish are high in iodine content. The leaves and flowers of plants have higher concentration of iodine than roots.

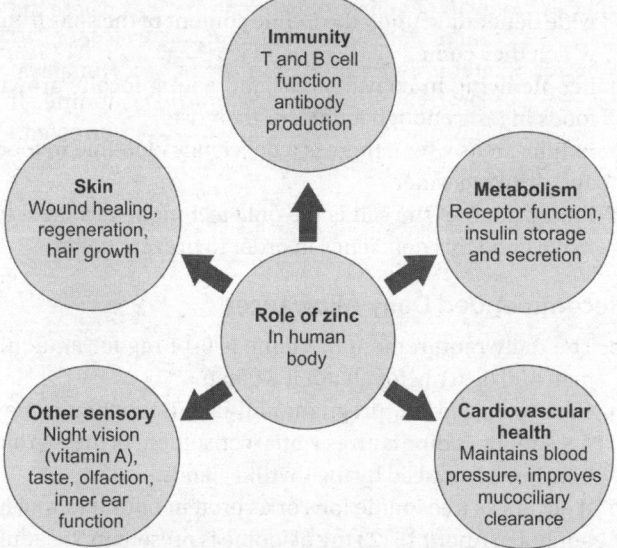

Fig. 6.13: Role of zinc in human body.

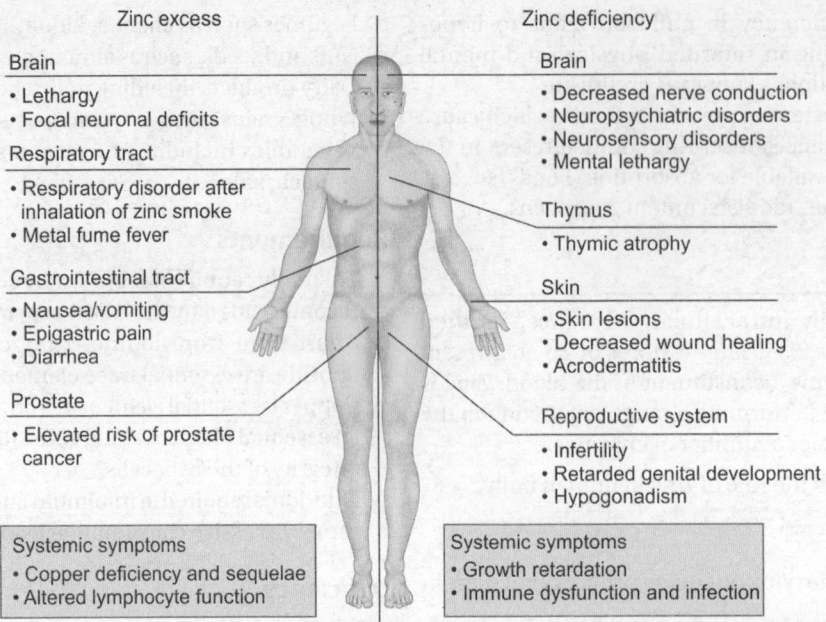

Fig. 6.14: Zinc deficiency and excess symptoms.

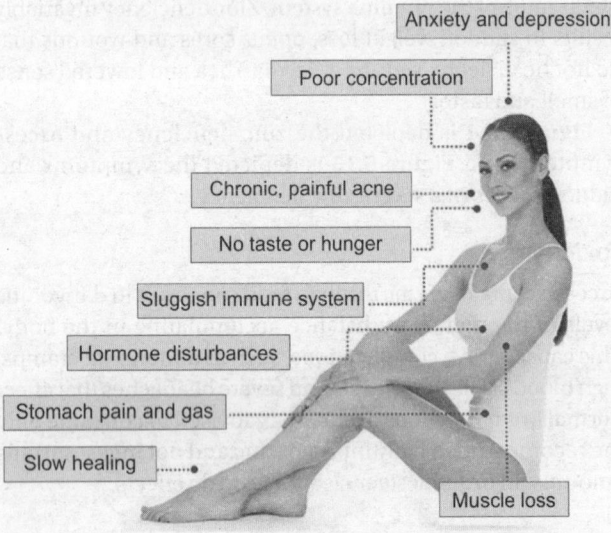

Fig. 6.15: Symptoms and hidden causes of a severe zinc deficiency.

- The recommended daily allowances of iodine have been reported to be about 100–150 mg.
- Prolonged deficiency of iodine not only develops goiter but also causes sterility in many cases. Development of goiter enlargement of thyroid gland, during pregnant indicates special requirement of iodine.

Figure 6.16 is depicted the health benefits of iodine.

Functions

- The only known function of iodine is as a constituent of thyroglobulin, a protein complex of several iodine-containing compounds.
- The thyroid hormone regulates the rate of oxidation within the cells and in doing so, regulates the physical and mental growth; the functioning of nervous and muscle tissues, circulating activity and the metabolism of all nutrients.

Figure 6.17 is depicted the iron deficiency.

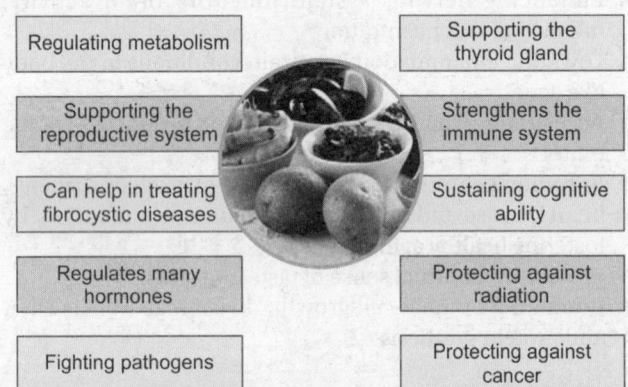

Fig. 6.16: Health benefits of iodine.

Food Sources

- Iodine is supplied by food and water; the variations are wide depending upon the iodine content of the soils from which they come.
- People living in coastal areas and eating locally grown foods ingests enough iodine for their use.
- In hilly areas where there is a deficiency of iodine in food and drinking water.
- Iodinization of the salt is the only technique available to make good this deficiency in order to prevent goiter.

Recommended Daily Allowances

- The daily requirement of iodine is 0.14 mg for an adult man and 0.10 mg for an adult woman.
- Growing children, pregnant and lactating women may need more. Iodine is an essential constituent of the thyroid hormone produced by the thyroid glands.
- It occurs as free iodide ions or as protein bound iodine in our body. About 15–23 mg of iodine is present in the adult human body.

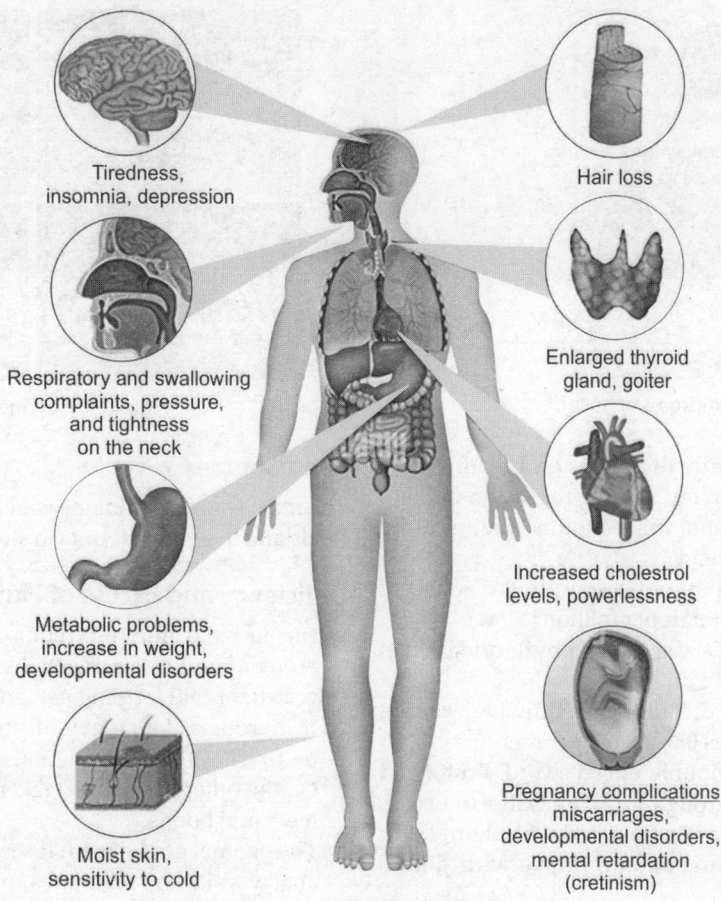

Fig. 6.17: Iron deficiency.

- The body store of iodine is predominantly present in thyroid gland and also in salivary gland, mammary glands, gastric glands and in kidneys to a certain extent.

  The amount of iodine you need each day depends on your age. Average daily recommended amounts are listed below in micrograms (µg).

Life stage	Recommended amount
Birth to 6 months	110 µg
Infants 7–12 months	130 µg
Children 1–8 years	90 µg
Children 9–13 years	120 µg
Teens 14–18 years	150 µg
Adults	150 µg
Pregnant teens and women	220 µg
Breastfeeding teens and women	290 µg

Iodine Deficiency Disorders

- Iodine deficiency disorders (IDD) is one of the biggest worldwide public health problems of today. Their effect is hidden and profoundly affects the quality of human life.
- Iodine deficiency occurs when the soil is poor in iodine, causing a low concentration in food products and insufficient iodine intake in the population. When iodine requirements are not met, the thyroid may no longer be able to synthesize sufficient amounts of thyroid hormone.
- The resulting low-level of thyroid hormones in the blood is the principal factor responsible for the series of functional and developmental abnormalities, collectively referred to as IDD.
- Iodine deficiency is a significant cause of mental developmental problems in children, including implications on reproductive functions and lowering of IQ levels in school-aged children.
- The consequence of iodine deficiency during pregnancy is impaired synthesis of thyroid hormones by the mother and the fetus.
- An insufficient supply of thyroid hormones to the developing brain may result in mental retardation. Brain damage and irreversible mental retardation are the most important disorders induced by iodine deficiency.

Figure 6.18 is depicted the symptoms of goiter.

FLUORIDE

Fluoride occurs normally in the body primarily as a Ca salt in the bones and teeth. It is not essential for life, but small amounts of fluoride bring about striking reductions in tooth decay.

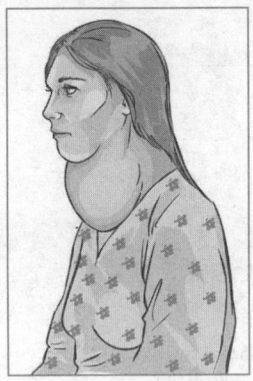

Fig. 6.18: Symptoms of goiter.

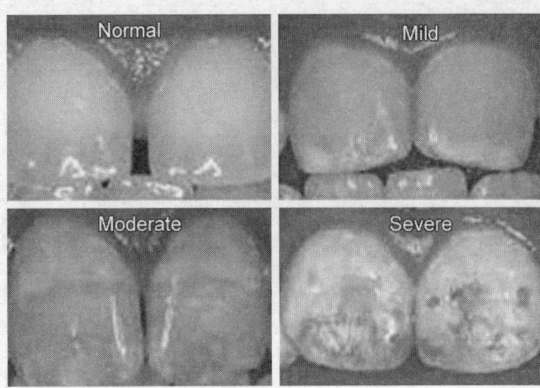

Fig. 6.19: Fluorine deficiency.

- Fluoride is found primarily the bones and teeth. Small amount fluoride brings about striking reduction in teeth decay because this mineral makes tooth enamel more resistant to the action of acid.
- Dental caries is reduced more resistant to the action of acid, water at the rate of 1 part per million (PPM).
- Source of fluoride: Food as well as water by fluoridation of the water at the rate of 1 PPM.
- The recommended level of fluorides in drinking water in this country is accepted as 0.5–0.8 mg per liter.
- Fluoride is often called double-edged sword. Prolonged ingestion of fluorides through drinking water in excess of the daily requirement is associated with dental and skeletal fluorosis and inadequate intake with dental caries.

Box 6.1 is depicted the fluorine.

Functions

A proper intake of fluoride is essential to prevent dental caries. It is required for normal mineralization of bones.

- As the enamel is developing in children's teeth, if fluoride is present, it replaces the OH (hydroxy-) part of hydroxyapatite, forming fluorapatite, which is harder and more resistant to decay.
- When the demineralization process is occurring in the presence of fluoride, again the newly formed enamel is stronger.
- Fluoride becomes concentrated inside the plaque bacteria, which reduces their ability to produce acid, so less demineralization of the teeth occurs.
- There is some evidence that children who grow up in areas where fluoride is present in the water have shallower grooves in the biting surfaces of their teeth, thus reducing the places where bacteria can lodge to form plaque.

> **Box 6.1:** Fluorine sources and RDA.
>
> **Source**
> - Source of fluorine is drinking water
> - The content of fluorine in water is dependent on the soil content of fluoride
>
> **RDA**
> - 1.5 to 4 mg/day or 1.2 ppm (since it is present in water, it is expressed as ppm)

Food Sources

The main source is drinking water. It occurs in traces in many foods and in good amounts in shellfish, cheese, etc.

Deficiency and Excess of Fluoride

- On one hand fluoride is required for deposition of fluorides on teeth and discourages the solubility of minerals and growth of acid forming bacteria.
- If there is a deficiency of fluoride during the growing period, it will result in dental caries and tooth decay.
- On the other hand when taken in excess it could damage teeth and bones.
- The enamel on the teeth loses its luster, becomes patchy, chalky white and pits appear on its surface. This condition is known as dental flurosis.

Figure 6.19 is depicted the fluorine deficiency.

■ SODIUM

An adult body contains approximately 120 g of sodium of which about 50% of the body's sodium is present in the extracellular fluid, 40% in bones and 10% or less in intracellular fluid. (Intracellular fluid refers to fluid inside the cell).

Functions

- **To conduct nerve impulses:** During the resting state, the sodium-potassium pump maintains a difference in charge across the cell membrane of the neuron, when signals come across the membrane, the sodium channel opens and they enter into the cell.
- **Contract/relax muscles:** To contract a muscle fiber, sodium rapidly flows into the cell, and simultaneously potassium comes out of the cell. These steps are reversed when a muscle relaxes means sodium moves out of the cell, and potassium back into the cells.
- Maintain a proper balance of water/minerals: It is one of the body's electrolytes and an important part of a very complex, fluid balance process. Our body keeps a record for loss of body water and the hypothalamus senses the sodium and water concentration in extracellular fluids and accordingly restores them. Most of the body's sodium resides in blood and the fluid that surrounds the cells.

Figure 6.20 is depicted the health benefits of sodium.

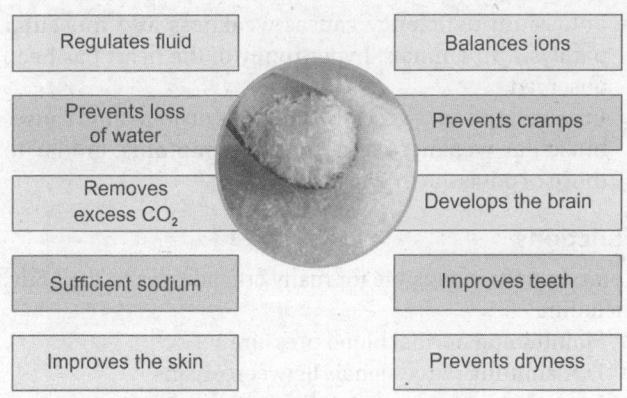

Fig. 6.20: Health benefits of sodium.

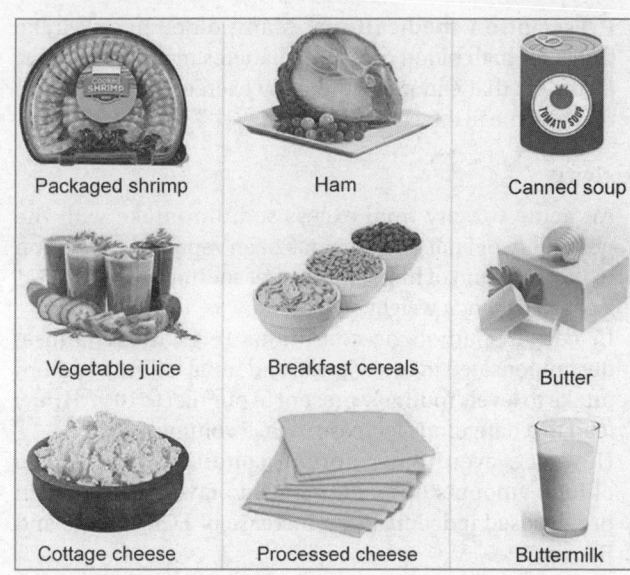

Fig. 6.21: Food sources.

Food Sources

- Common salt or sodium chloride is the chief source of sodium in the diet. One teaspoon of salt provides almost 2,000 mg sodium. It universally used to flavor the food we eat and is also used for preserving food for long periods.
- Numerous sodium compounds are used in food processing and preparation; baking soda, baking powder, sodium alginate, sodium propionate, sodium citrate.
- Sodium is basically ingested into the body as salt, i.e., sodium chloride, via processed foods and the table salt or iodized salt used in cooking and seasoning.
- While only negligible amounts of sodium are absorbed by means of salt used in preparing dishes or flavoring salads, soups, the major proportion of sodium consumed as part of diet actually comes from packaged foods and enriched products.
- These comprise bread, pizza, frozen meat, oily and fried fast food, as well as spicy snacks and savouries such as chips, popcorn, crackers, cookies, sauces, dips and ketchup.
- The recommended daily intake of sodium for healthy adults is 2,300 mg per day. Adults with high blood pressure should further limit salt quantities to less than 1,500 mg per day.

Figure 6.21 is depicted the food sources.

Recommended Daily Allowances

5–10 g of salt (sodium chloride) is sufficient for an average adult. An individual doing hard labor may need more.

Sodium Imbalance

- Osmotic pressure and the pH are seriously affected when there is a disturbance in the concentrations of sodium in the extracellular fluid of the body tissues.
- When there is retention of sodium in the tissue, edema occurs. In cardiac and renal failure sodium excretion gets reduced.
- Excess sodium losses occur during the hot weather causing muscular weakness, cramps, fatigue, vomiting and loss of appetite. In this case, a small amount of salt may be added to liquid intake.

Deficiency Diseases

- Hyponatremia is a deficiency disease wherein sodium concentrations in the body are very low.
- A normal blood sodium level is between 135 and 145 milliequivalents per liter (mEq/L). Hyponatremia occurs when the sodium in your blood falls below 135 mEq/L.
- Hyponatremia usually develops when the body retains too much fluid, as in the case of heart failure or liver disease. It is very commonly observed in people who drink too many fluids regularly, as well as those on diuretic medicines, to resolve the health issue of kidneys not functioning optimally.

Imbalance in Sodium Levels and Risk of Hypertension

As people age, the body is less able to maintain fluid and sodium balance for several reasons, such as:

- **Unhealthy diet:** Consuming processed, deep-fried foods regularly, as well as snacking often on salted nuts, chips and biscuits.
- **Decreased thirst:** As people age, they sense thirst less quickly or less intensely and thus may not drink fluids when needed.
- **Changes in the kidneys:** Aging kidneys may become less able to reclaim water and electrolytes from the urine and as a result, more water may be excreted in the urine.
- **Less fluid in the body:** In older people, the body contains less fluid. Only 45% of body weight is fluid in older people, compared with 60% of younger people. This change means that a slight loss of fluid and sodium, as can result from a fever or from not eating and drinking enough, can have more serious consequences in older people.
- **Inability to obtain water:** Some older people have physical problems that prevent them from getting something to drink when they are thirsty. Others may have dementia, which may prevent them from realizing they are thirsty or from saying so. These people may have to depend on other people to provide them with water.

- **Prescription medications:** Many older people take drugs for high blood pressure, diabetes mellitus, or heart disorders that can make the body excrete excess fluid or magnify the ill effects of fluid loss.

Toxicity

- An acute toxicity from excess sodium intake with the possibility of fatal outcome has been reported in relation to the ingestion of huge amounts of sodium, such as 0.5–1 g of salt/kg body weight.
- In certain pathologic conditions (e.g., heart failure, decompensated liver cirrhosis, and renal failure), sodium intake to levels routinely present in our diet (≥10 g/d) may lead to a dangerous increase in ECF volume.
- However, even under normal conditions, the intake of high amounts of sodium tends to favor, especially in predisposed individuals, an increase of ECF volume and BP.

■ POTASSIUM

Potassium is an essential mineral that is needed by all tissues in the body. It is sometimes referred to as an electrolyte because it carries a small electrical charge that activates various cell and nerve functions. Potassium is found naturally in many foods and as a supplement. Its main role in the body is to help maintain normal levels of fluid inside our cells. Sodium, its counterpart, maintains normal fluid levels outside of cells. Potassium also helps muscles to contract and supports normal blood pressure.

Figure 6.22 is depicted the health benefits of potassium.

An adult body contains about 250 g of potassium of which about 97% of the potassium in the body is in intracellular fluid (intracellular fluid refers to fluid inside the cells), while the remainder being in the extracellular fluid compartments (extracellular fluid refers to fluid outside the cells).

- The adult human body contains about 250 g potassium, which is present almost in the cells of different tissues, muscle, etc.
- The functions of potassium is regulation of pH of cell contents, regulation of the osmotic pressure of cell contents and potassium ion increases the relaxation of heart muscle which is antagonized by calcium ion.
- Potassium deficiency causes weakness and muscular paralysis. In animals, hypertrophy of the heart has been observed.
- In consumption of excessive amounts of potassium causes muscular weakness and apathy; symptoms similar to those of potassium deficiency.

Functions

Potassium is responsible for many crucial roles in the body, including:
- Maintaining normal blood pressure
- Transmitting nerve signals between organs
- Controlling muscle contractions
- Ensuring optimal water balance within the system
- Balancing pH in the body between acidity and alkalinity
- Upholding accurate heart rate, i.e., pulse
- Regulating proper digestion processes
- Preventing stroke and heart disease
- Sustaining regular heart muscle activity

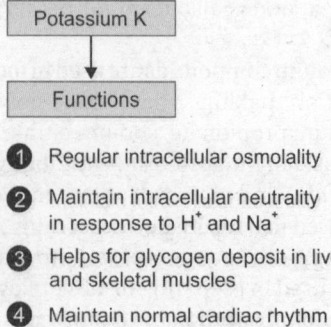

1. Regular intracellular osmolality
2. Maintain intracellular neutrality in response to H^+ and Na^+
3. Helps for glycogen deposit in liver and skeletal muscles
4. Maintain normal cardiac rhythm
5. Maintain smooth muscles and skeletal muscles contraction

Food Sources

- Potassium is widely distributed in foods. Meat, poultry and fish are good sources.
- Fruits, vegetables and whole grain cereals are especially high in potassium. Banana, potatoes, tomatoes, carrots orange juice, grapefruit juice are rich sources.
  - Winter squash, cubed, 1 cup, cooked: 896 mg
  - Sweet potato, medium, baked with skin: 694 mg
  - Potato, medium, baked with skin: 610 mg
  - White beans, canned, drained, half cup: 595 mg
  - Yogurt, fat-free, 1 cup: 579 mg
  - Halibut, 3 ounces, cooked: 490 mg
  - 100% orange juice, 8 ounces: 496 mg
  - Broccoli, 1 cup, cooked: 457 mg
  - Cantaloupe, cubed, 1 cup: 431 mg
  - Banana, 1 medium: 422 mg
  - Pork tenderloin, 3 ounces, cooked: 382 mg
  - Lentils, half cup, cooked: 366 mg
  - Milk, 1% low fat, 8 ounces: 366 mg
  - Salmon, farmed Atlantic, 3 ounces, cooked: 326 mg
  - Pistachios, shelled, 1 ounce, dry roasted: 295 mg
  - Raisins, quarter cup: 250 mg
  - Chicken breast, 3 ounces, cooked: 218 mg
  - Tuna, light, canned, drained, 3 ounces: 201 mg

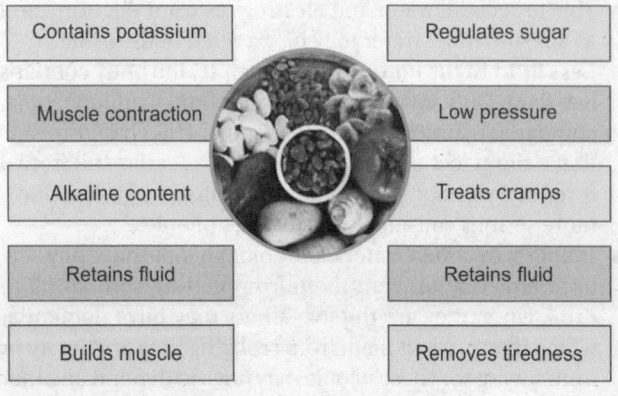

Fig. 6.22: Health benefits of potassium.

Food type	Amount of potassium (mg)	Percentage of daily value
A half-cup of dried apricots	1,101	23%
1 cup of cooked lentils	731	16%
A half-cup of dried prunes	699	15%
1 cup of mashed acorn squash	644	14%
A medium baked potato, no skin	610	13%
1 cup of canned kidney beans	607	13%
1 cup of orange juice	496	11%
A half-cup of boiled soybeans	443	9%
A medium banana	422	9%
1 cup of 1% milk	366	8%

Recommended Daily Allowance

The exact amount of potassium required is not known. A normal diet provides this mineral in sufficient amount.

Age	Male	Female
0–6 months	400 mg/day	400 mg/day
7–12 months	860 mg/day	860 mg/day
1–3 years	2,000 mg/day	2,000 mg/day
4–8 years	2,300 mg/day	2,300 mg/day
9–13 years	2,500 mg/day	2,300 mg/day
14–18 years	3,000 mg/day	2,300 mg/day
19+ years	3,400 mg/day	2,600 mg/day

The adequate intake during pregnancy is 2,900 mg, and it is 2,800 mg while breastfeeding or chest feeding.

Deficiency

Primarily the deficiency of potassium is not seen. Impaired appetite, severe malnutrition, chronic alcoholism and burn injuries can disturb the acid base balance and lower osmotic pressure.

- The normal body levels of potassium lie in the range of 3.5–5 mmol per liter of blood serum. When potassium levels drop significantly below this range, i.e., lower than 2.5 mmol/liter, a deficiency disorder arises, termed as hypokalemia.
- A person with hypokalemia displays prominent external indications including exhaustion, extreme fatigue even after resting, soreness in muscles and problems with digestion, such as bloating, flatulence and constipation.
- As the quantities of blood potassium fall dangerously low, much below 2.5 mmol per liter, then the severity of symptoms is much higher. The affected individual exhibits partial paralysis in certain muscles and even breathing difficulties and must be given prompt medical care.
- It is hence advised to go for regular health checks, at least once every 6 months, to obtain current blood test results and ensure that bodily potassium levels are at optimal range.

Toxicity

Too much potassium in the blood is called hyperkalemia. In healthy people the kidneys will efficiently remove extra potassium, mainly through the urine. However, certain situations can lead to hyperkalemia—advanced kidney disease, taking medications that hold onto potassium in the body (including NSAIDs), or people who have compromised kidneys who eat a high-potassium diet (more than 4,700 mg daily) or use potassium-based salt substitutes. Symptoms of hyperkalemia:
- Weakness, fatigue
- Nausea, vomiting
- Shortness of breath
- Chest pain
- Heart palpitations, irregular heart rate

■ MAGNESIUM

The amount of magnesium in the body is much smaller than that of calcium and phosphorus, i.e., about 20–35 g in the adult body. Of this about 60% are carbonates and phosphates at the surfaces of the bones. Most of the remaining magnesium is within the cells.
- Magnesium is a constituent of bones and is present in all body cells.
- Human adult body contains about 25 g of magnesium of which about half is found in the skeleton.
- It appears that magnesium is essential for the normal metabolism of calcium and potassium
- Magnesium deficiency may occur in chronic alcoholic, cirrhosis of liver, toxemias of pregnancy, protein-energy malnutrition and malabsorption syndrome.
- The principal clinical features attributed to magnesium deficiency are irritability, tetancy, hyperreflexia and occasionally hyporeflexia.
- The requirements are estimated to be about 200–300 mg/day for adults.

Figure 6.23 is depicted the functions of magnesium in human body.

Functions

- Magnesium is required for numerous biological reactions involving the release of energy.
- It is a constituent of bone. It is involved in bone mineralization.
- It is also essential for normal metabolism of calcium and phosphorus.
- Its presence in the extracellular fluids regulates the transmission of nerve impulses..
- It activates the enzyme responsible for breakdown of glycogen.

Food Sources

Dairy products excluding butter provide enough magnesium. Flour and cereals products, dry beans, soybeans, peas and nuts are good sources of magnesium. Green leafy vegetables are excellent sources because magnesium is a part of chlorophyll. Some of the foods rich in magnesium content are:

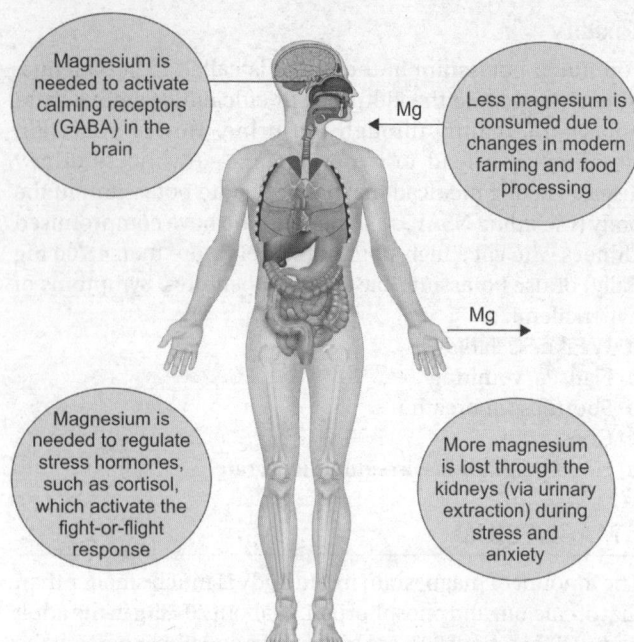

Fig. 6.23: Functions of magnesium in human body.

- Nuts and seeds like almonds and pumpkin seeds
- Dark green leafy vegetables, such as spinach and kale
- Whole wheat bread, oatmeal
- Fruit, such as figs, avocado, banana and raspberries
- Legumes including black beans, chickpeas and kidney beans
- Vegetables, such as peas, broccoli, cabbage, green beans, artichokes, asparagus, brussels sprouts
- Raw cacao
- Dark chocolate
- Tofu

Recommended Intakes

Intake recommendations for magnesium and other nutrients are provided in the Dietary Reference Intakes (DRIs) developed by the Food and Nutrition Board (FNB) at the Institute of Medicine of the National Academies (formerly National Academy of Sciences). DRI is the general term for a set of reference values used to plan and assess nutrient intakes of healthy people. These values, which vary by age and sex, include:

- **Recommended dietary allowance (RDA):** Average daily level of intake sufficient to meet the nutrient requirements of nearly all (97-98%) healthy individuals; often used to plan nutritionally adequate diets for individuals.
- **Adequate intake (AI):** Intake at this level is assumed to ensure nutritional adequacy; established when evidence is insufficient to develop an RDA.
- **Estimated average requirement (EAR):** Average daily level of intake estimated to meet the requirements of 50% of healthy individuals; usually used to assess the nutrient intakes of groups of people and to plan nutritionally adequate diets for them; can also be used to assess the nutrient intakes of individuals.

Table 6.1: Recommended dietary allowances (RDAs) for magnesium.

Age	Male	Female	Pregnancy	Lactation
Birth to 6 months	30 mg*	30 mg*		
7–12 months	75 mg*	75 mg*		
1–3 years	80 mg	80 mg		
4–8 years	130 mg	130 mg		
9–13 years	240 mg	240 mg		
14–18 years	410 mg	360 mg	400 mg	360 mg
19–30 years	400 mg	310 mg	350 mg	310 mg
31–50 years	420 mg	320 mg	360 mg	320 mg
51+ years	420 mg	320 mg		

*Adequate Intake (AI)

- **Tolerable upper intake level (UL):** Maximum daily intake unlikely to cause adverse health effects.

Table 6.1 is depicted the recommended dietary allowances (RDAs) for magnesium.

Effect of Imbalances

- Under normal conditions of health and food intake magnesium deficiency is not likely to occur.
- A deficiency of it may result from malabsorption syndrome, chronic alcoholism and toxemia of pregnancy or after intake of diuretics.
- Deficiency of magnesium results in neuromuscular irritability, tetanic convulsions, twitching, tremors and convulsions.
- In excess, it results in extreme thirst, excessive heat in the body, decrease in neuromuscular.

Figure 6.24 is depicted the magnesium deficiency.

Deficiency:

- Most healthy children and adults do not suffer from a low intake of magnesium in the diet. However, in instances of magnesium deficiency, symptoms such as nausea, vomiting, fatigue, muscle cramps do occur in the person.
- Severe deficiency of magnesium is rare but in such cases, immediate medical care needs to be provided, as abnormal heartbeat and brain disorders are triggered in the individual.

Figure 6.25 is depicted the symptoms of magnesium deficiency.

Toxicity

- Most of the magnesium consumed in the diet is flushed out by means of urine.
- Situations of magnesium accumulating in the body to toxic levels do not occur often. Nevertheless, when magnesium toxicity is detected in a person, grave complications like kidney problems, central nervous system malfunctioning and cardiac arrest can occur. Hence, prompt medical treatment is required in such cases, for normalizing body functions in the person.

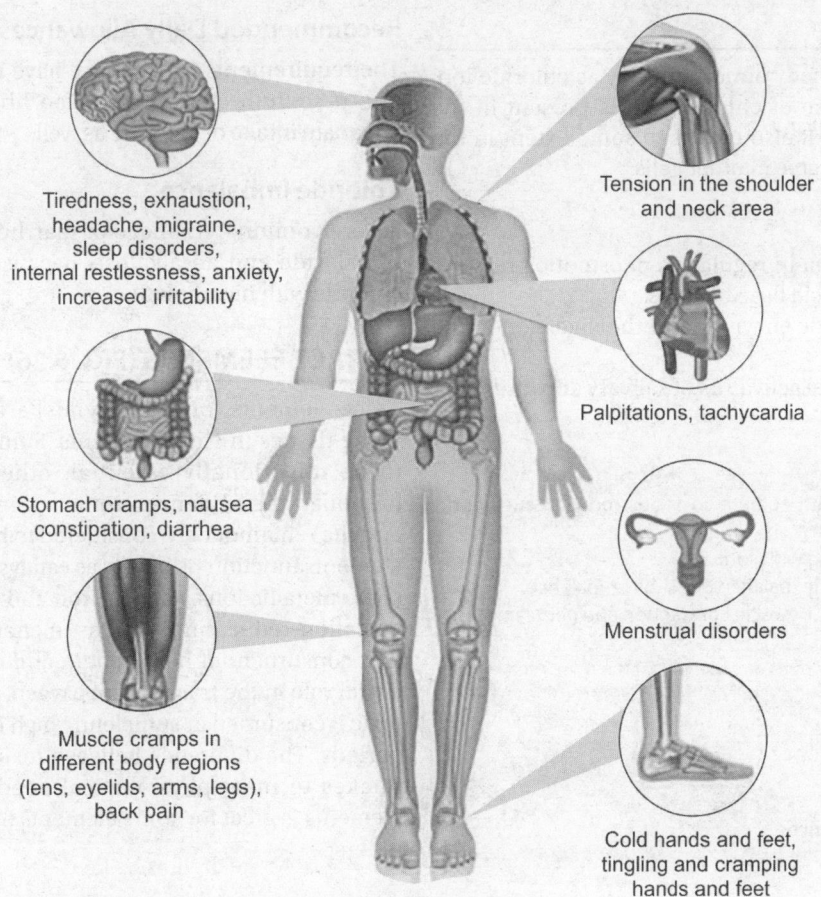

Fig. 6.24: Magnesium deficiency.

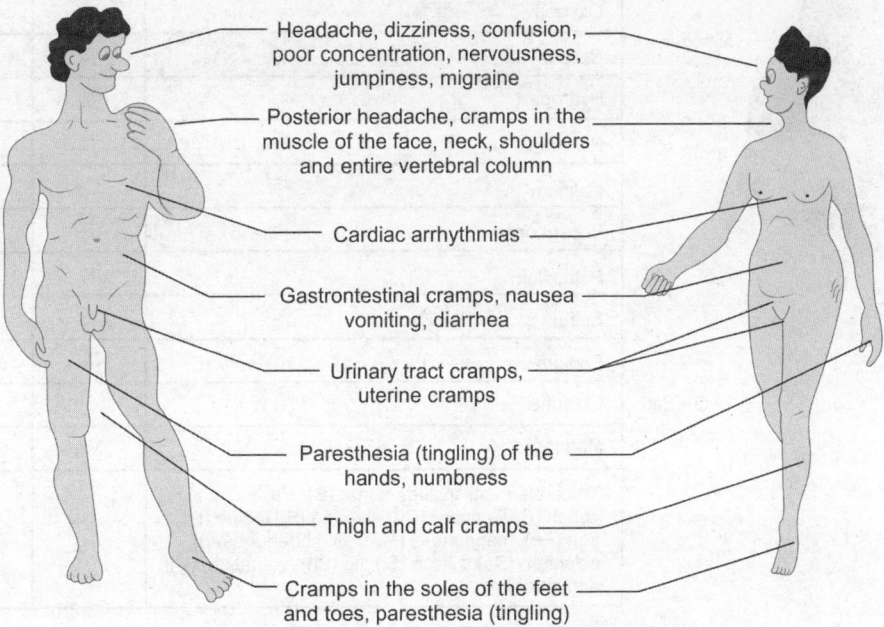

Fig. 6.25: Symptoms of magnesium deficiency.

CHLORINE

Chlorine exists in the body almost entirely as chloride ion. Most of the 100 g or so of chloride ion is present in the extracellular fluid, but it also occurs to some extent in the RBCs and to a lesser degree in other cells.

Functions

- Chlorine is important in regulation of osmotic pressure, water balance and acid base balance.
- It activates the gastric enzymes and the digestion in the stomach.
- It is one of the several activators of salivary amylase.

> **Chloride (Cl)**
> - An essential anion
> - Closely connected with sodium in foods, body tissues and fluids and excretions
> - Readily absorbed along with sodium
> - Important for osmotic balance, acid-base balance, in the formation of gastric HCl, muscle contraction and nerve impulse transmission

> **Deficiency of chloride**
> - Hypochloremic alkalosis
> - Hypovolemia
> - Pernicoious vomiting
> - Psychomotor disturbances

Recommended Daily Allowances

The requirements for chlorine have not been ascertained, but, if sodium chloride is taken liberally, it ensures the adequate intake of chloride as well.

Chloride Imbalance

Severe vomiting, drainage or diarrhea leads to large loses of chloride and an alkalosis because the replacement of chloride with bicarbonate.

TRACE ELEMENTS (FIG. 6.26)

Trace elements (or trace metals) are minerals present in living tissues in small amounts. Some of them are known to be nutritionally essential, others may be essential (although the evidence is only suggestive or incomplete), and the remainder are considered to be nonessential. Trace elements function primarily as catalysts in enzyme systems; some metallic ions, such as iron and copper, participate in oxidation-reduction reactions in energy metabolism. Iron, as a constituent of hemoglobin and myoglobin, also plays a vital role in the transport of oxygen. All trace elements are toxic if consumed at sufficiently high levels for long enough periods. The difference between toxic intakes and optimal intakes to meet physiological needs for essential trace elements is great for some elements but is much smaller for others.

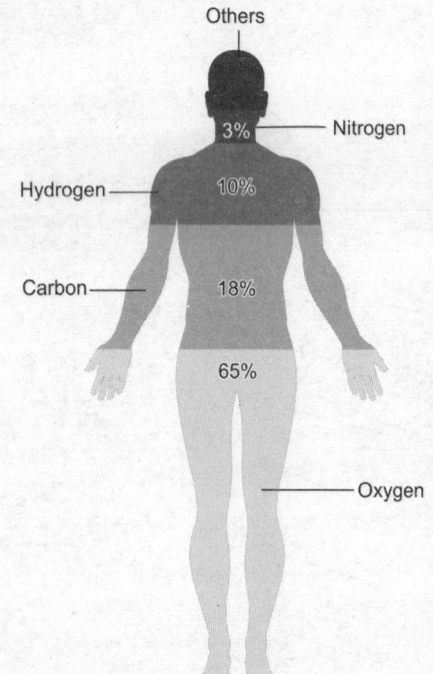

Element	Symbol	Percentage in body
Oxygen	O	65.0
Carbon	C	18.5
Hydrogen	H	9.5
Nitrogen	N	3.2
Calcium	Ca	1.5
Phosphorus	P	1.0
Potassium	K	0.4
Sulfur	S	0.3
Sodium	Na	0.2
Chlorine	Cl	0.2
Magnesium	Mg	0.1
Trace elements include boron (B), chromium (Cr), cobalt (Co), copper (Cu), fluorine (F), iodine (I), iron (Fe), manganese (Mn), molybdenum (Mo), selenium (Se), silicon (Si), tin (Sn), vanadium (V), and zinc (Zn).		less than 1.0

Fig. 6.26: Trace elements.

Trace Minerals (Microminerals)

The body needs trace minerals in very small amounts. Note that iron is considered to be a trace mineral, although the amount needed is somewhat more than for other micro minerals.

Trace minerals		
Mineral	**Function**	**Sources**
Iron		
Iron	Part of a molecule (hemoglobin) found in red blood cells that carries oxygen in the body; needed for energy metabolism	Organ meats; red meats; fish; poultry; shellfish (especially clams); egg yolks; legumes; dried fruits; dark, leafy greens; iron-enriched breads and cereals; and fortified cereals
Zinc	Part of many enzymes; needed for making protein and genetic material; has a function in taste perception, wound healing, normal fetal development, production of sperm, normal growth and sexual maturation, immune system health	Meats, fish, poultry, leavened whole grains, vegetables
Iodine	Found in thyroid hormone, which helps regulate growth, development, and metabolism	Seafood, foods grown in iodine-rich soil, iodized salt, bread, dairy products
Selenium	Antioxidant	Meats, seafood, grains
Copper	Part of many enzymes; needed for iron metabolism	Legumes, nuts and seeds, whole grains, organ meats, drinking water
Manganese	Part of many enzymes	Widespread in foods, especially plant foods
Fluoride	Involved in formation of bones and teeth; helps prevent tooth decay	Drinking water (either fluoridated or naturally containing fluoride), fish, and most teas
Chromium	Works closely with insulin to regulate blood sugar (glucose) levels	Unrefined foods, especially liver, brewer's yeast, whole grains, nuts, cheeses
Molybdenum	Part of some enzymes	Legumes; breads and grains; leafy greens; leafy, green vegetables; milk; liver

Other trace nutrients known to be essential in tiny amounts include nickel, silicon, vanadium, and cobalt.

Copper

Copper is a cofactor for certain enzymes involved in energy production, connective tissue formation, and iron metabolism. Copper deficiency can be caused by poor nutrition, poor absorption, or excessive zing intake. The RDA of copper is 800 micrograms for adults. Copper is found in shellfish, nuts, seeds, and whole grains.

- The healthy human adult body contains about 100–150 mg of copper. Copper present in the blood in the form of copper protein complex hemocuprin in RBCs ad ceruloplasmin in plasma.
- Anemia produced in infants fed exclusively on milk can be cured only by giving copper salts along with iron. The estimated of average daily intakes in adult diets range from 2 to 3 mg.
- The high intake in Indian diets may due to contamination of copper from brass vessels used in cooking.

Zinc

Zinc plays multiple roles in the body. It is involved in many cellular metabolic processes and is used in growth and development, the immune system, neurological function, and reproduction. It also forms a structural part of cell membranes and is a component of the zinc finger proteins, which act as transcription factors. The RDA for zinc is 11 mg for men and 8 mg for women.

- Zinc (Zn) is active in the metabolism of glucides and proteins, and is required for the synthesis of insulin by the pancreas and for the immunity function.
- Zinc is present is small amount in all tissues. Zinc plasma level is about 96 mg/100 mL for healthy adults and 89 mg/100 mL for healthy children.
- The average adult body contains 1.4–2.3 g of Zn. Zinc deficiency in the diet has been reported to the cause of anemia, growth retardation and delayed genital maturation. (Dwarfism) in children.
- Zinc is a constituent of insulin; the hormone present in the Islets of Langerhans of pancreas.

Cobalt

Cobalt is present in the body as a part of vitamin B_{12}, which is involved in manufacture of blood cells and nervous system function.

- Cobalt occurs in small amounts in all tissues, highest concentration occurring in liver and kidneys. Most of the cobalt is present in vitamin B_{12}.
- It is suggested that cobalt may be necessary for the first stage of hormone production. Cobalt may interact with iodine and affect its utilization

Iodine

Iodine is a critical mineral in the body. It is a component of the thyroid hormone and is required for normal thyroid function. Iodine is found naturally in seafood, dairy products, grains, eggs, and poultry. Iodine deficiency can cause brain damage, mental retardation, hypothyroidism, goiter, and other health problems. The US RDA of iodine is 150 micrograms.

Chromium

- The chromium content of an adult human body is estimated to be 6 mg. Most adult tissues contain 0.02–0.4 ppm of chromium on dry basis. The blood contains about 0.009–0.055 ppm.
- Chromium plays an important role in carbohydrate, lipid and protein metabolism.
- Chromium deficiency is characterized by impaired growth and disturbances in glucose, lipid and protein metabolism.

Selenium

Selenium functions in the body in the form of selenoproteins, which have many metabolic functions. The US RDA for selenium is 55 micrograms. Foods rich in selenium include Brazil nuts, tuna, oysters, pork, beef, chicken, whole wheat bread, and milk. Deficiency of selenium does not usually result in obvious clinical illness, but may contribute to Keshan disease and Kashin-Beck disease.

- Selenium administration to children with kwashiorkor resulted in significant weight increase.
- Studied indicate that human selenium deficiency may occur in protein-energy malnutrition.
- Selenium deficiency especially when combined with vitamin E deficiency reduces production.

CONCLUSION

The body needs many minerals; these are called essential minerals. Essential minerals are sometimes divided up into major minerals (macrominerals) and trace minerals (microminerals). These two groups of minerals are equally important, but trace minerals are needed in smaller amounts than major minerals. The amounts needed in the body are not an indication of their importance. Mineral salts are responsible for structural functions involving the skeleton and soft tissues and for regulatory functions including neuromuscular transmission, blood clotting, oxygen transport, and enzymatic activity. Calcium, phosphorus, and magnesium are required in relatively large amounts and are designated as macrominerals.

BIBLIOGRAPHY

1. Abrams SA, et al. A micronutrient-fortified beverage enhances the nutritional status of children in Botswana. Journal of Nutrition. 2003; 133:1834 -40.
2. Banerjee S. Studies in Energy Metabolism, Indian Council of Medical Research Special Report Series no. 43, 1962.
3. Latham MC, et al. Micronutrient dietary supplements -a new fourth approach. Archivos Latinoamericanos de Nutricion. 2001;51(1 Suppl 1):37 -41.
4. Leverton RM. Food Becomes You: Better Health through Better Nutrition, Doubleday Publishing, Boston, USA, 1980.
5. Martin EA, Ardath A. Coolidge: Nutrition in Action, 4th edition. Holt Rinehart and Winston, New York; 1978.
6. Patwardhan VN. Nutrition in India, 2nd edition. Indian Journal of Medical Sciences, New Delhi; 1961.

REVIEW QUESTIONS

Long Essays

1. Define minerals, explain the classifications of minerals.
2. Describe the difference between macro- and micro-minerals.

Short Essays

1. Define calcium and explain the functions, dietary sources and deficiencies of calcium.
2. Explain the functions, dietary sources and deficiencies of phosphorus.
3. Enumerate the functions, dietary sources and deficiencies iron.
4. Enlist trace minerals, describe the functions and deficiencies of copper and zinc.
5. Define sodium and explain the functions, dietary sources and deficiencies of sodium.

Short Answers

1. Factors influencing calcium absorption.
2. Iodine.
3. Functions of potassium.
4. Dietary sources of magnesium.
5. Functions of chloride.
6. Selenium.

CHAPTER 7

Water and Electrolytes

CHAPTER OUTLINE

- Water Requirement and Regulation
- Water Metabolism and Distribution
- Maintenance of Fluid and Electrolyte Balance
- Dehydration, Over Hydration and Water Intoxication
- Electrolyte Imbalance

TERMINOLOGY

- **Homeostasis**: The ability of a system or living organism to adjust its internal environment to maintain a stable equilibrium; such as the ability of warm-blooded animals to maintain a constant temperature.
- **Electrolyte**: Any of the various ions (such as sodium or chloride) that regulate the electric charge on cells and the flow of water across their membranes.
- **Sodium**: A chemical element with symbol Na and atomic number 11. It is a soft, silvery white, highly reactive metal and is a member of the alkali metals.
- **Alkalotic**: A condition that reduces the hydrogen ion concentration of arterial blood plasma (alkalemia). Generally, alkalosis is said to occur when the blood pH exceeds 7.45.
- **Potassium**: A chemical element with the symbol K and the atomic number 19. Elemental potassium is a soft, silvery white, alkali metal that oxidizes rapidly in the air and is very reactive with water—it can generate sufficient heat to ignite the hydrogen emitted in the reaction.
- **Acidosis**: An increase in acidity of the blood and other body tissue (i.e., an increased hydrogen ion concentration). If not further qualified, it usually refers to the acidity of the blood plasma.
- **Calcium**: A chemical element, atomic number 20, that is an alkaline earth metal and occurs naturally as carbonate in limestone and as silicate in many rocks.
- **Parathyroid hormone**: A polypeptide hormone that is released by the chief cells of the parathyroid glands and is involved in raising the levels of calcium ions in the blood.
- **Vitamin D**: A fat-soluble vitamin that is required for normal bone development and that prevents rickets; it can be manufactured in the skin on exposure to sunlight.
- **Hyperphosphatemia**: An elevated amount of phosphate in the blood.
- **Hypochloremia**: An electrolyte disturbance caused by an abnormally depleted level of chloride ions in the blood.
- **Hypophosphatemia**: An electrolyte disturbance caused by an abnormally low level of phosphate in the blood.
- **Bicarbonate buffer system**: Sodium bicarbonate and carbonic acid are the body's major chemical buffers.
- **Carbon dioxide**: The major compound controlled by the lungs is CO_2, and the respiratory system can very rapidly compensate for too much acid and too little acid by increasing or decreasing the respiratory rate, thereby altering the level of CO_2.
- **Bicarbonate**: Bicarbonate ions are basic components in the body, and the kidneys are key in regulating the amount of bicarbonate in the body.
- **Measurement of arterial blood gas**: The pH level and amounts of specific gases in the blood indicate if there is more acid or base and their associated values.
- **Respiratory acidosis**: Respiratory acidosis occurs when breathing is inadequate and $PaCO_2$ builds up.
- **Respiratory alkalosis**: Respiratory alkalosis occurs as a result of hyperventilation or excess aspirin intake.
- **Metabolic acidosis**: In metabolic acidosis, metabolism is impaired, causing a decrease in bicarbonates and a buildup of lactic acid.
- **Metabolic alkalosis**: Metabolic alkalosis occurs when bicarbonate ion concentration increases, causing an elevation in blood pH.

INTRODUCTION

Water and electrolyte balance is crucial for body homeostasis and is one of the most protected physiological mechanisms in the body. While we can survive for months without food, without water intake we die very quickly. Similarly the body has very strong mechanisms to control salt and water balance, an understanding of which has major implications in clinical practice.

WATER REQUIREMENT AND REGULATION

Water requirements: Water is vital for human existence. We can live without food for extended periods of time, but without water will result in death. Water is colorless, calorie less compound of hydrogen and oxygen that virtually every cell in the body needs to survive.

Figure 7.1 is depicted the water needs.

- Water is closer being a universal solvent than any other compound. To maintain good health and proper body functions, the amount of water in the body should remain relatively constant.
- The amount of water lost daily must be replaced by an equivalent amount of daily water intake to maintain the proper balance.
- It is important to keep in mind that water requirements can vary from one person to another and depend on several factors—physical activity, ambient temperature, health status (fever, diarrhea, and bleeding injury), physiological condition (pregnancy, lactation), age and gender, among other things.

A sedentary adult with normal physiological conditions in a temperate climate (18°–20°C), loses on average 2.5 liters of water a day (1). This water loss is due mainly to:

- The kidneys, through urine excretion (1.5 L per day)
- The lungs by breathing (0.35 L)
- The skin by perspiring (0.45 L)
- The intestines in the form of feces (0.2 L)
- To avoid dehydration we need to ingest as much water as we lose.

Functions (Box 7.1 and Fig. 7.2)

- It is an essential constituent of all the cells of the body and the internal environment.
- Serves as a transport medium by which most of the nutrients pass into the cells and removes excretory products.
- Water is a medium for most biochemical reactions within the body and sometimes a reactant.
- It is a valuable solvent in which various substances, such as electrolytes, non-electrolytes, hormones, enzymes, vitamins are carried from one place to another.
- Plays a vital role in the maintenance of body temperature. Heat is produced when food is burnt for energy. Body temperature must be kept at 80°–108°F
- Fahrenheit for higher or lower body temperature will cause death. Body heat is lost through the skin, lungs, urine and feces.
- It forms a part of fluids in body tissues; (e.g.) the amniotic fluid surrounds and protects the fetus during pregnancy.
- Saliva is about 99.5% water. In healthy individuals, it makes swallowing easier by moistening the food.
- Water helps in maintaining the form and texture of the tissues.

Box 7.1: Functions of water in human body.

- Transports nutrients and oxygen into cells
- Regulates body temperature
- Detoxifies
- Moisturizes the air in lungs
- Helps with metabolism
- Protects vital organ
- Helps with metabolism
- Protects vital organ
- Helps organs to absorb nutrients
- Protects and moisturizes our joints

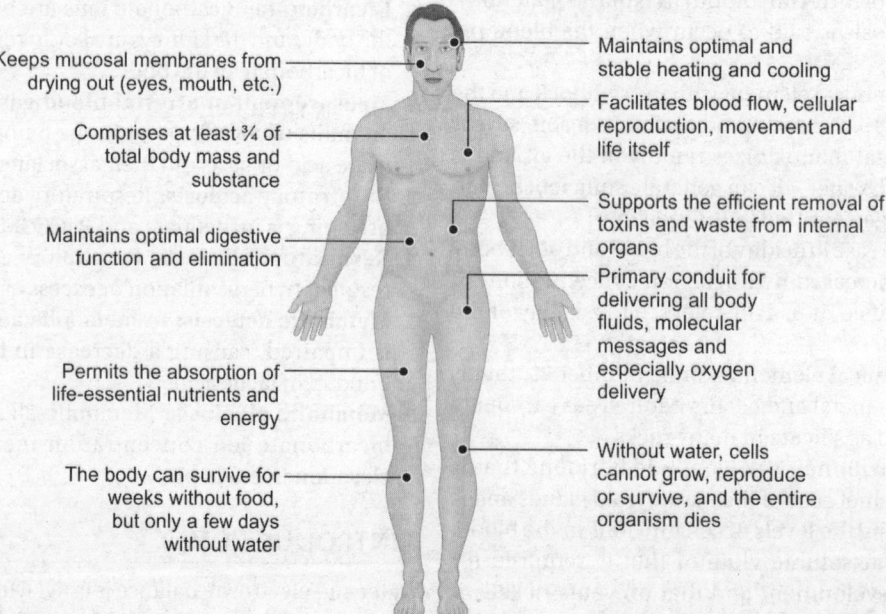

Fig. 7.1: Water needs.

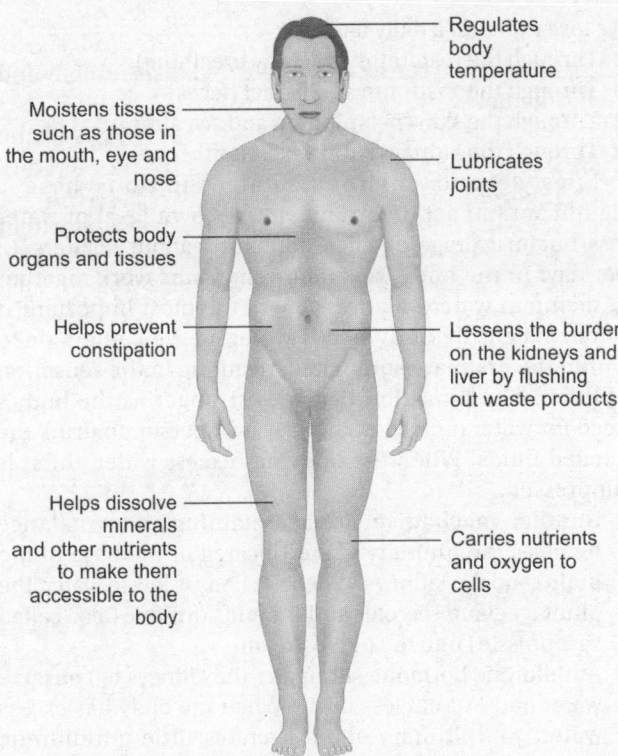

Fig. 7.2: Functions of water in human body.

- Water is essential for the maintenance of acid base and electrolyte balance. It should be noted that pure water consists of hydrogen ion (H^+) and hydroxyl ion (OH^-). Substances dissolve in water as ions with positive and negative charge. They are called electrolytes. The common electrolytes in our body are sodium, potassium and chloride.

Changes in electrolyte balance causes accumulation or depletion of water in intracellular and extracellular fluid. The balance between the positively and negatively charged ions is essential for water flow and maintains osmolarity between the cells. This is called electrolyte balance. Acid base balance is the dynamic state of equilibrium of hydrogen ion concentration. When pH falls below 7, it is termed acidity and when it increases above 7, it is termed alkalinity. Extremes of both cases results in death. The pH of the body should be maintained near neutrality. Enzymatic action depends on the pH. The digestion, absorption and utilization of nutrients are dependent on pH. Most body fluids are near neutral with the exception of gastric juice.

Water Consumption and Utilization in the Body

- Water in food: 0.7 l
- Metabolic water (which is produced in the body during biochemical reactions): 0.3 l
- Drinking: 1.5 additional liters.

Water is the preferred drink to hydrate the body. Water is an essential nutrient for healthy hydration without bringing any other elements into the body. An over-consumption of sugar sweetened beverages can lead to excessive calorie intake; substitution of sugary beverages by water is one of the healthy habits which help to fight against overweight/obesity risk.

Water requirements of water vary with climate, dietary constituents, activities and surface area of the body. As a rule a person should take enough water to excrete about 1200–1500 mL of urine per day. In tropics because of greater water loss through perspiration increased water intake is required to maintain urine volume. Normal intake of water ranges between 8–10 glasses per day.

- **Daily water input:** In tropical countries, such as India, the daily water input amounts to 2400–3000 mL of water through food, as fluid drinks and as metabolic water.
  - As fluid drinks—water, tea, coffee, milk soups 1500–1750 mL
  - Water intake through solid food 600–900 mL
  - Oxidation of carbohydrate, fat, 300–350 mL proteins (metabolic water)
  - Total 2400–3000 mL
- **Daily output of water**
  - Urine 1200–1500 mL (kidney)
  - Perspiration 700–900 mL (Skin)
  - Respiration 400 mL (lung)
  - Feces 100–200 mL (intestine)
  - Total 2400–3000 mL

Figure 7.3 is depicted the body water intake and output.

Therefore, the water intake and output is fairly kept constant. This is called water balance. The average adult metabolizes 2.5–3.00 liters of water and a constant balance is maintained between intake and output. Inadequate water intake disturbs water equilibrium resulting in decreased urinary output, thereby causing changes in extracellular fluid (ECF) and intracellular fluid (ICF). The water equilibrium is maintained by kidneys, lungs, intestine and pituitary gland. The water balance coordinates with both electrolyte and acid base balance.

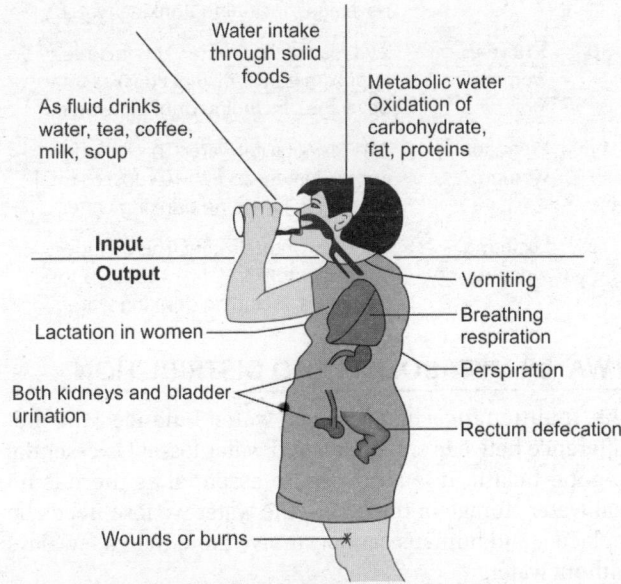

Fig. 7.3: Body water intake and output.

Adequate intake for total water table: An adequate intake for total water (from a combination of drinking water, beverages, and food) is set to prevent deleterious, primarily acute, effects of dehydration, which include metabolic and functional abnormalities.

Sl. No.	Age, gender and additional information	Adequate intake for total water
1.	0–6 months infants	0.7 L/day of water, assumed to be from human milk.
2.	7–12 months infants	0.8 L/day of total water, assumed to be from human milk, complementary foods and beverages. This includes approximately 0.6 L (≈ 3 cups) as total fluid, including formula or human milk, juices, and drinking water.
3.	1–3 years children	1.3 L/day of total water. This includes approximately 0.9 L (≈ 4 cups) as total beverages, including drinking water.
4.	4–8 years children	1.7 L/day of total water. This includes approximately 1.2 L (≈ 5 cups) as total beverages, including drinking water.
5.	9–13 years boys	2.4 L/day of total water. This includes approximately 1.8 L (≈ 8 cups) as total beverages, including drinking water.
6.	14–18 years boys	3.3 L/day of total water. This includes approximately 2.6 L (≈ 11 cups) as total beverages, including drinking water.
7.	9–13 years girls	2.1 L/day of total water. This includes approximately 1.6 L (≈ 7 cups) as total beverages, including drinking water.
8.	14–18 years girls	2.3 L/day of total water. This includes approximately 1.8 L (≈ 8 cups) as total beverages, including drinking water.
9.	>18 years men	3.7 L/day of total water. This includes approximately 3.0 L (≈ 13 cups) as total beverages, including drinking water.
10.	>18 years women	2.7 L/day of total water. This includes approximately 2.2 L (≈ 9 cups) as total beverages, including drinking water.
11.	Pregnant women	3.0 L/day of total water. This includes approximately 2.3 L (≈ 10 cups) as total beverages, including drinking water.
12.	Lactating women	3.8 L/day of total water. This includes approximately 3.1 L (≈ 13 cups) as total beverages, including drinking water.

WATER METABOLISM AND DISTRIBUTION

The maintenance of a correct water balance (the net difference between water gain and water losses) is essential to good health. It is all the more essential as there is no real water storage in the body—the water we lose needs be replaced, and humans cannot survive more than a few days without water.

We lose water on a daily basis.
- Through the respiratory tract (by breathing)
- Through the gastrointestinal tract (feces)
- Through the skin (perspiration and sweating)
- Through the kidneys (urine excretion)

Lifestyle and environmental conditions have a significant impact on an individual's own level of water loss, but on average, a typical adult loses about 2.6 liters (L) per day. In the body, several mechanisms work together to maintain water balance. One of the most important is thirst. When the body needs water, nerve centers deep within the brain are stimulated, resulting in the sensation of thirst. The sensation becomes stronger as the body's need for water increases, motivating a person to drink the needed fluids. When the body has excess water, thirst is suppressed.

- Another mechanism for maintaining water balance involves the pituitary gland (located at the base of the brain) and the kidneys. When the body is low in water, the pituitary gland secretes antidiuretic hormone (also called vasopressin) into the bloodstream.
- Antidiuretic hormone stimulates the kidneys to conserve water and excrete less urine. When the body has excess water, the pituitary gland secretes little antidiuretic hormone, enabling the kidneys to excrete excess water in the urine.
- The body can move water from one area to another as needed. When water loss is severe, the amount of water in the bloodstream decreases, so the body moves water from inside the cells to the bloodstream until it can be replaced through increased intake of fluids.
- When the body has excess water, the amount of water in the bloodstream increases, so the body moves water from the bloodstream into and around the cells. In this way, blood volume (the amount of blood, both blood cells and fluids, including water, circulating in the body) and blood pressure can be kept relatively constant.

Physiology of Body Fluids

- The primary body fluid, i.e., water is the most important nutrient of life. Whereas life can be sustained for many days without food, but it can be sustained for only a few days without water.
- Water comprises 60% of the body weight of an average adult, although the percentage is lower in obesity, since adipose tissue contains less water than lean tissue. The total body water is divided functionally into the extracellular (ECF = 20% of body weight) and the intracellular fluid spaces (ICF = 40% of body weight) separated by the cell membrane with its active sodium pump, which ensures that sodium remains largely in the ECF.
- The cell, however, contains large anions, such as protein and glycogen, which cannot escape and, therefore, draw in K^+ ions to maintain electrical neutrality (Gibbs-Dornan equilibrium). These mechanisms ensure that Na^+ and its balancing anions, Cl^- and HCO_3^-, are the mainstay of ECF osmolality, and K^+ has the corresponding function in the ICF.

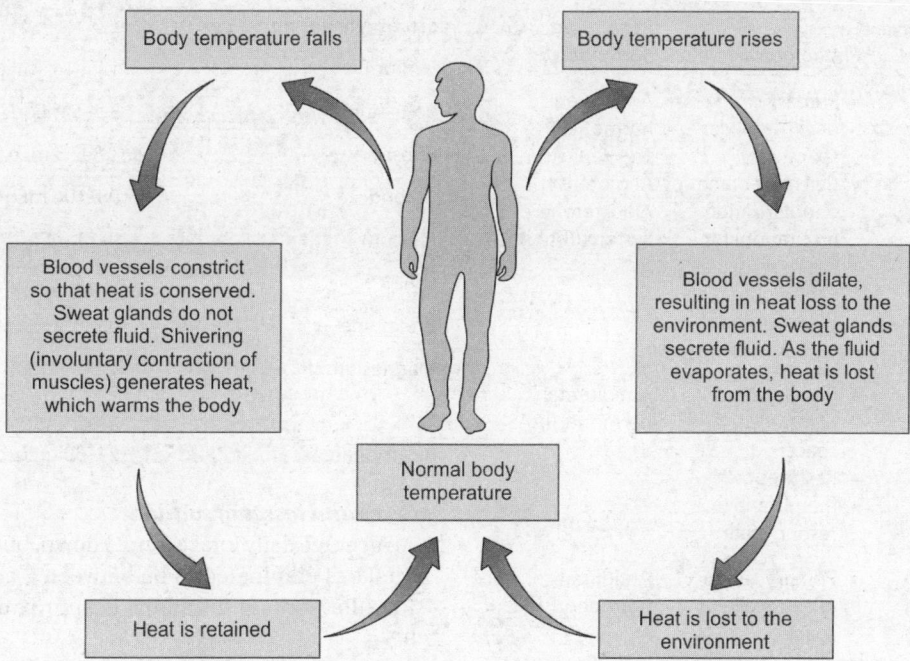

Fig. 7.4: Regulation of body temperature on fluid balance.

The Primary Functions of Water in the Body are as Follows:

- Provides a medium for transporting nutrients to cells and wastes from cells and transporting substances such as hormones, enzyme, blood platelets, and red and white blood cells
- Facilitates cellular metabolism and proper cellular chemical functioning
- Acts as a solvent for electrolytes and nonelectrolytes
- Helps to maintain normal body temperature
- Facilitates digestion and promotes elimination
- Acts as a tissue lubricant.

Figure 7.4 is depicted the regulation of body temperature on fluid balance.

ELECTROLYTES: TYPE, SOURCES AND CONSUMPTION OF BODY FLUIDS

Electrolytes are substances whose molecules dissociate or split into ions when placed in water. These substances are found in ECF and ICF that dissociate into electrically charged particles known as 'ions'. 'Cations' are positively charged ions. For example, sodium (Na), potassium (K), calcium (Ca^2) and magnesium (Mg), hydrogen (Hf) ions.

Figure 7.5 is depicted the main electrolytes in body fluid.

'Anions' are negative charged ions. For example, bicarbonates (HCO_3^-), chloride (Cl^-) and phosphate (PO_4^{3-}) ions and proteins. The ionic charge is termed 'valence'. Cations and anions combine according to their valency. The concentration of electrolytes can be expressed in mol per deciliter (mol/dL), millimole per liter (mmol/L) or milliequivalent per liter (mEq/L). See the normal level of electrolytes in appendix. The role of electrolytes in cellular functions includes the following:

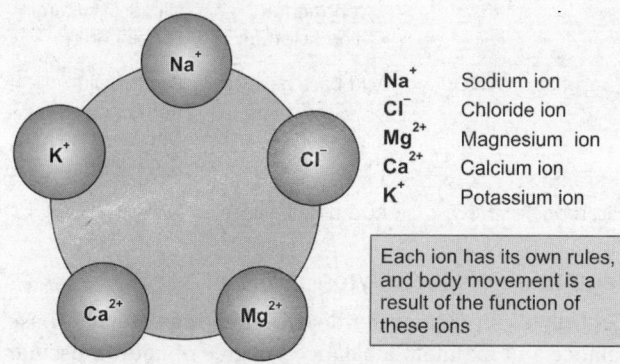

Fig. 7.5: Main electrolytes in body fluid.

- Regulation of water distribution, and osmolality.
- Regulation of acid-base balance.
- Transmission of nerve impulses, i.e., neuromuscular activity.
- Contraction of muscles.
- Clotting of blood.
- Enzyme reaction.

Definition

Electrolytes are charged particles (ions). These particles exist dissolved in the various fluid compartments of the body (intravascular, interstitial, and intracellular) and perform a variety of functions in the total physiology of the human body. The electrolytes of importance at this point in the course are: (1) Sodium; (2) Potassium; (3) Calcium; (4) Hydrogen; and (5) Bicarbonate.

Electrolyte	Chemical symbol	Physiological role	Regulating hormone(s)
Sodium	Na^+	• Primary cation of extracellular space • Cell membrane depolarization (excitation) for neuro muscular action potentials • Blood volume and pressure	Antidiuretic hormone, The Renin-Angiotensin-Aldosterone System (RAAS)
Potassium	K^+	• Primary cation of intracellular space • Restores cell membrane to resting state	Antidiuretic hormone, RAAS
Chloride	Cl^-	• Primary cation of extracellular space • Blood volume	Antidiuretic hormone, RAAS
Calcium	Ca^{2+}	• Bone structure • Muscle contraction • Blood clotting	Parathyroid hormone, Dihydroxyvitamin D, Calcitonin
Phosphate	HPO_4^{2+}	Acid-base balance	Parathyroid hormone, Dihydroxyvitamin D, Calcitonin
Bicarbonate	HCO_{3+}	Acid-base balance	N/A

Electrolyte normal values	
Sodium	135–145 mEq/L
Potassium	3.5–5 mEq/L
Phosphorus	1.8–2.3 mEq/L
Chloride	98–106 mEq/L
Calcium	9–11 mEq/L
Urea	20–40 mEq/L
Creatinine	0.7–1.2 mEq/L
Magnesium	1.5–3 mEq/L
CO_2	22–26 mEq/L
Bicarbonate	24–30 mEq/L

Regulation of Electrolytes

Electrolytes regulate water distribution, regulate acid-base balance and maintain a balanced degree of neuromuscular excitability. There are many different kinds of electrolytes in the body. These include sodium (Nat), potassium (K), calcium (Ca), magnesium (Mg^2), chloride (Cl), bicarbonate (HCO_3), phosphate (PO_4^{3-}), etc.

I. Sodium

Sodium is the chief electrolyte of ECF. It moves easily between intravascular and interstitial spaces and moves across cell membrane by active transport. Many chemical reactions in the body are influenced by sodium, particularly in nervous tissue cells and muscle tissue cells.

The functions of sodium are as follows:

- It controls and regulates the volume of body fluids
- It maintains water balance throughout the body
- It is the primary regulator of ECF volume
- It influences ICF volume
- It participates in the generation and transmission of nerve impulses
- It is an essential electrolyte in the sodium-potassium pump.

Sources and losses of sodium

- An average daily intake is not known, but the average adult intake is eliminated to be between 6 and 15 mg and the RDA for sodium for adults is approximately 500 mg for 0.5 g
- Sodium is found in many foods, particularly bacon, ham, sausage, catsup, mustard, relish, processed cheese, canned vegetables, bread, cereal, and salted snack food. It is found in table salt (NaCl) which has about 46 percent sodium
- Sodium excess are eliminated primarily by the kidneys, small amounts are lost in feces and perspiration.

Regulation of sodium

- Sodium normally is maintained in the body within a relatively narrow range, and deviations quickly result in a serious health problem
- Salt intake regulates sodium concentrations
- Sodium is conserved through reabsorption in the kidneys, a process of stimulation by aldosterone
- The normal extra cellular concentrations of sodium is 135 to 145 mEq/L (mmol/L).

II. Potassium

Potassium is the major cation of ICF. Potassium and sodium work reciprocally. For example, an excessive intake of sodium results in an excretion of potassium and vice versa. The functions of potassium are as follows:

- It is the chief regulator of cellular enzyme activity and cellular water content.
- It plays a vital role in such process as the transmission of electric impulses, particularly in nerve, heart, skeletal, intestinal, and lung tissue; protein and carbohydrate metabolism and cellular building.
- It assists in regulation of acid—base balance by cellular exchange with H.

Sources and losses of potassium

An average daily requirement of K is not known; but an intake of 50 to 100 mEq daily maintains potassium balance

- A well-balanced diet contains adequate quantities of potassium. Major sources include bananas, peaches,

kiwi, figs, dates, apricots, oranges prunes, melons, raising, broccoli, and potatoes. Meat and dairy products also provide adequate amounts of potassium.
- Potassium excreted primarily by the kidneys. The kidneys have no effective method of conserving potassium. Therefore, deficits develop readily if excreted in excess amount without being replaced simultaneously
- Gastrointestinal secretions contain potassium in large quantities. Some is also found in perspiration and saliva.

> - **Hyponatremia** refers to a serum sodium level that is less than 135 mEq/L
> - **Hypernatremia** is a serum sodium level higher than 145 mEq/L.
> - **Hypokalemia** usually indicates a deficit in total potassium stores.
> - **Hyperkalemia** refers to a potassium level greater than 5.0 mEq/L.
> - **Hypocalcemia** are serum levels below 8.6 mg/dL.
> - **Hypercalcemia** is calcium level greater than 10.2 mg/dL.
> - **Hypomagnesemia** refers to a below-normal serum magnesium concentration.
> - **Hypermagnesemia** are serum levels over 2.3 mg/dL.
> - **Hypophosphatemia** is indicated by a value below 2.5 mg/dL.
> - **Hyperphosphatemia** is a serum phosphorus level that exceeds 4.5 mg/dL in adults.

Regulation of K
- Cellular potassium is conserved by the sodium pump when sodium is excluded
- The kidneys conserve potassium when cellular K is decreased
- Aldosterone secretions trigger potassium excretion in urine
- The normal range for serum potassium is 3.5 to 5 mEq/L.

III. Calcium

Calcium is the most abundant electrolyte in the body. Up to 99% of the total amount of calcium in the body is found in bones and teeth in ionized form. There is close link between concentration of calcium and phosphorus.

The functions of calcium are as follows:
- It is necessary for nerve impulse transmissions and blood clotting.
- It is catalyst for muscle contraction. Strength of contractions (especially cardiac muscle contraction) is directly related to the serum concentration of calcium ions.
- It is needed for vitamin B_{12} absorption and for its use by body cells.
- It acts as a catalyst for many cell chemical activities.
- It is necessary for strong bones and teeth.
- It establishes thickness and strength of cell membrane.

Sources and losses of calcium
- The average daily requirements for calcium is about 1 g for adults. Higher amounts are required according to body weight; for children, for pregnant and lactating women, and postmenopausal women
- Calcium is found in milk, cheese and dried beans. Some calcium is present in meats and vegetables
- Use of calcium is stimulated by vitamin D. The most active form of vitamin D (calcitriol) promotes calcium absorption and limits calcium excretion when levels are inadequate
- It leaves bones and teeth to maintain normal blood calcium levels, if necessary.
- It is excreted in urine, feces, bile, digestive secretion and perspiration.

Regulation of Calcium
- When ECF calcium levels decrease, the parathyroid glands increase the secretions of PTH, which acts on bones to increase the release of calcium into the blood and acts on the kidney, tubules and the intestinal mucosa to increase the absorption of calcium from the kidneys and the intestine chloride.
- A high serum phosphate concentration increases serum calcium; a low serum phosphate concentration decreases serum calcium.
- Calcitonin, a hormone secreted by the thyroid gland has an opposite effect on calcium than PTH. Increase in calcitonin reduces the serum calcium concentration primarily by opposing osteoclast bone resorption.

IV. Magnesium

Most of the cation magnesium is found within body cells. It is present in heart, bone, nerve, and muscle tissues. Magnesium is the second most important cation of ICF.

The functions of magnesium are as follows:
- It is important for the metabolism of carbohydrates and proteins.
- It is important for many vital reactions related to the body's enzymes.
- It is necessary for protein and DNA synthesis, DNA and RNA transcription, and translation of RNA.
- It maintains normal intracellular levels of potassium.
- It serves to help or maintain electric activity in nervous membranes and muscle membranes.

Sources and losses of magnesium:
The average daily adult requirement for magnesium is about 18 to 30 mEq. Children are required larger amount magnesium is found in most foods but especially in vegetables, nuts, fish, whole grains, peas and beans.

Regulation of magnesium:
Magnesium is absorbed by the intestines and secreted by the kidneys Plasma concentration of magnesium range from 1.3 to 2.1 mEq/L with about one third of that amount bound to plasma proteins.

V. Chloride

Chloride the chief extracellular anion is found in blood, intestinal fluid, and lymph and in minute amounts in intracellular fluid.

The functions of chlorides are as follows:
- It acts with sodium to maintain the osmotic pressure of the blood
- It plays a role in the body's acid-base balance

- It is important in buffering action when O_2 and CO_2 exchange in RBCs.
- It is essential for the production of HCl in gastric juices.
- The average daily requirement of chlorides is unknown. It is found in foods rich in sodium, in dairy products and meat. Regulation of Chloride.
- It is normally paired with sodium and excreted and conserved with sodium by the kidneys.
- Chloride deficit leads to potassium deficit and vice-versa.
- Normal serum chloride levels range from 95 to 105 mEq/L.

VI. Bicarbonate

The bicarbonate molecule is an anion. It is the major chemical base buffer within the body and is found in both ECF and ICF. It is essential for acid—base balance. Bicarbonate and carbonic acid constitute the body's primary buffer systems.

VII. Phosphate

The phosphate ion is the major anion in body cells. It is a buffer anion in both ICF and ECF.

The functions of phosphate are as follows:
- It helps maintain acid—base balance
- It is involved in important chemical reactions in the body. For example, it is necessary for many B vitamins to be effective; helps promote nerve and muscle action, and plays role in carbohydrate metabolism

It is important for cell division and for the transmission of heredity or hereditary traits. An average daily requirement for phosphorus is similar to those for calcium. It is found in most foods by especially in beef, pork, and dried peas and beans. It is metabolized in the same manner as calcium.

Phosphate is regulated by PTH and by activated vitamin D. Calcium and phosphates are inversely proportional and one results in a decrease in the other. The normal range of phosphate is 2.5 to 4.5 mEq/L (mmol/L).

MAINTENANCE OF FLUID AND ELECTROLYTE BALANCE

The kidneys are essential for regulating the volume and composition of bodily fluids. This page outlines key regulatory systems involving the kidneys for controlling volume, sodium and potassium concentrations, and the pH of bodily fluids. A most critical concept for you to understand is how water and sodium regulation are integrated to defend the body against all possible disturbances in the volume and osmolarity of bodily fluids. Simple examples of such disturbances include dehydration, blood loss, salt ingestion, and plain water ingestion.

Water Balance

- Water balance is achieved in the body by ensuring that the amount of water consumed in food and drink (and generated by metabolism) equals the amount of water excreted.
- The consumption side is regulated by behavioral mechanisms, including thirst and salt cravings. While almost a liter of water per day is lost through the skin, lungs, and feces, the kidneys are the major site of regulated excretion of water.
- One way the kidneys can directly control the volume of bodily fluids is by the amount of water excreted in the urine. Either the kidneys can conserve water by producing urine that is concentrated relative to plasma, or they can rid the body of excess water by producing urine that is dilute relative to plasma.
- Direct control of water excretion in the kidneys is exercised by vasopressin, or anti-diuretic hormone (ADH), a peptide hormone secreted by the hypothalamus. ADH causes the insertion of water channels into the membranes of cells lining the collecting ducts, allowing water reabsorption to occur. Without ADH, little water is reabsorbed in the collecting ducts and dilute urine is excreted.

ADH secretion is influenced by several factors (note that anything that stimulates ADH secretion also stimulates thirst):
- By special receptors in the hypothalamus that are sensitive to increasing plasma osmolarity (when the plasma gets too concentrated). These stimulate ADH secretion.
- By stretch receptors in the atria of the heart, which are activated by a larger than normal volume of blood returning to the heart from the veins. These inhibit ADH secretion, because the body wants to rid itself of the excess fluid volume.
- By stretch receptors in the aorta and carotid arteries, which are stimulated when blood pressure falls. These stimulate ADH secretion, because the body wants to maintain enough volume to generate the blood pressure necessary to deliver blood to the tissues.

Sodium Balance (Fig. 7.6)

- In addition to regulating total volume, the osmolarity (the amount of solute per unit volume) of bodily fluids is also tightly regulated. Extreme variation in osmolarity causes cells to shrink or swell, damaging or destroying cellular structure and disrupting normal cellular function.
- Regulation of osmolarity is achieved by balancing the intake and excretion of sodium with that of water. (Sodium is by far the major solute in extracellular fluids, so it effectively determines the osmolarity of extracellular fluids.)
- An important concept is that regulation of osmolarity must be integrated with regulation of volume, because changes in water volume alone have diluting or concentrating effects on the bodily fluids.
- For example, when you become dehydrated you lose proportionately more water than solute (sodium), so the osmolarity of your bodily fluids increases. In this situation the body must conserve water but not sodium, thus stemming the rise in osmolarity.
- If you lose a large amount of blood from trauma or surgery, however, your loses of sodium and water are proportionate to the composition of bodily fluids. In this situation the body should conserve both water and sodium.
- As noted above, ADH plays a role in lowering osmolarity (reducing sodium concentration) by increasing water

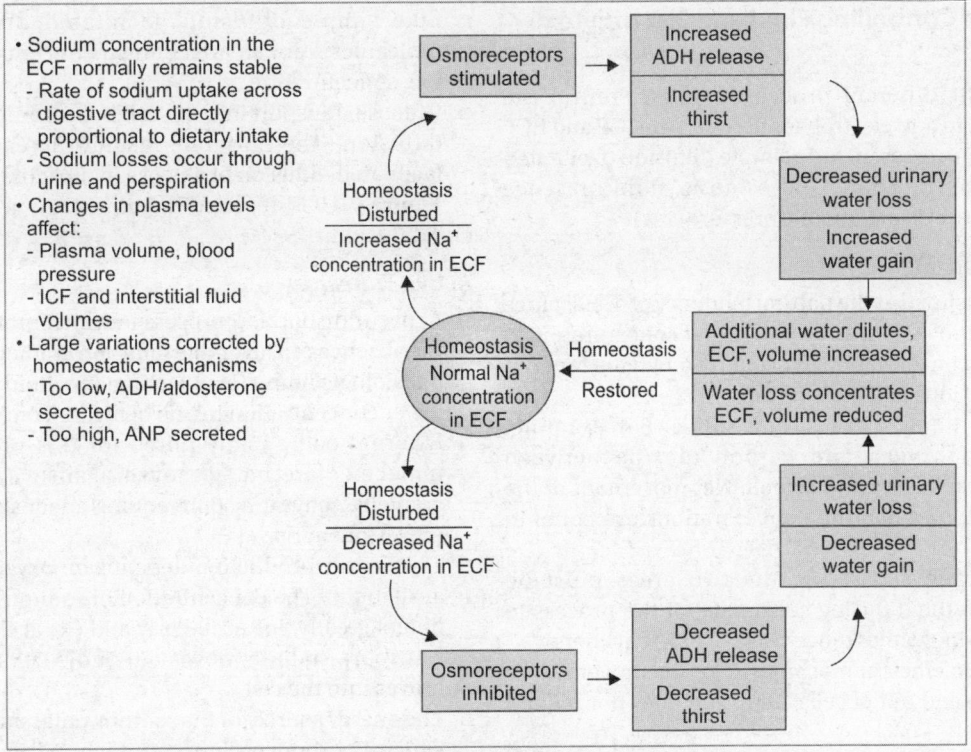

Fig. 7.6: Sodium balance.

reabsorption in the kidneys, thus helping to dilute bodily fluids.
- To prevent osmolarity from decreasing below normal, the kidneys also have a regulated mechanism for reabsorbing sodium in the distal nephron. This mechanism is controlled by **aldosterone**, a steroid hormone produced by the adrenal cortex.

Aldosterone Secretion is Controlled Two Ways

- The adrenal cortex directly senses plasma osmolarity. When the osmolarity increases above normal, aldosterone secretion is inhibited.
- The lack of aldosterone causes less sodium to be reabsorbed in the distal tubule. Remember that in this setting ADH secretion will increase to conserve water, thus complementing the effect of low aldosterone levels to decrease the osmolarity of bodily fluids.
- The net effect on urine excretion is a decrease in the amount of urine excreted, with an increase in the osmolarity of the urine.
- The kidneys sense low blood pressure (which results in lower filtration rates and lower flow through the tubule). This triggers a complex response to raise blood pressure and conserve volume.
- Specialized cells (juxtaglomerular cells) in the afferent and efferent arterioles produce renin, a peptide hormone that initiates a hormonal cascade that ultimately produces angiotensin II.
- Angiotensin II stimulates the adrenal cortex to produce aldosterone. Note that in this setting, where the body is attempting to conserve volume, ADH secretion is also stimulated and water reabsorption increases.
- Because aldosterone is also acting to increase sodium reabsorption, the net effect is retention of fluid that is roughly the same osmolarity as bodily fluids.
- The net effect on urine excretion is a decrease in the amount of urine excreted, with lower osmolarity than in the previous example.

Figure 7.7 is depicted the organs involved in fluid control.

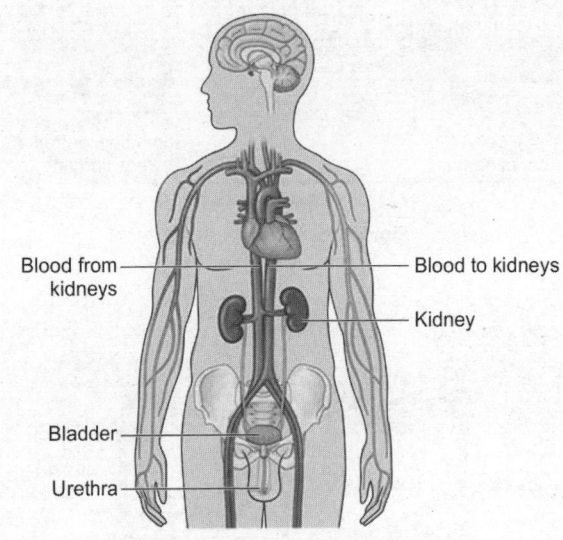

Fig. 7.7: Organs involved in fluid control.

Mechanism of Controlling Fluid and Electrolyte Movement

There are many different processes which control the movement of fluid and electrolytes between the ICF and ECF spaces. These processes include simple diffusion, facilitated diffusion, active transport, and osmosis, fluid presence (hydrostatic pressure and oncotic pressure).

Simple Diffusion (Fig. 7.8)

- Diffusion is defined as the natural tendency of a substance or solutes to move from an area of higher concentration to that of lower concentration. It occurs through the random movement of ions and molecules.
- It occurs in liquids, gases, and solids. For example, exchange of oxygen and carbon dioxide between pulmonary capillaries and alveoli. Net movement of the molecules stops when the concentrations are equal in both areas.
- The membrane separating the two areas must be permeable to the diffusing substance for the process to occur. These molecules move without external energy.
- Diffusion is an efficient mechanism for the movement of molecules in and out of cells. Diffusion does not require energy.

Facilitated Diffusion (Fig. 7.9)

- Some molecules diffuse slowly into the cell because of the composition of cellular membrane. However, when they are combined with a specific carrier molecule, the rate of diffusion accelerates.
- Like simple diffusion, facilitated diffusion moves molecules from an area of high concentration to one of low concentration.
- Glucose transport into the cell is an example of facilitated diffusion. The hormone insulin increases the rate of facilitated diffusion of glucose in most tissues.

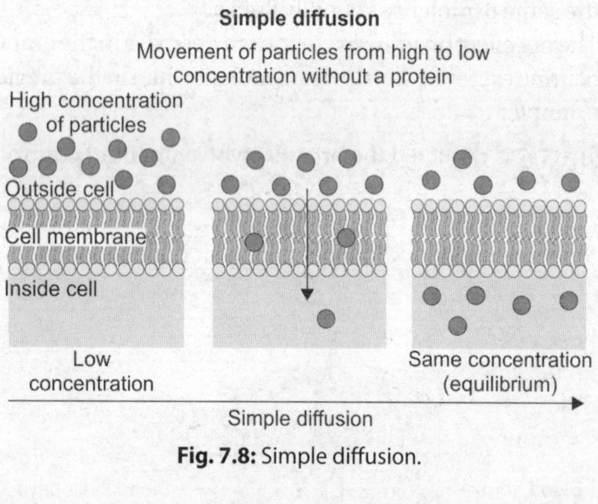

Figure 7.10 is depicted the difference between osmosis and diffusion.

Active Transport

- Active transport is a process in which molecules move in the absence of a favorable diffusion gradient. In which, the physiologic pump (Naik) that moves fluid from an area of lower concentration to one of higher concentration.
- External energy is required for this process because molecules are being moved against a concentration gradient. Active transport requires adenosine triphosphate (ATP) for energy.
- The energy production depends on oxygen and glucose availability. The concentration of sodium and potassium differs greatly, intracellularly and extracellular. By active transport, sodium moves out of the cell and potassium moves into the cell.
- The energy source for the sodium-potassium pump is ATP which is produced in the mitochondria. By definition, active transport implies that energy expenditure must take place for the movement to occur against a concentration of gradient.

Osmosis

- Osmosis, a special type of diffusion, is the flow of water between too compartments separated by a membrane permeable to water but not to solute. Here the movement of fluid across a semi permeable membrane from an area of low solute concentration to an area of high solute concentration.
- This process stops when the solute concentrations are equal on both sides of the membrane. In this, water moves from the compartments that is more dilute (has more water) to the side that is more concentrated (has less water).
- The semipermeable membrane prevents movement of solute particles.
- Osmosis requires no outside energy sources and stops when concentration differences disappear. In addition to

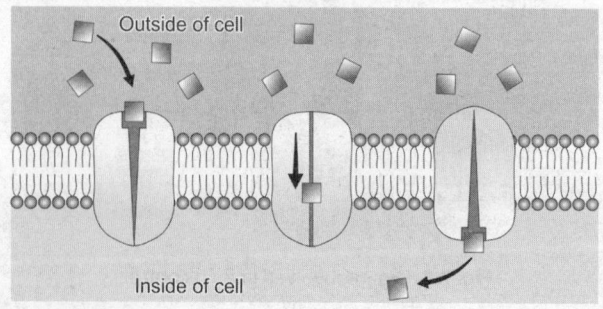

Fig. 7.8: Simple diffusion.

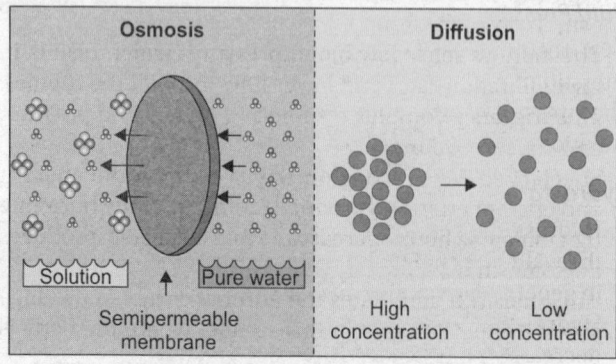

Fig. 7.10: Difference between osmosis and diffusion.

Fig. 7.9: Facilitated diffusion.

diffusion, osmosis is very important for maintaining the chemical stability of body cells.

Osmotic Pressure or Force

- Osmotic pressure is a term used to describe the movement of water by the process of osmosis. It can be described as a pulling of water.
- Osmotic pressure is an important factor in the movement of water between fluid compartments. 'Osmolarity' and 'osmolality' both are measurements of osmotic pressure.

Osmolality

- It measures the osmotic force of solute per unit of weight of solvent. It reflects the concentration of fluid that affects the movement of water between fluid compartments by osmosis.
- It measures the solute concentration per kilogram in blood and urine. It is measured in milliosmole per kg of water (mosm/kg). The normal osmolality of body fluids is between 275 and 295 mmol/kg or mosm/kg.
- The major determinants of osmolality are sodium, glucose, and urea with sodium.
- Increased in the concentration of these substances in the plasma causes fluid movement into plasma because of its increased osmotic pressure.

Osmolarity

- It measures the total milliosmole of solutes per unit of a total volume of solution.
- The number of osmoles, the standard unit of osmotic pressure per liter of solution. It is expressed as milliosmole per liter (mosm/L) used to describe the concentration of solutes or dissolved particles.
- In clinical practice, osmolality is used most frequently. Serum osmolality may be measured directly through laboratory tests or estimated at the bedside by doubling the serum sodium level or by utilizing the following formula: In osmotic movement of fluid, cells are affected by the osmolality of the fluid that surrounds them. Where fluids are added to the body those that have same osmolality as cell interior are "isotonic".
- Solutions that contain more water than the cell are "hypotonic" (hypoosmolar), those with less water than the cell are hypertonic (hyperosmolar).

Fluid Pressure

As a result of pressure, body fluids shift between the interstitial space and the vascular space within the capillary. The pressure in the body fluids are either hydrostatic or oncotic.

Hydrostatic Pressure

- Hydrostatic pressure is the force exerted by a fluid against the walls of its container. The heart is a main component in generating pressure in blood vessels.
- Hydrostatic pressure in the vascular system gradually decreases as the blood moves through the arteries until it is about 40 mm Hg at the arterial end of a capillary.
- Because of the size of the capillary bed and fluid movement into the interstitial, the pressure decreases to about 10 mm Hg at the venous end of the vessel.
- Hydrostatic pressure in the capillaries tends to filter fluid out of the vascular compartment into the interstitial fluid.

Oncotic Pressure (Colloidal Osmotic Pressure)

- Oncotic pressure is an osmotic pressure exerted by colloidal, in solution. In plasma, proteins and molecules attract water and contribute to the total osmotic pressure in the vascular system.
- Unlike electrolytes, the large molecular size prevents proteins from leaving the vascular space through pores in capillary walls.
- Plasma oncotic pressure is approximately 25 mm Hg. Some patients are found in the interstitial space, and they exert an oncotic pressure of approximately 1 mm Hg.

Figure 7.11 is depicted the pressure regulation in the blood vessels.

Filtration

- The movement of the fluid through a capillary via the above stated two pressures (hydrostatic and oncotic) is called 'filtration'.
- An example of filtration is the passage of water and electrolytes from the arterial capillary bed to the interstitial fluid.
- In this instance, the hydrostatic pressure is furnished by the pumping action of the heart. Through filtration, absorption or reabsorption, and resorption will take place.

Absorption

It usually refers to the initial movement of substances, such as end products of digestion or medications from organ, such as GI tract or tissues, such as the muscle, subcutaneous or dermal tissue, buccal or pharyngeal tissues, into the vascular system.

Reabsorption

- It refers to movement of water, electrolytes, vitamins, amino acids, glucose, lactate or other essential substances from one compartment, such as the interstitial or renal tubules, back into vascular capillaries.
- Resorption refers to the process of calcium salts leaving the bone and moving to the blood in an form.

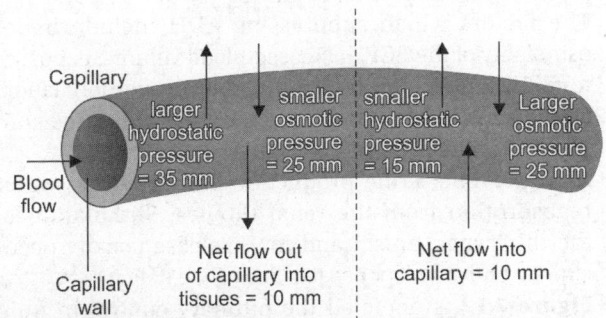

Fig. 7.11: Pressure regulation in the blood vessels.

Regulation of Fluids and Electrolytes or Homeostatic Mechanism:

The body is equipped with remarkable homeostatic mechanisms to keep the composition and volume of body fluid within narrow limits of normal. Organs involved in the homeostatic mechanism or regulation of fluid and electrolytes include hypothalamus, pituitary gland, adrenal gland, kidney, GI tract, parathyroid gland, heart and blood vessels, lungs, etc.

Hypothalamus

- Water ingestion in the conscious client is regulated by the thirst receptors located in the hypothalamus.
- The thirst mechanism is stimulated by the hypotension and increased serum osmolality. In addition thirst may result from polyuria, fluid volume depletion as small as 0.5%, excess sodium intake, hypertonic feedings, and hypertonic IV fluids.
- Thirst can be reported and is an important clinical manifestation of fluid imbalances; it is not a true indicator of fluid balance in all persons. The thirst mechanism is depressed in the elderly.
- The desire to consume fluids is also affected by social and psychological factors not related to fluid balance.
- A dry mouth will cause the client to drink, even when there is no measurable body water deficit.
- Water ingestion will equal water excretion in the individual who has free access to water, a normal thirst and ADH mechanism and normally-functioning kidneys.

Pituitary Gland

- The hypothalamus manufactures a substance known as antidiuretic hormone (ADH) which is stored in vesicle in the posterior pituitary gland and released as needed. ADH regulates water retention by kidneys.
- The distal tubules and collecting ducts in the kidneys respond to the ADH by becoming more permeable in water so that water is absorbed into the blood and not excreted.
- When there is a normal plasma osmolality and normal circulating plasma volume, continued ADH secretion is called "syndrome inappropriate to antidiuretic hormone (SIADH)". ADH is released in response to many conditions
- An increase in plasma osmolality, ECF volume depletion, pain, stress, and use of certain medications, such as narcotics, barbiturates, and anesthetics-stress may be physiologic or psychologic.
- The factors which suppressing ADH include hypo-osmolality of the ECF, increased blood volume, exposure to cold, acute alcohol ingestion, carbon dioxide inhalation, administration of some diuretics, lithium and some anti-psychotic medications.
- ADH prevents urine production and promotes water reabsorption from the renal tubules. Stimulation of the thirst mechanism and ADH release usually occur concurrently in response to a body fluid deficit.

Figure 7.12 is depicted the pituitary control in fluid regulation.

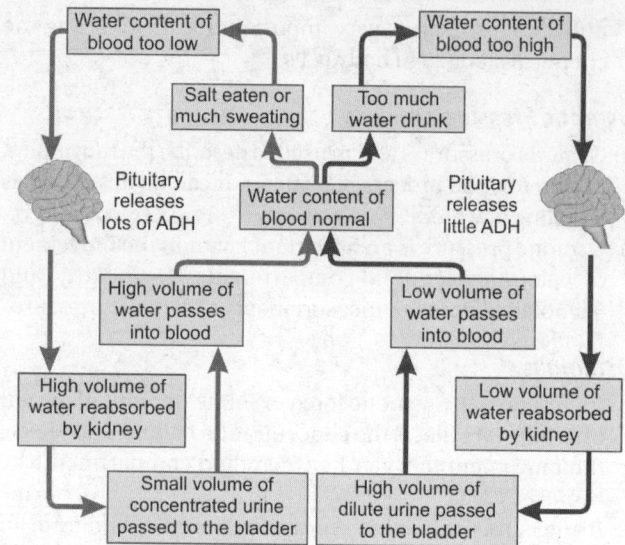

Fig. 7.12: Pituitary control in fluid regulation.

Adrenal Gland

- Adrenal gland fluid volume is maintained by combinations of hormonal influences. ADH only water reabsorption.
- Hormones released by the adrenal cortex helps to regulate both water and electrolytes. Two groups of hormones secreted by the adrenal cortex include glucocorticoids and mineral corticoids.
- Extra-cellularcoids primarily have an anti-inflammatory effect and increase serum glucose; whereas mineral affects corticoids (e.g., aldosterone) enhances sodium retention and potassium excretion.
- When sodium is reabsorbed, water follows as a result of osmotic charges. "Cortisol" is most common hormone. Which has both gluco and mineralocorticoids properties.
- Adrenocorticotropic hormone (ACTH) from the anterior pituitary is necessary for aldosterone secretions. Hypovelemia is a common clinical condition in which aldosterone is secreted to maintain homeostasis.

Kidneys

- The kidneys maintain fluid volume and concentration of urine by filtering the ECF through the glomeruli.
- Reabsorption and excretion of ECF occur in the renal tubules in response to ADH, aldosterone and ANP (atrial natriuretic peptides).
- ANP released from the atria in response to atrial distention, vasoconstriction, or direct cardiac failure. These factors increase the excretion of sodium and water and results in vasodilatation.
- Renal prostaglandins and renal renin-kinin system also increases sodium excretion.

The major functions of kidneys in maintaining normal fluid balance include the following:

- Regulation of ECF volume and osmolality by selective retention and excretion of body fluids
- Regulation of electrolytes level in the ECF by selective retention of needed substances and excretion of unneeded substances

- Regulation of pH of ECF by retention of hydrogen ions
- Excretion of metabolic wastes and toxic substances.

Parathyroid Gland
- The parathyroid glands embedded in the corners of thyroid gland; regulate calcium and phosphate balance by means of parathyroid hormone (PTH).
- PTH influences bone resorption, calcium absorption from the intestine and renal tubules.

Gastrointestinal Tract
- Daily water intake and output are between 2000 mL and 3000 mL. The gastrointestinal tract accounts for the most of the water intake.
- Water intake includes fluids, water from foods metabolism and water present in solid goods.
- Lean meal has approximately 70% water whereas the water content of many fruits and vegetables approaches 100%.
- Most of the body water is excreted by kidneys. A small amount of water eliminated by GI tract is feces.

Lungs
- The lungs are also vital in maintaining homeostasis. Insensible water loss, which is unavoidable vaporization from the lungs and skin assists in regulating body temperature.
- Normally, about 900 mL of water per day is lost. The amount of water loss is increased by accelerated body metabolism, which occurs with increased body temperature and exercise.
- Through exhalation, the lungs remove approximately 300 mL of water daily in the normal adult.

Heart and Blood Vessels
- The pumping action of the heart circulates blood through the kidneys under sufficient pressure for urine to form.
- Failure of the pumping action interferes with renal perfusion and thus with water and electrolytic regulation.

Neural Mechanism
In addition, neural mechanisms also contribute to the balance of water and sodium. Mechanoreceptors and baroreceptors are nerve receptors involved in neural mechanism.

DEHYDRATION, OVER HYDRATION AND WATER INTOXICATION

Dehydration
When water is constantly lost from the body as in severe vomiting, diarrhea, excessive sweating or excessive urine formation due to treatment with diuretics, the total water content of the body is reduced. Extracellular and intracellular cellular fluid decreases leading to dehydration.

Figure 7.13 is depicted the clinical feature of dehydration.

Effects of Dehydration
- Tongue is dry.
- Pinch test is done by raising and releasing the skin. Slow return of skin to original position indicates decreased ECF.
- Decrease in plasma volume reduces cardiac output and may lead to cardiac failure.

Prevention of Dehydration
Dehydration can be prevented by taking sufficient amounts of water as fluids. The correction of dehydration is called rehydration.

Oral rehydration therapy:
It is the administration of fluid to prevent or correct dehydration.

Oral rehydration salt:
- WHO, UNICEF formula consist of the NaCl—3.5 g, $NaHCO_3$—2.5 g, KCl—1.5 g and glucose—20 g to be dissolved in one liter of potable drinking water.
- The glucose present aids in the absorption of sodium chloride and potassium chloride apart from giving energy.
- This mixture is administered through the oral route at frequent intervals until the normal state is attained. Potable water is that water which is safe and wholesome. It should be:
  - Free from pathogenic agents
  - Free from harmful chemical substance
  - Pleasant to taste; free from color and odor
  - Usable for domestic purpose.

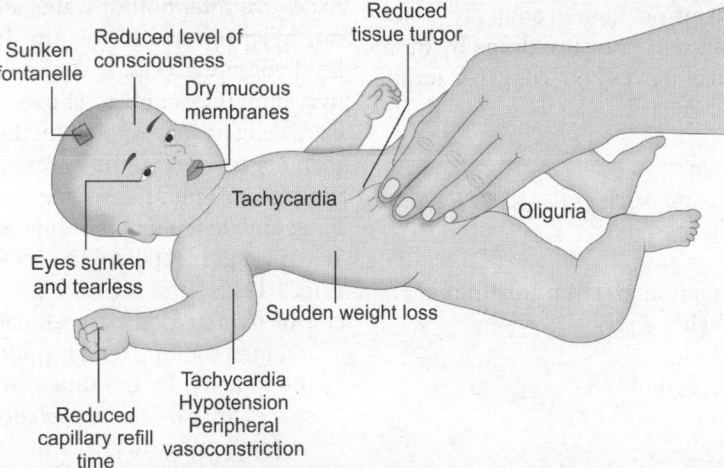

Fig. 7.13: Clinical feature of dehydration.

Fluid Volume Deficit (FVD)

Fluid volume deficit can be caused by a deficiency in the amount of both water and electrolytes in ECF, but the water and electrolytes proportions remain near normal. The state is commonly known as 'hypovolemia'. Both osmotic and hydrostatic pressure changes force the interstitial fluid into intravascular space. As the interstitial space is depleted, its fluid becomes hypertonic, and cellular fluid is then drawn into the interstitial space, leaving cells without adequate fluid of function properly.

Fluid volume deficit results from the loss of body fluids, especially if fluid intake is simultaneously decreased.

Lab values for fluid and electrolyte status		
Test	Usual reference range	SI units
Serum sodium	135–145 mEq/L	135–145 mmol/L
Serum potassium	3.5–5.3 mEq/L	3.5–5.3 mmol/L
Total serum calcium	8.6–10. mg/dL (approx. 50% in ionized form)	2.15–2.5 mmol/L
Serum magnesium	1.3–2.5 mEq/L	0.65–1.25 mmol/L
Serum phosphorus	2.5–4.5 mg/dL	0.87–1.45 mmol/L
Serum chloride	97–107 mEq/L	97–107 mmol/L
Carbon dioxide content	22–30 mEq/L	22–30 mmol/L
Serum osmolality	280–300 mOsm/kg H_2O	280–300 mmol/kg H_2O
Blood urea nitrogen (BUN)	5–20 mg/dL	1.8–7.1 mmol/L
Serum creatinine	Females: 0.5–1.1 mg/dL	44–97 mmol/L
	Males: 0.6–1.2 mg/dL	53–105 mmol/L

The main characteristics of fluid volume deficits are as follows:
- Weight loss over short period (except in third space losses)
- Decreased skin and tongue turgor
- Dry mucous membranes
- Urine output less than 30 mL per hour in adult
- Postural hypotension (systolic pressure drops by more than 15 mm Hg when client moves from lying to standing or sitting position)
- Weak, rapid pulse
- Slow-filling peripheral veins
- Decreased body temperature, such as 95° to 98°F (38° to 36.7°C) unless infection is present
- CVP less than 4 cm H_2O
- BUN elevated out of proportion to serum creatinine
- Specific gravity (urine) high
- Hematocrit elevated
- Flat neck veins in supine position
- Marked oliguria, late
- Altered sensorium

Nursing Intervention for FVD
- Assess for presence or worsening of FVD.
- Administer oral fluids if indicated.
- Consider the client's likes and dislikes when offering fluids
- If the client is reluctant to drink because of oral discomfort select fluids that are non-irritating to the mucosa, and provide frequent mouth care (offer saline gargle and apply lubricant to lips).
- Offer fluids at frequent intervals
- Explain the need for fluid replacement to the client
- Administer PRN medications if nausea is present, to provide relief before fluids are offered.
- Consider the following interventions for clients with impaired swallowing **(Fig. 7.14)**.
- Assess gag reflex and ability to swallow water before offering solid foods; have a suction apparatus on hand.
- Position the client in an upright position with head and neck flexed slightly forward during feeding (tilting the head backward during swallowing predisposes to aspiration because this position opens the airway).
- Provide thick fluids or semisolid foods (such as pudding or gelatine). These are more easily swallowed because of their consistency and weight than are thin liquids.
- If the client is unable to eat and drink, discuss possibility of tube feeding or TPN with the physician.
- Monitor response to fluid intake, either orally or parenterally.
- Monitor clients with tendency for abnormal fluid retention (such as renal or cardiac problems) for signs of overload during aggressive fluid replacement.
- Turn client frequently, apply moisturizing agents on the skin.

Sometimes dehydration is used as synonym for hypovolemia; technically it is wrong. Dehydration refers only to a decreased volume of water; but water is not decreased without electrolyte charges also. Hydration is the union of a substance with water and is often used to indicate that there is normal water volume in the body.

Fluid Volume Excess (FVE)

Excessive retention of water and sodium in ECF in near-normal proportions results in a condition termed as fluid volume excess. It is also called "hypervolemia". Over hydration refers only to above-normal amounts of water in extra cellular spaces. Malfunction of the kidneys causing an inability to excrete, the success and failure of the heart to function as a pump resulting in accumulation of fluid in the lungs and dependant parts of the body, are common causes. When water is retained in excessive amount, so as sodium **(Fig. 7.15)**.
- Due to increased extracellular osmotic pressure from the retained sodium, fluid is pulled from the cells to equalize the tonicity. By the time intracellular and extracellular spaces are isotonic to each other, an excess of both water and sodium are in ECF, while the cells are nearly depleted.

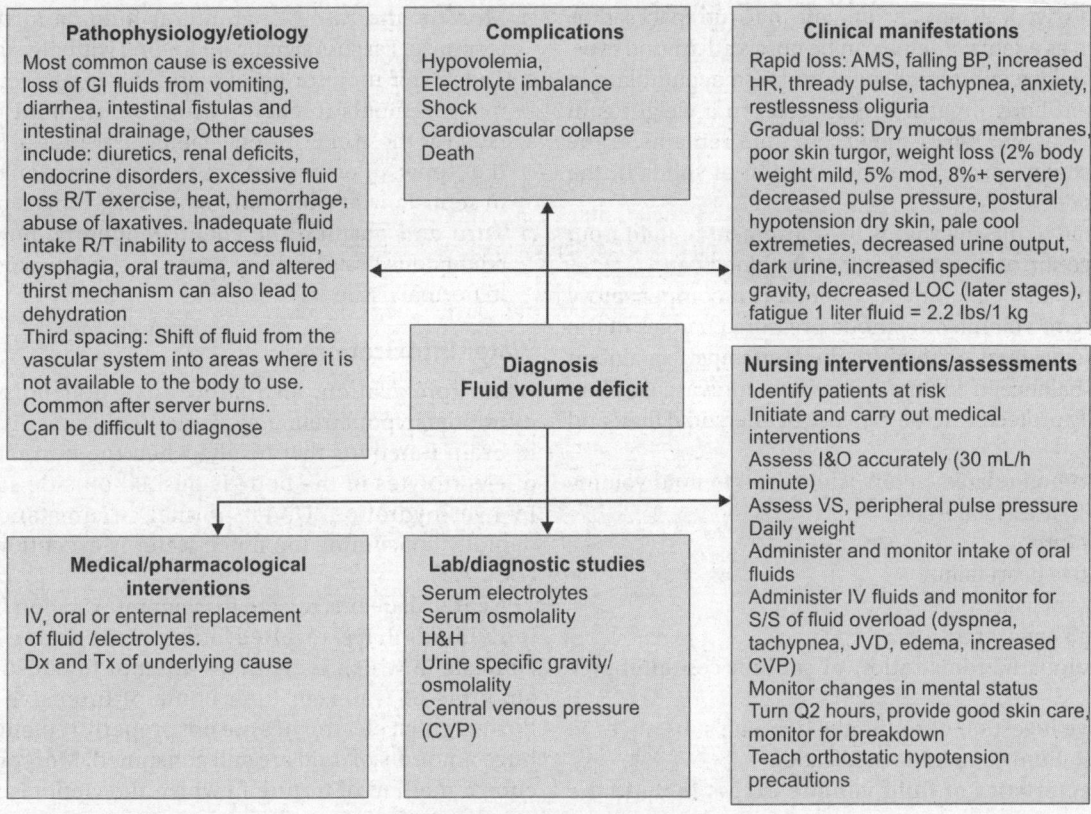

Fig. 7.14: Diagnosis of fluid volume deficit.

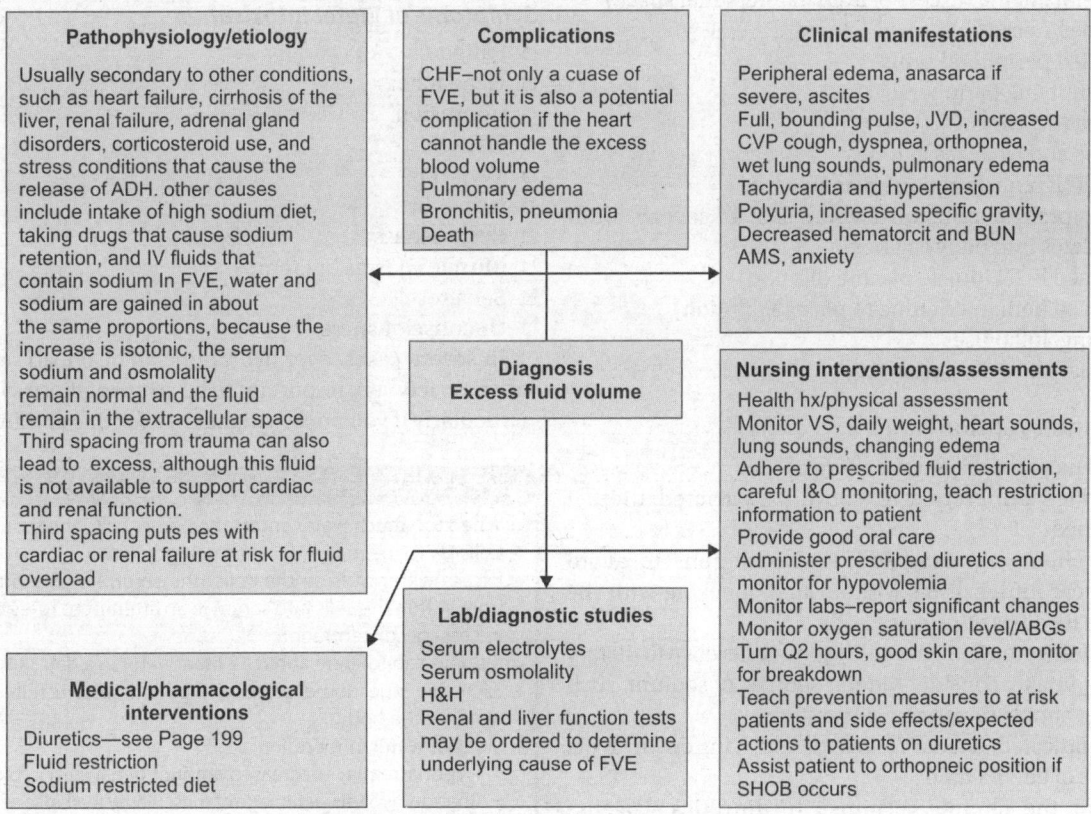

Fig. 7.15: Diagnosis of excess fluid volume.

- The excessive ECF may accumulate in tissue spaces, thus is known as edema: Edema can be observed around eyes, fingers ankles and sacral space and also accumulate in or around body organs. It may result in a weight gain in excess of 5%. When the excess fluid remains in the intravascular space, the concentration of solids in the blood is decreased.
- Interstitial to plasma shift is the movement of fluid from the space surrounding the cells to the blood.
- The shift, also called hypervolemia is a compensatory response to volume or osmotic pressure changes of the intravascular fluid. Although the body attempts to maintain normal balance in all fluid spaces, the intravascular fluid is usually protected at the expense of interstitial fluid and ICF.

The common related factors which lead to fluid volume excess (FVE) are as follows:
- Renal failure
- Congestive heart failure
- Cirrhosis of liver
- Cushing's syndrome
- Overzealous administration of sodium containing IV fluids
- Excessive ingestion of sodium containing substances in diet or sodium containing medication

The characteristics of fluid volume excess include the following:
- Weight gain over short period
- Peripheral edema (excess of fluid in interstitial space)
- Distended neck veins
- Distended peripheral veins
- Slow-emptying peripheral veins
- CVP over 11. cm H_2O
- Crackles and wheezes in lungs
- Polyuria (if renal function normal)
- Ascites, pleural effusion (when FVE is severe, fluid transudates into body cavities)
- Decreased BUN (due to plasma dilution)
- Decreased hematocrit (due to plasma dilution)
- Bounding, full pulse
- Pulmonary edema, if severe.

Nursing Intervention for FVE

- Assess the presence or worsening of FVE
- Encourage adherence to sodium restricted diet, if prescribed
- Teach client requiring sodium restrictions to avoid over-the-counter drugs without first checking with the healthcare adviser/nurse
- When fluid retention persists despite adherence to dietary sodium intake, consider hidden sources of sodium, such as water supply or use of water softener
- When indicated, encourage rest period, lying down favors diuresis of edema fluid
- Monitor the client's response to diuretics. Discuss significant findings with physician
- Monitor the rate of parenteral fluids and the client response. Discuss significant finding with physician
- Teach self-monitoring of eight and intake and output measurements to clients with chronic fluid retention (such as those of ECF, renal failure, cirrhosis of liver)
- If dyspnea or orthopnea are present, position the client in semi-Fowler's position to facilitate lung expansion.
- Turn and position the client frequently, beware that edematous tissue is more prone to skin breakdown than in normal tissue.

Water Intoxication

Water intoxication, also known as water poisoning or dilutional hyponatremia, is a potentially fatal disturbance in brain functions that results when the normal balance of electrolytes in the body is pushed outside safe limits by over-hydration. Under normal circumstances, accidentally consuming too much water is exceptionally rare (Box 7.2).

Nearly all deaths related to water intoxication in normal individuals have resulted either from water drinking contests in which individuals attempt to consume large amounts of water, or long bouts of intensive exercise during which electrolytes are not properly replenished, yet huge amounts of fluid are still consumed. Moreover, water cure, a method of torture in which the victim is forced to consume excessive amounts of water, can cause water intoxication.

Symptoms of Water Intoxication

- Fatigue
- Headache
- Confusion
- Nausea
- Vomiting
- Irritability
- Restlessness
- Muscle spasms or cramps
- Seizures
- Unconsciousness

In severe cases, over hydration can also lead to coma or death, so it is very important to be aware of these symptoms-particularly if you are at a higher risk for this condition.

Box 7.2: Hyperhydration-water intoxication.

- When too much water enters the body's cells, the tissues swell
- Cells try to maintain concentration gradient
- Excess water outside the cells (the serum) draws out sodium from within the cells into serum in an attempt to re-establish the necessary concentration
- Kidneys can tolerate about 17 liters water in a day
- Excessive ingestion of water and other liquids resulted in extra work for the body
- Signs of water intoxication:
  - Hyponatremia—decreased amount of natrium in blood)
  - Rhabdomyolysis—damage of muscularity (collapse of skeleton), acute incompetence of kidneys

Pathophysiology

- The onset of this condition, fluid outside the cells has an excessively low amount of solutes (such as sodium (hyponatremia) and other electrolytes) in comparison to that inside the cells causing the fluid to shift through (via osmosis) into the cells to balance its concentration.
- This causes the cells to swell. In the brain, this swelling increases intracranial pressure (ICP).
- It is this increase in pressure which leads to the first observable symptoms of water intoxication: headache, personality changes, and changes in behavior, confusion, irritability, and drowsiness.
- These are sometimes followed by difficulty breathing during exertion, muscle weakness and pain, twitching, or cramping, nausea, vomiting, thirst, and a dulled ability to perceive and interpret sensory information.
- As the condition persists, papillary and vital signs may result including bradycardia and widened pulse pressure.
- The cells in the brain may swell to the point where blood flow is interrupted resulting in vertebral edema.
- Swollen brain cells may also apply pressure to the brain stem causing central nervous system dysfunction.
- Both cerebral edema and interference with the central nervous system are dangerous and could result in seizures, brain damage, coma or death.

Treatment

- For mild hyponatremia, a reduction in the intake of fluids is often sufficient for solving the problem.
- Eating a small amount of salty foods can also be helpful if you have lost excessive electrolytes by sweating. Keep a close eye on your symptoms to make sure that they don't worsen.
- With more severe cases of hyponatremia, you may need to take medications to offset the feelings of nausea and headaches.
- If symptoms worsen, you may need to visit the hospital in order to receive intravenous (IV) fluids to even out the electrolyte levels in your body.
- Chronic cases of hyponatrema may require hormone therapy depending on the causes behind the condition. In some cases, hormone replacements can be used to keep electrolytes balanced.

■ ELECTROLYTE IMBALANCE

Human body contains quite large volume of water as ICF and ECF and the fluid contains several inorganic ions, such as sodium, potassium, chloride, bicarbonate, sulfate, phosphate, calcium and magnesium. The complex mechanism of human life maintains the concentration and volume of the body fluids at a constant level and in general, it is not influenced by dietary intake and metabolism, while kidneys play a vital role in maintaining the balance. When clients present with deficit or excesses of sodium, potassium, calcium, magnesium or phosphate, special nursing care is required. A brief description of the common electrolyte imbalances are as follows:

Normal range	Causes of elevation	Causes of decline
Sodium (Na): 135–145 mEq/L	**IHypernatremia:** Excessive loss of water through GI system, lungs, or skin; fluid restriction, certain diuretics, hypertonic IV solutions, tube feeding; hypothalamic lesions, hyperal dosteronism, cortioosteroid use, Cushing's syndrome, diabetes insipidus	**Hyponatremia:** Congestive heart failure, cirrhosis, nephrosis, excess fluid intake, syndrome of inappropriate antidiuretic hormone secretion (dilutional hyponatremia); sodium depletion, loss of body fluids without replacement, diuretic therapy, laxatives, nasogastric suctioning, hypoaldosteronism, cerebral salt-wasting disease
Potassium (K): 3.5–5.0 mEq/L	**Hyperkalemia:** Aldosterone deficiency, sodium depletion, acidosis, trauma, hemolysis of red blood cells, potassium-sparing diuretics	**Hypokalemia:** Lack of dietary intake of potassium, vomiting, nasogastric suctioning, potassium-depleting diuretics, aldosteronism, salt-wasting kidney disease, major GI surgery, diuretic therapy with inadequate potassium replacement
Calcium (Ca): 8..5–10.5 mg/dL	**Hypercalcemia:** Excessive vitamin D, immobility, hyperparathyroidism, potassium-sparing diuretics, ACE inhibitors, malignancy of bone or blood	**Hypocalcemia:** Hypoparathyroidism, malabsorption, insufficient or inactivated vitamin D or inadequate intalke of calcium, hypoalbuminemia, diuretic therapy, diarrhea, acute pancreatitis, bone cancer, gastric surgery
Magnesium (Mg): 1.5–2.5 mg/dL	**Hypermagnesemia:** Excessive use of magnesium-containing antacids and laxatives, untreated diabetic ketoacidosis, excessive magnesium infusions	**Hypomagnesemia:** Malabsorption related to GI disease, excessive loss of GI fluids, acute alcoholism/cirrhosis, diuretic therapy, hyper- or hypothyroidism, pancreatitis, preeclampsia, nasogastric suctioning, fistula drainage

Hyponatremia

Hyponatremia refers to a sodium deficit in ECF caused by loss of sodium or a gain of water. It is a condition on lowered level of plasma volume. In this condition, osmotic pressure changes result in ECF, moving into the cells. When this occurs, an examiner's fingerprints tend to remain on the client's skin over the sternum where pressure is applied with the fingers.

The Related Factors Leading to Hyponatremia are as follows:

- Loss of sodium as in—loss of CI fluids, use of diuretics; adrenal insufficiency
- Gains of water as in: excessive administration of D5W, diseases associated with SIADH; pharmacological agents that impair renal water excretion
- Hyponatremia or sodium depletion occurs from loss of body fluids through sweating, vomiting, diarrhea, intestinal fistula, and dialysis and from aspiration of gastric contents
- Chronic pyelonephritis, chronic uremia, diuretic phase of acute renal failure, diabetic ketoacidosis, cystic diseases of the kidney, and excessive or prolonged use of diuretics result in excessive loss of sodium through urine
- Endocrine diseases show as myxedema, Addison's disease, hyperaldosteronism, and uncontrolled diabetes mellitus also lead to sodium depletion
- Excessive loss of sodium can also occur through the skins as in extensive burns, generalized dermatitis and, etc., in children with cystic fibrosis.

Sodium is mainly an extracellular ion, and its depletion causes migration of water in the intracellular compartments, making the extra cellular fluid hypotonic. Consequently, plasma becomes hypo-osmolar and plasma volume falls.

Figure 7.16 is depicted the hyponatremia clinical features.

Main Characteristics

- Anorexia
- Fingerprint over sternum
- Nausea and vomiting
- Muscular twitching
- Lethargy
- Seizures
- Confusion
- Coma
- Muscle cramps
- Serum sodium below 135 mEq/L.

This condition presents with tiredness, lethargy, muscular weakness, mental confusion, and in severe cases, convulsions and coma. The skin appears cold, pale and inelastic. Tongue is dry. Reduction in plasma volume causes reduction in cardiac output and results tachycardia, fall of blood pressure and raising pulse rate. The eyeballs become soft due to reduced intraocular pressure, urine output is reduced and soon oliguria supervenes and finally leads to uremia. When the plasma serum concentration falls exaggeratedly to 120 mmol/L of blood or less, muscle cramps occur. It can produce acidosis and circulatory failure as complication.

Treatment

Mild cases are treated with frequent drink of water with added sodium chloride or with isotonic (0.9%) saline solution by IV injection. In other cases, 2–4 liters of isotonic saline solution is given IV infusion over 6–12 hours. More severe cases are treated with 2–3 liters of IV isotonic solution in first 2–3 hours, followed by further 2–5 liters within 24–48 hours. If there is associated water intoxication, water intake is restricted to 500–1000 mL in 24 hours. In addition, the client is given treatment for the underlying condition.

Nursing Intervention

- Identify clients at risk for hyponatremia
- Monitor fluid losses and gains. Look for loss of sodium containing fluids, particularly in conjunction with low sodium intake
- Monitor presence of gastrointestinal symptoms, such as anorexia, nausea, vomiting, and abdominal cramping
- Monitor laboratory date for serum sodium levels less than normal
- Check specific gravity of urine
- With clients able to consume a general diet, encourage foods and fluids with high sodium content
- Be familiar with the sodium content of commonly used parenteral fluids. Monitor client with cardiovascular disease receiving sodium-containing fluids closely for sign of circulatory overload, such as moist rales in the lungs
- Use extreme caution when administering hypertonic saline solution (3 to 5% NaCl). Beware that these fluids can be lethal if infused carelessly.
- Avoid giving large water supplements to clients receiving isotonic tube feedings, particularly if routes of abnormal sodium loss are present or water is being retained abnormally.

Hypernatremia

Hypernatremia or sodium excess refers to surplus of sodium in ECF that can result from excess water loss or overall excess of sodium. Because of the increased extracellular osmotic pressure, fluids move from the cells, leaving them without sufficient fluid. It is a condition which excess of sodium occurs in the ECF, giving rise to cellular dehydration.

Figure 7.17 is depicted the organs affected due to hyponatremia and **Figure 7.18** is depicted the hyponatremia: The model.

The related factors which lead to hyponatremia are as follows:

- Deprivation of water, most common in those unable to perceive or respond to thirst

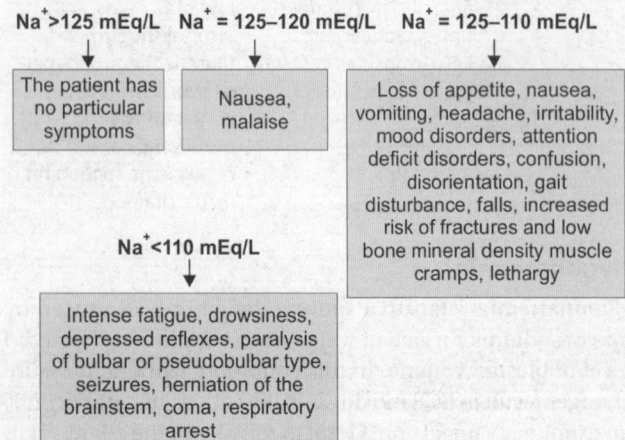

Fig. 7.16: Hyponatremia clinical features.

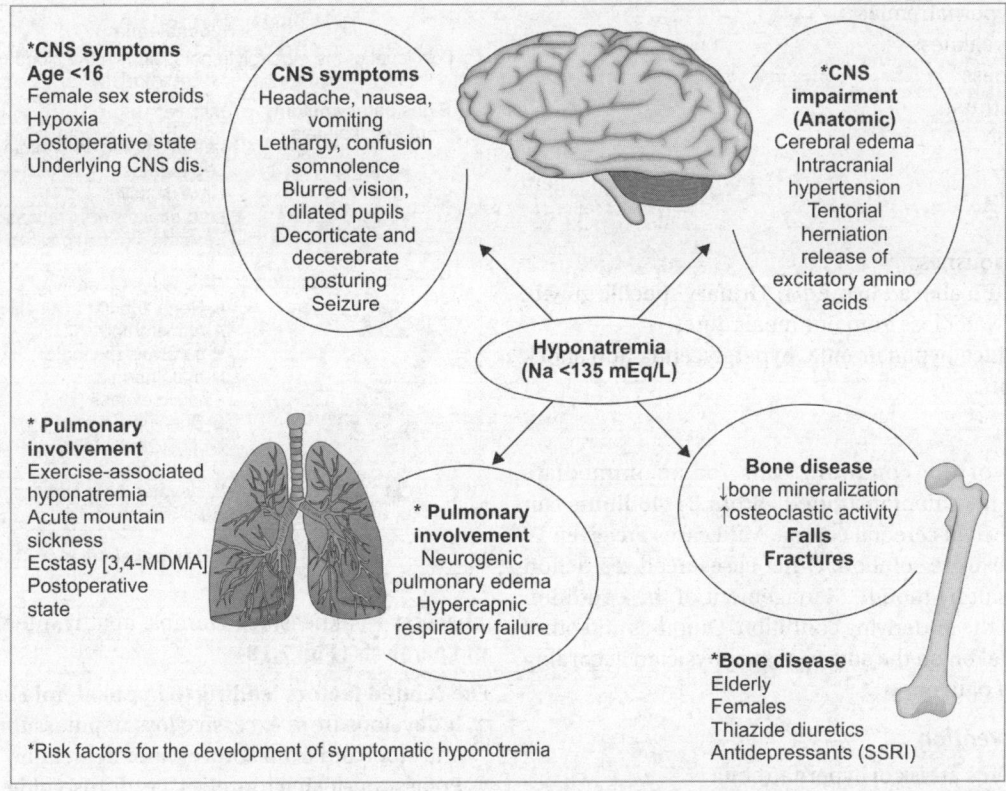

Fig. 7.17: Organs affected due to hyponatremia.

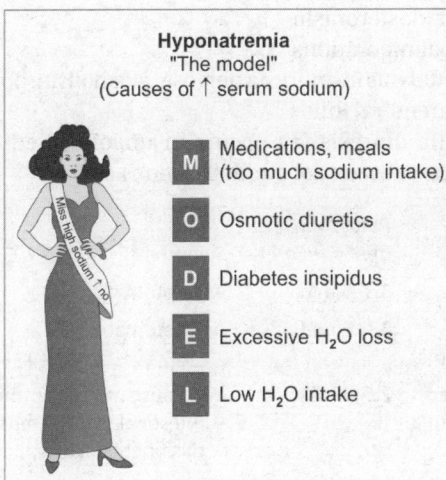

Fig. 7.18: Hyponatremia: The model.

- Hypertonic tube feeding with inadequate water supplements
- Increased insensible water loss (as in hyperventilation)
- Ingestion of salt in unusual amounts
- Excessive parenteral administration of sodium-containing solution:
- Hypertonic saline (3 or 5% NaCl)
- 7.5% sodium bicarbonate
- Isotonic saline
- Profuse sweating
- Diabetes insipidus
- Heat stroke

Box 7.3: Symptoms of hypernatremia.

- Initial symptoms include lethargy, weakness and irritability
- Can progress to twitching, seizures, obtundation or coma
- Resulting decrease in brain volume can lead to rupture of cerebral veins leading to hemorrhage
- Severe symptoms usually occur with rapid increase to sodium concentration of 158 mEq or more
- Sodium concentration greater than 180 mEq are associated with high mortality

- Drowning in sea water
- Hypernatremia also occurs when water losses of the body exceed sodium loss as that is seen in diabetes insipidus, marked glycosuria, hypercalcemia, hypokalemia, chronic renal failure, and recovery phase of acute renal failure. **Box 7.3** is depicted the symptoms of hypernatremia.
- Sodium excess may occur along with water excess when due to inadequate clearance of the kidneys both sodium and water accumulate in the extracellular space, leading to edema, for example, nephrotic syndrome, cardiac failure, nutritional or thiamine deficiency, cirrhosis of liver, and in cases of usage of drugs, such as corticosteroids, androgens, phenylbutazone, oral contraceptive and carbenoxelone. It causes retention of sodium, increased volume of ECF and edema in the interstitial compartment.

Main Characteristics

- Thirst
- Elevated body temperature
- Tongue dry and swollen, sticky mucous membranes

- In severe hypernatremia:
  - Muscle weakness
  - Restlessness
  - Extreme thirst
  - Confusion
  - Lethargy
  - Irritability
  - Seizures
  - Unconsciousness

Serum sodium above 145 mEq/L. Urinary specific gravity .015 provided water loss from nonrenal route.

It may produce hyponatremia, hyperglycemia and shock as complication.

Treatment

Management of the condition calls for an immediate attention and treatment instituted within 24–48 hours can avoid occurrence of cerebral edema. Mild cases are given IV infusion 5% dextrose solution. Other cases need restriction of water and salt by mouth. Management of the condition depends upon the underlying condition. Diuretics and other measures are taken on the advice of the physician according to condition of patient.

Nursing Intervention

- Identify clients at risk of hypernatremia
- Monitor fluid losses and gains. Look for abnormal losses of water or low water intake; and for large gains of sodium as might occur with ingestion of proprietory drugs with high sodium content. And also consider that prescription drugs may have high sodium content. Of course one should look for excessive intake of high sodium foods
- Monitor changes in behavior, such as restlessness, disorientation and lethargy
- Look for excessive thirst, and elevated body temperature. If present, evaluate in relation to other signs
- Monitor serum sodium level
- Prevent hyponatremia in debilitated clients unable to perceive or respond to thirst by offering them fluids at regular intervals. If fluids intake remains inadequate, consult the physician in order to plan and alternate route for intake, either by tube feedings or by the parenteral route
- If tube feedings are used, give sufficient water to keep the serum sodium and the BUN level within normal limits. Beware that the higher the osmolity of the feeding, the greater the need for water supplements.

Hypokalemia

Hypokalemia refers to a potassium deficit in ECF. When the extra cellular potassium level falls, potassium moves from the cell, creating an intracellular potassium deficiency. Sodium and hydrogen ions are then retained by the cells to maintain isotonic fluids. These electrolyte shifts influence normal cellular functioning, the pH of ECF, and function of most of the body systems. Skeletal muscles are generally the first to demonstrate a potassium deficiency. It is a condition associated with depletion of potassium characterized by

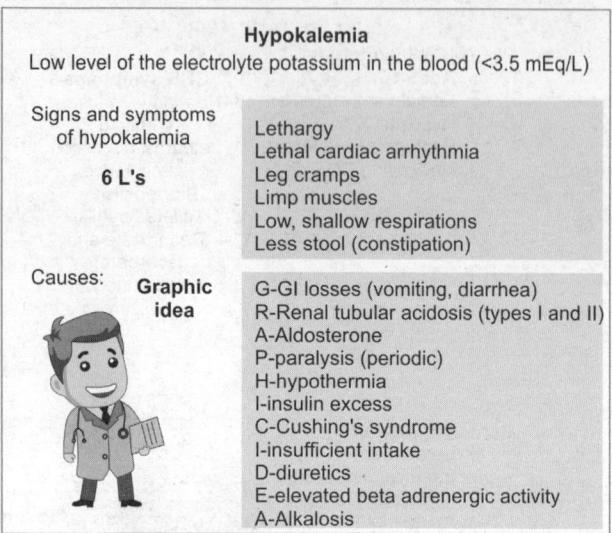

Fig. 7.19: Hypokalemia.

muscular weakness, leg cramps, apathy, mental confusion and paralysis (**Fig. 7.19**).

The related factors leading to hypokalemia are as follows:
- It develops from excessive loss of potassium in the urine and stool and from severe water depletion
- Potassium-losing diuretics, i.e., furosemide, thiazide, etc.
- Steroid administration
- Use of carbenicillin, sodium penicillin, amphotericin B
- Hyperaldosteronism
- Hyper alimentations
- Poor intake as in anorexia nervosa, alcoholism, potassium-free parenteral fluids
- Osmotic diuresis (as occurs in uncontrolled diabetes mellitus or mannitol administration).

	Potassium level (mM = mEq/L)	Symptoms
Normal	3.5–5 mM	Asymptomatic
Mild hypokalemia	3–3.5 mM	Asymptomatic
Moderate hypokalemia	2.5–3 mM	May cause mild symptoms • Intestinal smooth muscle dysfunction causes ileus
Severe hypokalemia	<2.5 mM	May cause severe symptoms • Muscle cramps • Weakness (classically ascending weakness, can involve diaphragm) • Torsacles de pointes, other arrhythmias • Heart failure • Rhabdomyolysis

Main Characteristics

- Fatigue
- Anorexia, nausea and vomiting
- Muscle weakness
- Decreased bowel motility (intestinal ileus)—paralytic ileus
- Cardiac arrhythmia

- Increased, i.e., sensitivity to digitalis
- Polyuria, nocturia, dilute urine (if hypokalemia prolonged)
- Mild hyperglycemia a serum K below 3.5 mEq/L
- Paresthesis or tender muscles
- ECG changes—flattened T waves, ST segment depressions
- Respiratory hyperventilation.

Treatment

Management of the condition requires adequate management of the underlying conditions.

- Beware of clients at risk for hypokelemia and monitor for its occurrence
- Assess digitalized clients at risk for hypokelemia especially closely for symptoms of digitalis toxicity
- Take measures to prevent hypokalemia when possible
- Prevention may take the form of encouraging extra potassium intake for at-risk patient (when the diet allows)
- When hypokalemia due to abuse of laxatives or diuretics education of the client may help alleviate the problems
- Administer oral potassium supplement when prescribed

Hypokalemia	Hyperkalemia
• Decreased dietary intake	• Increased dietary intake
• Excess fluid loss	• Rapid infusion of potassium containing solution
• Kidney losses (diuretics, steroids, diuretic phase of acute kidney	• Salt substitutes (potassium chloride)
• Nausea, vomiting, diarrhea	• Decreased kidney function
• Laxative abuse or overuse	• Release of potassium from tissue trauma, burns, crush injuries, catabolism, and hemolysis
• Shift of potassium from extracellular fluid to cells (hypothermia, sodium polystyrene sulfonate, insulin and sodium bicarbonate administration)	• Shift of potassium from cells to the extracellular fluid (beta-blockers, acidosis)

- Beware that clients may not need potassium supplements if they are using salt substitutes because these substances usually contain sizable amounts of potassium
- Be thoroughly familiar with the critical facts related to administering potassium intravenously.

Hyperkalemia

Hyperkalemia refers to a condition with excess of potassium in ECG, characterized by conduction defect in the heart and myoneural junction of the muscle.

The related factors which lead to hyperkalemia are as follows:
- Decreased potassium excretions as in:
- Oliguric renal failure
- Potassium-conserving diuretic usage
- Hypoaldosteronism.
- High potassium intake, especially in presence of renal insufficiency:
- Improper use of oral potassium supplements
- Rapid excessive administration of IV potassium
- High-dose potassium penicillin
- Foods high in potassium (such as dried apricots).
- Shift of potassium out of cells due to acidosis, tissue trauma, and malignant cell lysis
- Potassium excess also occurs in acute renal failure, severe crush injuries and burns. Severe hemorrhages and adrenal insufficiency
- It is also seen in diabetic ketoacidosis.

Main Characteristics

- Vague muscular weakness is usually first sign
- Cardiac arrhythmias, bradycardia and heart block can occur
- Paresthesias of face, tongue, feet and hands
- Flaccid muscle paralysis (spreads from legs to trunk and arms, respiratory muscle may be affected)
- Gastrointestinal symptoms, such as nausea, intermittent intestinal colic, or diarrhea may occur
- ECG changes falls, peaked T waves, absent P wave's widened QRS complex
- Serum K, above 5.0 mEq/L (mmol/L).
- It can produce cardiac arrest, metabolic acidosis and respiratory acidosis as complications.

Figure 7.20 is depicted the signs and symptoms of hyperkalemia.

Treatment

Management of the condition is done by replacements of water loss and correction of electrolyte imbalance. The client is given diet with restricted protein but with as much as fat and carbohydrate and also managing the underlying condition.

Nursing Intervention

- Beware of clients at risk for hyperkalemia and monitor for its occurrence. Hyperkalemia is life-threatening; it is imperative to detect it easily
- Follow rules for safe administration of potassium
- Avoid administration of potassium con serving diuretics, potassium supplements or salt substitutes to client with renal insufficiency
- Caution client to use salt substitute sparingly if they are taking other supplementary form of potassium or taking potassium-conserving diuretics (e.g., spironolactone, triamterene, and amiloride)

Caution hyperkalemic clients to avoid foods high in potassium content. Some of these are coffee, cocoa, tea, dried fruits, dried beans, whole grain breads.

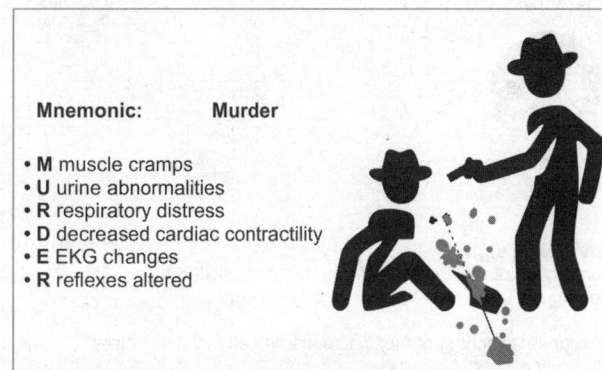

Fig. 7.20: Signs and symptoms of hyperkalemia.

Hypocalcemia

Hypocalcemia refers to a calcium deficit in ECF. If the condition is prolonged calcium is taken from bones. This results in osteomalacia, which is characterized by soft and pliable bones. Common signs and symptoms for hypocalcaemia include numbness and tingling of fingers, muscle cramps and tetany.

Box 7.4 is depicted the common causes of hypocalcemia.
The related factors leading to hypocalcemia are as follows:
- Surgical hypoparathyroidism (may follow thyroid surgery or radical neck surgery for cancer)
- Malabsorption
- Vitamin D deficiency
- Acute pancreatitis
- Excessive administration of citrated blood
- Primary hypothyroidism
- Alkalitic states (decreased ionized calcium)
- Hyperphosphatemia
- Medullary carcinoma of thyroid
- Hypoalbuminemia (as in cirrhosis, nephrotic syndrome and starvation)
- Hypomagnesemia
- Increased/decreased ultraviolet exposure.

Figure 7.21 is depicted the hypocalcemia.

Box 7.4: Common causes of hypocalcemia.
- Hypoparathyroidism
- Vitamin D deficiency or insufficiency
- Altered vitamin D metabolism due to medication usage
- Diseases affecting the klidneys and/or the liver
- Pseudohypoparathyroidism
- Hypomagnesemia or hypermagnesemia
- Hungry bone syndrome
- Infusion of phosphate
- Rapid citrated blood transfusion
- Medications

Trousseau's sign
Induction of carpopedal spasm by inflation of a sphygmomanometer above SBP for 3 minutes

Response: Carpopedal spasm characterized by
- Adduction of the thumb
- Flexion of the metacarpophalangeal joints
- Extension of the interphalangeal joints
- Flexion of the wrist

Chvostek's sign
Contraction of the ipsilateral facial muscles elicited by tapping the facial nerve just anterior to the ear

Response: twitching of the lip to spasm of all facial muscles

Fig. 7.21: Hypocalcemia.

Main Characteristics
- Numbness, tingling fingers, circumoral region and toes
- Cramps in the muscle of extremities
- Hyperactive deep tendon reflexes (such as patellar and triceps)
- Trousseau's sign
- Chvostek's sign
- Mental changes, such as confusion and alteration in mood and memory
- Convulsions, usually generalized but may be focal
- Spasm of laryngeal muscles
- ECG shows prolonged QT interval
- Spasms of muscles in abdomen (can simulate acute abdo-emergency)
- Total calcium level below 8.5 mg/dL or ionized level below normal (below 50%)
- Hypocalcemic state occurs when calcium loss occurs causing a fall in serum calcium level. This may eventually cause tetany and teeth.
- It is usually asymptomatic and the neurological manifestation develop slowly.
- It then gives rise to diffuse encephalopathy, depression and psychosis.
- In severe cases, there may be laryngospasm and general convulsion.
- It may also give rise to papilledema and cataract.

Figure 7.22 is depicted the signs and symptoms of hypercalcemia.

Treatment
Most cases respond well to adequate or supplement calcium and phosphorus. The patient may be given calcium carbonate, 2.52 to 3.78 g daily orally or calcium gluconate 0.5–1.5 g along with calciferol 15.45 mg daily orally. Otherwise, 10 mL of 10% calcium gluconate is given by slow IV. Adequate management and control of predisposing causes can prevent the occurrence of the condition.

Nursing Interventions
- Beware of clients at risk for hypocalcemia and monitor its occurrence
- Be prepared to take seizures precautions
- Monitor condition of airway closely because laryngeal stridor can occur
- Take safety precautions if confusion is present
- Beware of factors related to the safe administration of calcium replacement salts

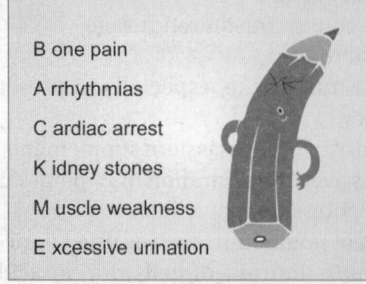

Fig. 7.22: Signs and symptoms of hypercalcemia: Nurse buff.

- Educate people in high-risk groups for osteoporosis (especially postmenopausal women not on estrogen therapy). If adequate amounts are not consumed in the diet (as is often the case), calcium supplements should be considered
- Educate people at risk for osteoporosis about the value of regular physical exercise in decreasing bone loss
- To prevent osteoporosis in later years, educate young women about the need for a normal diet to ensure adequate calcium intake. Also discuss the calcium-losing aspects of alcohol and nicotine use.

Hypercalcemia

Hypercalcemia refers to an excess of calcium in ECF. It presents an emergency situation because this condition often leads to cardiac arrest. It is a condition of excess of calcium and is characterized by polyuria, polydipsia, skeletal muscle weakness and hypertension.

	Mild (corrected calcium 10.5–11.9 mg/dL)	Moderate (corrected calcium 12.0–13.9 mg/dL)	Severe (corrected calcium >14.0 mg/dL)
Neuropsychiatric	Anxiety, depression	Cognitive dysfunction	Lethargy, confusion, stupor, coma
Gastrointestinal	Anorexia, nausea, constipation	Anorexia, nausea constipation	Pancreatitis
Renal	Polyria	Dehydration	Renal insufficiency, dehydration
Cardiac	Shortened QT interval	Shortened QT interval	Arrhythmia, ventricular tachycardia
Musculoskeletal	None	Weakness	Weakness

The related factors that lead to hypercalcemia are as follows:
- Hyperparathyroidism
- Malignant neoplastic disease
- Prolonged immobilization
- Large doses of vitamin D
- Overuse of calcium containing antacids or calcium supplements thiazide diuretics
- Milk-alkali syndromes
- Sarcoidosis
- It is also seen in person with Paget's disease, myxoedema, Addison's disease and osteoporosis in aged persons.

Main Characteristics

- Muscle weakness
- Tiredness, restlessness, lethargy
- Constipation
- Anorexia, nausea, and vomiting
- Decreased memory span, decreased attention span, and confusion
- Polyuria, and polydipsia
- Renal stones
- Neurobic behavior progressing to frank psychosis may occur (reversible with correction of hypercalcemia)

Symptoms	Signs
Fatigue or lethargy	Altered mental state
Confusion	Polyuria (if diabetes insipidus)
Thirst	Oliguria (if acute kidney injury)
Muscle pain	Renal angel tenderness or hematuria (if renal calculi)
Abdominal pain	Myopathy
Nausea or vomiting	Reduced bowel sounds
Anorexia	Arrhythmia (also demonstrates short QT interval on ECG)
Constipation	Dehydration
Palpitations	Band keratopathy

(ECG: electrocardiography)

- Cardiac arrest may occur in hypercalcemic crisis
- ECG shows shortened QT interval
- Serum calcium over 10.5 mg/dL
- It may produce renal failure, shock and death in complication.

Treatment

In mild cases, adequate rehydration is often effective. Management of the condition also includes management of the underlying conditions. In other cases, intravenous infusion of isotonic saline is given to promote calciuria. Calcium is also eliminated or maintained in the lower level by giving sodium phosphate 1–2 g orally daily, and client is encouraged to take more fluids.

Nursing Intervention

- Beware of clients at risk for hypercalcemia and monitor its occurrence
- Increase client mobilization when feasible
- Encourage the oral intake of sufficient fluids to keep the client well hydrated
- Discourage excessive consumption of milk products and other high calcium foods
- Encourage adequate bulk in the diet to offset the tendency for constipation
- Take safety precautions if confusion or other mental symptoms by hypercalcemia are present
- Beware that cardiac arrest can occur in clients with every hypercalcemia be prepared to deal with this emergency
- Beware that bones may fracture more easily in clients with chronic hypercalcemia because bone resorption has been excessive, weakening the bony structure. Transfer clients cautiously
- Educate home-bound oncology clients with a predisposition for hypercalcemia and their families, to be alert for symptoms that occur with this condition and to report them to the healthcare providers before they become severe
- Be alert for signs of digitalis toxicity when hypercalcemia occurs in digitalized clients

- Help prevent formation of calcium renal stones in clients with longstanding hypercalcemia or immobilization by:
- Forcing fluids to maintain dilute urine, thus avoiding super saturation of precipitates
- Encouraging fluids that yield an acid ash (prune or cranberry milk) because a urinary pH less than 6.5 favors calcium deposits
- Preventing urinary stasis by turning the immobilized client, elevating head of the bed and having the client sit up if this can be tolerated.

Hypomagnesmia (Fig. 7.23)

Magnesium is an important and plentiful cation, and is essential for many enzymatic system associated with protein, carbohydrate and lipid metabolism. Hypomagnesemia refers to magnesium deficit. It is condition of low plasma concentration of magnesium, characterized by neuromuscular and CNS hyperirritability

The related factors which lead to hypomagnesemia are as follows:
- Chronic alcoholism
- Intestinal malabsorption syndrome
- Diarrhea
- Nasogastric suction-prolonged
- Aggressive refeeding after starvation (as in TPN)
- Prolonged administration of magnesium-free IV fluids
- Uncontrolled diabetes mellitus-diabetic ketoacidosis
- Hyperaldosteronism
- Drugs-prolonged use of: Diuretics, aminoglycoside, antibiotics (e.g., gentamycin), cisplatin
- Excessive dose of vitamin-D or calcium supplements
- Citrate preservative in blood products pancreatitis, thyrotoxicosis, hyperparathyroiders
- Severe osteitis fibrosa, PEM.

Figure 7.24 is depicted the symptoms of magnesium deficiency.

Main Characteristics

- It presents with multiple metabolic and nutritional deficiency
- It gives rise to anorexia, lethargy, vomiting, weakness, and tetany

Neuromuscular Irritability

- Increased reflex
- Course tremors
- Positive Chvostek's and Trousseau's signs
- Convulsions

Cardiac Manifestations will include:

- Tachyarrhythmias
- Increased susceptibility to digitalis toxicity

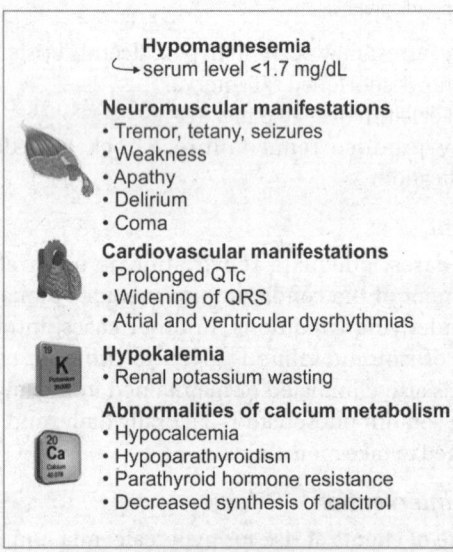

Fig. 7.23: Hypomagnesemia.

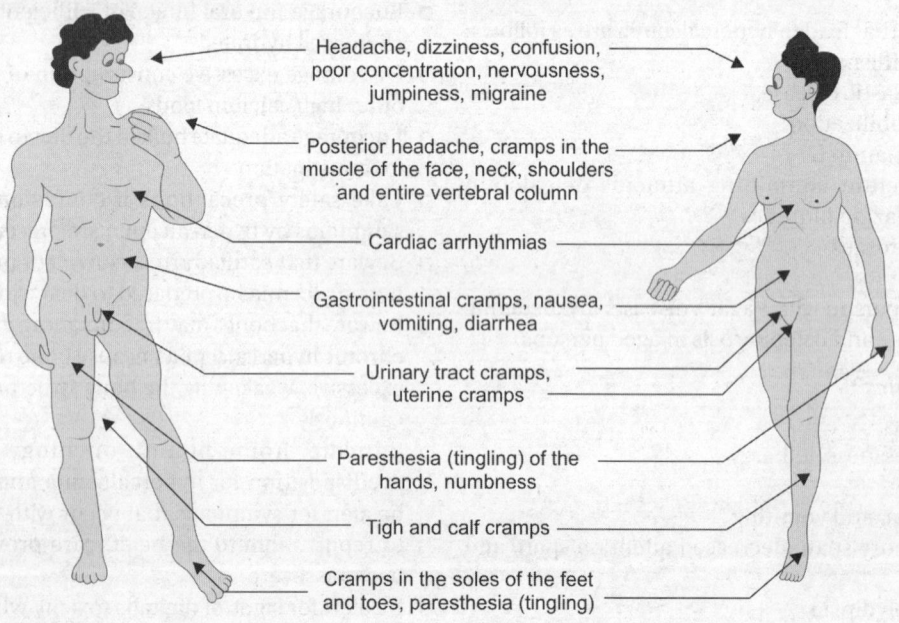

Fig. 7.24: Symptoms of magnesium deficiency.

- ECG changes in severe cases, PR and QT interval prolongation, widened QRS complex, ST segment depression and T-wave inversion.
- Mental changes
- Disorientation in memory
- Mood changes
- Intense confusion
- Hallucination
- Serum magnesium level below 1.3 mEq/L.

Treatment
Repletion of the cases is done through magnesium sulfate and chloride. It is customary to give double the amount required because half of magnesium given excreted by the kidneys. The repletion is done gradually and is given orally or intravenously; in severe cases, IV only.

Nursing Intervention
- Beware, client at risk for hypomagnesemia, especially closely for symptoms of digitalis toxicity because a deficit of magnesium predisposes to toxicity
- Be prepared to take seizure precautions when hypomagnesemia, especially closely for symptoms of digitalis toxicity, because a deficit of magnesium predisposes to toxicity
- Monitor condition of airway, because laryngeal stridor can occur
- Take safety precautions if confusion presents be familiar with magnesium replacement salts and factors related to this safe administration
- Beware that magnesium-depleted clients may experience difficulty in swallowing
- When magnesium deficit is due to abuse of diuretics in laxatives, educating the client may help alleviate problem
- Beware that most commonly used IV fluids have either no magnesium or relatively small amount. When indicated, discuss the need for magnesium replacement with physicians
- For clients experiencing abnormal losses, but able to consume a general diet, encourage intake of magnesium-rich foods (such as green-leafy vegetables, nuts, legumes and fruits such as bananas, oranges, and grape fruits).

Hypermagnesemia
Hypermagnesemia refers to a magnesium excess. It can occur especially in end stage renal failure. When kidneys fail to excrete magnesium and excessive amounts are administered therapeutically. It is a condition associated with excess of magnesium and is characterized by muscular weakness and ECG changes.

The related factors which lead to hypermagnesemia are as follows:
- Renal failure (particularly when magnesium containing medications are administered)
- Adrenal insufficiency
- Excessive magnesium administration during treatment of eclampsia
- Hemodialysis with excessively hard water or with dialysate inadvertently high in magnesium content.
- Magnesium has a direct action on the myoneural junction. Its excess produces blockage causing impairment of neuromuscular transmission and that results diminished excitability of the muscle cells.

Table 7.1 is depicted the interpreting magnesium levels.

Table 7.1: Interpreting magnesium levels.

	mg/dL	mM	mEq/L	Clinical significance
Severe hypermagnesemia	>~12 mg/dL	>~5 mM	>~10 mEq/L	Severe symptoms • Muscle weakness • Respiratory distress, apnea • Heart block, severe bradycardia • Delirium, coma
Moderate hypermagnesemia	5–12 mg/dL	2–5 mM	4–10 mEq/L	Hyporeflexia Mild symptoms • Lethargy, confusion • Nausea, vomiting • Bradycardia
Therapeutic target during Mg infusion	3.6–4.9 mg/dL	1.5–2 mM	3–4 mEq/L	Should be asymptomatic
Normal	1.7–3 mg/dL	0.7–1.2 mM	1.4–2.4 mEq/L	Normal. May consider targeting Mg >2 mg/dL (or >0.8 mM) to avoid arrhythmias in patients at increased risk
Moderate hypomagnesemia	1.2–1.7 mg/dL	0.5–0.7 mM	1–1.4 mEq/L	May see: • Neuromuscular irritability • Tremor • Hypocalcemia • Hypokalemia
Severe hypomagnesemia	<1.2 mg/dL	<0.5 mM	<1 mEq/L	May see: • Tetany • Nystagmus • Seizures • Psychosis • Arrhythmia

Main Characteristics

- Early signs (serum level of mg of 3 to 5 mEq/L)
- Flushing and a sense of skin warmth (due to peripheral vasodilation)
- Hypotension (due to blockage of sympathetic ganglia)
- Depressed respiration
- Drowsiness, hypoactive reflexes and muscular weakness
- Cardiac abnormalities—cardiac arrest may develop
- Weak or absent cry in newborn
- ECG shows prolonged PR interval, widened QRS complex and elevated T-wave amplitude
- Elevated serum magnesium level

Figure 7.25 is depicted the hypermagnesemia.

Treatment

In severe cases and also in other cases cardiac and respiratory support is given by IV injection of 10–20 mL of 10% calcium gluconate. Maintenance of adequate hydration is essential. The client is also given frusemide by IV injection to promote excretion of magnesium. In more severe cases, hemodialysis is done.

Nursing Intervention

- Beware of client at risk for hypomagnesemia and assess for its presence. When it is suspected assess the following parameters:
  - Vital signs: Look for low blood pressure and shallow respirations with periods of apnea
  - Level of consciousness: Look for drowsiness, lethargy and coma
- Do not give magnesium containing medication to clients with renal failure or compromised renal function
- Be particularly careful in following 'standing order' for bowel preparation for X-ray because some of these include the use of magnesium citrate
- Caution clients with renal disease to check with their healthcare providers before taking over the counter medication
- Beware of factors related to safe parenteral administration of magnesium salts.

Hypophosphatemia (Fig. 7.26)

Hypophosphatemia refers to a below normal serum concentration of inorganic phosphorus. It is a clinical

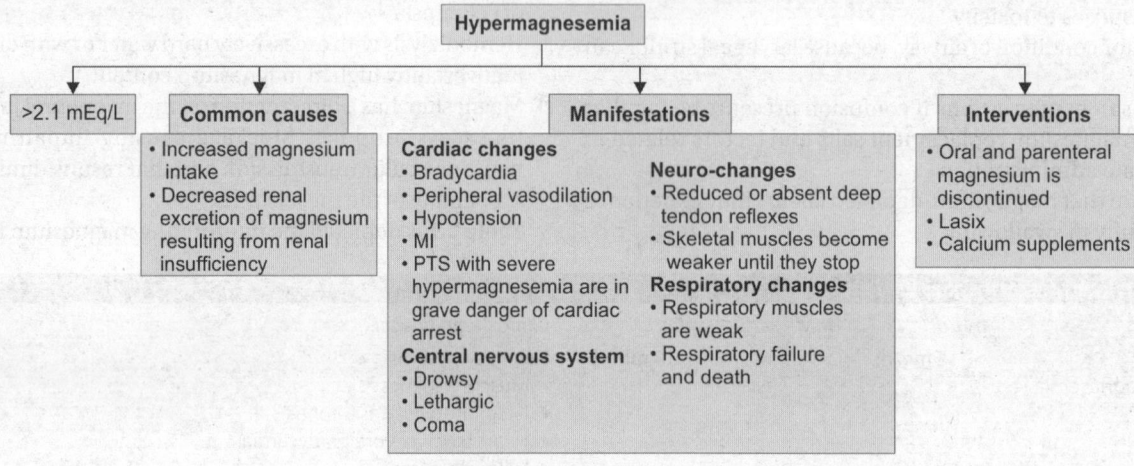

Fig. 7.25: Hypermagnesemia.

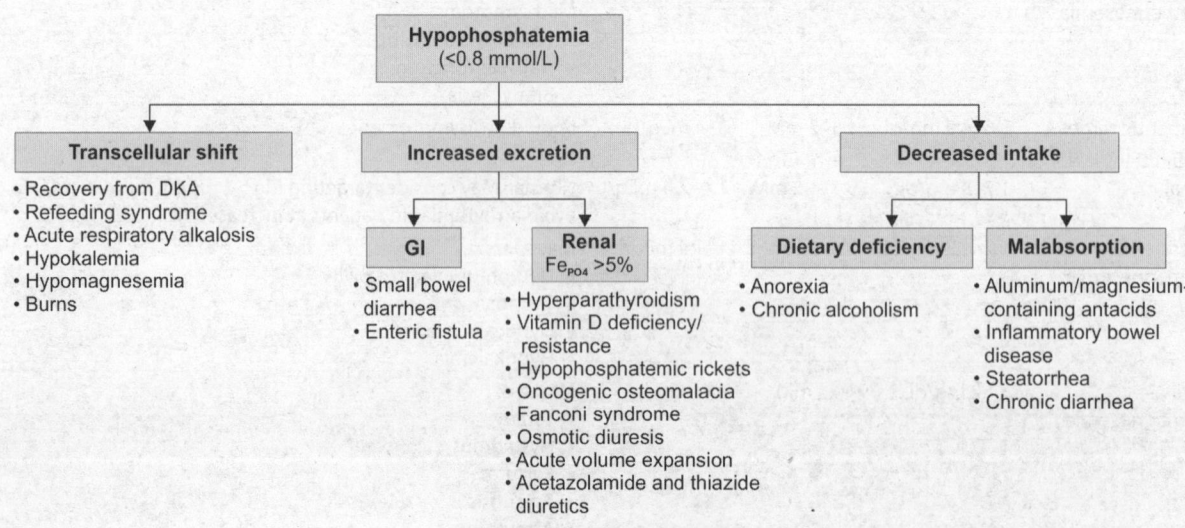

Fig. 7.26: Hypophosphatemia.

manifestation of phosphate depletion, characterized by progressive encephalopathy and osteomalacia.

The related factors which lead to hypophosphatemia are as follows:
- Inadequate intake or absorption of phosphorus-malabsorption
- It is associated with vomiting and diarrhea
- Prolonged injection of aluminum hydroxide or bicarbonate

Main Characteristics
- Progressive encephalopathy
- Paresthesias
- Muscle weakness
- Muscle pain and tenderness
- Mental changes, such as apprehension, confusion, delirium coma
- Cardiomyopathy
- Acute respiratory failure
- Seizures
- Decreased tissue oxygenation
- Joint stiffness
- Serum phosphate below 2.5 mg/dL
- Phosphate compounds are present in all normal foods and are essential for metabolism of carbohydrate, protein and fat. They are also responsible for changes, transfer, or depletion occurs from prolonged negative phosphate balance and form chronic malnutrition.

Treatments
Management of the condition includes treatment of the underlying cause, repletion of phosphate, and maintenance of body fluids.

Nursing Intervention
- Identify clients at risk for hypophosphatemia
- Severely malnourished clients
- Alcoholic clients
- Clients with diabetic ketoacidosis
- Monitor clients at risk for the presence of hypophosphatemia
- Beware that severely hypophosphatemic clients are thought to be greater risk for infection because of changes in WBCs
- Administer IV phosphate products cautiously
- Beware that in adults the usual maintenance dose of phosphorus is 10 to 15 mmol/L of TPN solution
- Beware of the need to introduce hyperalimentation gradually in clients who are malnourished
- Because it is possible to give too much phosphorus when administering phosphate solutions, monitor for signs of hyperphosphatemia and of the salt in which it is administered
- Monitor for diarrhea in clients taking oral phosphorus supplements; consult physician if it persists or is severe
- Powdered oral phosphorus supplements with chilled or ice water to make them more palatable.

Hyperphosphatemia (Fig. 7.27)
Hyperphosphatemia refers to above normal serum concentrations of inorganic phosphorus. It is a condition associated with increased level of phosphate and is characterized by hypocalcemia.

The related factors which lead to hyperphosphatemia are as follows:
- Excessive intake of phosphate
- Hypervitaminosis D-large vitamin D intake
- Chronic renal insufficiency
- Chemotherapy, particularly for acute lymphoblastic leukemia and lymphoma
- Large intake of milk
- Use of cow's milk in infants
- Excessive intake of phosphate containing laxatives
- Overzealous administration of phosphorus supplements (oral or IV)
- Excessive use of Fleet's phospho-soda as enema solution particularly in children and people with slow bowel elimination
- Hypoparathyroidism
- Hyperthyroidism

Main Characteristics
This condition by itself does not give rise to any symptoms but manifested with that of hypocalcaemia. This includes:
- **Short-term consequences:** Symptoms of tetany, such as tingling of fingertips and around mouth, numbness and muscle spasms
- **Long-term consequences:** Precipitation of calcium phosphate in nonosseous sites; such as kidney, joints, arteries, skin to cornea
- Serum phosphate above 4.5 mg/dL.

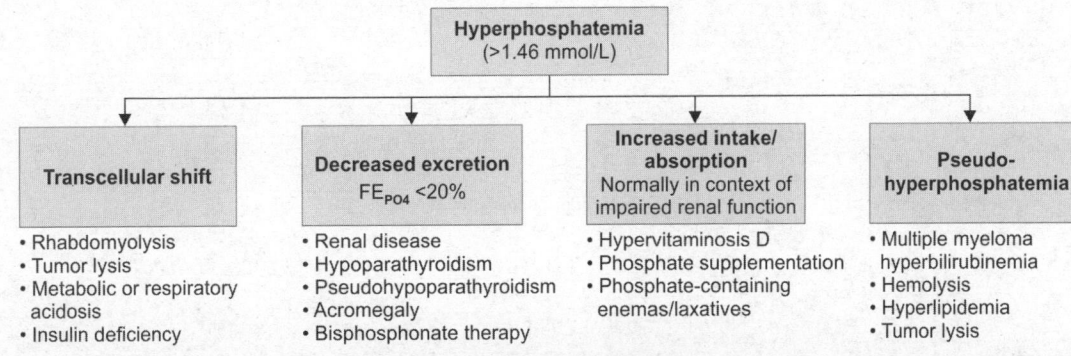

Fig. 7.27: Hyperphosphatemia.

Treatment

Management of the condition requires correction of underlying condition.

Nursing Intervention

- Identify clients at risk for hyperphosphatemia
- Monitor signs of tetanus and other features of hypocalcemia
- Beware that soft-tissue calcification can be long-term complication of a chemically elevated serum phosphate level. Calcification may occur in site such as kidney, arteries, joints, etc.
- Administer prescribed oral or IV phosphate supplements cautiously and monitor serum phosphorus levels periodically during their use.
- When appropriate, instruct clients that use of phosphate, containing laxatives may result in acute phosphate poisoning.
- Beware that phosphate-containing enema can result in hyperphosphatemia if used injudiciously, particularly in children and those with slow bowel emptying, instruct clients accordingly
- When low-phosphorus diet is prescribed, instruct clients to avoid foods high in phosphorus content. Such foods include hard cheese or cream, nuts and nut products; whole grain cereals (e.g., bran and oatmeal), dried fruits, dried vegetables; special meats, such as kidneys, sardines, and sweet breads and desserts made with milk.

CONCLUSION

Body fluids are mainly water and electrolytes, and the three main organs that regulate fluid balance are the brain, the adrenal glands and the kidneys. One-third of the total is circulatory fluid, sometimes known as extracellular fluid (ECF); the remainder is intracellular fluid (ICF) contained within cells. The anatomy and physiology of homeostasis are covered in part one of this series.

A client's condition can change rapidly if she develops a fluid and electrolyte imbalance. The nurse must be able to recognize signs and symptoms of fluid and electrolyte imbalances, prevent possible complications due to these imbalances, evaluate lab work critically, and implement appropriate nursing interventions.

BIBLIOGRAPHY

1. Adrogue H, Madias N. Management of life threatening acid base disorders. N Engl J Med. 2008;338:26-34.
2. Gennari F. Serum osmolality. N Engl J Med. 2004;310:102-5.
3. Joshi SA. Nutrition and Dietetics, Tata McGraw Hill, New Delhi, India, 1992.
4. Kobrin S, Goldfarb S. Hypocalcemia and hypercalcemia. In adrogue H acid base and electrolyte disorders. Newyork, Churchill, living stone. 1999; pp69-96.
5. Lutz CA, Karen RP. Nutrition and Diet Therapy, 4th edition. Davis FA, Philadelphia, USA, 1995.
6. Patwardhan VN. Nutrition in India, 2nd edition. Indian Journal of Medical Sciences. New Delhi, 1961.
7. Pestana C. Fluids and electrolytes in surgical patients, 2nd edition. Baltimore, Williams and wilkins. 2001; pp101-44.

REVIEW QUESTIONS

Long Essays

1. Explain electrolytes: Type, sources and consumption of body fluids.
2. Describe water requirement and regulation.
3. Explain in detail about water metabolism and distribution.

Short Essays

1. Electrolyte imbalance.
2. Maintenance of fluid and electrolyte balance.
3. Regulation of electrolytes.
4. Dehydration, over hydration and water intoxication.
5. Fluid volume deficit (FVD).

Short Answers

1. How is water distributed in the body?
2. What is over hydration and water intoxication?
3. Define dehydration.
4. Explain ORT/ORS.
5. What is the daily requirement of water?
6. What is electrolyte imbalance?
7. What are normal ranges of plasma electrolyte?

CHAPTER 8

Balanced Diet

CHAPTER OUTLINE

- ❖ Balanced Diet
  - Definition, Principles, Steps
  - Food Guides—Basic Four Food Groups
  - RDA—Definition, Limitations, Uses
  - Food Exchange System
  - Calculation of Nutritive Value of Foods
  - Dietary Fiber
- ❖ Nutrition Across Life Cycle
  - Meal Planning/Menu Planning—Definition, Principles, Steps
  - Infant and Young Child Feeding (IYCF) Guidelines—Breastfeeding, Infant Foods
- Diet Plan for Different Age Groups—Children, Adolescents and Elderly
- Diet in Pregnancy—Nutritional Requirements and Balanced Diet Plan
- Anemia in Pregnancy—Diagnosis, Diet for Anemic Pregnant Women, Iron and Folic Acid Supplementation and Counseling
- Nutrition in Lactation—Nutritional Requirements, Diet for Lactating Mothers, Complementary Feeding/Weaning

TERMINOLOGY

- **Balanced diet:** A diet consisting of adequate amounts of all the necessary nutrients recommended for healthy growth and for efficient daily activities and functions. A balanced diet contains the proper quantities and proportions of the needed nutrients to maintain good health.
- **Recommended dietary allowances** (RDAs) are the levels of intake of essential nutrients that, on the basis of scientific knowledge, are judged by the Food and Nutrition Board to be adequate to meet the known nutrient needs of practically all healthy persons.
- **EAR** (Estimated Average Requirement): The intake that meets the estimated nutrient need of 50% of the individuals in that group.
- **RDA** (Recommended Dietary Allowance): The intake that meets the nutrient need of almost all (97 to 98%) individuals in that group.
- **AI** (Adequate Intake): Observed or experimentally derived intake by a defined population or subgroup that, in the judgment of the DRI Committee, appears to sustain a defined nutritional state, such as normal circulating nutrient values, growth, or other functional indicators of health.
- **UL:** The highest level of daily nutrient intake that is likely to pose no risk of adverse health effects to almost all individuals in the general population. As intake increases above the UL, the risk of adverse effects increases.
- **Optimum nutrition:** Optimum nutrition is also known as adequate nutrition or good nutrition.
- **Good nutrition:** Good nutrition thus provides all essential nutrients in correct balance which are further utilized to promote the highest level of physical and mental health. Such a state of nutrition can be attained through balanced diets.
- **Balanced diet:** Balanced diet can be defined as one which contains different types of foods (from all food group) in such quantities and proportions that needs for all the nutrients are adequately met and a small extra allowance is made as a margin of safety.
- **Digestion:** Mechanical and chemical process in which food is broken down in the gastrointestinal (GI) tract, releasing nutrients in forms the body can use.
- **Absorption:** Process in which released nutrients are taken into the cells lining the GI tract.
- **Metabolism:** The sum of the body processes involved in converting food necessary for energy, tissue building, and metabolic controls.

INTRODUCTION

There is not one single food or type of food that provides all the nutrients that the human body needs to function efficiently. A balanced diet will depend on the types of food eaten over a period of time and the nutritional needs of the particular individual. The wider the variety of foods eaten, the more nutrients will be provided by them. It is now known that some health problems are caused by dietary intake, such as too much fat causing heart disease and too much salt contributing to strokes. Balanced diet is one that contains different types of foods, such as cereals, pulses and vegetables in such quantities and proportions so that the need for calories, proteins, minerals, vitamins and other nutrients is adequately met and a small provision is made for extra nutrients to withstand short duration of leanness. A balanced diet should provide around 60—70% of total calories from carbohydrate, 10–12% from protein and 20–25% from fat.

DEFINITION

Balanced diet is a diet consisting of adequate amounts of all the necessary nutrients recommended for healthy growth and for efficient daily activities and functions. A balanced diet contains the proper quantities and proportions of the needed nutrients to maintain good health.

MEANING OF BALANCED DIET

- Healthy eating increases energy, improves the way the body functions, strengthens the immune system and prevents weight gain.
- Eating a balanced diet is key in maintaining good health and keeping your body in optimum condition. A balanced diet does not cut out food groups; it consists of a wide variety of foods to support your body and keep you energized, motivated and healthy.
- A balanced diet is a diet that contains differing kinds of foods in certain quantities and proportions so that the requirement for calories, proteins, minerals, vitamins and alternative nutrients is adequate.
- Opting for a balanced, adequate and varied diet is an important step towards a happy and healthy lifestyle.
- Vitamins and minerals in the diet are vital to boost immunity and healthy development.
- A healthy diet can protect the human body against certain types of diseases, in particular noncommunicable diseases, such as obesity, diabetes, cardiovascular diseases, some types of cancer and skeletal conditions.
- Healthy diets can also contribute to an adequate body weight.
- Healthy eating is a good opportunity to enrich life by experimenting with different foods from different cultures, origins and with different ways to prepare food.
- The benefits of eating a wide variety of foods are also emotional, as variety and color are important ingredients of a balance diet.

Figure 8.1 is depicted the balanced diet.

ELEMENTS OF BALANCED DIET (FIG. 8.2)

The food pyramid divides the foods we eat into the categories of grains, vegetables, fruits, milk, meat and beans, oils and discretionary calories.

Grain

- Grains, including wheat, rice and oats, can be either whole grains, which contain the entire grain kernel, or refined grains, in which the bran and germ have been removed.
- Refined grains lack the rich fiber, iron and vitamin content of whole grain.
- The USDA recommends making whole grains at least half of your daily grain intake.
- Recommended daily amounts vary depending on age, sex and level of physical activity; recommended servings range from three daily for toddlers to eight servings daily for young men.

Vegetables

- Vegetables are a crucial component of a well-balanced diet. The USDA divides vegetables into the categories

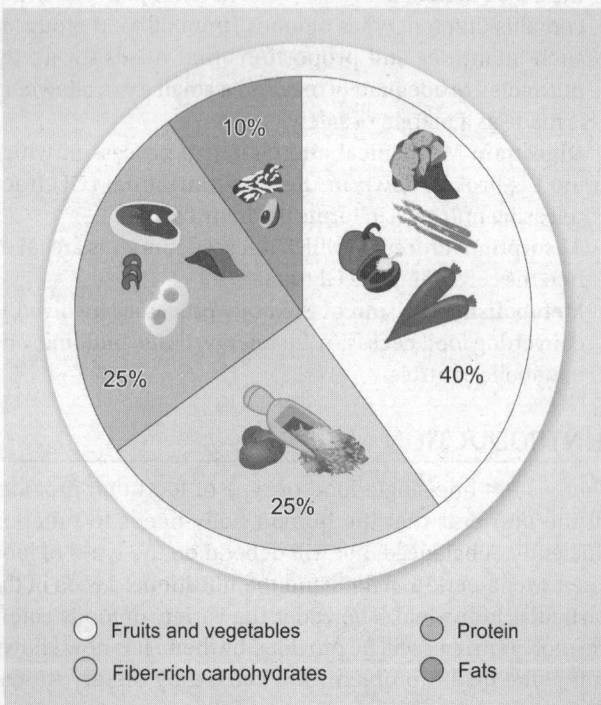

Fig. 8.1: Balanced diet.

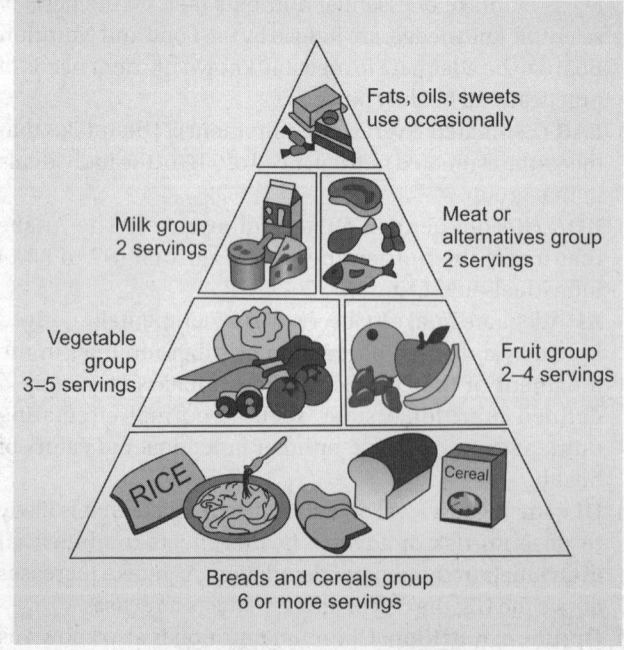

Fig. 8.2: Elements of balanced diet.

of dark-green vegetables, orange vegetables, starchy vegetables, other vegetables and dry beans and peas.
- Incorporating more fruits and vegetables into your diet may reduce the risk of some chronic diseases.
- Vegetables are a rich source of many important nutrients, including potassium, dietary fiber, folate and vitamins A, E and C.
- Vegetables are low in calories and can help in weight management. Young women should strive to eat at least 2½ cups of vegetables daily, and women 51 or older should aim for 2 cups.
- Men should eat 3 cups and then aim for 2½ cups once they turn 51. Over the course of a week, people should eat vegetables from all categories.

Fruits

- Fruits are cholesterol-free and low in fat, sodium and calories. Such as, vegetables, fruits are important sources of a number of key nutrients, including potassium, dietary fiber, vitamin C and folate.
- Fruit juice is a good way of incorporating fruit into the diet, but it lacks the dietary fiber found in whole fruit.
- Fruits that is particularly rich in potassium, which can help control blood pressure, include bananas, prunes, cantaloupe and honeydew.
- Young men and women should eat at least 2 cups of fruit daily. When women turn 31, this can be cut back to 1½ cups daily.

Table 8.1 is depicted the basic four food groups.

Milk, Yogurt and Cheese

- As with all the food groups, daily dairy needs vary by age. Dairy products provide calcium, vitamin D and potassium.

Table 8.1: Basic four food groups.

Food groups	Main nutrient
1. Cereal millets and pulses: Rice, wheat, ragi, bajra, maize, rice flakes Pulses and legumes: Bengal gram, black gram, green, red gram, rajmah	Energy, protein, invisible fats, vitamin B1, B2, folic acid, iron, fiber energy, proteins, invisible fats, vitamin B1, B2, folic acid, calcium, iron fiber
2. Milk and animal products: Milk, curd, skimmed milk, cheese, chicken, liver, fish, egg, meat	Protein, fat, vitamin B2, calcium
3. Fruits and vegetables: Mango, guava, tomato, papaya, orange, etc. Green leafy vegetables: Amaranth, spinach, coriander leaves, fenugreek leaves, drumstick leaves Other vegetables: Carrot, brinjal, beans, onions, etc.	Carotenoids, vitamin C, vitamin B2, iron, folic acid, fiber Carotenoids, vitamin B2, folic acid, fiber Carotenoids, folic acid, calcium
4. Oils, fats and nuts	

- Calcium is important in building and maintaining bone mass, and consuming dairy products is important to help prevent osteoporosis later in life.
- For men, women and children age 9 and up, recommended daily dairy intake is 3 cups. Children younger than 9 should consume 2 cups.

Meat and Beans

- Nutrients found in meat, poultry, fish, dry beans and peas, eggs, nuts and seeds include protein, B vitamins, vitamin E, iron, zinc and magnesium.
- Fatty meats and eggs should be eaten in limited amounts, as they can raise cholesterol levels. This recommendation is echoed by the American Heart Association's guidelines for a heart-healthy diet.
- Fish, nuts and seeds are good sources of monounsaturated and polyunsaturated fatty acids.
- The USDA recommends six-and-a-half daily servings from this group for young men and five-and-a-half daily servings for young women.
- After age 31, women should consume five servings, and men should eat six. Men 51 and older should cut back even further to five-and-a-half servings daily.

Oils

- The USDA recommends getting most of your dietary fat from fish, nuts and vegetable oils.
- Most oils have high levels of monounsaturated or polyunsaturated fats and low levels of saturated fat.
- Oils from plant sources, such as vegetable and nut oils, are cholesterol-free.
- Daily intake recommendations range from 3 teaspoon for toddlers to 7 teaspoon for young men.

Discretionary Calories

- In the USDA pyramid plan, discretionary calories are allotted based on your food choices.
- These discretionary calories can be used to eat more foods from any food group than the food guide recommends, eat higher-calorie forms of foods, add fats or sweeteners to foods or consume items, such as, candy, soda, wine and beer.
- For a physically active young man, discretionary calories should make 410 to 510 calories of a 2,600 to 3,000-calorie diet.

RDA—DEFINITION, LIMITATIONS, USES

The Recommended Dietary Allowance (RDA) is the average amount of a nutrient a healthy person should get each day. RDAs vary by age, gender, and whether a woman is pregnant or breastfeeding. The RDA is the value to be used in guiding individuals to achieve adequate nutrient intake. RDAs are given separately for specified life stage groups and by gender if applicable; they are intended to apply to healthy individuals. Due to the large variation in intakes, the RDAs are seldom appropriate for planning diets for or assessing the nutrient intakes of free-living groups.

Definition
Recommended dietary allowances RDA is defined as the nutrients present in the diet which satisfy the daily requirement of nearly all individuals in a population.

Factors that Affects RDA
RDA of an individual depends on many factors, such as:
- Age
- Sex
- **Physical work:**
  - Sedentary
  - Moderate
  - Hard (Heavy)
- **Physiological stress:**
  - Pregnancy
  - Lactation

This implies addition of safety factor amount to the estimated requirement to cover
- Variation among individuals
- Losses during cooking
- Lack of precision in estimated requirement

Recommended dietary allowances = Requirements + Safety factor

Figure 8.3 is depicted the recommended dietary allowances (RDA).

Uses
- Recommended dietary allowances are on nutrition facts labels on all of the foods you eat. Food manufacturers are required to list the percent daily value of RDAs for certain nutrients, including vitamin A, vitamin C, calcium and iron.
- Some manufacturers may list other nutrients if they desire and enrich their products to boost nutritional value.
- Additionally, schools, prisons, hospitals and other institutions use recommended dietary allowances to create nutritious recipes and healthful meals.

Other Guidelines
- The recommended dietary allowances are a part of the dietary reference intakes, or DRIs. These guidelines include recommended intake for macronutrients, adequate intakes, tolerable upper intake levels and recommended dietary allowances.
- Adequate intakes, called AI for short, are recommended intake levels for certain food components and nutrients that do not have a recommended dietary allowance.
- For example, fiber has an adequate intake of 14 g per 1,000 calories, according to the Dietary Guidelines for Americans 2010.
- This is an adequate amount of fiber you need to consume to support normal digestion. Adequate intakes are listed when recommended dietary allowances cannot be established.

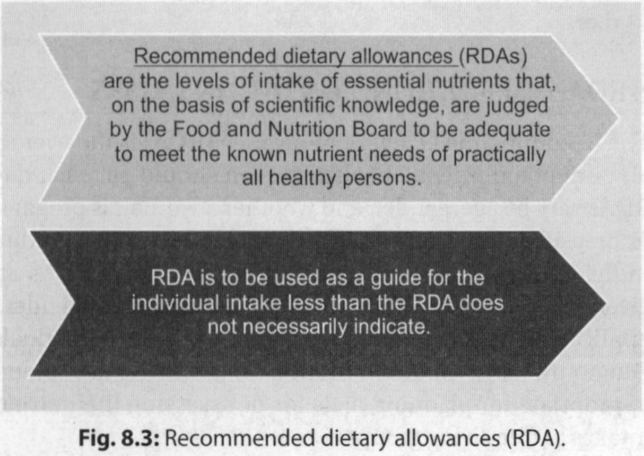

COMPONENTS OF HEALTHY BALANCED DIET (FIG. 8.4)

Dairy
- This includes cheese, milk and yogurt. Dairy foods are usually high in saturated fat so to reduce fat and calories it is best to choose low fat or fat free varieties.
- Dairy is essential in the diet to provide calcium for strong bones as well as protein and vitamin D.
- For those who do not consume dairy products it is essential to use a replacement, such as soy or nut based milks or supplement calcium in the diet.

Protein
- This is the main protein containing food group and includes lean meat and poultry with visible fat and skin removed, as well as fish, beans, lentils, peas, nuts and seeds, eggs and soy proteins, such as tofu and tempeh.
- Meat and poultry are high in iron, whilst legumes are a rich source of fiber and eggs provide a multitude of vitamins and minerals.
- Fish should be included regularly, particularly oily fish high in omega three fatty acids such as salmon and sardines.
- Cooking methods should be low fat such as grilling, poaching, dry frying or steaming to minimize extra fat added during the cooking process.
- It is also important to avoid processed meats, such as sausages and sandwich meats where possible as these are high in fat and sodium

Fruit
- Fruit is virtually fat free, low in calories, high in fiber and very nutritious. Aim to include a variety of fruits to get a wide range of vitamins and minerals.

Recommended dietary allowances (RDAs) are the levels of intake of essential nutrients that, on the basis of scientific knowledge, are judged by the Food and Nutrition Board to be adequate to meet the known nutrient needs of practically all healthy persons.

RDA is to be used as a guide for the individual intake less than the RDA does not necessarily indicate.

Fig. 8.3: Recommended dietary allowances (RDA).

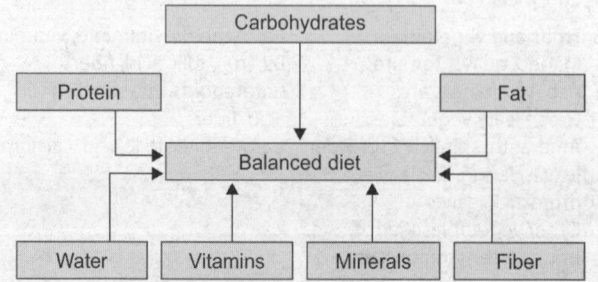

Fig. 8.4: Components of balanced diet.

- This could also include dried fruits 100% and fruit juices, however, it is important to choose unsweetened varieties.
- Both dried fruit and juices are concentrated sources of calories, so make sure portion sizes are controlled.

Vegetables

- These generally contain the least calories and the most vitamins and minerals, hence they are an excellent option for filling up on. Make sure to include a wide variety in your meals as different vegetables are rich in different vitamins.
- Try to use low fat cooking methods such as steaming or grilling. About 100% vegetables juices can also be included, and are a great way to get a few serves of vegetables into your diet.
- If you struggle to include enough vegetables in your day to day meals, try adding grated of finely chopped vegetables to mixed dishes, such as pasta sauces, burger mince or lasagnes, chances are you would not even notice the difference.

Grains

- This group is the major carbohydrate source in a balanced diet and includes bread, cereals, pasta and rice. Try to choose whole-grain varieties as these are higher in fiber and contain more B vitamins than white versions.
- Enriched cereals and breads, for example with iron, calcium or omega 3 can also be a good way to add some extra nutrition to your diet.
- Avoid sugary or toasted breakfast cereals and sweetened breads made with refined flour as these contain little fiber and are higher in calories and fat.

Fats and Oils

- Whilst some fat is necessary in our diets for the body to function correctly, it is important that these are the right types of fats.
- Saturated and trans fats should be minimized as these are unhealthy for the heart.
- These should be replaces with vegetable fats, such as canola, olive, or sunflower oil or spreads.
- All fats do contain a high amount of calories however, so it is important to keep added fats to a minimum in order to maintain a healthy body weight.
- Opt for light or low-fat salad dressings and mayonnaise, and use vegetable oils for cooking and baking. Other good sources of unsaturated fats include nuts, avocado and fish.

Treats and 'Sometimes' Foods

- Foods that do not fit into the above groups are generally considered to provide no or little nutritional benefit and are therefore not required in a balanced diet.
- Foods, such as candy, chocolate, cakes, chips, and other 'junk' foods should be avoided. If you do indulge in a treat, try to choose one that is less than 145 calories.

Figure 8.5 is depicted the balanced diet according to the age group.

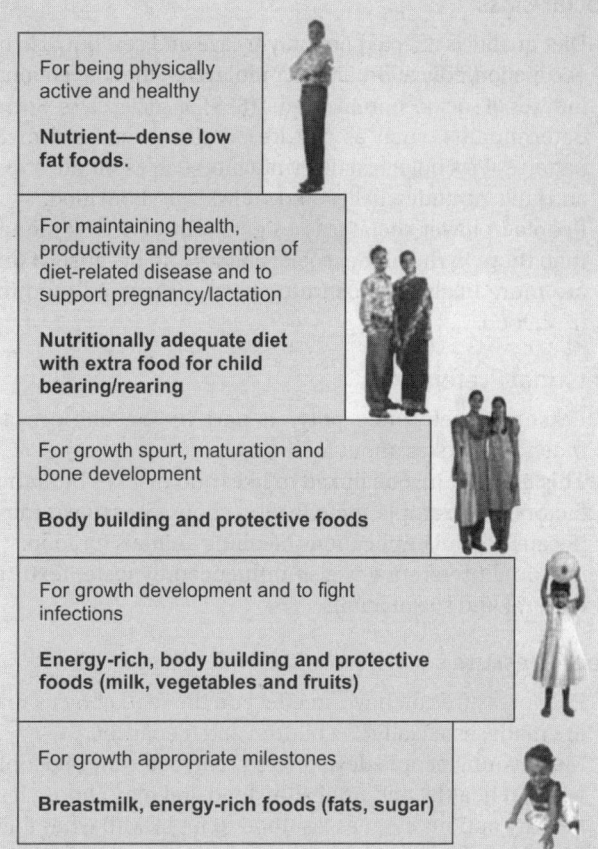

Fig. 8.5: Balanced diet according to the age group.

FACTORS INFLUENCING BALANCED DIET

Dietary needs will vary for each individual. As you have seen from the information above, dietary needs will differ according to age, but other factors will come into play. Such factors include:
- The level of exercise taken
- The type of job a person does
- Religious or cultural decisions
- Likes and dislikes
- A person's health
- Availability of food

Religion/Culture

- Religion and culture will play a large part in the food that people eat. Various foods are forbidden in certain religions. In general, Jews and Muslims do not eat pork, Hindus do not eat beef and Buddhists are vegetarian.
- Asian groups, particularly teenage girls, may be deficient in vitamin D, which is known as the sunshine vitamin. Because their religion requires them to cover most of their body, they do not get the opportunity to expose their skin to the sunlight.
- This can result in conditions known as rickets and osteomalacia. The most common sign of this is bowed legs.
- They should ensure that they eat a diet that is high in vitamin D. They may also be more at risk of becoming anemic as a traditional Asian diet may not provide enough iron.

Social Class

- Diet quality is affected not only by age and sex, but also by occupation, education, and income levels—the conventional indexes of socioeconomic status (SES) or social class. Social determinants, such as culture, family, peers and meal patterns. Psychological determinants such as mood, stress and guilt. Attitudes, beliefs and knowledge about food.
- People in lower social classes generally earn less money than those in the higher social classes and because of this are more likely to substitute cheap, processed food for fresh food.

Personal Preference

- Personal preference plays a part in the choices an individual makes about food.
- This may not just be linked to likes and dislikes but other factors, for example, people who choose not to eat meat because of the implications of killing animals for food.
- Personal preference is also influenced by taste, texture, cultural and social habits.

Peer Pressure

- Peer pressure can have an effect on the food choices that are made, especially by children and teenagers.
- Many young people develop a stereotyped view of people who eat healthy and unhealthy food and may choose less healthy options such as fast food to fit in with what their friends eat because they do not want to seem different.

The Media

- Information publicized in the media can be another factor that influences food choice.
- Food scares can often be caused by reporting of facts in the press and in news bulletins. Two examples of this were the egg scare in 1988 and 'mad cow disease' in 1995.
- In 1988, a junior health minister, Edwina Curry, said that the majority of eggs in the UK were contaminated with Salmonella. This had a huge impact on the sale of eggs—400 million eggs and 4 million chickens were destroyed.
- In 1996, beef exports to Europe were banned when a link between eating beef and a brain disease, Creutzfeld Jacob Disease, was established. Again, this had a huge impact on beef sales and consumption of beef, and beef was banned from school menus.

Position in Family

- There is little evidence available to suggest that there is a difference in food choice depending on the position you hold in the family, but it is known that mothers will often give more protein or fruit and vegetables or larger quantities to their husband/partner or children.
- They will then fill up on lower quality food and their nutritional status may suffer as a result.
- Choice may also be related to who in the family does the shopping and cooking. If you do most of the family shopping and do not like a particular food, even if others in the family do like it you are less likely to buy it.

Geographic Location

- Where you live will have an effect on the diet you have. Although there is enough food in the world, it is not evenly distributed.
- More wealthy countries can afford to buy food and so have a greater variety than countries that are poor.
- Food that is grown in poor soil will contain fewer minerals and so the quality of the diet will be poorer.

Availability of Food

- Many developing countries suffer from poor soil conditions, flooding and drought, which result in repeated years of lost harvests.
- People have access to restricted diets that are high in carbohydrates and not so rich in protein and fats. This can lead to under nutrition.
- In developed countries, people have access to a good variety of food.
- Much of it is home grown and the increase in air travel means that most foods are available all year round. As a result, the population of developed countries is more likely to suffer from over nutrition.
- Other factors influenced by geographical location will be where people live and how easily they can get food.
- Greater variety is available in large supermarkets generally situated on the outskirts of large towns.
- Small corner shops in rural areas tend to have less variety and less fresh fruit and vegetables.

Financial Resources

- The ability to afford food is linked to social class (see above). People who are in the higher social classes have more money to spend on food and tend to buy better quality food and eat out more.
- People who have low incomes are more likely to buy food that is high in salt, fat and sugar and provide concentrated sources of energy.

■ IMPORTANCE OF BALANCED DIET

A balanced diet is important to maintain health and a sensible body weight. No single food will provide all the essential nutrients that the body needs to be healthy and function efficiently. A balanced diet should contain protein, fats, carbohydrates and fiber in the form of fresh vegetables and fresh fruit, all in the right amounts, providing you with a good supply of essential amino acids, essential fatty acids, vitamins, minerals, and of course fresh drinking water. In addition, the nutritional value of a person's diet depends on the overall mixture, or balance, of food that is eaten over a period of time, as well as on the needs of the individual. A diet that includes a variety of different foods is most likely to provide all the essential nutrients.

Health Benefits of Balanced Diet

- Healthy eating increases energy, improves the way your body functions, strengthens your immune system and prevents weight gain. The other major benefits are:

- **Meets your nutritional need:** A varied, balanced diet provides the nutrients you need to avoid nutritional deficiencies.
- **Prevent and treat certain diseases:** Healthful eating can prevent the risk of developing certain diseases such as diabetes, cancer and heart disease. It is also helpful in treating diabetes and high blood pressure.
- Following a special diet can reduce symptoms, and may help you better manage an illness or condition.
- **Feel energetic and manage your weight:** A healthy diet will assist you to feel higher, provide you with more energy, and help you fight stress.
- Food is the mainstay of many social and cultural events. Apart from nutrition properties, it helps facilitate connections between individuals.

Figure 8.6 is depicted the benefits of balanced diet.

General Guidelines for Healthy Eating

- The most important rule of healthy eating is not skipping any meal. Skipping meals lowers your metabolic rate. Normal eating includes 3 major meals and 2 snacks between meals. Also, never skip breakfast. It is the foremost vital meal of the day.
- Learn simple ways to prepare food. Healthy eating does not have to mean complicated eating. Keep meal preparation easy, eat more raw foods such as salads, fruits and vegetable juices, and focus on the pleasure of eating healthy food rather than the calories.
- It is important to stop when you feel full. This will help you maintain your weight to an extent. This also will help you remain alert and feeling your best.
- Drink lots of water. Keep a bottle of water near you while working, watching TV, etc.
- Variety of foods should be used in the menu. No single food has all the nutrients.
- To improve the cereal and pulse protein quality, a minimum ratio of cereal protein to pulse protein should be 4:1. In terms of the grains, it will be eight parts of cereals and one part of pulses.
- Eat five portions of fruit and vegetables every day.
- Keep a supply of healthy snacks to hand. This will stop you from eating an unhealthy snack when hungry.
- Remove all visible fat from food before you cook it—take the skin off chicken and trim the white fat off any meat.
- Limit stimulants, such as caffeine, alcohol and refined sugar.
- Limit the number of times you eat out to once a week. Take your own packed lunch to work.
- Only eat things you like the taste of—find what works for you and do not force yourself to eat things just because they are good for you.

CALCULATION OF BALANCED DIET

Steps in planning balanced diet:
1. **Identify the individual and his/her specific characteristics:**
   - Age
   - Sex
   - Activity level (for adults)
   - Income, socioeconomic status
   - Religion
   - Region where residing

   The above-mentioned information will help decide the kind of diet to be planned. The background of income, socioeconomic status, religion and region will decide the kind of foods to be included in the plan. The age and sex play very important role in deciding the number of calories and proteins to be given.

   Figure 8.7 is depicted the balanced diet calculator.

   The diet must suit the pocket of the person.

   Religion is a sensitive issue and should not be ignored while planning diet. Different regions of the country have different staple foods which the planner must be aware of, keeping in mind not to include foods that are not available in local markets.

2. **Consult the recommended dietary intake (RDI) for energy and protein:** Generally, if the diet contains required amount of energy and protein as per the RDIs, it provides sufficient amounts of other nutrients as well. Careful selection of foods with inclusion of rich sources of vitamins and minerals will help meet the needs.

3. **Decide the total amounts of specific food groups:** The selection of specific foods will depend on the income, personal preferences. The foods should be selected from each food group as mentioned earlier. The amount and selection of foods should be done carefully so as to meet the requirement of energy and protein.

4. **Decide on number of meals to be consumed:** Meal frequency is influenced by various factors, such as income, occupation, school timings and convenience. People of more affluent society have more meals. The number of

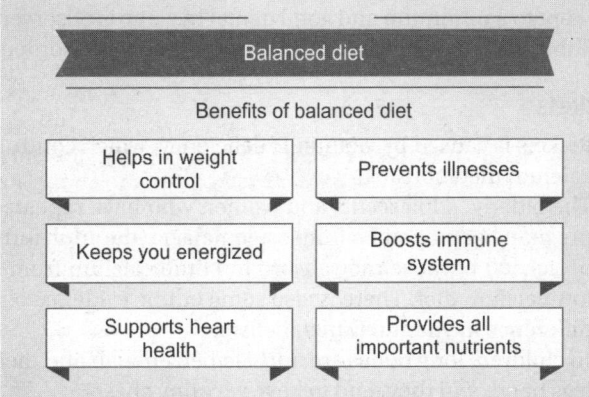

Fig. 8.6: Benefits of balanced diet.

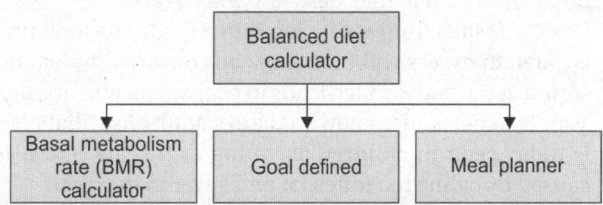

Fig. 8.7: Balanced diet calculator.

meals consumed may be a three meal, a four meal, a five meal or a seven to eight meal pattern. Traditionally most regions in India, follow three to five meal pattern which include three major meals (breakfast, lunch and dinner) and two small meals (mid-morning and late afternoon). The frequency of meals may vary according to the age.

5. **Distribute total amounts decided between meals:** The total amounts of foods from each food group should be distributed over the day's meal.
6. **Decide the items and their amounts within each group for each meal:** In other words, plan the menu. The dishes to be included from each food group must be decided. This means selecting specific foods for a particular dish or a meal.
7. **Check day's diet for inclusion of each food group and the amounts decided:** In step, 6 the menu was planned. In this step, we must check whether all the food items decided in step 3 are included or not.

EFFECTS OF UNBALANCED DIETS

Diets based either on a small amount of fat, either on a small amount of carbohydrates, either on clear vegetable soup or on the consumption of fruit juices days and weeks in a row, are unbalanced and have unwanted effects on health status. Where there are no medical conditions that require special diets without fats or with a small amount of carbohydrates, things can seriously degenerate. Even short periods of unbalanced eating can have negative consequences in the long run.

Malnutrition

- A balanced diet is based on the consumption of appropriate amounts of nutrients and energy.
- Malnutrition can result from people eating too much or too little of some nutrients over a period of time.
- Insufficient intake can result in under nutrition or starvation and excessive intake can result in over nutrition and obesity.

Over Nutrition

- There are some conditions that are related to eating too much of a certain nutrient. Coronary heart disease occurs as a result of eating too many foods such as animal proteins that are high in saturated fats.
- Fatty deposits build up in the coronary arteries in the heart and this can lead to the formation of a clot that will stop the supply of blood to part of the heart muscle which then dies. This is known as a heart attack.
- Symptoms of a heart attack can include shortness of breath and pain in the chest, jaw and left arm.
- Obesity results from eating too much food. Any food that is eaten in excess will ultimately be converted to fat and stored in the body, which leads to overweight and obesity.
- Type 2 diabetes, also known as late or adult onset diabetes, is today seen in children as young as 9 years old. It is caused by eating too much fat and sugar in the diet.

> **Box 8.1:** Long-term effects of a balanced diet.
>
> ❖ **Raised immunity:** The body's immune system helps to protect against diseases. Fresh fruit and vegetables will contain vitamins A and E and foods, such as garlic and honey can help to maintain a healthy immune system. Foods high in zinc and omega-3 fatty acids also boost the immune system.
> ❖ **Energy levels:** People who are over weight often lack in energy, completing exercise can be a struggle as large amounts of energy are used. Although we need to eat carbohydrates to give us energy, it is important to have a balance and choose to eat carbohydrates that realize energy slowly. Eating healthy will boost energy levels.

- The pancreas is either unable to produce enough insulin to allow the cells to absorb glucose from the blood or the body becomes resistant to the insulin that is produced. Symptoms of Type 2 diabetes include thirst, excessive urination and extreme tiredness.

Box 8.1 is depicted the long-term effects of a balanced diet.

Under Nutrition

- Under nutrition can result from a general lack of nutrients, particularly protein and energy, or from a lack of a particular nutrient.
- Two conditions that are seen in underdeveloped countries and that particularly affect children are kwashiorkor and marasmus.

SPECIFIC NUTRITIONAL DEFICIENCIES

Anemia: Anemia is caused by iron deficiency. Iron is used for making red blood cells and in the body's use of oxygen. Symptoms include:
- Fatigue/lack of energy
- Weakness
- Brittle fingernails
- Tooth decay

Tooth decay or dental caries cannot be strictly be described as under nutrition, as it is caused by an excess of sugar in the diet. Sticky deposits called plaque are deposited on the teeth. Plaque is acid and over time it will dissolve the enamel on teeth, causing cavities. If they remain untreated, they can kill the tooth's nerve and blood supply and eventually the whole tooth will die. It is important that sugary foods and drinks are kept to a minimum and good dental hygiene is observed.

Table 8.2 is depicted the nutritional deficiencies disorders.

Rickets

- Rickets is caused by vitamin D deficiency, which controls calcium metabolism.
- The elderly, adolescents and women who have repeated pregnancies may suffer from osteomalacia (the adult form of rickets) because they absorb too little calcium from a low calcium diet. There is also some ethnic evidence of a difference in vitamin D metabolism.
- In children, long bones are not calcified enough and their legs bend, and they tend to have very tiny chests.

Table 8.2: Nutritional deficiencies disorders.

Vitamins	Deficiency disease	Symptoms
Vitamin A	Loss of vision	Poor vision, loss of vision in darkness
Vitamin B1	Beriberi	Weak muscles and very little energy to work
Vitamin C	Scurvy	Bleeding gums
Vitamin D	Rickets	Bones are bent
Calcium	Weak bone and tooth decay	Weak bone and tooth decay
Iodine	Goiter	Gland in neck
Iron	Anemia	Weakness

- The four main plates of the skull are not ossified—this is known as the hot-cross bun sign in newborn babies.

Night Blindness

- Night blindness is caused by a lack of vitamin A. It is also known as xerophthalmia or dry eye.
- In its early stages, it can be cured by providing sufferers with vitamin A supplements such as palm oil or other foods high in vitamin A. However, in its later stages it is incurable and leads to complete blindness and in some cases death.

Beriberi: Beriberi is vitamin B1 or thiamin deficiency—this vitamin is needed to metabolize carbohydrates.

Scurvy

- Scurvy is known as vitamin C deficiency and only occurs when fresh food, especially citrus fruits, is not available.
- Symptoms include swelling of gums and teeth falling out, bleeding and slow wound healing.

CONDITIONS WITH SPECIFIC DIETARY REQUIREMENT

Coronary Heart Disease

People who suffer from coronary heart disease should modify their diet in order to prevent further damage to the heart. Sufferers should be advised to make the following changes to their diet:

- Eat at least five portions of fruit and vegetables a day.
- Reduce the total amount of fat in the diet and substitute saturated fats for poly- and mono-unsaturated fats such as vegetable and olive oils.
- Eat oily fish such as mackerel, sardines, herring, tuna, and salmon two to three times a week.
- Introduce nuts and seeds into the diet.
- Maintain a healthy weight.
- Reduce the amount of salt in the diet to a maximum of 6 grams per day.
- Drink alcohol in moderation—1–2 units per day.
- Take exercise—a minimum of 30 minutes three times a week.

Obesity: The best way to combat obesity is to maintain a diet low in fat and sugar and high in complex carbohydrates and fruit and vegetables. Regular exercise will also help to burn up any excess energy intake.

Type 2 diabetes:
1. People who suffer from Type 2 diabetes can do a lot to help the levels of blood glucose by maintaining a diet low in fat and sugar.
2. Complex carbohydrates should form a part of the diet, as low carbohydrate diets can be high in fat. There is a relatively high incidence of coronary heart disease in diabetics sufferers in the UK.

Lactose Intolerance

- Lactose intolerance is an inability to digest lactose, the sugar found in milk and milk products.
- It is particularly common in people of African and Asian origin and can lead to digestive disturbance such as cramps, diarrhea and wind.
- Milk should be avoided in the diet, but often sufferers can tolerate yoghurt and cheese because the lactose is converted to lactic acid during manufacture.

Food Allergies

- Allergic reactions to food vary in intensity, and similar symptoms and illnesses can be triggered by different allergens as well as the same allergens causing very different reactions in different people.
- Symptoms can include eczema, asthma, urticaria (hives) and other health problems.
- Anaphylaxis is an extreme reaction which must be treated by adrenaline injections.
- Failure to treat this promptly can result in death. Avoidance of food that causes allergies is the only way to prevent the onset of symptoms.

Genetic Disorders

- Certain genetic disorders can cause problems that can be relieved by diet. Cystic fibrosis is a disorder that causes thick, sticky mucous to coat the pancreatic duct.
- Pancreatic enzymes needed to digest food cannot pass into the small intestine and sufferers are given these enzymes in powdered form sprinkled onto their food.
- Phenylketonuria is a rare inherited condition in which there is a buildup of phenylalanine in the body.
- Phenylalanine is an amino acid—a building block of protein. A low-protein diet is essential for sufferers and has to be supplemented with artificial protein that does not contain phenylalanine. If this diet is not followed, learning difficulties can result.

Religion/Culture

- The main dietary rules for some world religions. Some people choose not to eat meat and become vegetarian or vegan.
- Vegetarians do not usually eat meat, poultry, game or fish. However, most will eat eggs and dairy products.

- Vegetarians will be healthy as long as they eat a varied diet and combine plant proteins.
- Vegans eat no animal foods at all and have to be careful about the plant proteins they eat to ensure that they have a balanced diet.
- There is a possibility that they may suffer from vitamin B12 deficiency as this is mainly found in animal products, although yeast extract is a good source.

Fundamentals of Balanced Diet

See Table 8.3.

Table 8.3: Basic food groups.

Group	Examples and serving size	Daily servings
Grains	Breakfast cereals, rice, pasta, bread, and noodles **Emphasize whole grains:** • 1 slice of bread or small muffin • 1 cup of dry cereal • ½ cup cooked cereal, rice, pasta	6–8 ounce equivalents The lower number is the servings for a 2000 calorie diet, higher number for 2400 calorie diet
Vegetables	Tomatoes, potatoes, carrots, green peas, squash, broccoli, spinach, green beans, sweet potatoes 1 cup raw leafy vegetables = ½ cup	2.5–3.5 cups
Fruits	Apricots, bananas, dates, grapes, grapefruit, oranges, orange juice, mangoes, melons, peaches, pineapples, plums, berries	1.5–2 cups
Dairy	Milk, yogurt, and cheese The following count as 1 cup: • 1½ ounces of natural cheese • 2 ounces of processed cheese	3 cups
Meat, eggs, nuts, and beans	Meat, poultry, fish, eggs, dry beans, and nuts • 1 ounces of cooked lean meat, poultry, or fish • 1 egg • ½ oz of nuts or seeds • 1 tablespoon peanut butter • ¼ cup cooked dried beans or tofu	5.5–6.5 ounce equivalents
Oils	Soft margarine, low-fat mayonnaise, light salad dressing, vegetable oil (olive, canola, safflower, corn)	27–31 g
Discretionary calorie allowance	After selecting nutrient dense foods from the list above there is room for a few more calories. Fat and added sugar is always counted as discretionary calories	267–362 calories

Nurses' Health Promotion Role

- Nurses have the expertise and responsibility to ensure that patients and clients' nutritional needs are met. Providing nutrition screening and appropriate nutrition advice is essential to improve healthy eating and subsequent health outcomes. Non-communicable diseases are often associated with modifiable risk factors.
- Nurses can talk to patients at the bedside and explain the special meals they have at the hospital that aid recovery, as many patients will be on special diets during their stay.
- Registered dietitians and nurses can work together to advice people on healthy eating. All nurses play a vital role in the promotion of healthy eating.
- Primary care nurses, in particular practice and school nurses are well placed to promote healthy eating.

■ FOOD EXCHANGE SYSTEM

The word exchange refers to the food items on each list which may be substituted with any other food item on the same list. One exchange is approximately equal to another in carbohydrate, calories, protein and fat within each food list. In 1950, the US Food Exchange list was developed by the American Dietetic Association, the American Diabetes Association and the US Public Health Service to target meal planning problems. The aim of this concept was to provide people with diabetes with the tools to incorporate consistency in their meal planning and include a wider variety of foods.

Table 8.4 is depicted the food pyramid and exchange list.

Definition and Meaning

- The word exchange refers to the fact that each item on a particular list in the portion listed may be interchanged with any other food item on the same list.
- An exchange can be explained as a substitution, choice, or serving.
- Each list is a group of measured or weighed foods of approximately the same nutritional value. Within each food list, one exchange is approximately equal to another in calories, carbohydrate, protein, and fat.

Table 8.4: Food pyramid and exchange list.

	Compression	
	Serving size	
Type of food	Food exchange	Pyramid
Vegetables	1/2 cup–1 cup	1 cup–2 cups
Milk	1 cup	1 cup
Cheese	30 g	45 g
Meat	1 oz	2 to 3 oz
Fruits	1 piece, 1/2–1 cup	1 C or 1 medium sized–1/2 cup
Starches	30 g–1/2 cup	30 g–1/2 cup
Rice	1/2 cup	1/3 cup
Fats	1 tablespoon, 1–2 tablespoons	1 tablespoon, 1–2 tablespoon

- To use the exchange lists, an individual needs an individualized meal plan that outlines the number of exchanges from each list for each meal and for snacks.
- The American Diabetes Association recommends that because of the complexity of nutrition issues, a registered dietitian, knowledgeable and skilled in implementing nutrition therapy into diabetes management and education, be the team member developing and implementing meal plans.
- The meal plan is developed in cooperation with the person with diabetes and is based on an assessment of eating changes that would assist the individual in achieving his or her target metabolic goals and of changes the individual is willing and able to make.
- Because of the accuracy and convenience of the exchange system, the exchange lists are used for weight management as well for diabetes management.

Principles and Importance

- The food exchange system is based on principles of good nutrition that apply to everyone. The food exchange system is updated as necessary
- The word exchange refers to the fact that each item on a particular list in the portion listed may be interchanged with any other food item on the same list. An exchange can be explained as a substitution, choice, or serving.

1500 Calories	Starch	Meat	Vegetable	Fruit	Fat	Milk
Breakfast	2	2	–	1	1	1
Snack	1	–	1	–	–	–
Lunch	2	1	–	1	1	–
Snack	–	–	1	1	–	–
Dinner	3	2	1	–	1	1

- The food exchange system includes six groups of food, each group of foods are placed in a food exchange list. The food exchange lists are—fruits, vegetables, milk, starches, fats, meats and meat substitutes. The foods in each individual group have a similar amount of calories and nutrients, such as carbohydrates, fat and protein.
- Many foods are made up of more than one food category, so they will not fall nicely in just one of the exchange lists. These types of foods are known as "combination foods".
- The number of servings, or "exchanges", from a group that you can consume each day depends on how many calories you need. A dietitian can help you determine your nutrition needs, including total calories and proportion of carbohydrates, protein, fats that you should consume.

Advantages of the food exchange system are:
- It provides a system in which a wide selection of foods can be included, thereby offering variety and versatility.
- It provides a framework to foods with similar carbohydrate, protein, fat, and calorie contents.
- It emphasizes important management concepts, such as carbohydrate amounts, fat modification, calorie control, and awareness of high-sodium foods.
- By making food choices from each of the different food exchange lists, a variety of healthful food choices can be assured.
- It provides a system that allows individuals to be accountable for what they eat.
- It provides an understanding of the nutrient composition of the exchange lists.
- Nutrient values from food labels can be used and understood.
- The ability to customize your menu whenever you want is especially important because many dieters return to their earlier unhealthy eating habits when they become bored or frustrated with restrictive or confusing diets.
- Diabetics that use the food exchange system can easily follow a healthier diet that helps to control their blood sugar and improve their health.
- The food exchange system is an easy way to begin counting carbohydrates for diabetics to help them regulate their blood sugar level.
- Because of the accuracy and convenience of the food exchange system is helpful not only in diabetes, but also for regulating weight and maintaining a balanced diet. Many popular diets are based on the food exchange system.

Advantages and Disadvantages

- An advantage of the food exchange system is that it provides a system in which a wide selection of foods can be included, thereby offering variety and versatility to the person with diabetes.
- Other advantages of the lists are: (a) they provide a framework to group foods with similar carbohydrate, protein, fat, and calorie contents; (b) they emphasize important management concepts, such as carbohydrate amounts, fat modification, calorie control, and awareness of high-sodium foods; (c) by making food choices from each of the different lists a variety of healthful food choices can be assured; and (d) they provide a system that allows individuals to be accountable for what they eat.
- Furthermore, with an understanding of the **nutrient** composition of the exchange lists, nutrient values from food labels can be used and a wider variety of foods can be incorporated accurately into a meal plan.

Helpful Hints for Using the Exchange Lists

- Cereals, grains, pasta, breads, crackers, snacks, starchy vegetables, and cooked beans, peas, and lentils are on the starch list. In general, one starch exchange is ½ cup cereal, grain, or starchy vegetable; one ounce of a bread product, such as one slice of bread; one-third cup rice or pasta; or three-fourths to one ounce of most snack foods.
- Fresh, frozen, canned, and dried fruits and fruit juices are on the fruit list. In general, one fruit exchange is—one small to medium fresh fruit, one-half cup of canned or fresh fruit or fruit juice, or one-fourth cup of dried fruit.
- Different types of milk and milk products, such as yogurt, are on the milk list. One cup (eight fluid ounces) or two-thirds cup (six ounces) of fat-free or low-fat flavored yogurt

sweetened with a non-nutritive sweetener are examples of one exchange.
- Vegetables are included in the carbohydrate group and are important components of a healthful diet. However, since three servings of vegetables are the equivalent of one carbohydrate serving, one or two servings per meal need not be counted. This was done to encourage consumption of vegetables and to simplify meal planning.
- Meat and meat substitutes that contain both protein and fat are on the meat list. In general, one exchange is—one ounce meat, fish, poultry, or cheese; or one-half cup beans, peas, lentils.
- In general, one fat exchange is—one teaspoon of regular margarine, mayonnaise, or vegetable oil; one tablespoon of regular salad dressings or reduced-fat mayonnaise; or two tablespoons of reduced-fat salad dressings.
- A free food is any food or drink that contains less than 20 calories or less than five grams of carbohydrate per serving. Foods with approximately 20 calories should be limited to three servings per day and spread throughout the day.
- Some foods are in one list, but they may fit just as appropriately in another list. For example, foods in the starch, fruit, and milk lists of the carbohydrate group each contribute similar amounts of carbohydrates and calories and may be interchanged. If fruits or starches are regularly substituted for milk, calcium intake may be decreased. Conversely, regularly choosing milk instead of fruits or starches may result in inadequate fiber intake. Foods from the other carbohydrate list of the carbohydrate group, the combination foods list, and the fast foods list are also interchangeable with the starch, fruit, and milk lists. However, most of the dessert-type foods on the other carbohydrate list are higher in sugars and fat and need to be eaten within the context of a healthful meal plan.
- Beans, peas, and lentils are included in the starch list of the carbohydrate group. The serving size (usually one-half cup) is counted as one starch and one very lean meat for vegetarian meal planning. If individuals are not practicing vegetarians, or use these foods less frequently and often as side dishes rather than main dishes, the very lean meat exchange does not need to be counted—one-half cup is equivalent to one starch.
- Skim and reduced-fat milks are recommended for adults and children over two years of age, rather than whole milk.
- Meat choices from the very lean or lean meat lists are encouraged. However, it is not necessary to add or subtract fat exchanges when using meat lists that differ from those ordinarily consumed.
- Whenever possible, monounsaturated or polyunsaturated fats should be substituted for saturated fats.

The exchange lists are updated periodically and a database is kept of the **macronutrient** composition of each food, thus assuring the accuracy of the lists. For health professionals, the macronutrient and calorie values of the exchange lists provide a useful and efficient tool for evaluating food records and for assessing nutrition adequacy.

DIETARY FIBER

Fiber or roughage consists of cellulose and hemicellulose. This part of carbohydrates is not digested by digestive juice. They are left unchanged after digestion. Dietary fiber is defined as that portion of plant material ingested in the diet that is resistant to digestion by gastrointestinal secretions.
- It consists of hemicellulose, cellulose, lignins, oligosaccharides, pectins, gums and waxes.
- Some bacteria in the large intestine can degrade some components of fiber releasing products that can be absorbed into the body and used as energy source. Two categories of fiber are found in food.
- Crude fiber (CF) is defined as the residue remaining after the treatment with hot sulfuric acid, alkali and alcohol. The major component of crude fiber is a polysaccharide called cellulose.
- CF is a component of dietary fiber. Several other carbohydrate and related compounds called pectins; hemicellulose and lignins are the second category found in plant foods and are also resistant to digestion. These together with cellulose are collectively known as dietary fiber.

Figure 8.8 is depicted the differences between insoluble fiber and soluble fiber.

Mechanism of Fiber
- Fiber refers to certain types of carbohydrates that our body cannot digest.
- These carbohydrates pass through the intestinal tract intact and help to move waste out of the body.
- Diets that are low in fiber have been shown to cause problems, such as constipation and hemorrhoids and to increase the risk for certain types of cancers, such as colon cancer.

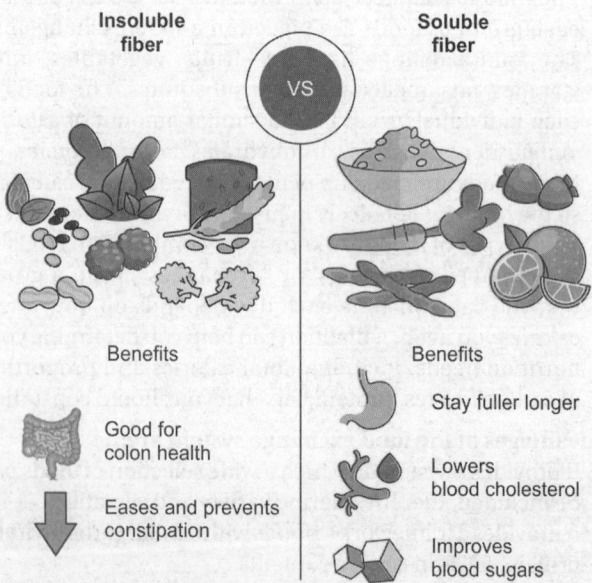

Fig. 8.8: Differences between insoluble fiber and soluble fiber.

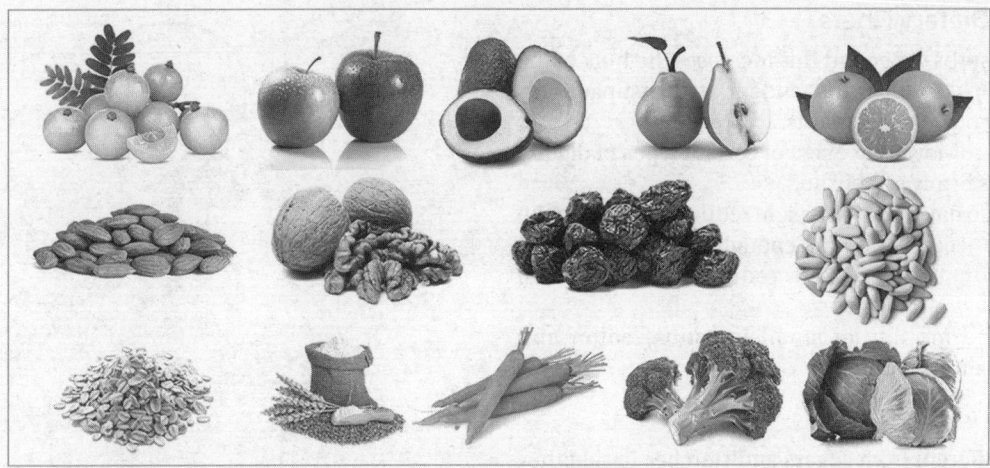

Fig. 8.9: Sources of dietary fiber.

- Diets high in fiber; however, have been shown to decrease risks for heart disease, obesity, and they help lower cholesterol.
- Foods high in fiber include fruits, vegetables, and whole grain products.

Figure 8.9 is depicted the sources of dietary fiber.

Role of Dietary Fibers

- Fibers are indigestible substance of plant foods, roughage not digested by human enzyme contribute bulk to the stool. Example of fibrous foods is whole cereals, fenugreek, cabbage and greens.
- Fiber part of the foods is cellulose hemicellulose and lignin. Dietary fibers, such as cellulose, hemicellulose, pectin, gum and mucilage are important carbohydrates for several reasons.
- Soluble dietary fibers, such as pectin, gum and mucilage pass undigested through the small intestine and are degraded into fatty acids and gases by the large intestine.
- The fatty acids produced in this way can either be used as a fuel for the large intestine or be absorbed into the bloodstream. Therefore, dietary fiber is essential for proper intestinal health.
- In general, the consumption of soluble and insoluble fiber makes the elimination of waste much easier. Since dietary fiber is both indigestible and an attractant of water, stools become large and soft.
- As a result, feces can be expelled with less pressure. However, not enough fiber consumption will change the constitution of the stool and increase the amount of force required during defecation.
- Excessive pressure during the elimination of waste can force places in the large intestine wall out from between bands of smooth muscle to produce small pouches called diverticula. Hemorrhoids may also result from unnecessary strain during defecation.

Table 8.5 is depicted the types of dietary fibers.

Table 8.5: Types of dietary fibers.

Dietary fiber			
Soluble fibers	Features	Sources	Health benefits
Pectin	It is been galacturonic acid, rhamnose, arabinose, the high content of galactose, intermediate laminate and on the primary wall	Whole grains, apple, legumes, cabbage, root vegetables	
Gum	Generally are composed monomers of hexose and pentose	Oatmeal, haricot beans, legumes	Reduce cholesterol glucose regulation
Mucilages	Componds which is synthesized in plants that it is contain of glycoprotein	Food additives	
Insoluble fibers			
Cellulose	It is the main component of cell walls which consisting of glucose Monomers	Whole grains, bran, peas, root vegetables, beans family of cruciferous, apple	
Hemi-celluloses	Primary and secondary the cell walls	Bran, whole grains Guava pomace	Water absorption Intestinal regulation
Lignin	It is been consist of aromatic alcohols and the components of other cell wall	Vegetables, flour	

Functions of Dietary Fibers

1. The fiber absorbs water and this increases the bulk of the stool and helps to reduce the tendency to constipation by encouraging bowel movements.
2. The cholesterol-lowering effect of certain types of dietary fiber appears firmly established.
3. Fiber may also have a role in weight reduction; people who eat well-balanced diets obtain enough roughage.
4. Prevents constipation and reduce the effects of carcinogens.
5. Increases the motility of small intestine, colon and decreases the transit time.

RDA of Dietary Fibers

- Fibers are different from sugars and starches in that they are not digested and absorbed in the small intestine and converted to glucose.
- Humans do not have the necessary enzymes to break down fibers into their constituent parts so that they can be absorbed into the body. Therefore, fibers pass from the small intestine into the large intestine relatively intact.
- There they can be fermented by the colonic microflora to gases such as hydrogen (H_2) and carbon dioxide (CO_2) and to short chain fatty acids.
- Although fibers are not converted to glucose as are sugars and starches, some of these short chain fatty acids are absorbed and can be used for energy in the body.
- Determining the amount of calories supplied by fiber is complex since it depends on such factors as the fermentability of the fiber, the individual's colonic microflora, how long fiber stays in the colon, etc.
- The IOM has set an Adequate Intake (AI) value for fiber of 14 g of fiber per 1,000 kcal.
- This AI is based on the totality of the evidence for fiber decreasing the risk of chronic disease and other health-related conditions, but the actual numbers for the AI were derived from the data supporting a decreased risk for the development of coronary heart disease (CHD).
- The major food sources of fiber are fruits, vegetables (particularly legumes), and grains. Milk does not contain fiber although certain milk-containing products may.

Adequate Fiber Intake (Fig. 8.10)

Food Intake
- Slows eating rate/reduces hunger
- Reduces food energy density (2 kcal/g vs 4 kcal/g refined carbohydrates)
- Increases food volume/bulk/viscosity

Stomach
- Delays emptying rate (w/bulking/viscosity)
- Increases satiety/satiation

Small Intestine
- Decreases postprandial absorption rate
- Increases release of satiety peptides

Pancreas
Lowers insulin response and β-cell activity

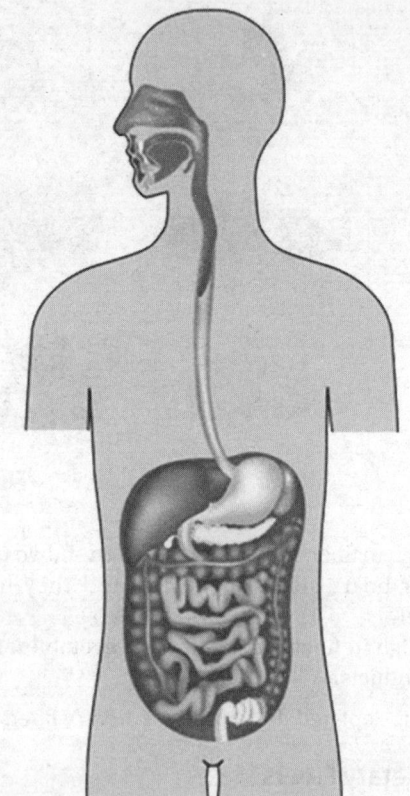

Fig. 8.10: Adequate fiber intake.

Colon
- Promotes colonic health (e.g., lower pH, better laxation, fermentation to SCFAs, calcium absorption, healthy microbiota)
- Stimulates release of glucagon-like peptide-1 neuropeptide
- Reduces endotoxin leakage into circulation
- Lowers risk of diverticula and colorectal polyps

Fecal Excretion
- Increases fecal macronutrient and bile acid excretion
- Lower net metabolizable energy

Circulatory System
- Lowers postprandial lipid, glucose, insulin and inflammatory markers
- Attenuates fasting glucose/insulin, systemic inflammation, LDL-cholesterol
- Promotes insulin sensitivity and adiponectin levels

Body Weight and Composition
- Reduces risk of weight gain/obesity
- Lowers risk of abdominal or visceral body fat

Liver
- Increases lipoprotein uptake and bile acid synthesis/secretion
- Decreases lipogenesis and inflammation

Figure 8.11 is depicted the dietary fiber health benefits.

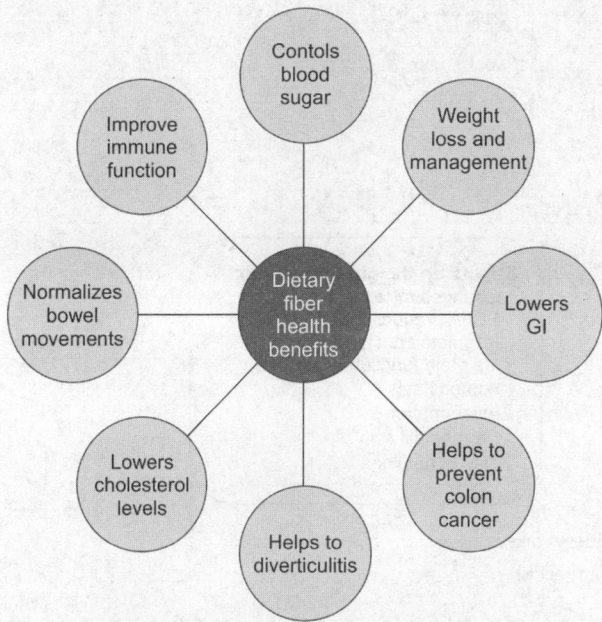

Fig. 8.11: Dietary fiber health benefits.

Role of Fibers in Disease Prevention

- The disease of having many diverticula in the large intestine is known as diverticulosis. Although diverticula is often asymptomatic, food particles become trapped in their folds and bacteria begin to metabolize the particles into acids and gases. Eventually, the diverticula may become inflamed, a condition known as diverticulitis.
- To combat the disease, antibiotics are administered to the patient to destroy the bacteria while the intake of fiber in the diet is decreased until the inflammation has subsided.
- Once the inflammation has been reduced, a high fiber diet is begun to prevent a relapse. Besides the prevention of intestinal disease, diets high in fiber have other health benefits.
- High fiber intake reduces the risk of developing obesity by increasing the bulk of a meal without yielding much energy. An expanded stomach leads to satisfaction despite the fact that the caloric intake has decreased.
- Beyond dieters, diabetics can also benefit from consuming a regular amount of dietary fiber. Once in the intestine, it slows the absorption of glucose to prevent a sudden increase in blood glucose levels.
- A relatively high intake of fiber will also decrease the absorption of cholesterol, a compound that is thought to contribute to atherosclerosis or scarring of the arteries.
- Serum cholesterol may be further reduced by a reduction in the release of insulin after meals. Since insulin is known to promote cholesterol synthesis in the liver, a reduction in the absorption of glucose after meals through the consumption of fiber can help to control serum cholesterol levels.
- Furthermore, dietary fiber intake may help prevent colon cancer by diluting potential carcinogens through increased water retention, binding carcinogens to the fiber itself and speeding the passage of food through the intestinal tract so that cancer-causing agents have less time to act.

Figure 8.12 is depicted the dietary fiber.

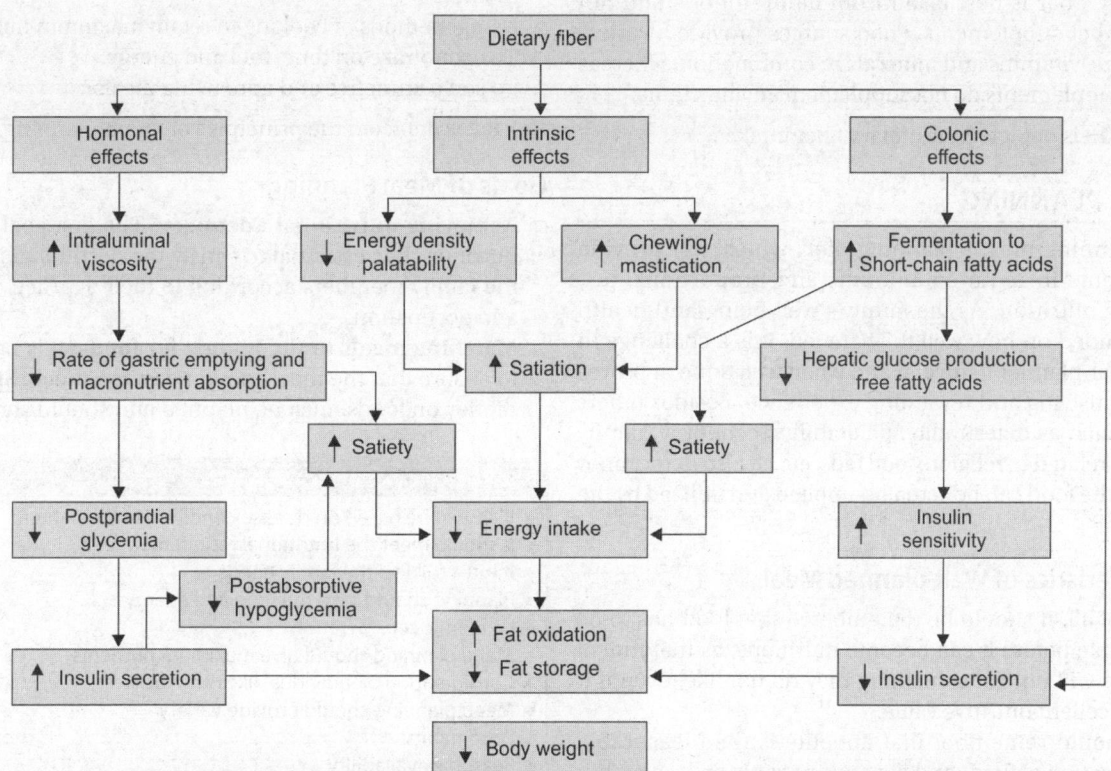

Fig. 8.12: Dietary fiber.

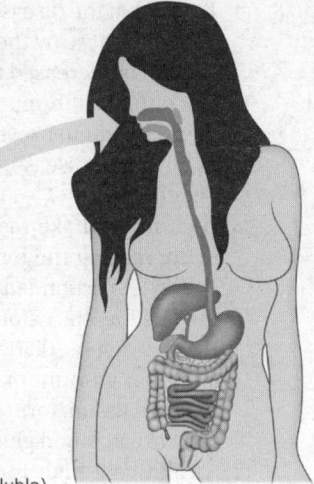

Fig. 8.13: Dietary fiber intake.
(SCFA: short-chain fatty acids)

Adverse Effects of Dietary Fibers

- Intestinal absorption of some minerals and trace elements is decreased.
- Intestinal bacteria ferment some fiber causing flatulence and abdominal discomfort.
- An excessive intake of fiber results in intestinal obstruction, if it is not accompanied by water.
- If fiber intake suddenly increased, complaints, such as cramping, diarrhea, excessive intestinal gas are common. To minimize these effects, fiber content of diet should be gradually increased over a period of several weeks.
- Dietary fiber is best taken from natural foods and not from fiber supplements. Food sources provide a variety of fibers, vitamins and minerals in combination, whereas fiber supplements do not supplement any nutrients.

Figure 8.13 is depicted the dietary fiber intake.

MEAL PLANNING

Meal planning means planning diets which will provide all nutrients in required amounts and proportions, i.e., adequate nutrition. As the family's well being and health are depended on how well they are fed. It is a challenge to every meal-planner to meet it and when well done, it proves to be a satisfying and rewarding experience. Besides others factors, such as digestibility, palatability, economy, family customs, related to religion, food fads, etc., it also determines whether the food can be actually supplied and utilized by the individual.

Characteristics of Well-planned Meal

- First of all, it should be remembered that food has to be palatable before it can become nutritious, as majority of people will not eat something they do not like, even if it has excellent nutritive value.
- We should remember that appetite is the pleasurable anticipation of foods and depends not only on hunger but also on taste, texture, appearance and attractiveness of the foods, pleasantness of the surrounding and a cheerful frame of mind.
- Meal planning thus is both an art and a science—an art in the skillful blending of colors, texture and flavor—and a science in the wise choice of food for optimum nutrition and digestion.

Objectives of Meal Planning

- To satisfy the nutritional needs of the family members.
- To keep expenditure within family food budget.
- To take into account the food preference of individual members.
- Using methods of cooking to retain maximum nutrients.
- To economize on time, fuel and energy.
- To serve attractive and appetizing meals.

Box 8.2 is depicted the principles of menu planning.

Goals of Meal Planning

- **Achieving nutritional adequacy:** The first goal is good nutrition. It is essential to satisfy the nutritional needs of the family members according to their age, activity level and occupation.
- **Matching meals to the budget for foods:** It is necessary to ensure that the meals do not cost too much. Spending money on foods must be planned and should stay within

---

Box 8.2: Principles of menu planning.

- It should be based on disease condition of the patient
- It should meet the nutritional requirement
- It must full feel the family needs
- Planning should save the time and energy
- Economic consideration
- Menu planning should give maximum nutrients
- Consideration of individual likes and dislikes
- Menu planning should provide variety
- Food habits
- Seasonal availability
- Psychological aspect

the family's food budget. Purchase foods from each food group.
- **Achieving meals the family wants and likes:** Meals must be so planned that it should be accepted, eaten, and enjoyed by the family members. The kind of meals we eat is influenced by ethnic background, family customs, region of residence, socioeconomic status, education, religion and the previous experiences. Family size must also be considered.
- **Matching meals to available time:** Meals must be planned according to the time and energy available. Time is required for planning and organizing the manual work of meal. Time and energy are required for shopping, meal preparation and clean-up after meals.

Importance of Meal Planning

The meal planning helps to make the best use of the material, time and financial resources. To obtain meals that meets the physical, social and psychological needs of the individual and families. It is very important to plan family meals in order to fulfill the nutritional requirement of the family members. This is essential to keep them strong, healthy, and free from any disease and deficiency of any kind.

- Meal planning is of utmost importance because it economizes on time, labor and fuel.
- While planning meals, the methods of working can be carefully throughout, so that there is maximum retention of nutrients and minimum losses.
- Meals can be planned according to the budget of the family. There can then be maximum utilization of money, if it is spent in the best possible way. Once can have a rich diet without buying expensive foods. Meal planning therefore, encourage one to plan within the family means
- Meal planning allows one to select different foods from the same food group and avoid monotony. Besides, use of variety of foodstuffs is important from nutritional points also.
- Meal planning determines the adequacy of the diet, the kinds of foods purchased, its quality and cost, the way it is stored, prepared and served.

Factors Affecting Meal Planning

Meal planning whether for the simplest family meal or for an elaborate company dinner, involve consideration of a number of factors. These are:

Nutritional Adequacy

- Meal pattern must fulfill the family needs, so that the nutrition requirement of each individual in the family are met. These requirements differ from person-to-person according to age, sex, activity and the physiological condition, therefore, due consideration should be given to each member of the family.

  Box 8.3 is depicted the factors affecting menu planning.
- The best way to ensure nutritional adequacy of a diet is to select the food from all the five food groups.
- The different requirements for different family members do not mean that separate cooking is to be done for all of

> **Box 8.3:** Factors affecting menu planning.
> - **Cultural food patterns**, regional food preferences, and age are related considerations.
> - Too often, menu planners are influenced by their own likes and dislikes of foods and food combinations rather than those of the customer.
>   - Food habits are the practices and associated attitudes that predetermine **what**, **when**, **why**, and **how** a person will eat.
>   - Food preferences express the degree of liking for a food item.
> - **Nutritional influence:** Nutritional needs of the customer should be a primary concern for planning menus for all foodservice operations, but they are a special concern when living conditions constrain persons to eat most of their meals in one place.

them. But the diet can be planned in such a way that while cooking the same food the nutritional requirements of all the members can be catered.
- By increasing or decreasing the amount of certain foodstuff by including some extra protein food for growth periods. For instance, the same salad can be used for both the overweight and the underweight members of the family if the dressing is omitted for the former.

Box 8.4 is depicted the factors influencing menu planning.

Economy

- The amount of money available, depending upon the socio-economic status also effects the meal planning.
- The major part of the income is spent on food. Therefore, one should spend economically to get maximum utilization. Although the budget of a family of moderate-income group may not provide for foods of the luxury class, it can still offer variety and opportunity for choice.
- Food budgets in lower income families permit even more limited choice and it may become increasingly necessary to depend on cereal foods for the main or substantial part of the meal.
- Then the problem faced is the supplementation of this cereal with foods necessary for a balanced diet. Although it may become difficult to plan, it is nevertheless possible.
- Thereby, it is very important to know the less expensive alternative for the more expensive recommended foods, having high nutritive value.
- Such recipes and foods should be included in meal preparation, such as using cereal pulse combination, e.g., khichri, paushitik roti, seasonal vegetables; butter milk; jaggery, pickle and chutney.

The facilities and help available:

- The time spent in cooking depends on other facilities and other help availability of servant, using readymade foods, using labor saving devices.

> **Box 8.4:** Factors influencing menu planning.
> - Customer preferences
> - Number of customer to be served
> - Nutritional needs based on age, gender, activity levels
> - Food habits
> - Season and availability
> - Pleasing combinations (gastronomic aspects)

- However, time like money needs to be budgeted for its best use. Time management in the preparation of foods is essential for the home maker who is also employed outside the home.

Satiety Value

- Any individual meal should provide enough satiety value, so that one does not feel hungry till it is time for the next meal.
- Proteins and fats have greater satiety value as compared to carbohydrates, e.g., a breakfast of just tea and toast will not provide enough satiety value till lunch, whereas, a breakfast of milk, cereal, eggs and fruit will provide enough satiety value till lunch.

Figure 8.14 is depicted the factors that make people for food habits.

Personal Likes and Dislikes

- The recommended dietary allowances for each of the classes of food should be followed; there is room for individual preference amongst the foods in each class.
- Some people make personal likes and dislike the only basis for the inclusion or exclusion of certain foods in their meals—the failure to include milk is a common practice.
- It is always better to change the form of the food rather than to completely omit it.
- For example, milk can be given in the form of curd, cheese, custard or other sweet dish, soybeans in the form of soya flour chapatis mixed with wheat flour.

Religion, Traditions and Customs

- They are important in determining the food included in the diet, type of meal and the dishes served to the individual of family. For instance, Muslims do not eat pork, whereas Hindus do not eat beef.
- Rice is considered an auspicious dish at festivals and marriages. Widows are generally not served fish in Bengal. Therefore, religion, traditions and customs should be kept in view while planning meals for a family.

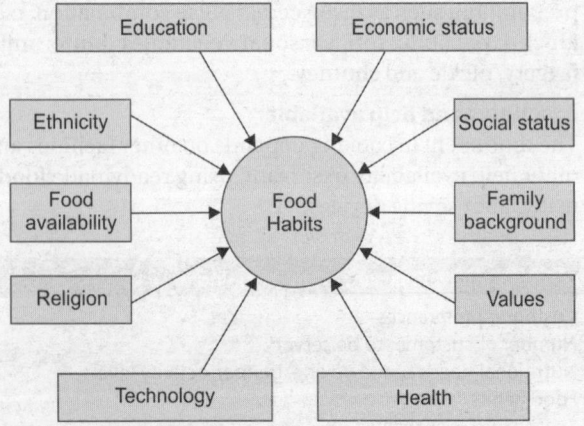

Fig. 8.14: Factors that make people for food habits.

Food Fads and Fallacies

It often receives more publicity than sound nutrition information. Therefore, while planning the meals, one must try and remove these foods fads, so that notorious meals are provided.

Availability of Foods Stuffs and Climate

- In earlier times, the dietary habits depended mainly upon the foods produced in a particular area or community, but today with improved methods of foods preservation and distribution, even the most perishable foods are available over large areas.
- The wide variation in dietary patterns throughout the world depends largely upon the available food supply and which depends on the climate. Thereby, only seasonal foods should be included in the diet.
- Also, the season of the year requires some consideration, for the type of dishes selected, e.g., inclusion of hot soups, etc., in cold winter days and chilly salads and juices in summers.

Figure 8.15 is depicted the factors affecting food choice.

Variety

- It is very important, because nobody likes to eat even his favorite food stuff over and over again. Therefore, to introduce variety, do not repeat same food items during day meal.
- Also variety in meal planning is the sum total of many kinds and classes of food served in pleasing color combinations, with judicious mixture of soft and crisp foods, blunt and sharp flavors, hot and cold dishes.
- It ensures better nutrition and also results in more interesting meals with an attractive variety of texture, color, taste and appearance which in turn stimulates appetite and pleases the palate.
- Various methods of working can also introduce a variety—a meal consisting of tandoori roti, dhal and seasonal green vegetable also with a crisp salad.

Schedules of Family Members

- When planning meals, one needs to think of the schedules (time table) of the family members—meal times and the number of meals eaten at home and those that are eaten away from home.
- If packed lunches are made, the menus need to be modified to ensure that the items can be packed and the menu is appetizing even when cold.

Family Size and Composition

- The family size affects the foods that can be served. It is known that the money spent for food per person decreases as the family size increases, when the family income remains constant.
- Staples, such as wheat and rice are bought in larger amounts but quantity of milk, vegetables and fruits is lowered. Thus, the quality of the diet is affected.
- Family composition affects the kind and amounts of mood needed and pattern of meals served.

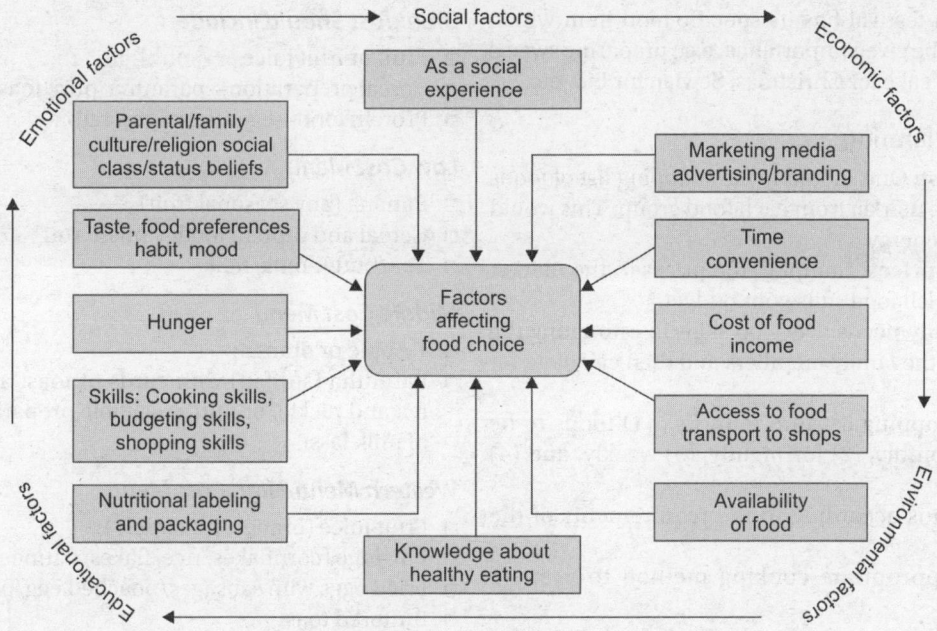

Fig. 8.15: Factors affecting food choice.

- For example, when children are below 5 years of age, more milk is required, the numbers of meals are more, as the child cannot take large amount at a time.
- As the child grows the meal pattern changes to accommodate the school hours and the need to pack lunch or snack may arise.
- Older members of the family may require change in consistency of food due to faulty teeth.

Figure 8.16 is depicted the factors affecting menu planning.

Meal Times

- It is also an important factor in meal planning. The meals should be planned according to the time for meal, i.e., whether it is breakfast, lunch or dinner.
- Normally while planning the meal for whole day, it is seen that 1/3rd of days requirement are met by lunch 1/3rd by dinner and 1/3rd by breakfast and evening tea.
- But this is not a rigid schedule and can be changed according to individual requirement. But as long as the total nutritional requirements are being met.

Occasion

- For daily meals, the first importance is given to nutritive value. However, for special occasion, special importance has to be given to color, appearance, number of dishes to be included, but at the same time nutritive value cannot be ignored.

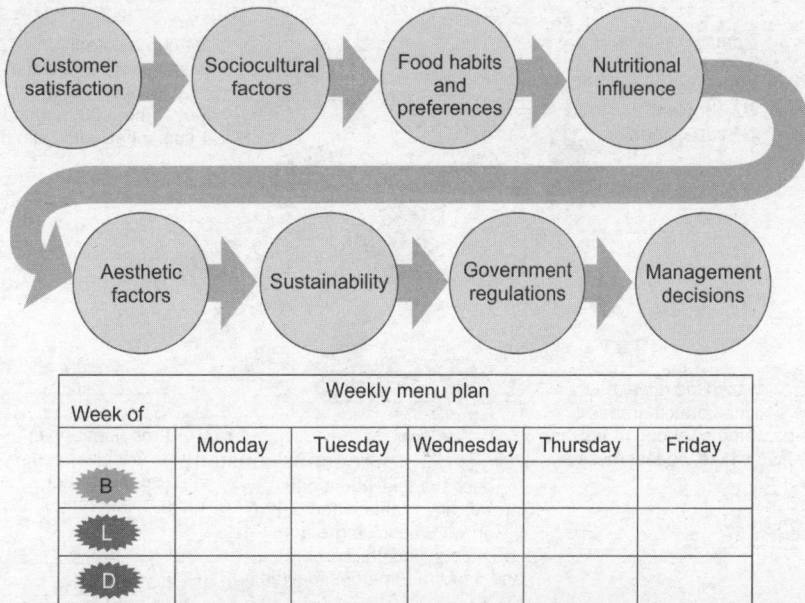

Fig. 8.16: Factors affecting menu planning.

- Similarly each festival has its specific food item which should always be given importance, e.g., preparing sweets for Deepawali, cake for Christmas, Sewian for Eid, etc.

Steps in Meal Planning

- **Preparing a list:** One should make shopping list of foods available in the market from each food group. This would save time and energy.
- **Compare the prices:** Compare the prices in the market and decide which food suits your budget.
- **Estimating daily needs:** Develop skills in estimating the daily needs of the family members and then calculate for the month.
- Divide the shopping list into four, i.e., (1) foods to be purchased monthly, (2) fortnightly, (3) weekly, and (4) daily.
- Planning menus according to the requirements of the family.
- Choose an appropriate cooking method to prepare meals.

MEAL PLANNING FOR DIFFERENT MEALS IN A DAY (FIG. 8.17)

Breakfast

It is very important meal as taken after 10–12 hours long gap between dinner and breakfast the next day. It should be well planned, nutritious attractive and should provide 1/3rd to 1/4th of the day's requirements, but do not make it very heavy which would lead to lethargy. The school children usually miss breakfast and as a result, they cannot concentrate on studies after some time.

Breakfast Should Include

- Fruit or fruit juice
- Cereal preparation—parantha, puri, toast, porridge
- Protein food—eggs, sausages, milk

Low Cost Menu

- Banana (any seasonal fruit)
- Cereal and protein food—'missi' roti
- Tea/butter milk/milk

Middle Cost Menu

- 1 Apple or orange
- Parantha (stuffed) with curds or toast and butter, milk/tea and pickle, or puri, vegetable preparation and a glass of milk lassi.

Western Menu/High Cost Menu

- Fruit juice (orange, pineapple)
- Porridge (cornflakes, rice, flakes, oatmeal, etc.) with milk
- Fried eggs with sausages/poached egg/panner-subzi
- Buttered toast
- Coffee/tea

Lunch

It is the main meal, hence an important meal. About 1/3rd of the total day's requirements should be provided. The members, who are not at home for the lunch, should be given packed lunch, which should be nutritious, easy to carry, attractive and with some variety.

Packed Lunch Menu (for School Children)

- Dal/paneer stuffed parantha
- Fruit, e.g., orange

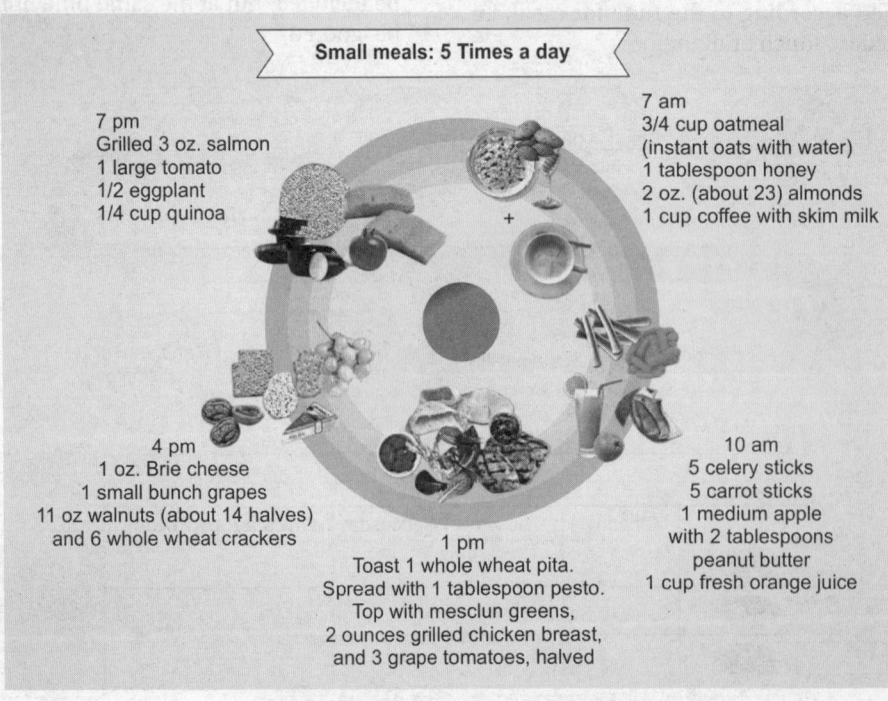

Fig. 8.17: Small meals: Five times a day.

- Piece of cake
        Or
- Sandwiches (paneer/egg/beans)
- Sweet (peanut chikki/besan ladoo/halwa/burfi)

For children food stuff should have variety, but it has to be handy too.

Packed Lunch Menu for (Adults)
- Paranthas/chapatis
- Dry vegetable
- Dry dal
- Salad/Fruit

However, on holidays when everyone is at home, menu with difference is prepared.

Normal Lunch Menu (on Holidays)
- Soup
- Cereal preparation—rice/pulao/chapati/puri/parantha
- Meat curry/egg curry/kabuli channas, pulse preparation, etc.
- Vegetable preparation—carrot, pea, subzi/koftas
- Curd preparation
- Salad
- Desert/fruit—custard/kheer/carrot—halwa/soufflé/pudding/fruit salad.

The selection of food items and number of dishes can vary according to the socioeconomic status.

On the other hand, where normally lunch is eaten at home, the menu should be simpler. Also dishes, such as curries, rice, curd, etc., can be included which are otherwise difficult to carry, some of the examples are:

- Moong whole, brinjal bhurtha, rice/chapatti, curd fruit
- Stuffed tandoori paranthe, curd, potato-pea curry, fruit
- Chapati, pea-paneer curry, pumkin subzi, curd fruit
- Rice, sambhar, sweet curd mixed with fruits

Figure 8.18 is depicted the kids school lunch foods.

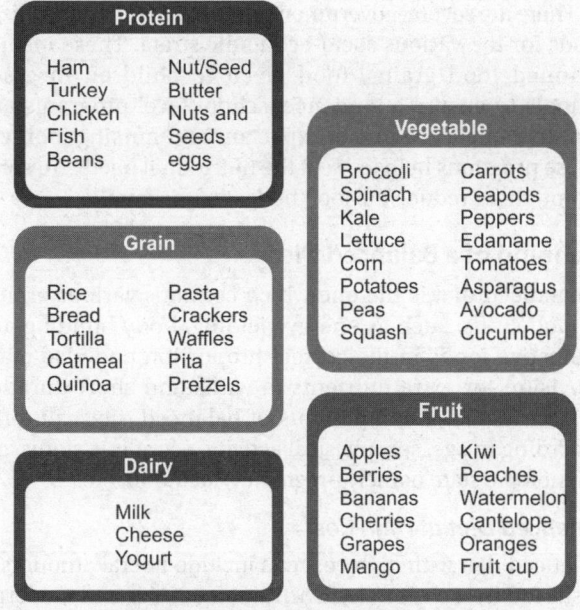

Fig. 8.18: Kids school lunch foods.

Evening Tea
It is generally light and usually includes snacks, sweets, pakoras, cutlets. For children something heavy should be given, such as sandwiches, ladoos, burfi, cakes, etc. It tea time is special occasion, 3–4 snacks and beverage can be served.

Normal Evening Tea Menu
- Pakoras, tea
- Tomato sandwich, tea
- Mathri, ladoo, tea
- Biscuit, vadas, tea
- Jalebi, wafers, tea

Evening Tea Menu (for Special Occasion)
- Rainbow sandwich, coconut rolls, cashew nuts fried, tea
- Cutlets, rasgullas, chirwa, biscuit, tea
- Chocolate burfi, samosa, pastry, wafers, tea
- Coconut burfi, khandwi, gulabjamun, dal-moth, tea
- Cashew nut burfi, peanut cutlets, chocolate cake, chirwa, tea

Dinner
It is also the main meal and should provide 1/3rd of day's requirements and should make up for all deficiencies in person's meal, e.g., if curd has not been taken in the morning, include it in the dinner.

Menu has to be elaborate when someone is invited. Otherwise, menu is like lunch. For festivals, prepare particular food according to sanity of festivals, e.g., various sweets on Deepawali, cake on Christmas, Sevian on Eid and Gujiya on Holi, etc.

Suggestions for Menu Planning
- Consider whole day as a unit rather than individual meals.
- Try to distribute carbohydrates, fats and proteins throughout the day, so that no meal has predominance of any kind of food stuff.
- Use seasonal foods because they are best in flavor and cheap, however, avoid giving the same food stuff and especially in the same meal, e.g., do not give tomato soup, tomato macaroni and tomato salad for the same meal. But, during the day things, such as cereals, butter, milk has to be repeated.
- Take care of color; flavor and texture by giving contrast in each meal, e.g., keep the color combination of dishes in mind while planning the meal. The dishes can be garnished to bring about more color in diet.
- Flavor of food should be blended with each other. There should also be some contrast in texture, e.g., some dishes can be soft and some dishes can be crisp, such as with the soup we can be given toasted bread, etc.
- There should be a balance between the dishes, such as some dishes should be light and some should be heavy, e.g., filling soup can be served with light main meal and vice versa.
- Include the favorite foods of the family at different meals, but at the same time do not be limited to only these foods and try to introduce new dishes, so that food habits can be expanded.

Money can be saved on food by following methods:
- Buying bigger packs
- Compare the prices before buying
- Wholesale markets are cheaper than retail ones
- Cook just the required amounts: if food is left over then make use of it by converting to another dish, etc.
- Use seasonal fruits and vegetables
- Keep accounts

Time can also be saved by following methods:
- Plan meal for several days at a time
- Buy dry ingredients together at least for a month
- Avoid going market during crowded hours
- Arrange things properly in kitchen so as to save the time while working
- Use pressure cooker
- Plan your time while working
- Use labor saving devices, e.g., mixer, but possible only in case the money is available to purchase them.

BUDGET FOR FOOD

Budgeting the food means, to provide budget for the nutritional requirements of an individual, a family or a community. The practice of family budget in India is almost non-existent because of lack of education and traditions. So much that, even during times of requirement, a cut in meals time and a cut in expenditure on diet is the tendency of people. Under these circumstances, food budgeting is difficult to imagine yet it cannot be underestimated. Budgeting of food is becoming important in view of the greater literacy percentage of women. Food budgeting is becoming an important factor in family budgeting in the service class or in fixed income group families **(Fig. 8.19)**.

Importance of Food Budget
- To decide the expenditure on food in relation to income.
- To receive subsidy in food planning. Fulfillment of special nutrition for vulnerable classes, e.g., in children, in pregnancy and in lactation and old age.
- Prebudgeting for contingencies, such as guests and parties.
- Possibility of changes in diet, keeping in mind the nutritional requirements as per budget.
- To raise the health status of the individual or the family by food budgeting, so as to minimize the spending on disease and treatment.

- Many factors influence the amount of money in your food budget
- Income
- Number of family members
- Age of family members
- Time and skill for food preparation
- How often meals are eaten outside the home
- The amount of food wasted
- The types of food you buy

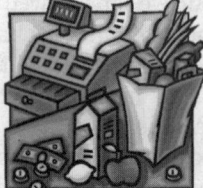

Fig. 8.19: Food budget.

Factors Affecting Food Budget
- Lack of nutrition education/less literacy
- Poverty/unemployment
- Less individual income or low per capita income
- Fluctuation in market prices of food, especially in dearness and inflation
- Lack of tradition of family and food budgeting
- Disturbances of family budget due to tradition of entertaining guests and arranging parties

Food Expenditure

The nutritionists are not unanimous on the percentage of expenditure on food budget, out of the family budget. There is no any definite principle, formula or ratio about this. However, 50% of total income should be spent on food. Higher classes spend more on.

Plans for Food Budget

In practice, one must make daily menus for a week and base the food purchase on them. This step is essential whether the plan is for a single person, a family or an institution. Food purchase is guided by nutrient needs and the food budget. Planning helps to make the best use of the available money to meet needs of the family. The food choices within a group can be guided by ones food budget. The steps which help to get the best returns for food money include:

- Buying the staple food, dhal and pulses in bulk, when the prices are competitive just after the harvest.
- Buying milk and milk products from government daily outlets.
- Buying fruits and vegetables from main markets at competitive rates.
- Buying seasonal vegetables and fruits.
- Buy sugar, jaggery in bulk from wholesale dealers.
- Buy oils from whole sale depots in bulk.
- Make butter and ghee at home.
- Buy spices in bulk and prepare the spices mix at home.

There are several government programs, which subsidized foods for the various socio-economic strata. These include rationed food grains, food given to children in grade schools to ensure attendance, school level programs and supplementary feeding of expectant and nursing mothers. These programs help to meet the nutritional needs. To some extent, these reduce the food budget of the family.

Planning of a Balanced Diet

A balanced diet is the one which contains various groups of food stuffs, such as energy yielding, body building and protective foods in the correct proportion and also make provision for extra nutrients to withstand short duration of leanness. The components of balanced diet will differ according to age, sex, physical activity, economic status and physiologic state namely pregnancy, lactation, etc.

Balanced Diet at High Cost

Balanced diet with high cost can include liberal amounts of costly foods, such as mile, fish, fruits, meat, egg and moderate amounts of cereals and pulses.

Balanced Diet with Moderate Cost

Balanced diet with moderate cost includes moderate amounts of cereals, pulses, nuts and green leafy vegetables.

Balanced Diet with Low Cost

Balanced diets of low cost will include large amounts of cereals, pulses and vegetables but small amounts of milk, eggs, fish and meat.

A balanced diet has become an accepted means to safeguard the population from nutritional deficiencies. Its goals are:
- The requirements of protein should be met which amounts to 15–20% of daily energy needs.
- Fat should be limited to 20–30% daily energy needs.
- Carbohydrates rich in natural fiber stored constitute the remaining food energy.

Ways to Save on Food Budget

- Eat meals at home or carry packed meals to work place whenever possible. Eating out in a restaurant is always more expensive than home cooked foods.
- Buy foods when they are in plenty. Take advantage of special offers, such as special of the week, buy one get one free, etc.
- Plan meals in advance and make use of food guides to ensure good nutrition.
- Plan meals according to the preference of the family. Introduce new varieties of dishes and serve attractively.
- Limit the use of ready-to-eat foods and prefer home-prepared foods from scratch.
- Limit the amount of money to be spent on snacks and aerated drinks. This will only increase the expenditure without providing any nutrients.
- Substitute foods with other foods of equal value if they are cheaper. Avoid impulsive buying.
- Read labels for dates and nutrition facts. Compare the prices.
- Try to purchase family packs as anything in bulk is always economical.
- Avoid food wastage at home by properly storing to maintain their freshness; avoid loss of nutrients by using appropriate cooking methods; and use leftovers within 24 hours.

Nutrition Across Life Cycle

- Meal planning/Menu planning—definition, principles, steps
- Infant and young child feeding (IYCF) guidelines—breastfeeding, infant foods
- Diet plan for different age groups—children, adolescents and elderly
- Diet in pregnancy—nutritional requirements and balanced diet plan
- Anemia in pregnancy—diagnosis, diet for anemic pregnant women, iron and folic acid supplementation and counseling
- Nutrition in lactation—nutritional requirements, diet for lactating mothers, complementary feeding/weaning

INFANT AND YOUNG CHILD FEEDING (IYCF) GUIDELINES—BREASTFEEDING, INFANT FOODS

Undernutrition is estimated to be associated with 2.7 million child deaths annually or 45% of all child deaths. Infant and young child feeding is a key area to improve child survival and promote healthy growth and development. The first 2 years of a child's life are particularly important, as optimal nutrition during this period lowers morbidity and mortality, reduces the risk of chronic disease, and fosters better development overall. Optimal breastfeeding is so critical that it could save the lives of over 820 000 children under the age of 5 years each year.

Figure 8.20 is depicted the infant and young child feeding.

Concept of IYCF

- Every infant and child has the right to good nutrition according to the "Convention on the Rights of the Child".
- Undernutrition is associated with 45% of child deaths.
- Globally in 2020, 149 million children under 5 were estimated to be stunted (too short for age), 45 million were estimated to be wasted (too thin for height), and 38.9 million were overweight or obese.
- About 44% of infants 0–6 months old are exclusively breastfed.
- Few children receive nutritionally adequate and safe complementary foods; in many countries less than a fourth of infants 6–23 months of age meet the criteria of dietary diversity and feeding frequency that are appropriate for their age.
- Over 820,000 children's lives could be saved every year among children under 5 years, if all children 0–23 months were optimally breastfed. Breastfeeding improves IQ, school attendance, and is associated with higher income in adult life.
- Improving child development and reducing health costs through breastfeeding results in economic gains for individual families as well as at the national level.

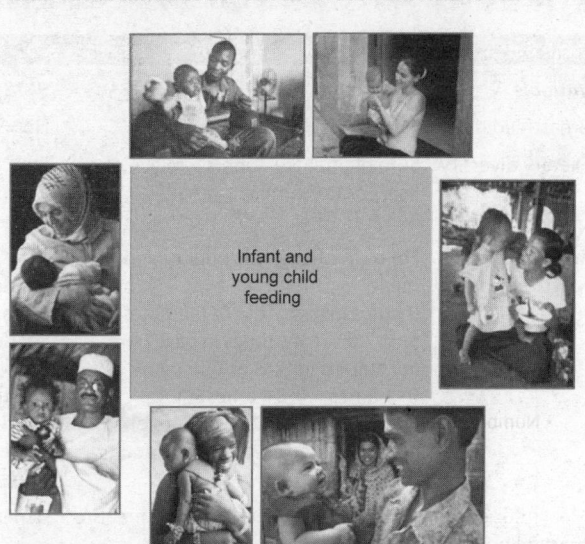

Fig. 8.20: Infant and young child feeding.

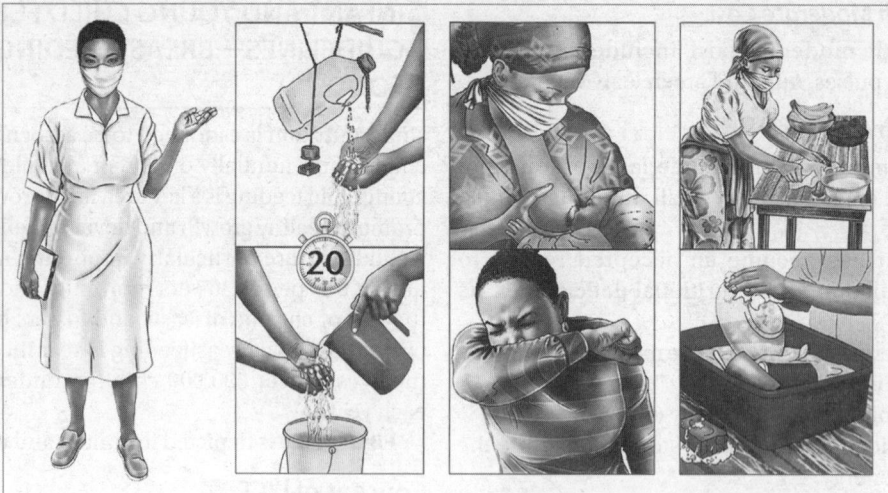

Fig. 8.21: Hygienic ways of handling food.

Figure 8.21 is depicted the hygienic ways of handling food and **Box 8.5** is depicted the objectives of the national guidelines on IYCF.

WHO and UNICEF Recommend

- Early initiation of breastfeeding within 1 hour of birth;
- Exclusive breastfeeding for the first 6 months of life; and
- Introduction of nutritionally-adequate and safe complementary (solid) foods at 6 months together with continued breastfeeding up to 2 years of age or beyond.

However, many infants and children do not receive optimal feeding. For example, only about 44% of infants aged 0–6 months worldwide were exclusively breastfed over the period of 2015–2020. Recommendations have been refined to also address the needs for infants born to HIV-infected mothers. Antiretroviral drugs now allow these children to exclusively breastfeed until they are 6 months old and continue breastfeeding until at least 12 months of age with a significantly reduced risk of HIV transmission.

Breastfeeding

Exclusive breastfeeding for 6 months has many benefits for the infant and mother. Chief among these is protection against gastrointestinal infections which is observed not only in developing but also industrialized countries.

Table 8.6 is depicted the scoring of the Child Feeding Index for IYCFPs.

> **Box 8.5:** Objectives of the national guidelines on IYCF.
>
> - To advocate IYCN and its improvement through optimal feeding practices
> - To disseminate widely the correct norms of BF and complementary feeding from policy making level to the public at large in different parts of the country in regional languages
> - To help plan efforts for raising awareness and increasing commitment of the concerned sectors of the government, NGOs and professional groups for achieving optimal feeding practices for infants and young children
> - To achieve the national goals for IYCF practices set by the planning commission for the 10th five year plan so as to achieve reduction in malnutrition levels in children.

Table 8.6: Scoring of the Child Feeding Index for IYCFPs.

Variable	6–9 months	9–12 months	12–24 months
Breastfeeding	No = 0; Yes = +2	No = 0; Yes = +2	No = 0; Yes = +2
Dietary diversity	Sum of (grains + tubers + milk + egg/fish/poultry + meat + other): 0 = 0; 1–3 = 1; 4+ = 2	Sum of (grains + tubers + milk + egg/fish/poultry + meat + other): 0 = 0; 1–3 = 1; 4+ = 2	Sum of (grains + tubers + milk + egg/fish/poultry + meat + other): 0 = 0; 1–3 = 1; 4+ 2
Food frequency (past 7 days)	For each of egg/fish/poultry and meat: 0 times in past 7 d = 0; 1–3 times in past 7 d = 1; 4+ times in past 7d = 2. For staples (grains or tubers): 0–2 times = 0; 3+ times = 1 Food group frequency = sum of scores for staples + egg/fish/poultry +meat	For each of egg/fish/poultry and meat: 0 times in past 7 d = 0; 1–3 times in past 7 d = 1; 4+ times in past 7 d = 2 For staples (grains or tubers): 0–2 times = 0; 3+ times = 1 Food group frequency = sum of scores for staples + egg/fish/poultry + meat	For each of egg/fish/poultry + meat: 0 times in past 7 d = 0; 1–3 times in past 7 d = 1; 4+ times in past 7 d = 2 For staples (grains or tubers): 0.2 times = 0; 3+ times = 1 Food group frequency = sum of scores for staples + egg/fish/poultry + meat
Meal frequency (past 24 hours)	0 meals/d = 0; 1 meal/d = 1; 2 meals/d = 2	0 meals/d = 0; 1 meal/d = 1; 2 meals/d = 2	0 meals/d = 0; 1 meal/d = 1; 2 meals/d = 2
Total score	0/+11 points	0/+11 points	0/+11 points

- Early initiation of breastfeeding, within 1 hour of birth, protects the newborn from acquiring infections and reduces newborn mortality.
- The risk of mortality due to diarrhea and other infections can increase in infants who are either partially breastfed or not breastfed at all.
- Breast-milk is also an important source of energy and nutrients in children aged 6–23 months.
- It can provide half or more of a child's energy needs between the ages of 6 and 12 months, and one third of energy needs between 12 and 24 months. Breast milk is also a critical source of energy and nutrients during illness, and reduces mortality among children who are malnourished.
- Children and adolescents who were breastfed as babies are less likely to be overweight or obese. Additionally, they perform better on intelligence tests and have higher school attendance.
- Breastfeeding is associated with higher income in adult life. Improving child development and reducing health costs results in economic gains for individual families as well as at the national level.
- Longer durations of breastfeeding also contribute to the health and well-being of mothers—it reduces the risk of ovarian and breast cancer and helps space pregnancies—exclusive breastfeeding of babies under 6 months has a hormonal effect which often induces a lack of menstruation.
- This is a natural (though not fail-safe) method of birth control known as the Lactational Amenorrhea Method.
- Mothers and families need to be supported for their children to be optimally breastfed.
  - Skin-to-skin contact between mother and baby immediately after birth and initiation of breastfeeding within the first hour of life
  Figure 8.22 is depicted the infant and young child feeding (IYCF) counseling.

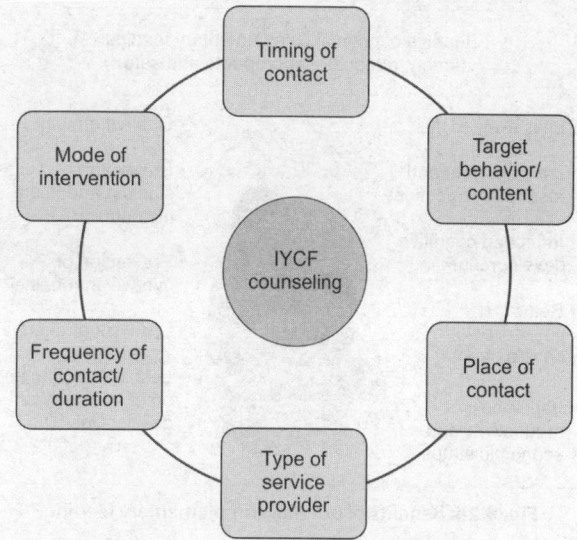

Fig. 8.22: Infant and young child feeding (IYCF) counseling.

- Breastfeeding on demand (i.e., as often as the child wants, day and night)
- Rooming-in (allowing mothers and infants to remain together 24 hours a day)
- Not giving babies additional food or drink, even water, unless medically necessary
- Provision of supportive health services with infant and young child feeding counseling during all contacts with caregivers and young children (**Fig. 8.23**), such as during antenatal and postnatal care, well-child and sick child visits, and immunization; and
- Community support, including mother support groups and community-based health promotion and education activities.

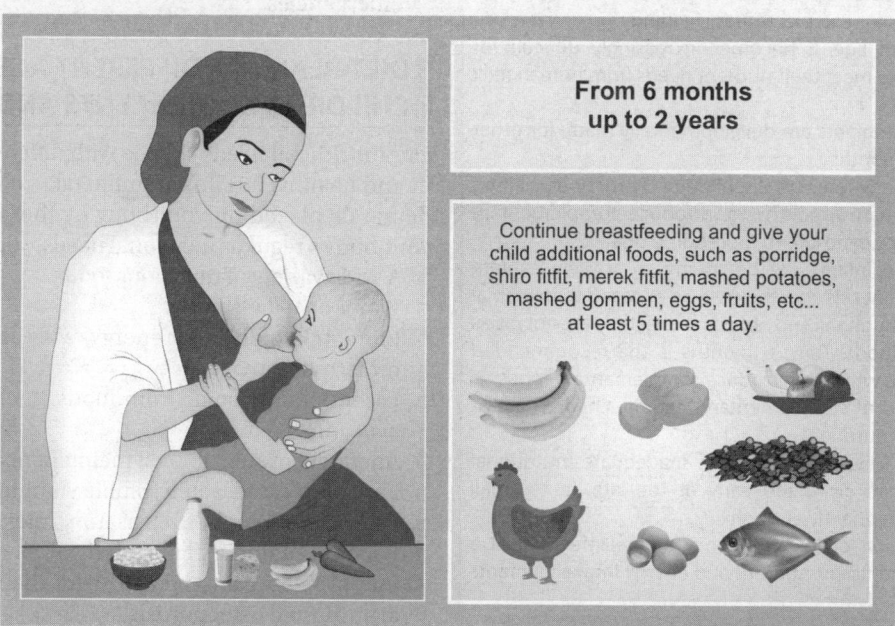

Fig. 8.23: Child feeding from 6 months up to 2 years.

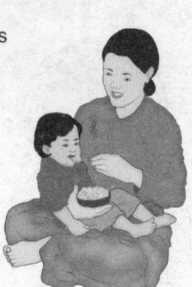

Fig. 8.24: Benefits of optimal complementary feeding.

Breastfeeding practices are highly responsive to supportive interventions, and the prevalence of exclusive and continued breastfeeding can be improved over the course of a few years.

Figure 8.24 is depicted the benefits of optimal complementary feeding.

Complementary Feeding (Box 8.6)

Around the age of 6 months, an infant's need for energy and nutrients starts to exceed what is provided by breast milk, and complementary foods are necessary to meet those needs. An infant of this age is also developmentally ready for other foods. If complementary foods are not introduced around the age of 6 months, or if they are given inappropriately, an infant's growth may falter. Guiding principles for appropriate complementary feeding are:

> **Box 8.6:** Complementary feeding.
> - Guiding principles for complementary feeding
> - After 6 months of age, it becomes increasingly difficult for breastfed infants to meet their nutrient needs from human milk alone
> - Furthermore most infants are developmentally ready for other foods at about 6 months
> - In settings where environmental sanitation is very poor, waiting until even later than 6 months to introduce complementary foods might reduce exposure to food-borne diseases
> - However, because infants are beginning to actively explore their environment at this age, they will be exposed to microbial contaminants through soil and objects even if they are not given complementary foods. Thus, 6 months is the recommended appropriate age at which to introduce complementary foods
> - During the period of complementary feeding, children are at high risk of under nutrition
> - Complementary foods are often of inadequate nutritional quality, or they are given too early or too late, in to small amounts, or not frequently enough
> - Premature cessation or low frequency of breastfeeding also contributes to insufficient nutrient and energy intake in infants beyond 6 months of age

- Continue frequent, on-demand breastfeeding until 2 years of age or beyond.
- Practice responsive feeding (for example, feed infants directly and assist older children. Feed slowly and patiently, encourage them to eat but do not force them, talk to the child and maintain eye contact).
- Practice good hygiene and proper food handling.
- Start at 6 months with small amounts of food and increase gradually as the child gets older.
- Gradually increase food consistency and variety.
- Increase the number of times that the child is fed—2–3 meals per day for infants 6–8 months of age and 3–4 meals per day for infants 9–23 months of age, with 1–2 additional snacks as required.
- Use fortified complementary foods or vitamin-mineral supplements as needed; and
- During illness, increase fluid intake including more breastfeeding, and offer soft, favorite foods.

Figure 8.25 is depicted the complementary feeding at 6 months.

Table 8.7 is depicted the ten steps to healthy feeding of infants younger than 2 years.

Feeding in Exceptionally Difficult Circumstances

Families and children in difficult circumstances require special attention and practical support. Wherever possible, mothers and babies should remain together and get the support they need to exercise the most appropriate feeding option available. Breastfeeding remains the preferred mode of infant feeding in almost all difficult situations, for instance:
- Low-birth-weight or premature infants;
- Mothers living with HIV in settings where mortality due to diarrhea, pneumonia and malnutrition remain prevalent;
- Adolescent mothers;
- Infants and young children who are malnourished; and
- Families suffering the consequences of complex emergencies.

DIET PLAN FOR DIFFERENT AGE GROUPS—CHILDREN, ADOLESCENTS AND ELDERLY

Our nutritional needs change with different life stages. To be fit and healthy, it is important to take into account the extra demands placed on your body by these changes. To meet your body's regular nutritional needs, you should consume:
- A wide variety of nutritious foods
- Water on a daily basis
- Enough kilojoules for energy, with carbohydrates as the preferred source
- Essential fatty acids from foods, such as oily fish, nuts, avocado
- Adequate protein for cell maintenance and repair
- Fat-soluble and water-soluble vitamins
- Essential minerals, such as iron, calcium and zinc
- Foods containing plant—derived phytochemicals, which may protect against heart disease, diabetes, some cancers, arthritis and osteoporosis.

Chapter 8: Balanced Diet

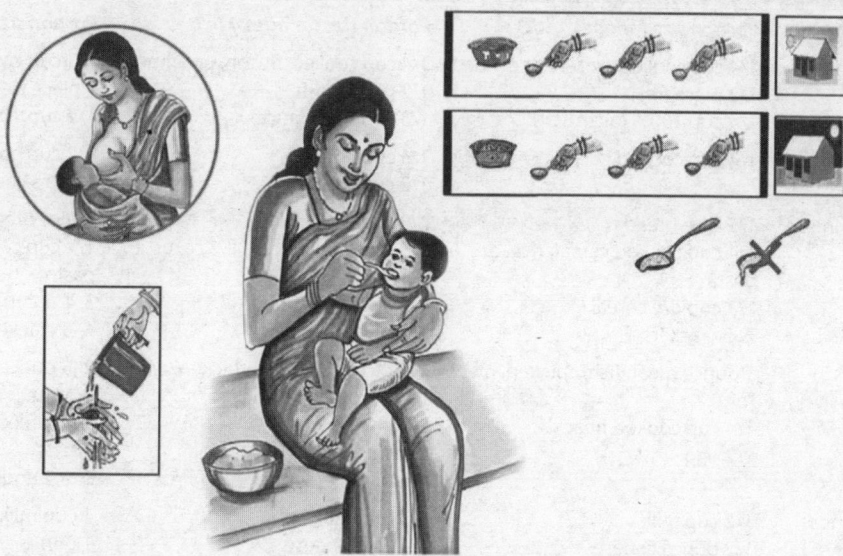

Fig. 8.25: Complementary feeding at 6 months.

Table 8.7: Ten steps to healthy feeding of infants younger than 2 years.	
Step 1	Feed the infant exclusively with human milk up to 6 months. Do not offer water, tea or any other kind of food
Step 2	After 6 months, gradually introduce other kinds of food. Keep providing human milk up to 2 years or longer
Step 3	After 6 months, give complementary food (cereals, vegetables, meat, fruits) three times a day if the child being breastfed, and five times a day if the child is no longer breastfed
Step 4	Complementary food must be offered on demand, always respecting the child's appetite
Step 5	Complementary food must be thick and it must be offered with a spoon; in the beginning it should have a pasty consistency (porridge/mashed food) and, gradually, it should get thicker up to the time when the child is able to eat a family meal
Step 6	Offer the child with different kinds of food throughout the day. A varied diet is colorful
Step 7	Stimulate the daily intake of fruits and vegetables
Step 8	Avoid sugar, coffee, canned food, fried food, soft drinks, candies, and treats in the first years of life. Use a moderate amount of salt
Step 9	Make sure to washed your hands before handing food; make sure the food is appropriately stored
Step 10	Stimulate the sick child to eat. Offer the usual and favorite meals and respect the child's appetite

Source: Brasil/ministério da Saúde/Organização Pan-Americana da Saúde. Guia alimentar para crianças menores de 2 anos. Serie A. Normas e manuais técnicos no 107. Brasília, DF, Ministério da Saúde; 2002.

Infancy—0 to 12 months

- Babies usually double their length and triple their weight between birth and one year of age.

- Breast milk generally supplies a baby with the required amounts of nutrients, fluids and energy up to about six months of age. It is recommended that infants be exclusively breastfed up to around six months of age.
- Solids should be introduced around six months of age to meet your baby's increasing nutritional and developmental needs. However, breastfeeding should continue until twelve months of age and beyond, or for as long as the mother and child desire **(Table 8.8)**.

Babies—Birth to Six Months of Age

- Babies usually double their length and triple their weight between birth and one year of age. Breast milk generally supplies a baby with the required amounts of nutrients, fluids and energy up to about six months of age.
- It is recommended that infants be exclusively breastfed up to around six months of age.

Table 8.8: A day's sample diet for a 5-year-old child.		
Meal	**Food**	**Amount**
Early morning	*Milk with sugar*	*200 mL*
Breakfast	Paratha with curd or Egg and bread	1 paratha 1 egg, 2 slice of bread
Mid morning	*Fruit or fruit juice*	*1 fruit/1 glass*
Lunch	Rice Mixed vegetables Curd Chapati	Small plate Small katori 1/2 katori 1–2
Evening tea	Milk+biscuit	150 mL, 4–6 biscuits
Dinner	Dal Chapati Salad	1 katori 2
Bed time	*Fruit custard*	*1 katori*

Table 8.9: Maintaining the nutrient body stores.

Food group	Servings per day	Portion size for ages 1 to 3	Portion size for ages 4 to 6	Portion size for ages 7 to 10
Fruits	2–3 servings	1/4 cup cooked, frozen, or canned 1/2 piece fresh 1/4 cup 100% juice	1/4 cup cooked, frozen, or canned 1/2 piece fresh 1/3 cup 100% juice	1/3 cup cooked, frozen, or canned 1 piece fresh 1/2 cup 100% juice
Vegetables	2–3 servings	1/4 cup cooked	1/4 cup cooked 1/2 cup salad	1/2 cup cooked 1 cup salad
Grains	6–11 servings	1/2 slice bread 1/4 cup cooked cereal, rice, or pasta 1/3 cup dry cereal 2–3 crackers	1/2 slice bread 1/3 cup cooked cereal, rice, or pasta 1/2 cup dry cereal 3-4 crackers	1 slice bread 1/2 cup cooked cereal, rice, or pasta 3/4–1 cup dry cereal 4–5 crackers
Meats and other proteins	2 servings	1 ounce meat, fish, chicken, or tofu 1/4 cup cooked beans 1/2 egg	1 ounce meat, fish, chicken, or tofu 1/3 cup cooked beans 1 egg	2–3 ounces meat, fish, chicken, or tofu 1/2 cup cooked beans 1 or 2 eggs
Dairy	2–3 servings	1/2 cup milk 1/2 ounce cheese 1/3 cup yogurt	1/2 cup milk 1 ounce cheese 1/2 cup yogurt	1 cup milk 1 ounce cheese 3/4–1 cup yogurt

- Breast milk is preferred to infant formula where possible, as it contains many protective and immunological factors that benefit the baby's development. Fruit juice is not recommended for babies under the age of six months.
- Breast milk or correctly prepared infant formula provides enough water for a healthy baby to replace any water losses. However, all babies need extra water once solid foods are introduced.

Food for Babies—six to 12 months of Age

Solids should be introduced around six months of age to meet your baby's increasing nutritional and developmental needs. However, breastfeeding should continue until twelve months of age and beyond, or for as long as the mother and child desire. Different societies have their own traditions about which food is more appropriate to start feeding a baby with. Culturally appropriate foods and preparation methods should be encouraged when these are nutritionally adequate. As a baby is gradually weaned from the breast or bottle and new solids are introduced, there may be reduced body stores of iron. Stores is depicted in the **Table 8.9**.

- Give your baby foods that are rich in iron and zinc, such as iron-enriched infant cereals, pureed meats and poultry dishes, cooked plain tofu and legumes/soy beans/ lentils. Iron-enriched rice-based cereals are frequently recommended as the first food to be introduced, as there is the additional benefit of a lower risk of an allergic reaction.
- Foods can be introduced in any order, provided the texture is suitable for your baby's stage of development. Foods range from fruits and vegetables (for vitamin and mineral content) to meat, poultry, fish and whole eggs..
- Do not add salt, sugar or honey to your baby's food. It is unnecessary.
- Avoid cow's milk as a drink in the first 12 months. Small amounts can be used in cereals and custards. All milk used should be pasteurized.
- Whole fruit is preferable to fruit juice. Avoid juices and sugar sweetened drinks.
- Put your baby to bed without a bottle, or take the bottle away when they have finished feeding to minimize long-term exposure of their teeth to sugar-containing liquids.
- Avoid whole nuts, seeds or similar hard foods to reduce the risk of choking.
- Introduce foods one at a time. Offer new foods once every three to four days to avoid confusion and to rule out food allergy and sensitivity.
- Feed babies during any illness and feed up after illness. Give ample liquids if your baby has diarrhea.

Table 8.10 is depicted the one day menu for an adult (sedentary work).

Table 8.10: One day menu for an adult (sedentary work).

- Energy—2875 kcal
- Protein—60 g (60 kg weight)

Meal	Food	Quantity
Early morning	Milk with sugar or tea	1 cup
Breakfast	Egg with bread or paratha with curd, coffee	1 egg, 2 bread, 2 paratha, 1
Mid-day	Fruit chaat or fruit juice or Tea with biscuits	1 cup, 4–6
Lunch	Vegetables, chapati, rice, curd, salad	1 katori, 2 1 plate, 1 katori, mixed
Evening tea	Tea with snacks	1 cup
Night dinner	Dal/rajama Vegetables Chapati	1 katori 1 katori 3
Bed time	Kheer/fruit	1 katori/fruit

Food for Young Children

Once a child is eating solids, offer a wide range of foods to ensure adequate nutrition. Young children are often picky with food, but should be encouraged to eat a wide variety of foods. Trying again with new foods may be needed for a child to accept that food. As many as eight to fifteen times may be needed. During childhood, children tend to vary their food intake (spontaneously) to match their growth patterns. Children's food needs vary widely, depending on their growth and their level of physical activity. Like energy needs, a child's needs for protein, vitamins and minerals increase with age.

Ideally, children should be accumulating stores of nutrients in preparation for the rapid growth spurt experienced during adolescence. Appropriate weight gain and development will indicate whether food intake is appropriate. Food-related problems for young children include overweight, obesity, tooth decay and food sensitivities.

Recommendations include:

- If a child is gaining inappropriate weight for growth, limit energy-dense, nutrient-poor snack foods. Increase your child's physical activity. You could also limit the amount of television watching.
- Tooth decay can be prevented with regular brushing and visits to the dentist. Avoid sugary foods and drinks, especially if sticky or acidic.
- Ensure your child has enough fluids, especially water. Fruit juices should be limited and soft drinks avoided.
- Reduced-fat milks are not recommended for children under the age of two, due to increased energy requirements and high growth rate at this age.
- Be aware of foods that may cause allergic reactions, including peanuts, shellfish and cow's milk. Be particularly careful if there is a family history of food allergy.

Box 8.7 is depicted the importance of diet during different stages of life.

Preschool and School-going Children

- Once a child is eating solids, offer a wide range of foods to ensure adequate nutrition.
- Young children are often picky with food, but should be encouraged to eat a wide variety of foods. Trying again with new foods may be needed for a child to accept that food. As many as eight to fifteen times may be needed.
- During childhood, children tend to vary their food intake (spontaneously) to match their growth patterns. Children's food needs vary widely, depending on their growth and their level of physical activity. Like energy needs, a child's needs for protein, vitamins and minerals increase with age.
- Ideally, children should be accumulating stores of nutrients in preparation for the rapid growth spurt experienced during adolescence. Appropriate weight gain and development will indicate whether food intake is appropriate.

Box 8.8 is depicted the nutrition advise for preschool children.

Adolescence

The growth spurt as children move into adolescence needs plenty of kilojoules and nutrients. For girls, this generally occurs around 10 to 11 years of age. For boys, it occurs later, at around 12 to 13 years.

Table 8.11 is depicted the recommended dietary allowance of nutrients for adolescents in 24 hours.

Factors Influencing Nutrition of Adolescents

- Lack of knowledge in the family and community about the importance of nutrition during adolescence
- Lack of food because of socioeconomic circumstances
- Inequitable distribution of food in the family wherein girls being denied nutritious food
- Poor dietary intake of food and vegetables rich in iron
- Poor bioavailability of iron in the diet
- Hookworm infestation
- Diseases, such as Malaria

Box 8.7: Importance of diet during different stages of life.

- **Senior citizens:** For being physically active and healthy require nutrient dense low fat foods.
- **Pregnancy:** For maintaining health, productivity and prevention of diet-related diseases and to support pregnancy/lactation require nutritionally adequate diet with extra food for child bearing/rearing.
- **Adolescent:** For growth spurt, maturation and bone development require body building and protective foods.
- **Child age:** For growth, development and to fight infections require energy, body building and protective food.
- **Infant:** For growth and appropriate milestones require breast milk, energy rich foods.

Box 8.8: Nutrition advise for preschool children.

The best nutrition advise to keep your child healthy includes encouraging her to:
- Eat a variety of foods
- Balance the food you eat with physical activity
- Choose a diet with plenty of grain products, vegetables and fruits
- Choose a diet low in fat, saturated fat, and cholesterol
- Choose a diet moderate in sugars and salt
- Choose a diet that provides enough calcium and iron to meet their growing body's requirements

Table 8.11: Recommended dietary allowance of nutrients for adolescents in 24 hours.

	Male			Female		
	10–12 Years	13–15 Years	16–18 Years	10–12 Years	13–15 Years	16–18 Years
Energy (Kcal)	2200	2500	2700	2000	2100	2100
Protein (g)	54	70	78	57	65	63
Calcium (mg)	600	600	500	600	600	500
Iron (mg)	34	41	50	19	28	30

Section 1: Applied Nutrition and Dietetics

- Bad cooking habits (over boiling vegetables and straining water, removing husk from wheat, eating polished rice and straining rice water, etc.)
- Perpetuation of a vicious cycle of malnutrition and infection, which might begin, even before birth and may have more serious consequences for the girl child.

Eating Right and Nutritious Food During Adolescence

- Food selection is based mainly on availability, convenience and time, rather than food value
- Influence of peers, mass media, and prevalent body image
- Personal self-esteem and body image guide the eating behavior
- Missing meals and snacking are very common
- Fast food joints are mainly patronized by adolescents. These spoil the appetite for regular meals and are high on calories and low on nutrients.
- Helps in achieving rapid growth and full growth potential
- Helps in timely sexual maturation
- Ensures adequate calcium deposition in the bones and helps in achieving normal bone strength
- Establishes good eating habits and sets the tone for a lifetime of healthy eating. This prevents obesity, osteoporosis (weak bones due to deficiency of calcium), and diabetes in later life.

Recommendations include:

- The extra energy required for growth and physical activity needs to be obtained from foods that also provide nutrients, instead of just 'empty calories'.
- Take away and fast foods need to be balanced with nutrient-dense foods, such as whole grain breads and cereals, fruits, legumes, nuts, vegetables, fish and lean meats.
- Milk, yogurt and cheese (mostly reduced fat) should be included to boost calcium intake—this is especially important for growing bones. Cheese should preferably be a lower salt variety.
- Adolescent girls should be particularly encouraged to consume milk and milk products.

Table 8.12 is depicted the IFA supplementation program and service delivery.

Young Adults

- Moving away from home, starting work or study, and the changing lifestyle that accompanies the late teens and early 20s can cause dietary changes that are not always beneficial for good health.
- Nutrients recommendations depend upon lifestyle and physical activity.

Old Age

Physical activity is not much during old age hence carbohydrates and fats need to be restricted. But there is muscle loss and fragility of bones is common, hence protein is required to make up for the loss and for maintaining growth of cells. Since teeth start falling off hence chewing becomes difficult and thus milk is a good option for old people.

Recommendations include:

- Be as active as possible to encourage your appetite and maintain muscle mass.
- Remain healthy with well-balanced eating and regular exercise.
- Eat foods that are nutrient dense rather than energy dense, including eggs, lean meats, fish, liver, low-fat dairy foods, nuts and seeds, legumes, fruit and vegetables, whole grain breads and cereals.
- If possible, try to spend some time outside each day to boost your vitamin D synthesis for healthy bones.
- Limit foods that are high in energy and low in nutrients, such as cakes, sweet biscuits and soft drinks.
- Choose foods that are naturally high in fiber to encourage bowel health.
- Limit the use of table salt, especially during cooking.
- Choose from a wide variety of foods and drink adequate fluids.
- Share mealtimes with family and friends.

Table 8.12: IFA supplementation program and service delivery.

Age group	Intervention/dose	Regime	Service delivery
6–60 months	1 mL of IFA syrup containing 20 mg of elemental iron and 100 µg of folic acid	Biweekly throughout the period 6–60 months of age and de-worming for children 12 months and above	Through ASHA Inclusion in MCP card
5–10 years	Tablets of 45 mg elemental iron and 400 mcg of folic acid	Weekly throughout the period 5–10 years of age and biannual de-worming	In school through teachers and for out-of-school children through Anganwadi center (AWC) Mobilization by ASHA
10–19 years	100 mg elemental iron and 500 µg of folic acid	Weekly throughout the period 10–19 years of age and biannual deworming	In school through teachers and for those out-of-school through AWC Mobilization by ASHA
Pregnant and lactating women	100 mg elemental iron and 500 µg of folic acid	1 tablet daily for 100 days, starting after the first trimester, at 14–16 weeks of gestation. To be repeatedly for 100 days post-partum	ANG/ANM/ASHA Inclusion in IMCP card
Women in reproductive age (WRA) group	100 mg elemental iron and 500 µg of folic acid	Weekly throughout the reproductive period	Through ASHA during house visit for contraceptive distribution

DIET IN PREGNANCY—NUTRITIONAL REQUIREMENTS AND BALANCED DIET PLAN (FIG. 8.26)

A pregnant woman should concentrate on increasing her nutrient intake, rather than her kilojoule intake, particularly in the first and second trimesters. In Australia, pregnant women are expected to gain about 10 to 13 kg during pregnancy. However, this depends on the pre-pregnancy weight of the mother. Recommendations include:

- No 'crash dieting', as this can have a negative impact on the baby.
- No 'eating for two', as this will lead to unnecessary weight gain. A healthy pregnancy only requires about an extra 1,400 to 1,900 kilojoules a day during the second and third trimester, which is equivalent to a glass of milk or a sandwich.
- Concentrate on diet quality rather than quantity.
- Accommodate cravings, but do not let them replace more nutritious foods.
- Nutrients for which there are increased requirements during pregnancy include folate, iron, vitamin B12 and iodine.
- Iron is required for oxygen transport in the body. Iron supplements can be advised by your doctor during pregnancy, but do not take them unless your doctor recommends them. Increasing vitamin C intake can help increase iron absorption from foods.
- Folate is important three months before and in the first trimester of pregnancy to avoid neural tube defects (such as spina bifida) in the baby. All women of child-bearing age should eat high-folate foods (such as green leafy vegetables, fruits and legumes). If planning for pregnancy, it is important to obtain 400 µg folate/day and if you are pregnant, this increases to 600 µg/day. This can be obtained from folate supplement and a diet high in folate-rich foods (remember to talk to your doctor first). It is now mandatory for all bread-making flour to be fortified with folic acid (a form of folate that is added to foods). This will help women reach their recommended intake of folate.
- Iodine is important for normal growth and development of the baby. Iodine supplements are often advised during pregnancy to meet the increased needs, as food sources (such as seafood, iodides salt and bread) are unlikely to provide enough iodine. Talk to your doctor about this.
- The recommended intake of calcium does not specifically increase during pregnancy. It is, however, very important that pregnant women do meet calcium requirements during pregnancy.

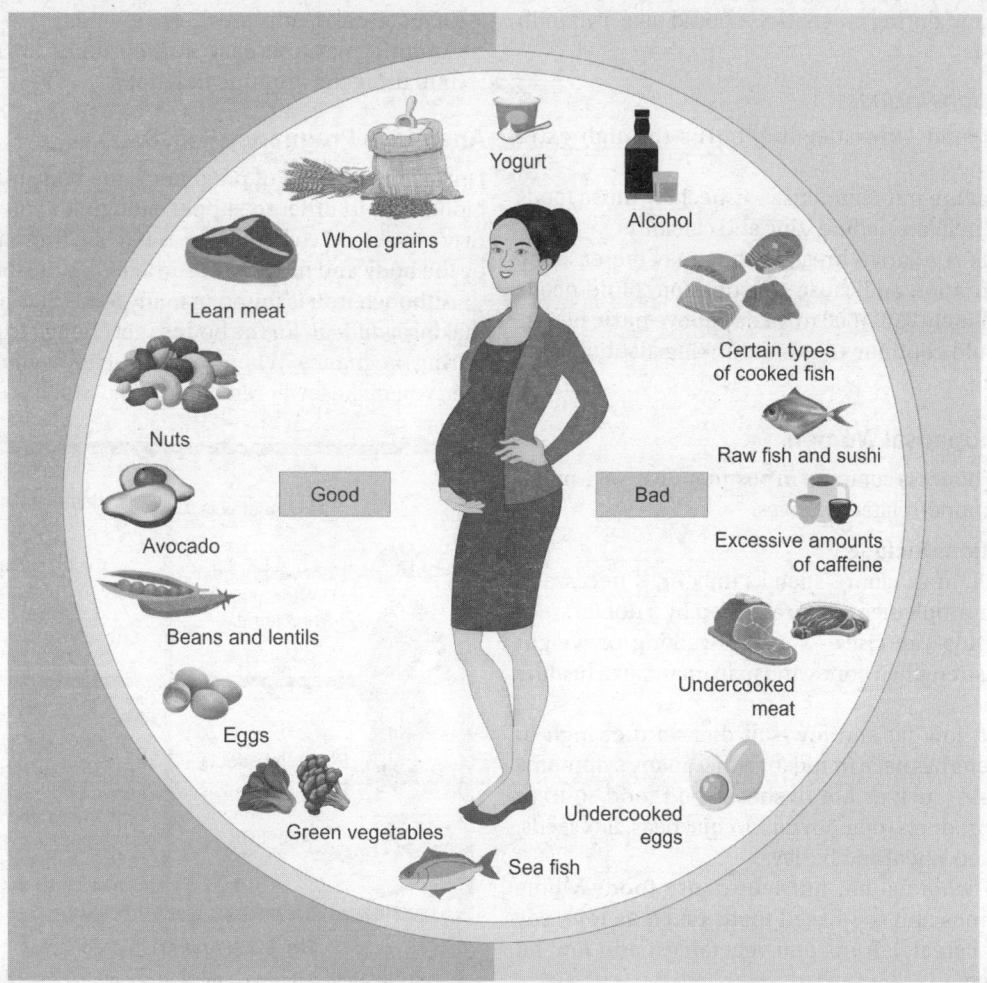

Fig. 8.26: Pregnant diet.

- No one knows the safe limit of alcohol consumption during pregnancy. Recommendations are to not drink at all.
- Pregnant women are advised to avoid foods that are associated with increased risk of the listeria bacteria (such as soft cheese and cold seafood) and to be careful with foods that are more likely to contain mercury (such as certain fish. such as flake). *Listeria* can seriously affect your growing baby.
- Being physically active has many benefits. If you are active and fit, and are experiencing a normal pregnancy, you can remain physically active during your pregnancy. Otherwise, consult your doctor for advice.
- Drink plenty of fluids.
- Do not smoke—both direct and passive smoking is associated with growth retardation, increased risk of spontaneous abortion, stillbirths, placental complications and low birth weight.

Food for Breastfeeding Mothers

Breastfeeding mothers need a significant amount of extra energy to cope with the demands of breastfeeding. This extra energy should come in the form of nutrient-dense foods to help meet the extra nutrient requirements that also occur when breastfeeding. Vegan mothers who are breastfeeding (and during pregnancy) should take a vitamin B12 supplement.

Recommendations Include

- Eat enough food—breastfeeding burns through extra kilojoules.
- Eat foods that are nutrient dense—especially those foods that are rich in folate, iodine, zinc and calcium.
- Eat and drink regularly—breastfeeding may increase the risk of dehydration and cause constipation. Fluid needs are approximately 750–1000 mL a day above basic needs.
- Women should continue to avoid drinking alcohol while breastfeeding.

Food for Menopausal Women

Thinning of the bones is common in postmenopausal women because of hormone-related changes.

Recommendations include:

- Eat foods rich in calcium—such as milk or, if necessary, take calcium supplements as prescribed by a doctor.
- Weight-bearing exercises—such as walking or weight training can strengthen bones and help maintain a healthy body weight.
- A high-fiber, low-fat and low-salt diet—a diet high in phytoestrogens has been found to reduce many symptoms of menopause, such as hot flushes. Good food sources include soy products (tofu, soymilk), chickpeas, flax seeds, lentils, cracked wheat and barley.
- A variety of whole grain, nutrient-dense food—whole grains, legumes and soy-based foods (such as tofu, soy and linseed cereals), fruits and vegetables, and low-fat dairy products.

ANEMIA IN PREGNANCY—DIAGNOSIS, DIET FOR ANEMIC PREGNANT WOMEN, IRON AND FOLIC ACID SUPPLEMENTATION AND COUNSELING

The need for iron increases with rapid growth and expansion of blood volume and muscle mass. As boys gain lean body mass at a faster rate than girls, they require more iron than girls. The onset of menstruation imposes additional needs for girls. Adolescents should be encouraged to consume iron rich foods (green leafy vegetables, jaggery, meat) complemented with a vitamin C source, such as citrus fruits (oranges, lemon) and Indian gooseberry (Amla). Adolescent girls need additional requirement of iron to compensate for menstrual blood loss.

Nutritional Anemia

Our blood contains a red pigment called hemoglobin, which carries oxygen and is rich in iron. Anemia is the loss of oxygen carrying capacity of the blood due to deficiency of hemoglobin in the red blood cells.

Iron deficiency anemia is a major nutritional problem in adolescent boys and girls in India. The ill effects of anemia can be seen as:

- Reduced capacity to work and thus decreased productivity
- Increased risk to pregnant girls/women. (In India, 20–40% of maternal deaths are due to anemia).
- Anemia may increase susceptibility to infections by impairing the immune functions.

Anemia in Pregnancy (Fig. 8.27)

During the last half of pregnancy, the body makes more red blood cells in order to supply enough for you and the baby. Every red blood cell uses iron as its core. Iron cannot be made by the body and must be absorbed from the foods you eat.

Although iron is found in many foods, it is hard to absorb, making it difficult for the body to get enough to meet its needs during pregnancy. When you do not have enough iron in the diet, you make fewer red blood cells, which is called anemia.

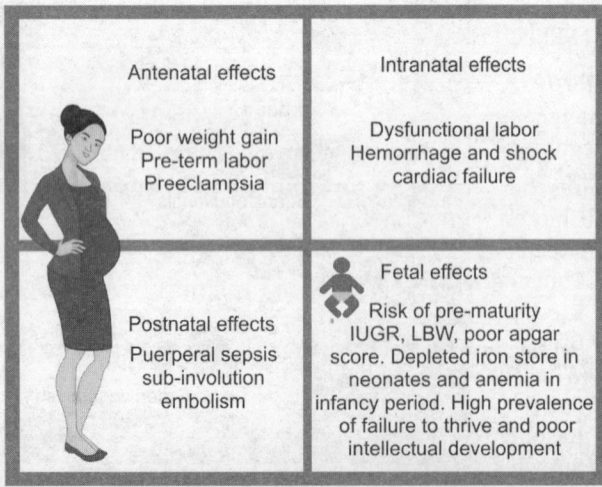

Fig. 8.27: Anemia in pregnancy.
(IUGR: intrauterine growth retardation; LBW: low birth weight)

Iron deficiency anemia is very common and is easy to correct. The body also needs a nutrient called folate to make healthy blood cells. Folate is easily absorbed and found in most green vegetables.

Causes of Anemia

- Poor intake of iron- and folate-rich foods
- Increased destruction of red blood cells that can occasionally occur during illness

Anemia Signs and Symptoms

Often, women with anemia do not have specific symptoms. If anemia is severe, you may feel tired and weak.

Preventing Anemia

- Eat iron-rich foods, such as meat, chicken, fish, eggs, dried beans and fortified grains. The form of iron in meat products, called heme, is more easily absorbed than the iron in vegetables. If you are anemic and you ordinarily eat meat, increasing the amount of meat you consume is the easiest way to increase the iron your body receives.
- Eat foods high in folic acid, such as dried beans, dark green leafy vegetables, wheat germ and orange juice.
- Eat foods high in vitamin C, such as citrus fruits and fresh, raw vegetables.
- Cooking with cast iron pots can add up to 80% more iron to your food.
- Take your prenatal multivitamin and mineral pill which contains extra folate.

Iron Supplements

- Because it is difficult to get enough iron from your diet, you may need to take an iron supplement. There usually is enough iron in your prenatal vitamin to prevent anemia, but your provider may prescribe an extra iron pill if you are anemic.
- If the iron tablet upsets your stomach, take it with a small amount of food.
- Do not take your iron tablet with dairy products or calcium supplements.

Iron-rich Foods

The recommended dietary allowance (RDA) of iron during pregnancy is 30 milligrams. Here are some foods rich in iron.

Foods that provide .5 to 1.5 milligrams of iron:

- Chicken, 3 ounces
- Green peas, 1/2 cup
- Tomato juice, 6 ounces
- Broccoli, 1/2 cup
- Brussels sprouts, 1/2 cup cooked
- Whole wheat bread, 1 slice
- Dried apricots, 5 halves
- Raspberries, 1 cup
- Strawberries, 1 cup

Foods that provide 1.6 to 3 milligrams of iron:

- Sirloin steak, 3 ounces
- Roast beef, 3 ounces
- Lean hamburger, 3 ounces
- Baked potato with skin
- Kidney beans, 1/2 cup cooked
- Lima beans, 1/2 cup cooked
- Navy beans, 1/2 cup cooked
- Oatmeal, 1 cup cooked
- Raisins, 1/2 cup

Foods that provide 3 to 12 milligrams of iron:

- Clams, 4 large or 9 small
- Oysters, 6 medium
- Spinach, 1/2 cup cooked
- Fortified cereal, 1 cup

Additional sources of iron:

- All-kinds of liver (except fish)—however, liver should not be eaten more than once a week
- Lean beef, veal, pork or lamb
- Greens, all kinds
- Beets
- Sauerkraut
- Tofu
- Lentils
- Soybean flour
- Enriched pastas
- Unrefined sugars, such as molasses
- Eat more food during pregnancy.
- Eat more whole grains, sprouted grams and fermented foods.
- Take milk/meat/eggs in adequate amounts.
- Eat plenty of vegetables and fruits.
- Avoid superstitions and food taboos.
- Do not use alcohol and tobacco. Take medicines only when prescribed.
- Take iron, folate and calcium supplements regularly, after 14–16 weeks of pregnancy and continue the same during lactation.

Nutrients that require special attention during pregnancy and lactation period.

The daily diet of a woman should contain an additional 350 calories, 0.5 g of protein during first trimester and 6.9 g during second trimester and 22.7 g during third trimester of pregnancy.

- Some micronutrients are especially required in extra amounts during these physiological periods.
- Folic acid, taken throughout the pregnancy, reduces the risk of congenital malformations and increases the birth weight.
- The mother as well as the growing fetus needs iron to meet the high demands of erythropoiesis (RBC formation).
- Calcium is essential, both during pregnancy and lactation, for proper formation of bones and teeth of the offspring, for secretion of breast-milk rich in calcium and to prevent osteoporosis in the mother.
- Similarly, iodine intake ensures proper mental health of the growing foetus and infant. Vitamin A is required during lactation to improve child survival.
- Besides these, nutrients, such as vitamins B12 and C need to be taken by the lactating mother.

Ways to meet the nutritional demands during pregnancy and lactation:

- The pregnant/lactating woman should eat a wide variety of foods to make sure that her own nutritional needs as well as those of her growing foetus are met.
- There is no particular need to modify the usual dietary pattern. However, the quantity and frequency of usage of the different foods should be increased.
- She can derive maximum amount of energy (about 60%) from rice, wheat and millets. Cooking oil is a concentrated source of both energy and polyunsaturated fatty acids.
- Good quality protein is derived from milk, fish, meat, poultry and eggs. However, a proper combination of cereals, pulses and nuts also provides adequate proteins.
- Mineral and vitamin requirements are met by consuming a variety of seasonal vegetables particularly green leafy vegetables, milk and fresh fruits.
- Bioavailability of iron can be improved by using fermented and sprouted grams and foods rich in vitamin C, such as citrus fruits.
- Milk is the best source of biologically available calcium.
- Though it is possible to meet the requirements for most of the nutrients through a balanced diet, pregnant/lactating women are advised to take daily supplements of iron, folic acid, vitamin B and calcium.

Importance of Eating Folate-rich Foods

- Folic acid is essential for the synthesis of hemoglobin.
- Folic acid deficiency leads to macrocytic anemia.
- Pregnant women need more of folic acid.
- Folic acid supplements increase birth weight and reduce congenital anomalies.
- Green leafy vegetables, legumes, nuts and liver are good sources of folic acid.
- 500 mg (0.5 mg) folic acid supplementation is advised pre-conceptionally and throughout pregnancy for women with history of congenital anomalies (neural tube defects, cleft palate).

Importance of Eating Iron-rich Foods

- Iron is needed for hemoglobin synthesis, mental function and to provide immunity against diseases.
- Deficiency of iron leads to anemia.
- Iron deficiency is common particularly in women of reproductive age and children.
- Iron deficiency during pregnancy increases maternal mortality and low birth weight infants.
- In children, it increases susceptibility to infection and impairs learning ability.
- Plant foods, such as green leafy vegetables, legumes and dry fruits contain iron.
- Iron is also obtained through meat, fish and poultry products.
- Iron bio-availability is poor from plant foods but is good from animal foods.
- Vitamin C-rich fruits, such as gooseberries (Amla), guava and citrus improve iron absorption from plant foods.
- Beverages, such as tea bind dietary iron and make it unavailable. Hence, they should be avoided before during or soon after a meal.
- Commonly consumed plant based diets provide around 18 mg of iron as against recommended intake of 35 mg per day. Therefore, supplementation of iron (100 mg elemental iron, 0.5 mg folic acid) is recommended for 100 days during pregnancy from 16th week onwards to meet the demands of pregnancy.

NUTRITION IN LACTATION—NUTRITIONAL REQUIREMENTS, DIET FOR LACTATING MOTHERS, COMPLEMENTARY FEEDING/WEANING

Nutrient needs during lactation depend primarily on the volume and composition of milk produced and on the mother's initial nutrient needs and nutritional status. Among women exclusively breastfeeding their infants, the energy demands of lactation exceed prepregnancy demands by approximately 640 kcal/day during the first 6 months postpartum compared with 300 kcal/day during the last two trimesters of pregnancy (NRC, 1989). In contrast, the demand for some nutrients, such as iron, is considerably less during lactation than during pregnancy.

Table 8.13 is depicted the nutrient requirements during breastfeeding and examples of food sources.

Table 8.13: Nutrient requirements during breastfeeding and examples of food sources.

Nutrient	RNI	Extra during breastfeeding	Examples of food sources
Energy	1,940 kcal	+330 kcal for exclusive breastfeeding	Good sources of energy include potatoes, bread, rice, pasta or other starchy carbohydrates—choosing whole grains where possible
Protein	45 g	+11 g (56 g in total)	Beans, pulses, fish, eggs, lean meat
Long chain omega 3	140 g (one portion of oily fish per week)	No extra requirement	Salmon, trout, mackerel, sardines
Vitamin A	600 µg	+350 µg	Eggs, cheese, fortified fat spreads, carrots, green leafy vegetables, orange-colored fruits and vegetables

Contd...

Contd...

Nutrient	RNI	Extra during breastfeeding	Examples of food sources
Vitamin B2 (riboflavin)	1.1 mg	+0.5 mg	Milk and milk products, eggs, fortified breakfast cereals, rice, mushrooms
Niacin	13.2 mg	+2.2 mg	Meat, fish, bread, pasta, eggs, milk and milk products
Vitamin B12	1.5 µg	+0.5 µg^c	Meat, fish, milk and milk products, eggs, yeast extract, some fortified breakfast cereals
Folate	200 µg	+60 µg	Green leafy vegetables, fortified breakfast cereals, bread, pulses, some other vegetables (e.g., peas, asparagus), some fruit (e.g., oranges, berries, bananas)
Vitamin C	40 mg	+30 mg	Fruit (e.g., citrus fruits, berries) and vegetables (e.g., peppers, Brussels sprouts)
Vitamin D	10 µg	Everyone, including pregnant and breastfeeding women, should consider taking a daily supplement containing 10 µg of vitamin D	Salmon, trout, mackerel, sardines, eggs, some fortified breakfast cereals, fortified fat spreads
Calcium	700 mg (for girls under 18 years, 800 mg)	+550 mg	Milk and milk products, bread, some vegetables (e.g., kale, okra, rocket), fortified dairy alternatives
Magnesium	270 mg	+50 mg	Some vegetables (e.g., spinach, okra), nuts, whole grains, dried fruit (e.g., apricots)
Iron	14.8 mg	No extra requirement	Red meat, fortified breakfast cereals, pulses, nuts/seeds, dried fruit, whole grain, green leafy vegetables
Selenium	60 µg	+15 µg	Brazil nuts, fish, meat and eggs
Zinc	7.0 mg	+6.0 (1–4 months) +2.5 (4+ months)	Meat, cheese, eggs, shellfish, whole grain cereals, nuts and seeds

WEANING

Weaning is a process by which food other than breast milk is introduced gradually into the baby's diet first to complement the breast milk and then to replace it with thicker feeds. Weaning practices are vulnerable to social pressures. Majority of nutritional problems in rural areas are due to faulty weaning practices.

When to Start

Following guidelines will be useful:
- Child is above 6 month age
- Child weighs 7 kg

What to Give

There are many weaning foods advised and available. Commercially available Farex, Cerelac, etc., have the advantage of palatability, convenience of preparation and fortification with vitamins and minerals. The disadvantage is the cost and improper use. Many mothers add a measure Farex to bottle of milk. This practice defeats the sole purpose of weaning. Mother gets the satisfaction of 'giving Farex' but child does not get the advantage of 'getting Farex'. So Farex should not be used as a drink, it is to be given in form of a paste.

The ideal advice would be to take:
- 2 teaspoon cooked rice,
- 2 teaspoon cooked dal,
- 2 teaspoon cooked vegetables (before adding chilli and spices)
- A piece of roti

Ground it to prepare a paste, such as 'chutni'. It is to be given initially twice a day, then thrice a day and then quantity is increased gradually. For a malnourished or a child above 1 years age still not weaned, 2 teaspoon of groundnut powder and 2 teaspoon of milk powder is to be added. This preparation overcomes the social, cultural, financial and nutritional restraints of successful weaning. There will not be any 'protein gap' or 'food gap'.

As a rule after 1 year, child should be offered full family diet.

Problems of Weaning: Problems with Child

Infections, malnutrition and refusal to accept food are major problems. Proper weaning advice can prevent infections and malnutrition. If a child does not accept food, following are the possibilities:
- As yet he does not know it is a food. Within weeks of starting it, child will develop a liking.
- He does not like taste or appearance of particular preparation.
- Child is being forced or rushed through a feed.
- Food is too hot.
- He wants a drink first.
- He is not hungry.
- He is uncomfortable due to heat, cold or a wet napkid.

☐ He wants his favorite cup or dist (s) He wants to feed himself.

Problem with Parent

Parents just do not know that child needs food. The religious ceremony required for 'Starting food' is many times postponed. Either parents do not get time or there is no motivation to perform the ceremony. Following slogan, if posted in the clinic, helps.

"Starting food ceremony should be performed in sixth months." Breastfeeding exclusively for first six months, timely and adequate supplementation, maintaining breast milk long enough to ensure its replacement by a safe and nutritious diet and discouraging a bottle are therefore extremely important measures to ensure a healthy start in life.

■ COMPLEMENTARY FEEDING

The staple cereal of the family should be used to make the first food for an infant. Porridge can be made with suji (semolina), broken wheat, atta (wheat flour) ground rice, ragi, millet, etc., by using a little water or milk, if available. Roasted flour of any cereal can be mixed with boiled water, sugar and a little fat to make the first complementary food for the baby and could be started after completion of 6 months of age.

☐ Adding sugar or jaggery and ghee or oil is important as it increases the energy value of the food. In the beginning, the porridge could be made a little thinner but as the child grows older the consistency has to be thicker.
☐ A thick porridge is more nutritious than a thin one. In case a family cannot prepare the porridge for the infant separately, pieces of half chapati could be soaked in half a cup of milk or boiled water, mashed properly and fed to the baby after adding sugar and fat.
☐ Soaked and mashed chapati could be passed through a sieve so as to get a soft semi-solid food for the infant.
☐ Fruits, such as banana, papaya, chikoo, mango, etc., could be given at this age in a mashed form. Infants could also be given reconstituted instant infant foods at this age.

Box 8.8 is depicted the infant's nutritional needs.

> **Box 8.8:** Infant's nutritional needs.
>
> ☐ Ensuring that infant's nutritional needs are met requires that complementary foods be:
> • Timely—meaning that they are introduced when the need for energy and nutrients exceeds what can be provided through exclusive breastfeeding
> • Adequate—meaning that they provide sufficient energy, protein and micronutrients to meet a growing child are nutritional needs
> • Safe—meaning that they are hygienically stored and prepared, and fed with clean hands using clean utensils and not bottles and teats
> • Properly fed—meaning that they are given consistent with a child's signals of appetite and satiety, and that meal frequency and feeding are suitable for age

Traditional Foods for Infants

☐ Once the child is eating cereal porridge well, mixed foods including cooked cereal, pulse and vegetable(s) could be given.
☐ Most traditional foods given to infants in different parts of the country are examples of mixed foods, such as khichidi, dalia, suji kheer, upma, idli, dokhla, bhaat-bhaji.
☐ Sometimes, traditional foods are given after a little modification so as to make the food more suitable for the child. For instance, mashed idli with a little oil and sugar is a good complementary food for the infant.
☐ Similarly bhaat can be made more nutritious by adding some cooked dal or vegetable to it. Khichidi can be made more nutritious by adding one or two vegetables in it while cooking.

Modified Family Food

☐ In most families, there is a cereal preparation in the form of roti or rice and a pulse or a vegetable preparation. For preparing a complementary food for the infant from the foods cooked for the family, a small amount of dal or vegetable preparation should be separated before adding spices to it.
☐ Pieces of chapatti could be soaked in half a katori of dal and some vegetable, if available.
☐ The mixed food could be mashed well and fed to the baby after adding a little oil. If necessary the mixture could be passed through a sieve to get a semi-solid paste. Thus, rice or wheat preparation could be mixed with pulse and/or vegetable to make a nutritious complementary food for the infant.
☐ Modifying your family's food is one of the most effective ways of ensuring complementary feeding of infants.

Instant Infant Foods

☐ Infant food mixes can be made at home from food grains available in the household. These mixes can be stored for at least a month and enable frequent feeding of infants.
☐ These are sattu-like preparations which are quite familiar in the Indian community. Take three parts of any cereal (rice/wheat) or millet (ragi, bajra jowar), one part of any pulse (moong/channa/arhar) and half part of groundnuts or white til, if available.
☐ The food items should be roasted separately, ground, mixed properly and stored in airtight containers.
☐ For feeding, take two tablespoons of this infant food mix, add boiled hot water or milk, sugar or jaggery and oil/ghee and mix well.
☐ Cooked and mashed carrot, pumpkin or green leafy vegetables could be added to the porridge, if available.
☐ The infant can be fed with this food whenever freshly cooked food is not available in the family.
☐ The infant food mix could also be made into preparations like halwa, burfi, upma, dalia, and given to the child.

Protective Foods

☐ Besides modified family food and reconstituted infant food mixes, protective foods, such as milk, curd, lassi, egg,

fish and fruits and vegetables are also important to help in the healthy growth of infants.
- Green leafy vegetables, carrots, pumpkin and seasonal fruits, such as papaya, mango, chikoo, banana, are important to ensure good vitamin A and iron status of the child.
- Baby needs all foods after completion of 6 months of age namely cereals, pulses, vegetables.
- Particularly green leafy vegetables, fruits, milk and milk products, egg, meat and fish if non-vegetarian, oil/ghee, sugar and iodized salt in addition to breastfeeding.
- In addition to breastfeeding, a diversified diet will also improve the micronutrients status of the child.

Energy Density of Infant Foods
- Low 'energy density' complementary foods given to young children and the low frequency of feeding can result in an inadequate intake of calories.
- Most of the foods are bulky and a child cannot eat more at a time. Hence, it is important to give small energy dense feeds at frequent intervals with a view to ensure adequate energy intake by the child.

Energy density in foods given to infants and young children can be increased in four different ways:
1. **By adding a teaspoonful of oil or ghee to the child's food:** Fat is a concentrated source of energy and substantially increases energy content of food without increasing the bulk. There is no reason to feel that a child cannot digest visible fat when added to food.
2. **By adding a teaspoonful of sugar or jaggery to the child's food:** Children need more energy and hence adequate amounts of sugar or jaggery can be added to their food.
3. **By giving malted foods:** Malting reduces the viscosity of foods and hence a child can eat more at a time. Malting is germinating whole grain cereals or pulses, drying it after germination and grinding. Infant food mixes prepared after malting the cereal or pulse will provide more energy. Flours of malted food when mixed with other foods help in reducing the viscosity of that food. Amylase Rich Flour (ARF) is the scientific name given to flours of malted foods and must be utilized in infant foods.
4. **By feeding thick but smooth mixtures:** Thin gruels do not provide enough energy. A young infant particularly during 6–9 months requires thick but smooth mixtures as hard pieces in the semi-solid food may cause difficulty if swallowed. Semi-solid foods for young infants can be passed through a sieve by pressing with a ladle to ensure that the mixed food is smooth and uniform without any big pieces or lumps.

CONCLUSION
A balanced diet includes foods from five groups and fulfills all of a person's nutritional needs. Eating a balanced diet helps people maintain good health and reduce their risk of disease. A balanced diet is one which provides all the nutrients in required amounts and proper proportions. It can easily be achieved through a blend of the four basic food groups. The quantities of foods needed to meet the nutrient requirements vary with age, gender, physiological status and physical activity. A balanced diet should provide around 50–60% of total calories from carbohydrates, preferably from complex carbohydrates, about 10–15% from proteins and 20–30% from both visible and invisible fat. Requirements are the quantities of nutrients that healthy individuals must obtain from food to meet their physiological needs. The recommended dietary allowances (RDAs) are estimates of nutrients to be consumed daily to ensure the requirements of all individuals in a given population. The recommended level depends upon the bioavailability of nutrients from a given diet. The term bioavailability indicates what is absorbed and utilized by the body.

BIBLIOGRAPHY
1. ICMR. Nutrient requirements and recommended dietary allowances for Indians. A report of the expert group of the Indian Council of Medical Research, National Institute of Nutrition, Hyderabad, India, 2010.
2. ICMR Dietary guidelines for Indians- A Manual. National Institute of Nutrition, Hyderabad, India, 2003.
3. Nair KM, Augustine LF. Basis of current allowances of nutrients in food fortification in India. Bull Nutr Foundation, India. 2016;37(3):1-5.
4. Nair KM, Augustine LF. Country specific nutrient requirements & recommended dietary allowances for Indians: Current status & future directions. Indian J Med Res. 2018;148:52230.
5. Nair KM, Augustine LF. Food synergies for improving bioavailability of micronutrients from plant foods. Food Chem. 2018;238:180-5.
6. Nutrition Advisory Committee of the Indian Research Fund Association (IRFA). A report of the twelfth meeting. New Delhi, India, 1944.
7. Rao BSN. Nutrient requirement and safe dietary intake for Indians. Bull Nutr Foundation India. 2010;31:1-5.

REVIEW QUESTIONS

Long Essays
1. Define balanced diet. What are the factors you would consider while planning a diet?
2. What is balanced diet? How do you plan a balanced diet for a pregnant woman?
3. What is therapeutic diet? What are the modifications in diet? Plan a menu for a diabetic person.
4. What are weaning foods? Explain the principles of weaning foods. What are the advantages of breastfeeding?
5. What is menu planning? Discuss in detail the steps involved in planning a menu.
6. Define therapeutic diets. Explain therapeutic diet for cardiovascular disease.
7. Write a detailed account of nutritive values of all food groups.
8. Write a detailed account of balanced diet and factors affecting it.
9. Discuss the nutritional requirements during pregnancy and lactation.
10. What are the concepts of a balanced diet? Discuss steps you would consider while planning a diet for an expectant mother.
11. Explain the nutritional requirements during Infancy.
12. Explain the nutritional requirements in old age and plan menu for them.

13. What is balanced diet? Discuss steps that you consider while planning for 70 years person.
14. Define diet plan. Describe the role of a nurse in planning a diet for an adult.
15. What is the calorie requirement of preschools? Prepare a diet plan for the preschools to meet the requirements.
16. What is the calorie requirement of schools age child? Prepare a diet plan for a 5-year-old school child.
17. Define balanced diet. Discuss the importance of balanced diet.
18. Discus the principles and points to be considered while planning balanced diet.
19. Discuss the dietary goals and guidelines for calculating individual nutrients.
20. Discuss the nutritional requirements of infant. Discuss various principles of weaning.
21. Explain various factors to be considered while planning balanced diet.
22. Define menu planning. Mention the principles of meal planning.
23. What is therapeutic diet? Enumerate various principles of therapeutic diet.
24. Enumerate different types of therapeutic diet and use of naturopathy diet in maintaining health.

Short Essays

1. What are the different food groups?
2. Define exclusive breastfeeding and advantages of breastfeeding.
3. Define weaning and explain the principles of weaning.
4. What is colostrum? Explain the advantages of breastfeeding.
5. How does economic status and food budget of the family affect menu planning?
6. Define diet consistency. Classify diets based on consistency.
7. Discuss various special feeding methods.
8. Explain role of nurse in balanced diet.
9. What are the factors affecting menu planning?
10. Prepare diet plan for a schooler.
11. What are objectives of planning a menu to an infant?
12. What are factors promoting adequate supply of breast milk?
13. What are the reasons for weaning of infants?
14. Define balanced diet.
15. Define weaning.
16. Diet for elderly.
17. Explain nurses role in importance of breastfeeding.
18. Importance's of breastfeeding.
19. Chemical composition of milk.
20. Explain the nutritional needs of teenagers
21. What are calcium requirements for a pregnant and lactating woman?
22. Precaution of introduction of weaning diet.
23. Define exclusive breastfeeding.

Short Answers

1. What is food pyramid?
2. Explain 5 food group systems.
3. Explain 11 food group systems.
4. Fruits and vegetables.
5. Cereals.
6. Pulses.
7. What is composition of milk?
8. Colostrum.
9. Explain naturopathy diet.
10. What is soft diet?
11. What is bland diet?
12. Explain intravenous feeding.
13. Explain tube feeding.
14. What are clear fluids?
15. What is liquid diet?
16. Breast milk.
17. Exclusive breastfeeding.
18. What is semisolid diet?
19. What are supplementary and complementary feeds?
20. What is beverage?
21. Mention the uses of iodized salt.
22. What is light diet?
23. What is protein diet?

CHAPTER 9

Nutritional Deficiency Disorders

CHAPTER OUTLINE

- **Protein-energy Malnutrition:** Magnitude of the Problem, Causes, Classification, Signs and Symptoms, Severe Acute Malnutrition (SAM), Management and Prevention and Nurses' Role
- **Childhood Obesity:** Signs and Symptoms, Assessment, Management and Prevention and Nurses' Role
- **Vitamin Deficiency Disorders:** Vitamin A, B, C and D Deficiency Disorders—Causes, Signs and Symptoms, Management and Prevention and Nurses' Role
- **Mineral Deficiency Diseases:** Iron, Iodine and Calcium Deficiencies—Causes, Signs and Symptoms, Management and Prevention and Nurses' Role

TERMINOLOGY

- **Protein-energy malnutrition** or PEM is the condition of lack of energy due to the deficiency of all the macronutrients and many micronutrients. It can occur suddenly or gradually. It can be graded as mild, moderate or severe.
- **Marasmic kwashiorkor:** Marked protein deficiency and marked calorie insufficiency signs present, sometimes referred to as the most severe form of malnutrition.
- **Electrolytes:** Salts and minerals that produce electrically charged particles (ions) in body fluids. Common human electrolytes are sodium chloride, potassium, calcium, and sodium bicarbonate. Electrolytes control the fluid balance of the body and are important in muscle contraction, energy generation, and almost all major biochemical reactions in the body.
- **Nutrient:** Substances in food that supply the body with the elements needed for metabolism. Examples of nutrients are vitamins, minerals, carbohydrates, fats, and proteins.
- **Osteoporosis:** Literally meaning "porous bones," this condition occurs when bones lose an excessive amount of their protein and mineral content, particularly calcium. Over time, bone mass and strength are reduced leading to increased risk of fractures.

PROTEIN-ENERGY MALNUTRITION

Protein-energy undernutrition (PEU), previously called protein-energy malnutrition, is an energy deficit due to deficiency of all macronutrients. It commonly includes deficiencies of many micronutrients. PEU can be sudden and total (starvation) or gradual. Severity ranges from subclinical deficiencies to obvious wasting (with edema, hair loss, and skin atrophy) to starvation. Multiple organ systems are often impaired. Diagnosis usually involves laboratory testing, including serum albumin. Treatment consists of correcting fluid and electrolyte deficits with IV solutions, then gradually replenishing nutrients, orally if possible.

Definition: Protein-energy malnutrition (PEM) is a potentially fatal body-depletion disorder. It is the leading cause of death in children in developing countries.

Classification and Etiology of PEU

PEU is graded as mild, moderate, or severe. Grade is determined by calculating weight as a percentage of expected weight for length or height using international standards (normal, 90 to 110%; mild PEU, 85 to 90%; moderate, 75 to 85%; severe, <75%).

PEU may be:
1. **Primary:** Caused by inadequate nutrient intake
2. **Secondary:** Results from disorders or drugs that interfere with nutrient use

Figure 9.1 is depicted the protein-energy malnutrition.

Primary PEU

Worldwide, primary PEU occurs mostly in children and older people who lack access to nutrients; although a common

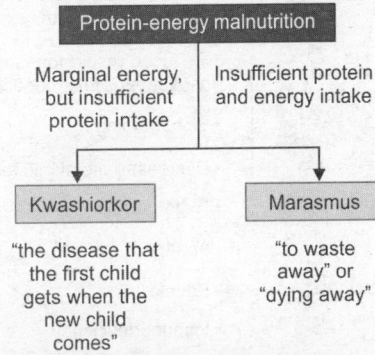

Fig. 9.1: Protein-energy malnutrition.

cause in older people is depression. PEU can also result from fasting or anorexia nervosa. Child or elder abuse may be a cause. In children, chronic primary PEU has 2 common forms:
1. Marasmus
2. Kwashiorkor

The form depends on the balance of nonprotein and protein sources of energy. Starvation is an acute severe form of primary PEU.
1. **Marasmus** (also called the dry form of PEU) causes weight loss and depletion of fat and muscle. In countries with high rates of food insecurity, marasmus is the most common form of PEU in children.
2. **Kwashiorkor** (also called the wet, swollen, or edematous form) is a risk after premature abandonment of breastfeeding, which typically occurs when a younger sibling is born, displacing the older child from the breast. So children with kwashiorkor tend to be older than those with marasmus.

Secondary PEU
This type most commonly results from the following:
1. **Disorders that affect gastrointestinal function:** These disorders can interfere with digestion (e.g., pancreatic insufficiency), absorption (e.g., enteritis, enteropathy), or lymphatic transport of nutrients (e.g., retroperitoneal fibrosis, Milroy disease).
2. **Wasting disorders:** In wasting disorders [e.g., AIDS, cancer, chronic obstructive pulmonary disease (COPD)] and renal failure, catabolism causes cytokine excess, resulting in undernutrition via anorexia and cachexia (wasting of muscle and fat). End-stage heart failure can cause cardiac cachexia, a severe form of undernutrition; mortality rate is particularly high. Factors contributing to cardiac cachexia may include passive hepatic congestion (causing anorexia), edema of the intestinal tract (impairing absorption), and, in advanced disease, increased oxygen requirement due to anaerobic metabolism. Wasting disorders can decrease appetite or impair metabolism of nutrients.

3. **Conditions that increase metabolic demands:** These conditions include infections, hyperthyroidism, pheochromocytoma, other endocrine disorders, burns, trauma, surgery, and other critical illnesses.

Figure 9.2 is depicted the clinical manifestations of PEM and **Table 9.1** is depicted the clinical signs of malnutrition.

Pathophysiology of PEU
- The initial metabolic response of PEU is decreased metabolic rate. To supply energy, the body first breaks down adipose tissue. However, later, when these tissues are depleted, the body may use protein for energy, resulting in a negative nitrogen balance.
- Visceral organs and muscle are broken down and decrease in weight. Loss of organ weight is greatest in the liver and intestine, intermediate in the heart and kidneys, and least in the nervous system.

Table 9.2 is depicted the difference between marasmus and kwashiorkor.

Clinical Features of Protein-energy Malnutrition
Early signs of protein-energy malnutrition in children include weight loss or poor weight gain, slowing of linear growth, fatigue, apathy at rest, and irritability when disturbed. Weight loss in adults may be masked by edema.

Table 9.1: Clinical signs of malnutrition.

Site	Signs
Face	Moon face (kwashiorkor), simian facies (marasmus)
Eye	Dry eyes, pale conjunctiva, Bitot's spots (vitamin A), periorbital edema
Mouth	Angular stomatitis, cheilitis, glossitis, spongy bleeding gums (vitamin C), parotid enlargement
Teeth	Enamel mottling, delayed eruption
Hair	Dull, sparse, brittle hair, hypopigmentation, flag sign (alternating bands of light and normal color), broomstick eyelashes, alopecia
Skin	Loose and wrinkled (marasmus), shiny and edematous (kwashiorkor), dry, follicular hyperkeratosis, patchy hyper- and hypopigmentation (crazy paving or flaky paint dermatoses), erosions, poor wound healing
Nail	Koilonychia, thin and soft nail plates, fissures or ridges
Musculature	Muscle wasting particularly buttocks and thighs. Chvostek or Trousseau signs (hypocalcemia)
Skeletal	Deformities usually a result of calcium, vitamin D or vitamin C deficiencies
Abdomen	Distended-hepatomegaly with fatty liver; ascites may be present
Cardiovascular	Bradycardia, hypotension, reduced cardiac output, small vessel vasculopathy
Neurologic	Global developmental delay, loss of knee and ankle reflexes, impaired memory
Hematological	Pallor, petechiae, bleeding diathesis
Behavior	Lethargic, apathetic, irritable on handling

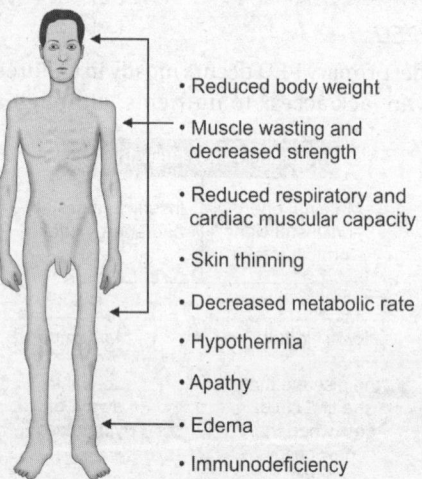

- Reduced body weight
- Muscle wasting and decreased strength
- Reduced respiratory and cardiac muscular capacity
- Skin thinning
- Decreased metabolic rate
- Hypothermia
- Apathy
- Edema
- Immunodeficiency

Fig. 9.2: Clinical manifestations of PEM.

Table 9.2: Difference between marasmus and kwashiorkor.

	Marasmus	Kwashiorkor
Welcome trust definition	<60% without edema stunting + wasting below 3rd centile	60–80% with edema
Physiological state	Catabolism	Very low anabolism
Theory		
Classical	Low energy → Fat and muscle wasting	Low protein → low oncotic pressure → edema
Gopalan's (Theory of dysadaptability)	Chronic adaptation to starvation	Inability to adapt to nutritional stress → edema and epithelial damage
Golden's theory (free radical imbalance)	Imbalance between production and disposal of free radical	Inability to produce protein
Signs and symptoms		
Appearance	Old man/monkey facies; Baggy pant appearance	Moon face appearance; Puffy sugar boy appearance
Age	Infants	1–5 years
Prevalance	More common	Less common
Limbs	Wasted Subcutaneous tissue emaciated	Wasted but masked by edema; Weak hypotonic limbs
Skin and hair	Hypopigmented hair and dry scaly skin	Flaky paint skin; Flag sign (alteranting hypo and hyper pigmentation of hair)
Abdomen	Distended but not ascetic	Hepatomegaly (fatty liver); Petechial rashes (liver damage, low clotting factor)
Infection	Low	High
Mental status	Alert	Apathetic and irritable
Appetite	Good	Poor
Others		
Serum albumin globulin ratio	Low	Very low
Response to treatment	Good	Poor

With time, loss of subcutaneous fat becomes prominent, muscle mass decreases, skin and hair become dry and fragile, bones protrude, and wound healing is impaired.

Symptoms of Protein-energy Malnutrition

The symptoms of protein-energy malnutrition or PEM are as follows:
- Apathy and irritability
- The patient becomes weak and inefficient
- Impaired cognition and consciousness
- Temporary lactose deficiency
- Diarrhea
- Gonadal tissues atrophy
- Causes amenorrhea in women
- Causes libido in both men and women
- Weight loss
- Shrinking of muscles
- Protrusion of bones
- The skin gets thin, pale, dry, inelastic and cold
- Hair fall
- Impaired wound healing
- Risk of hip fractures and ulcers increases in elderly patients
- Heart size and cardiac output decreases in severe cases
- A decrease in respiratory rate and vital capacity
- Liver, kidney or heart failure
- Acute PEM might also prove fatal

Clinical Features of Marasmus
- Dry loose wrinkled skin
- Marked loss of subcutaneous fat and muscle wasting
- Triangular 'monkey' face due to loss of fat pads in the cheeks

Clinical Features of Kwashiorkor
- Edema—peripheral and facial
- Moon 'bulldog' face
- Pot belly due to abdominal muscle wasting
- Skin, hair, and nail changes
  - *'Flaky paint skin'*: Dark, dry skin which splits when stretched or peels to leave pale areas; begins in friction sites such as the groin, behind the knees, buttocks, and elbows; if severe can affect any skin site; 'dermatosis of kwashior'
  - *Hair:* Red-yellow to gray-white scalp hair; dry, brittle, sparse or lost, decurled, easily pluckable; alternating transverse pale bands in dark hair ('hair flag sign') due to alternating periods of adequate- and under-nutrition.

Diagnosis
When the physician suspects PEM, A thorough physical examination is performed, and these areas assessed:
- Eating habits and weight changes
- Body-fat composition and muscle strength
- Gastrointestinal symptoms
- Presence of underlying illness
- Developmental delays and loss of acquired milestones in children
- Nutritional status

Doctors further quantify a patient's nutritional status by:
- Comparing height and weight to standardized norms
- Calculating body mass index (BMI)
- Measuring skin fold thickness or the circumference of the upper arm

Treatment
- Treatment is designed to provide adequate **nutrition** restore normal body composition, and cure the condition that caused the deficiency.

- Tube feeding or intravenous feeding is used to supply nutrients to patients who cannot or will not eat protein-rich foods.
- In patients with severe PEM, the first stage of treatment consists of correcting fluid and electrolyte imbalances, treating infection with **antibiotics** that do not affect protein synthesis, and addressing related medical problems.
- The second phase involves replenishing essential nutrients slowly to prevent taxing the patient's weakened system with more food than it can handle.
- Physical therapy may benefit patients whose muscles have deteriorated significantly.

Prognosis
- Most children can lose some of their body weight without side effects, but losing more than 40% is usually fatal.
- Death usually results from heart failure, an electrolyte imbalance, or low body temperature. Patients with certain symptoms, including semiconsciousness, persistent diarrhea, jaundice and low blood sodium levels, have a poorer prognosis than other patients.
- Recovery from marasmus usually takes longer than recovery from kwashiorkor.
- The long-term effects of childhood malnutrition are uncertain. Some children recover completely, while others may have a variety of lifelong impairments, including an inability to properly absorb nutrients in the intestines, as well as mental retardation.
- The outcome appears to be related to the length and severity of the malnutrition, as well as to the age of the child when the malnutrition occurred.

Prevention
- Breastfeeding a baby for at least six months is considered the best way to prevent early-childhood malnutrition. Talking to a doctor before putting a child on any kind of diet, such as vegan, vegetarian, or low-carbohydrate, can help assure that the child gets the full supply of nutrients that he or she needs.
- Every child being admitted to a hospital should be screened for the presence of illnesses and conditions that could lead to PEM.
- The nutritional status of patients at higher-than-average risk should be more thoroughly assessed and periodically reevaluated during extended hospital stays.

SEVERE ACUTE MALNUTRITION

Severe acute malnutrition (SAM) is caused by a significant imbalance between nutritional intake and individual needs. It is most often caused by both quantitative (number of kilocalories/day) and qualitative (vitamins and minerals, etc.) deficiencies.

Figure 9.3 is depicted the clinical forms of acute malnutrition.

Children Over 6 months of Age

The two principal forms of SAM are:
1. **Marasmus:** Significant loss of muscle mass and subcutaneous fat, resulting in a skeletal appearance.
2. **Kwashiorkor:** Bilateral edema of the lower limbs/edema of the face, often associated with cutaneous signs (shiny or cracked skin, burn-like appearance; discolored and brittle hair).

The two forms may be associated (marasmic-kwashiorkor).
1. In addition to these characteristic signs, SAM is accompanied by significant physiopathological disorders (metabolic disturbances, anemia, compromised immunity, leading to susceptibility to infections often difficult to diagnose, etc.).
2. Complications are frequent and potentially life-threatening.
3. Mortality rates may be elevated in the absence of appropriate medical management.

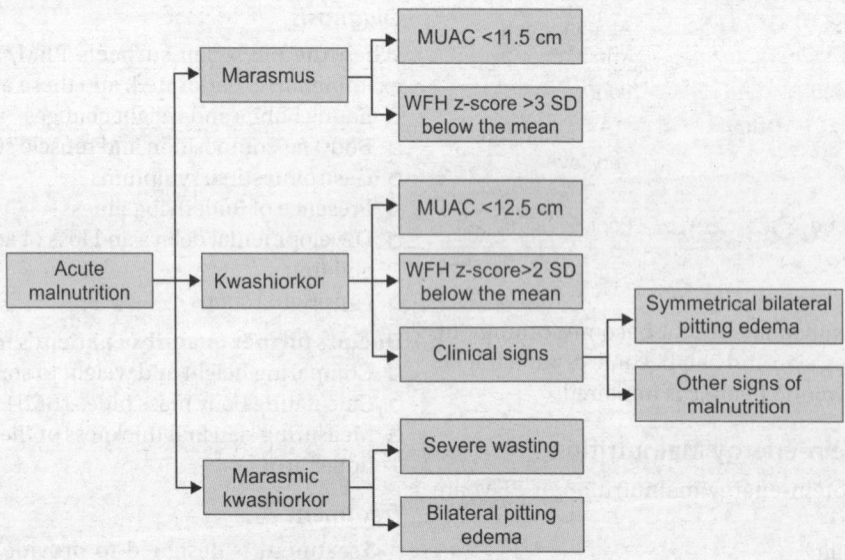

Fig. 9.3: Clinical forms of acute malnutrition.
(MUAC: mid-upper-arm circumference; WFH: weight for height; SD: standard deviation)

4. Admission and discharge criteria for treatment programs for SAM are both anthropometric and clinical:
   - Mid-upper arm circumference (MUAC) is the circumference, measured in mid-position, of the relaxed left upper arm, taken in children of 6 to 59 months (65 to 110 cm in height). MUAC measures the degree of muscle wasting. A MUAC of <115 mm indicates SAM and significant mortality risk.
   - Weight for height (W/H) index assesses the degree of weight loss by comparing the weight of the SAM child with non-malnourished children of the same height. Severe malnutrition is defined as a W/H index of < − 3 Z-score with reference to the new WHO child growth standards
   - The presence of bilateral edema of the lower limbs (when other causes of edema have been ruled out) indicates SAM, regardless of the MUAC and W/H.
5. Usual admission criteria are—MUAC <115 mm (MUAC is not used as an admission criterion in children older than 59 months or taller than 110 cm) or W/H < −3 Z or presence of bilateral edema of the lower limbs.
6. Usual discharge (cure) criteria are—W/H > −2 Z and absence of bilateral edema (2 consecutive assessments, one week apart) and absence of acute medical problems.
7. Medical management (hospitalization or ambulatory care) is based on the presence or absence of associated serious complications:
   - Children exhibiting anorexia, or significant medical complications, such as severe anemia, severe dehydration or severe infection (complicated acute malnutrition) should be hospitalized
   - Children without significant medical complications (uncomplicated acute malnutrition) may undergo treatment on an ambulatory basis, with weekly medical follow-up.

Figure 9.4 is depicted the acute nutrition.

Treatment

Nutritional treatment

Nutritional treatment is based on the use of therapeutic foods enriched with vitamins and minerals:

Therapeutic milks (for use exclusively in hospitalized patients):

- F-75 therapeutic milk, low in protein, sodium and calories (0.9 g of protein and 75 kcal per 100 mL) is used in the initial phase of treatment for patients suffering from complicated SAM. It is used to cover basic needs while complications are being treated. It is given in 8 daily meals.
- F-100 therapeutic milk, in which the concentration of protein and calories is higher (2.9 g of protein and 100 kcal per 100 mL), replaces F-75 after several days, once the patient is stabilized (return of appetite, clinical improvement; disappearance or reduction of edema). The objective is to facilitate rapid weight gain. It can be given with, or be replaced by, RUTF.
- RUTF (ready-to-use therapeutic food), i.e., foods which are ready for consumption (for example, peanut paste enriched with milk solids, such as Plumpy'nut®), are used in children treated in both hospital and ambulatory settings.
- The nutritional composition of RUTF is similar to F-100, but the iron content is higher. It is designed to promote rapid weight gain (approximately 500 kcal per 100 g). RUTF are the only therapeutic foods which can be used in ambulatory treatment.
- Furthermore, it is important to give drinking water, in addition to meals, especially if the ambient temperature is high or the child has a fever.

Breastfeeding should continue in children of the appropriate age.

Figure 9.5 is depicted the clinical features of malnutrition.

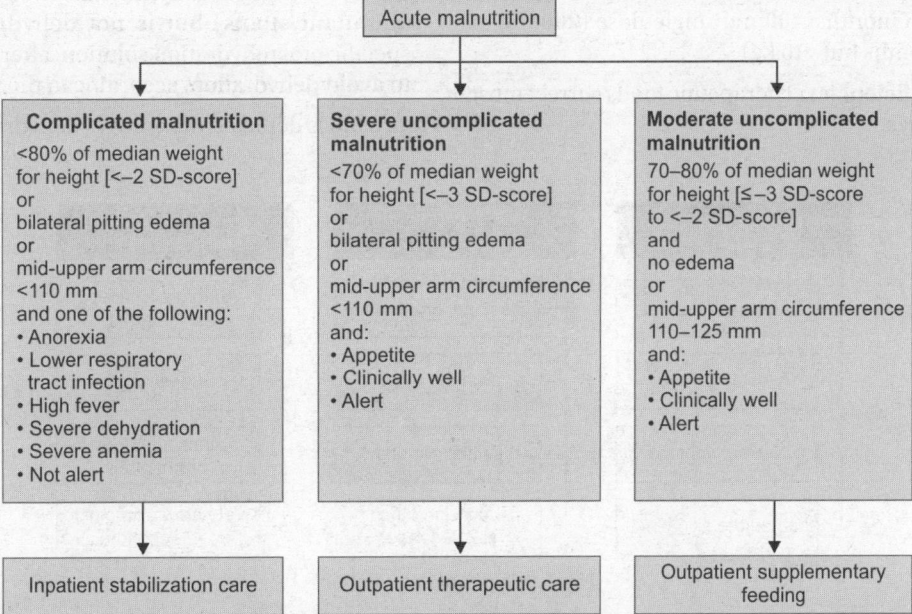

Fig. 9.4: Acute nutrition.

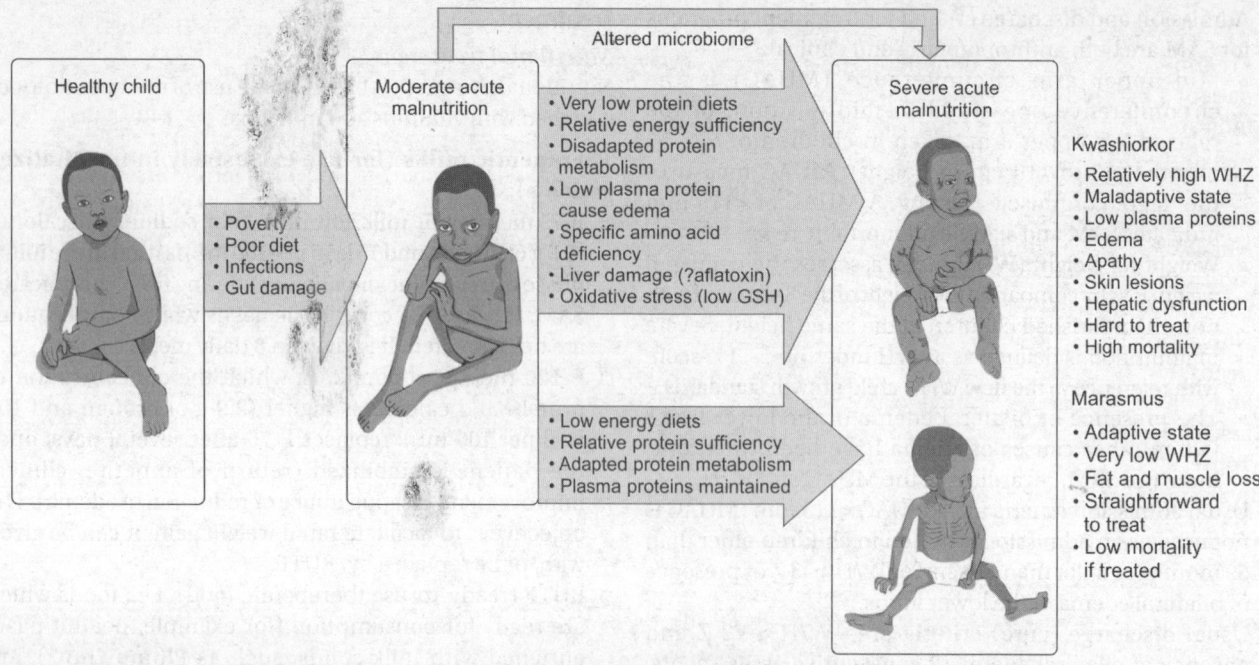

Fig. 9.5: Clinical features of malnutrition.

Routine Medical Treatment

In the absence of specific medical complications, the following routine treatments should be implemented in both ambulatory and hospital settings:

Infections

- Measles vaccination on admission.
- Broad spectrum antibiotherapy starting on D1 (**amoxicillin** PO: 50 mg/kg 2 times daily for 5 days).
- **In endemic malaria areas:** Rapid test on D1, with treatment in accordance with results. If testing is not available, give malaria treatment.
- **Treatment for intestinal worms on D8:** Albendazole PO children >6 months: 400 mg single dose (200 mg in children >6 months but <10 kg)

Micronutrient deficiencies: Therapeutic foods correct most of these deficiencies.

Management of Common Complications

Diarrhea and dehydration

- Diarrhea is common in malnourished children. Therapeutic foods facilitate the recovery of gastrointestinal mucosa and restore the production of gastric acid, digestive enzymes and bile.
- Amoxicillin, administered as part of routine treatment, is effective in reducing bacterial load. Diarrhea generally resolves without any additional treatment.
- Watery diarrhea is sometimes related to another pathology (otitis, pneumonia, malaria, etc.), which should be considered.
- If a child has a significant diarrhea (very frequent or abundant stools) but is not dehydrated, administer specific oral rehydration solution, after each watery stool, to avoid dehydration, according to the WHO.

Figure 9.6 is depicted the types of dehydration.

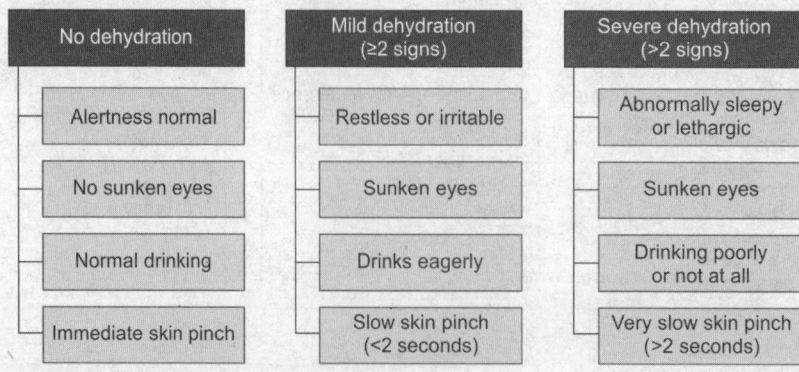

Fig. 9.6: Types of dehydration.

Nurses role to Treat Malnourished Patients

- Treatment options vary depending on the cause of a patient's malnutrition. The severity of malnourishment indicates whether patients should be treated in a hospital or at home.
- The primary treatment for patients who can eat on their own is to make dietary changes.
- Nurses educate patients about the nutritional content of food and how to make healthy choices. If patients will not or cannot eat, nurses may need to feed them intravenously.
- Nurses have a responsibility to address patient nutritional needs by conducting screenings, performing assessments and administering interventions. But, malnutrition is not just a problem for patients.

Table 9.3 is depicted the signs and management of dehydration.

Table 9.3: Signs and management of dehydration.

Signs	Classify as	Identify treatment (urgent pre-refferal treatments are in bold)
Two of the following signs: • Lethargic or unconscious • Sunken eyes • Not able to drink or drinking poorly • Skin pinch goes back very slowly	Severe dehydration	• **If child has no other severe classification:** Give fluid for severe dehydration (Plan C) Or • **If child also has another severe classification:** Refer urgently to hospital with mother giving frequent sips of ORS on the way. Advise the mother to continue breastfeeding • If child is 2 years or older, and there is cholera in your area, give antibiotic for cholera
Two of the following signs: • Restless, irritable • Sunken eyes • Drinks eagerly, thirsty • Skin pinch goes back slowly	Some dehydration	• Give fluid, zinc supplements and food for some dehydration (Plan B) • **If child also has a severe classification:** Refer urgently to hospital with mother giving frequent sips of ORS on the way. Advise the mother to continue breastfeeding • Advise mother when to return immediately • Follow-up in 5 days if not improving • If confirmed/symptomatic HIV, follow-up in 2 days if not improving
• Not enough signs to classify as some or severe dehydration	No dehydration	• Give fluid, zinc supplements and food to treat diarrhea at home (Plan A) • Advise mother when to return immediately • Follow-up in 5 days if not improving • If confirmed/symptomatic HIV, follow-up in 2 days if not improving

Direct nutrition interventions: All can be provided by health workers interventions that encourage changes in behavior to improve nutrition:
- Promote breastfeeding for newborns within one hour of delivery
- Promote exclusive breastfeeding for the first 6 months
- Promote a good complementary diet for children aged 6 to 24 months
- Encourage hand washing or other interventions for good hygiene.

For infants and children:
- Increase the intake of zinc by giving supplements,
- Give zinc to treat diarrhea
- Give vitamin A supplements every six months
- Use iodized salt in food for children >2 years and mothers

For pregnant or breastfeeding mothers:
- Improve nutrient intake by taking multiple micronutrients supplements
- Providing iodine through iodization of salt
- Provide iron and folate supplements
- Provide calcium supplements

Therapeutic feeding interventions: Treat children with severe acute malnutrition using special foods

CHILDHOOD OBESITY

Childhood obesity is now an epidemic in India. With 14.4 million obese children, India has the second-highest number of obese children in the world, next to China. The prevalence of overweight and obesity in children is 15%. In private schools catering to upper-income families, the incidence has shot up to 35–40%, indicating a worrying upward trend.

Figure 9.7 is depicted the childhood obesity medical complications.

Definition

Childhood obesity is a serious medical condition that affects children and adolescents. It is particularly troubling because the extra pounds often start children on the path to health problems that were once considered adult problems—diabetes, high blood pressure and high cholesterol. Childhood obesity can also lead to poor self-esteem and depression.

Causes of Childhood Obesity (Fig. 9.8)

The fundamental cause of childhood obesity is an imbalance between calories consumed and energy spent. Indians are genetically predisposed to obesity. However, the rapid increase in childhood obesity is largely due to environmental influences. Economic prosperity leads to a change in diet from traditional to 'modern' foods, rich in fat and sugar. Urbanization leads to an increase in sedentary lifestyles and a decline in physical activity.

Reasons why more and more children are becoming obese include:
- **Behavioral factors:** Eating bigger portions, eating foods that are calorie-rich but nutrient poor (junk foods), spending lots of time in front of the television or computer, and spending too little time doing physical activities

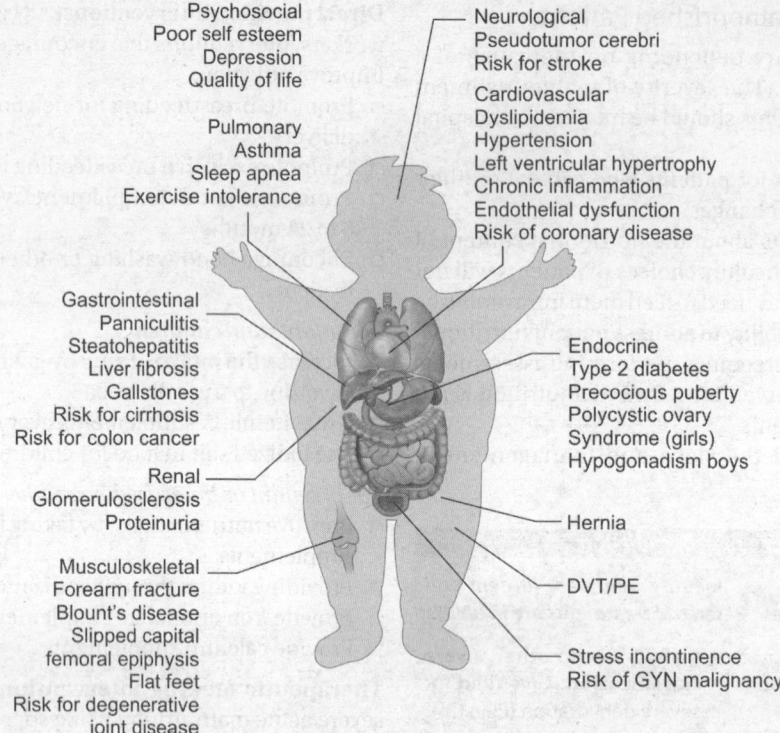

Fig. 9.7: Childhood obesity medical complications.

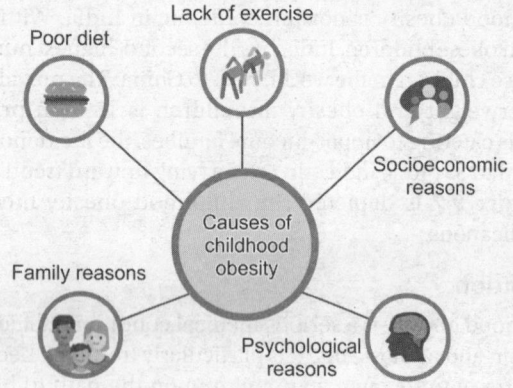

Fig. 9.8: Causes of childhood obesity.

- **Environmental factors:** Easy access to high-calorie junk foods, few opportunities for physical activity, lack of parks and playgrounds in some communities
- **Genetic factors:** A child is at increased risk for obesity when at least one parent is obese. However, genes do not necessarily mean a child is destined to be overweight—there are several steps a child can take to lower his risk.
- **Medications:** Steroids, some antidepressants, and others
- **Medical conditions:** Genetic syndromes, such as Prader-Willi, and hormonal conditions, such as hypothyroidism are among the medical disorders that can cause obesity.

The "body weight set point theory" suggests that weight is determined by complex interactions of genetic, hormonal, and metabolic factors.

Symptoms of Childhood Obesity

Each child may experience different symptoms but some of the most common include:

- **Appearance:** Stretch marks on hips and abdomen; dark, velvety skin (known as acanthosis nigricans) around the neck and in other areas; fatty tissue deposition in breast area (an especially troublesome issue for boys).
- **Psychological:** Teasing and abuse; poor self-esteem; eating disorders
- **Pulmonary:** Shortness of breath when physically active; sleep apnea
- **Gastroenterological:** Constipation, gastroesophageal reflux
- **Reproductive:** Early puberty and irregular menstrual cycles in girls; delayed puberty in boys; genitals may appear disproportionately small in males
- **Orthopedic:** Flat feet; knock knees; dislocated hip

Health Implication of Childhood Obesity

- Childhood obesity has serious health implications. Obese children are at increased risk of hypertension, osteoarthritis, high cholesterol and triglycerides, Type 2 diabetes, coronary heart disease, stroke, gallbladder disease, respiratory problems, emotional disturbances, and some cancers.
- Two in three obese children will remain obese as adults and at risk for adult lifestyle diseases. India is projected to become the diabetes capital in the world.

Complications

Childhood obesity often causes complications in a child's physical, social and emotional well-being (**Fig. 9.9**).

Physical Complications

Physical complications of childhood obesity may include:

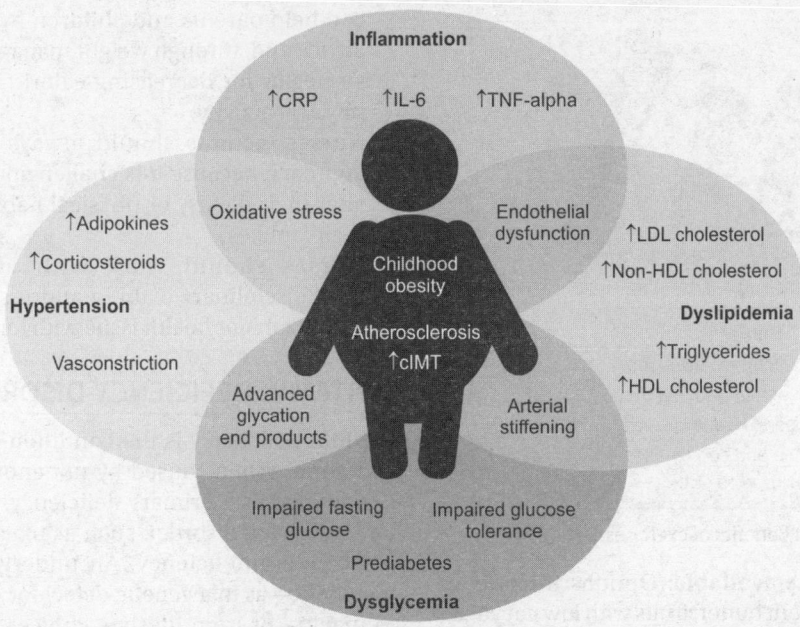

Fig. 9.9: Complications of childhood obesity.

- **Type 2 diabetes:** This chronic condition affects the way your child's body uses sugar (glucose). Obesity and a sedentary lifestyle increase the risk of type 2 diabetes.
- **High cholesterol and high blood pressure:** A poor diet can cause your child to develop one or both of these conditions. These factors can contribute to the buildup of plaques in the arteries, which can cause arteries to narrow and harden, possibly leading to a heart attack or stroke later in life.
- **Joint pain:** Extra weight causes extra stress on hips and knees. Childhood obesity can cause pain and sometimes injuries in the hips, knees and back.
- **Breathing problems:** Asthma is more common in children who are overweight. These children are also more likely to develop obstructive sleep apnea, a potentially serious disorder in which a child's breathing repeatedly stops and starts during sleep.
- **Nonalcoholic fatty liver disease (NAFLD):** This disorder, which usually causes no symptoms, causes fatty deposits to build up in the liver. NAFLD can lead to scarring and liver damage.

Social and Emotional Complications

Children who have obesity may experience teasing or bullying by their peers. This can result in a loss of self-esteem and an increased risk of depression and anxiety.

Figure 9.10 is depicted the factors that contribute to childhood obesity and consequences of childhood obesity.

Prevention

To help prevent excess weight gain in your child, you can:
- **Set a good example:** Make healthy eating and regular physical activity a family affair. Everyone will benefit and no one will feel singled out.

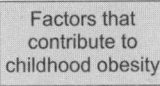
Factors that contribute to childhood obesity

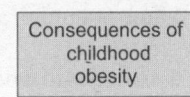
Consequences of childhood obesity

- Family eating habits
- Food advertising
- Unhealthy taste preferences
  (Juice, soft drink, noodles, chips, fried food)
- Exposure to unhealthy food
- Availability of food
- Physical inactivity
- Increased sitting time (watching TV, computer)
- Lack of fruits and vegetables
- Depression
- Skipping breakfast
- Eating adult portion sizes
- Obese parents (due to both lifestyle and genetics)

Childhood obesity = adult obesity

Increased risk of:
- Early onset diabetes
- Early onset heart disease
- Increased risk of lifestyle related cancers, such as breast and colorectal cancers
- Bullying
- Depression
- Poor self esteem
- Increased risk of asthma attacks
- Early puberty
- Increased risk of death in early adulthood

Fig. 9.10: Factors that contribute to childhood obesity and consequences of childhood obesity.

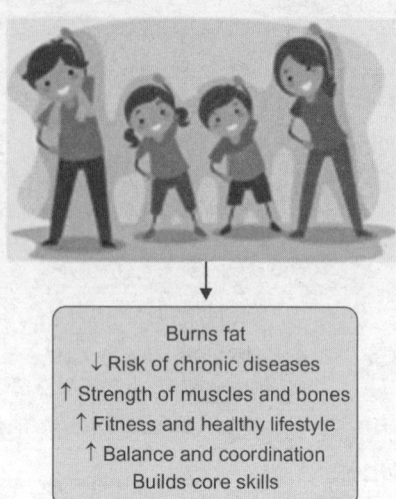

Fig. 9.11: Benefits of exercises.

- **Have healthy snacks available:** Options include air-popped popcorn without butter, fruits with low-fat yogurt, baby carrots with hummus, or whole-grain cereal with low-fat milk.
- **Offer new foods multiple times:** Do not be discouraged if your child does not immediately like a new food. It usually takes multiple exposures to a food to gain acceptance.
- **Choose nonfood rewards:** Promising candy for good behavior is a bad idea.
- **Be sure your child gets enough sleep:** Some studies indicate that too little sleep may increase the risk of obesity. Sleep deprivation can cause hormonal imbalances that lead to increased appetite.

According to WHO, childhood obesity is one of the most serious public health challenges of the 21st century. Prevention of childhood obesity is vital, especially since we know that the treatment of obesity is extremely difficult.

Proven and simple strategies to prevent obesity include:
- Increase fruit and vegetable intake.
- Reducing TV viewing. Eating while viewing TV is a major cause of excess food intake. TV commercials lead children towards fast foods,
- Reduce sugar intake. Sugar is now called the new 'tobacco' and must be limited at all ages. Water is encouraged instead of sweetened drinks.
- Encourage physical activity. It is a struggle to ensure active lives in children, due to limited time and academic pressures. Parents need to facilitate physical activity in young children, and 60 minutes of daily vigorous physical activity in older children.

Figure 9.11 is depicted the benefits of exercises.

Nurses Role

- Obesity is a significant long-term health problem that is common among children and adolescents in Western countries. Being overweight or obese (extremely overweight) can contribute to type 2 diabetes in childhood and increase the risk of cardiovascular disease in adulthood.
- Primary prevention of obesity prevents the development of serious secondary complications in adulthood. Nurses can help parents and children by providing nutritional advice and, through weight management programs, offer strategies for decreasing caloric intake and increasing physical activity.
- Nurses' actions should always take a whole-family approach because it is challenging for obese children to alter their dietary or physical habits if not supported by their families.
- Nurses should work with all members of the multidisciplinary team in addressing childhood obesity as it is a major health issue with long-term morbidities.

VITAMIN DEFICIENCY DISORDERS

Vitamin deficiency is the condition of a long-term lack of a vitamin. When caused by not enough vitamin intakes it is classified as a primary deficiency, whereas when due to an underlying disorder, such as malabsorption, it is called a secondary deficiency. An underlying disorder may be metabolic—as in a genetic defect for converting tryptophan to niacin—or from lifestyle choices that increase vitamin needs, such as smoking or drinking alcohol. Government guidelines on vitamin deficiencies advise certain intakes for healthy people, with specific values for women, men, babies, the elderly, and during pregnancy or breastfeeding. Many countries have mandated vitamin food fortification programs to prevent commonly occurring vitamin deficiencies.

VITAMIN A DEFICIENCY

Vitamin A deficiency results from a dietary intake of vitamin A that is inadequate to satisfy physiological needs. It may be exacerbated by high rates of infection, especially diarrhea and measles. It is common in developing countries, but rarely seen in developed countries.

Causes of Vitamin A Deficiency

Vitamin A deficiency may be caused by prolonged inadequate intake of vitamin A. This is especially so when rice is the main food in your diet (rice does not contain any carotene). Vitamin A deficiency may also occur when your body is unable to make use of the vitamin A in your diet. This may occur in a variety of illnesses, including:
- Celiac disease
- Crohn's disease
- Giardiasis—an infection of the gut (bowel).
- Cystic fibrosis
- Diseases affecting the pancreas.
- Liver cirrhosis
- Obstruction of the flow of bile from your liver and gallbladder into your gut.

Symptoms of a Vitamin A Deficiency

Symptoms of a vitamin A deficiency can differ in severity. Some people may have more serious complications than others. Below are several possible symptoms you may experience:
- **Night blindness:** This causes you to have trouble seeing in low light. It will eventually lead to complete blindness at night.

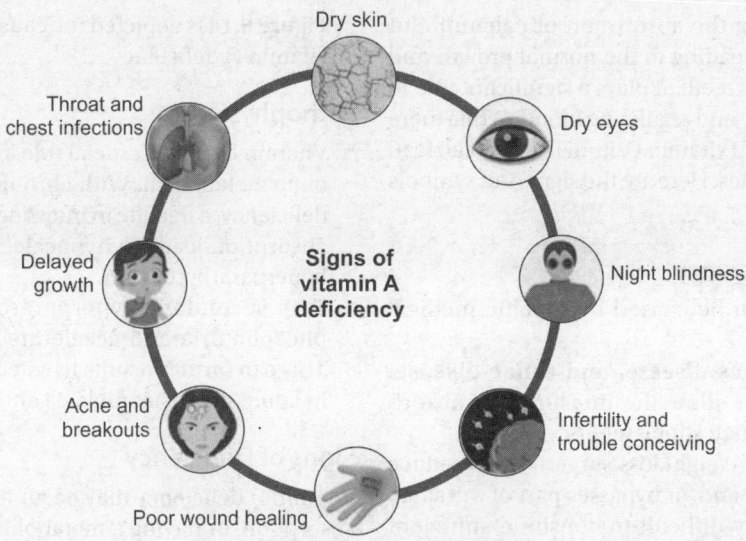

Fig. 9.12: Signs of vitamin A deficiency.

- **Xerophthalmia:** With this condition, the eyes may become very dry and crusted, which may damage the cornea and retina.
- **Infection:** A person with a vitamin A deficiency can experience more frequent health concerns as they will not be able to fight off infections as easily.
- **Bitot spots:** This condition is a buildup of keratin in the eyes, causing hazy vision.
- **Skin irritation:** People experiencing vitamin A deficiency could have problems with their skin, such as dryness, itching, and scaling.
- **Keratomalacia:** This is an eye disorder involving drying and clouding of the cornea—the clear layer in front of the iris and pupil.
- **Keratinization:** This is a process by which cells become filled with keratin protein, die, and form tough, resistant structures in the urinary, gastrointestinal and respiratory tracts.
- **Stunted growth:** Not having enough vitamin A could delay growth or cause children to experience slow bone growth or stunted growth.
- **Fertility:** A deficiency in vitamin A may cause challenges when trying to conceive a child, and in some cases, infertility.

Figure 9.12 is depicted the signs of vitamin A deficiency.

Figure 9.13 is depicted the deficiency of vitamin A leads to dry skin.

Vitamin A Deficiency Treatment

The treatment for mild forms of vitamin A deficiency includes eating vitamin A-rich foods. For more severe forms, a doctor may recommend eating more foods containing vitamin A in combination with taking vitamin supplements.

Foods Contain Vitamin A

- **Liver:** This type of food contains large amounts of vitamin A. One helping of liver contains more than the recommended minimum intake of vitamin A for a week.

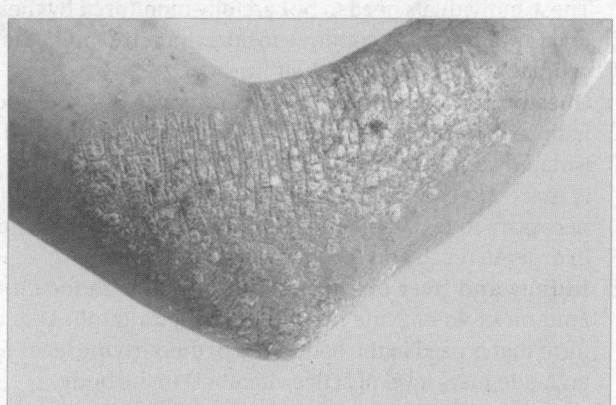

Fig. 9.13: Deficiency of vitamin A leads to dry skin.

- **Fish:** Oily fish, shellfish, and cod liver oil all contain quite a bit of vitamin A and can be eaten with meals or consumed as vitamin supplements.
- **Vegetables:** Orange vegetables have the highest level of vitamin A. The most common ones include sweet potato, pumpkin, carrot, and squash. Other green leafy vegetables, such as spinach, greens, and lettuce are also great options. Experts recommend cooking or processing these veggies to get the full benefit of vitamin A so that it is easier for the body to digest and absorb its nutritional value.
- **Dairy products:** Milk is generally a good source of vitamin A, although the amount in skim milk is lower than in full cream milk. Many soft cheeses may contain vitamin A as well, although cheddar cheese contains more than others.
- **Fruits:** Common fruits with the highest level of vitamin A are often orange—ripe mango, papaya, cantaloupe melon, and apricots—which can be consumed dried or fresh.

Vitamin A is most readily absorbed in fat particles in the gut or intestine, so it is helpful to incorporate some healthy fats into your meals.

VITAMIN D DEFICIENCY

Vitamin D plays a significant role in keeping our bones healthy, reducing anxiety and improving immune function.

It also helps in regulating the absorption of calcium and phosphorus in the body, leading to the normal growth and development of bones and teeth. It plays a significant role in reducing stress and anxiety and regulating mood. While there are wide-ranging benefits of vitamin D, its deficiency can lead to some serious health issues. Here are the signs and symbols of vitamin D deficiency.

Causes Vitamin D Deficiency

Vitamin D deficiency can be caused by specific medical conditions, such as:

- **Cystic fibrosis, Crohn's disease, and celiac disease:** These diseases do not allow the intestines to absorb enough vitamin D through supplements.
- **Weight loss surgeries:** Weight loss surgeries that reduce the size of the stomach and/or bypasses part of the small intestines make it very difficult to consume sufficient quantities of certain nutrients, vitamins, and minerals. These individuals need to be carefully monitored by their doctors and need to continue to take vitamin D and other supplements throughout their lives.
- **Obesity:** A body mass index greater than 30 is associated with lower vitamin D levels. Fat cells keep vitamin D isolated so that it is not released. Vitamin D deficiency is more likely in obese people. Obesity often makes it necessary to take larger doses of vitamin D supplements in order to reach and maintain normal D levels.
- **Kidney and liver diseases:** These diseases reduce the amount of an enzyme needed to change vitamin D to a form that is used in the body. Lack of this enzyme leads to an inadequate level of active vitamin D in the body.

Figure 9.14 is depicted the causes and associated diseases of Vitamin D deficiency.

Pathophysiology

- Vitamin D plays a crucial role in calcium homeostasis and bone metabolism. With chronic and/or severe vitamin D deficiency, a decline in intestinal calcium and phosphorus absorption leads to hypocalcemia leading to secondary hyperparathyroidism.
- This secondary hyperparathyroidism then leads to phosphaturia and accelerated bone demineralization. This can further results in osteomalacia and osteoporosis in adults and osteomalacia and rickets in children.

Signs of Deficiency

Vitamin D deficiency may occur from a lack in the diet, poor absorption, or having a metabolic need for higher amounts. If one is not eating enough vitamin D and does not receive enough ultraviolet sun exposure over an extended period, a deficiency may arise. People who cannot tolerate or do not eat milk, eggs, and fish, such as those with a lactose intolerance or who follow a vegan diet, are at higher risk for a deficiency. Other people at high-risk of vitamin D deficiency include:

- People with inflammatory bowel disease (ulcerative colitis, Crohn's disease) or other conditions that disrupt the normal digestion of fat. Vitamin D is a fat-soluble vitamin that depends on the gut's ability to absorb dietary fat.
- People who are obese tend to have lower blood vitamin D levels. Vitamin D accumulates in excess fat tissues but is not easily available for use by the body when needed.

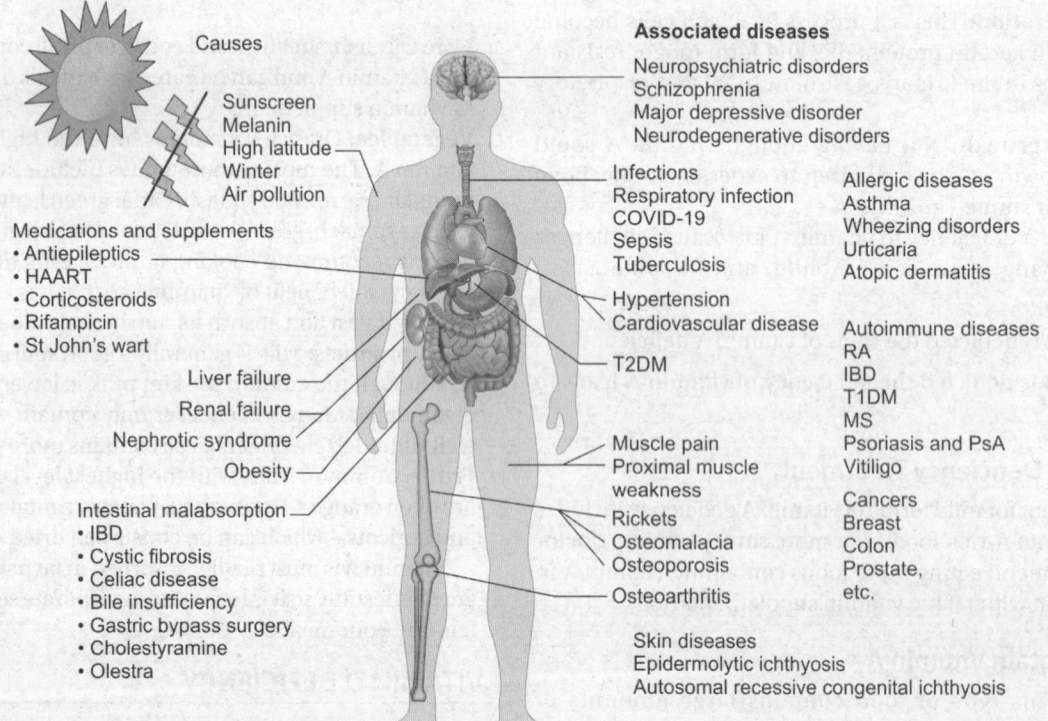

Fig. 9.14: Causes and associated diseases of vitamin D deficiency.

- Higher doses of vitamin D supplementation may be needed to achieve a desirable blood level. Conversely, blood levels of vitamin D rise when obese people lose weight.
- People who have undergone gastric bypass surgery, which typically removes the upper part of the small intestine where vitamin D is absorbed.

Conditions Resulting from Prolonged Vitamin D Deficiency

- **Rickets:** A condition in infants and children of soft bones and skeletal deformities caused by failure of bone tissue to harden.
- **Osteomalacia:** A condition in adults of weak and softened bones that can be reversed with supplementation. This is different than osteoporosis, in which the bones are porous and brittle and the condition is irreversible.

Diet Management

In order to prevent vitamin D deficiency, doctors recommend getting as much access to sunlight as possible (with adequate precautions to prevent sunburn) and ensuring that one maintains a balanced diet which includes regular intake of sources of vitamin D.

Foods which contain or are commonly fortified with vitamin D include:

- **Oily fish:** Trout, salmon, herring, sardines, pilchards, kippers, tuna.
- **Cod liver oil:** This contains a large amount of vitamin D and should not be taken in conjunction with supplements containing vitamin D.
- **Fortified dairy products:** Dairy-based spreads and cheese can be fortified with vitamin D. Check the nutritional information on the packet to ascertain the vitamin D content of individual products. Infant formula is generally fortified with vitamin D.
- **Fortified soy products:** Soy-based products, such as soy milk and soy yoghurt can be fortified with vitamin D. Check the nutritional information on the packet to ascertain the vitamin D content of individual products.
- **Natural animal products:** Raw milk, meat and egg yolk are sources of vitamin D.

Good to know: It is important to note that the vitamin D content of animal products will vary according to the season. Animal products contain more vitamin D during the spring and summer months because the livestock—and the plant material they feed on—is exposed to more sunlight and thus has greater potential to synthesize vitamin D.

Management of Vitamin D Deficiency

The amount of vitamin D required to treat the deficiency depends largely on the degree of the deficiency and underlying risk factors.

- Initial supplementation for 8 weeks with Vitamin D3 either 6,000 IU daily or 50,000 IU weekly can be considered. Once the serum 25-hydroxyvitamin D level exceeds 30 ng/mL, a daily maintenance dose of 1,000 to 2,000 IU is recommended.
- A higher-dose initial supplementation with vitamin D3 at 10,000 IU daily may be needed in high-risk adults who are vitamin D deficient (African Americans, Hispanics, obese, taking certain medications, malabsorption syndrome). Once serum 25-hydroxyvitamin D level exceeds 30 ng/mL, 3,000 to 6,000 IU/day maintenance dose is recommended.
- Children who are vitamin D deficient require 2,000 IU/day of vitamin D3 or 50,000 IU of vitamin D3 once weekly for 6 weeks. Once the serum 25(OH)D level exceeds 30 ng/mL, 1,000 IU/day maintenance treatment is recommended. According to the American Academy of Pediatrics, infants who are breastfed and children who consume less than 1 L of vitamin D-fortified milk need 400 IU of vitamin D supplementation.
- Calcitriol can be considered where the deficiency persists despite treatment with vitamin D2 and/or D3. The serum calcium level shall be closely monitored in these individuals due to an increased risk of hypercalcemia secondary to calcitriol.
- Calcidiol can be considered in patients with fat malabsorption or severe liver disease.

Figure 9.15 is depicted the vitamin D deficiency.

Prevention

The best ways to prevent a vitamin D deficiency are to eat foods that are rich in this nutrient and to spend some time outside each day. Some tips for avoiding a deficiency include:

- **Maintaining a healthy body weight:** Cycling or walking can provide both exercise and exposure to sunlight.
- **Treating medical conditions:** People with health conditions that affect the absorption of nutrients may find that treating the underlying condition helps boost their levels of certain nutrients, including vitamin D.

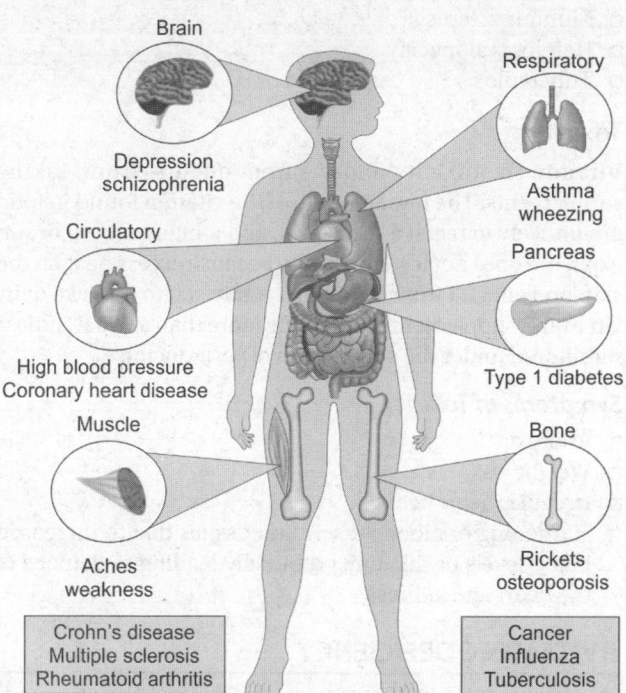

Fig. 9.15: Vitamin D deficiency.

- **Being proactive about preventive health:** People with a family history of osteoporosis or vitamin D deficiency may wish to consider speaking to their doctor about screening.

Complications of Vitamin D Deficiency

It is important to consult a healthcare professional if one suspects vitamin D deficiency, because the condition increases the likelihood of developing certain problems. The most commonly experienced problems related to vitamin D deficiency are skeletal disorders; diseases related to the growth and strength of one's bones. In children, vitamin D deficiency can cause rickets, a condition involving the weakening and softening of the bones. In adults, the equivalent to rickets is known as osteomalacia (soft bones).

Being deficient in vitamin D can also render the body less robust and heighten the likelihood of accidents occurring:
- Vitamin D deficiency increases the likelihood of breaking a bone in people of any age
- Elderly people with hypovitaminosis D are more likely to fall, trip or stumble

Health complications which are associated with vitamin D deficiency include: Osteomalacia (softening of the bones in adults) and osteoporosis (increased fragility of the bones)—
- Rickets (softening of the bones in children)
- Mental health conditions, such as seasonal affective disorder (SAD) and depression
- Increased susceptibility to infections and illnesses
- Glucose intolerance and type 1 and type 2 diabetes
- Obesity
- Cardiovascular diseases (conditions affecting the heart) such as hypertension, heart failure and ischemic heart disease
- Cancer of the colon, breast or prostate
- Rheumatoid arthritis
- Multiple sclerosis
- Hair loss (alopecia)
- Tuberculosis

Toxicity

Vitamin D toxicity most often occurs from taking supplements. The low amounts of the vitamin found in food are unlikely to reach a toxic level, and a high amount of sun exposure does not lead to toxicity because excess heat on the skin prevents D3 from forming. It is advised to not take daily vitamin D supplements containing more than 4,000 IU unless monitored under the supervision of your doctor.

Symptoms of Toxicity
- Anorexia
- Weight loss
- Irregular heart beat
- Hardening of blood vessels and tissues due to increased blood levels of calcium, potentially leading to damage of the heart and kidneys

VITAMIN C DEFICIENCY

Vitamin C cannot be made by the human body and so is an essential component of the diet. It is needed for the health and repair of various tissues in your body, including skin, bone, teeth and cartilage. Persistent lack of vitamin C in your diet can lead to a condition called scurvy. Symptoms of scurvy include easy bruising, easy bleeding and joint and muscle pains. Vitamin C deficiency can be treated with supplements of vitamin C and a diet rich in vitamin C (**Fig. 9.16**).

Cause of Vitamin C Deficiency

As already mentioned, the primary cause of vitamin C deficiency is an imbalanced diet. This is because the human body does not naturally synthesise vitamin C, and it has to be supplied via external sources. This primarily concerns food intake, including vegetables, fruits, and fortified foods. This is why most causes of deficiency of vitamin C involve an improper diet. Some of these are as follows:
- A diet lacking vitamin C-rich fresh vegetables and fruits
- A restrictive diet due to health conditions, such as weak digestive system, allergies, etc.
- Mental health issues and other disorders, such as anorexia
- Old age

Besides, there can be a number of other causes for lack of vitamin C. These include treatments, health conditions, and habits that limit the body's ability to absorb nutrients. Some of them are as follows:
- Ulcerative colitis
- Intake of illegal drugs and high amounts of alcohol
- Chemotherapy
- Crohn's disease
- Smoking

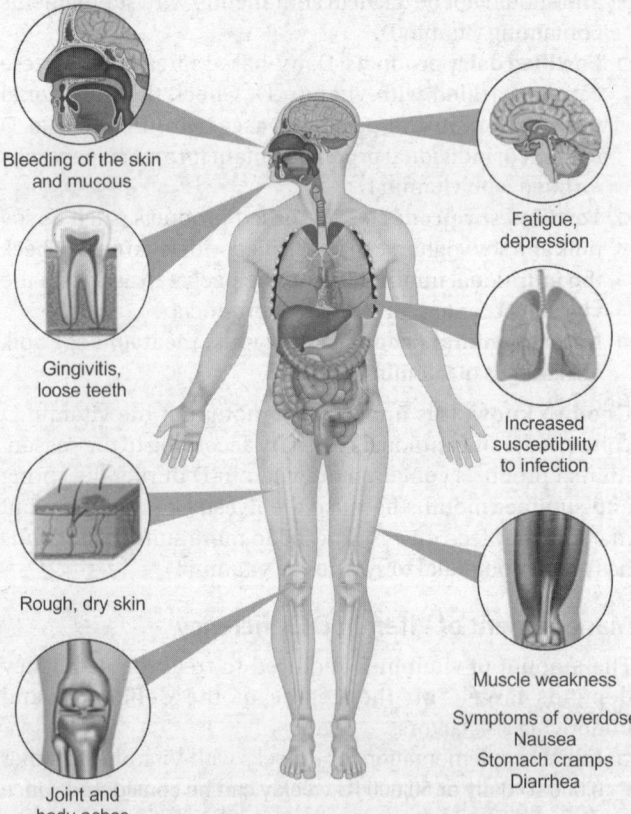

Fig. 9.16: Vitamin C deficiency.

- Hyperthyroidism
- Pregnancy
- Prolonged diarrhea
- Surgery

These factors can lead to a long-term condition of vitamin C deficiency, which might lead to detrimental side effects.

Pathophysiology

- As a clinical manifestation of severe vitamin C deficiency, scurvy is caused by ascorbic acid's role in collagen synthesis. Collagen type IV is the main constituent of blood vessel walls, skin, and specifically, the basement membrane zone separating the epidermis from the dermis.
- Vitamin C allows hydroxylation and cross linking of pro-collagen catalyzed by lysyl hydroxylase. Lack of vitamin C decreases transcription of pro-collagen.
- Additionally, a lack of ascorbic acid leads to epigenetic DNA hypermethylation and inhibits the transcription of various types of collagen found in skin, blood vessels, and tissue.
- Finally, the key feature of scurvy is hemorrhage which can occur in almost any organ. Further, bone formation is altered and becomes brittle.

Diseases Caused Due to Vitamin C Deficiency

The deficiency of vitamin C causes scurvy. Scurvy is characterized by the following symptoms:
- Gingivitis or gum disease
- Loss of teeth
- Skin problems
- Anemia
- Weak immunity
- Shortness of breath
- Corkscrew hairs

These signs occur along with the previously mentioned vitamin C deficiency symptoms.

In the long run, lack of vitamin C causes untreated scurvy, which can be life-threatening and may lead to the following conditions:
- Severe jaundice
- Neuropathy
- Hemolysis or destruction of RBCs
- Generalized edema

Since pregnant women are at increased risk of developing this deficiency due to the body's high nutrient requirement, scurvy in them may affect fetal brain development. To prevent the adverse eventualities of this nutrient deficiency, you must ensure all necessary precautions are followed, including a balanced diet.

Symptoms of Vitamin C Deficiency

There are a number of clear telltale signs of deficiency of vitamin C. If you suffer from any of the following symptoms, chances are that you may suffer from the lack of vitamin C:

Nosebleeds

- Nosebleeds are not nice, that is for sure. If you get them often, it could be an indication that the blood vessels in your nose are naturally weaker, or it could be a sign of vitamin C deficiency.
- Vitamin C helps your body produce collagen, which helps to strengthen your blood vessels.
- The less vitamin C you have in your body, the more likely you are to have weaker blood vessels.
- A case of regular nosebleeds could be a strong indication of weaker blood vessels as a result of vitamin C deficiency.

Sore, Bleeding or Swollen Gums

Such as in the case of nosebleeds, collagen is something your gums also need to stay healthy, and vitamin C directly plays a role in the production of collagen. If your body lacks collagen, your gums would not heal properly. Vitamin C also has antioxidant properties, so it will combat the swelling and inflammation in the gums.

Anemia or Iron Deficiency

- Iron is an important nutrient that has a variety of functions. It is essential for making red blood cells (RBCs) and transporting oxygen throughout the body.
- Vitamin C plays an important role in absorbing iron from your diet.
- It assists in converting iron that is poorly absorbed, such as plant-based sources of iron, into a form that is easier to absorb.
- Vitamin C is critical for individuals on a meat free diet as meat is one of the sources of iron.

Other symptoms of vitamin C deficiency include:
- Dry skin
- Splitting hair
- Swelling and discoloration of your gums
- Sudden and unexpected bleeding from your gums
- Nosebleeds
- Poor healing of wounds
- Problems fighting infections
- Bleeding into joints, causing severe joint pains
- Changes in your bones
- Tooth loss
- Weight loss

Tests for Vitamin C Deficiency

Testing for vitamin C deficiencies is a relatively simple process. In most cases, a doctor will advise the following pathology tests:
- **A blood test** is a simple yet effective way to test vitamin C deficiency.
- **An iron deficiency test** can confirm low iron (or anemia) which is a symptom of vitamin C deficiency.
- **An X-ray test** can detect low bone density which is a strong indication of vitamin C deficiency.

Side Effects of Vitamin C Deficiency

Unchecked early symptoms of lack of vitamin C can include some of the following persistent health issues:
- Bleeding from nose and gums
- Subperiosteal hemorrhage or bleeding between joints
- Loose teeth
- Improper and delayed wound healing
- Weak bones

Other severe persistent symptoms due to lack of vitamin C include fever, nerve problems, shortness of breath, and convulsions.

Individuals suffering from the same might not be able to identify these as a result of a specific nutrient deficiency. However, a lack of vitamin C can lead to severe diseases.

Treatment for Vitamin C Deficiency

Treatment for vitamin C deficiency can be either through replacing the vitamin C in your diet or by supplements.
- **Intake of foods rich in vitamin C:** This is perhaps the most natural and recommended way to treat vitamin C deficiency.
- **Through vitamin C supplements:** Supplements are another way to treat vitamin C deficiency. Supplements are a great way to achieve temporary relief. Nonetheless, in the long-run it is best to maintain a balanced diet.

Prevent of Vitamin C Deficiency

The best and easiest way to prevent vitamin C deficiency is by increasing intake of foods rich in the vitamin. The recommended intake for preventing vitamin C deficiency is:
- 75 g orally once a day for women
- 90 g orally once a day for men
- An additional 35 mg/day for smokers

Five servings of fruits and vegetables (mentioned above) will ensure that you attain the recommended level through the day. Preventing vitamin deficiency will also go a long way in helping to keep many other diseases at bay.

Prevent and Overcome Vitamin C Deficiency

The best way to prevent vitamin C deficiency is to ensure a diet rich in vitamin C. Some of the most prominent food sources of this nutrient are as follows (**Fig. 9.17**):

Fruits
- Kiwi fruit
- Lemons
- Strawberries
- Papaya
- Blackberries
- Guava
- Oranges

Vegetables
- Carrots
- Spinach
- Bell peppers
- Tomatoes
- Broccoli
- Cabbage
- Potatoes

Other Eatables
- Oysters
- Paprika

Note that vitamin C can disintegrate under the effect of heat during storage. This is why, it is advisable to consume raw and fresh fruits and vegetables as much as possible. On the other hand, if you have already been diagnosed with a

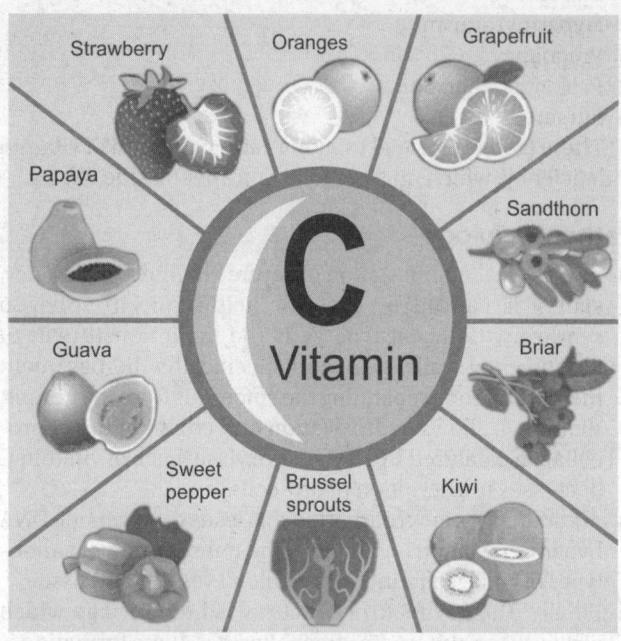

Fig. 9.17: Prominent food sources of vitamin C.

vitamin C deficiency, you will need to consult a dietician who might suggest the following treatment methods:
- Oral vitamin C supplements
- Vitamin C injections

The healthcare professional will recommend the ideal dosage, depending on your deficiency level.

VITAMIN B1 DEFICIENCIES (FIG. 9.18)

Thiamine Deficiency

Thiamine deficiency is a medical condition of low levels of thiamine (vitamin B1). A severe and chronic form is known

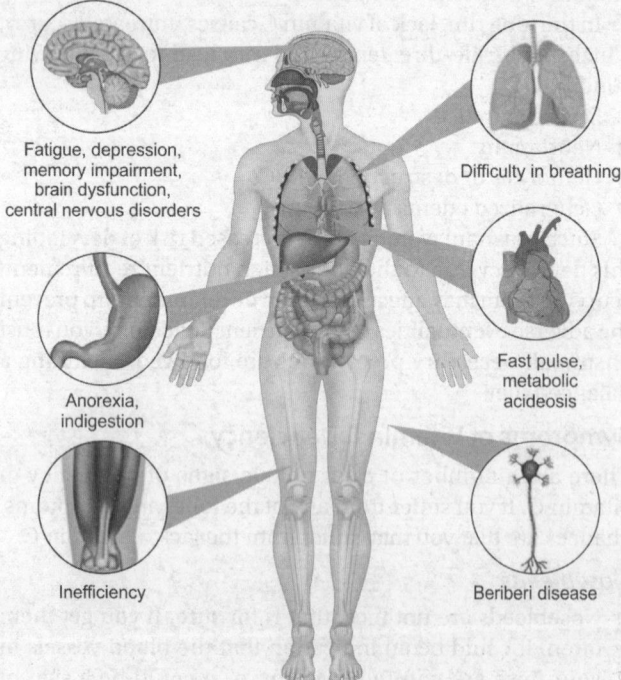

Fig. 9.18: Vitamin B1 deficiency.

as beriberi. The two main types in adults are wet beriberi and dry beriberi. Wet beriberi affects the cardiovascular system, resulting in a fast heart rate, shortness of breath, and leg swelling.

- Thiamin deficiency is usually associated with a low-calorie intake. But frank thiamin deficiency is usually not seen. Thiamin deficiency ultimately causes beriberi in humans.
- Gastrointestinal disturbances and severe diarrhea vomiting may cause thiamin deficiency.
- The efficiency symptoms may also be seen in febrile conditions or surgery when the intake is inadequate.
- The symptoms of thiamin deficiency include anorexia, indigestion and severe constipation, lack of gastric muscle tone and lack of hydrochloric acid secretion.
- Alcoholics are especially susceptible to thiamin deficiency. The deficiency of thiamin also affects cardiac muscles and the central nervous system (CNS) also.
- With continued deficiency cardiac muscles weaken and results in cardiac failure. The functioning of CNS depends on glucose for energy.
- Thiamin helps fulfill this need. Inadequate thiamin affects nerve activity, reflex responses are reduced and general weakness and fatigue results.
- Prolonged thiamin deficiency hinders lipogenesis and degeneration of myelin sheaths occurs.
- The symptoms include progressive nerve irritation, pain and prickly sensations. If the severe deficiency state is left untreated, paralysis results.
- Adequate amounts of TPP in muscle tissue, results in chronic, painful musculoskeletal condition known as fibromyalgia.

Symptoms

- Deficiency affects the gastrointestinal, cardiovascular and peripheral nervous systems.
- Early symptoms include fatigue, lack of interest, emotional instability, irritability depression, anger and fear and loss of appetite, loss of weight and loss of strength.

Table 9.4 is depicted the water-soluble vitamins.

- As the deficiency progresses, the symptoms become more marked, which include indigestion, constipation, headache, insomnia (inadequate sleep), tachycardia (rapid heartbeat), feeling of heaviness and weakness of the legs, cramps of the calf muscles and burning and numbness of the feet (peripheral neuritis).
- Eventually muscle degeneration and lack of coordination occurs. This is often referred to as 'dry beriberi'.
- B1 deficiency also leads to cardiomegaly, tachycardia, mental confusion and muscle wasting. This condition of the disease is known as 'wet beriberi' because it is associated with edema.

Table 9.4: Water-soluble vitamins.

B complex vitamins

Vitamin B1 (thiamine): A coenzyme in carbohydrate metabolism; essential for energy production	RDAs Females 14–18 years, 1 mg 19 years and older, 1.1 mg Pregnancy, 1.4 mg Lactation, 1.4 mg Males 14 years and older, 1.2 mg Children 1–3 years, 0.5 mg 4–8 years, 0.6 mg 9–13 years, 0.9 mg Infants (Als) 0–6 months, 0.2 mg 7–12 months, 0.3 mg	Meat, poultry, fish, egg, yolk, dried beans, whole grain cereal products, peanuts	Mild deficiency; fatigue, anorexia; retarded growth; mental depression; irritability; apathy, lethargy Severe deficiency (beriberi): Peripheral neuritis; personality disturbances; heart failure; edema Wernicke-Korsakoff syndrome in alcoholics	Not established
Vitamins B2 (riboflavin): A coenzyme in metabolism; necessary for growth; may function in production of corticosteroids and red blood cells an in gluconeogenesis	RDAs Females 14–18 years, 1 mg 19 years and older, 1.1 mg Pregnancy, 1.4 mg Lactation, 1.6 mg Males 14 years and older, 1.3 mg Children 1–3 years, 0.5 mg 4–8 years, 0.6 mg 9–13 years, 0.9 mg Infants (Als) 0–6 months, 0.3 mg 7–12 months, 0.4 mg	Milk, cheddar and cottage cheeses, meat, eggs, green leafy vegetables	Seborrheic dermatitis; glossitis; stomatitis; eye disorders (burning, itching, lacrimation, photophobia, vascularization of the cornea)	Not established

Contd...

Contd...

B complex vitamins				
Biotin Part of the vitamin B2 complex; essential in fat and carbohydrate metabolism	Females 14–18 years, 25 µg 19 years and older, 30 µg Pregnancy, 30 µg Lactation, 35 µg Males 14–18 years, 25 µg 19 years and older, 30 µg Children 1–3 years, 8 µg 4–8 years, 12 µg 9–13 years, 20 µg Infants 0–6 months, 5 µg 7–12 months, 6 µg	Meat, egg yolk, nuts, cereals, most vegetables	Anorexia, nausea; depression; muscle pain; dermatitis	Not established
Vitamin B3 (niacin) Essential for glycolysis, fat synthesis, and tissue respiration. It functions as a coenzyme in many metabolic processes (after conversion to nicotinamide, the physiologically active form)	RDAs Females 14 years and older, 14 mg Pregnancy, 18 mg Lactation, 17 mg Males 14 years and older 16 mg Children 1–3 years, 6 mg 4–8 years, 8 mg 9–13 years, 12 mg Infants (AIs) 0–6 months, 2 mg 7–12 months, 4 mg	Meat, poultry, fish, peanuts	Pellagra: Erythematous skin lesions; GI problems (stomatitis, glossitis, enteritis, diarrhea); CNS problems (headache, dizziness, insomnia, depression memory loss) Severe deficiency; delusions, hallucinations, impairment of peripheral motor and sensory nerves	Flushing, pruritus, hyperglycemia, increased liver enzymes, uricemia
Vitamin B5 (pantothenic acid) Essential for metabolism of carbohydrate, fat, and protein (e.g., release of energy from carbohydrate, fatty acid metabolism, synthesis of cholesterol, steroid hormones, and phospholipids)	AIs Females 14 years and older, 5 mg Pregnancy, 6 mg Lactation, 7 mg Males 14 years and older 5 mg Children 1–3 years, 2 mg 4–8 years, 3 mg 9–13 years, 4 mg Infants 0–6 months, 1.7 mg 7–12 months, 1.8 mg	Eggs, liver, salmon, yeast, cauliflower, broccoli, lean beef, potatoes, tomatoes	No deficiency state established	Not established
Vitamin B6 (pyridoxine) A coenzyme in metabolism of carbohydrate, protein, and fat; required for formation of tryptophan to conversion of tryptophan to niacin; helps release glycogen from the liver and muscle tissue; functions in metabolism of the central nervous system; helps maintain cellular immunity	DRLs Females 14–18 years, 1.2 mg 19–50 years, 1.3 mg 51–70 years, and older, 1.5 mg Pregnancy, 1.9 mg Lactation, 2 mg Males 14–50 years, 1.3 mg 51–70 years and older 1.7 mg Children 1–3 years, 0.5 mg 4–8 years, 0.6 mg 9–13 years, 1 mg Infants (AIs) 0–6 months, 0.1 mg 7–12 months, 0.3 mg	Yeast, wheat germ, liver and other glandular meats, whole grain cereals, potatoes, legumes	Skin and mucous membrane lesions (seborrheic dermatitis, intertrigo, stomatitis, glossitis); neurologic problems (seizures, peripheral neuritis, mental depression)	Not established

Contd...

B complex vitamins

Vitamin B12 (cyanobacterium) Essential for normal metabolism of all body cells, normal red blood cells, normal nerve cells, growth, and metabolism of carbohydrate, protein, and fat	RDAs Females 14 years and older, 2.4 µg Pregnancy, 2.6 µg Lactation, 2.8 µg Males 14 years and older 2.4 µg Children 1–3 years, 0.9 µg 4–8 years, 1.2 µg	Meat, eggs, fish, cheese	Pernicious anemia decreased numbers of RBCs; large, immature RBCs; fatigue; dyspnea Severe deficiency; leukopenia, infection, thrombocytopenia, cardiac dysrhythmias, heart failure Neurologic signs and symptoms	Not established

Infantile Beriberi

- Infants in the Far East are especially prone to this deficiency because their mothers had decreased thiamin intake and the milk produced by them for the infants contains very small amounts of thiamin.
- Onset is sudden and is characterized by pallor, facial edema, irritability, vomiting, abdominal pain, loss of voice and convulsions.
- The progression of the disease is so fast that the infant may die within a few hours, but with thiamin treatment, recovery is remarkable.

Treatment: Thiamin deficiency can be treated with B-complex vitamins rather than thiamin alone. Along with B-complex vitamins, a high-calorie and high-protein diet is prescribed.

Toxicity

- Little is known about thiamin toxicity. However, mega doses of 1,000 times more than the RDA of commercial preparation have caused the suppression of respiratory center and ultimately cause death.
- Studies have further reported that the parenteral doses of thiamin of 100 times more than the recommended levels have produced weakness headache, convulsions, muscular weakness, cardiac arrhythmia and allergic reactions.

RIBOFLAVIN

Riboflavin (also known as vitamin B2) is one of the B vitamins, which are all water soluble. Riboflavin is naturally present in some foods, added to some food products, and available as a dietary supplement. This vitamin is an essential component of two major coenzymes, flavin mononucleotide (FMN; also known as riboflavin-5'-phosphate) and flavin adenine dinucleotide (FAD). Riboflavin deficiency is prevalent mainly among the low income groups particularly the vulnerable group and the elderly adults.

Etiology

- Riboflavin deficiency can result from inadequate dietary intake or by endocrine abnormalities. Riboflavin deficiency also correlates with other vitamin B complexes.
- Riboflavin naturally occurs in some food, such as eggs, dairy products, meats, green vegetables, and grains.
- The main antioxidant riboflavin works as is glutathione. Glutathione works to destroy free radicals and detox the liver, as free radicals can cause to develop several diseases.
- Riboflavin deficiency can also result from chronic diarrhea, liver disorder, alcoholism, and hemodialysis.

Riboflavin deficiency is characterized by:
- Soreness and burning of the mouth and tongue
- Lesions at the angles of the mouth called angular stomatitis
- The inflammation of the tongue called glossitis
- Dry chapped appearance of the lip with ulcers termed cheilosis
- The skin becomes dry and results in seborrheic dermatitis
- Photophobia, lacrimation, burning sensation of the eyes and visual fatigue
- Decreased motor coordination
- Normocytic anemia.

Figures 9.19A and B are depicted the riboflavin deficiency and vitamin B2 deficiency.

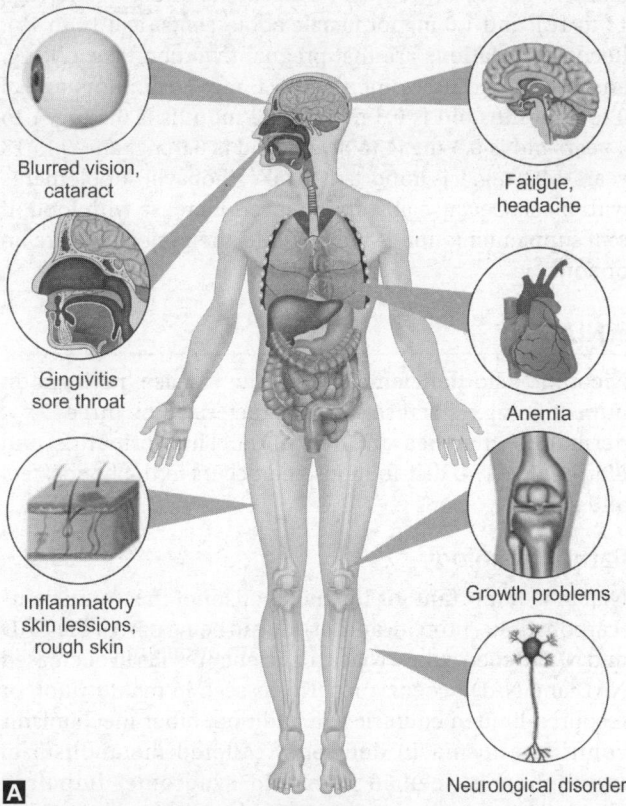

Fig. 9.19A

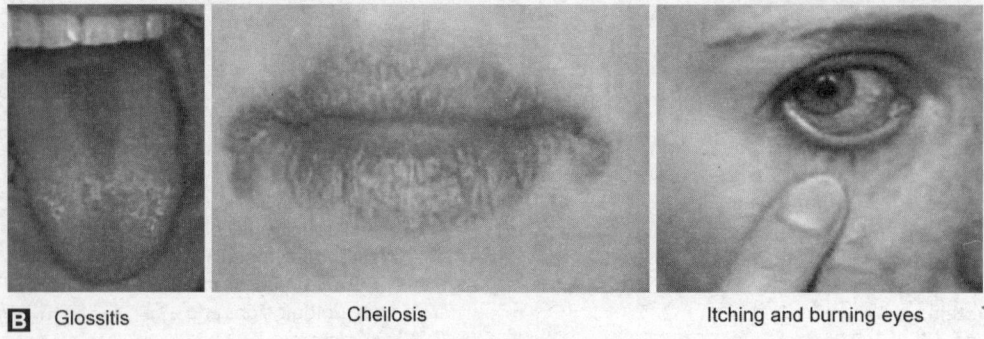

Fig. 9.19B
Figs. 9.19A and B: (A) Riboflavin deficiency; (B) Vitamin B2 deficiency.

History and Physical

- Riboflavin deficiency can cause fatigue, swollen throat, blurred vision, and depression. It can affect the skin by causing skin crack, itching, and dermatitis around the mouth.
- Hyperemia and edema around the throat, liver degeneration, and hair loss can also occur along with reproductive issues.
- Usually, people with riboflavin deficiency also have deficiencies of other nutrients.
- In most cases, riboflavin deficiency is reversible unless it is anatomical changes such as cataracts.

Treatment/Management

Riboflavin supplements come in 25 mg, 50 mg, and 100 mg tablets. According to the National Institutes of Health, the recommended daily nutrient intake of riboflavin is 1.3 mg for men, 1.1 mg for women, 1.3 mg for male adolescents (age 14 to 18), and 1.0 mg for female adolescents (age 14 to 18). Recommendations are that pregnant women take 1.4 mg, and breastfeeding women take 1.6 mg. For infants age of 0 to 6 months old is 0.3 mg, 7 to 12 months is 0.4 mg, 1 to 3 years old is 0.5 mg, 4 to 8 years old is 0.6 mg, and 9 to 13 years is 0.9 mg. It is important to take riboflavin supplements with meals because absorption levels increase with food. If oral supplementation is not possible, then injections are an option.

■ NIACIN

Nicotinic acid deficiency causes the disease 'pellagra' in human being. This disease is characterized by three D's—dermatitis, diarrhea and dementia. The dermatitis and diarrhea are two distributions and occurs in the hands, feet and neck.

Pathophysiology

Niacin is important for the metabolism of macronutrients (carbohydrate, protein, and fat), due to being part of the NAD and NADP coenzymes. Niacin deficiency results in decreased NAD and NADP coenzymes. This is seen in malnutrition or resource-limited countries. In addition, other mechanisms contribute to niacin deficiency. Altered metabolism of tryptophan is seen in carcinoid syndrome, impaired absorption of tryptophan is seen in the autosomal recessive condition Hartnup disease, and prolonged use of certain medications may decrease the production of tryptophan (isoniazid) or inhibit the conversion of tryptophan to. niacin (azathioprine, 6-mercaptopurine, or 5-fluorouracil)

Figure 9.20 is depicted the vitamin B3 deficiency.

- **Dermatitis:** Pellagra comes from **'pelle means skin'** and **'agra means rough'**. Marked changes occur in the skin especially in the skin exposed to sun and friction areas, such as elbows, surfaces of arms, knees. Lesions are symmetrically distributed in the affected parts. At first there is reddening, thickening and pigmentation of the skin. Later on there is exfoliation leading to ultimately parchment of skin-butterfly-like appearance.
- **Diarrhea:** Diarrhea enhances the deficiency state. There are structural and absorptive defects in the small intestine. Tongue appears raw and mucous membrane of the tongue is inflamed.

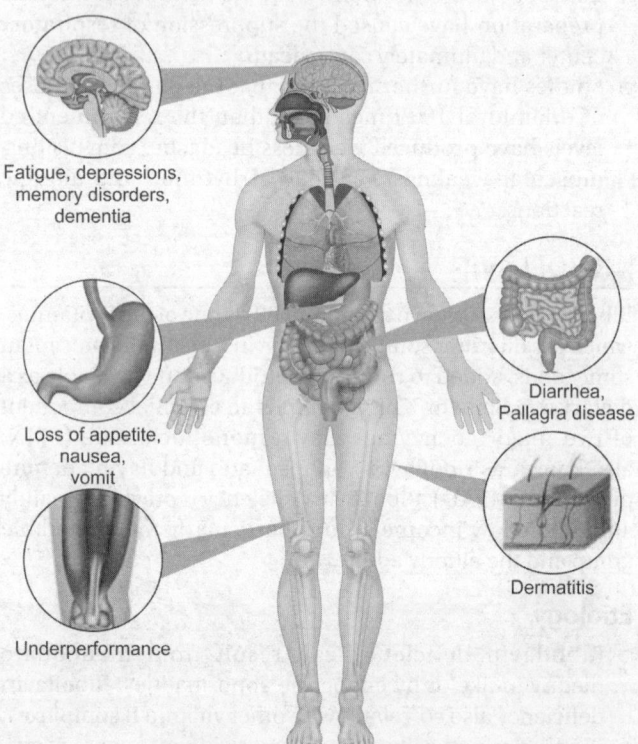

Fig. 9.20: Vitamin B3 deficiency.

☐ **Dementia:** Dementia is irritability, depression, poor concentration and loss of memory. Delirium is a common mental disturbance.

Pellagra is another disease that led to the discovery of a vitamin. Pellagra is caused by a deficiency of vitamin B3 (niacin).

The common symptoms of pellagra are:
☐ Hair loss
☐ Dermatitis and swelling of the skin
☐ Inflamed tongue
☐ Insomnia
☐ Diarrhea
☐ Weakness
☐ Ataxia
☐ Confusion
☐ Aggression
☐ Dilated cardiomyopathy
☐ Dementia

A lack of niacin in the diet leads to decreased production of nicotinamide adenine diphosphate (NAD). NAD is required for a number of critical metabolic functions in the body. If untreated, it can lead to death in four to five years.

Treatment/Management
☐ Pellagra can be reversed by giving niacin accompanied by a high energy diet that is rich in all other B-vitamins, zinc, and magnesium that are important for optimum metabolic reactions in the body.
☐ Avoidance of sun exposure is helpful in the management of skin rash, and having a liquid diet temporarily is needed in the setting of difficulty swallowing related to glossitis.
☐ Nicotinamide 300 mg daily in divided doses is recommended for a total of 3 to 4 weeks. Nicotinamide is better tolerated than niacin (fewer side effects).
☐ Referral to a nutritionist, psychiatrist, or neurologist may be needed.
☐ To ensure sufficient intakes of niacin, several countries fortified some of the staple food items, such as wheat flour, milk, maize flour, cornmeal, and/or rice with niacin.

Figure 9.21 is depicted the nicin deficiencies.

Toxicity

Toxicity when eating foods containing niacin is rare, but can occur from long-term use of high-dose supplements. A reddened skin flush with itchiness or tingling on the face, arms, and chest is a common sign. Flushing occurs mainly when taking high-dosage supplements in the form of nicotinic acid, rather than nicotinamide. Other signs:
☐ Dizziness
☐ Low blood pressure
☐ Fatigue
☐ Headache
☐ Upset stomach
☐ Nausea
☐ Blurred vision
☐ Impaired glucose tolerance and inflammation of liver in severe cases (at very high doses of 3,000–9,000 mg daily for several months/years).

▌PYRIDOXINE

Vitamin B6 is one of the central molecules in the cells of living organisms. Water-soluble vitamin B6 is widely present in many foods, including meat, fish, nuts, beans, grains, fruits, and vegetables. Additionally, B6 is present in many multivitamin preparations for adults and children and is added to foods as a supplement to foods, power bars, and powders.

Figure 9.22 is depicted the symptoms of vitamin B6 deficiency.

Deficiency: The clinical symptoms of vitamin B5 deficiency include:
☐ **Anemia:** Certain types of anemia's, such as hypochromic (deficient content of RBCs) and microcytic (smaller than normal erythrocytes and less circulating hemoglobin) occur even when the serum iron levels are high or adequate.
☐ **Central nervous system disorder (CNS):** Pyridoxine controls neurological conditions related to brain activity. Due to the deficiency of the vitamin CNS disorders show abnormal electroencephalogram (EEG) readings. In infants, the deficiency of vitamin B6 causes hyperirritability, which progresses to convulsive seizures. This condition arises in infants who are fed commercial milk formula because most of the pyridoxine is destroyed by high-temperature autoclaving.
☐ **Drugs:** Isoniazid used for tuberculosis is an antagonist to pyridoxine.
☐ **Pregnancy:** Along with maternal metabolic demands, fetal growth increases the pyridoxine requirement.
☐ **Oral contraceptives:** Women who are on estrogen-progestin oral contraceptives require more vitamin B6. It causes abnormal tryptophan metabolism, which contributes to the increased requirement.

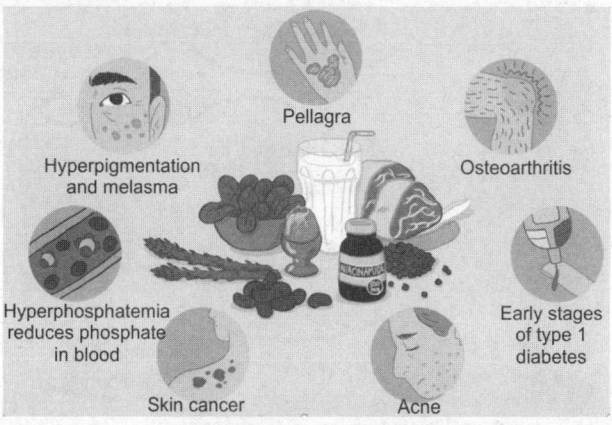

Fig. 9.21: Nicin deficiencies.

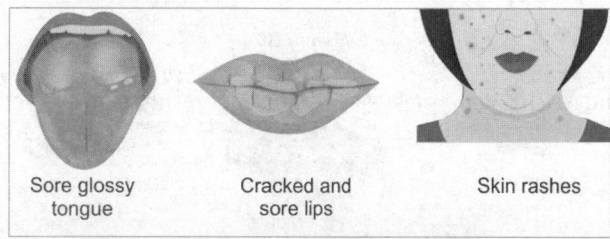

Fig. 9.22: Symptoms of vitamin B6 deficiency.

Pathophysiology

- Vitamin B6 is predominantly absorbed in the small intestine jejunum and is metabolized at the cellular level in the mitochondria and cytosol to active forms in the liver.
- The phosphorylated form of the vitamin is converted in dephosphorylated form and the pool of free vitamin B6 in jejunum by passive diffusion.
- Excretion of excess B6 occurs in the kidney and is albumin-bound in plasma. The half-life elimination exceeds 15 to 20 days.
- Vitamin B6 deficiency may present with seizures in the young. Severely deficient adults commonly present with rashes and mental status changes.
- Additional clinical findings of deficiency may include normocytic anemia, a nonspecific pruritic rash, cheilitis with scaly lip skin and cracks in the corner of the mouth, and glossitis (swelling of the tongue). Depression is associated with a severe B6 deficiency as well.

Figure 9.23 is depicted the food sources of vitamin B6.

Treatment/Management

- In vitamin B6-deficient states and illnesses, treatment dosage is variable and depends on the severity of symptoms. The vitamin is available therapeutically in both oral and parenteral formulations.
- Neonates with B6 deficiency seizures may require 10 to 100 mg intravenous (IV) for effective treatment of active seizures. Less serious or less acute presentations can be supplemented with doses ranging from 25 mg to 600 mg per day orally depending on symptom complex.
- Importantly, Vitamin B6 therapy can be life-saving in refractory INH overdose-induced seizures.
- The dose is equal to the known amount of INH ingested or a maximum of 5 g and is dosed 1 to 4 g IV as the first dose, then 1 g IM or IV every 30 minutes.
- In ethylene glycol overdose, vitamin B6 is recommended at 50 to 100 mg IV every 6 hours to facilitate shunting the metabolism of ethylene glycol to nontoxic pathways leading to glycine (nontoxic) instead of toxic pathways leading to toxic metabolites, such as formate.
- Additional, less common uses are in hydralazine overdose, where the recommended dose of vitamin B6 is 25 mg/kg, the first third administered intramuscularly, and the remainder as a 3-hour IV infusion.
- Gyromitra (mushroom) toxicity treatment is at 25 mg/kg infused IV over 30 min.
- Hyperemesis gravidarum may respond to vitamin B6 at a dosage of 25 mg orally every 8 hours.

PANTOTHENIC ACID

Vitamin B5 deficiency is rare, but may include symptoms, such as fatigue, insomnia, depression, irritability, vomiting, stomach pains, burning feet, and upper respiratory infections. Vitamin B5 is a medication used in the management and treatment of nutrient deficiencies. It is in the dietary supplement class of medications. This activity reviews the indications, actions, and contraindications for vitamin B5 as a valuable agent in treating nutritional deficiencies. This activity will highlight the mechanism of action, adverse event profile, and other key factors in the treatment of patients with nutritional deficiencies and related conditions.

High Cholesterol/High Triglycerides

- Several small, double-blind studies suggest that pantethine may help reduce triglycerides, or fats, in the blood in people who have high cholesterol.
- Some of these studies show that pantethine helped lower LDL (bad) cholesterol and raise HDL (good) cholesterol.
- In some open studies, pantethine seems to lower levels of cholesterol and triglycerides in people with diabetes. But not all studies agree. Larger studies are needed to see whether pantethine has any real benefit.

Figure 9.24 is depicted the vitamin B5 deficiency.
Figure 9.25 is depicted the vitamin B5 rich foods' benefits.

Skin Care and Wound Healing

- Preliminary research suggests that vitamin B5 has moisturizing effects on the skin; however, researchers are not clear why it works.

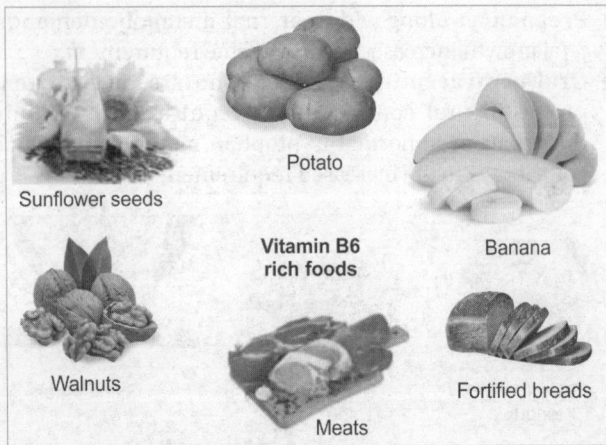

Fig. 9.23: Food sources of vitamin B6.

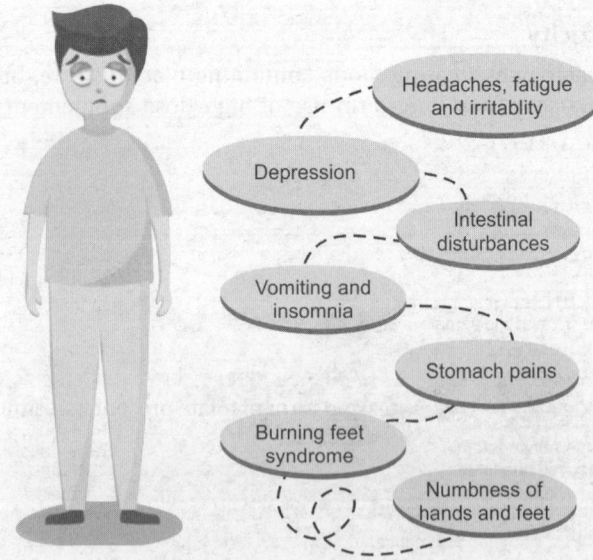

Fig. 9.24: Vitamin B5 deficiency.

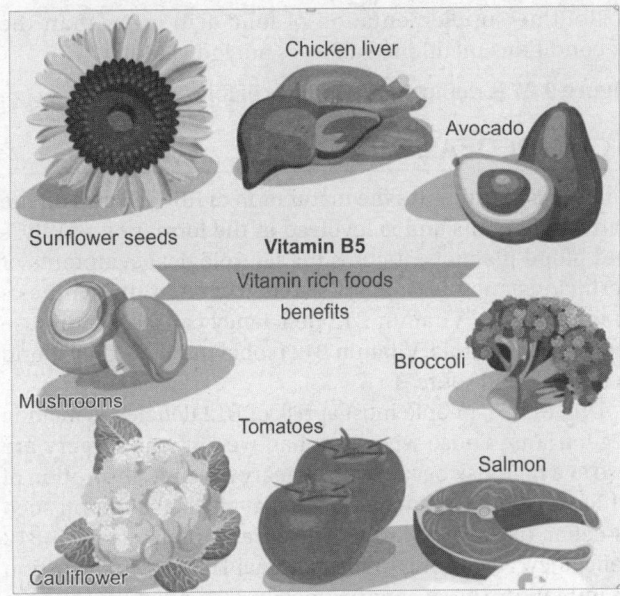

Fig. 9.25: Vitamin B5 rich foods' benefits.

Folate (vitamin B9) is an important vitamin that works with other B vitamins to metabolize proteins, and synthesize both blood cells DNA. Green leafy vegetables, legumes, grains, meats, and organ meats are high in folate. The vitamin is not stored in the body, so levels of folate in the body can become low after just a few weeks of eating a folate-deficient diet. As with other deficiency syndromes above, disorders of the digestive system and alcoholism can contribute to folate deficiency. Additionally, certain medications, hemolytic anemia, and kidney dialysis can result in folate deficiency.

- Overcooking destroys much of folic acid and thus contributes of folate deficiency in man.
- Nutritional megaloblastic anemia in adults, the classical studies of Wills (1931) in India showed that the megaloblastic anemia prevalent in pregnant women of the low-income groups substituting on poor vegetarian diets.
- Megaloblastic anemia has been reported to occur among malnourished children in the developing countries.

Symptoms of folate deficiency include fatigue, irritability, diarrhea, poor growth, and a smooth or tender tongue. In pregnant women, a deficiency of folate can also increase the risk of neural tube defects in the developing fetus.

For most people, a healthy diet high with a variety of meats, grains, fruits, and vegetables is enough to prevent a deficiency of B complex vitamins. Women who expect to become pregnant are advised to take folate supplements. Older people or those with medical conditions that increase the risk of B vitamin deficiency may also benefit from taking a daily supplement.

Figure 9.26 is depicted the folic acid deficiency.

- Other studies, mostly in test tubes and animals but a few on people, suggest that vitamin B5 supplements may speed wound healing, especially following surgery. This may be particularly true if vitamin B5 is combined with vitamin C.

Rheumatoid Arthritis

- Preliminary evidence suggests that pantothenic acid might improve symptoms of rheumatoid arthritis (RA), but the evidence is weak.
- One study found that people with RA may have lower levels of B5 in their blood than healthy people, and the lowest levels were associated with the most severe symptoms.
- Other studies show that calcium pantothenate improves symptoms of RA, including morning stiffness and pain. More studies are needed to confirm these findings.

Toxicity

It is highly unlikely to have toxicity in the case of vitamin B5. The Recommended Dietary Intake of vitamin B5 is 5 mg for adults. It is extremely necessary to get consulted with a doctor or health supervisor before taking Vitamin B5 in supplement form as an over dosage might cause diarrhea, stomach trouble, headache, excessive stress and might also increase the risk of bleeding, etc. Vitamin B5 supplements are mostly prescribed to be taken with water, preferably after eating.

FOLIC ACID

Folate is an essential water-soluble vitamin, naturally present in food, especially in fruits, green leafy vegetables, and liver. Folic acid is the synthesized form of folate present in fortified foods and supplements and has a higher bioavailability than naturally occurring folate. Folate has been added to grains to prevent congenital disabilities, especially neural tube defects, as it is necessary for the formation of several coenzymes in many metabolic systems and maintenance in erythropoiesis.

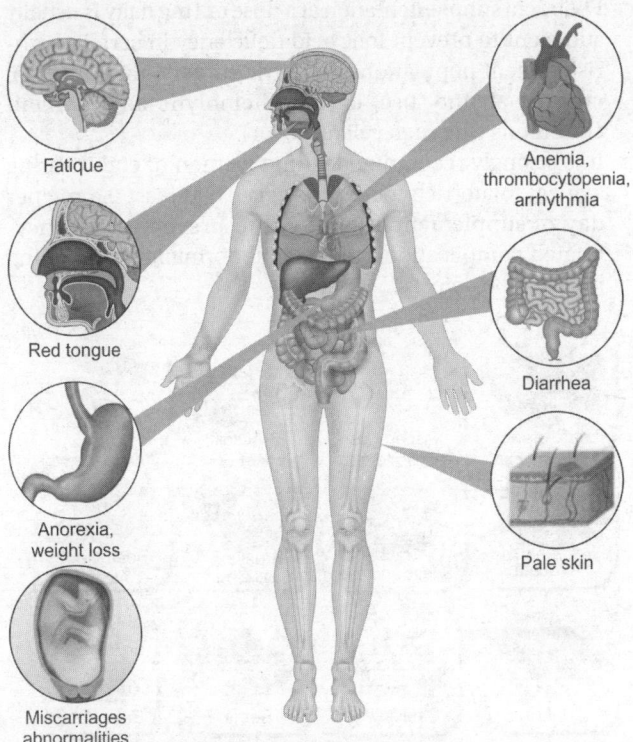

Fig. 9.26: Folic acid deficiency.

Treatment/Management

- All patients with folate deficiency should be offered supplemental folic acid for the correction of the deficiency. Typically, oral folic acid (1 to 5 mg daily) suffices to treat folate deficiency.
- Intravenous, subcutaneous, or intramuscular formulations of folic acid can be used for patients unable to tolerate oral medications.
- Folinic acid (also called leucovorin), a reduced form of folate, is primarily used to prevent the toxicities of methotrexate.
- The duration of therapy depends on whether the cause of the initial deficiency persists. Patients with malabsorption or short gut syndromes may typically require long-term treatment.
- In patients who have a concomitant vitamin B12 deficiency, it is imperative to replete vitamin B12 as well.
- Folate treatment alone does not improve neurological symptoms and signs due to B12 deficiency, which, if untreated may likely progress and cause permanent neurological damage

Complications

- Untreated folic acid deficiency can lead to megaloblastic anemia and pancytopenia. In addition, it can cause glossitis, angular stomatitis, and oral ulcers.
- Neuropsychiatric manifestations, including depression, irritability, insomnia, cognitive decline, fatigue, and psychosis, are also known to occur with folic acid deficiency

Patient Education

- Patients with folic acid deficiency should be encouraged to eat a diet rich in green leafy vegetables and fruits.
- Folic acid supplementation at a dose of 1mg daily is usually sufficient to prevent folic acid deficiency in certain high-risk patient populations (bariatric surgery, malnutrition, chronic alcohol use, chronic hemolytic anemia, and conditions with high cell turnover).
- It is strongly recommended that women of childbearing age eat folate-rich foods, and receive at least 0.4 mg per day of supplemental folic acid to prevent pregnancy-related complications and fetal abnormalities, including neural tube defects.
- Routine supplementation of folic acid other than the conditions mentioned above is not indicated.

Figure 9.27 is depicted the sources of folic acid.

CYANOCOBALAMIN

Vitamin B12 promotes the maturation of RBCs. It acts on the narrow elements and is involved in the formation of WBCs and blood platelets. It cures the neurological symptoms of pernicious anemia. It acts as a coenzyme in the synthesis of methionine. Vitamin B12 deficiency causes the disease 'pernicious anemia'. Vitamin B12 (cobalamine) is only found in animal food sources.

Due to this, people most at risk of B12 deficiency include vegetarians. Those who have had weight loss surgery are also at a high risk because the surgery disrupts absorption of B12 from food. Other conditions that affect absorption such as celiac disease or Crohn's disease, can also lead to B12 deficiency. According to the National Health and Nutrition Examination Survey, approximately 3.2% of adults over the age of 50 have a B12 deficiency, and up to 20% may have levels of B12 that are borderline.

Figure 9.28 is depicted the vitamin B12 deficiency.
- Pernicious anemia is the major problem arising from an inadequate amount of vitamin B12.
- Pernicious anemia is a condition characterized by very large, immature RBCs with normal amounts of hemoglobin.

The primary symptoms of B12 deficiency are:
- Numbness or tingling in hands, legs, and feet
- Difficulty walking
- Anemia

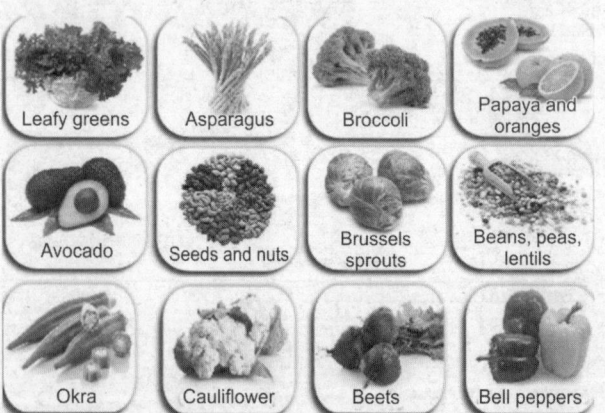

Fig. 9.27: Sources of folic acid.

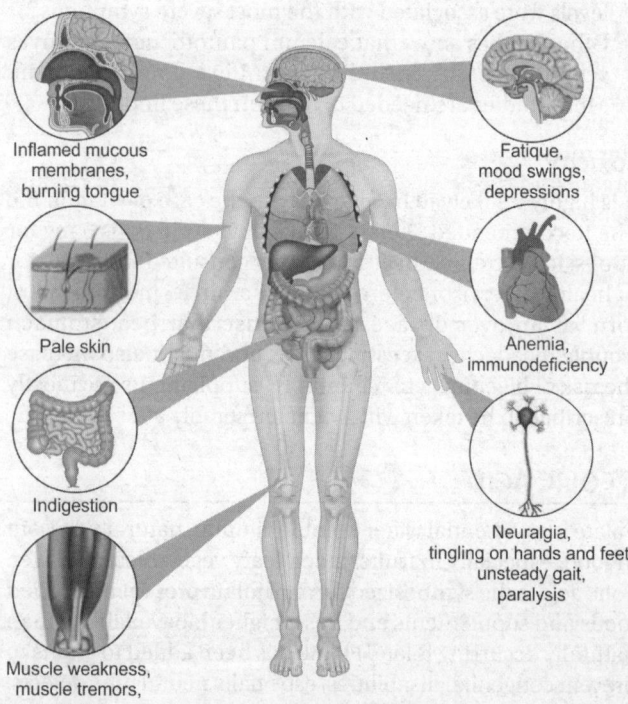

Fig. 9.28: Vitamin B12 deficiency.

- A swollen tongue
- Jaundice
- Cognitive changes
- Hallucinations
- Paranoia
- Weakness
- Fatigue

Toxicity

Cyanocobalamin secretion is usually in bile. With higher doses of cyanocobalamin, it undergoes rapid elimination in the urine. No over dosage occurs with cyanocobalamin. There is no antidote to vitamin B12.

Adverse Effects

Cyanocobalamin, though only a vitamin, can cause several adverse effects. Patients with sensitivity can even experience life-threatening anaphylactic reactions. Apart from that, allergic reactions, such as itching, erythema, wheals may appear. Other common adverse effects include:
- Shortness of breath (even with mild exertion), swelling, rapid weight gain
- Pulmonary edema, congestive heart failure; peripheral vascular thrombosis
- Hypokalemia—leg cramps, irregular heartbeats, tingling/numbness, muscle weakness, or limp feeling
- Numbness or tingling and joint pain
- Fever
- Swollen tongue
- Itching or rash
- Polycythemia (cyanocobalamin can unmask the underlying polycythemia)

MINERAL DEFICIENCY DISEASES

Mineral deficiency is a lack of the dietary minerals, the micronutrients that are needed for an organism's proper health. The cause may be a poor diet, impaired uptake of the minerals that are consumed, or a dysfunction in the organism's use of the mineral after it is absorbed. These deficiencies can result in many disorders including anemia and goitre. Examples of mineral deficiency include, zinc deficiency, iron deficiency, and magnesium deficiency.

Table 9.5 is depicted the types of minerals and their deficiencies.

Definition: Mineral deficiency is a reduced level of any of the minerals essential to human health. An abnormally low mineral concentration is usually defined as a level that may impair a function dependent on that mineral.

Calcium

- Essential for strong bones and teeth, healthy gums, and bone growth and mineral density in children.
- Calcium helps regulate the heart rate and nerve impulses, lower cholesterol, prevent atherosclerosis, develop muscles, and prevent muscle cramping.
- Calcium is an important component of blood clotting. Calcium and phosphorus are closely related minerals that should be balanced.
- About 99% of calcium and 85% of phosphate occur in the skeleton as crystals of calcium phosphate.
- Both nutrients occur in a variety of foods, such as milk, eggs, and green, leafy vegetables.
- Calcium deficiency due to lack of dietary calcium occurs only rarely and is often due to vitamin D deficiency, because vitamin D is required for efficient absorption of dietary calcium. Significant depletion of calcium stores can lead to osteoporosis.

Magnesium

- Assists in the utilization of calcium and potassium, and functions in enzyme reactions to produce energy.
- Magnesium protects the lining of arteries and helps form bones. It helps prevent cardiovascular disease, osteoporosis, and some cancers.
- By acting with vitamin B6, magnesium can help prevent or dissolve calcium oxalate kidney stones, the most common kind of stones. Dietary magnesium deficiency is uncommon, but may occur in chronic alcoholics, persons taking diuretic drugs, and as a result of severe, prolonged diarrhea.

Sodium

- Sodium deficiency (hyponatremia) is a serious deficiency, arising most often after excessive losses of body fluid (**dehydration**) during prolonged and severe diarrhea or **vomiting**.
- Sodium and potassium are electrolytes that must be balanced in the body. Since most people get more than enough salt in the diet, potassium may be needed to balance it.
- Together, these minerals control fluid balance through a mechanism called "the sodium/potassium pump." Prolonged imbalances in sodium and potassium can contribute to heart disease.

Potassium

- Important for a healthy nervous system and a steady heart rate, helps to prevent stroke, and, with sodium, is critical in maintaining fluid balance.

Table 9.5: Types of minerals and their deficiencies.

Mineral	Major deficiency disorders
Iodine	Goiter, hypothyroidism, iodine deficiency disorders, increased risk of stillbirth, birth defects infant mortality, cognitive impairment
Calcium	Decreased bone mineralization, rickets, osteoporosis
Iron	Iron deficiency anemia, reduced learning and work capacity, maternal and infant mortality, low birth weight
Zinc	Poor pregnancy outcome, impaired growth (stunting), genetic disorders, decreased resistance to infectious diseases
Fluoride	Increased dental decay, affects bone health
Selenium	Cardiomyopathy, increased cancer and cardiovascular risk

- Potassium, an electrolyte, must be balanced with sodium. Potassium deficiency is usually associated with sodium deficiency and both are associated with dehydration stemming from excessive losses of body fluid.

Phosphorus

- Helps form bones and teeth, supports cell growth, and regulates heart muscle contraction and kidney function.
- Phosphorus converts food to energy and supports the utilization of vitamins.
- Deficiency is rare because phosphate is plentiful in plant and animal foods and is efficiently absorbed from the diet.
- Phosphorus is closely related to calcium and the two minerals should be in balance with each other and with magnesium.
- Deficiency in one will affect all and will ultimately have an unwanted effect on body function.
- Calcium and phosphorus are stored in the bones as crystals of calcium phosphate. Milk, eggs, and green, leafy vegetables are rich in calcium and phosphate.

Trace minerals essential for human health include:
- **Boron:** Required for healthy bones, brain function, alertness, and the metabolism of bulk minerals, such as calcium, phosphorus, and magnesium. Deficiencies are rare except in aging, when supplementation may help absorb calcium. A deficiency in boron is associated with vitamin D deficiency. Boron supplements can improve calcium levels as well as vitamin D levels, and can help prevent osteoporosis in postmenopausal women by promoting calcium absorption.
- **Chromium:** Required for maintaining energy levels. Chromium helps metabolize glucose and stabilize glucose levels. It helps the body manufacture and use cholesterol and protein.
- **Copper:** Helps form healthy bones, joints, and nerves as well as hemoglobin and red blood cells. Copper contributes to healing, energy production, taste, and hair and skin color. It is essential in forming collagen for healthy bones and connective tissue, and helps prevent osteoporosis. Except in osteoporosis, copper deficiency is rare, although dramatic changes in copper metabolism occur in two serious genetic diseases, Wilson disease and Menkes' disease.
- **Germanium:** Helps improve the delivery of oxygen to tissues and remove toxins and poisons from the body. Germanium gives garlic its natural antibiotic properties.
- **Iodine:** Helps promote healthy physical and mental development in children. Iodine is required for thyroid gland function and metabolizing fats. Iodine deficiency is a public health problem in parts of the world that have iodine-deficient soils. Iodine is needed to make thyroid hormone, which has a variety of roles in human embryo development. A deficiency during pregnancy can cause serious birth defects. Deficiency in adults can result in an enlarged thyroid gland (goiter) in the neck.
- **Iron:** Critical in the production of hemoglobin, the oxygen-carrying protein in red blood cells, and myoglobin found in muscle tissue. Iron is essential for important enzyme reactions, growth, and maintaining a healthy immune system. In the blood, iron is found in larger amounts than any other mineral. Iron deficiency causes anemia (low hemoglobin and reduced numbers of red blood cells), which results in tiredness and shortness of breath because of poor oxygen delivery.
- **Manganese:** Essential for metabolizing fat and protein, regulating blood glucose, and supporting immune system and nervous system function. Manganese is necessary for normal bone growth and cartilage development. It is involved in reproductive functions and helps produce mother's milk. Along with B vitamins, manganese produces feelings of well-being. Deficiency can lead to convulsions, vision and hearing problems, muscle contractions, tooth-grinding and other problems in children; and atherosclerosis, heart disease, and **hypertension** in older adults.
- **Molybdenum:** Found in bones, kidneys, and liver. Only extremely small amounts are needed to metabolize nitrogen and promote proper cell function. Molybdenum is present in beans, peas, legumes, whole grains, and green leafy vegetables. A diet low in these foods can lead to mouth and gum problems and cancer.
- **Selenium:** An important antioxidant that works with vitamin E to protect the immune system, heart, and liver, and may help prevent tumor formation. Selenium deficiency occurs in regions of the world where soils are selenium-poor and low-selenium foods are produced. Premature infants are naturally low in selenium with no known serious effects.
- **Silicon:** Helps form bones and connective tissue, nails, skin, and hair. Silicon is important in preventing cardiovascular disease.
- **Sulfur:** Disinfects the blood and helps to rid the body of harmful bacteria and toxic substances.
- **Vanadium:** Vital to cell metabolism, and helps reduce cholesterol and form healthy bones and teeth. Vanadium functions in reproduction. Deficiencies may be associated with heart and kidney disease and reproductive disorders. Vanadium deficiency may be associated with infant mortality.
- **Zinc:** Important in the growth of reproductive organs and regulation of oil glands. Zinc is required for protein synthesis, immune system function, protection of the liver, collagen formation, and wound healing. A component of insulin and major body enzymes, zinc helps vitamin absorption, particularly vitamins A and E. Deficiency is rare.

Nutritional Concerns

- A balanced diet includes fresh vegetables and fruits, legumes, whole grains (cereal, bread, rice, pasta, and other grains), eggs, dairy products, fish, fowl, and lean meat as preferred.
- A diet high in refined foods, prepared foods, sugars, and fats will not provide sufficient quantities of essential minerals.

- Water delivers nutrients throughout the body; it is essential to drink enough clean water daily to maintain fluid balance and distribute nutrients.

IRON DEFICIENCY (FIG. 9.29)

Iron deficiency occurs most often because of poor iron intake and poor absorption. In children, iron deficiency is due to periods of dietary deficiency and heavy demands for iron during rapid growth. Human milk and cow's milk both contain low levels of iron; however, the iron in human milk is in a highly absorbable form.

- Infants are at risk for acquiring iron deficiency because their rapid rate of growth needs a corresponding increased supply of dietary iron, for use in making blood and muscles.
- Cow's milk formula is fortified with iron. Human milk is a better source of iron than cow's milk, since about half of the iron in human breast milk is absorbed by the infant's digestive tract. In contrast, only 10% of the iron in cow's milk is absorbed by the infant.
- Toddlers who drink excessive whole cow's milk are at risk for iron deficiency. Iron deficiency can also be caused by excess phosphorus in the diet, chronic intestinal bleeding, poor digestion and absorption, prolonged illness, ulcers, and the use of antacids.
- In women and teenage girls, blood loss through menstruation can result in iron deficiency. Symptoms of iron deficiency include anemia and resulting fatigue and weakness, especially during physical exertion.
- Fragile bones, brittle hair and nails, hair loss, spoon-shaped fingernails or ridges from the base of the nails to the ends, difficulty swallowing, nervousness, paleness, and lagging mental responses are also possible iron deficiency symptoms

Iron Deficiency Anemia

Anemia is a condition in which the body does not have enough healthy red blood cells. Red blood cells provide oxygen to body tissues. There are many types of anemia. Iron deficiency anemia occurs when your body does not have enough iron. Iron helps make red blood cells. Iron deficiency anemia is the most common form of anemia.

Figure 9.30 is depicted the iron deficiency and iron-deficiency anemia.

Causes

Iron deficiency anemia relates directly to a lack of iron in the body. The cause of the iron deficiency varies, however.

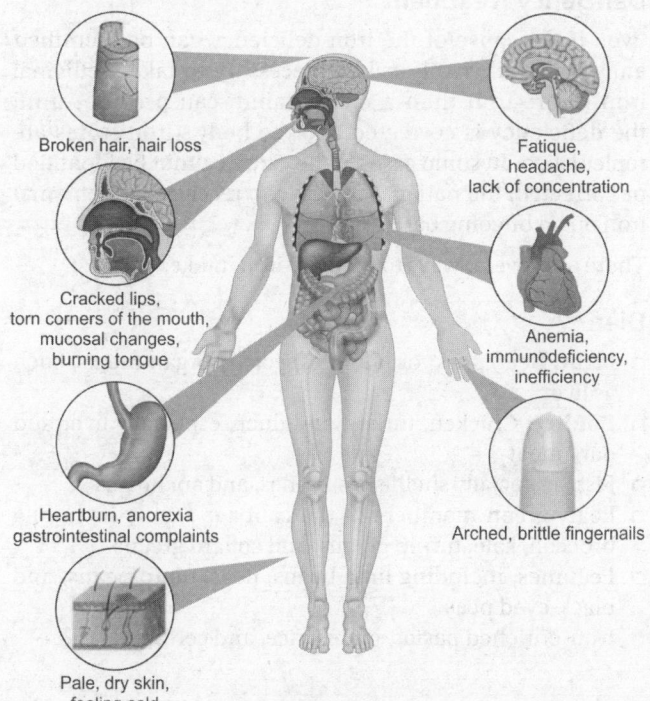

Fig. 9.29: Iron deficiency.

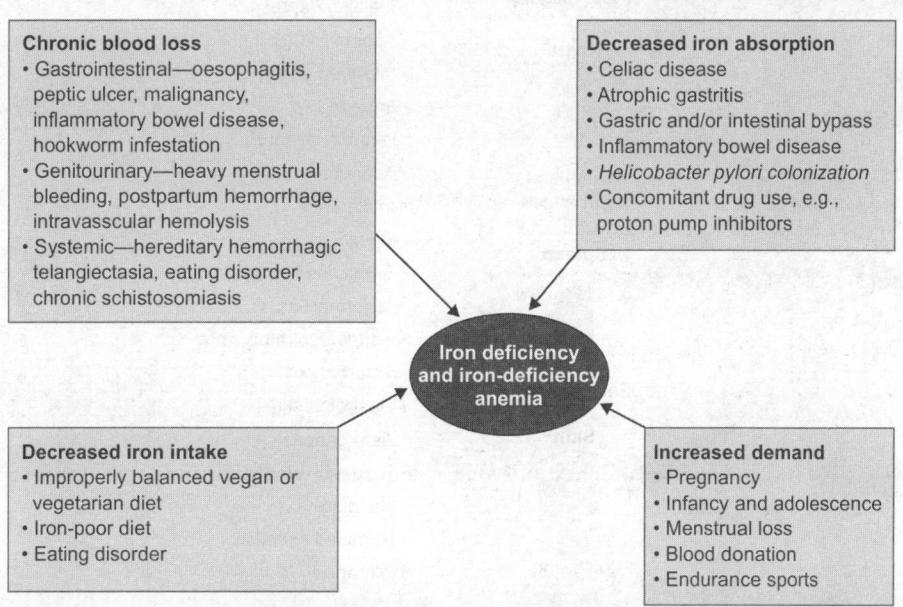

Fig. 9.30: Iron deficiency and iron-deficiency anemia.

Some common causes include:
- Poor diet or not enough iron in the diet
- Blood loss
- A decreased ability to absorb iron
- Pregnancy

Poor diet: Diets that lack iron are a leading cause of iron deficiency. Foods rich in iron, such as eggs and meat, supply the body with much of the iron it needs to produce hemoglobin. If a person does not eat enough to maintain their iron supply, an iron deficiency can develop.

Blood loss: Iron is found primarily in the blood, as it is stored in red blood cells. An iron deficiency may result when a person loses a lot of blood from an injury, giving birth, or heavy menstruation. In some cases, slow loss of blood from chronic diseases or some cancers can lead to an iron deficiency.

Decreased ability to absorb iron: Some people are not able to absorb enough iron from the food they eat. This may be due to a problem with the small intestine, such as celiac disease or Crohn's disease, or if a portion of the small intestine has been removed.

Pregnancy: Low iron levels are a common problem for pregnant women. The growing fetus needs a lot of iron, which can lead to an iron deficiency.

Also, a pregnant woman has an increased amount of blood in her body. This larger volume of blood demands more iron to meet its needs.

Signs and Symptoms of Iron-deficiency Anemia

Symptoms of iron-deficiency anemia are related to decreased oxygen delivery to the entire body and may include:
- Being pale or having yellow "sallow" skin
- Unexplained fatigue or lack of energy
- Shortness of breath or chest pain, especially with activity
- Unexplained generalized weakness
- Rapid heartbeat
- Pounding or "whooshing" in the ears
- Headache, especially with activity
- Craving for ice or clay—"picophagia"
- Sore or smooth tongue
- Brittle nails or hair loss

Figure 9.31 is depicted the symptoms of anemia.

Figure 9.32 is depicted the signs and symptoms of iron-deficiency anemia and **Figure 9.33** is depicted the cognitive impairments of iron deficiency anemia.

Deficiency Treatment

Even if the cause of the iron deficiency can be identified and treated, it is still usually necessary to take medicinal iron (more iron than a multivitamin can provide) until the deficiency is corrected and the body's iron stores are replenished. In some cases, if the cause cannot be identified or corrected, the patient may have to receive supplemental iron on an ongoing basis.

There are several ways to increase iron intake:

Diet

- **Meat:** Beef, pork, or lamb, especially organ meats, such as liver
- **Poultry:** Chicken, turkey, and duck, especially liver and dark meat
- Fish, especially shellfish, sardines, and anchovies
- Leafy green members of the cabbage family including broccoli, kale, turnip greens, and collard greens
- Legumes, including lima beans, peas, pinto beans, and black-eyed peas
- Iron-enriched pastas, grains, rice, and cereals

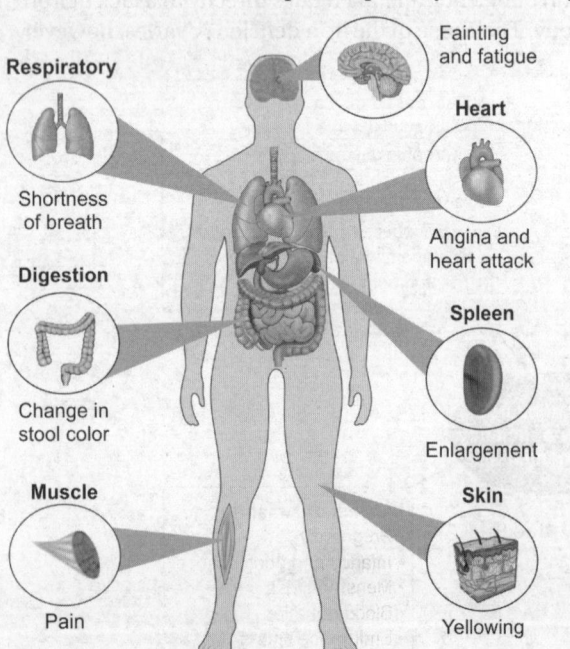

Fig. 9.31: Symptoms of anemia.

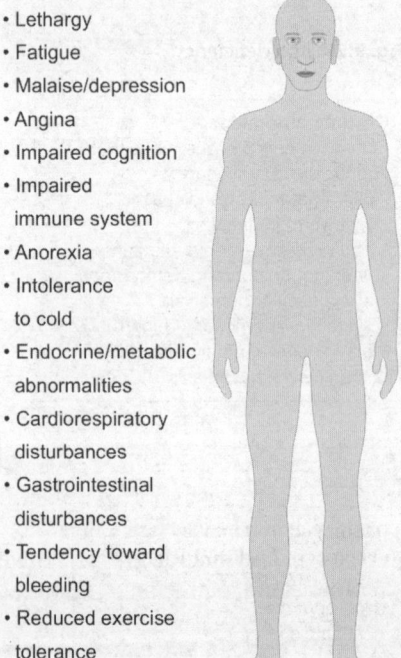

Fig. 9.32: Signs and symptoms of iron-deficiency anemia.

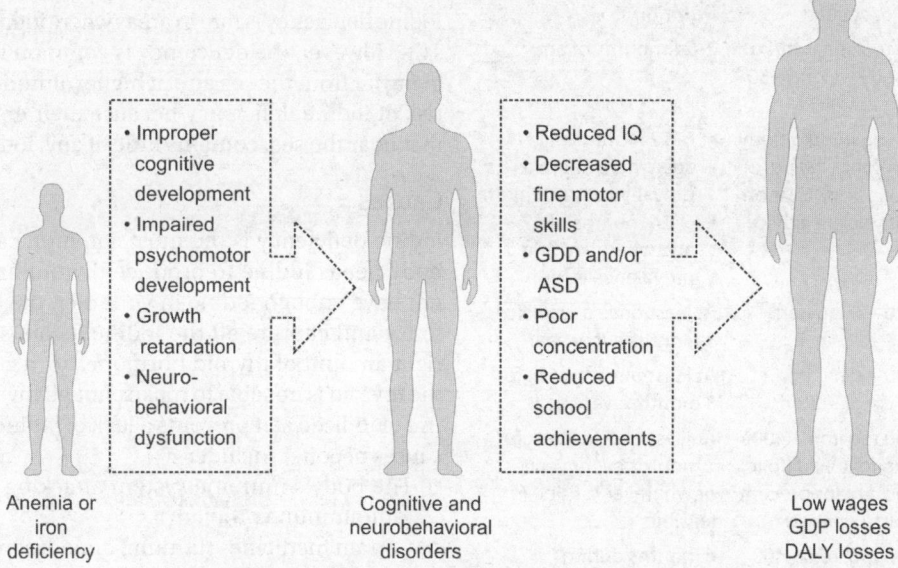

Fig. 9.33: Cognitive impairments of iron deficiency anemia.

Medicinal Iron

- The amount of iron needed to treat patients with iron deficiency is higher than the amount found in most daily multivitamin supplements.
- The amount of iron prescribed by your doctor will be in milligrams (mg) of elemental iron.
- Most people with iron deficiency need 150–200 mg per day of elemental iron (2 to 5 mg of iron per kilogram of body weight per day).

Intravenous Iron

In some cases, your doctor may recommend intravenous (IV) iron. IV iron may be necessary to treat iron deficiency in patients who do not absorb iron well in the gastrointestinal tract, patients with severe iron deficiency or chronic blood loss, patients who are receiving supplemental erythropoietin, a hormone that stimulates blood production, or patients who cannot tolerate oral iron. If you need IV iron, your doctor may refer you to a hematologist to supervise the iron infusions. IV iron comes in different preparations:

1. Iron dextran
2. Iron sucrose
3. Ferric gluconate

Large doses of iron can be given at one time when using iron dextran. Iron sucrose and ferric gluconate require more frequent doses spread over several weeks. Some patients may have an allergic reaction to IV iron, so a test dose may be administered before the first infusion. Allergic reactions are more common with iron dextran and may necessitate switching to a different preparation. Severe side effects other than allergic reactions are rare and include urticaria (hives), pruritus (itching), and muscle and joint pain.

Blood Transfusions

- Red blood cell transfusions may be given to patients with severe iron-deficiency anemia who are actively bleeding or have significant symptoms such as chest pain, shortness of breath, or weakness.
- Transfusions are given to replace deficient red blood cells and will not completely correct the iron deficiency.
- Red blood cell transfusions will only provide temporary improvement. It is important to find out why you are anemic and treat the cause as well as the symptoms.

Complications

In milder cases of iron deficiency anemia, a person is unlikely to have more than the normal symptoms described above. However, additional complications can occur if the iron deficiency anemia is left untreated.

Possible complications include:

- Slow growth and developmental delays in children and infants
- Heart problems, including heart failure or an enlarged heart due to it compensating for lack of oxygen
- Pregnancy complications, including low birth weights and an increased risk for premature birth

Preventing Iron Deficiency and Anemia

Control bleeding by encouraging women to:

- Be delivered by a trained birth attendant or at a maternity unit if there is a risk of complications.
- Start breastfeeding within ½ hour of birth. Breastfeeding makes the mother's uterus tighten and reduces bleeding.
- Wait two minutes after birth before clamping the umbilical cord so the baby gets more blood from the placenta.

Give Prophylactic Supplements (Table 9.6)

- Give oral iron and folic acid supplements to pregnant and lactating women, to females of reproductive age and to low birth weight babies.

Table 9.6: Prophylactic supplements of iron.

Group	Dosage/day	Duration
Low birth weight infants <2500 g	1 to 2 mg iron/kg body weight + 50 µg folic acid	2–24 months of age
Children 6–24 months	2 mg iron/kg body weight + 50 µg folic acid[b]. Give on physician's advice	• 6–12 months of age where anemia prevalence is not high • 6–24 months of age where anemia prevalence is high
Children 24–59 months	20–30 mg iron	At least once a week for 3 months every year
Children 6–11 years	30–60 mg iron	At least once a week for 3 months every year
Adolescents and women of reproductive age	60 mg iron + 400 µg folic acid (folic acid helps prevent birth defects)	At least once a week for 3 months every year—or whatever routine is feasible
Women pregnant and lactating	60 mg iron + 400 µg folic acid	6 months during pregnancy and 3 months postpartum

- Do not give routine prophylactic iron or folic acid to children in malaria endemic areas as it may increase adverse effects and mortality unless they are proven to be iron-deficient.
- Explain the importance of taking supplements regularly for the full duration and how to deal with possible side effects.

To prevent iron deficiency advise families to:
- Eat more meat (of any kind), fish, poultry and organ meats—the darker red the food the more hem iron it contains. These foods must be well cooked to kill parasites and pathogens.
- Eat more fresh vegetables and fruits (to increase absorption of non-hem iron from other foods in a meal). Foods high in non-hem iron include egg yolk, dark green vegetables, millet, sorghum and legumes.
- Avoid drinking tea or coffee with or soon after meals. Do not give tea and coffee to children.
- Eat fermented porridges and germinate/malt cereals and legumes to reduce phytates.
- Eat foods fortified with iron if feasible, such as some wheat flours. Families can use home fortification products if available.
- Breastfeed babies exclusively for 6 months and then to include iron-rich foods, such as suitably prepared meat or fish in their diets.
  • Iron tablets usually contain 60 mg iron and folic acid tablets 400 µg folic acid. Iron syrup usually contains 20 mg iron/mL. Check before prescribing.
  • Do not give folic acid if the person is taking sulfur-based drugs including sulfadoxine-pyrimethamine (Fansidar) for malaria as it may interfere with the action of the antimalarial.
  • A pregnant woman should stop taking folic acid for one week after taking a dose of Fansidar.

IODINE DEFICIENCIES

Iodine deficiency is rare in areas where iodine is added to table salt. However, the deficiency is common worldwide. People living far from the sea and at higher altitudes are at particular risk of iodine deficiency because their environment, unlike that near the sea, contains little, if any, iodine.

Causes

Iodine deficiency is the most common cause of goiter. The body needs iodine to produce thyroid hormone. If you do not have enough iodine in your diet, the thyroid gets larger to try and capture all the iodine it can, so it can make the right amount of thyroid hormone. So, a goiter can be a sign the thyroid is not able to make enough thyroid hormone. The use of iodized salt prevents a lack of iodine in the diet. Other causes of goiter include:
- The body's immune system attacking the thyroid gland (autoimmune problem)
- Certain medicines (lithium, amiodarone)
- Infections (rare)
- Cigarette smoking
- Eating very large amounts of certain foods (soy, peanuts, or vegetables in the broccoli and cabbage family)
- Toxic nodular goiter, an enlarged thyroid gland that has a small growth or many growths called nodules, which produce too much thyroid hormone

Symptoms of Iodine Deficiency (Fig. 9.34)

Many people do not know they have an iodine deficiency. However, some people who do not have enough iodine develop a goiter or enlargement of the thyroid gland in the neck. Iodine deficiency can also lead to hypothyroidism, (underactive thyroid, where there is too little of the thyroid hormone). This can cause symptoms including:
- Constant tiredness
- Muscle weakness
- Unexpected weight gain
- Difficulty learning and remembering

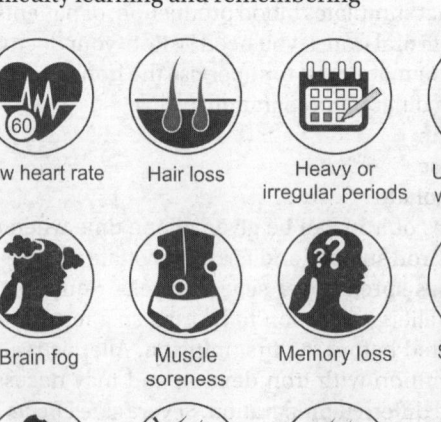

Fig. 9.34: Symptoms of iodine deficiency.

- Constipation
- Weak, slow heartbeat
- Dry skin
- Hair loss
- Puffy face
- Feeling cold

Diagnosis of Iodine Deficiency

- Assessment of thyroid structure and function
- Diagnosis of iodine deficiency in adults and children is usually based on thyroid function tests, examination for goiter, and imaging tests identifying abnormalities in thyroid function and structure.
- All neonates should be screened for hypothyroidism by measuring the TSH level.

Dietary Treatment

According to the National Institutes of Health Source, the following are good sources of iodine:
- Seaweed, 1 sheet dried: 11 to 1,989% of RDI (recommended daily intake)
- Cod, 3 ounces or 85 g: 66% of the RDI
- Yogurt, plain, 1 cup: 50% of the RDI
- Iodized salt, 1/4 teaspoon or 1.5 g: 47% of the RDI
- Shrimp, 3 ounces or 85 g: 23% of the RDI
- Egg, 1 large: 16% of the RDI
- Tuna, canned, 3 ounces or 85 g: 11% of the RDI
- Dried prunes, 5 pieces: 9% of the RDI

A person needs to consume 150 µg of iodine each day to maintain a healthy level for their body.

Treatment of Iodine Deficiency

- Iodide with/without levothyroxine
- Infants with iodine deficiency are given levothyroxine 3 µg/kg orally once/day for a week plus iodide 50 to 90 µg orally once/day for several weeks to quickly restore a euthyroid state.
- Children are treated with iodide 90 to 120 µg once/day and are given levothyroxine until able to synthesize T4.
- Adults are given iodide 150 µg once/day. Iodine deficiency can also be treated by giving levothyroxine.
- Women who are pregnant or breastfeeding should ingest iodide 250 µg once/day.
- Serum TSH levels are monitored in all patients until the levels are normal (i.e., <5 µgIU/mL).

CALCIUM DEFICIENCIES

Hypocalcemia, also known as calcium deficiency disease, occurs when the blood has low levels of calcium. A long-term calcium deficiency can lead to dental changes, cataracts, alterations in the brain, and osteoporosis, which causes the bones to become brittle. A calcium deficiency may cause no early symptoms. It is usually mild, but without treatment, it can become life threatening. By definition, hypocalcemia is the condition used to describe a calcium deficiency (Fig. 9.35).

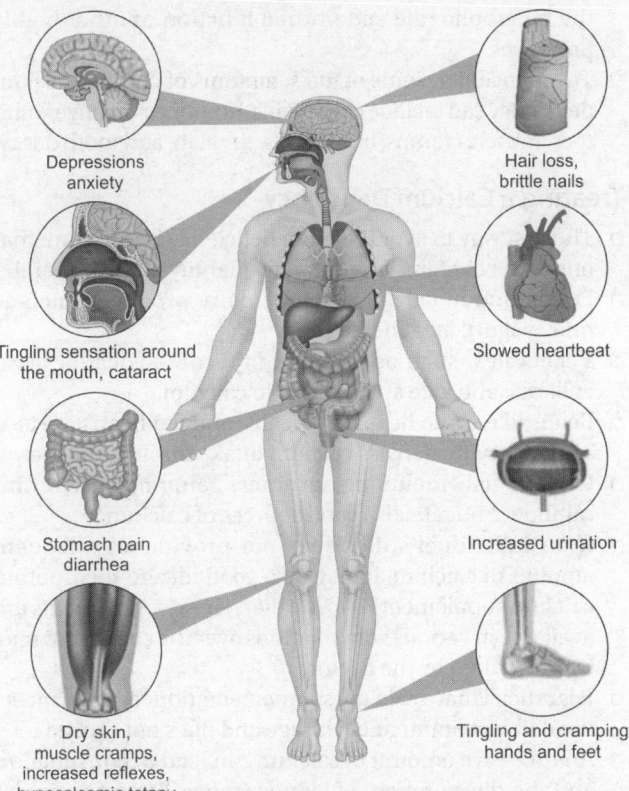

Fig. 9.35: Calcium deficiency.

Causes of Calcium Deficiency

- There are a number of reasons as to why blood calcium levels decline. For example, a lack of vitamin D, which is required for the absorption of calcium, can arise when people stay indoors for extended periods of time.
- Hypoparathyroidism is another reason for calcium deficiency. This condition can occur post-surgery or due to an autoimmune disease or genetic reasons.
- Renal disease and liver problems may also result in vitamin D deficiency and consequent calcium deficiency.
- Other conditions that may cause a calcium deficiency include pseudohypoparathyroidism, hypomagnesemia, hypermagnesemia, sclerotic metastases, and Fanconi syndrome.
- Any illness affecting the thyroid and parathyroid glands will also result in a general mineral deficiency that will therefore include calcium.

Symptoms of Calcium Deficiency

- A calcium deficiency often occurs in babies who are barely a few days old as a result of the often high levels of phosphate present in formula products that can reduce calcium levels in the blood.
- Some of the primary symptoms of hypocalcemia include irritability, muscle twitching, jitters, tremors, lethargy, and seizures. Aside from infants, a calcium deficiency can occur at any age.
- Chronic calcium deficiency can result in rickets, osteoporosis, and osteopenia, as well as disruptions in

the metabolic rate and normal function of other bodily processes.
- Taken together, some of the symptoms of chronic calcium deficiency can include chest pains, numbness in fingers and toes, muscle cramps, brittle nails, dry skin, and tooth decay.

Treating a Calcium Deficiency
- The first way to avoid calcium deficiency is to ensure that one's diet contains an adequate quantity of the mineral.
- Foods rich in calcium include dairy products, such as milk, yogurt, and cheese.
- Vegetables, such as spinach, broccoli, avocado, okra, collards, and kale are also rich in calcium.
- Beans like white beans, soybeans, and flat beans are also a good way to increase calcium intake through the diet.
- Certain fish including sardines, salmon, perch, and rainbow trout are also good sources of calcium.
- If an individual's diet does not provide an adequate amount of calcium, it may be a good idea to incorporate calcium supplements into the diet. These supplements are available in various combinations over the counter or may be prescribed by the doctor.
- It is crucial that a calcium supplementation regimen meets the daily recommended dosage and does not exceed it.
- An excessive amount of calcium can lead to constipation and the development of kidney stones. The presence of caffeine, alcohol, and extra sodium in the body will also decrease the body's ability to absorb calcium.

Figure 9.36 is depicted the calcium rich foods.

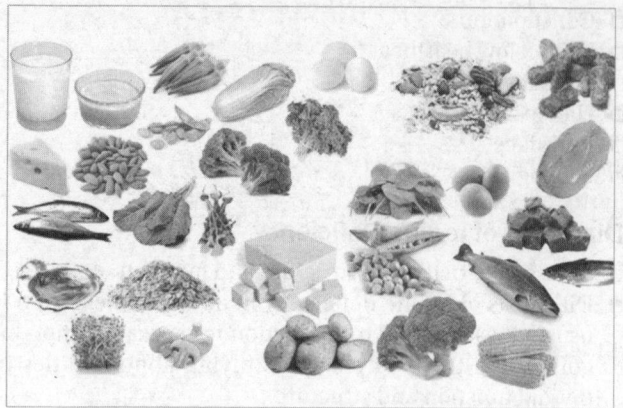

Fig. 9.36: Calcium rich foods.

Daily Recommended Calcium Intake
- Age is the main factor in determining an individual's daily recommended intake of calcium. Babies up to 6 months of age should get about 1000 mg of calcium per day, whereas infants between the ages of 7 and 12 months will require a daily intake of 1500 mg.
- Children between the ages of 1 and 8 years are advised to consume 2500 mg, whereas children between 9 to 18 years should consume 3000 mg of calcium daily.
- For adults between the ages of 19 to 50 years, the daily recommended calcium intake is 2500 mg. However, by the age of 51 and beyond, 2000 mg of calcium should be consumed daily.
- There may be a different requirement for special conditions. For example, pregnant women should have at least 2500 mg daily, no matter how old they are.
- A pregnant teenager, who may have to breastfeed later, will require 3000 mg of calcium daily.
- Other medical conditions, such as osteoporosis may benefit from calcium supplementation, in addition to vitamin D, to ensure that the body absorbs the calcium from the supplements.

Role of Nurse in Dealing with Nutritions Disorders
- Monitor food/fluid ingested and calculate daily caloric intake, as appropriate
- Monitor appropriateness of diet orders to meet daily nutritional needs, as appropriate
- Determine in collaboration with the dietician, the number of calories and types of nutrients needed to meet nutritional requirements, as appropriate
- Determine food preferences with consideration of the patient's cultural and religious preferences
- Encourage nutritional supplements, as appropriate
- Provide patients with nutritional deficits high-protein, high-calorie, nutritious finger foods and drinks that can be readily consumed, as appropriate
- Determine need for enteral tube feedings in collaboration with a dietician
- Administer enteral feedings, as prescribed
- Administer parenteral nutrition, as prescribed
- Structure the environment to create a pleasant and relaxing meal atmosphere
- Present food in an attractive, pleasing manner, giving consideration to color, texture, and variety
- Provide oral care before meals
- Assist the patient to a sitting position before eating or feeding
- Implement interventions to prevent aspiration in patients receiving enteral nutrition
- Monitor laboratory values, as appropriate
- Instruct the patient and family about prescribed diets
- Refer for diet teaching and planning, as appropriate
- Give the patient and family written examples of prescribed diet

CONCLUSION

Nutrition disorders are diseases that occur when a person's dietary intake does not contain the right amount of nutrients for healthy functioning, or when a person cannot correctly absorb nutrients from food. Nutritional deficiency occurs when the body is not getting enough nutrients such as vitamins and minerals. There are a number of conditions that are caused by nutritional deficiency such as anemia. The body requires vitamins to stay healthy and function properly. These include, but are not limited to, Protein Energy Malnutrition,

Scurvy, Rickets, Beriberi, Hypocalcemia, Osteomalacia, Vitamin K Deficiency, Pellagra, Xerophthalmia, and Iron Deficiency. To reduce the risk of nutritional deficiency, eat a balanced diet rich in nutritious foods. Crash diet or fad diet to reduce body weight can cause nutritional deficiency because they may lack essential vitamins and minerals. Following a restricted diet can result in nutritional deficiency because of consumption of improper nutrition.

BIBLIOGRAPHY

1. Calcium Requirements WHO Tech. Report Series 230, Geneva, 1962.
2. Control of Nutrition Anemia with Special Reference to Iron Deficiency, Tech. Report Series 580, Geneva, 1975.
3. Food Composition Tables for International Use, FAO Nutritional Studies No. 11, FAO, Rome, 1954.
4. Jelliffe DB. Assessment of Nutritional Status for the Community, WHO, 1966.
5. Mudambi SR, Rao SM, Rajagopal MV. Food Science, 2nd edition. New Age International, New Delhi, 2005.
6. Nutrition and Working Efficiency FFHC Basic Study No. 5, 1962.
7. Peckman GC, Jeanne H. Freeland-Graves: Foundations of Food Preparation, 5th edition. Macmillan, New York, 1987.
8. Potter NN, Birch GG. Food Science, Westport, Conn, USA, 1986.
9. Requirements of Ascorbic Acid, Vitamin D, Vitamin B-12, Folate and Iron, WHO Tech. Report Series 452, Geneva, 1975.
10. Vitamin A Deficiency and Xerophthalmia, Tech. Report Series 590, Geneva, 1976.

REVIEW QUESTIONS

Long Essays
1. Explain in detail about protein-energy malnutrition.
2. Discuss in detail about childhood obesity.
3. Describe vitamin deficiency disorders.
4. Explain mineral deficiency diseases.

Short Essays
1. Clinical features of protein-energy malnutrition.
2. Nurses role to treat malnourished patients.
3. Diarrhea and dehydration.
4. Severe acute malnutrition.
5. Folic acid deficiency.
6. Thiamine deficiency.
7. Symptoms of vitamin C deficiency.
8. Vitamin D deficiency.
9. Iron deficiency.
10. Iodine deficiencies.
11. Calcium deficiencies.

Short Answers
1. Electrolytes.
2. Marasmic kwashiorkor.
3. Nutrient.
4. Clinical features of kwashiorkor.
5. Iron deficiency anemia.
6. Infantile beriberi.
7. Causes of childhood obesity.
8. Causes of vitamin A deficiency.

CHAPTER 10

Therapeutic Diets

CHAPTER OUTLINE

- Definition, objectives, principles
- Modifications—consistency, nutrients,
- Feeding techniques
- Diet in diseases—obesity, diabetes mellitus, CVD, underweight, renal diseases, hepatic disorders constipation, diarrhea, pre and postoperative period

GLOSSARY

- **Therapeutic diet:** Means a diet ordered by a licensed practitioner or other licensed professional with prescriptive authority as part of the treatment for disease, clinical conditions, or increasing or decreasing specific nutrients in the food consumed by the client.
- **Absorption:** The process by which nutrients pass through the cells of the intestinal tract into the circulatory system to be utilized by the body.
- **BRAT diet**: Diet commonly recommended for nausea and vomiting that contains bananas, rice, applesauce and toast. They are easier to digest and give the GI tract a rest.
- **Complementary protein:** The combining of two protein sources, so that all of the essential amino acids are present.
- **Comprehensive care:** Plan developed by the interdisciplinary team addressing the multifaceted needs of the client.
- **Dentition:** The development of teeth in the gums of a human, their arrangement, and the function of those teeth in the process of digestion.
- **Diet manual:** Standardized document that specifies therapeutic diets and their application; each facility will specify the diet manual they intend to use.
- **Diet order:** Diet prescribed by the physician (or other authorized healthcare professional) for an individual client.
- **Dietary supplement:** A product that is intended to supplement the diet, to increase the total daily intake of a particular substance.
- **Empty calories:** Foods that are not nutrient dense and may contain many calories.
- **Energy-yielding nutrients:** Nutrients that provide energy or calories to the body, such as carbohydrates, fats and protein.
- **Enteral nutrition:** Feeding of formula, by mouth or by tube, into the gastrointestinal tract.
- **Essential nutrients:** Nutrients that cannot be made in the body or cannot be made in the quantity needed by the body. Humans must get them via food.
- **Fixed menu:** A menu that offers the same foods every day.
- **Food allergy:** The adverse allergic reaction resulting in acute (mild) to chronic (severe) symptoms. The immune system mistakenly targets a harmless food protein—an allergen—as a threat and attacks it, causing a reaction.
- **Food intolerance:** The intake of food that cannot be tolerated or digested properly (seen in the case of lactose or gluten intolerance). Food intolerance does not generally produce an immune response.
- **Food record:** A diary of food and beverages consumed, usually for a given number of days.
- **Medical nutrition therapy (MNT):** Nutrition assessment and treatment of clients with an illness, disease-related condition or injury, in order to benefit the health of the client.
- **Nutrition assessment:** A comprehensive approach by a Registered Dietitian Nutritionist using multiple data sources to determine nutrition status.
- **Nutrition care process:** A method of documenting nutrition data with five steps—nutrition assessment, nutrition diagnosis, nutrition intervention, nutrition monitoring and evaluation.
- **Nutrition care protocols:** Documents that outline a care process related to a specific medical condition.
- **Nutrition screening:** A component of nutrition assessment meant to identify potential nutrition problems.
- **Nutrition support:** A general term describing the provision of foods and liquids to improve nutrition status and good medicine.
- **Parenteral nutrition:** Administration of simple, essential nutrients into a vein.
- **Protein-calorie malnutrition:** A name for a group of diseases characterized by protein and energy deficiency.
- **Selective menu:** An adaptation of a cycle menu, that allows clients to choose foods in advance of meal service.

- **SMART objective:** A learning objective that is specific, meaningful, affordable, reasonable and timed.
- **Tube feeding:** Enteral feeding given through a feeding tube.

INTRODUCTION

The term "diet therapy" refers to a modification in food intake for the purpose of improving health. Balanced nutrition is essential to overall wellness, but medical nutrition therapy (MNT) describes an intervention that adjusts both the quantity and quality of food to treat a disease or its symptoms. Diet therapy is devised and monitored by a certified healthcare provider, such as a physician or a registered dietitian. Dietetics is concerned with planning of diets in maintaining health and in prevention and treatment of disease. It is a science as it uses the rudiments of principles of nutrition and it is an art as it is concerned with the aesthetics of food service. When designing a diet therapy menu, a dietitian will take into consideration a number of factors. These include the age of the patient, the specific illnesses to be treated and the functional ability of the patient to achieve success with a therapeutic diet.

CONCEPT AND MEANING OF DIET THERAPY

Diet therapy also refers to nutrient modification for therapeutic purposes. A diet type described as "low" would minimize a certain nutrient or nutrients. A low-fiber diet, for example, might be prescribed for a patient after stomach or intestinal surgery to reduce the amount of digestion taking place after a meal. Other diet therapy types that minimize nutrients include a low-cholesterol diet, a low-sodium diet or a low-oxalate diet.
- The type of diet therapy prescribed will include modifications of three general factors—texture, nutrients to minimize and nutrients to maximize. Certain medical conditions require a modification in the texture of a diet because of swallowing or chewing difficulties.
- A liquid diet, for example, would be prescribed for a post-surgical patient who needs easily digested nutrition or a person who has had oral surgery and is unable to consume larger chunks of food.
- A puréed or blended diet would be provided for an elderly nursing home patient who is unable to chew food to a safe consistency for swallowing. When a soft diet is prescribed, tough meats are either chopped or ground and served with a sauce or gravy for easier chewing and swallowing. Foods, such as corn on the cob or nuts are eliminated from a soft diet.
- Certain conditions require an increase in nutrient intake. Pregnancy diets are prescribed to supply the mother and fetus with extra calories, protein, iron and folate.
- A high-fiber diet might be recommended for patients suffering from constipation, which is a side effect of many pain medications.
- A comprehensive diet plan, prescribed for patients with multiple issues, might increase certain nutrients and minimize others.
- Patients who suffer from heart disease, diabetes or obesity might be prescribed a plan that reduces the amount of calories, fats and sugars in the diet but increases fiber and protein intake for satiety.
- For a person to ensure that a diet therapy regimen is sound and appropriate for a particular medical condition, it is important for him/her discuss nutritional intake, including the use of alternative therapies, such as dietary supplements, with a licensed healthcare provider.

Figure 10.1 is depicted the nurse serving diet in the hospital and **Figure 10.2** is depicted the role of nutrition in maintaining health.

DEFINITION

- **Dietetics:** It is the branch of science that deals with the practical application of the principles of nutrition in health which is required to the human body.
- **Therapeutic diet:** Means a diet prescribed by a physician, which may include modifications in nutrient content, caloric value and consistency, methods of food preparation, content of specific foods or a combination of these modifications.

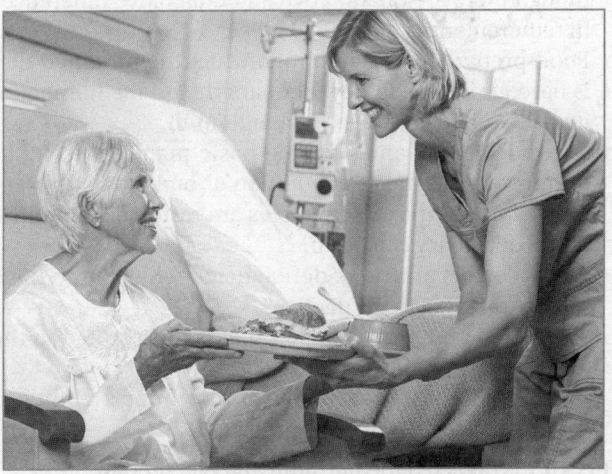

Fig. 10.1: Nurse serving diet in the hospital.

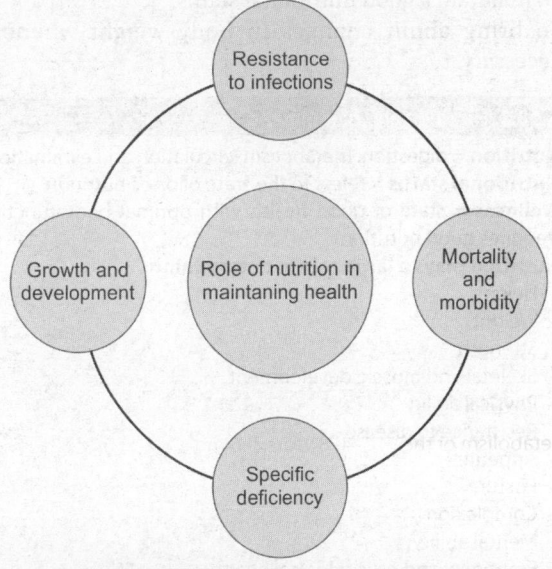

Fig. 10.2: Role of nutrition in maintaining health.

- **Therapeutic diet:** Means a diet ordered by a physician or practitioner as part of treatment for a disease or clinical condition or to eliminate or decrease specific nutrients in the diet, (e.g., sodium) or to increase specific nutrients in the diet (e.g., potassium) or to provide food the resident is able to eat (e.g., mechanically altered diet).

DIET AS A THERAPEUTIC AGENT

Diet therapy is concerned with the modification of normal diet to meet the requirements of the sick individual. Diet therapy means use of diet (food and drink) not only in the care of the sick, but also in the prevention of disease and maintenance of health. Diet therapy in most instances is not a remedy in itself but is a measure which supplements or makes the medical or surgical treatment more effective. Therapeutic nutrition begins with the normal diet.

Advantages of using normal diet as the basis for therapeutic diets are:
- It emphasizes the similarity of psychological and social needs of those who are ill and those who are well, even though there are quantitative and qualitative differences in requirements.
- Food preparation is simplified when the modified diet is based upon the family diet pattern and the number of items required is reduced to a minimum.
- The calculated values for the basic plan are useful in finding out the effects of addition or omission of certain foods, for example, if vegetables are restricted vitamin A and C deficiency can occur.
  - To correct nutrient deficiencies which may have occurred due to the disease?
  - To plan and provide a diet that is most suited to the disease condition.
  - To adjust the food intake to the body's ability to metabolize the nutrients in sickness.

Box 10.1 is depicted the nutrition and diet therapy.

The general objectives of diet therapy are:
- To maintain a good nutritional status.
- To bring about changes in body weight whenever necessary.

Box 10.1: Nutrition and diet therapy.
- **Nutrition** = digestion, metabolism, circulation and elimination
- **Nutritional status** = refers to the state of one's nutrition
- **Wellness** = state of good health with optimal body function (requires good nutrition)
- **Nutrition plays a large role in determining:**
  - Height
  - Weight
  - Strength
  - Skeletal and muscle development
  - Physical agility
  - Resistance to disease
  - Appetite
  - Posture
  - Complexion
  - Mental ability
  - Emotional and psychological health

Modification of Normal Diet

The alteration of the normal diet requires an appreciation of:
- The underlying disease conditions which require a change in the diet.
- The possible duration of the disease.
- The factors in the diet therapy which must be altered to overcome these conditions.
- The patient's tolerance for food by mouth.
- In planning meals for a patient his economic status, his food preferences and his occupation, time of meals and effect on family should be considered.

The normal diet may be modified:
- To provide change in consistency as in fluid and soft diets.
- To increase or decrease the energy value.
- To include greater or lesser amounts of one or more nutrients, for example, high protein, low sodium, etc.
- To increase or decrease bulk-high and low fiber diets.
- To provide foods bland in flavor,

PRINCIPLES OF DIET THERAPY

Diet therapy is concerned with the modification of the normal diet to meet the requirements of the sick individual. Its purposes are:
- To maintain good nutritional status.
- To correct deficiencies this may have occurred.
- To afford rest to the whole body or to ascertain body's ability to metabolize the nutrients.
- To bring about changes in body weight whenever necessary. Therapeutic nutrition begins with the normal diet. Advantages of using normal diet, as the basis for therapeutic diets are:
  - It emphasizes the similarity of psychological and social needs of those who are ill and those who are well even though there are quantitative and qualitative differences in requirements.
  - Food preparation is simplified when the modified diet is based upon the family pattern and the number of items required in special preparation is reduced to a minimum.
  - The calculated values for the basic plan are useful in finding out the effects of addition or omission of certain foods, for example, if vegetables are restricted vitamin A and C deficiency can occur.

Figure 10.3 is depicted the therapeutic diet.

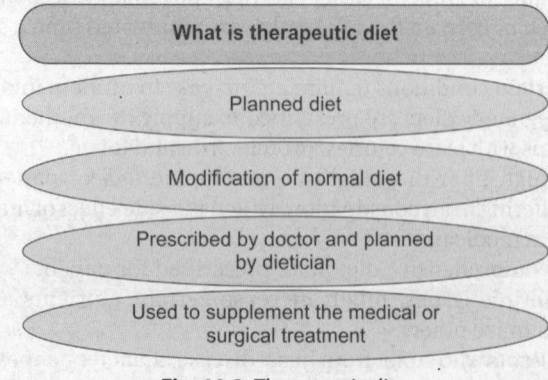

Fig. 10.3: Therapeutic diet.

FACTORS TO CONSIDER IN PLANNING THERAPEUTIC DIETS

The alteration of the normal diet requires an appreciation of:
- The underlying disease conditions which require a change in the diet.
- The possible duration of the disease.
- The factors in the dietary which must be observed.
- The patient's tolerance for food by mouth.

In planning meals for a patient his economic status, his food preferences and his occupation and time of meals should also be considered.

Figure 10.4 is depicted the purposes of therapeutic diets and **Figure 10.5** is depicted the team involves in diet therapy.

MODIFICATION OF NUTRIENTS IN THERAPEUTIC DIETS

The normal diet may be modified:
- To provide change in consistency as in fluid and soft diets.
- To increase or decrease the energy value.
- To include greater or lesser amount of one or more nutrients, for example, high protein, low sodium, etc.
- To increase or decrease bulk-high and low fiber diets.
- To provide foods bland in flavor.

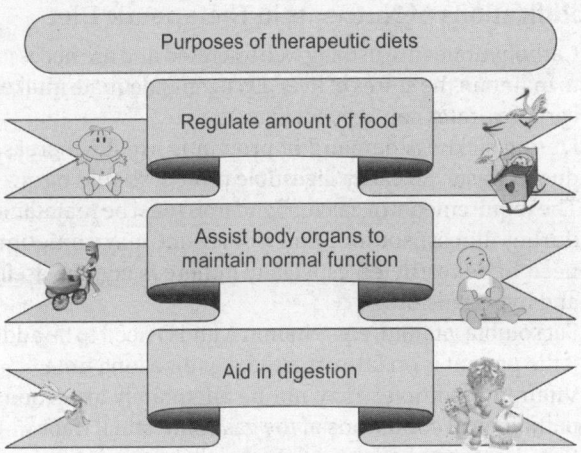

Fig. 10.4: Purposes of therapeutic diets.

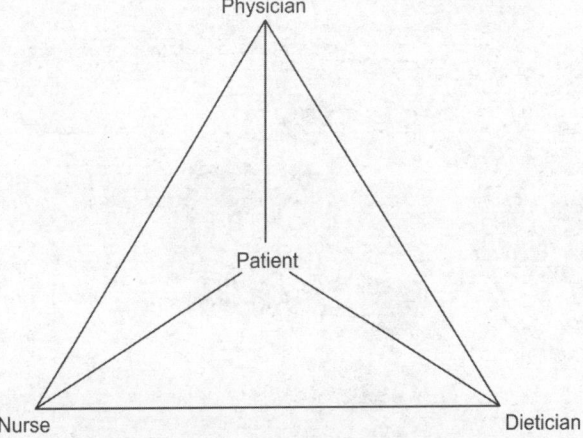

Fig. 10.5: Team involves in diet therapy.

TEAM APPROACH

These health professionals are primarily involved in the nutritional care. However, at times, the services of other health professionals, such as social worker, physiotherapist, etc., may also be directly involved. The physician, while prescribing the diet, should also explain to the patient why modified diet has been prescribed. In order to meet the nutritional needs of the patient, physician, nurse and dietician.

Responsibilities of a Dietician

- The dietician, after receiving the written diet prescription translates it to practicality in terms of food.
- The dietician assesses and formulates the nutritional status of the patient.
- She formulates nutrition care plan.
- She plans individualized meal pattern according to the patient's food habits and modification needed.
- If patient is on enteral formula, she recommends appropriate proprietary formulas, if needed.
- She counsels the patients and their family regarding the therapeutic diet prescribed and its importance.

Role of a Nurse

- Nutrition not only deals with food and its components but it is also a multidisciplinary field which deals with social, economic, cultural, psychological implications of foods.
- Nutrition is a discipline intimately related with medicine. It is also closely related with physiology and biochemistry.
- As nurses you should have a thorough understanding of these fields of studies in order to give better care to the patients.
- As nurses you may choose to work in a large hospital, community health centers or nursing homes. Irrespective of your place of work, you have a crucial role to play in ensuring the medical and nutrition success of therapy.

Nurses Role in Nutritional Care in Hospital Setup

I. **Keeping in touch with the doctor and dietician** regarding the patient's medical and dietary needs:
   - Obtaining a diet prescription if there is one and arranging food for the patient. Nowadays dietary facilities are available in most of the hospitals. In such cases food can be arranged from hospital itself.
   - Communicate with the dieticians regarding the patient's response to the diet.
   - Serve as a mediator between the patient, physician and the dietician.

II. **Assisting the patient at meal time:**
   - To prepare the patient for the meals and educate him/her about the importance of nutrition.
   - Assist the patient in feeding especially if the patient is unconscious or unable to feed himself. Tube feeding, may it be enteral or parenteral, must be done by the nurses.
   - Teach and encourage the handicapped patients to feed themselves.

- Encourage and support the patient at meal time.
- Must make the meal time a pleasant and relaxed affair.

III. **Help the dieticians in special tasks:**
- Interpret the diet to the patient. A nurse should explain why the modified diet is being given. The patient should also be told what to expect with reference to diet therapy.
- Observe, record and report the patient's response to diet. She should communicate with the patient regarding his food habits, likes and dislikes and attitude towards the diet or specific foods.
- Note the intake of foods according to the diet prescription.
- Reporting patient's response to dietician and physician for any weight loss or gain.

IV. **Plan for home care**
- Before patient leaves the hospital, it is the duty of a nurse to arrange for diet counseling to be followed at home.
- Along with the patients, members of the family must also be counseled for home care.

A nurse can be of great help in community set up. She can perform the duties of a dietician in health centers. She can give nutrition education through various methods to prevent nutritional deficiency diseases. The government of India has launched various nutritional programs to eradicate malnutrition where a nurse plays a crucial role.

DIET IN SICKNESS (FIG. 10.6)

Diet is as important as medicine in the treatment of diseases. A modification in the diet or in the nutrients can cure certain diseases. Nutrition during illness should be adequate to prevent weight loss and weakness. An acutely ill or injured patient is in danger of malnutrition.

Purpose
- To meet the metabolic needs of human body..
- To prevent dehydration.
- To improve the appetite.
- To provide adequate nutrition.
- It is necessary for the growth and maintenance of bones and other tissues.

General Rules of Treatment
- The diet must be planned in relation to changes in metabolism occurring as a result of the disease.
- The diet must be planned to agree as nearly as possible with the patients food habits, his likes and dislikes and the amount of exercise he takes.
- Changes should be made gradually adequate explanation must be when given, it is necessary to make dietary changes gradually.
- There should be plenty or variety in the diet, hot food should be served hot and cold foods cold.

Problems During Sickness
- There will be disturbance of gastrointestinal function
- Anorexia (loss of appetite)
- Defective digestion and absorption
- Lack of exercise decreases need for energy
- The process of anabolism and catabolism are not normal in sickness.
- Vomiting and diarrhea are problems in which intravenous fluid administration is required.
- In some kinds of illness, protein requirements are more while in some others, both protein and carbohydrate are needed in large amounts.

Modifications of Nutrients in Therapeutic Diet
- Carbohydrates are usually well tolerated and are necessary to maintain the stores of liver glycogen. Adequate intake of carbohydrates can prevent ketosis.
- During sickness demand of protein is usually increased due to waste. So easily digestible protein should be given.
- The requirements of calcium and iron must be maintained during illness, sodium and potassium may sometimes need to be restricted especially if there is edema, ascites and hypertension.
- Fat soluble vitamin, e.g., vitamin A and D need to be added if the patient is on fat-restricted diet for a long time.
- Vitamin B complex may not be adequately absorbed in pathological conditions of the gastrointestinal tract.
- Requirement of vitamin C is greatly increased in fevers and is especially necessary for the healing of wounds after surgery.

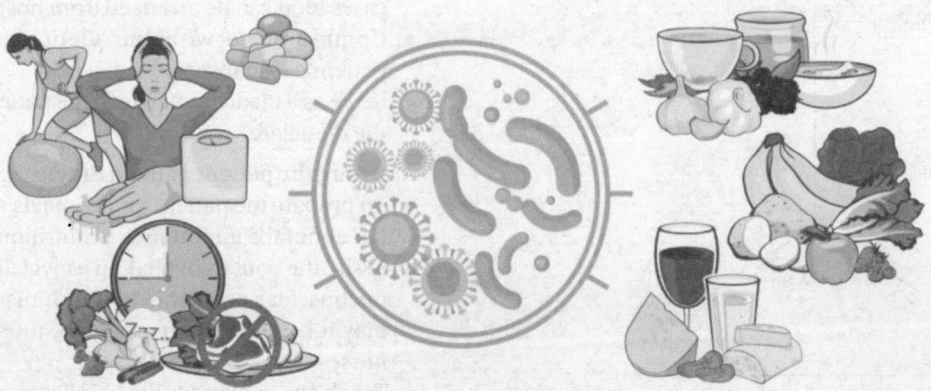

Fig. 10.6: Diet in sickness.

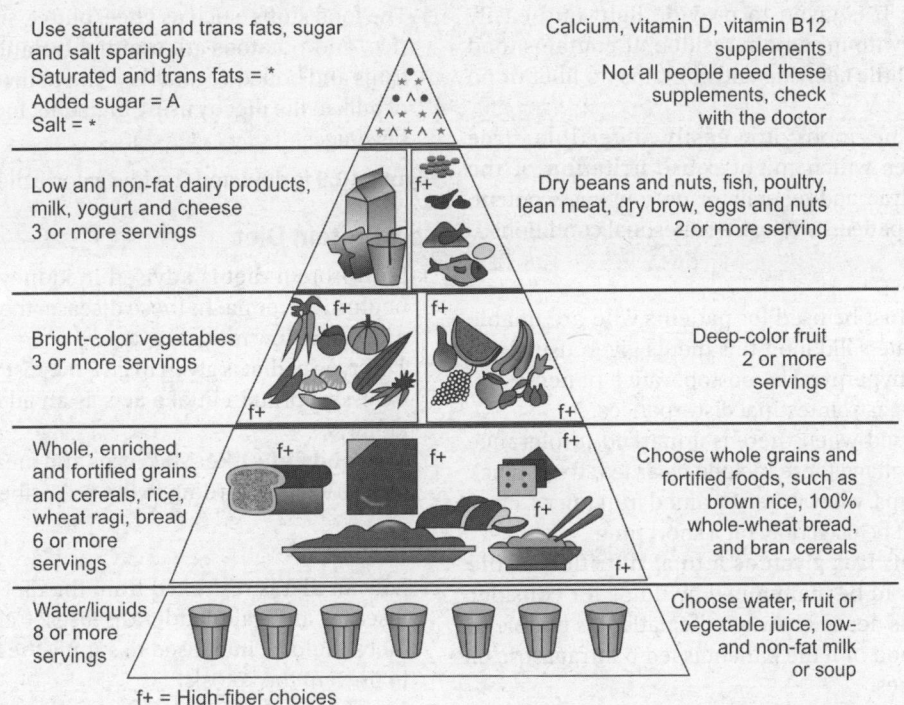

Fig. 10.7: Pyramid of diet therapy.

- Fluids are very important to prevent dehydration especially in conditions, such as high fevers, diarrhea and vomiting, in such conditions the fluid intake within 24 hours should be 2,500 mL to 3,000 mL
- If adequate fluids cannot be given by mouth, they must be given intravenous maintain fluid balance by maintaining accurate intake output chart
- Infants require a higher amount of fluid compared to adult requirements they need 150 mL of fluid per kg of body weight.

Figure 10.7 is depicted the pyramid of diet therapy.

THERAPEUTIC DIET

Diet in disease must be planned as part of the complete care of the patient. Many modifications may have to be made according to the disease and the condition of the patient.

Objective

- To improve the general health
- To meet the metabolic needs
- To promote healing
- To prevent dehydration
- To facilitate tissue repair and growth.

Box 10.2 is depicted the diet therapy.

Principals Involved in Diet Therapy

- The diet must be planned in relation to changes in metabolism occurring as a result of disease
- The diet must be planned according to the habits of the patient based on culture, religion, socioeconomic status, personal preferences, physiological and psychological conditions.

> **Box 10.2:** Diet therapy.
>
> **Principle of diet therapy:**
> - The total daily caloric contents of diet should be reduced
> - The total daily fat intake should be reduced <30% of total calories
> - Carbohydrates intake should represent >55% of total calories
> - Protein intake should be <15% of total calories
> - The daily cholesterol should be <300 mg/day
> - Daily fiber intake should be (20–30) g/day
> - The initial calories intake should be reduced by 500 kcal/day
> - For the patient with BMI >35, the daily calories should be reduced by 500–1000 calories
> - The principle of weight reduction during the next 6 months should be about 10 kg of the original weight (i.e., 500 g/week)

- As far as possible, changes in the diet should be brought gradually and adequate explanations are given with the changes made, if any.
- In short and acute illness, the food should not be forced because his appetite is very poor but le may soon recover the normal appetite.
- Whatever the diet prescribed, there should be variety of for selection.
- Small and frequent feeds are preferred to the usual three meals
- Hot foods should be served hot and cold foods should be served cold.

REGULAR DIET

- **Full diet:** It is a regular well balanced diet. It is vegetarian or non-vegetarian, this is for patients who do not need any special modification

Section 1: Applied Nutrition and Dietetics

- **Soft light diet:** It is given to provide light and easily digestible food with minimum residue. It contains food which requires little chewing and contains no fiber or no seasoning
- **Bland diet:** The foods are easily digestible, free from substances which might cause irritation of the gastrointestinal tract and generally or low roughage content, used mainly for patients with gastrointestinal conditions.

Liquid Diets

- **Liquid diets:** Must be used for patients who are unable to take or tolerate solid food this diet is given usually to patient having hyperpyrexia, postoperative patients and patients having gastrointestinal disturbances.
- **Clear fluids:** Used when there is a marked intolerance to food and roughage these include clear tea, weak black coffee, clear soups, whey water, strained fruit juices, clear fluid diet should be used only for a short time.
- **Full liquid diet:** It is given as a total nutrition of the patient and has to be maintained by fluids for considerable time. This is necessary when the patient is unable to swallow solid food or if the patient is fed b intragastric or gastrostomy tubes.

Figure 10.8 is depicted the liquid diet chart.

Low Calorie Diet

- The total calorie intake is reduced to less than the body's requirements so that the remainder of the calories required can be derived from the stored fat.
- The aim of this diet is to slow steady loss of weight over a period of several weeks or even months. This diet is advised obese patients.
- The food stuffs, such as ghee, butter, sugar, sweets bread, rice, and potatoes are omitted from the diet. Use salads fruits and boiled vegetables. The patient must have plenty of bulk in the diet by using high fiber foods and low calorie beverages.

Figure 10.9 is depicted the low calorie diet chart.

Low Protein Diet

- Low protein diet is advised in kidney diseases, such as nephritis, uremia. In these disease, the protein is avoided or given in low moderate type
- This type of diet is given to give the rest to kidneys because excessive protein intake acts as an additional load to the kidneys.
- **The foodstuffs like:** Milk; eggs and meat, etc., are omitted or restricted according to the prescribed protein intake.

Low Fat Diet

- Low fat diet is restricted from the diet patients with liver diseases and gallbladder diseases. Carbohydrates in the diet should be increased to supply the liver with glycogen to prevent the ketosis.
- **No fried food:** Ghee, butter or other fat is allowed in the diet, only rice chapattis bread, fruits, dali, vegetables.

Figure 10.10 is depicted the low fat diet chart.
Figure 10.11 is depicted the low sodium diet chart.

Salt Free Diet

- Sodium is totally or partially restricted; the restriction of sodium depends on the severity of the condition of the patient.

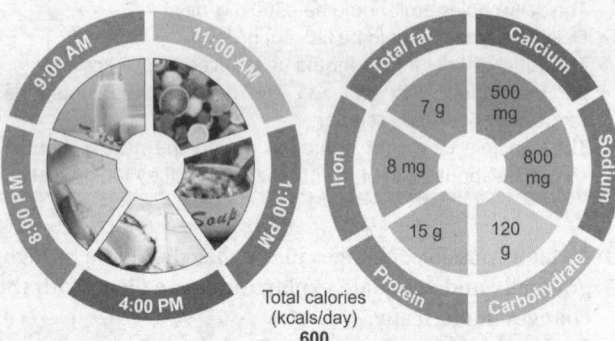

Fig. 10.8: Liquid diet chart.

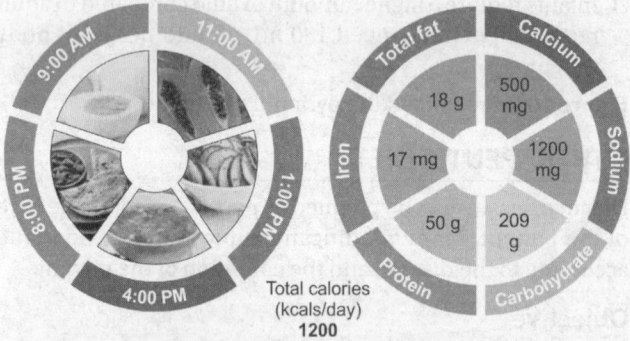

Fig. 10.9: Low calorie diet chart.

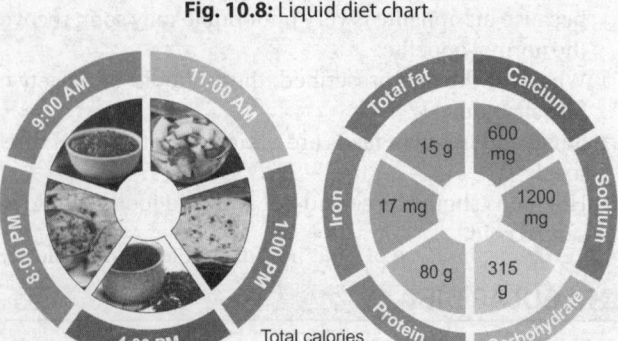

Fig. 10.10: Low fat diet chart.

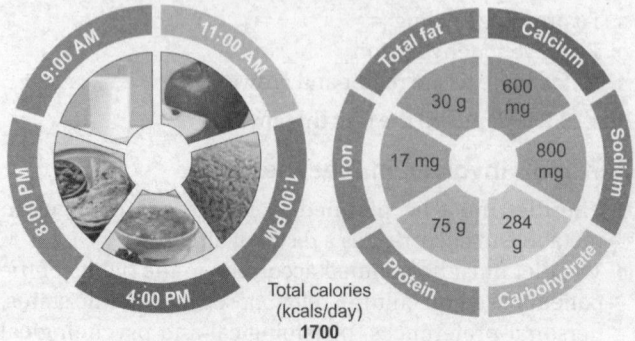

Fig. 10.11: Low sodium diet chart.

- The patients with heart diseases, hypertension, kidney diseases, etc., are given salt restricted diet or low salt diet. The necessity of the restriction should be carefully explained to the patient and relatives.
- The following foods are totally avoided—salt, baking powder, pappads, canned foods, cheese, and pickles, salted—hips and biscuits, etc.

High Protein Diet

- **High protein diet:** The protein intake should be average from 75 to 100 g per day for adult. In protein energy malnutrition cases easily digestible and high nutritive value protein, e.g., milk protein should be given.
- High protein diet is given to the patients, such as operated cases, tuberculosis accident, burns, and nephritic syndrome and decided cases.
- The food stuffs contains rich protein are milk and milk proteins, eggs, fish meat, broth, dhals, dahi beans, soybean and ground nuts.

Figure 10.12 is depicted the high protein diet chart.
Figure 10.13 is depicted the diabetic diet chart.

Diabetic Diet

- In diabetes mellitus, the metabolism of carbohydrate, fat and protein are affected. Diabetes is lifelong disease which can be treated but not cured. The dietary treatment depends upon the severity of the condition.
- The purpose of diabetic diet is to keep the patient in good health to keep the blood sugar level within normal level and to keep urine free from sugar.

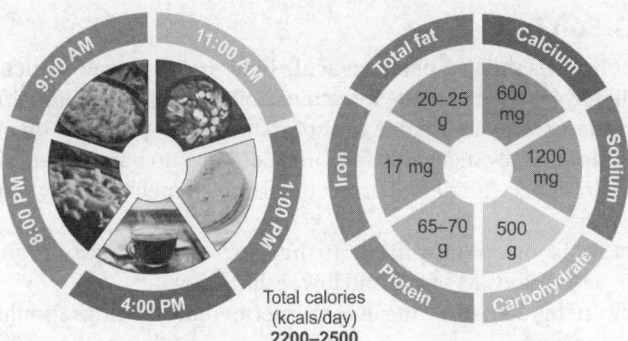

Fig. 10.12: High protein diet chart.

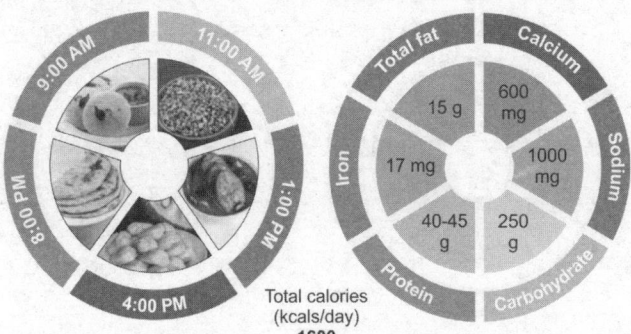

Fig. 10.13: Diabetic diet chart.

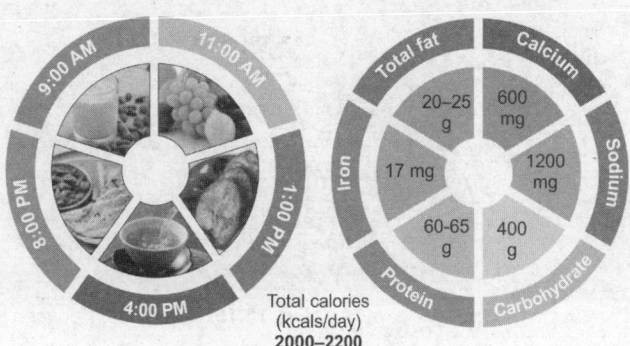

Fig. 10.14: Iron deficiency anemia diet chart.

- The diet should be balanced but there should be restriction of carbohydrates, e.g., rice, biscuits, s Igor, jams, sweets, honey, carrots, and sweet potatoes. The patient should have egg, milk raw salads all types of green leafy vegetables.
- The total calories required 20 to 25% should be from protein 40% from carbohydrates and 40 percent from fat.

Figure 10.14 is depicted the iron deficiency anemia diet chart.

Diet in Anemia

- This type of patient requires the diet which is high in protein, high in iron and high in vitamins. The diet should provide necessary nutrients for the formation of new red blood cells or hemoglobin.
- The main purposes are to provide necessary nutrients for blood cell formation and to remove the cause of anemia.
- The food stuffs recommended are liver, meat, eggs, spinach drumstick leaves, ragi, jaggery, etc.

TYPES OF DIET USED IN HOSPITALS

1. Clear-fluid diet
2. Full-fluid diet
3. Soft diet
4. Normal diet

1. Clear-fluid Diet

Whenever an acute illness or surgery produces a marked intolerance for food as may be evident by nausea. Vomiting, anorexia, distention and diarrhea, it is advisable to restrict the intake of food.

Figure 10.15 is depicted the differences between low-residual diet and clear liquid diet.

- In acute infection, in acute inflammatory conditions of the intestinal tract, following operations upon the colon or rectum when it is desirable to prevent evacuation from the bowel, clear fluid diet is suggested.
- This diet is also given to relieve thirst, to supply the tissues with water, to aid in the removal of gas.
- The diet is made up of clear liquids that leave no residue, and it is non-gas forming action.
- This diet is entirely inadequate from a nutritional standpoint. Since it is deficient in protein, minerals, vitamins, and calories. It should not be continued for more than 24 to 48 hours.

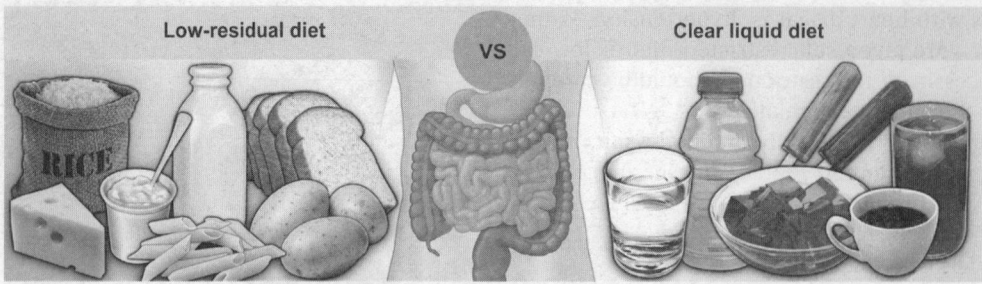

Fig. 10.15: Differences between low-residual diet and clear liquid diet.

- The amount of fluid is usually restricted to 30 to 60 mL per hour at first, with gradually increasing amounts being given as the patients tolerance improves.
- This diet can meet the requirement of fluids and some minerals and can be given in 1 to 2 hour intervals.

Figure 10.16 is depicted the commonly followed full-liquid diet regimens.

Conditions necessitating the use of clear liquid diet:
- Preoperative period, e.g., as a preparation for bowel surgery.
- Prior to colonoscopic examination.
- Postoperative phase, e.g., in the initial recovery phase after abdominal surgery or after a period of intravenous therapy.
- Acute illness and infections as in acute gastrointestinal disturbances, such as acute gastroenteritis, when fluid and electrolyte replacement is desired to compensate for losses from diarrhea.
- As the first step in oral alimentation of a nutritionally debilitated person.
- In temporary food intolerance.

2. Full-fluid Diet

This diet bridges the gap between the clear fluid and soft diet. It is used following operations in acute gastritis, acute infections and in diarrhea. This diet is also suggested when milk is permitted and for patients not requiring special diet but too ill to eat solid or semisolid foods.

- In this diet, foods which are liquid or which readily become liquid on reaching the stomach are given.
- This diet may be made entirely adequate and may be used over an extended time without fear of deficiencies developing, provided it is carefully planned. This diet is given at 2–4 hours interval.

Conditions necessitating the use of full fluid diet:
- Postoperative phase when progressing from clear liquids to solid foods.
- Acute gastritis and infections.
- Following oral surgery or plastic surgery of face or neck area.
- In chewing and swallowing dysfunction.
- In esophageal or stomach disorders causing intolerance to solid food intake.

3. Soft Diet

It bridges the gap between acute illness and convalescence. It may be used in acute infections, following surgery, and for patients who are unable to chew. The soft diet is made up of simple, easily digestible food and contains no harsh fiber.

- Patients with dental problems are given mechanically soft diet.
- It is often modified further for certain pathologic conditions as bland and low residue diets.
- In this diet, three meals with intermediate feedings should be given.

Figure 10.17 is depicted the soft food diet chart.

Breakfast
- Vegetable juice
- one bowl gelatin
- One glass pulp-less fruit juice
- One cup coffee or tea
- Water
- Supplement with honey

Lunch
- Glass pulp-less fruit juice
- Vegetable juice
- One bowl gelatin
- Broth
- Cream soup
- Beverage
- Water
- Ice cream

Supper
- Glass pulp-less fruit juice
- Vegetable juice
- One bowl gelatin
- Broth
- Coffee/tea
- Supplement with honey/nector

Fig. 10.16: Commonly followed full-liquid diet regimens.

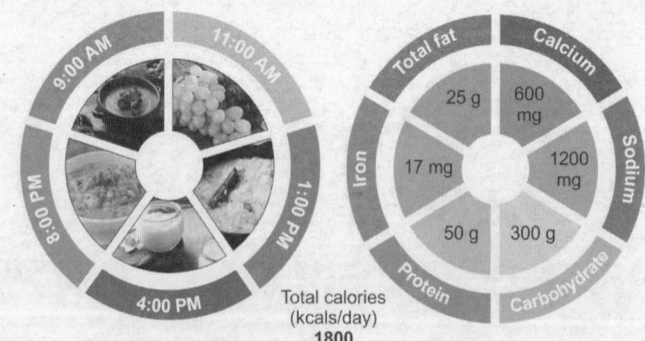

Fig. 10.17: Soft food diet chart.

Conditions necessitating the use of soft diet:
- While progressing from full fluid diet to general diet.
- During postoperative phase when a patient is unable to tolerate normal diet.
- Gastrointestinal problems, e.g., diarrhea.
- General debilitation and inadequate dentition.
- Convalescence.
- Transition from acute phase of illness to convalescence.
- Acute infections.

A soft diet can be modified as mechanical soft diet.

Mechanical soft diet: Many people require a soft diet simply because they have no teeth and such a diet is known as mechanical or a dental soft diet. It is not desirable to restrict the patient to the food selection of the customary soft diet and the following modifications to the normal diet may be made:
- Vegetables may be chopped or diced before cooking.
- Hard raw fruits and vegetables are to be avoided; tough skins and seeds to be removed.
- Nuts and dried fruits may be used in chopped or powdered forms.
- Meat to be finely minced or ground.

Figure 10.18 is depicted the balanced diet.

4. Normal Diet

It is used for ambulatory and bed patients whose conditions do not necessitate a special diet as one of the routine diets. Many special diets progress ultimately to a regular diet. The regular hospital diet is simple in character and preparation, easy of digestion and calculated to afford maximum nourishment with minimum effort to the body.

- The diet is well balanced, adequate in nutritional value and attractively served to stimulate a possible poor appetite.
- A normal diet is defined as one which consists of any and all foods eaten by a person in health. It is planned keeping the basic food groups in mind so that optimum amounts of all nutrients are provided. As there is no restriction of any kind of food, this diet is well balanced and nutritionally adequate.
- Since the patient is hospitalized and/or is at bed rest, a reduction of 10% in energy intake should be made and too many fatty foods and fried foods be avoided as they are difficult to digest.
- The proteins are slightly increased (+10%) to counteract a negative nitrogen balance. All other nutrients are supplied in normal amounts.

SPECIAL FEEDING METHODS (MANAGEMENT OF SPECIAL DIETS)

Oral feeding is the best for the nourishment of a patient. But in the following conditions it is not possible to give the feeding orally:
- Those who cannot swallow due to paralysis of the muscles of swallowing (diphtheria, poliomyelitis), etc., or cancer of the oral cavity or larynx.
- Those who cannot be persuaded to eat.
- Those with persistent anorexia requiring forced feeding.
- Semiconscious or unconscious patients.
- Severe malabsorption requiring administration of unpalatable formula.
- Short bowel syndrome.
- Those who are undernourished or at risk of becoming so.
- Those that cannot digest and absorb.
- After surgery.
- Patients with neurological and renal disorders or have continued fevers or diabetes.
- Babies of very low birth weight.

Figure 10.19 is depicted the nasogastric tube feeding by continuous controlled pump.

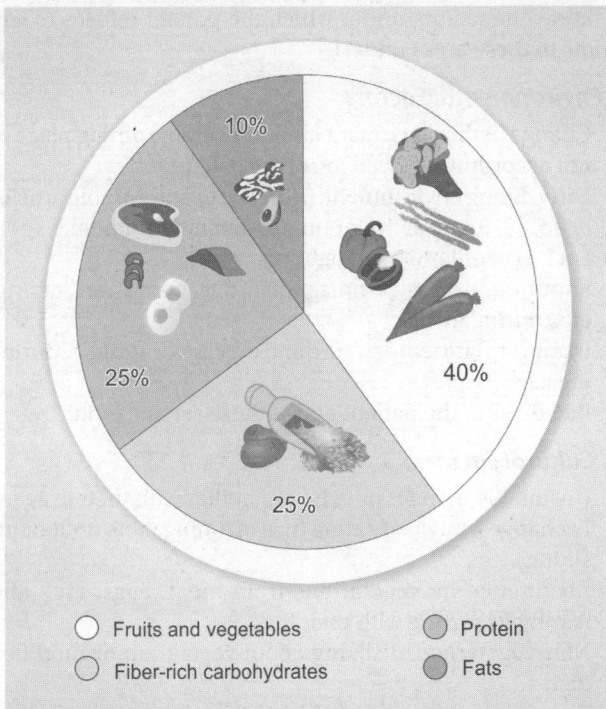

Fig. 10.18: Balanced diet.

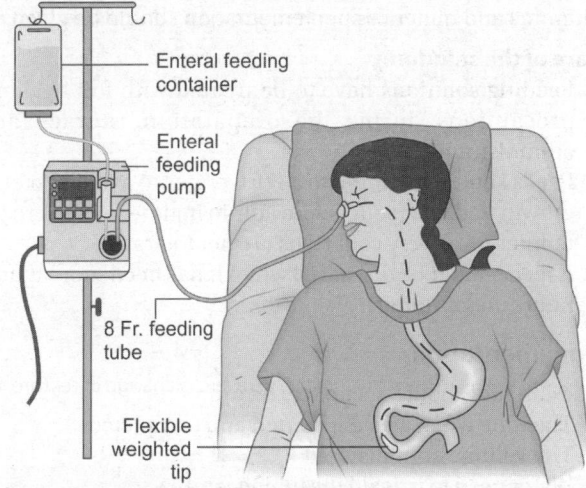

Fig. 10.19: Nasogastric tube feeding by continuous controlled pump.

TUBE FEEDING

This is done by passing a tube into the stomach or duodenum through the nose which is called nasogastric feeding or directly by surgical operation known as gastrostomy and jejunostomy feeding. A satisfactory tube feeding must be:
- Nutritionally adequate
- Well tolerated by the patient so that vomiting is not induced.
- Easily digested with no unfavorable reactions, such as distension, diarrhea or constipation.
- Easily prepared, and
- Inexpensive.

Nutrition supplied through the tube may be:
- Natural liquid foods.
- Blenderized to make liquid food.
- Commercially supplied polymeric mixtures or elemental diet (predigested diet).

Feeding Requirements

A concentration of about 1 kcal per milliliter is satisfactory. Lesser concentration increases the volume which must be given to meet the nutrient and energy needs and greater concentration are more likely to produce diarrhea and may be too thick to pass through a nasogastric tube.
- The feeding is started through a continuous drip at a rate of 50 mL per hour.
- The rate is increased by 20 mL every 24 hours until the required volume is achieved.
- Usually with 100-120 mL per hour. The concentration or rate of flow may have to be reducing, if there is vomiting, abdominal cramps or diarrhea.
- Feeding requirements are based on previous nutritional status and other feeds given to the patient.
  - Fluids—30 mL/kg
  - Energy—32 kcaL/kg
  - Protein—1 g/kg body weight
  - Sodium—30-40 mmoL/(Provided there are no external losses)
  - Potassium—1 mmoL/g of protein

Vitamins and minerals supplementation should be given.

Care of the solution:
- Feeding solutions have to be treated with full hygienic precautions during the preparation, storage and administration.
- Feeds should be stored in a refrigerator to avoid bacterial growth and taken out before admin in time to reach room temperature; very cold feeds are not tolerated.
- A feed should be discarded when it has been more than 2 hours out of storage.

Documentation

Nursing staff should accurately record:
- The time when a feed is started and completed.
- The volume administered.
- Water used to irrigate the tubing, and
- The patients output of urine. Careful monitoring is needed to see that the patient is in fluid balance.

PARENTERAL FEEDING

- Here the nutrient preparations are given directly into a vein. This method may be used to supplement normal feeding by mouth but can provide all the nutrients necessary to meet patient's requirements.
- Then, it is known as Total Parenteral Nutrition or TPN. The same process is called hyper alimentation when at least 150% of the daily requirements are provided to produce a positive nitrogen balance for gain in weight.
- Partial parenteral nutrition provides 30-50% of daily requirements.

DIETARY MODIFICATIONS

Meal frequency modifications often, especially in GI-related disorders; small frequent meals will be used rather than three larger meals. Perhaps as many as six to eight small meals or snacks may be consumed daily. By eating smaller meals, the work load placed on the GI tract and cardiovascular system is less than that with a large meal. Small frequent meals may be used for GI disorders, such as Hiatal hernia and epigastric distress, during periods of nausea or indigestion, for esophageal reflux and in pancreatitis. They may also be prescribed after MI and in CHF.

Importance Factors Involves

Ordinarily, meal is a pleasant experience for every person. But under diseased condition, the digestion mechanism is affected. His hunger may be reduced or may end. He has no interest towards meals. Absence from eating or refusal to eat is a common behavior of the patients during illness. Refusal to eat becomes a problem. Hence, it is necessary for the nurse to know the factors under which the patient refuses to eat. Some of these areas under:

I. Environmental Factors
- Change in the place of meals or unsuitable dining place or not according to the liking of the patient.
- Dirty dining environment, presence of undesirable articles or scene, unattractive or unpleasant environment.
- Lack of ventilation and lighting.
- Shouting, excessive noise, disorder, confusion, crying, etc., during meals.
- Inappropriate temperature and excessive humidity during meals.
- Bad dress of the patient and of those serving food.

II. Cultural Factors
- Unsuitable utensils or to be unfamiliar with their usage.
- Exchange in style of eating (use of dining table or floor for sitting).
- Abstinence by vegetarians from meat, eggs, etc., and fearing its mixing with their food.
- Non-vegetarians disliking about vegetarian or modified diet.
- To condemn some vegetables, fruits or diets.
- Timing of meals not suitable with religious beliefs (Jams do not eat during night).

- Irregular timing or excessive punctuality.
- Not getting food cooked or prepared by desired persons as per religious beliefs or the method of cooking not according to their religious belief.
- Not getting an opportunity to pray before meals or to follow some religious practices.

III. Psychological Factors
- Meals not according to the liking or taste of the patient.
- Physical and mental exhaustion.
- Unattractive flavor and color of meals.
- Feeling fear, worries or confusion, while eating or serving food.
- Personal experience of the patient not favorable, while eating.
- Unfavorable behavior of doctor, nurse or those serving meals with the patient.
- The patient being in a state of worry. Anger, emotion or remembering his household affairs during eating.
- Unclean or unprotected serving utensils.

IV. Other Factors
- Physical weakness of patient.
- Full rejection of diet by patient.

In this manner, the patient can create problems or non-cooperation in accepting diet for various reasons. Sometimes, it becomes difficult to find that due to what unknown fear, doubt or event the patient is not accepting diet. Hence, the nurse, based on her knowledge and previous experience, should skillfully motivate and encourage the patient for accepting food, by removing all the hurdles.

Kilocalorie Modifications

The body requires a specific amount of energy each day to carry out its tasks. Energy intake includes foods and beverages consumed daily. Energy output includes energy used for:
- Basal metabolic rate (BMR)
- Physical activities
- Digestion of food

Energy balance is achieved when energy intake equals output. During energy balance, weight should remain constant if energy intake is greater than output, positive energy balance results causing weight gain. On the other hand if intake is less than output, negative energy balance occurs leading to weight loss.

HIGH-CALORIE AND HIGH-PROTEIN DIETS

During times of physiological stress, such as after surgery, bone fractures, sepsis, burns, cancer and some other disease states, the body's energy and protein needs are increased. Medical trauma can greatly increase the BMR, so that if energy needs are not met by diet, negative energy balance will result. The patient will lose protein stored and weight.
- Many trauma and cancer patients suffer from anorexia or lack of appetite and may also have difficulty with the eating process. This further complicates the problem of nutritional inadequacies.

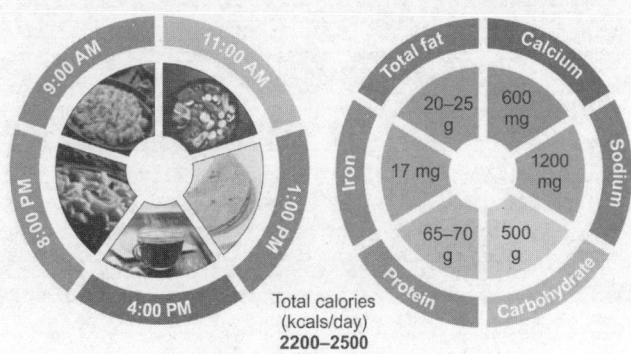

Fig. 10.20: High protein diet chart.

- Dietary treatment should aim at restoring energy balance in the normal weight patient or creating a positive energy balance in the underweight patient.
- High-calorie and high-protein diets should provide increased amounts of kcal and problem in a small volume.
- Commercially prepared liquid supplements may be used.

Figure 10.20 is depicted the high protein diet chart.

Suggestions to Increase Kilocalorie and Protein
- Add milk powder to milkshakes, beverages, soups, puddings and cooked cereals
- Spread peanut butter on crackers, fruits or celery
- Add cheese to casseroles, soups and sauces
- Use extra meat, chicken or fish in casseroles and soups
- Add sugar to foods, where reasonable (this only adds kcal)
- Use generous amounts of dense foods, such as butter, margarine, mayonnaise, cream cheese, sour cream and cream in recipes, as spreads or as dips, which are rich in kilocalorie
- Have snacks available at all times
- Encourage the patient to eat high-calorie foods first and eat the low-calorie foods, if still hungry.

Of course, the diet should still provide a balance of foods from all the food groups. It should be kept in mind that, the appearance of the food and how it is served may determine whether it is eaten or not. That serving foods should do so with a positive attitude and encouragement. The meals should be as attractive as possible. Beverages, especially liquid supplements should be served in glasses, not in cans. Foods should be served at the correct temperature, meals should be served promptly and snacks and supplements should be refrigerated, if necessary. If a patient is not able to consume adequate kcal or refuses to eat, then nutritional support in the form of tube feedings or intravenous (IV) feedings may be considered.

KILOCALORIE-CONTROLLED AND LOW-KILOCALORIE DIETS

Obesity is the condition of having an abnormally large amount of fat on the body. Ideally obesity should be determined by using measures of body composition. Methods of measuring body composition includes hydrostatic weighing (submerging the body in a tank of water and measuring displacement),

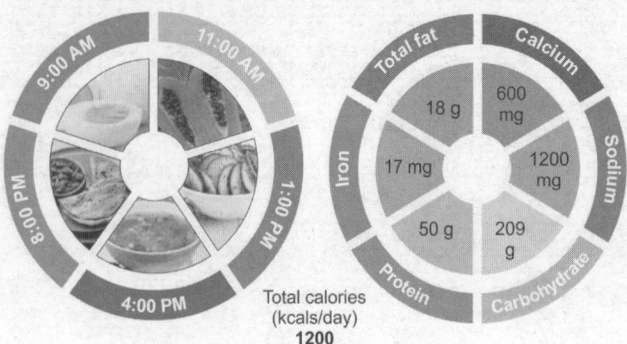

Fig. 10.21: Low calorie diet chart.

skin fold thickness measures (measuring the pinch of skin using skin fold calipers) and electrical impedance tests a small electrical current is transmitted through the body and its resistance is measured).

Figure 10.21 is depicted the low calorie diet chart.

- These methods measure percent of body fat and are better suited for determining obesity; however, they are not always available and nor are they as simple as using a weight scale.
- The cause of obesity is difficult to explain. Many factors may contribute to the positive energy balance that leads to obesity.
- Most experts agree that both heredity and lifestyle contribute to obesity. Regardless of cause, obesity is a major health problem, particularly in well-developed countries.
- Obese people have a higher incidence of non-insulin-dependent diabetes mellitus (NIDDM), high blood lipid levels, hypertension, coronary heart disease, post-surgical complications, gynecological irregularities, pregnancy-induced hypertension and gout.
- Excess weight exacerbates arthritis and some respiratory problems. It can lead to varicose veins and abdominal hernia.
- Obesity is resistant to treatment. Some studies have shown that if 'cure' from obesity is defined as reduction to ideal weight and maintenance of that weight for 5 years, a person is more likely to recover from many forms of cancer than from obesity.
- Treatment of obesity has ranged from diets, medications and psychotherapy to surgery.
- The goal of any treatment is to cause a negative energy balance resulting in weight loss. B far, the most common treatment and probably the safest is a low-calorie diet and exercise.
- Low-calorie diet must be based on the exchange lists for meal planning discussed later on under the heading of diabetes mellitus.
- A successful weight reduction program should incorporate three major components.

They are:
- A low-calorie diet.
- Exercise and physical activity.
- Behavior modification and other lifestyle changes.

The program should help and prepare patients to control weight throughout life and not just on a temporary basis. Diet should be not less than 1,200 kcal/day and weight loss should occur at the' rate of approximately 1 to 2 lb/week. Diets that require the purchase of specially prepared foods, supplements or magic diet aids should be avoided. Person who is trying to lose weight must learn to take charge of their own life and not rely on expensive products for weight control. Individuals consuming less than 1,500 kcal/day may need to take a multivitamin/minor supplement providing approximately 100% of the recommended dietary allowance (RDA).

VERY LOW-CALORIE DIET

Very low-calorie diet (VLCD) programs, sometimes called liquid fasts, are being used increasingly in many hospital outpatient clinics and doctors' offices. These diets consist of a low-calorie and nutritionally balanced. Liquid diet provides 300 to 500 kcal/day. Throughout the liquid fast, patients are monitored by their physician and other health professionals.

- They should receive dietary and behavioral counseling and should be involved in an exercise program.
- The patient continues on the liquid fast for a given period, eating the other foods and then begins a gradual refeeding program and is instructed on a diet for weight maintenance.
- Long-term results of VLCDs prove disappointing, showing a higher percentage of dieters regaining over half of the weight lost on the program.
- With VLCDs as with any weight reduction regimen, the principles of weight management still apply. Unless exercise continues, food intake is controlled and dietary habits are changed, weight loss will be only temporary.

Table 10.1 is depicted the differences between very low calorie diet (VLCD) and low calorie diet (LCD).

CARBOHYDRATE MODIFIED DIETS

Diabetes Mellitus

Probably the most common type of carbohydrate-modified diet is the diabetic diet used for that person with diabetes mellitus. In diabetes mellitus, beta cells in the pancreas do not produce.

Figure 10.22 is depicted the managing diabetes with healthy food.

Table 10.1: Differences between very low calorie diet (VLCD) and low calorie diet (LCD).

Very low calorie diet (VLCD)	Low calorie diet (LCD)
• Diet <800 kcal/d	• Hypocaloric meal plan <800 kcal/d
• Defined by NHLBI and European Expert Panel	• Easier to comply (for some people)
• Meal replacements	• Meal replacements and/or regular food
• Rapid weight loss (2–5 pounds/week)	• More moderate weight loss
• Requires medical monitoring	• Does not require close medical monitoring

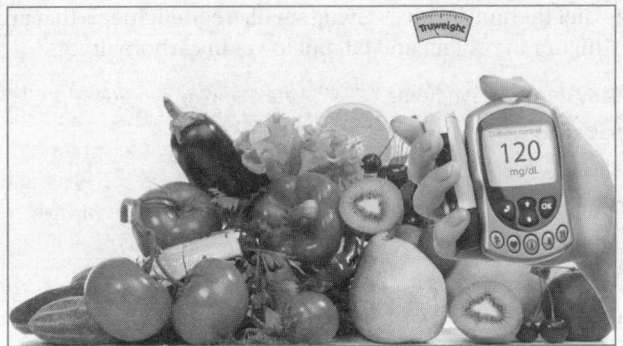

Fig. 10.22: Managing diabetes with healthy food.

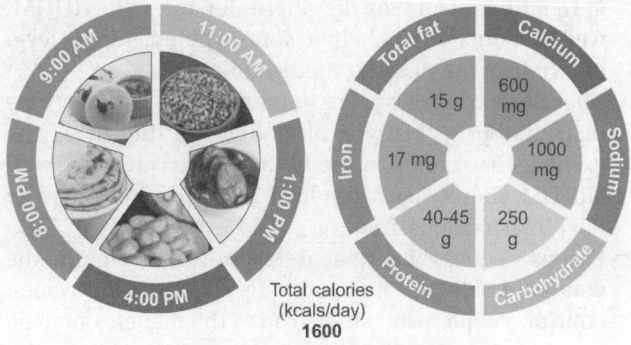

Fig. 10.23: Diabetic diet chart.

- Insulin is the hormone, which is necessary to move glucose from the blood stream into the cells, where it is used for energy.
- Without insulin, glucose builds up in the blood stream, leading to hyperglycemia (elevated blood glucose).
- Diabetes also may affect fat metabolism and increase levels of blood lipids (cholesterol and triglycerides) over time, elevated blood glucose and lipid levels may cause serious long-term complications.
- Perhaps not enough emphasis has been placed on the role of diet in the management of diabetes
- Proper diet is essential for blood glucose control and may help to reduce insulin needs, if strictly followed. By keeping blood glucose levels relatively constant and in an appropriate range, the risk of diabetic complications may be lessened.
- Persons with diabetes should continually be encouraged to follow their individualized meal plan.
- Dietary goals differ somewhat depending on the type of diabetes being treated.

Insulin-dependent Diabetes Mellitus (IDDM)

- It occurs most often in children and adolescents. Those with DDM do not produce insulin; their body cannot use glucose for energy and begins to burn the fat.
- When fat is burned for energy in the absence of glucose with the production of wastes called ketones.
- Ketones builds up in the blood and lead to a life-threatening condition called ketoacidosis. People with IDDM must take insulin to avoid this condition.
- The most important principle for those with IDDM is consistency. Meals and snacks should be eaten at about the same time each day.
- The types and amounts of foods eaten should be similar from day to day. This s necessary because the carbohydrate eaten must balance the insulin administered each day.
- Carbohydrate intake should be distributed evenly throughout the day to provide adequate amounts of glucose for the available insulin to move from the blood stream to the cells. This is called carbohydrate distribution.
- The patient should be given a meal, plan to follow that specified number of food choices (exchanges) to be consumed at each meal and snack.
- Carbohydrate is distributed among the meals to correspond with insulin dosage.
- If a person taking insulin fails to consume adequate carbohydrate, blood glucose levels may drop, causing hypoglycemia (low blood glucose).
- Symptoms of hypoglycemia may include headache, confusion, weakness, perspiration, shallow breathing, nervousness, visual disturbances and vertigo and also may lead to unconsciousness.
- Sometime the person experiencing hypoglycemia may be mistakenly judged to be intoxicated. Proper medical identification should be worked to prevent such a mistake.
- Hypoglycemia should be treated with immediate administration of glucose in a readily available form, such as orange juice, followed by food containing both carbohydrate and protein. If juice is not available, sugar or hard candy may be eaten. In the event of unconsciousness, glucose should be administered intravenously.
- In times of illness, the patient with diabetes may not want to eat the usual foods on the meal plan. In such cases, it is essential to provide carbohydrates in the diet to correspond with insulin dosage.
- Carbohydrate containing beverages, such as juices and punch, should be offered. Popsicles, flavored gelatin, crackers, puddings and ice milk provide carbohydrate and may be better accepted during illness.

Figure 10.23 is depicted the diabetic diet chart.

Non-insulin-dependent Diabetes Mellitus (NIDDM)

- It usually occurs in adults, many of whom are overweight. People with NIDDM produces insulin, but either there is not enough insulin or the body is unable to use it properly.
- This type of diabetes often may be controlled by diet and exercise. Some people with NIDDM use oral hypoglycemic agents, medications that stimulate insulin production and use.
- In some instances, insulin injections may be needed to help to regulate blood glucose levels. Whenever insulin is administered, the dietary principles for IDDM should be used.
- Many people with NIDDM are overweight and one of the major dietary goals with this type of diabetes

is weight control. For the obese person with NIDDM, weight reduction can help to control blood glucose level and reduce the need for medication.

- Kilocalorie control is more important than carbohydrate distribution in this type of diabetes. A diet using the exchange lists is an ideal method of weight control. As with NIDDM, simple sugar should be restricted and adequate fiber intake emphasized.
- Exercise reduces blood glucose levels. This is helpful in the control of blood glucose and is also important or weight control. People with either type of the diabetes may be able to reduce insulin or medication needs with regular exercise.
- Diet can also be adjusted to compensate for exercise. If a patient with NIDDM is to be involved in a physical activity that he/she is not accustomed to some carbohydrate containing food (milk, fruits, vegetables or starches) may be added to the meal just before engaging in the activity. In this way, the extra carbohydrate will provide more glucose to satisfy the demands of exercise.

DUMPING SYNDROME

Dumping syndrome may occur after surgery, where a portion of all of the stomach is removed (partial or total gastrectomy). After partial or total gastrectomy, the stomach contents may empty too rapidly into the jejunum.

Figure 10.24 is depicted the pathophysiology of dumping syndrome.
- The body reacts by sending water to the intestinal tract, thus blood pressure is reduced.
- The load on the intestinal tract increases peristalsis (contractions that move food through the GI tract), leading to diarrhea.
- Symptoms occur 15 to 30 minutes after meals and include cramping, weakness, diaphoresis, vertigo, nausea and possibly vomiting.

- Diet therapy involves giving small, frequent meals that are higher in protein and fat, but lower in carbohydrates.

Early dumping syndrome	Late dumping syndrome
Sweating	Sweating
Blush	Tachycardia
Tonture	Hunger
Tachycardia	Somnolence
Abdominal pain	Unconsciousness
Diarrhea	Tremor
Swelling	Irritability
Nausea	

- Concentrated sweets should be avoided and fluids should be taken 30 to 60 minutes before or after a meal.
- The dumping syndrome diet may be needed only temporarily until the body adjusts to the changes caused by surgery.

LACTOSE INTOLERANCE

Lactose intolerance occurs as a result of lack of the digestive enzyme, lactase, Because of this, the GI tract is unable to breakdown lactose (milk sugar). Symptoms occur after ingestion of milk products and include nausea, cramps, bloated feeling, flatulence and diarrhea.
- Diet for lactose intolerance excludes milk and milk products, such as ice cream, puddings, cheese, and powdered milk.
- Food with milk added, such as biscuit or muffin mixes, some soups and other prepared foods, they need to be avoided.

Some individuals have a deficiency rather than a total absence of lactase. These individuals may be able to tolerate small amount of milk products.

Figure 10.25 is depicted the lactose intolerant people's reactions to lactose.

Yogurt and cheese are often well tolerated. Lactase enzyme-containing preparations are available and can be added to milk before drinking.

FAT-MODIFIED DIETS

Dietary fat intake may also be modified in the treatment of disease.

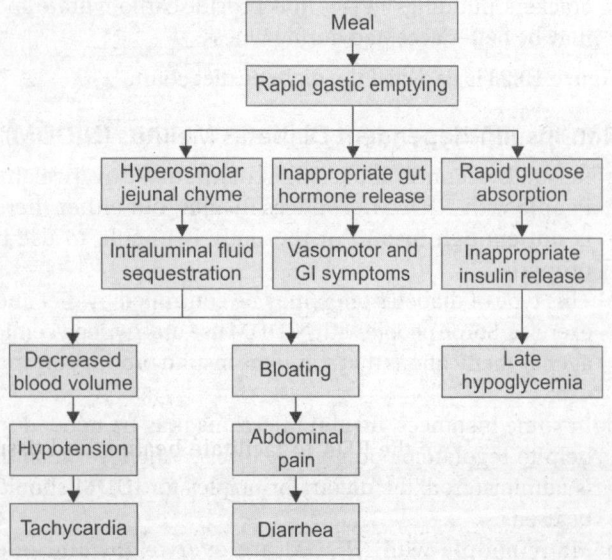

Fig. 10.24: Pathophysiology of dumping syndrome.

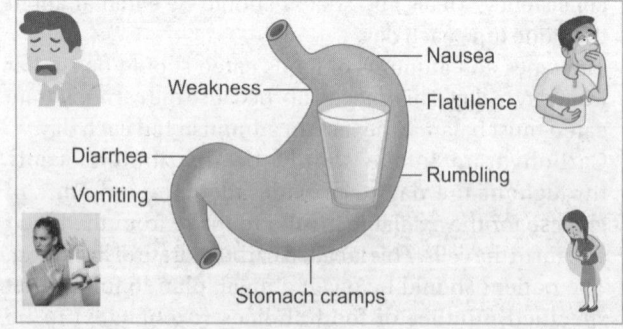

Fig. 10.25: Lactose intolerant people's reactions to lactose.

Fat-controlled Diets

- A fat-controlled diet is desirable for the treatment of atherosclerosis, heart disease and hyperlipidemias.
- Diabetic diets also incorporate fat control. A fat-controlled diet limits both total fat and saturated fat intake.
- Usually when saturated fat intake is reduced, cholesterol intake also drops, since it is often found in foods containing saturated fat. The individual who is reducing saturated fat in the diet should choose low-fat dairy products, lean meats, skinless poultry and fish.
- Eggs should be limited to three per week and organ meats, such as liver, limited to one serving per week or less.
- Visible fats, such as butter, margarine, mayonnaise, cream, sour cream, nuts and rich desserts, should be limited.
- Cooking methods may need to be altered as well. Patients should be encouraged to bake, boil or poach the food, rather than to fry and add bread or butter to it. Foods should be eaten without the addition of sauces, gravies or dips that are high in fat.
- When fat is necessary in food preparation, unsaturated fats (monounsaturated and polyunsaturated) should be used in place of saturated fats.

Low-Fat Diets

- Some medical conditions warrant the use of a low-fat diet. It differs from fat-controlled diets in which all fate is limited, regardless of saturation. Any time fat malabsorption occurs, dietary fat should be limited.
- GI diseases that involve malabsorption of fat include cystic fibrosis, inflammatory bowel disease, and pancreatitis and snort-bowel syndrome secondary to bowel resection.
- Gallbladder disease often requires a low-fat diet. The gallbladder stores bile and contracts whenever fat is present in the intestinal tract. If gallstones are present or inflammation of the gallbladder exists, contraction may be painful.
- A low-fat diet may alleviate some discomfort. After the gallbladder is removed (cholecystectomy), as low-fat diet is no longer required.
- Some patients with gallbladder disease may be overweight or obese. Weight reduction is indicated for these individuals and may reduce symptoms of gallbladder disease.

Figure 10.26 is depicted the low fat diet chart.

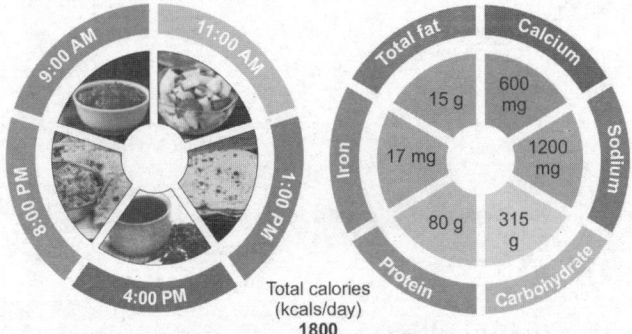

Fig. 10.26: Low fat diet chart.

PROTEIN, ELECTROLYTE AND FLUID-MODIFIED DIETS

Protein–restricted Diets

- In disease states, increased protein needs are often considered to facilitate healing. However, in the presence of defects in protein metabolism or excretion, protein intake should be reduced or controlled.
- One such case is during renal failure or may progress slowly (end-stage renal disease). Acute renal failure is often temporary, whereas end-stage renal disease is irreversible.
- The kidney normally functions to excrete wastes, concentrate urine and conserve needed electrolytes.
- During renal failure, the nephrons (working units of the kidney) fail to maintain normal function so that oliguria (decreased urine output) or anuria (no urine output) may result.
- Urea and other nitrogenous wastes, the end products of protein metabolism, build up in the blood steam, leading to a condition known as azotemia.
- Many electrolytes, particularly potassium, sodium and phosphorus are retained and increased blood levels of these nutrients may occur. Because of the buildup of protein waste products, dietary protein should be restricted.
- A therapeutic diet for renal failure limits the amount of protein consumed; the degree of limitation depends on the extend of renal failure.
- Patients are encouraged to consume moderate amounts of only high-quality or complete proteins found in milk, meat, fish, poultry and eggs.
- Incomplete proteins, those found in plant products, contribute to uremia, so that it should be restricted.
- Other dietary modification in renal failure includes the restriction of potassium, sodium, phosphorus and fluids. Vitamin and mineral supplements are generally prescribed.
- Cirrhosis is a chronic, degenerative disease of the liver. It is most often seen secondary to alcoholism, but my also be seen as a result of hepatitis A and B or other infection.
- Scar tissue develops in the liver, hampering its effectiveness in removing waste products from the blood stream. In this case, ammonia, which is a waste product of protein metabolism, builds up in the blood stream. If not controlled, high ammonia levels may contribute to hepatic coma (coma secondary to liver disease), brain damage and death.
- Ascites, a condition characterized by an accumulation of fluid in the abdominal cavity, may occur. If the liver is unable to produce bile, fat malabsorption also may take place.
- In the presence of cirrhosis, protein intake should initially be at or above the RDA to facilitate healing and tissue regeneration. However, if blood ammonia levels become elevated and signs of impending coma are present, such as confusion, apathy and drowsiness, a strict low-protein diet should be followed.

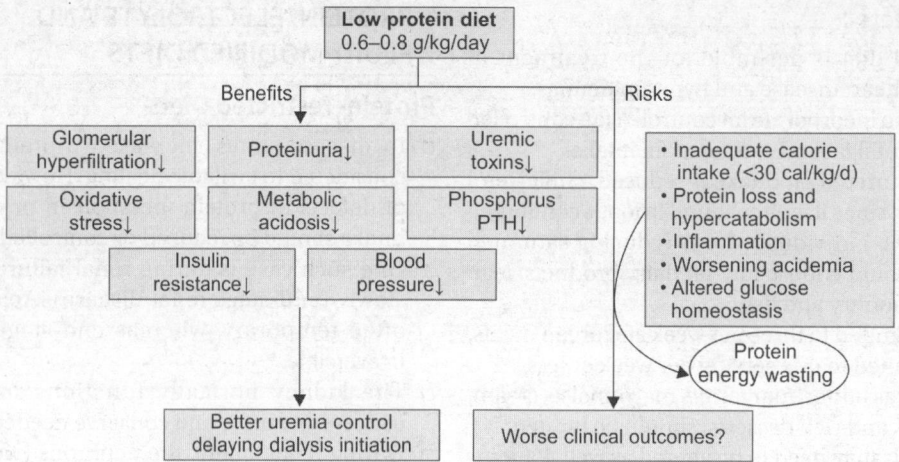

Fig. 10.27: Low protein diet.

- The low-protein diets for cirrhosis restrict milk and milk products, meats, fish, poultry, cheese, eggs, legumes and nuts.
- Special nutritional support formulates with modified protein content have also been developed for hepatic coma.
- The veins at the lower end of the esophagus may become enlarged and tortuous during cirrhosis, this condition known as esophageal varices.
- Esophageal varices are painful and the use of a soft or liquid diet may be beneficial in this case.
- Other dietary modifications for cirrhosis include total abstinence from alcohol and may require restriction if malabsorption is present. Vitamin and mineral supplements are also given.

Figure 10.27 is depicted the low protein diet.

Sodium-restricted Diets

Sodium restrictions may be used to treat a number of medical conditions. Hypertension is often responsive to a lowered sodium intake. It is estimated that 20% of the population is 'sodium sensitive', i.e., they have a genetic sensitivity to sodium that leads to hypertension. In such individuals, sodium reduction appears beneficial in controlling blood pressure.

- Sodium is also restricted when water retention or edema is present. In the presence of congestive heart failure (CHF), sodium intake should be decreased to alleviate pulmonary and peripheral edema.
- Directly after a myocardial infarction (MI) sodium fluid, kcal and fat restrictions may be implemented. These restrictions are to minimize the work load on the heart. As recovery progresses, the diet will be liberalized as individual condition permits.
- If cirrhosis is accompanied by ascites, sodium intake should be reduced and in renal failure, if anuria or oliguria exists, sodium should be restricted.
- Sodium-restricted diets vary in degree of restriction. The no-added-salt diet is the least restrictive, allowing 2000 to 3,000 mg of sodium/day. This diet allows the use of most foods with the exception of highly salted snack foods and prepared foods.
- Patients following this diet should read nutrition labels to assess the sodium content of food products and determine which would be appropriate for their diet. No salt should be added in cooking or at the table.
- Other sodium restricted diets range from 2,000 mg (2 g) sodium to as little as 250 mg of sodium/day. In the presence of cystic fibrosis, the sweat glands produce excessive amounts of sodium and chloride.
- In uses special condition, sodium intake is not restricted, but generous amounts of sodium and salt are encouraged to compensate for the excess losses of sodium.

Figure 10.28 is depicted the low sodium diet chart.

Potassium-modified Diets

- Potassium is considered to play a role in blood pressure control. Evidence indicates that populations with higher potassium intakes have less incidence of hypertension.
- Increased potassium intake from foods may be' beneficial for blood pressure control.
- Many patients with hypertension or other conditions that cause water retention may get potassium-wasting diuretics.
- An increased intake of potassium is needed to counteract the loss of potassium caused by the diuretic.

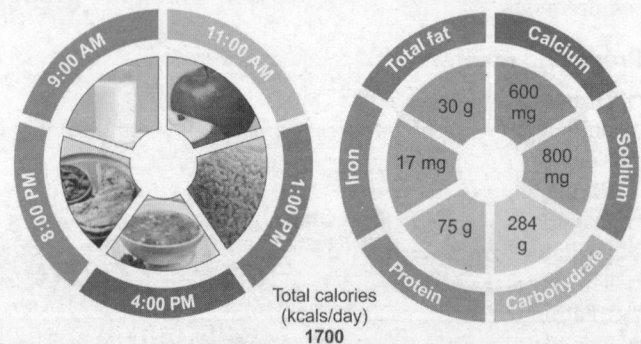

Fig. 10.28: Low sodium diet chart.

- In end-stage renal diseases and other kidney diseases, potassium intake may need to be restricted to as little as 1,500 to 2,000 mg/day.

Fluid-modified Diets

Fluid is found in the diet in a number of forms. Of course, all beverages, milk, juices, coffee and tea add fluid to the diet. Other dietary fluid sources include gelatins, ice cream, sherbet, puddings, popsicles, fruit ices and soups.

- During end-stage renal disease and other kidney disease with oliguria and anuria fluid is restricted to 400 to 500 mL/day plus an amount equal to daily urine output, if any.
- Fluid restrictions may also be implemented during CHF, directly after MI or in hepatic coma or ascites.
- During fluid restrictions, patients may experience excessive thirst. Some suggestions to help alleviate thirst include rinsing the mouth with cold mouthwash, putting lemon into cold water to make it more refreshing, freezing fluid so it takes longer time to consume, eating cold fruits and raw vegetables, chewing gum, sucking to breath mints or hard candies (in moderation) and brushing teeth often can helps to alleviate thirst.
- Increased fluid intake is a common dietary treatment for renal calculi (kidney stones) a urinary tract infection.
- Additional fluid helps to dilute the urine and increases urinary output. Fluid needs are also increased during periods of diarrhea, vomiting or malabsorption, such as in inflammatory bowel disease. Care should be taken to replace fluids that are lost, to prevent dehydration.
- The burn victim loses a large volume of fluids from the wounds, immediately after a severe burn, fluids, electrolytes and protein are given intravenously rather than orally, because bum patients experience a temporary loss of bowel function.
- Once bowel activity resumes, adequate fluids should be a part of dietary treatment. Most conditions requiring diet therapy involve combinations of therapeutic diets.

■ NURSES RESPONSIBILITIES IN FOOD SERVING

The Nurse's Responsibilities in Serving Food to the Patient are as Follows

It is necessary to plan different diets for different patients considering the physical and mental condition of the patient, his social and cultural background, the treatment requirements, availability of food and the economic aspects.

Preparing Environment for Meals

- Dressing and other such painful procedures should be ended, one hour before serving meal.
- Keep the dining place clean (while serving food on bed, dining table/cardiac table/small stool should be used).
- Provide privacy to the patient (if no separate room is available, curtains can be used).
- The meal hours should be fixed. Avoid the rounds, treatment formalities and visitors during meal time.
- The articles disliked by the patient or causing nausea, e.g., appliances, such as bedpan, urine pot, dirty dressing, dreadful equipment, dirty substances, refuse, etc., should be removed before serving meal.
- Try to save the patient from the cry of other patients, noise and confusion, etc., at the time of meals.
- Arrange for proper lighting and temperature.
- Keep the patient clean (if necessary, his clothes be changed before meals).
- Attempts should be made to reduce the patient's physical and mental fatigue. Diversional technique, soft melodious music, flower arrangement give pleasant environment for meals.

Box 10.3 is depicted the nurse's role in nutrition care.

> **Box 10.3:** Nurse's role in nutrition care.
>
> If you think dietitians alone are responsible for patients' nutrition care, think again. In the early part of nursing's modern era, nurses were responsible for preparing patients' meals and assessing and monitoring the impact of nutrient intake (or lack thereof) on their recovery and well-being.
>
> Today, nurses still play a key role in nutritional care. Although we are no longer responsible for overseeing food preparation and delivery, nutrition continues to be an essential domain of nursing practice.
>
> All nurses who provide patient care are responsible for addressing patients' nutritional needs. This can take the form of:
> - Conducting nutrition screening
> - Performing assessment and intervention
> - Providing mealtime assistance and nutrition support therapy
> - Monitoring, managing, or evaluating the impact of nutrient and dietary therapies.

Serving Food

- Keep the patient in fowler's or comfortable position (as far as possible the patient should be encouraged to eat in sitting posture).
- Mouth and hands of the patients should be washed.
- Serve the food in an attractive manner through covered and cleaned utensils.
- Motivate the patient to eat meals.
- Direct the patient to use spoons or take small morsels (weak patient should be fed by nurse herself).
- Engage the patient in entertaining conversation during meals.
- Give sufficient time to patient for mastication.
- Give water whenever required.

After Care and Other Precautions

- The patient should be provided comfortable position after washing his hands and mouth, following meals.
- The quality of food consumed by the patient and any abnormality if observed should be noted.
- Food hygiene should be followed, right from cooking to consumption.
- The cooperation offered by the patient while consuming food should be appreciated, so that his morale goes up.
- The opportunity of serving food should be fully utilized for giving nutrition education.

Figure 10.29 is depicted the nurses role in dietary care.

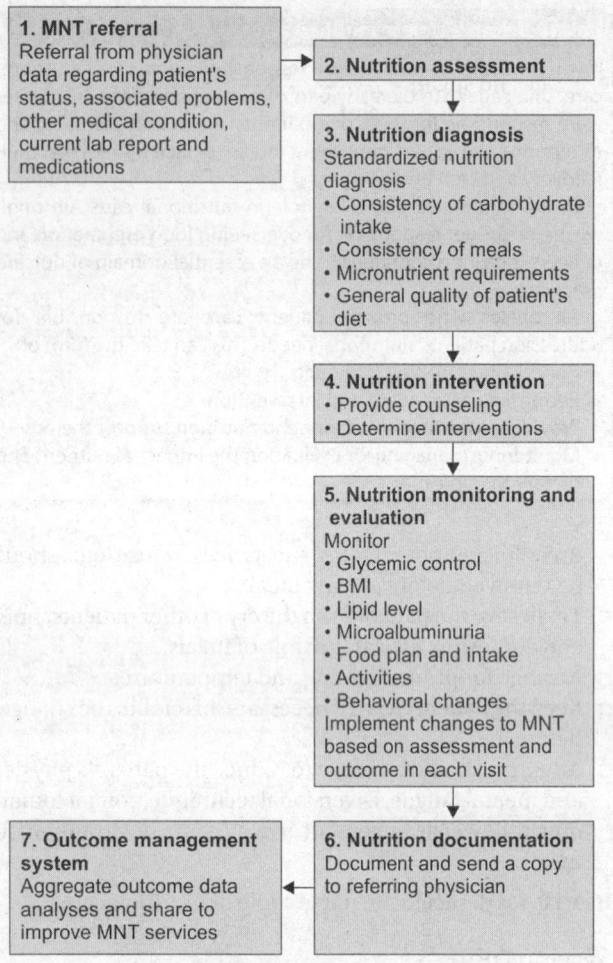

Fig. 10.29: Nurses role in dietary care.

DIET THERAPY FOR PERIOPERATIVE CONDITIONS (FIG. 10.30)

Malnutrition has long been recognized as a risk factor for postoperative morbidity and mortality. Traditional metabolic and nutritional care of patients undergoing major elective surgery has emphasized preoperative fasting and re-introduction of oral nutrition 3–5 d after surgery. Attempts to attenuate the consequent nutritional deficit and to influence post-operative morbidity and mortality have included parenteral, enteral and oral sip feeding. Recent studies have emphasized that an enhanced rate of recovery can be achieved by a multi-modal approach focused on modulating the metabolic status of the patient before (e.g., carbohydrate and fluid loading), during (e.g., epidural anesthesia) and after (e.g., early oral feeding) surgery).

Pre- and Postoperative Diet

- Good nutrition prior to and following surgery ensures fewer postoperative complications better wound healing.
- Short convalescence, lower mortality, and chronic diseases increase the nutritional requirements.
- Malnutrition can lead to weight loss, poor wound healing, decreased intestinal motility, anemia, edema or dehydration and ulcers.
- The circulating blood volume and the concentration of the serum proteins hemoglobin and electrolytes maybe reduced.

Preoperative Nutritional Assessment

The objectives in the dietary management of surgical conditions are:

- To improve the preoperative nutrition whenever the operation is not of an emergency nature.
- To maintain correct nutrition after operation or injury as far as possible, and
- To avoid harm from injudicious choice of foods.

A satisfactory state of protein nutrition ensures:

- Rapid wound healing.
- Increases the resistance to infection.
- Exerts a protective action upon the liver against the toxic effects of anesthesia, and
- Reduces the possibility of edema at the site of the wound. The level of protein to be used in preoperative and postoperative diets depends on the previous state of nutrition, the nature of the operation and the extent of the postoperative losses. Intake of 1.0 to 1.5 per kilogram of body weight or about 100 g of protein is necessary as a rule.

Energy: With 2500 to 3000 kcal patients make progress. Obesity constitutes a hazard in surgery. Whenever possible

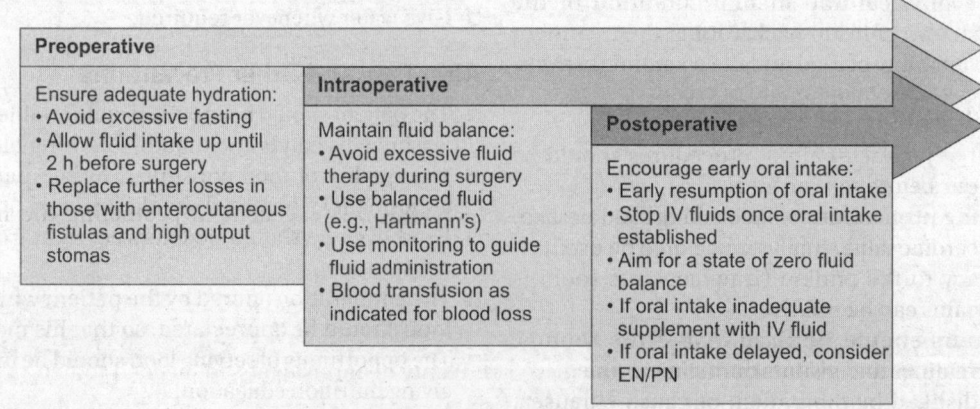

Fig. 10.30: Diet therapy for perioperative conditions.

it should be corrected. Rapid weight loss results in loss of lean body mass and should be avoided.

Minerals: A liberal intake of protein and ascorbic acid and administration of iron salt is necessary.

Fluid: A patient should not go to operation in a stage of dehydration since the subsequent dangers of acidosis are great. If the patient is unable to ingest sufficient liquid by mouth, parental fluids are administered.

Vitamins: Vitamin C is important for wound healing. Loss of vitamin K results in bleeding. Hemorrhage is especially likely to occur in patients who have diseases of the liver.

Postoperative Diet

Following minor surgery, liquids are often tolerated within a few hours and rapid progression to a normal diet is made after major surgery, oral intake may be delayed for days. Complete nutritional support is provided by conventional intravenous feedings, catheter jejunostomy, total parenteral nutrition, tube feedings or semisynthetic fiber free diets.

The success of the surgery depends on following a modified textured diet for the next eight to 10 weeks. Below is an idea of the timescale for this:
- Weeks 1 to 3—liquid diet only
- Weeks 4 to 6—puree diet
- Weeks 7 to 8—soft mashable diet
- Weeks 8 and onward—resume solid food

Step 1—for the first 3 weeks consume a liquid diet only: To ensure an adequate intake of protein, calcium and other nutrients to help you heal, the liquid diet must be based on milk. Ideally low fat milk which can be flavored with milk shake powder or low calorie hot chocolate. If you have diabetes, then a milkshake may not be appropriate for you.

Aim to have two pints of milk per day. If you do not like milk choose an alternative, such as soya milk but make sure it is enriched with calcium. You may find very hot or very cold drinks difficult to tolerate, in this case drink fluids at room temperature.

Other fluids allowed:
- Slimming drinks, e.g., slim fast or chemists/supermarket own brands
- Complan or 'Build up' soups and shakes
- Yoghurt drinks and smoothies
- Still mineral water and still low calorie fruit squash
- Clear low calorie soups
- Smooth soups, e.g., cream of tomato or cream of chicken
- Tea and coffee without sugar
- Unsweetened fruit juice
- Marmite or Bovril drinks

Be cautious with the quantities of fluid you drink over the first few days until you establish how much liquid you can tolerate. Do not drink fizzy drinks at any time as they will cause bloating and increase stomach size.

Some people find they experience constipation in the first few weeks. This is due to the low intake of fiber in the diet. The weetabix in the meal plan may help but make sure it's liquidized to a thin smooth liquid.

Step 2—for week's 4–6 progress to a pureed diet: Gradually introduce pureed foods. These should be high in protein and low in fats and sugars.
- A pureed diet means your food should be the consistency of baby food or apple sauce-many people find a hand held blender most suited to pureeing small quantities of food.
- Eat 4–5 small meals per day (about 1–2 tablespoons at each)
- Eat slowly and stop as soon as you feel full.
- If a food makes your feel nauseous avoid it for a few days and then try again.

Step 3—for weeks 7–8 progresses to a moist soft mashed diet: This is similar to the puree diet but food simply needs to be soft and moist and mashed with a fork. Adding sauces and gravies can be helpful.

Step 4–8 weeks and lifelong-returning to a normal diet: You will now begin to include normal texture foods. Crispy textures may be better tolerated at first. For example, crisp breads and breadsticks rather than bread.

Aim for three meals per day. You can include healthy snacks between meals but try to avoid high fat and sugary foods, such as chocolate. These foods can still be included as treats but not as meal replacements.

Diet for Pre- and Postoperative Surgery

Start with a healthy liver:
- In the case of operations involving a general anesthetic, the liver is the organ that takes the hardest knock from the drugs used.
- A good form of preparation for an operation would therefore involve restoring the liver to optimum health prior to undergoing surgery. Avoid alcohol and saturated fats.
- Wake up to a cup of hot water with the juice of half a lemon squeezed into it.
- Eat grapefruit with your breakfast and plenty of fresh fruit with lemon juice squeezed over it.
- Eat lots of fresh, raw or lightly steamed vegetables, especially the colorful varieties.
- Drink plenty of juiced carrots, beetroot or any other vegetable juices you can tolerate. These will very effectively detoxify your liver.

Sulfur containing foods best:
- To prevent the after-effects of anesthetics, such as hepatitis, eat foods rich in the sulfur-containing amino acid, methionine, such as free-range eggs, Brazil nuts, fish and meat.
- St Mary's thistle which contains the active ingredient, silymarin, is excellent in protecting the liver against anesthetics and so is dandelion root. These also help to regenerate liver cells if there is damage to the liver.

Antioxidants
- Plenty of antioxidants are needed to neutralize the free-radicals which result from all the chemicals in anesthetics and other drugs that may be prescribed.

- Mopping up of these free-radicals depends upon your levels of beta carotene, vitamin A, C and E as well as zinc, manganese and copper levels.
- Take a good plant-based green leaf multivitamin and mineral supplement, such as AIM's
- BarleyLife for a few weeks before the operation. Your surgeon may insist you stop all vitamin supplements just prior to and immediately after the surgery. This is fine; however do try to get back onto them as soon as possible to give your body a fighting chance against infection. Prior to surgery eat plenty of pawpaw, beetroot, carrots, broccoli, apricots, all citrus, even the pith, and green, yellow and red peppers.

Figure 10.31 is depicted the natural painkillers.

Preventing Blood Clots

- For at least a month before your operation take a pharmaceutical grade fish oil capsule daily to keep your blood thin and prevent clotting after surgery. You will need to tell your surgeon you are taking these as he may wish to put you on a blood-thinning drug, such as:
- Warfarin and the two should not be taken together as this may cause excessive bleeding during surgery. Continue with fish oil capsules as soon after surgery as possible.

Healing of Wounds

- Build up the liver stocks of beta carotene a week prior to surgery with carrot and beetroot juice which will also detox the liver.
- Beta carotene converts to vitamin A in your body and will improve wound tensile strength, thus preventing possible tearing.
- Eat lots of apricots and watermelon if in season. Vitamin E promotes healing of ulcerated tissue and helps prevent hard scar formation.
- Use it mainly as an ointment rubbed on the scar after the wound has closed but the vitamin E in your plant-based multivitamin supplement will also be of great benefit.

Vitamin C

- Vitamin C promotes elastogen and collagen formation and prevents pressure sores. Mouth ulcers, common after surgery or chemotherapy, heal faster with 250 g vitamin C at meals and 500 mg at bedtime.
- Eat broccoli, pawpaw, kiwi fruit and oranges pre- and post-surgery. Throw in bioflavonoids to strengthen the integrity of mucous membranes and zinc for the correct formation of collagen and elastogen, particularly for leg ulcers.

Cancer Patients

- Cancer patients should try to avoid infections after any surgery as infections will only hinder recovery.
- Supplement with buffered Vitamin C, 2 g per day in divided doses, 20 mg zinc, 2 g bioflavonoids). This same program may be used by all patients going for surgery.

Bromelain

- Bromelain, an enzyme found in pineapple, reduces edema and inflammation. Either eat lots of pineapple or take bromelain in supplement form.
- If undergoing plastic surgery you could minimize bruising by using vitamin C, bioflavonoids and zinc before surgery and bromelain after.

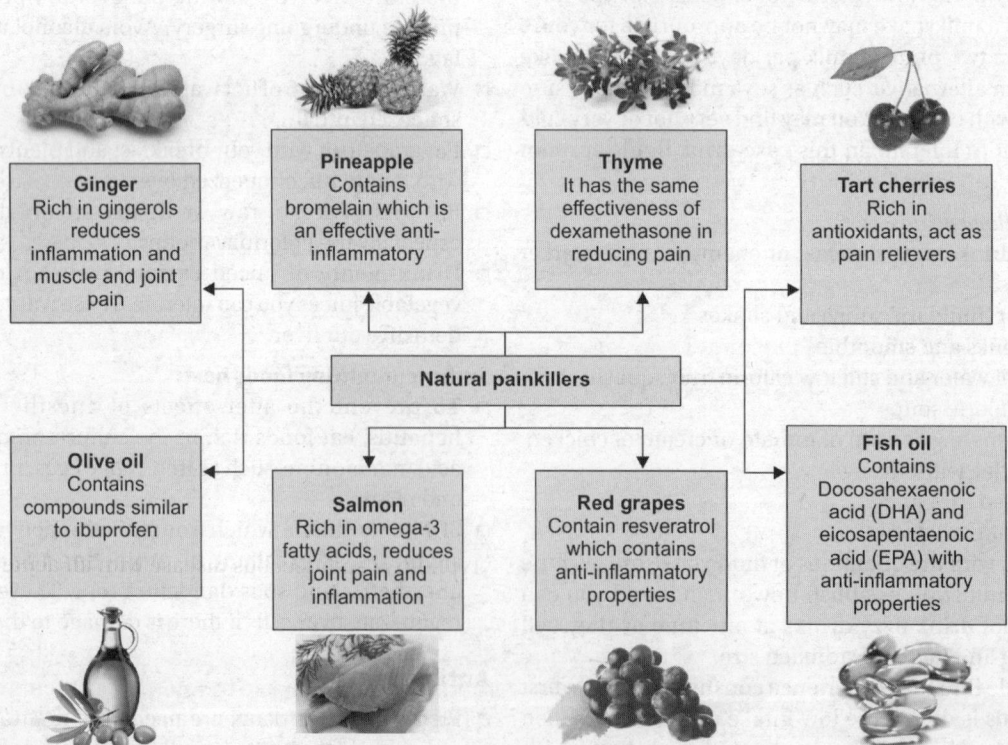

Fig. 10.31: Natural painkillers.

DIET THERAPY IN FEVERS

Fever is a common symptom which is associated with a host of infectious and chronic conditions. Fever is a natural response of the body, to destroy virus or pathogens in the blood, by raising the body's natural metabolic rate. There are various dietary measures that have been suggested to improve and hasten recovery after a fever. Though the dietary modalities will differ depending upon the cause of the fever, however there are certain basic guidelines that have been found to be highly beneficial Fever is an elevation in body temperature above the normal which may occur due to exogenous and endogenous factors.

Figure 10.32 is depicted the diet chart in fever.

Diet for Common Fever

There are certain simple dietary recommendations that can help hasten the recovery from fever. Eating right and getting enough rest is essential when trying to avoid illnesses and this includes the prevention of fevers.

- To begin with the patient should be put on a juice and water diet for a couple of days. A glassful of orange juice every three hours is considered beneficial for health. Orange juice is a great source of energy and is also loaded with vitamin C which helps enhance immunity and natural ability of the body to fight infection.
- Following the juice diet, an all fruit diet is recommended. Fruits are easier to digest and loaded with essential vitamins and minerals which hasten the process of recovery.
- Fresh fruits including grapes, apple, oranges, peach, pineapple, lemons, etc., should be included in the diet. Fresh fruit juices are also recommended. Avoid tinned or canned fruit juices as they are loaded with preservatives and can delay the recovery process.
- Always ensure that you consume about three liters of water each day, especially during fever. Water helps flush the toxins out of the body system and hastens recovery.
- Once the fever subsidizes, opt for a soft diet. A soft diet may comprise of boiled eggs, steamed vegetables vegetable soups, porridge and yoghurt. These foods are easier to digest and supply with loads of energy which is essential to hasten the recovery process.
- Rice porridge with ginger and made with vegetable broth is good to have when you have a fever. This diet is easy to digest. Further ginger has strong anti-inflammatory properties which are beneficial in resolving the fever at the earliest.

A healthy lifestyle practice is considered to be beneficial in reducing the incidence of fevers. Increase the intake of water, green vegetables, fresh fruits and low fat dairy products. These foods are loaded with essential vitamins and enhance the overall immunity of the body. These dietary measures can help improve the body's natural immune system and can also help in preventing the occurrence of infections.

General Dietary Considerations

- **Energy:** The caloric requirement may be increased as much as 50%, if the temperature is high and the tissue destruction is great. The patient may be able to ingest only 600 to 1,200 kcal daily, but this should be increased as rapidly as possible.
- **Protein:** About 100 g protein or more is prescribed for the adult when a fever is prolonged. High protein beverages may be used as supplements to the regular meals.
- **Carbohydrates:** Glycogen stores are replenished by a liberal intake of carbohydrates. Glucose which is readily absorbed is preferred.
- **Fats:** The energy intake may be rapidly increased through the judicious use of fats but fried foods and rich pastries are to be avoided.
- **Minerals:** A sufficient intake of NaCl is accomplished by the use of salty broth and soups and by liberal sprinklings of salt on food. Fruit juices and milk are relatively good sources of minerals.
- **Vitamins:** Fevers apparently increase the requirement for vitamin A and vitamin C just as the B complex vitamins are needed at increased levels.
- **Fluids:** Daily 2500–5000 mL is necessary including beverages, soups, fruit juices and water.
- **Ease of digestion:** Bland readily digested food should be used to facilitate digestion and rapid absorption. The food may be soft or of regular consistency. Fluid diets can be used initially.
- **Intervals of feeding:** Small quantities of food at interval of 2 to 3 hours will permit adequate nutrition without overtaking the digestive system at anytime. During an acute fever the patient's appetite is often very poor and small feedings of soft or liquid foods as desired should be offered at frequent intervals. Sufficient intake of fluids and salt is essential. If the illness persists for more than a few days high protein, high calorie foods will be needed.

Figure 10.33 is depicted the diet during fever.

Typhoid Fever

Typhoid is an infectious disease with an acute fever of short duration and occurs only inhuman. *Salmonella typhi* causes typhoid. Feces and urine of the patients or carriers of the disease are the source of infection. Drinking water or milk and food contaminated by intestinal contents of the patients or carriers or by flies often transmit the disease. The disease is characterized by a continued and high inflammation of the intestine. Formation of intestinal ulcers, hemorrhage and

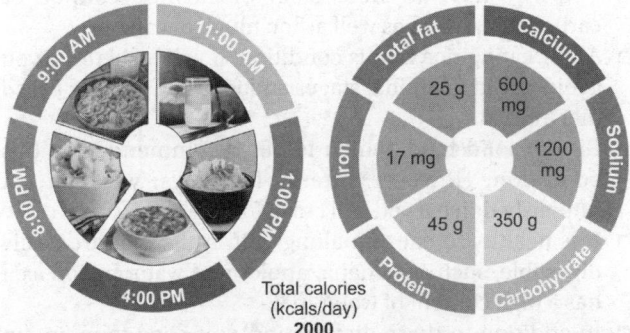

Fig. 10.32: Diet chart in fever.

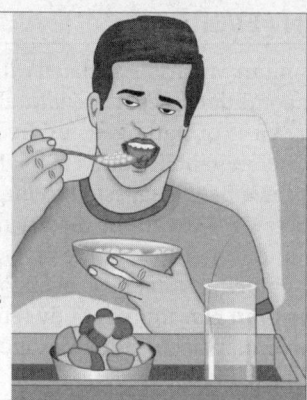

Fig. 10.33: Diet during fever.

enlargement of spleen can occur. The patient may complain of diarrhea or constipation and severe stomach ache. Abdominal absorption of nutrients can cause headache.

Figure 10.34 is depicted the typhoid diet chart.

Principles of Dietary Therapy

- A high calorie, high protein, high carbohydrates, low fat, high fluid, low fibre and bland diet are suggested for typhoid patents.
- At first clear fluid diet is given followed by full fluid and soft diet is suggested because of the intestinal inflammation.
- Great care must be exercised to eliminate all irritating fibers and spices in the diet.
- Refined cereals, bread, eggs, boiled potato and simple desserts, such as custards, porridges can be given.
- Adequate nutrition reduces convalescence period.

Guidelines for Dietary Treatment

- High calorie diet is prescribed to maintain the weight or to gain weight. Caloric requirement may be as high as 2500–3000 kcal per day.
- Daily requirement of protein ranges from 80–120 g to make up for tissue wasting. Good quality proteins, such as egg and milk should be incorporated.
- Minerals especially calcium, iron and phosphorus is to be provided liberally as they help in regeneration of cells, blood and body fluids.
- Diet must be planned judiciously to provide good dose of vitamins especially vitamin A and vitamin C as these are essential for the regenerative purpose.

- High fluid and soft diet in small frequency is recommended.
- Food must be appetizing and made after considering the likes and dislikes of the patient.
- Fatty, highly fibrous and very spicy foods should be avoided as they are hard to digest.

Treatment-diet

- It is essential to have a healthy, hygienic diet if someone suffers from typhoid fever.
- There is a need to keep the body hydrated enough in this condition. So please drink plenty of fluids, such as unsweetened lime water, clear soups, fresh juices (which you are sure is safe and uncontaminated), and especially boiled and filtered water.
- As for food, you must eat food items that provide plenty of calories, protein and carbohydrates. When a person gets fever, his metabolic rate becomes high, hence calorie intake has to be increased.
- Protein is also essential in curing a fever, so consume plenty of eggs and milk to fulfill the requirement.
- Carbohydrates also meet the new needs that your body develops due to typhoid fever. These elements are known to be effective to this disease.

Care-digestible Diet

- It is absolutely necessary for food to be thoroughly cooked and easily digestible for a typhoid fever patient. Avoid raw food in any form. You will also have to control the urge to eat outside food, as it is likely to be unhygienic.
- You also have to steer clear of alcohol, canned or carbonated drinks as well as too much of caffeine.
- As for eating rice in this condition, it will be better if you avoid rice in the initial stages and focus on a liquid based diet instead.
- Rice is solid food, which is not recommended in this condition. However, after a few days, you can eat unpolished rice if you still crave for rice.
- It is healthy to eat that along with fruits that are easily digestible, such as banana, apples and water melon as it has a high content of water in it.
- In addition to these dietary tips, you need to maintain proper hygiene to avoid typhoid fever.

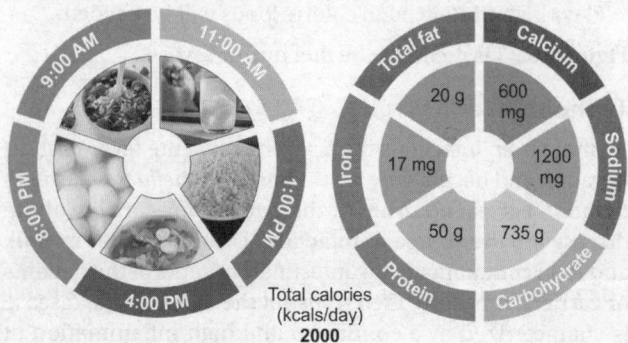

Fig. 10.34: Typhoid diet chart.

Foods to be included: Fruit juices with glucose, coconut water, barley water, milk, milk shakes if there is no diarrhea, custards, thin dal curries, eggs, baked fish, minced meat, curds, cottage cheese, cereals, gruels, steamed vegetable juices, milk puddings, vegetable puree.

Foods to be avoided: Butter, ghee, vegetable oil, no irritating fibrous food, chilies and other spices, rich pastries, fried foods, heavy puddings and cream soups.

DIET THERAPY FOR GASTROINTESTINAL DISORDERS

Diet therapy through the elimination of offending foods, such as wheat gluten or lactose, or inclusion of specialized products, such as medium chain triglycerides or elemental formulas, can sustain nutritional status. Dietary components, such as insoluble fiber appear to have physiologic effects, while soluble fibers may have metabolic effects important to diabetes and cardiovascular disease. There is a high potential for malnutrition in Crohn's disease during active and remittent phases. Elemental enteral formulas or TPN are used during the active phase to ensure optimal nutritional status and bowel rest. Hyperalimentation using the GI tract during remittent stage maintains this.

DIARRHEA

This is the passage of stools with increased frequency, fluidity or volume compared to the usual for a given individual. Diarrhea is a symptom of underlying functional or organic disease and is acute or chronic in nature.
- **Chemical toxins:** Such as arsenic, lead, mercury or cadmium.
- **Bacterial toxins:** Such as *Salmonella* or staphylococcal food poisoning.
- **Bacterial infections:** Such as *Streptococcus, E. coli.*
- **Drugs:** Such as quinidine, neomycin.
- **Psychogenic factors:** Such as emotional instability.
- **Dietary factors:** Such as food sensitivity or allergy.

Chronic Type

- Malabsorptive lesions of anatomic, mucosal or enzymatic origin.
- Metabolic diseases, such as diabetic neuropathy, uremia.
- Alcoholism
- Carcinoma of small bowel or colon
- Post-irradiation to small bowel or colon
- Cirrhosis
- Laxative abuses

Figure 10.35 is depicted the diarrhea diet chart.

Nutritional Considerations in Diarrhea

Fluid electrolyte and tissue protein losses are usually severe if diarrhea is prolonged.
- **Fluids:** Losses of fluids should be replaced by a liberal intake to prevent dehydration, especially in susceptible age groups.

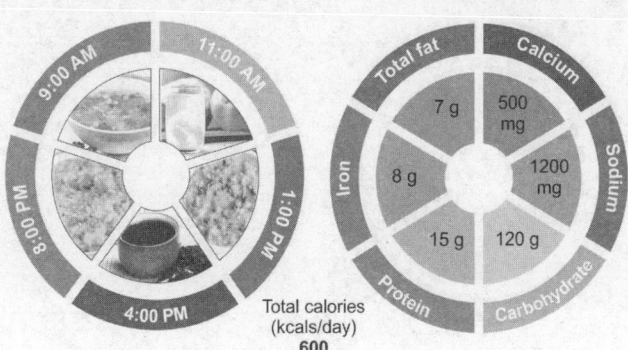

Fig. 10.35: Diarrhea diet chart.

- **Electrolytes:** Losses of sodium, potassium and others with severe diarrhea. Potassium loss is detrimental as potassium is necessary for normal muscle tone of the gastrointestinal tract. Losses can be replaced by liberal fluids, such as fruit juices that are high in potassium.

Nutrient Malabsorption

- Long continued diarrhea may result in depletion of tissue, proteins and decreased serum protein levels.
- Fat losses are considerable in certain disorders with consequent loss of calories and fat soluble vitamins.
- Intake of calories as high as 3000 with 100 to 150 g protein, 100 to 120 g fat and the remainder as carbohydrates.
- Vitamin deficiencies frequently seen in chronic diarrhea are related to the decreased intake of vitamins and the increased requirements because of losses in the stools.
- Iron deficiency owing to the increased losses of iron in the feces, the occasional blood losses and the reduced intake of iron rich foods because of fear that some foods might aggravate an existing lesion.

Dietary Considerations

- In acute diarrhea, current recommendations include oral intake of glucose electrolyte solutions for those able to drink with progression to foods as tolerated in small frequent feedings as appetite improves.
- Many patients with chronic diarrhea do not tolerate milk or foods high in fat or fiber content.
- Generally speaking, however the need is for a diet high in protein and calories with adequate amounts of vitamin and minerals and liberal amounts of fluids.

CONSTIPATION

In this condition, there is the duodenum and introvert or difficult evacuation of feces from the intestine. Insufficient or infrequent emptying of the bowel may lead to malaise, headache, coated tongue, foul breath and lack of appetite. These symptoms usually disappear after satisfactory evacuation has taken place. Correction of constipation depends in large measure on establishing regularity in habits, eating, rest, exercise and elimination.

Figure 10.36 is depicted the constipation diet plan.

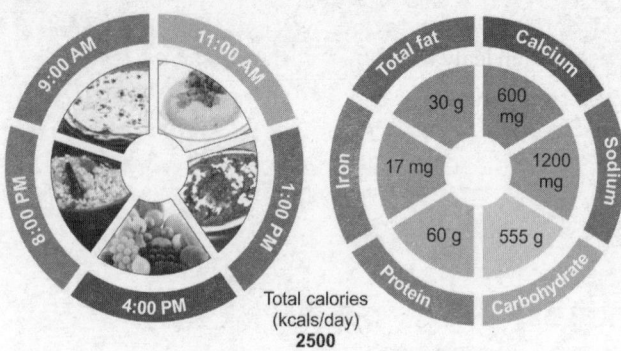

Fig. 10.36: Constipation diet plan.

Requirements for Normal Defecation

- Moist bulky fecal bolus
- Stimulus capable of transporting bolus to distal colon
- Normal colon
- Rectum capable of reasonable degree of distension
- Normal internal and external sphincters
- Normal peripheral nervous system to send afferent impulses
- Normal CNS response to send efferent impulses
- Conducive physical and psychological environment
- Appropriate posture, valsalva maneuver
- Desire and ability to evacuate bolus

Causes of Constipation

Dietary
- Low fiber intake
- Reduced food intake
- Reduced fluid intake

Functional
- Reduced physical inactivity
- Weakness
- Immobility
- Depression
- Disorientation
- Physical disability
- Repeated suppression of urge to defecate

Secondary Causes
- Metabolic, endocrine disorders
- Neuromuscular disorders
- Colonic obstruction

Medication
- Aluminum/calcium antacids
- Anticholinergics
- Antidepressants
- Antihypertensives
- Antiparkinsonian drugs
- Antispasmodics
- Bismuth-containing drugs
- Diuretics
- Narcotic analgesics
- Opiates

Dietary Considerations

- The diet should contain sufficient fibre to induce peristalsis and to contribute bulk to the intestine.
- A regular diet with an abundance of both raw and cooked fruits and vegetables is suitable for such patients.
- Whole grain cereals should be substituted for refined ones. Bran is useful but excesses are to be avoided since it may act as an irritant to sensitive intestinal tracts.
- Fat containing foods are useful because of the stimulating effect of the fatty acids on the mucous membranes.
- Excesses may cause diarrhea and should be avoided. Mineral oil, if used should not be taken at mealtime because of its interference with the absorption of fat soluble vitamins.
- A fluid intake of 8 to 10 glasses a day is useful in keeping the intestinal contents in a semisolid state for easier passage along the tract.
- Some individuals find that 1 or 2 glasses of hot or cold water plain or with lemon are helpful in initiating peristalsis when taken before breakfast.

Energy: Normal calories according to age, sex and occupation.

Proteins: About 60–80 g protein/day.

Fats: Fats stimulate the flow of bile and lubricate the bowel. Fried foods should be avoided.

Carbohydrates: Adequate bulk should be supplied in the form of bran, vegetables and whole fruits which are rich in unabsorbable cellulose. Bran is made more palatable by adding cooked fruits and vegetables.

Vitamins: B group vitamins help to regulate the bowel function.

Minerals: Acutely ill or bed ridden patients require potassium in the form of vegetable soup and fruit juice to prevent constipation.

Fluids: A liberal amount of fluids, about 10 glasses per day is advised. Warm fluid taken early morning on an empty stomach helps in the evacuation of bowel.

Fiber: The intake of dietary fiber should be increased by eating whole cereals and increasing consumption of fruits and vegetables. The most important factor is the water holding capacity of the fiber.

Oranges, carrots and cabbage fibers hold water more effectively. Whole grain breads and cereals should be used instead of refined cereals, e.g., whole wheat flour instead of maids.

PEPTIC ULCER

The term peptic ulcer is used to describe any localized erosion of the mucosal lining of those portions of the alimentary tract that come in contact with gastric juice. The majority of ulcers are found in the stomach although they also occur in the duodenum, jejunum or any other part of the GI tract exposed to the gastric juice.

- **Dietary management:** It was customary to suggest bland diet for ulcer patients. Bland diet is a diet which is mechanically, chemically and thermally nonirritating.

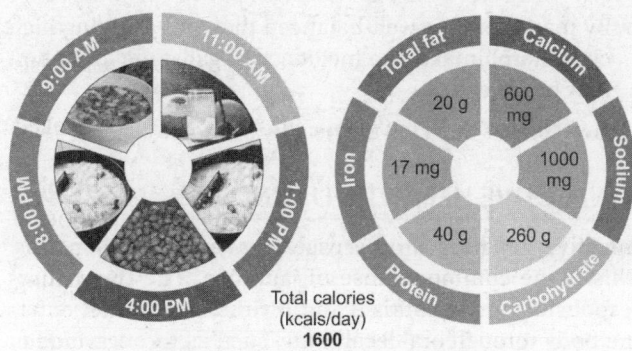

Fig. 10.37: Peptic ulcer diet chart.

flakes, puffed rice, margarine, well cooked cereal, semolina, cooked green leafy vegetables, custards, malted drinks.

Food to be avoided: Alcohol, strong tea, coffee, cola, beverages, gravies, soups, pickles, spices, curries, condiments, all fried foods, pastries, cakes, heavy sweets, such as halwa, barfi, raw unripe fruits, raw vegetables, such as cucumber, onions, radish and tomatoes.

- **Protein foods:** Milk and protein foods do have some buffering effect but they also evoke gastric secretions more than carbohydrates and fats. Milk should be included as a source of nutrients factors for healing purposes. Protein provides the necessary amino acids for synthesis of tissue proteins which helps in healing ulcer.

Figure 10.37 is depicted the peptic ulcer diet chart.

Fat

- Moderate amounts of the fat help to suppress gastric secretion and motility though the enterogastrone mechanism.
- Foods believed to be chemically irritating because of their stimulatory effect on gastric secretion include meat extractives, caffeine, alcohol, citrus fruits and juices and some spicy foods.
- Mechanically irritating foods include those with indigestible carbohydrates, such as whole grains and most raw fruits and vegetables.
- Foods believed to be thermally irritating are those ordinarily served at extremes of temperatures, such as very hot or iced liquids.
- In addition, certain foods traditionally forbidden include strongly flavored vegetables, such as cabbage, cauliflower, onions and turnips and fried foods.
- Restriction of these foods is based on subjective evidence from patients who experience distress following ingestion of these items including good food.

Figure 10.38 is depicted the duodenal ulcer diet chart.

Food to be included: Diary products, such as milk, cream, butter, milk cheese and eggs (not fried) steamed fish, rice, rice

Dietary Guidelines

- Whether a patient is on bland diet or regular diet, the patient and the family need to know which foods are needed for a nutritionally adequate diet and the importance of including these daily.
- The patient should select foods from the basic five food groups, omitting those foods known to irritate the mucosa.
- Small and frequent meals at regular intervals are essential.
- Patient should consume moderate quantities of food, as heavy foods tend to exert antral pressure against the stomach wall stimulating gastric secretion through the gastrin mechanism.
- The cultural pattern, economic status, preferences of the patient, and effect on the family has to be taken into consideration while planning the diet.
- Meals should be eaten in a relaxed atmosphere.
- A short rest before and after meals may be conducive to greater benefit of meals.
- Food should be eaten slowly and chewed well as fast eating provokes gastric feeding reflex.

MODIFICATION OF DIET IN BLEEDING ULCER

- The degree of dietary modification in bleeding ulcer depends on the peculiarities of the individual case.
- The severe hemorrhage, it is customary to give no food until the bleeding has been controlled and the patient's conditions are stabilized.
- If hemorrhage is not severe and if nausea and vomiting are not a problem, the patient may desire food and tolerate it well. Initial dietary treatment consists of mild alternated at 2 hours interval with small feedings of easily puddings toast and tender cooked fruits and vegetables.
- Gradual progression in amounts and types of foods is made as the patient improves.

DIET THERAPY FOR LIVER DISEASES

The liver is one of the main organs of nutritional metabolism, including protein synthesis, glycogen storage, and detoxification. These functions become damaged to a greater or lesser extent in patients with liver diseases, resulting in various metabolic disorders, and their disturbed nutritional condition is associated with disease progression. Therefore, dietary counseling and nutritional intervention can support other medical treatments in some liver diseases.

Figure 10.39 is depicted the liver disease diet chart.

- It is vitally important that patients with liver disease maintain a balanced diet, one which ensures adequate

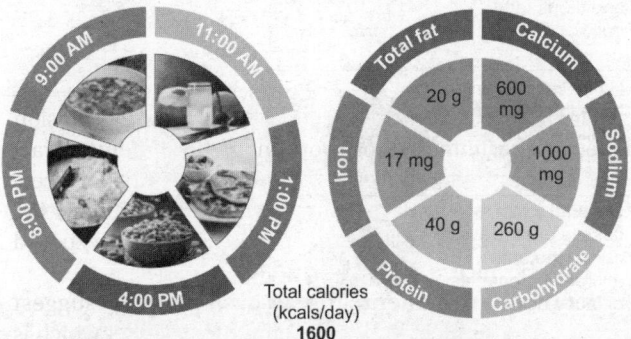

Fig. 10.38: Duodenal ulcer diet chart.

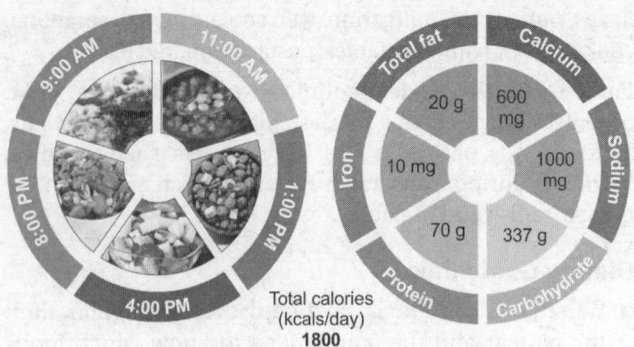

Fig. 10.39: Liver disease diet chart.

calories, carbohydrates, fats and proteins. Such a diet will aid the liver in the regeneration of liver cells.
- Nutrition that supports this regeneration is a means of treatment of some liver disorders.
- Patients with cirrhosis, who are malnourished, require a diet rich in protein and providing 2,000–3,000 calories per day to help the liver re-build itself. However, some cirrhotic patients have protein intolerance.
- Too much protein will result in an increased amount of ammonia in the blood, while too little protein can reduce healing of the liver.
- Doctors must carefully prescribe a specific amount of protein that will not elevate the blood ammonia. Lactulose and neomycin are two drugs that help keep the ammonia down.
- It is believed that the risk of gallbladder disorders can be reduced by avoiding high fat and cholesterol foods and preventing obesity.
- The gallbladder is a storage sac for the bile produced by the liver. During digestion, the gallbladder releases bile into the small intestine through the common bile duct.
- Most gallbladder problems are caused by gallstones and 80–90% of all gallstones are produced from excessive cholesterol which crystallizes and forms stones.
- By maintaining a well-balanced diet and avoiding high cholesterol intake, the incidence of gallstone formation may be lowered.

Figure 10.40 is depicted the healthy liver diet.

INFECTIVE HEPATITIS (JAUNDICE)

Infective hepatitis is otherwise known as viral hepatitis. This is the common cause of jaundice. The two viruses responsible are hepatitis A and B virus. The former enters the body through oral fecal route, such as through food or water, while the latter is passed through by using infected blood products from carriers, use of unsterilized needles and through sexual contact.

Jaundice may be produced due to the following factors/reasons
- Obstructive jaundice results from the interference of the flow of bile by the formation of stone and tumors.
- Hemolytic jaundice results from an abnormally large destruction of red blood cells as in hemolytic anemia.
- Toxic jaundice originates from poisons, drugs or viral infection.

Symptoms: Anorexia, fever, headache, rapid weight loss, loss of muscle tone and abdominal discomfort.

Figure 10.41 is depicted the jaundice diet chart.

Dietetic Management

Energy: In nasogastric feeding stage about 1000 kcal are supplied. In severe cases, 1600 kcal to 2000 kcal are suggested.

Protein: For the liver cells to regenerate an adequate supply of proteins is needed. Protein requirements vary according to the severity of the disease with severe jaundice 40 g. while in mild jaundice 60–80 g of protein is permitted with hepatic precoma and coma, protein containing foods are withheld and only high carbohydrate containing foods are given.

Foods that detox	Foods that protect
Cauliflower, cabbage, broccoli, beetroot and carrot clear heavy metal deposits and purify blood	Watermelon banana, oranges for fiber, vitamins and enzymes
Garlic and onions are a rich source of essential amino acid, methionine it detoxes mercury and other heavy metals	Yogurt stabilizes blood sugar levels and stops fatty build-up in liver
Freshly squeezed lemon juice in a cup of boiled water first thing in the morning cleanses the liver and stimulates bile flow	Haldi and dalchini have the healing qualities required to protect against liver damage
Legumes, such as peas, beans and lentils provide protein, fatty acids, fiber, minerals hormones, B vitamins and stimulate bite flow	Coconut water flushes out the liver due to the anti-microbial properties of lauric acid

Fig. 10.40: Healthy liver diet.

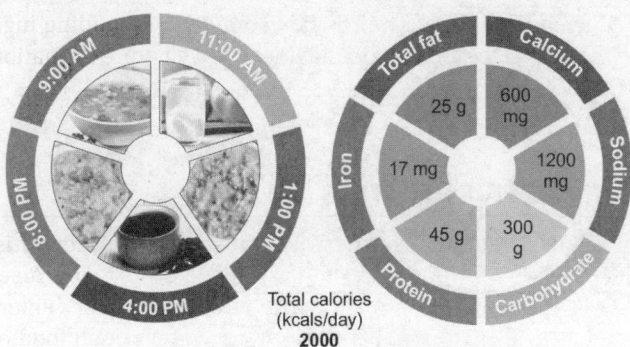

Fig. 10.41: Jaundice diet chart.

Fats: During hepatic precoma and coma due to severe liver failure, fats are not metabolized by the liver and so fat is restricted, in severe jaundice 30 g and in moderate jaundice 50–60 g. A high protein, high carbohydrate, moderate fat diet is recommended. Small attractive meals at regular intervals are better tolerated.

Carbohydrates: High carbohydrate content in the diet is essential to supply enough calories so that tissue proteins are not broken down for energy.

Vitamins: They are essential to regenerate liver cells—500 mg of vitamin C along with 10 mg vitamin K and supplements of vitamin B.

Minerals: Oral feeds of fruit juice, vegetable and meat soups with added salt, given orally or through a nasogastric tube help in maintaining the electrolyte balance.

Food to be included: Cereal porridge, soft chapattis, bread, rice, skimmed milk, tapioca, potato, yam, fruit, fruit juices, sugar, jaggery, honey, biscuits, soft custards without butter cream and non-stimulant beverages.

Foods to be avoided: Pulses, beans, meat, fish, chicken, egg, soups, sweet preparations where ghee, butter or oil are used, bakery products, dried fruits, nuts, spices, papads, chutney, alcoholic beverages, fried preparations, whole milk creams.

CIRRHOSIS OF LIVER

Cirrhosis is a condition in which there is destruction of the liver cell due to necrosis, fatty infiltration and fibrosis. The cirrhotic process may commence many years before it becomes clinically obvious and usually the patient when first seen is at a very late stage with complications, such as ascites, ruptured esophageal varices or hepatic coma. Almost 85–90% of liver damage also does not produce symptoms. The initial change in cirrhosis is wide spread liver cell necrosis due to viral hepatic, alcohol, etc.

Causes

- Viral infection by hepatitis A and B viruses
- Alcohol
- Nutrition mainU 1t 10h 1
- Toxins of food, aflatoxin, Bush tea.

Symptoms: The onset of cirrhosis may be gradual with gastrointestinal disturbances, such as anorexia, nausea, vomiting, pain and distension. As the disease progresses jaundice and other serious changes occur.

Ascites is the accumulation of abnormal amounts of fluids in the abdomen.

Principles of Diet

A high calorie, high protein, high carbohydrate, moderate or restricted fat, high vitamin diet helps in regeneration of liver and helps to prevent the formation of ascites.

Low fat with supplements of fat soluble vitamin and minerals should be given. Sodium should be restricted only when there is ascites. When there is danger of esophageal varices or portal hypertension, fiber should be restricted.

Figure 10.42 is depicted the cirrhosis diet chart.

Figure 10.43 is depicted the eatable and avoidable food in liver cirrhosis condition.

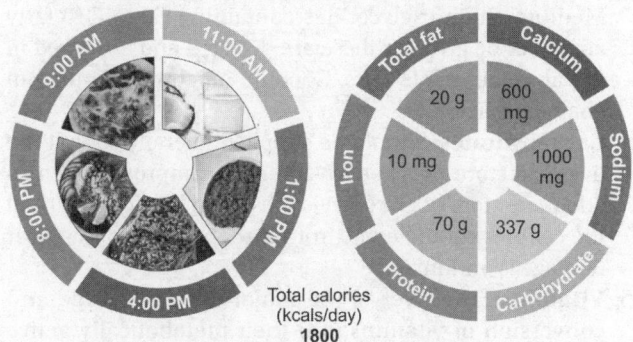

Fig. 10.42: Cirrhosis diet chart.

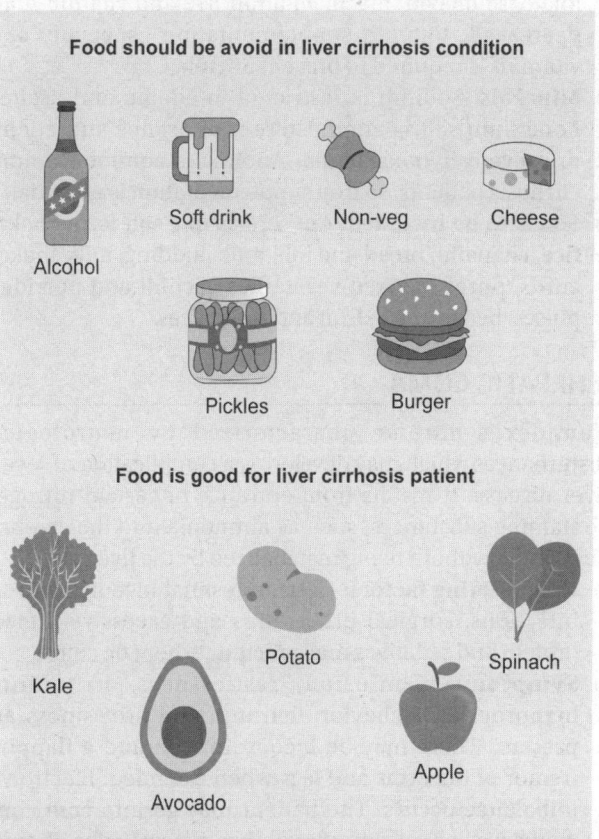

Fig. 10.43: Eatable and avoidable food in liver cirrhosis condition.

Dietary Treatment

- **Energy:** Consumption of food is difficult because of anorexia and ascites. The patients are usually emaciated and require highly nutritious food, i.e., high calorie diet is necessary because of prolonged undernourishment. The calorie requirement should be between 2000–2500 kcal.
- **Proteins:** A high protein diet is helpful for regeneration of the liver. In the absence of hepatic coma a high intake of proteins about 1.2 g/kg of body weight can be given. If the patient is in precoma or coma, proteins should be withheld till the patient tides over the crisis. Vegetable proteins containing more valine are beneficial in preventing encephalopathy.
- **Fats:** About 1 g of fat/kg of body weight is given. Even if fatty changes are present in the liver, fats should be given provided adequate amounts of protein is supplied. Medium chain triglycerides containing C8 to C10 fatty acids can be given as these are digested and absorbed in the absence of bile salts. Coconut oil contains medium chain fatty acids.
- **Carbohydrates:** Should be supplied liberally so that the liver may store glycogen. Liver function improves when an adequate store of glycogen is present in liver cells. 60% of the calories should come from carbohydrate so that liver damage is minimized.
- **Vitamins:** The liver is the major site of storage and conversion of vitamins into their metabolically active form. In cirrhosis, the liver concentration complex of folate, riboflavin, niacin, vitamin B12 and vitamin A are decreased. Vitamin supplementation especially of B vitamins is required to prevent anemia,
- **Minerals:** Sodium is restricted in edema and ascites. Potassium salt is administered for ascites and edema to prevent hypokalaemia. Anemia is common among cirrhosis patients, so iron supplementation is essential.
- **Foods to be included:** Are cereals in a soft form cooked rice, chapathi, bread and idli, milk pudding, milk shakes, curds, puree, cooked vegetables, kichidi and porridge, pulses, beans, meat, fruit and fruit juices.

HEPATIC COMA

Complex syndrome characterized by neurological disturbances which may develop as a complication of severe liver disease. It results from entrance of certain nitrogen containing substances, such as ammonia into the cerebral circulation without being metabolized by the liver.

- **Precipitating factors:** Gastromtestinal bleeding, severe infections, surgical procedures and excessive dietary protein and sedatives may precipitate hepatic coma.
- **Symptoms:** Confusion, restlessness, irritability, inappropriate behavior, delirium and drowsiness are present. There may be incoordination and a flapping tremor of the arms and legs when extended. Electrolyte imbalance occurs. The patient may go into coma and may have convulsions. Breath has a faceal odor. Prompt treatment is imperative or death occurs.

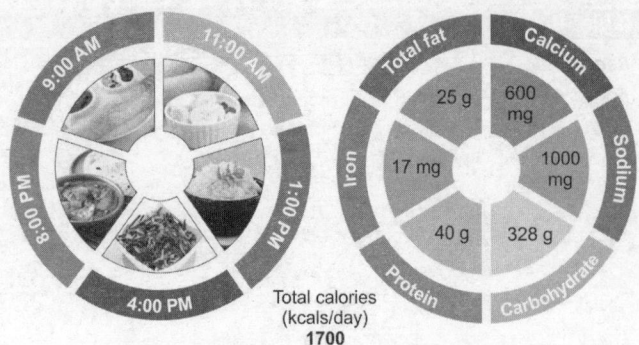

Fig. 10.44: Hepatic encephalopathy diet chart.

Figure 10.44 is depicted the hepatic encephalopathy diet chart.

Treatment

- Dietary protein restriction.
- Cleansing of the bowel with enemas or laxative to reduce the nitrogenous load or antibiotics to suppress bacterial growth.
- Administration of lactulose to increase motility. This is a synthetic disaccharide containing galactose and fructose, which is metabolized by colonic bacteria to acetic, and lactic acids and which lowers the pH of the colon, thereby favoring diffusion of ammonia from blood to the colon.
- Oral or intravenous administration of branched-chain amino acids or their keto analogs improve both the plasma amino acid pattern and the encephalopathy. Branched chain amino acids are believed to decrease the transport of aromatic amino acids into the brain and also serve as an energy in muscle, thereby lessening efflux of amino acids into the circulation.

Table 10.2 is depicted the diet in hepatic coma.

Dietary modifications: Low protein diet should be given. At the same time, catabolism of tissue proteins must be avoided.

Energy: About 1500 to 2000 kcals are needed to prevent breakdown of tissue proteins for energy and are provided chiefly in the form of carbohydrates and fats. Although anorexia may occur attempts should be made to keep the calorie intake as high as is practical to minimize tissue breakdown.

Protein: First 2 or 3 days protein is completely omitted or 20–30 g/day are given. As the patient improves the protein intake is gradually increased to 1 g/kg of body weight. Nitrogen balance can be achieved on protein intake as low as 35 g/day, if high quality protein is used and calorie intake is adequate.

Dietary Management

- These patients pose problems in feeding because of anorexia and behavioral patterns ranging from apathy, and drowsiness and hyper excitability.
- The protein free diet consisting of commercial sugar, fat emulsions, a butter sugar mixture or glucose in beverages

Table 10.2: Diet in hepatic coma.

	Regular diet		Vegetarian diet		Vegan diet
Breakfast	• 1 cup oatmeal with 1 tsp brown sugar and 1 tbsp chopped walnuts • 1 cup milk • 1 hard boiled egg • 1 Banana	Breakfast	• 1 cup oatmeal with 1 tsp brown sugar and 1 tbsp chopped walnuts • 1 cup milk • 1 hard boiled egg • 1 Banana	Breakfast	• 1 cup oatmeal with 1 tsp brown sugar and 1 tbsp chopped walnuts • 1 cup soy milk • 1 oz scrambled tofu • 1 Banana
	570 calories, 25 g protein		570 calories, 25 g protein		557 calories, 22 g protein
AM snack	Oral nutrition Supplement/beverage	AM snack	High protein Supplement/beverage	AM snack	Vegan high protein supplement/beverage
	350 calories 13 g protein		350 calories 13 g protein		222 calories, 16 g protein
Lunch	Whole wheat sandwich made with 2 slices of bread, 2 or low sodium turkey, 1 slice cheese, 2 tsp mayonnaise, lettuce, tomato 1 cup low sodium chicken noodle soup 10 saltine crackers, unsalted	Lunch	Whole wheat sandwich made with 2 slices of bread, 2 Tbsp peanut butter, 1 tbsp grape jelly 1 cup low sodium tomato soup with 1 oz shredded cheese 10 saltine crackers, unsalted	Lunch	Whole wheat sandwich made with 2 slices of bread, 2 tbsp peanut butter, 1 tbsp grape jelly 1 cup low sodium tomato soup 10 saltine crackers, unsalted 1 cup soy milk
	601 calories, 27 g protein		689 calories, 19 g protein		709 calories, 21 g protein
PM snack	1 medium apple, 2 tbsp peanut butter	PM snack	1 medium apple 1 oz almonds	PM snack	1 medium apple 1 oz almonds
	285 calories, 7 g protein		259 calories, 6 g protein		259 calories, 6 g protein
Dinner	3 oz grilled chicken breast 1 medium baked sweet potato with 2 tsp margarine 1 cup steamed broccoli 1 cup 2% milk	Dinner	Black bean burger patty 1 medium baked sweet potato with 2 tsp margarine 1 cup steamed broccoli	Dinner	Black bean burger patty 1 medium baked sweet potato with 2 tsp margarine 1 cup steamed broccoli
	468 calories 35 g protein		491 calories, 31 g protein		491 calories, 31 g protein
Night time snack	1/2 cup vanilla yogurt 1 cup fruit cocktail	Night time snack	6 oz yogurt 1 cup fruit cocktail	Night time snack	6 oz soy yogurt 1 cup fruit cocktail
	333 calories 5 g protein		333 calories 5 g protein		395 calories 6 g protein
Totals	2607 calories, 112 g protein	Totals	2692 calories, 99 g protein	Totals	2633 calories, 102 g protein

or fruit juices may be used initially through oral or tube feeding.

❑ With improvements, the diets providing 20, 40 and 60 g protein may be gradually introduced.

CHOLELITHIASIS

The function of the gallbladder and bile ducts is to concentrate, store and deliver bile into the duodenum at appropriate times to assist digestion—hormonal and nervous factors play a part in this process. The stimulus for this activity is the entry of food into the small intestine. This causes the mucosa of the duodenum and jejunum to secrete a hormone, cholecystokinin, which is carried in the blood to the gallbladder and causes it to contract. Fats and foods rich in fats are especially effective for this purpose.

❑ The bile is concentrated in the gallbladder and when it is super saturated gallstones are likely to form.
❑ Super saturation arises when there is insufficient amount of solubilizing agents, such as bile acids and to a lesser extent lecithin to keep cholesterol and bile pigments in solution.
❑ By far the most common gallstones are mixed stones composed of cholesterol, bile pigment and various calcium salts including calcium palmitate.
❑ Gallstones are more common in women than in men. Advanced age, repeated pregnancies and sedentary life and use of oral contraceptives are the contributing factors.
❑ In man, it has been suggested that high cholesterol diets, lack of dietary fibre and an insufficiency of polyunsaturated fats predispose to gallstones.

Energy: Excess calorie intake appears to be a risk for development of gallbladders disease. The disease is more common in obese persons.

Fat: The patient receives no food initially during attacks of cholecystitis.

Progression to a 20 to 30 g fat diet is made. If this is tolerated the fat can then be increased to 50 to 60 g per day.

Figure 10.45 is depicted the gallbladder stones diet chart.

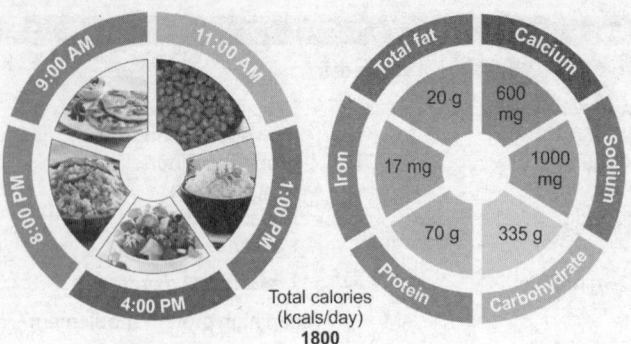

Fig. 10.45: Gallbladder stones diet chart.

■ DIETARY RESTRICTION FOR LIVER DISEASES

Beyond the maintenance of a good, well-balanced diet, several conditions that develop in the later stages of cirrhosis require specific dietary management.

Hepatic Encephalopathy

- Hepatic encephalopathy is a condition of impaired mental function due to altered liver function. It is often seen when scar tissue formation (cirrhosis) in the liver prevents the normal flow of blood through the liver.
- The blood which contains toxins is "shunted" or redirected, back to the central circulation and into the brain without first going through the liver for detoxification.
- Cirrhosis with portal hypertension (an elevation of the portal pressure due to the obstruction of blood flow through the liver) may be treated surgically by shunting some of the blood around the liver, connecting the portal system with the systematic circulation.
- This "shunted" blood contains high concentrations of amino acids and ammonia and probably other, as yet unidentified, toxic substances that may cause altered mental function in some patients.
- The treatment for hepatic encephalopathy is aimed at reducing toxins that cause this disorder. Just as patients with cirrhosis who have protein intolerance must restrict protein intake, so must patients with hepatic encephalopathy reduce the amount of protein in their diet.
- Severe protein restriction (to 20 g a day or less) is impractical for long term therapy.
- Most physicians will encourage their patients to take approximately 40 g of protein a day and will prescribe lactulose and neomycin to decrease the production of ammonia in the intestines.
- Certain specific amino acids (hepatamine) may be less likely to cause hepatic encephalopathy and have even been suggested as therapy.
- Certain foods (vegetables, milk) contain protein, rich in these amino acids and are preferred to meat as a source of protein in affected patients.
- A dietary supplement rich in these amino acids (hepatic-aid) is available and is in use in many liver centers.

Ascites and Edema

- Ascites is the accumulation of fluid in the abdominal cavity. Edema is fluid built up in the tissues, usually the feet, legs or back. Both conditions result from abnormal accumulation of sodium associated with portal hypertension and liver disease. Most affected patients will not require strict fluid restriction.
- Sodium intake is often restricted for patients with cirrhosis to avoid retention of fluids in the body. Such a diet would allow only 2–4 g of sodium and would exclude canned soups and vegetables, cold cut meats, condiments, such as mayonnaise and ketchup, dairy products, cheese and ice cream.
- Most fresh foods are low in sodium. The best salt substitute is lemon juice (which is salt free).

Cholestasis

- Cholestasis is an inability of the liver to excrete bile. This may result in steatorrhea (fat malabsorption due to inadequate amounts of bile which dissolve fat in the intestines).
- Steatorrhea may go unnoticed by the patient or can be associated with weight loss due to lost calories. Stools may be foul smelling and float.
- Fat supplements are available; the most commonly used being medium chain triglycerides (MCT oil) and safflower oil which are absorbable with less dependence upon bile.
- They may be used as a caloric supplement. MCT oil is used like any other cooking oil, in salad dressings or in cooking.
- Patients with steatorrhea may also have difficulty absorbing fat soluble vitamins. However, water soluble vitamins are absorbed normally.
- Supplementing the diet with fat soluble vitamins is possible, though it should only be carried out under the guidance of a physician.

Wilson Disease

- There is a defect in copper metabolism. Patients affected by this disorder have an abnormal build-up of copper in the body due to the inability of the liver to excrete it.
- This inability allows the copper to accumulate in several organs: first the liver and then, usually the brain and the cornea of the eye.
- Treatment involves the use of a de-coppering agent, penicillamine, which removes the excess copper from the body.
- Dietary therapy for this disease includes the avoidance of copper-containing foods, such as chocolate, nuts, shellfish and mushrooms.

Hemochromatosis

- It is a disease in which there is an inappropriate absorption of iron from the intestine.
- The excessive iron then accumulates in the liver, pancreas and other organs in the body. Patients with this disease should not be given iron supplements.

- Aside from this precaution, those with hemochromatosis may follow a normal diet. Treatment is achieved by frequent removal of blood from a large vein.

Fatty Liver
- It is related to alcohol, obesity, starvation, some drugs and other factors. It is not caused by eating fat and it should be treated with a well-balanced diet or the removal of the responsible chemical substance or drug.
- Finally, patients with liver disease should be wary of supplements to the diet, particularly fad foods or packaged "nutritional" aids.
- Such foods can contain a lot of salt, potassium or inappropriate protein mixtures. Those that are safe should be taken only under a physician's guidance.

DIET FOR METABOLIC DISORDERS

Hyperthyroidism
Hyperthyroidism is a disturbance in which there is an excessive secretion of the thyroid gland with a consequent increase in the metabolic rate. It is believed to be an autoimmune disease occurring in genetically predisposed persons.

Figure 10.46 is depicted the hyperthyroidism diet chart.
- The disease is also known as exophthalmic goiter, thyrotoxicosis, Graves disease, or Basedow's disease.
- The chief symptoms are weight loss, sometimes to the point of emaciation, excessive nervousness, prominence of the eyes and a generally enlarged thyroid gland. Increased appetite, weakness, and signs of cardiac failure are also present.
- The increased level of energy metabolism increases the requirement of B vitamins.
- The excretion of calcium and phosphorus is greatly increased in hyperthyroidism. 125 g protein.
- Frequent feedings will help satisfy hunger. A liberal calcium intake is desirable and may be provided in addition to the liberal use of milk.

Hypothyroidism
Decreased production or activity of the thyroid hormone or hypothyroidism is a relatively common problem.
- Obesity is a problem for some patients with hypothyroidism, since they may continue in their earlier patterns of eating even though the energy metabolism has been significantly reduced.
- In other patients, the appetite may be so poor that under nutrition results. For overweight persons, reduction of calories is necessary.
- Reduction of dietary cholesterol may be indicated. Adequate fluids and foods high in dietary fiber are needed to overcome constipation.

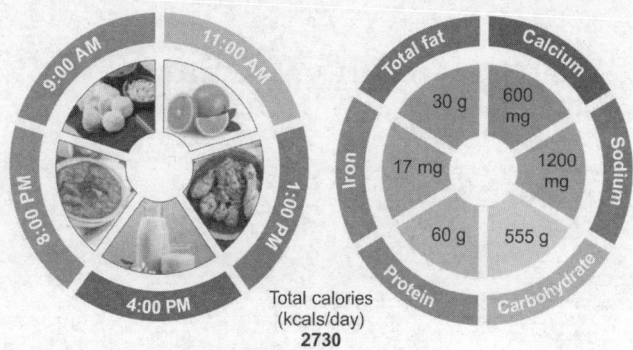

Fig. 10.47: Thyroid diet chart.

Figure 10.47 is depicted the thyroid diet chart.

Rheumatoid Arthritis
Rheumatoid arthritis is a highly inflammatory and very painful condition having its onset in young women. This is characterized by fatigue, pain, stiffness, deformity which may be severe and limited function.

Figure 10.48 is depicted the rheumatoid diet chart.

Dietary Counseling
- Arthritic patients require the same amount of calories as other persons need.
- Obesity is a common problem in osteoarthritis. Weight loss should be brought about in order to bring down the added stress on weight bearing joints.
- Many patients with rheumatoid arthritis have lost weight and are in poor nutritional status. A high calorie high protein diet is given.

GOUT

Gout, an inherited disease more often occurring in men, is due to abnormal uric acid metabolism. About five percent of

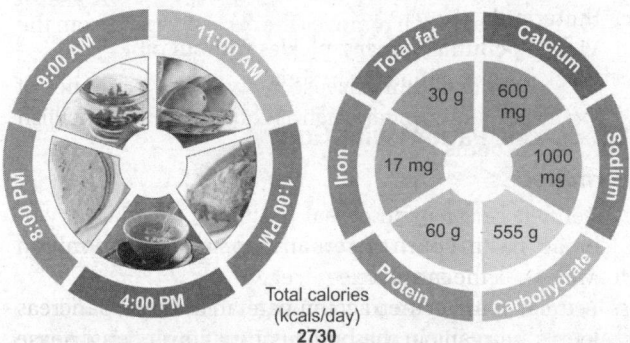

Fig. 10.46: Hyperthyroidism diet chart.

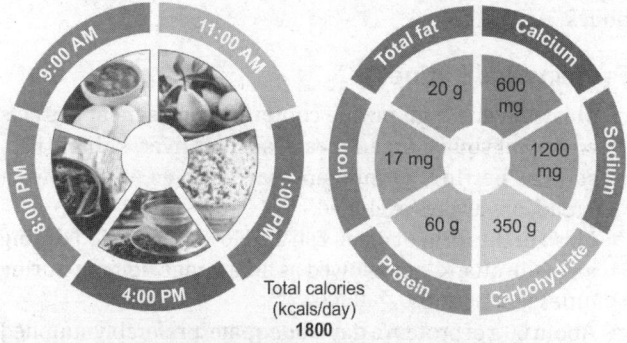

Fig. 10.48: Rheumatoid diet chart.

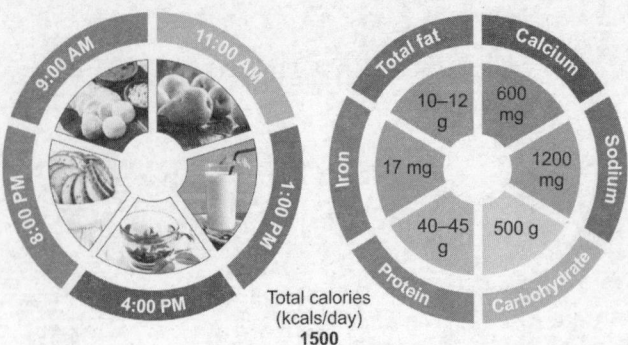

Fig. 10.49: Uric acid diet chart.

patients with gout are women; about 80% of them are post-menopausal at the time of onset.
- Excretion of the uric acid precursors- hypoxanthine and xanthine by the kidneys is reduced.
- The disturbance of purine metabolism is of similar magnitude in women as in men. Serum uric acid is raised, with deposition of urate (uric acid salt) in the cartilages and articular cartilages of the joints.
- There are recurrent attacks of pain and swelling of the joints, frequently of the metatarsophalangeal joint of the big toe, though other joints may also be affected. Joints vulnerable to injury are most liable to be involved.

Figure 10.49 is depicted the uric acid diet chart.

Dietary Management
- The dietetic treatment of gout has undergone a great deal of reorientation due to changing concepts of the disease.
- High-purine diet alone used to be implicated at one time. The knowledge that uric acid can be synthesized from endogenous sources, and that in some patients an abnormality of excretion of uric acid exists, has focused attention on the role of heredity. However, in a susceptible person, an attack of gout can be precipitated by purine-rich foods.

Principles of diet: A low-purine, low-protein, easy digestible diet with a liberal fluid intake is advised.

Calories: Obese persons may be more prone to gout. The body weight should be reduced to normal, not only to prevent recurrence of gout, but also to prevent changes in the weight-bearing joints that occur in the obese. A heavy meal supplying high calories should be avoided, as it tends to precipitate an attack.

Proteins and Purines
- Meats having high purine content, such as meat extracts and meat soups, organ meats, such as liver, kidney, fish, such as herring, salmon and sardines, as well as sweet bread, are always excluded.
- Flesh in the form of meat, fish and fowl is excluded during an acute attack, but allowed as an average helping during quiescent periods.
- About 60 g of protein a day is adequate, preferably supplied as vegetable or milk proteins.

Fats: Fat consumption is restricted, partly because its ingestion tends to cause retention of urates by the kidney, and partly to prevent obesity.

Carbohydrates: During an attack of gout, the main source of calories should be carbohydrate, because of its 'protein-sparing effect', which reduces endogenous protein breakdown.

Fluids: Liberal intake of fluid should be advised to ensure a daily excretion of about 2000 mL of urine.

Beverages: Tea and coffee contain methyl purines, which are not converted by the body into uric acid. About two or three cups a day are permitted.

Alcohol: There appears to be individual susceptibility to an attack of gout after ingestion of alcohol. Stopping alcohol may prevent attack of gout in such people. Otherwise, patients with gout usually tolerate a couple of ounces of white wine or whisky, but not beer, stout, or red wines.

Foods to be Avoided
- **Organ meat:** Liver, heart, kidney, brain
- Fatty meats, also sausages, bacon, salami, fatty beef, pork
- Shell fish, lobsters, oysters, shrimps, prawns, crabs
- Egg yolk
- Sauces containing egg yolk, also puddings containing egg custards
- Chocolate, cake, pastries, ice-cream, honey, sugar, jam, jelly, jaggery
- Cream, butter, ghee, fish liver oil, lards
- Concentrated milk preparations, khoa, sweets, etc.
- Alcoholic drinks and sweet soft drinks
- Nuts and dry fruits
- **Root vegetables:** potato, yam, colacassia, beetroot (limited quantities permitted)
- **Fruits:** mangoes, bananas, sapota, seetaphal. (Limited quantities permitted)

Free Foods
- Green leafy vegetables
- Tomato
- Cucumber
- Radish
- All gourds (e.g., ridge gourd, bitter gourd, etc.)
- Lime
- Clear soups
- Buttermilk
- Vinegar, chutney, spices, pickles without oil
- Black tea and coffee, plain soda.

Foods for a Patient with Gout
Permitted
- Refined cereals and cereal products; cornflakes, white bread, pasta, flour, arrowroot, sago, tapioca and cakes.
- Milk, milk foods and cheese, eggs.
- Lettuce, tomatoes and green vegetables (except all beans, lentils, peas, spinach, asparagus, cauliflower, mushrooms).
- Vegetables and cream soups made from vegetables.

Excluded: The following foods contain purine and are best avoided during an acute attack:

- Sugar and sweets, gelatin.
- Butter, polyunsaturated margarine, and fats of any kind.
- Fruit, nuts, peanut butter.
- Beverages—fruit juice, cordials, carbonated drinks, tea, coffee and cocoa may be taken if uric acid in the urine is to be measured by uricase method.
- Beans, peas, lentils, spinach, oatmeal, asparagus, cauliflower, mushrooms.
- Fish, sea food, sardines, herrings, anchovies.
- Meats, poultry or other flesh, meat extract, gravies, marmite.
- Liver, kidney, heart, sweet bread, brains.
- Yeast and beer products, beer, alcohol.

DIET THERAPY FOR URINARY DISORDERS

Glomerulonephritis

It is an inflammatory process affecting the glomeruli, the small blood vessels in the head of the nephron, most common in its acute form in children 3 to 10 years of age.

Symptoms: Hematuria, proteinuria, edema, shortness of breath, tachycardia and elevated BP anorexia. There may be oliguria or anuria.

Principles of the Diet

Fluids: The fluid intake will be adjusted to output including losses in vomiting or diarrhea. Daily fluid replacement should be 1000 mL plus daily amount excreted in the urine.

Insensible water loss is:
- 30 mL/kg body weight for infants
- 20 mL/kg body weight for older children
- 10 mL/kg body weight for adults.

Energy: Sufficient calories are given without increasing the protein intake by means of sugar, honey, glucose.

Figure 10.50 is depicted the renal diet chart.

Protein: Usually the diet contains 0.5 g of protein/kg body weight for older children and 1 to 1.5 g/kg per day for younger children. A low protein diet is recommended so as to give rest to the kidney. An intake of 20–40 g/day is considered sufficient. Out of the recommended protein 50 should be from animal protein.

Sodium: The restriction of sodium varies with the degree of oliguria and hypertension. If renal function is impaired the sodium will be restricted to 500 to 1000 mg/day. If edema is present, Na is restricted.

Potassium: When the kidneys do not work properly, potassium builds up in the body and causes heart to beat uneven and stop suddenly.

Phosphorus: Eating foods high in phosphorus will raise the phosphorus in the blood and this can cause Ca to be pulled from the bones. This will make bones weak and cause them to break easily.

NEPHROSIS (DEGENERATIVE BRIGHT'S DISEASE)

- **Symptoms:** Heavy proteinuria, hypoalbuminemia and peripheral edema.
- **Principles of diet:** High protein, high calorie, high carbohydrate, salt restricted moderate fat with restricted fluid are recommended. Vitamin supplements especially vitamin C are given.
- **Dietary treatment:** To ensure protein use for tissues synthesis, sufficient kcals must always be provided. About 200 kcals is suggested. About 100 to 120 g of protein should be provided. A high protein diet is required to meet the heavy loss of albumin and protein depletion of the tissues.

Sodium is restricted to prevent accumulation of edema fluid and prevent hypertension.

Special Instructions

- Since Ca and K deficiency may accompany severe proteinuria, bone refraction and hypokalemia are common and hence.
- The diet has to be soft.
- Low quality proteins, such as pulses should be mixed with cereals or milk to improve quality of protein, high quantity proteins like egg, meat are preferred.
- Vitamin supplements especially vitamin C are essential.

ACUTE RENAL FAILURE

There is a sudden shutdown of renal function following metabolic or traumatic injury to normal kidneys.

Symptoms: Anuria or oliguria-low urine volume, i.e., 20 to 200 mL/day.

Accumulation of waste products of protein metabolism in blood, excretion of K is diminished. There is also increased phosphate and sulphate with decreased Na, Ca and base bicarbonate. Lethargic, anorexia, nausea, vomiting, blood pressure, uremia.

Figure 10.51 is depicted the kidney failure diet chart.

Dietary Management

- **Energy:** A minimum of 600–100 kcal is necessary. A high calorie intake is desired mainly form carbohydrate and fats.

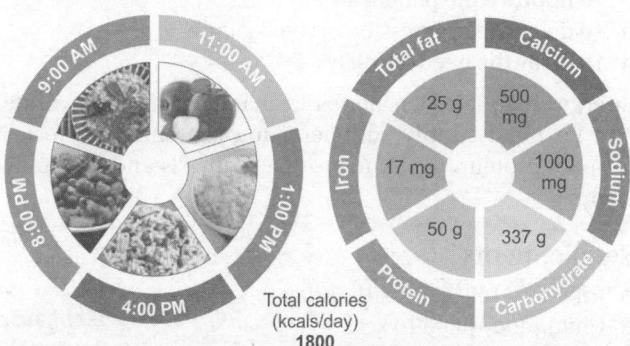

Fig. 10.50: Renal diet chart.

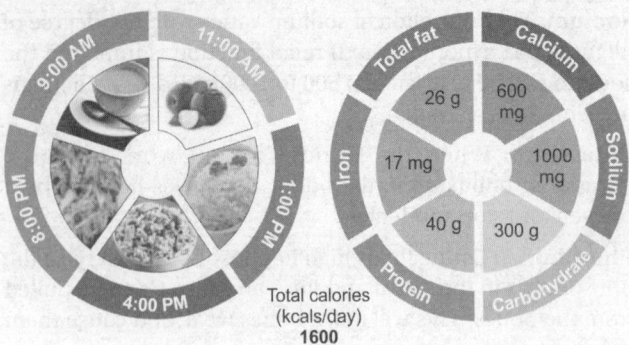

Fig. 10.51: Kidney failure diet chart.

- **Protein:** All foods containing protein is stopped if the patient is under conservative treatment and blood urea nitrogen is rising. However, 40 g is allowed when he is on hemodialysis or peritoneal dialysis.
- **Carbohydrates:** A minimum of 100 g/day is essential to minimize tissue protein breakdown.
- **Fluids:** The total fluid permitted is 500 mL + losses through urine and gastrointestinal tract with visible perspiration an additional 500 mL may be necessary.
- **Sodium:** Na loss through urine is measured and replaced. Na restriction is also judged based on Na loss in the urine.
- **Potassium:** Hyperkalemia occurs with a daily se of 0.7 mEq, Serum potassium. It has deleterious effects on heart,

CHRONIC RENAL FAILURE

It is also known as uremia as the level of urea in blood is very high when 90% if function renal tissue is destroyed, uremia occurs. It may be the end result of acute glomerulonephritis, pyelonephritis and nephritic syndrome.

Figure 10.52 is depicted the kidney (renal) failure basics for non-specialists.

Causes

- Progression of acute nephritis or nephrotic syndrome.
- Chronic infection of the urinary tract.
- Kidney stones.
- High blood pressure.
- Exposure to toxic substances.

Once chronic renal failure occurs, the normal functions of the kidneys, such as regulation of body fluids, electrolytes, pH and excretion of metabolites are disrupted.

Symptoms: In chronic renal failure, symptoms appear when the glomerular filtration rate (GFR) is inadequate to excrete nitrogenous wastes. When the GFR is less than 10 mL per minute (normal: 120 mL per minute) and the blood urea nitrogen (BUN) is more than 90 mg/dL (normal—8–18 mg/dL), dietary modification brings about improvement. As GFR falls, daily protein intake is restricted.

- The symptoms of the gastrointestinal tract are nausea or vomiting. The breath has an ammoniacal odor. Ulcerations of the mouth and hiccups interfere with food intake.
- The nervous system—patients are drowsy, irritable and sink to coma.

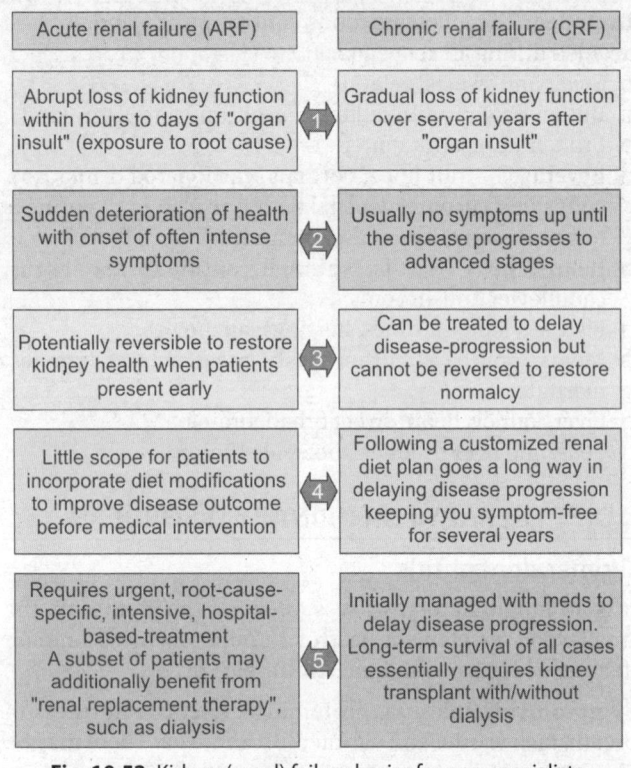

Fig. 10.52: Kidney (renal) failure basics for non-specialists.

- If there is hypertension—headache, dizziness, muscular twitching and failing vision occur.
- The functioning of the heart is seriously disturbed.
- Death results when hyperkalemia (elevated serum potassium) blocks the contraction of the heart.
- Dehydration, sodium depletion, high serum potassium, acidosis and increased susceptibility to infection are the most general manifestations.

Dietary Management

Diet should be palatable, must have varieties, adjusted according to altered biochemistry and physiology (hyperphosphatemia and hypertension) adequate enough for growth in children.

The objectives of treatment are:
- To maintain optimal nutritional status
- To minimize uremic toxicity
- To prevent protein catabolism
- To improve the patient's well-being
- To delay the progression of renal failure
- To delay the need for dialysis

Energy: Adequate kilocalories are mandatory. Carbohydrate and fat must supply sufficient non-protein kilocalories to spare protein for tissue protein synthesis and to supply energy.

Requirements

- Infancy—100–120 kcal/kg/day
- Childhood—80–110 kcal
- Adults—35–50 kcal

Protein: Failing kidney need to be given rest. Protein intake can be reduced to 0.5 g/kg of body weight per day.

Fluid: The usual fluid permitted is volume of daily urine plus 500 mL.

Sodium: 1 to 2 mmol/kg of body weight for infants. About 40–60 mmol/day for older children. Strict restriction is necessary only if hypertension and edema are present.

Potassium: This has to be restricted to 1 mmol/kg of body weight. Double boiling and draining excess water reduces potassium content.

UROLITHIASIS OR URINARY CALCULI

Urinary calculi (kidney stones) may be found in the kidney, ureter, bladder or urethra. About 90% of all renal stones contain calcium. The occurrence of kidney stones may be due to an outcome of different nutritional status, dietary habits and environmental factors, such as temperature and humidity.

In warm climates, the urine volume is low and concentrated with urates, oxalates and calcium salts. Frequent urinary tract infection may contribute to the formation of stones. In India, the most common type of calculi is calcium oxalate.

The diet should be low in oxalic acid and purine. Intake of calcium and phosphates should be reduced. Large amounts of fluid should be taken to increase urine output. A dilute urine prevents the formation of stones. Foods rich in calcium, phosphates. When stones are composed of calcium, magnesium, phosphates and carbonates the urine is alkaline and acid-ash diet is used. The acid-ash diet should maintain the urine pH between 4.5 and 5 and with an alkaline-ash diet, a urinary pH of 7.6—8 is maintained.

Figure 10.53 is depicted the kidney stones diet chart.

Causes

- **Climate:** In warm climate the urine volume is low.
- **Occupation:** People working under the sun and perspire a lot and pass concentrated urine.
- **Infection of urinary tract:** Frequent infection of urinary tract may be contributory in that pus cells and epithelial cells may form a focus around which the stone may be formed.
- **Dietary habits:** Foods rich in oxalates, calcium, purines and phosphate may predispose to formation of renal calculi.
- **Heredity.**
- **Vitamin A and B complex deficiency.**
- **Hyperthyroidism.**

Types of Calculi

1. Calcium phosphate
2. Calcium oxalate—mostly found in India
3. Uric acid
4. Magnesium ammonium phosphate.

Dietary Management

- **Planning acid-ash diet**
  - A liberal fluid intake
  - Salt in moderation
  - The fruits and vegetables so selected should not contribute more than 25 mL of base daily.
- **Planning alkaline:** Ash diet if stones of uric acid or cystine type occur, the diet should give alkaline ash, alkaline producing foods, such as fruits, vegetables and milk while acid producing foods use meat, eggs and cereals are restricted.
- **Planning low oxalate diets:** An acid or alkaline reaction of the diet is of little value for oxalate urolithiasis. Sources of oxalates should be omitted which include beans, beet greens, chocolate, cocoa, dried figs, plums, potatoes, spinach, tea and tomatoes.

Fluid: About 0.2 to 2.5 liters should be given. Water coconut and barley water, fruits

Table 10.3 is depicted the types of acid and alkali producing foods.

Acid producing foods	Alkali producing foods	Neutral foods
Bread, especially whole wheat	Milk	Butter
Cereals	Fruits	Coffee
Cheese	Vegetables	Tea
Corn	Almonds	Fats
Eggs	Dried apricots	Sugar
Lentils	Beans	Tapioca
Macaroni, spaghetti	Beet greens	
Noodles	Dates	
Meat, fish and poultry	Figs	
Peanuts	Dried peas	
Rice	Raisins	
Walnuts	• Spinach • Foods prepared with baking powder or baking soda	

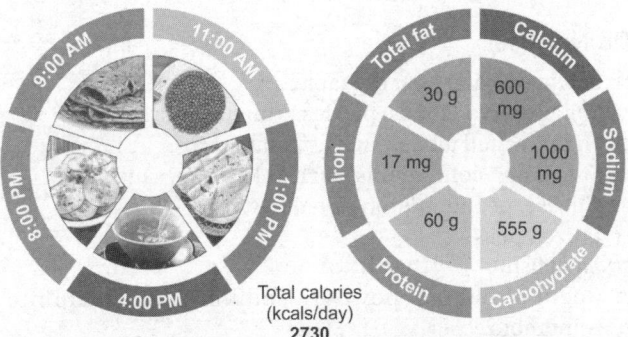

Fig. 10.53: Kidney stones diet chart.

DIET THERAPY FOR CARDIOVASCULAR DISORDERS

Cardiovascular diseases are characterized by a thickening of the arterial valves and their loss of elasticity.

Types

- **Atherosclerosis:** It is a degenerative disease of the arteries and consists of focal accumulation in the intimal lining of arteries of a variable combination of lipids, complex carbohydrates blood and blood products, fibrous tissue and Ca deposits.
- **Coronary heart disease:** It is syndrome arising from failure of the coronary arteries to supply sufficient blood to the myocardium. Also known as IHD (Ischemic Heart Diseases).
- **Myocardial infarction:** Necrosis or destruction of part of the heart muscle due to failure of blood supply and may lead to sudden death.
- **Angina pectoris:** Pain in the chest, exercise or excitement provokes severe chest pain and so limits patient's physical activities.

Dietary Management

Objectives

- Maximum rest for the heart
- Prevention or elimination of edema
- Maintenance of good nutrition
- Acceptability of the program

Principles of Diet

Low calories, low fat particularly low saturated fat, low cholesterol, high in PUFA (polyunsaturated fatty acids), low carbohydrate and normal protein, minerals and vitamins, high fiber diet is also recommended.

- **Energy:** Usually a 1000 to 1200 calorie diet is suitable for an obese patient in bed. Those patients with desirable level are permitted a maintenance level of calories during convalescence and their return to activity.
- **Fat:** The first step involves restriction of fats to no more than 30% of the total calories consumed. Levels as low as 20% are tolerated without side effects.

Total fat 30% met by saturated 10% monounsaturated vegetable oil.

Normal Allowances

- **Duration of meal:** 3 or 4 smaller meals are suggested instead of two big meals. The evening meals must be two hours before retiring to bed.
- **Sodium:** It is restricted when there is hypertension.
- **Fluid:** The restriction of fluid is not required as long as Na is not restricted.
- **High fiber diet:** Increasing fiber will serve to reduce cholesterol.

HYPERTENSION

Elevation of the blood pressure above normal is a symptom which accompanies many cardiovascular and renal diseases. High BP of unknown cause is known as essential hypertension.

Causes: Cardiovascular diseases, renal diseases, tumors of the brain or adrenal glands, hyperthyroidism or diseases of ovaries and pituitary may cause hypertension.

Types
1. **Mild hypertension:** Diastolic pressure is 90 to 104 mm Hg.
2. **Moderate hypertension:** Diastolic pressure is 105 to 119 mm Hg.
3. **Severe hypertension:** Diastolic pressure is 120 to 130 mm Hg.

Symptoms: Headache, dizziness, impaired vision, failing memory, shortness of breath, pain over the heart and gastrointestinal disturbance, unexplained tiredness.

Principles of diet: Low calorie, low fat, low sodium diet with normal protein intake is prescribed.

Energy: Obese patient must be reduced to normal body weight with low calorie diet.

Protein: A diet of 50 g protein is necessary to maintain proper nutrition.

Fats: About 40 g fat, partly as vegetable oil is permitted.

Sodium: Restrictions for moderate low sodium diet (1000 mg).

Sodium restricted diets:

The normal diet contains about 3 to 6 g of sodium daily. The normal diet is modified for its sodium content.

- **Extreme sodium restriction** (200 to 300 mg/day). No salt is used in cooking. Low sodium foods are selected. This diet is used in cirrhosis of the liver with ascites and congestive heart failure.
- **Severe sodium restriction** (500 to 700 mg/day). No salt is used in cooking. Careful selection of foods is necessary. This level is used for severe congestive heart failure.
- **Moderate restriction** (1000 to 1500 mg/day). No salt is used in cooking. Low sodium foods are selected. Measured amount of salt is used. This level is suggested for those with a strong family history of hypertension and patients with borderline hypertension.
- **Mild sodium restriction** (2000 to 3000 mg/day). Some salt is used in cooking, but no salty foods are permitted. No salt is used at the table. This level is used as a maintenance diet in cardiac and renal disease.

Do Not Use

- Salt in cooking or at the table.
- Salt preserved foods, pickles, canned foods.
- Highly salted foods, such as potato chips.
- Spices and condiments, such as ketchup, sauce.
- Cheese, peanut butter, salted butter.
- Frozen peas.
- Shell fish.
- Regular baking powder, sodium metabisulphite, Ajinomoto.
- Prepared mixture.

Figure 10.54 is depicted the high blood pressure diet chart.

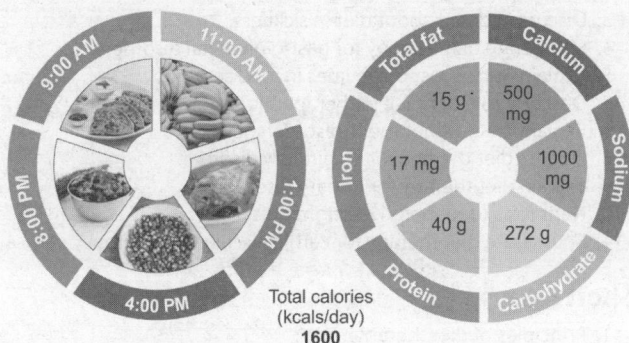

Fig. 10.54: High blood pressure diet chart.

DIET THERAPY FOR RESPIRATORY DISORDER

Tuberculosis

Tuberculosis is an infectious disease caused by the bacillus *Mycobacterium tuberculosis*. It affects the lungs most often but may also be localized in other organs, such as the lymph nodes or kidneys or it may be generalized.

Pulmonary tuberculosis is accompanied by wasting of tissue, exhaustion, cough, expectoration and fever. The acute phase resembles pneumonia with high fever and increased circulation and respiration. As the disease progresses, the patient begins to exhibit loss of appetite, pain in the chest, worsening cough.

Figure 10.55 is depicted the tuberculosis diet chart.
- **Principles of diet:** A high calorie, high protein, high vitaminized and mineralized, high fluid, soft diet is recommended.
- **Energy:** Since the metabolic rate is not as high as in other fevers, satisfactory weight can be maintained with 2500 to 3000 kcals.
- **Protein:** A protein intake somewhat in excess of normal requirements is necessary in tuberculosis. The daily requirement may be from 80 to 120 g.
- **Minerals:** Calcium, especially should be provided liberally, since, it is essential for the healing of tuberculosis lesion. At least 1 liter of milk should be taken daily. The iron needs may also be increased if there has been hemorrhage. Calcium, iron and phosphorus help in regeneration of cells, blood and fluids.
- **Vitamins:** The metabolism of vitamin A is adversely affected in tuberculosis.

Ascorbic acid deficiency is present with slight tuberculosis. Vitamin C is essential for many regenerative purposes.

Dietary Management

- Many patients with tuberculosis have very active peristalsis so that the selection of food should be from those bland in flavor, non-stimulating and easily digested.
- Since patients have poor appetite, food must be appetizing and patients likes and dislikes must be considered.
- During the acute stage, a high calorie fluid and soft diet are prescribed followed by high calorie soft regular diet.
- Initially small quantities of fluid diet should be given once in 3 hours when the fever comes down the interval can be increased to every 4 hours.
- In meeting, the protein requirement, good quality protein, such as eggs should be included.
- Fatty foods, highly fibrous foods, very spicy foods which are hard to digest should be avoided.

ROLE OF NURSE IN THERAPEUTIC DIET

Good nutrition is essential not only to promote health and well-being, but also to aid recovery from trauma, surgery or disease. Yet there is growing evidence that malnutrition is common among hospital patients. Many hospital patients do not receive enough food and in some wards up to 60% do not eat enough calories or protein.

Poor nutritional status is known to be associated with delayed recovery and adverse outcomes of illness and injury. Nurses have an important role to play in the prevention of malnutrition. Primarily, they should identify those at risk of malnutrition and plan for the care to meet their needs. In addition, they have a role in ensuring those who are initially well-nourished do not become malnourished, while in hospital. Appropriate and ongoing assessment is a key factor.

Figure 10.56 is depicted the role of nurse in therapeutic diet.

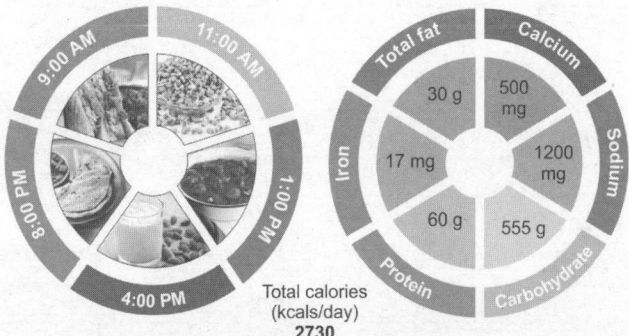

Fig. 10.55: Tuberculosis diet chart.

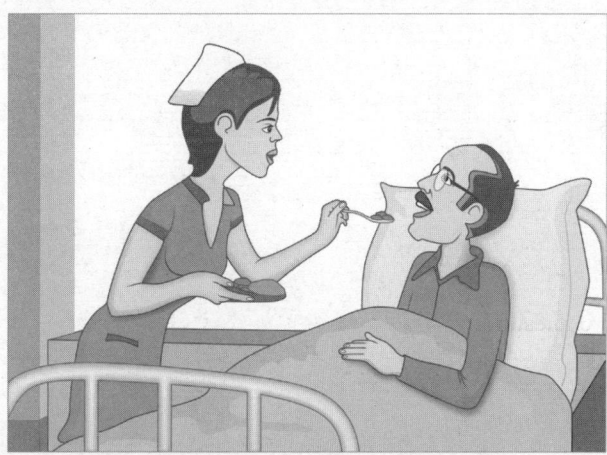

Fig. 10.56: Role of nurse in therapeutic diet.

CONCLUSION

Diet therapy is the treatment of disease. It involves modifying diets in such a way as to meet the requirements created by disease or injury. A diet used as a medical treatment is called a therapeutic diet. If a patient needs a special diet, the physicians prescribe the diet and write the diet order in a medical record. The therapeutic diet is planned by the dietician and usually served and monitored by the nurse. Nurses and other health professionals should consult with the physician when conditions may necessitate a change in diet order.

BIBLIOGRAPHY

1. McDivitt ME, Sumati RM. Human Nutrition—Principles and Applications in India, Revised Edition, Prentice Hall, New Delhi, 1973.
2. Patwardhan VN. Nutrition in India 2nd ed. Indian Journal of Medical Sciences, New Delhi, 1961.
3. Robinson CH, Lawler MR, Wanda LC, Garwick AE. Normal and Therapeutic Nutrition, 17th edition. Macmillan Publishing Co. New York, USA, 1996.
4. Shils MS, Benjamin CA, Catherine R, Robert JC. Modern Nutrition in Health and Disease, 10th edition. Lippincott, Williams & Wilkins, Baltimore, USA, 2005.
5. Swaminathan M. Essentials of Food and Nutrition, Volume I and II, 2nd edition. Ganesh, Madras, India, 1985.
6. Wardlaw GM, Insel PM. Perspectives in Nutrition, 2nd edition. Mosby Year Book Inc, St Louis, USA, 1996.
7. Williams SR. Basic Nutrition and Diet Therapy, 1st edition. Elsevier Science, New York, 1999.

REVIEW QUESTIONS

Long Essays

1. Explain diet as a therapeutic agent.
2. Describe therapeutic diet.
3. Discuss in detail about diet in sickness.
4. Enumerate diet therapy for gastrointestinal disorders.
5. Explain nurses responsibilities in food serving.
6. Describe role of nurse in therapeutic diet.
7. Explain diet for metabolic disorders.
8. Discuss diet therapy for respiratory disorder.
9. Explain diet therapy for urinary disorders.
10. Nephrosis (degenerative bright's disease).
11. Enumerate diet therapy for cardiovascular disorders.

Short Essays

1. Principles of diet therapy.
2. Concept and meaning of diet therapy.
3. Factors to consider in planning therapeutic diets.
4. Regular diet.
5. Postoperative diet.
6. Types of diet used in hospitals.
7. Dumping syndrome.
8. Tube feeding.
9. Diet therapy in fevers.
10. Protein, electrolyte and fluid-modified diets.
11. Fat-modified diets.
12. Lactose intolerance.
13. High-calorie and high-protein diets.
14. Dietary modifications.
15. Dietary restriction for liver diseases.
16. Modification of diet in bleeding ulcer.

Short Answers

1. Nutrition assessment.
2. Parenteral nutrition.
3. Medical nutrition therapy.
4. Dietary supplement.
5. Brat diet.
6. Therapeutic diet.
7. Parenteral feeding.
8. Diabetic diet.
9. Liquid diets.
10. Dietetics.

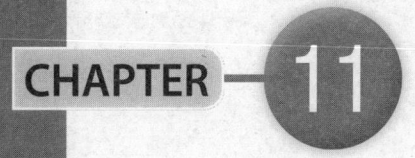

CHAPTER 11

Cookery Rules and Preservation of Nutrients

CHAPTER OUTLINE

- Cooking: Methods, Advantages and Disadvantages
- Preservation of Nutrients
- Measures to Prevent Loss of Nutrients During Preparation
- Safe Food Handling and Storage of Foods
- Food Preservation
- Food Additives and Food Adulteration
- Prevention of Food Adulteration (PFA) Act
- Food Standards

TERMINOLOGY

- **Boiling:** Cooking in water at its boiling point 100°C is known as boiling. Most of the vegetables are cooked by this method.
- **Simmering:** This method includes cooking below the boiling point, i.e, 85°C. Meat and fish are best cooked by simmering because cooking at high temperature hardens the fibers of meat. It helps in preserving the essential vitamins and minerals.
- **Steaming:** Cooking in this method involves direct heat steaming. Temperature is high and pressure is maintained. Pressure cooker is used to cook things by steam under pressure. This method is effective as it preserves nutrients, fuel and time.
- **Stewing:** This method included boiling in smaller amount of liquid for a prolonged, low degree of heat about 80°C. Here a pan is used which has well fitted lid to prevent evaporation.
- **Roasting:** Food is smeared with a little fat and exposed directly to heat or flame. This makes the food tender. Chicken and tender mutton may cooked by this method.
- **Frying:** Frying is a means of heat transfer that works by both conduction (direct contact) and convection (the natural movement of molecules in a fluid). Such as broiling, boiling, and baking, frying is a method of cooking, but unlike water-based cooking (boiling, braising, or steaming), frying uses dry heat. Oil wicks moisture away from food surfaces.
- **Baking:** Baking is cooking food by dry heat. It is done in a hot air oven. Temperature required for baking is 250–500°C. Baking is expensive form and slow process of cooking. Foods cooked by this method are bread, pastry, cakes, etc.
- **Grilling:** This is direct heat cooking method. Here direct heat flame, grill or pans are used to cook. It is quick method of cooking for tender foods like cheese, brinjals and tomatoes.
- **Solar cooking:** Here solar energy is used to cook foods. It takes a longer time for cooking by this method. It is simplest and traditional form of cooking. Solar cooker and closed containers are used which absorb maximum solar energy.
- **Bacteria:** Single-celled organisms without nuclei, some of which are infectious.
- **Bactericidal:** A state that prevents growth of bacteria.
- **Bateriostatic:** A substance that kills bacteria.
- **Carcinogen:** A cancer-causing substance.
- **Enrichment:** The addition of vitamins and minerals to improve the nutritional content of a food.
- **Fermentation:** A reaction performed by yeast or bacteria to make alcohol.
- **Fortification:** The addition of vitamins and minerals to improve the nutritional content of a food.
- **Leavening:** Yeast or other agents used for rising bread.
- **Microorganism:** Bacteria and protists; single-celled organisms.

INTRODUCTION

Cooking is an art (**Fig. 11.1**). It is linked with the dietary and cultural pattern of people. Almost all foods consumed need some form of cooking and processing before they are fit for serving and consumption. Fruits and some vegetables used in salad or chutneys are consumed uncooked. Food preparation is an important step in meeting the nutritional needs of the family. Food has to be pleasing in appearance and taste in order to be consumed. Foods like fruits, vegetables and nuts can be eaten raw but most foods are cooked to bring about desirable changes.

The process of subjecting food to the action of heat is termed as cooking. In cooking, there are some basic methods of cooking that are used. These commonly used basic cooking methods are divided into two general groups. The groups are: Dry heat cookery methods and moist heat cookery methods. The methods of cooking are divided into these two groups

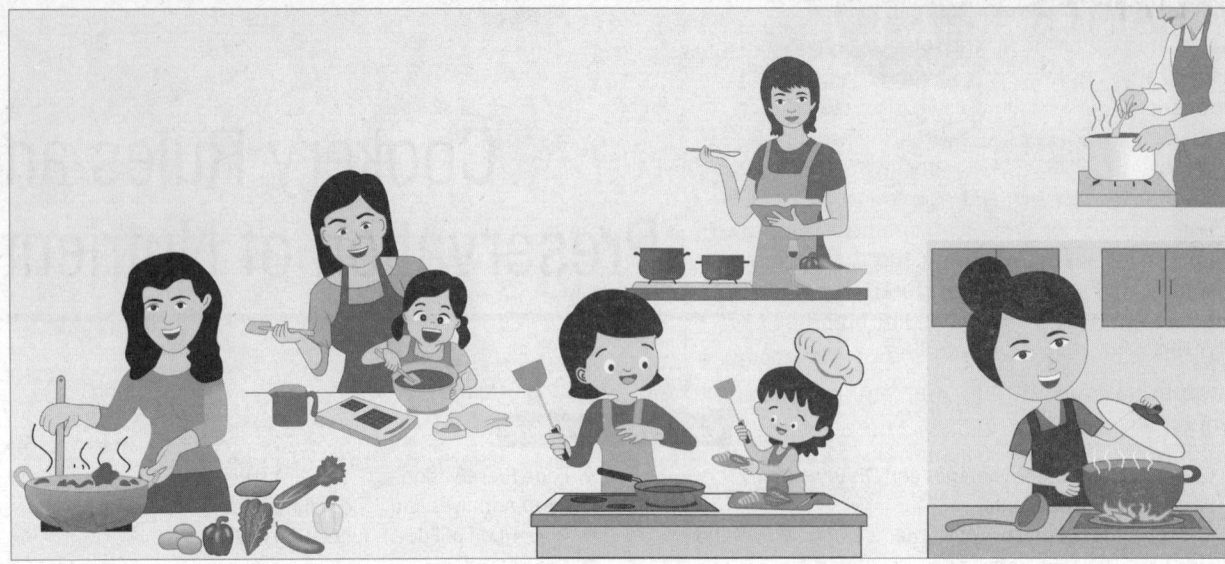

Fig. 11.1: Cooking as an art.

because of the way food is cooked and the type of heat that is used.

OBJECTIVES OF COOKING

- **Cooking sterilizes food:** Above 40°C the growth of bacteria decreases rapidly. Hence food is made safe for consumption.
- **Cooking softens the connective tissues** of meat and the coarse fiber of cereals, pulses and vegetables so that the digestive period is shortened and the gastrointestinal tract is less subjected to irritation.
- **Palatability and food quality is improved by cooking:** Appearance, flavor, texture and taste of food are enhanced while cooking.
- **Introduces variety:** Different dishes can be prepared with the same ingredients. For example, rice can be made into biriyani and kheer.
- **Increases food consumption:** Cooking brings about improvement in texture and flavor thereby increasing consumption of food.
- **Increases availability of nutrients:** Example, in raw egg, avidin binds biotin making it unavailable to the body. By cooking, avidin gets denatured and biotin is made available.

Box 11.1 summarizes aims and objectives of cooking.

> **Box 11.1:** Aims and objectives of cooking.
>
> - To make the food get cooked.
> - While cooking, it undergoes some chemical and physical changes to become acceptable.
> - Cooking enhances its ability to get digested, i.e., after cooking, the food can be digested by the system easily.
> - There is change in texture, which makes the mastication easier
> - It breaks down the cellulose, soften the connective tissues of meat and also breaks down the starch.
> - Cooking sterilizes the food to a good extent.
> - Cooking introduces variety. Different dishes can be prepared with the same ingredients.

Benefits of Cooking

- Cooking increases palatability of the food
- It makes mastication easier and renders the food easy to digest
- It sterilizes food by killing microorganism
- Adds new flavor and stimulates digestive juices
- Good cooking increases the acceptability of food
- It improves the appearance of food

COOKING METHODS

Heat is transferred to the food during cooking by conduction, convection, radiation or microwave energy. Cooking takes place by moist and dry heat. Moist heat involves water and steam. Air or fat are used in dry heat.

Moist Heat Methods

Boiling (Fig. 11.2)

This is the most common method of cooking and is also the simplest. With this method of cooking, enough water is

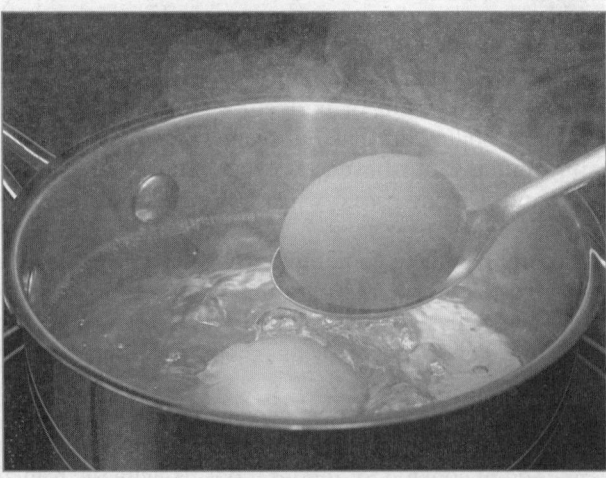

Fig. 11.2: Boiling.

added to food and it is then cooked over the fire. The action of the heated water makes the food to get cooked. The liquid is usually thrown away after the food is cooked. In the case of cooking rice, all the water is absorbed by the rice grains to make it get cooked. During the heating process, the nutrients can get lost or destroyed and the flavor can be reduced with this method of cooking. If you overcooked cabbage, all the nutrients can get lost. Boiling is a method of cooking foods by just immersing them in water at 100°C and maintaining the water at that temperature till the food is tender. Rice, egg, dal, meat, roots and tubers are cooked by boiling.

Merits
- **Simple method:** It does not require special skill and equipment.
- Uniform cooking can be achieved.

Demerits
- Continuous excessive boiling leads to damage in the structure and texture of food.
- Loss of heat labile nutrients, such as B and C vitamins if the water is discarded.
- Time consuming: Boiling takes more time to cook food and fuel may be wasted.
- Loss of color—water-soluble pigments may be lost.

Stewing (Fig. 11.3)

In the process of cooking using the stewing method, food is cooked using a lot of liquid. Different kinds of vegetables are chopped, diced or cubed and added to the pot. Sometimes pieces of selected meat, fish or chicken is also chopped and added to the stew. The liquid is slightly thickened and stewed food is served in that manner.

Box 11.2 depicts stewing process.

- This method is also used when preparing fruits that are going to be served as desserts. With this cooking method, every food is cooked together at the same time in one pot.
- The flavor, colors, shapes and textures of the different vegetables that are used, makes stewing a handy method of cooking.
- The only disadvantage is that some of the vegetables might be overcooked and thus the nutrient content becomes much less.
- It is therefore important that the vegetables that take the longest to cook to be put into the pot first and the ones that need least cooking to be put in last.
- In this way much of the nutrient contents of the food does not get lost.
- It refers to the simmering of food in a pan with a tight fitting lid using small quantities of liquid to cover only half the food.
- This is a slow method of cooking. The liquid is brought to boiling point and the heat is reduced to maintain simmering temperatures (82–90°C).
- The food above the liquid is cooked by the steam generated within the pan. Apple, meat along with roots, vegetables and legumes are usually stewed.

Merits
- Loss of nutrients is avoided as water used for cooking is not discarded.
- Flavor is retained.

Demerits
The process is time consuming and there is wastage of fuel.

Steaming

To steam food, water is added to a pot and then a stand is placed inside the pot. The water level should be under the stand and not above it. There is no contact between the food and the water that is added to the pot. Food is then placed on the stand and heat is applied. The hot steam rising from the boiling water acts on the food and the food gets cooked.

- It is the hot steam that cooks the food, as there is no contact between the food and the water inside the pot.
- This method of cooking for vegetables is very good as the food does not lose its flavor and much of the nutrients are not lost during the cooking.
- It is a method of cooking food in steam generated from vigorously boiling water in a pan.
- The food to be steamed is placed in a container and is not in direct contact with the water or liquid. Idli, custard and idiappam are made by steaming. Vegetables can also be steamed **(Fig. 11.4)**.

Merits
- Less chance of burning and scorching.
- Texture of food is better as it becomes light and fluffy, e.g., Idly.
- Cooking time is less and fuel wastage is less.
- Steamed foods like idly and idiappam contain less fat and are easily digested and are good for children, aged and for therapeutic diets.
- Nutrient loss is minimized.

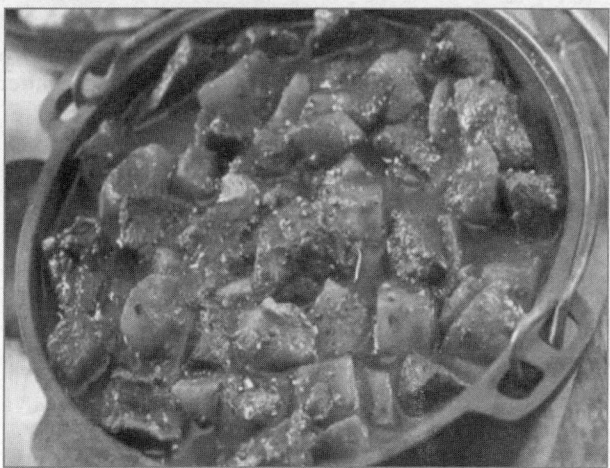

Fig. 11.3: Stewing.

Box 11.2: Stewing.
- Similar to braising
- Prepreparation different
- Cut into bite-sized pieces
- Sear or blanch meat/veggies
- Cover completely with liquid
- Cover pot and simmer
- Examples: Chili or beef stew

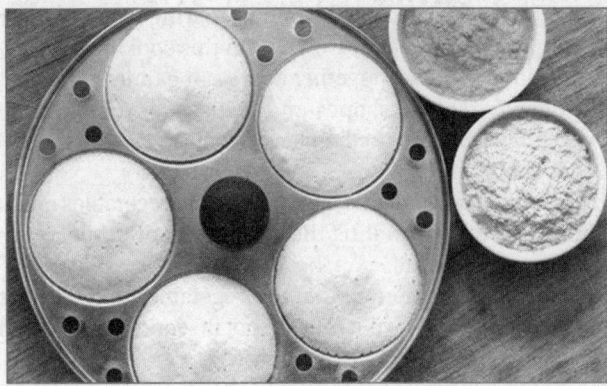

Fig. 11.4: Steaming.

Demerits
- Steaming equipment is required.
- This method is limited to the preparation of selected foods.

Pressure Cooking
When steam under pressure is used the method is known as pressure cooking and the equipment used is the pressure cooker. In this method the temperature of boiling water can be raised above 100° C. Rice, dal, meat, roots and tubers are usually pressure cooked **(Fig. 11.5)**.

Merits
- Cooking time is less compared to other methods.
- Nutrient and flavor loss is minimized.
- Conserves fuel and time as different items can be cooked at the same time.
- Less chance for burning and scorching.
- Constant attention is not necessary.

Demerits
- The initial investment may not be affordable to everybody.
- Knowledge of the usage, care and maintenance of cooker is required to prevent accidents.

- Careful watch on the cooking time is required to prevent overcooking.

Poaching
Poaching is an incredibly versatile cooking method; just about everything from fruits to meats can be cooked using this technique. Poaching is merely simmering food in liquid until it is cooked through. As with baking, the density of the food will determine the cooking duration time; fish is cooked for a short amount of time in liquid that is gradually heated, while denser meats cook longer starting with a cold liquid **(Fig. 11.6)**.

- The key to poaching meats and proteins is to make sure that your stove temperature is not too high, as this will cause the meat to break down, resulting in a greasy meal.
- Because eggs cook quickly, the liquid is first brought to a boil then turned off. Then, the eggs are added and covered until cooked to the desired doneness.
- This involves cooking in the minimum amount of liquid at temperatures of 80°–85°C that is below the boiling point. Egg and fish can be poached.

Merits
- No special equipment is needed.
- Quick method of cooking and therefore saves fuel.
- Poached foods are easily digested since no fat is added.

Demerits
- Poached foods may not appeal to everybody as they are bland in taste.
- Food can be scorched if water evaporates due to careless monitoring.
- Water soluble nutrients may be leached into the water.

Blanching
In meal preparation, it is often necessary only to peel off the skin of fruits and vegetables without making them tender.

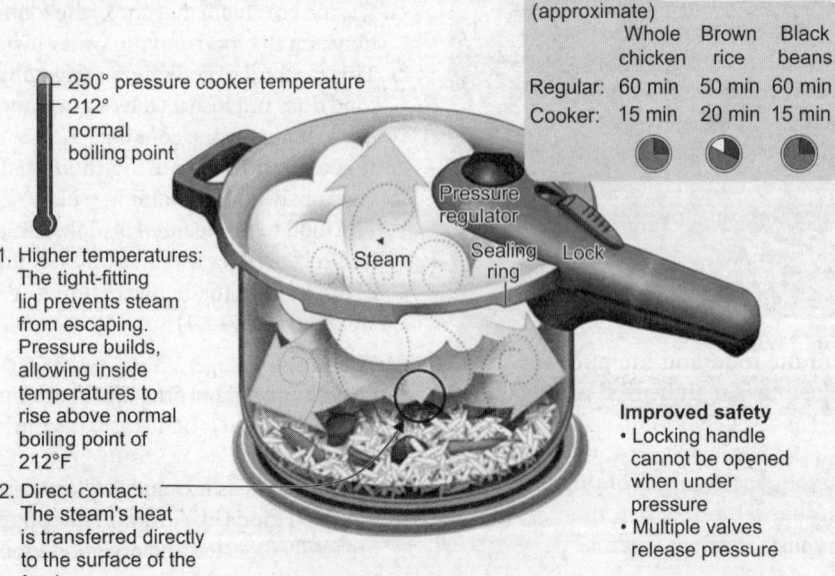

Fig. 11.5: Pressure cooking.

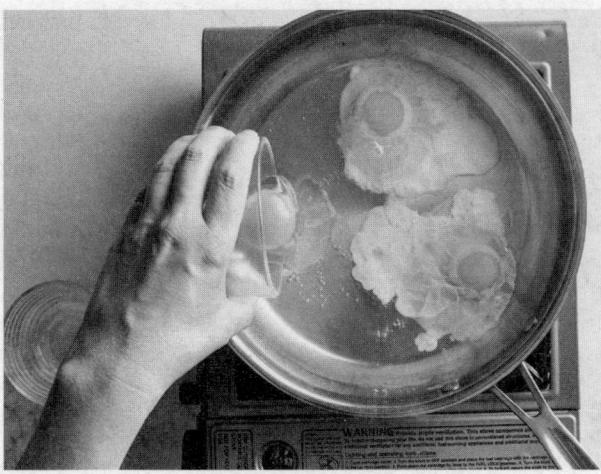

Fig. 11.6: Poaching.

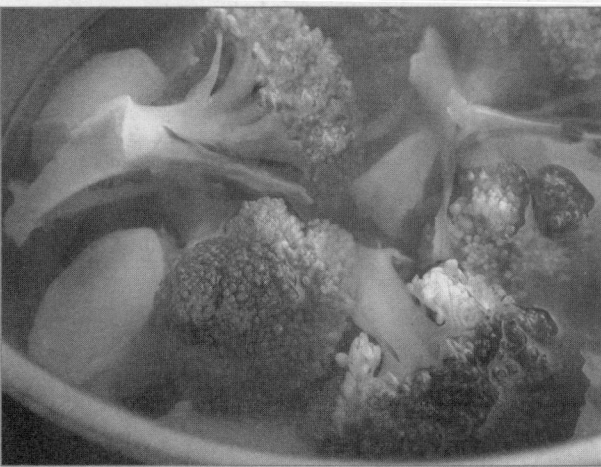

Fig. 11.7: Blanching.

This can be achieved by blanching. In this method, food is dipped in boiling water for 5 seconds to 2 minutes depending on the texture of the food. This helps to remove the skin or peel without softening food (**Fig. 11.7**).

Blanching can also be done by pouring enough boiling water on the food to immerse it for some time or subjecting foods to boiling temperatures for short periods and then immediately immersing in cold water. The process causes the skin to become loose and can be peeled off easily.

Merits
- Peels can easily be removed to improve digestibility.
- Destroys enzymes that bring about spoilage.
- Texture can be maintained while improving the color and flavor of food.

Demerits
Loss of nutrients if cooking water is discarded.

Dry Heat Methods

In dry heat cooking methods, the food being cooked does not use water to cook the food. The food is left dry and heat is applied to cook the food. Such methods of cooking are: baking, steaming, grilling, and roasting. When heat is applied to the food, the food cooks in its own juice or the water added to the food during its preparation evaporates during the heating process and this cooks the food. Heat is applied directly to the food by way of convection thus making the food to get cooked. The action or movement of air around the food cooks it.

Roasting

With roasting, direct heat is applied to the food. The heat seals the outside part of the food and the juice inside the food cooks the food. Roasting is mainly used when cooking fleshy food like fish, meat or chicken. When heat is applied to the outer covering of the food, it seals it up thereby trapping all the juices inside the food. The action of direct heating, heats up the juices inside the food, which then cooks the food. Again there is very little nutrient lost and the flavor is not spoilt (**Fig. 11.8**).

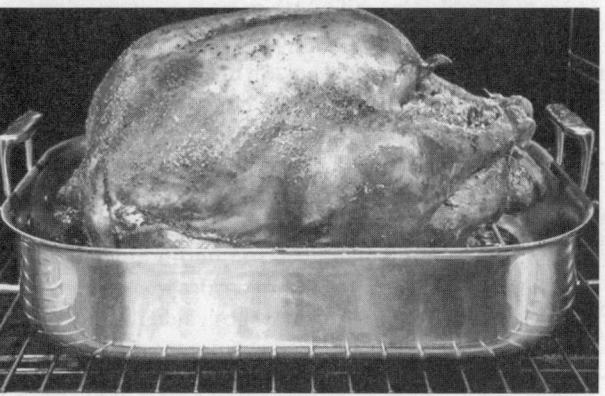

Fig. 11.8: Roasting.

Food is frequently rotated over the spit so that there is even heating applied to all parts of the food. This is so that heat is applied evenly to the food to make it get cooked properly. In this method food is cooked in a heated metal or frying pan without covering it, e.g., groundnut.

Merits
- Quick method of cooking.
- It improves the appearance, flavor and texture of the food.
- Spices are easily powdered if they are first roasted.

Demerits
- Food can be scorched due to carelessness.
- Roasting denatures proteins reducing their availability.

Grilling

There are two methods of grilling that are used these days. One type of grilling is the one that is commonly used by the people in the village. This is when food is cooked over hot charcoal on an open fire. The food is placed on top of the burning charcoal. Sometimes people improvise by using wire mesh and place it over the open fire to grill fish or vegetables (**Fig. 11.9**). The other method is using grills that are inbuilt in stoves.
- In this method, the griller, which has a tray, is heated up and the food is placed on the grill tray to cook. The heat

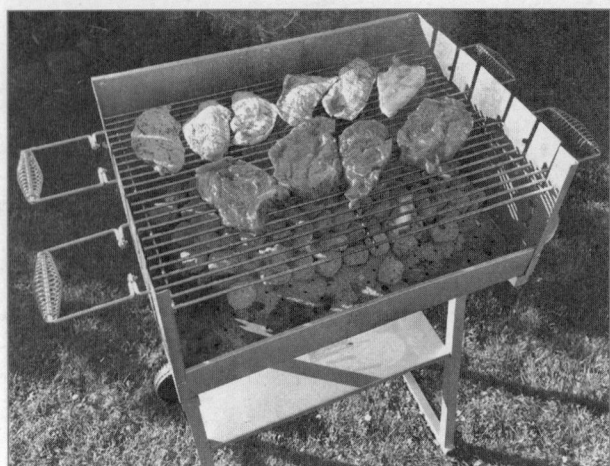

Fig. 11.9: Grilling.

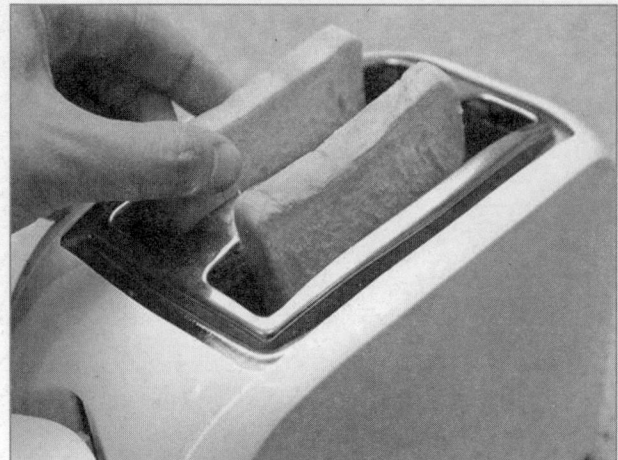

Fig. 11.10: Toasting.

can be gas-generated or electric-generated depending on the type of stove used.
- The food is again left to cook on the grill with the doors of the grill open. People who can afford to buy a stove would use the grilling part to grill their food. What happens in this type of cooking is the heat seals the outside part of the food and the juice inside the food cooks it.
- The flavor of the food is not lost and much of the nutrients are not lost either. Food is frequently turned over to prevent it from burning and to ensure that equal heating and cooking time is applied to both sides of the food. By doing this, the food is cooked evenly and thoroughly.
- Grilling or broiling refers to the cooking of food by exposing it to direct heat.
- In this method food is placed above or in between a red hot surface. Papads, corn, phulkas, chicken can be prepared by this method.

Merits
- Enhances flavor, appearance and taste of the product.
- It requires less time to cook.
- Minimum fat is used.

Demerits
Constant attention is required to prevent charring.

Toasting

This is a method where food is kept between two heated elements to facilitate browning on both sides. Bread slices are cooked by toasting (**Fig. 11.10**).

Merits
- Easy and quick method.
- Flavor improved.

Demerits
- Special equipment required.
- Careful monitoring is needed to prevent charring.

Baking

In baking method of cooking, the food is cooked using convection heating. The food is put into an enclosed area where heat is then applied and the movement of heat within

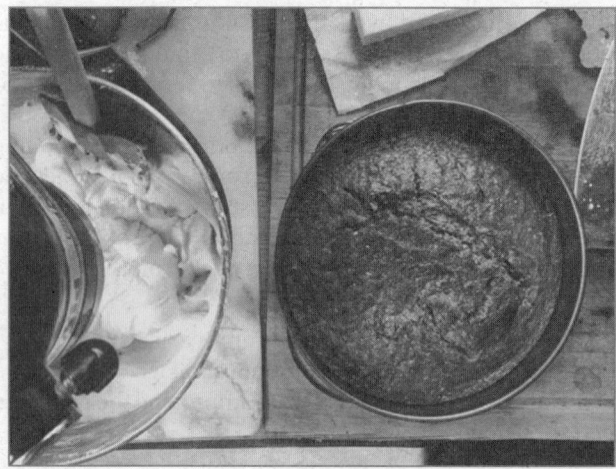

Fig. 11.11: Baking.

the confined space, acts on the food that make it get cooked. In this method, the food gets cooked in an oven or oven like appliance by dry heat. The temperature range maintained in an oven is 120–260°C (**Fig. 11.11**).

The food is usually kept uncovered in a container greased with a fat coated paper. Bread, cake, biscuits, pastries and meat are prepared by this method.

Merits
- Baking lends a unique baked flavor to foods.
- Foods become light and fluffy-cakes, custards, bread.
- Certain foods can be prepared only by this method—bread, cakes.
- Uniform and bulk cooking can be achieved, e.g., bun, bread.
- Flavor and texture are improved.
- Variety of dishes can be made.

Demerits
- Special equipment like oven is required.
- Baking skills are necessary to obtain a product with ideal texture, flavor and color characteristics.
- Careful monitoring needed to prevent scorching.

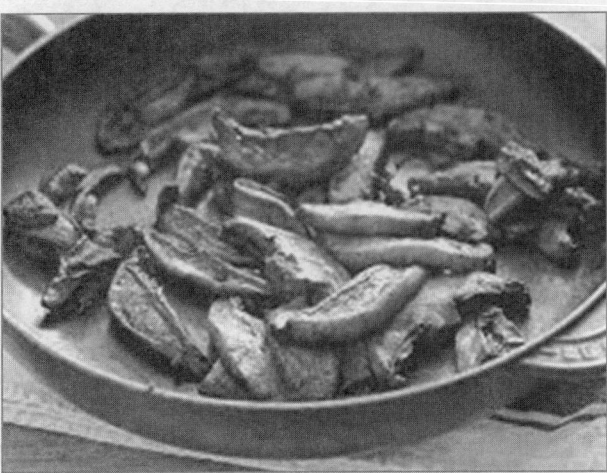

Fig. 11.12: Sauteing.

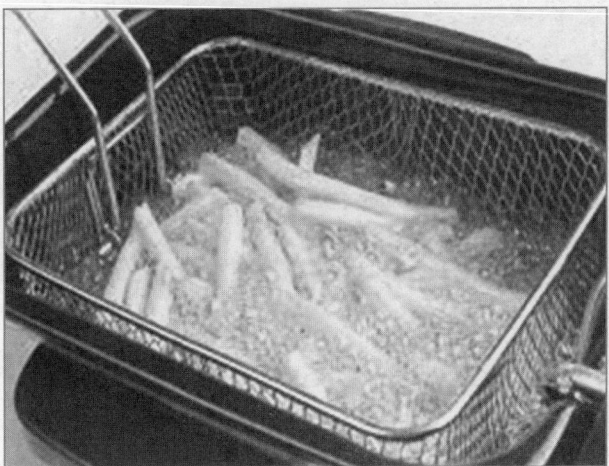

Fig. 11.13: Frying.

Sauteing

Sauteing is a method in which food is lightly tossed in little oil just enough to cover the base of the pan. The pan is covered with a lid and the flame or intensity of heat is reduced. The food is allowed to cook till tender in its own steam. The food is tossed occasionally, or turned with a spatula to enable all the pieces to come in contact with the oil and get cooked evenly (**Fig. 11.12**).

The product obtained by this method is slightly moist and tender but without any liquid or gravy. Foods cooked by sauteing are generally vegetables which are used as side dishes in a menu. Sauteing can be combined with other methods to produce variety in meals.

Merits
- Takes less time
- Simple technique
- Minimum oil is used

Demerits
Constant attention is needed as there is chance of scorching or burning.

Frying

In this method, the food to be cooked is brought into contact with larger amount of hot fat. When food is totally immersed in hot oil, it is called deep fat frying (**Fig. 11.13**). Samosa, chips, pakoda are examples of deep fat fried foods. In shallow fat frying, only a little fat is used and the food is turned in order that both sides are browned, e.g., omlette, cutlets, parathas. When food is fried using oil or solid fat it is important that you observe some rules in handling oil or fat.

Simple rules to follow when frying:
- Make sure there is enough oil or fat put in the frying pan or a deep frying pan.
- The food to be cooked must not have water dripping from it. This is because when water comes into contact with hot oil or fat, you will have the oil sizzling and spitting out of the pan, which could burn your skin if you are not careful.
- Put the food into the hot oil carefully. Try not to make a big splash as the oil could burn your skin.
- The oil of fat should be heated to the right temperature before putting food into the pan to be fried. If the food is put in when the oil or fat is not heated to the right temperature, the food will soak up the oil and you will have food that is all oily or greasy. If the oil or fat is overheated, you will end up with food that is burnt. Sometimes the food especially doughnuts will turn brown on the outside but the dough inside is uncooked. To cook food using the frying method, there are two ways of doing it. There is the shallow frying and the deep frying methods.

Shallow frying
- In shallow frying, food is cooked in a frying pan with a little amount of oil or fat.
- The oil or fat is heated to the correct amount and the food is put into the heated oil.
- The food is turned over a few minutes or is stirred around a couple of times before it is cooked and dished out.
- If patties, potato chips or coated foods are fried, it is best to put a piece of brown paper or paper napkin inside the tray to soak up any oil from the food before serving it.

Deep frying (Fig. 11.14)
- This is when a lot of oil or fat is used in cooking the food. The oil or fat is usually put into a deep pan and is heated to boiling point.
- Food is then put into the hot boiling oil and is cooked in that way. Such food as fish fingers, potato chips, meat balls, and doughnuts to name a few, is cooked using the deep frying method.

Merits
- Very quick method of cooking.
- The calorific values of food are increased since fat is used as the cooking media.
- Frying lends a delicious flavor and attractive appearance to foods.
- Taste and texture are improved.

Demerits
- Careful monitoring is required as food easily gets charred when the smoking temperature is not properly maintained.

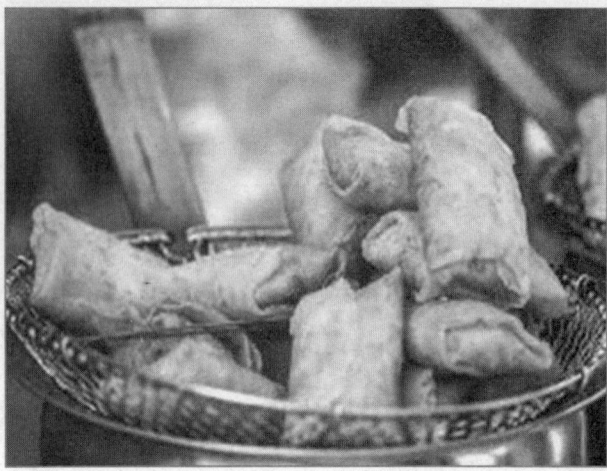

Fig. 11.14: Deep frying.

- The food may become soggy due to too much oil absorption.
- Fried foods are not easily digested.
- Repeated use of heated oils will have ill effects on health.

COMBINATION OF COOKING METHODS

Braising

Braising is a combined method of roasting and stewing in a pan with a tight fitting lid (**Fig. 11.15**). Flavorings and seasonings are added and food is allowed to cook gently. Food preparations prepared by combination methods are:
- **Uppuma:** Roasting and boiling.
- **Cutlet:** Boiling and deep frying.
- **Vermicilli payasam:** Roasting and simmering.

Microwave Cooking

Microwaves are electromagnetic waves of radiant energy with wavelengths in the range of 250×10^6 to 7.5×10^9 Angstroms. The most commonly used type of microwave generator is an electronic device called a magnetron which generates radiant energy of high frequency (**Fig. 11.16**).
- A simple microwave oven consists of a metal cabinet into which the magnetron is inserted.
- The cabinet is equipped with a metal fan that distributes the microwave throughout the cabinet. Food placed in the oven is heated by microwaves from all directions.
- Moist foods and liquid foods can be rapidly heated in such ovens. Food should be kept in containers made of plastic, glass or china ware which do not contain metallic substances.

These containers are used because they transmit the microwaves but do not absorb or reflect them.

Merits
- Quick method—10 times faster than conventional method. So loss of nutrients can be minimized.
- Only the food gets heated and the oven does not get heated.
- Food gets cooked uniformly.
- Leftovers can be reheated without changing the flavor and texture of the product.
- Microwave cooking enhances the flavor of food because it cooks quickly with little or no water.

Demerits
- Baked products do not get a brown surface.
- Microwave cooking cannot be used for simmering, stewing or deep frying.
- Flavors of all ingredients do not blend well as the cooking time is too short.

Solar Cooking

Solar cooking is a very simple technique that makes use of sunlight or solar energy which is a nonconventional source of energy. Solar cooker consists of a well insulated box which is painted black on the inside and covered with one or more transparent covers (**Fig. 11.17**).

The purpose of these transparent covers is to trap heat inside the solar cooker. These covers allow the radiation from the sun to come inside the box but do not allow the heat from the hot black absorbing plate to come out of the box. Because of this, temperature up to 140°C can be obtained which is adequate for cooking.

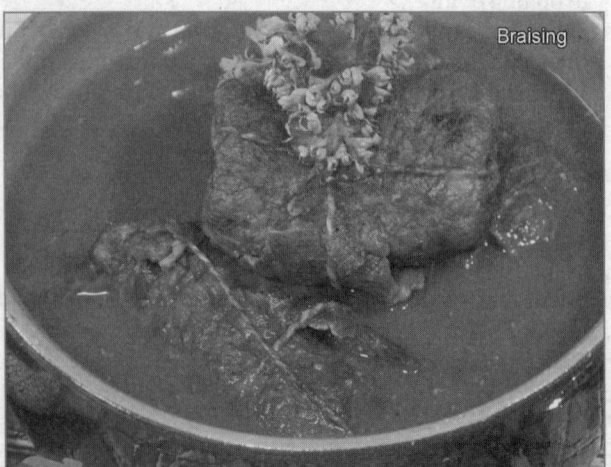

Fig. 11.15: Braising.

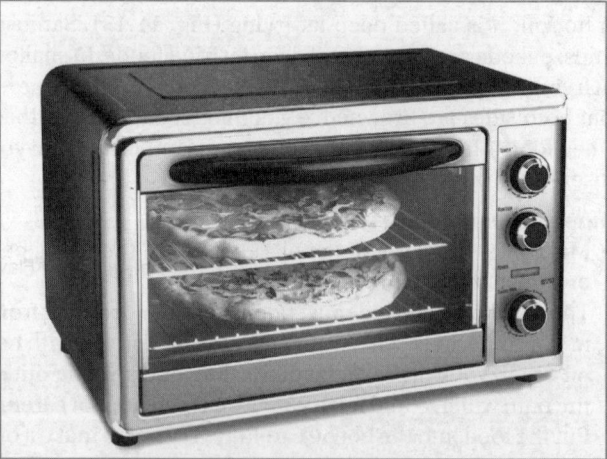

Fig. 11.16: Microwave.

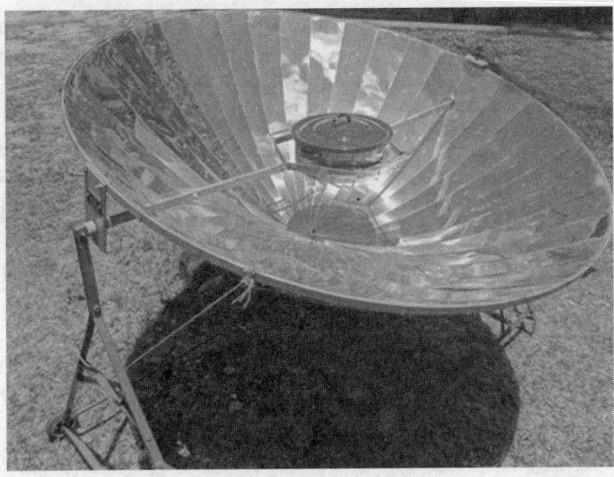

Fig. 11.17: Solar cooking.

Merits
- Simple technique—requires no special skill.
- Cost effective as natural sunlight is the form of energy.
- Original flavor of food is retained.
- There is no danger of scorching or burning.
- Loss of nutrients is minimum as only little amounts of water is used in cooking.

Demerits
- Special equipment is needed.
- Slow cooking process.
- Cannot be used in the absence of sunlight—rainy season, late evening and night

Figure 11.18 is depicted the common problems in cooking.

PRESERVATION OF NUTRIENTS

The various vitamins and minerals are susceptible to destruction by air, light, water, acid, alkali, heat, time and the action of enzymes in the foods themselves. However, you can cut losses and significantly increase your nutrient intake by the care you take in choosing, storing and cooking foods.

- Lean meats, skinless poultry and low-fat dairy products have more nutrients per calorie than their fattier versions.
- Whole grains (for example, whole wheat pasta, oatmeal and brown rice) have more nutrients than foods made from refined grains, even if they are enriched.
- Whole grain foods leavened with yeast have less phytate, which can inhibit the absorption of calcium, iron and zinc.
- Parboiled, or converted, white rice is more nutritious than regular white rice.
- Dark green leafy vegetables and deep-yellow vegetables have more vitamin A than lighter-colored ones.
- Fresh or frozen fruits and vegetables have more nutrients than canned ones (canning may reduce the amount of some vitamins by half).
- But fresh is not necessarily better than frozen, since frozen foods are usually processed soon after picking whereas fresh foods may spend days in transport and storage (both in the store and at home) before being consumed. If you cannot shop often, frozen produce may be more nutritious than fresh.
- Cooked vegetables that are reheated after being kept in the refrigerator for two or three days lose more than half their vitamin C.

Tips to Retain Nutrients While Cooking

Here are 10 simple tips which will help you retain nutrients while cooking. So that you can ensure highly nutritious food being served to your loved ones.

1. When peeling the skin of vegetables do peel as thinly as possible. The nutrients in vegetables and fruits are concentrated just below the skin, so peeling before boiling increases the loss of vitamin C, folic acid and other B vitamins. The peels of carrot, radish, gourd and ginger can be scraped instead of peeling. Peel only when absolutely necessary.
2. Do not cut vegetables into very small cubes as the surface area of vegetable increases that comes in contact with oxygen, destroying more.
3. Don't soak vegetables in water to prevent discoloration. Almost 40% of water-soluble vitamins and minerals are

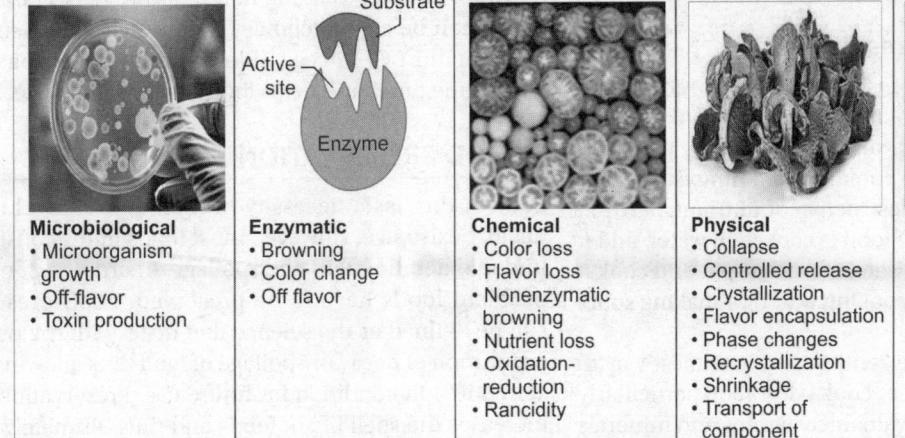
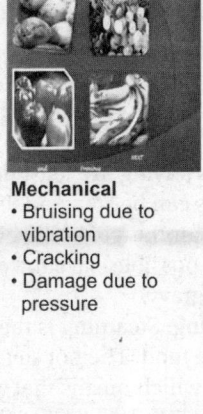

Fig. 11.18: Common problems in cooking.

lost in the water. If you must soak, use up the soaking water to knead the dough, prepare soups and gravies.
4. Salads should be prepared just before serving and should be served in closed dishes to avoid excessive exposure to air.
5. Do not throw away the excess water drained after boiling rice or vegetables. When preparing cottage cheese, the water left over after curdling (called whey) is extremely rich in good quality proteins and vitamins and should be used up in preparing gravies, kneading dough or simply had as a refreshing drink after flavoring with lemon juice, salt and pepper.
6. Do not keep milk open or exposed to light, as a considerable destruction of riboflavin can occur.
7. It is preferable to cook vegetables in a minimum amount of water keeping the vessel covered and to consume it as soon as possible. Reheating cooked vegetables further destroys vitamins.
8. Root vegetables should be boiled with skins on and then peeled after boiling. This helps the nutrients to migrate to the center of the vegetables, helping better retention of its nutrients. Do eat with skin on whenever possible.
9. Baking soda makes cooking water alkaline and thus helps retain the color of vegetables as well as speed up the cooking process, but it destroys thiamine and vitamin C.
10. Deep frying and heating for a long time or heating at a high temperature should be avoided during cooking. If food material is heated above 70°C for a long duration, proteins become hard and coagulated. In this form, they are not easily absorbed by the body. Thus, overcooking results in loss of precious nutrients.

Measures to Prevent Loss of Nutrients During Preparation

Many vitamins are sensitive to heat and air exposure – vitamin C, all B vitamins and folates in particular. This loss of nutrients increases with longer cooking times and higher temperatures. But there are many cooking methods that minimize cooking time, temperature and the amount of water needed. Learn more about cooking methods that preserve nutrients so that all the healthy vitamins stay for dinner (**Fig. 11.19**).

Techniques of Nutrient Preservation

The three R's for nutrient preservation are to reduce the amount of water used in cooking, reduce the cooking time and reduce the surface area of the food that is exposed. Waterless cooking, pressure cooking, steaming, stir-frying and microwaving are least destructive of nutrients. Frozen vegetables can be steamed. If food is cooked in water, add it to a small amount of boiling water, cover the pot and cook it rapidly. If possible, save the cooking water for making soup, sauces or gravy.
- **Steaming:** Steaming is the gentlest and healthiest way to prepare food. The hot steam cooks your food particularly gently, which means that valuable vitamins and minerals are preserved. Flavors can fully develop and vegetables retain their color.

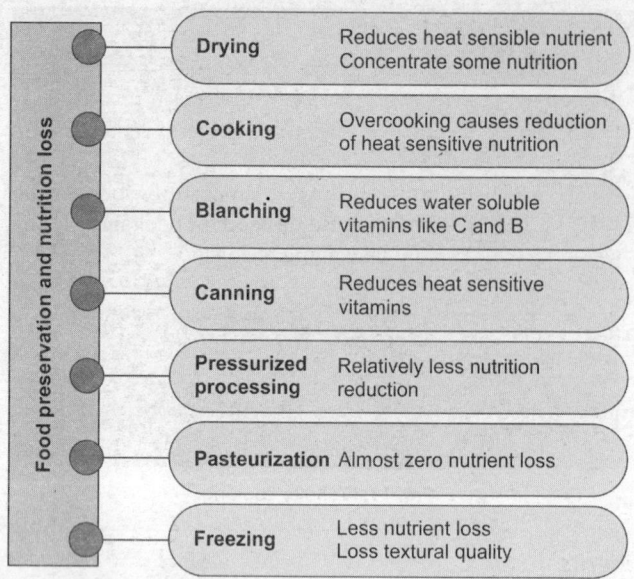

Fig. 11.19: Food preservation and nutrition loss.

- **Grilling:** Grilling lets you get maximum nutritional value from your vegetables and helps food retain its truest flavor. To preserve as many nutrients as possible, it's important not to overheat them. Place your vegetables on a grilling tray and coat them with olive oil. This helps break down the plant-cell walls, releasing more antioxidants while the olive oil also helps your body absorb carotenoids.
- **Baking or roasting:** Baking or roasting your vegetables is a great option for getting rich flavor out of them. Coat them in olive or canola oil before baking and enjoy valuable nutrients from vegetables like carrots, potatoes, and onions.
- **Sautéing:** A method of cooking food that uses a small amount of oil or fat in a shallow pan over relatively high heat—can be a good choice for certain vegetables. Kale, for example, contains polyphenols, which are preventative micronutrients, and carotenoids, which are powerful antioxidants. These are preserved when sautéing but lost when steaming or boiling.
- **Microwaving:** Cooking in a microwave isn't only faster but can be a good choice for preserving nutrients, such as vitamin C, in vegetables. Microwaving boasts short cooking times and helps food retain its full taste.

FOOD PRESERVATION

Food is the basic necessity of man and is invaluable for healthy existence. However, most foods fit for consumption undergo deterioration and spoilage. In order to combat this problem foods have to be preserved. Food preservation can be defined as the science that deals with the process of prevention of decay or spoilage of food thus allowing it to be stored in a fit condition for future use. Preservation of food increases the shelf life of foods and thus ultimately ensures its supply during times of scarcity and natural drought (**Fig. 11.20**).

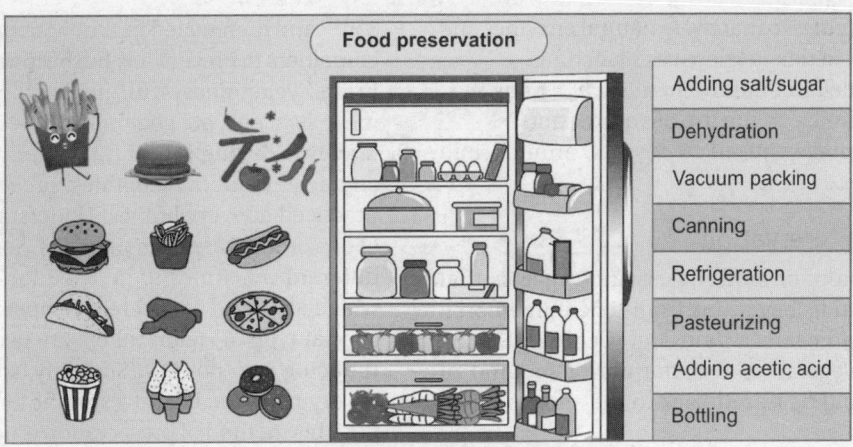

Fig. 11.20: Food preservation.

FOOD SPOILAGE

Food spoilage is a state in which food is deprived of its good or effective qualities. Deterioration or spoilage starts from the time food is harvested slaughtered or manufactured and results in undesirable changes in the physical and chemical characteristics of food.

Causes of Food Spoilage

- Growth and activity of microorganisms, such as bacteria, yeast and moulds.
- Activities of food enzymes and other chemical reactions within the food.
- Inappropriate temperatures for a given food.
- Gain or loss of moisture.
- Reaction with oxygen and light.
- Physical stress or abuse.
- Insects and rodents.
- Nonenzymatic reactions in food, such as oxidation and mechanical damage.

Principles of Food Preservation (Fig. 11.21)

I. **Prevention or delay of microbial decomposition:**
   - By keeping out microorganisms (asepsis)
   - By removal of microorganisms (e.g., filtration)
   - By hindering the growth and activity of microorganisms, e.g., refrigeration, dehydration, addition of chemical preservatives.
   - By killing microorganisms, e.g., boiling, irradiation.

II. **Prevention or delay of self-decomposition of food:**
   - By destruction or inactivation of enzymes, e.g., by blanching. The steaming or boiling of fruits or vegetables

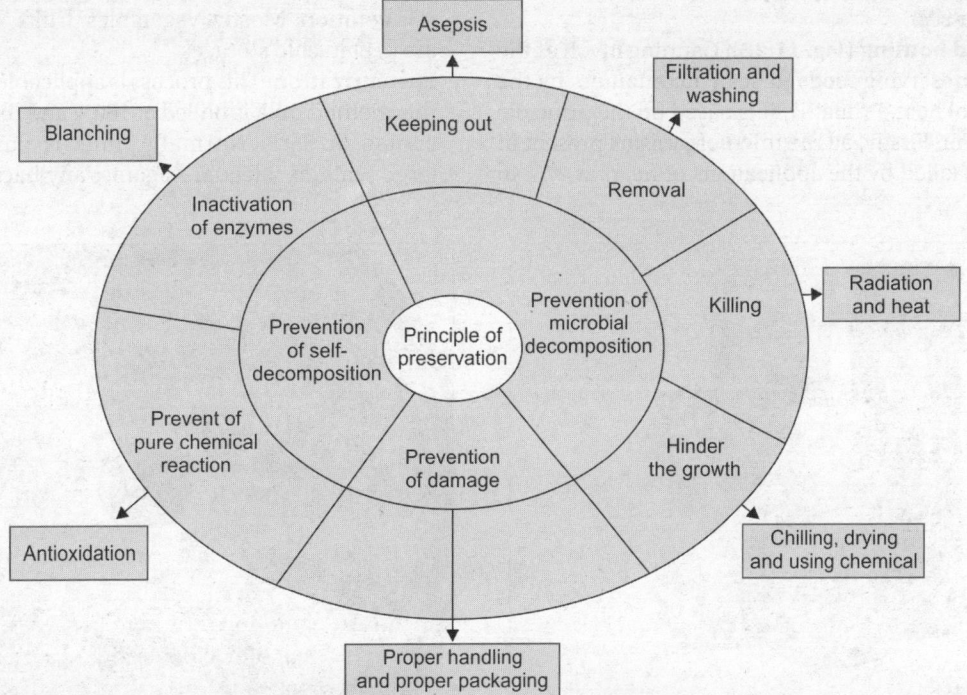

Fig. 11.21: Principles of preservation.

in water for few minutes to inactivate natural enzymes and facilitates removal of skin is known as blanching.
- By prevention or delay of purely chemical reactions, e.g., prevention of oxidation by the use of antioxidants.
- Prevention of damage caused by insects, animals and mechanical causes.

Methods of Food Preservation

A perusal of the history of food preservation reveals that food preservation had its beginning from time immemorial and could be traced to nearly a thousand years ago. Salting of meat, fish, and vegetables was the oldest method of preservation and could be traced back to the ancient Egypt and Greek civilizations.
- Pickling in salt and vinegar, sun-drying and preservation of fruits and vegetables in sugar and honey were among the other methods used.
- Storage of food in frozen conditions was also practiced for centuries in places where freezing temperatures were recorded.
- The discovery of canning as a standard technique of preserving foods in sealed containers subject to high temperature was established in 1810 by Nicholas Appert. Around 1860, Louis Pasteur discovered that microbes were the main cause of spoilage and introduced a heat treatment known as pasteurization to the world.
- All methods used for food preservation are based on preventing or retarding the cause of spoilage. When growth of microorganism is only retarded, preservation is temporary. When spoilage organisms are completely destroyed a more permanent preservation is achieved.

Commercial Methods of Preservation

Commercial, the food preservation technique depicts the following processes:
1. **Canning and bottling (Fig. 11.22):** Canning involves the process of preserving foods in sealed containers by the application of heat. Primarily, it is based on the principle of sterilization. Firstly, all the microorganisms present in the food are killed by the applications of heart at 275° to 350°F and then sealed in simultaneously sterilized air tight containers to prevent any further attack of microorganism. Fruits, vegetables, fruit juices, pickles, cheese, butter, meat, fish, etc., are generally canned or bottled.
2. **Machine drying (Fig. 11.23):** Dehydration in sunlight is an ancient and the lengthiest process of preserving food practiced at every homes. Understanding the difficulties of this process of preserving food, Scientists have invented different machines to be used for different food stuffs, which are dried at different temperatures. Commercially special type of steam rollers are used for drying milk for reducing it to powder. Similarly, special ovens are sued for drying vegetables at a specific temperature. It is found that this method of preservation is better than those of the traditional method of drying foods in sunlight.
3. **Freeze drying (Fig. 11.24):** This method of preserving food is adopted to overcome the difficulties of machine or sunlight drying. During drying vegetables or fruits by sunlight or by machine foods are too much squeezed, and do not take the original shape when it is in use. In order to overcome this defect, the process of freeze drying was invented.

   In this process, food stuffs are kept at a temperature of -20°C for about 12 hours, so that the water content of the food stuffs are converted to ice particles. Then it is dried up by machine under low pressure. When it is to be used, it is dipped in hot water. This method retains the shape of the food stuffs, which is damaged by machines drying process.
4. **Cold storage (Fig. 11.25):** This system has become one of the most popular methods of preserving food-stuffs in rural and urban areas of today. Many seasonal fruits and vegetables are stored in cold storages and according to the demand of the market are carried to the place of requirement. This method is based on the principle of refrigeration. Mostly, vegetables, fruits, eggs, meat, fish are kept in cold storages.
5. **Pasteurization:** This process is applicable to milk only. In this method milk is boiled at 160°F and then immediately cooled at 55°F. Normally, milk is pasteurized on a large scale to safeguard against any bacterial infection.

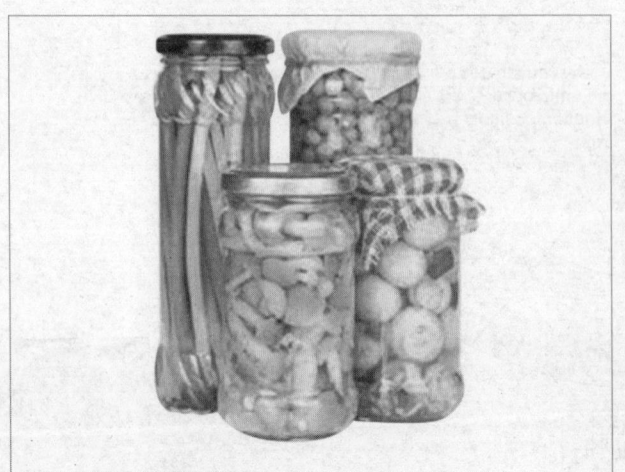

Fig. 11.22: Canned and bottling.

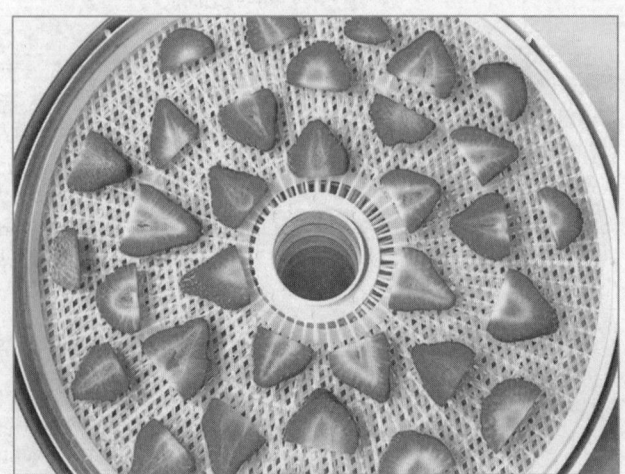

Fig. 11.23: Machine drying.

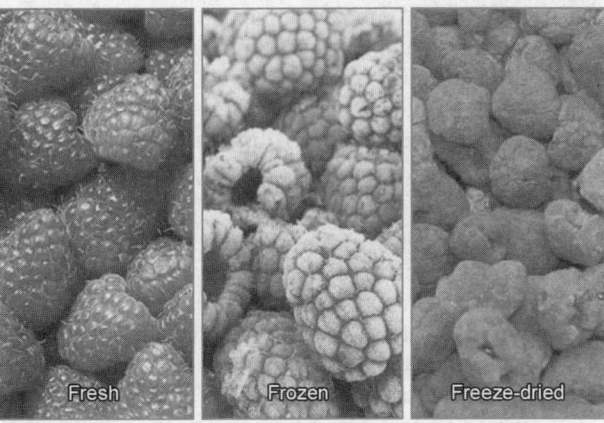

Fig. 11.24: Freeze drying.

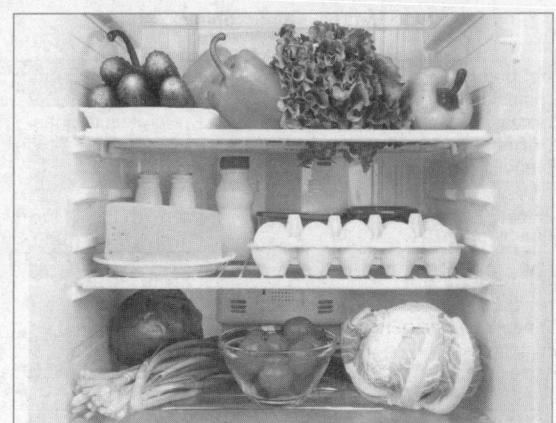

Fig. 11.25: Cold storage.

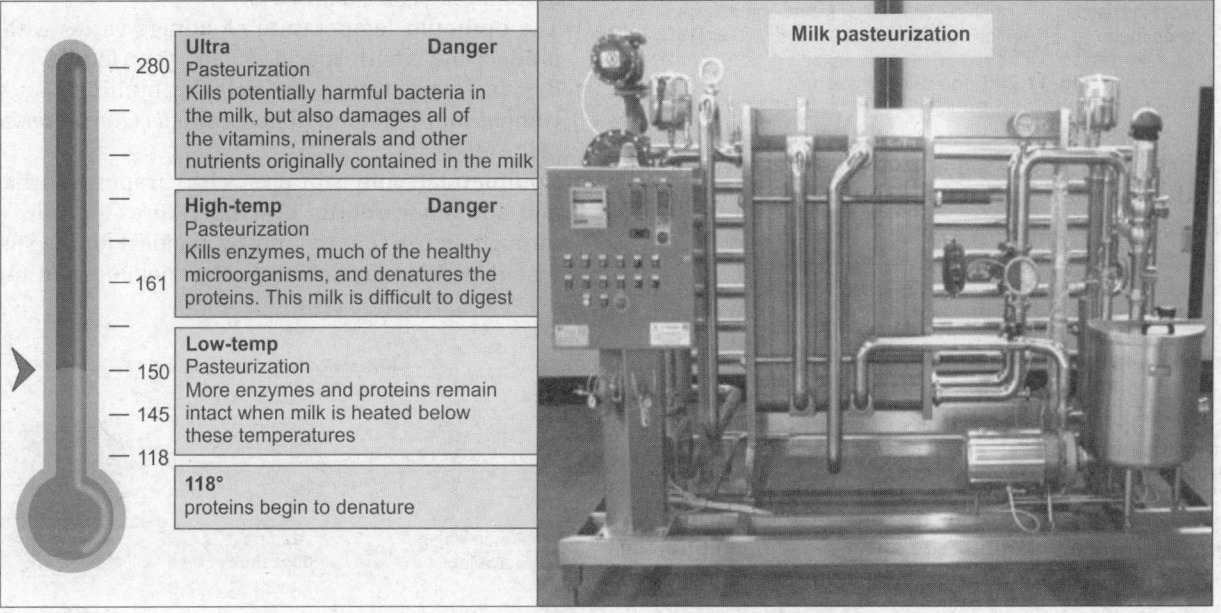

Fig. 11.26: Milk pasteurization.

The process aims at destroying the bacteria and inactivating the rest ones. The pasteurized milk is filled in sterilized bottles which are sealed. It could be preserved for 5–6 days and the color and flavor of pasteurized milk does not change in the process, as happens with the boiled milk **(Fig. 11.26)**.

6. **Irradiation:** This is a new technique of preservation, which is at the stage of experimentation. The WHO has advised the use of this process only in the case of wheat, onions and potatoes **(Fig. 11.27)**.

In this process, gamma rays or high speed electrons are used to destroy microorganism. These radiations are termed as ionizing radiations. The best advantage of this process is that the food can be stored without refrigeration.

7. **Use of antibiotics:** This is another method of preservation now under study. Use of antibiotics in food stuffs have

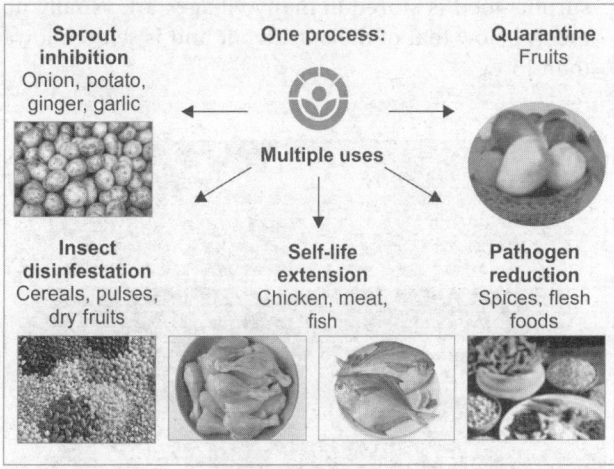

Fig. 11.27: Irradiation.

Section 1: Applied Nutrition and Dietetics

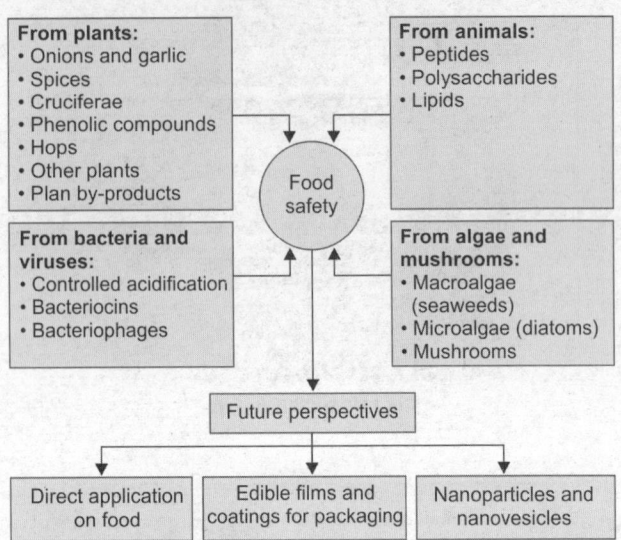

Fig. 11.28: Food safety measures.

considerably, increased during these days. When fish and poultry are treated with antibiotics, their self-life increases two to three times because of the reduced growth of the microorganisms. Similarly antibiotics are used in the ice crush, which is used for packing raw fish and shell fish.

Figure 11.28 is depicted the food safety measures.

USES OF TEMPERATURES

Use of Low Temperatures

Microbial growth and enzyme reaction are retarded in foods stored at low temperatures. The lower the temperature, the greater the retardation. The low temperatures employed can be:

Cellar storage temperatures (about 15°C) (Fig. 11.29):
- Temperatures in cellars (under ground rooms) where surplus food is stored in many villages are usually not much below that of the outside air and is seldom lower than 15°C.
- The temperature is not low enough to prevent the action of many spoilage organisms or of the plant enzymes.
- Decomposition is however, slowed down considerably. Root crops, potatoes, onions, apples and similar foods can be stored for limited periods during the winter months.

Refrigerator or chilling temperature (0°C to 5°C) (Fig. 11.30):
- Chilling (refrigerator), temperatures are obtained and maintained by means of ice or mechanical refrigeration.
- Fruits and vegetables, meats, poultry, fresh milk and milk products, fish and eggs can be preserved from two days to a week when held at this temperature.
- In addition to the foods mentioned above, foods prepared for serving or left over are may also be stored in the household refrigerator.
- The best storage temperature for many foods, eggs, for example, is slightly above 0°C.
- The optimum temperature of storage varies with the product and is fairly specific for any given food.
- Besides temperature, the relative humidity and the composition of the atmosphere can affect the preservation of the food.
- Commercial cold storages with proper ventilation and automatic control of temperatures are now used throughout the country (mostly in cities) for the storage of semi perishable products, such as potatoes and apples.

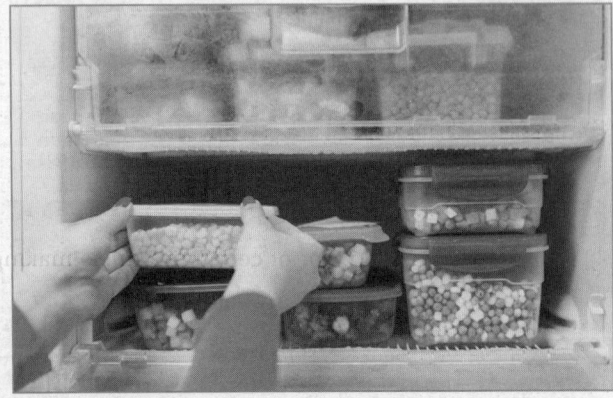

Fig. 11.29: Cellar storage temperature (about 15°C).

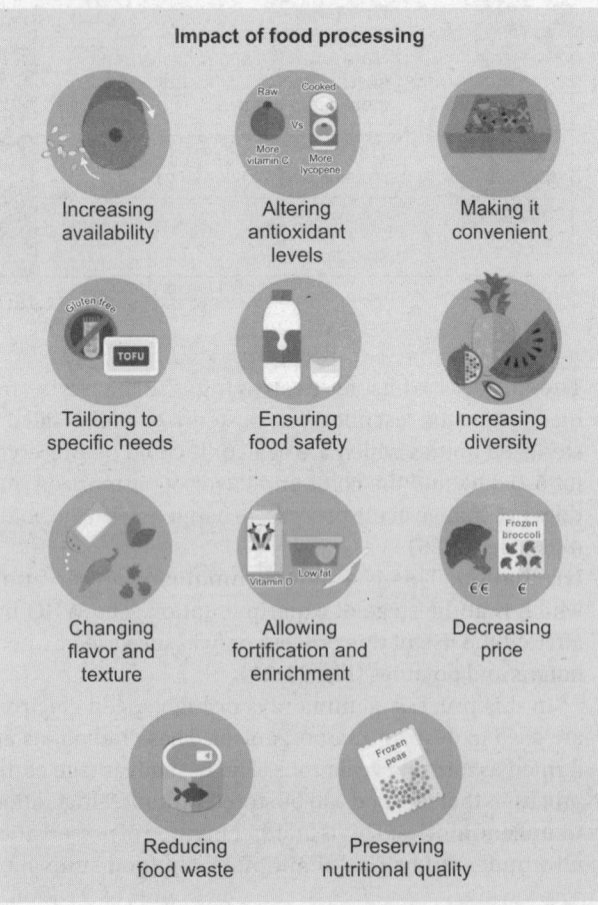

Fig. 11.30: Refrigerator or chilling temperature (0°C to 5°C).

- This has made such foods available throughout the year and has also stabilized their prices in these cities.
- Low temperatures chiefly inhibit the growth of microorganisms although freezing may result in the destruction of some microorganisms.

Freezing temperature:
- Freezing may preserve foods for long periods of time provided the quality of the food is good to begin with and the temperature of storage are far below the actual freezing temperature of food.
- Some microorganisms are destroyed during freezing preservation. The chief preservative effect of freezing temperatures lies in the inability of microorganisms to grow at freezing temperature.
- In vegetables, enzyme action may still produce undesirable effects on flavor and texture during freezing.
- The enzymes therefore must be destroyed by heating before the vegetables are frozen.

Slow Freezing Process
- It is also known as sharp freezing. In this method, the foods are placed in refrigerated cabinets at temperatures ranging from -4°C to -29°C.
- This method is adopted in home-freezers. Freezing may require from 3 to 72 hours under such conditions.

Quick Freezing Process
- The lower temperatures used -32°C to -40°C freeze foods so rapidly that fine crystals are formed and the time of freezing is greatly reduced over that required in sharp freezing.
- The fine crystals formed by quick freezing have a lesser effect on breaking up plant and animal cells than do methods of slow freezing that produce coarser ice crystals. In quick freezing, large quantity of food can be frozen in a short period of time.

Dehydro Freezing
- Dehydro freezing of fruits and vegetables consists of drying the food to about 50% of its original weight and volume and then freezing the food to preserve it.
- The quality of dehydro frozen fruits and vegetables is equal to that of fruits and vegetables frozen without preliminary drying.
- The cost in packing, freezing, storing and shipping of such foods is less because of the reduction in weight and volume of foods during dehydro freezing.
- The following figure depicts the relationship between bacterial growth and temperature. The rapid growth of bacteria occurs in the temperature zone of 60° F –120° F.

Uses of Heat or High Temperature

The destruction of microorganisms by heat is due to the coagulation of the protoplasm. The temperature and time used in heat processing a food depend upon the nature of the food and what other methods are combined with heat.

The various degrees of heating used in preservation of food can be classified into three: (a) Pasteurization, (b) Heating up to 100°C or 212°F and (c) Heating above 100°C.

Pasteurization
- The time and temperature used in the pasteurization process depend upon the product treated and the method used.
- In pasteurization, most of the spoilage organisms are killed but a few survive and hence must be inhibited by low temperatures or some other method, if spoilage is to be prevented.
- There are two methods of pasteurization: (1) flash method and (2) holder method.
- In flash method, otherwise called high temperature short time method, a high temperature for a short time is used, while in the holder method or low-temperature long-time method, a lower temperature for a longer time is used.
- There are slight variations in the time and temperature used for pasteurizing different foods, like milk, cream, ice cream mix and wines.

Heating up to a Temperature of About 100°C
- Most methods of cooking come under this. This temperature can be obtained by boiling any liquid food, by immersing a container in boiling water or by exposure to steam.
- Before the use of pressure cookers and autoclaves, canning was done at 100°C and this killed all bacteria except spores.

Heating above 100°C (212°F):
- Temperatures above 100°C are obtained by means of steam under pressure as in a pressure cooker or autoclave.
- Sterilization of foods can be brought about at 121°C for 15 minutes under moist conditions.

CANNING PROCEDURE

The details of canning procedures vary with the nature of the food to be canned, but there are certain important operations common to canning of all foods:

1. **Cleaning:** The first step in canning, whether done in the home or on a large scale in factories, is the thorough cleaning of the raw food to be preserved. By this means most of spoilage organisms are removed. On a large scale, cleaning is done with the help of various kinds of washers. The raw materials may be subjected to high pressure sprays or strong flowing streams of water, while passing along a moving belt.

2. **Blanching:** Blanching consists of the immersion of raw food materials, especially vegetables and fruits, into hot water or exposure to live steam.

    Blanching serves as an additional hot water wash. It softens fibrous plant tissues, inhibits the action of enzymes and fixes the natural color of certain products making them more attractive in appearance.

3. **Exhausting:** Gases are expelled by passing the open can containing the food through an exhaust box in which hot water or steam is used to expand the food and expel air and other gases from the contents and the head space area of

the can. After the gases are expelled, the can is immediately sealed, heat processed and cooled. In the case of certain products, exhausting is done by mechanical means, rather than by the use of heat. There are special machines which withdraw the air from the cans and they seal them at the same time—"vacuum packing".

4. **Sealing the container:** Each container must be sealed properly before it is subjected to the heat process, since recontamination of the contents must be prevented.
5. **Sterilizing the sealed container with its contents by heat processing:** This is meant to bring about complete sterilization to prevent spoilage of the food by microorganisms. This is usually done by the application of steam under pressure.

   The temperature and time used for heat processing depend on the kind of food, on the pH of the medium and other factors. It should however be remembered that an excessive period of heating at higher temperatures than necessary will spoil the product.

   A longer exposure to a relatively low temperature should be preferred to a short exposure at a higher temperature.
6. **Cooling the container:** The containers should be cooled rapidly to check the action of heat and prevent unnecessary softening of the food or change in color of the contents. Cooling can be done by means of air or water.

DRYING METHOD OF PRESERVATION

Microorganisms need moisture to grow. When exposed to sunlight or subjected to dehydration, the moisture in the food is removed and the concentration of water is brought below a certain level. This prevents the growth of microorganisms and thereby spoilage of food. Food preservation by drying is one of the oldest methods practiced from ancient times. This method consists of exposing food to sunlight and air until the product is dry **(Fig. 11.31)**.

Factors to be Considered in Drying Foods

- The temperature employed, which will vary with the food and the method of drying.
- The relative humidity of the air. It usually is higher at the start of drying than later.
- The velocity of the air.
- The duration of drying.

Treatment of Foods Before Drying

- Selection and sorting for size, maturity and wholesomeness.
- Washing, especially of fruits and vegetables.
- Peeling of fruits and vegetables by hand, machine or abrasion.
- Subdivision into halves, slices, shreds or cubes.
- Blanching or scalding of vegetables and some fruits like apricots and peaches.
- Sulfuring of light colored fruits and vegetables. Fruits are sulfured by exposure to sulfur dioxide gas produced by the burning of sulfur to a level of 1,000 to 3,000 ppm.

Methods of Drying

1. **Sun drying:** It is limited to regions with hot climates and a dry atmosphere and to certain fruits, such as raisins, prunes, figs, apricots, pears and peaches. It is a slow process. Many Indian foods are preserved by sun drying. Papads and vathals are made using this principle. Vegetables like cluster beans and curd chilli and fruits like jack fruit are preserved by this method. Fish and meat are also sun dried.
2. **Drying by mechanical driers:** Most methods of artificial drying involve the passage of heated air with controlled relative humidity over the food to be dried or the passage of the food through such air.

   Fruits, vegetables, nuts, fish and meat can be successfully preserved by this method. In the dehydration process, artificial drying methods (e.g., spray drier) are used for drying foods. Although it is expensive when compared to natural sun-drying procedures, it is very advantageous because the temperature and relative humidity can be manipulated **(Fig. 11.32)**.
3. **Spray drying:** Milk and egg are dried to a powder in spray driers in which the liquid is atomized and sprayed into a hot air stream for almost instant drying.
4. **Foam mat drying:** Foam mat drying may be used commercially with orange and tomato juice. In this process a small amount of edible foam stabilizer, such as monoglycerides or a modified soyabean protein with methyl cellulose is added to the liquid and stiff foam is produced by whipping. The foam is spread in a thin layer and dried in a stream of hot air. The product separates easily into small particles on cooling.

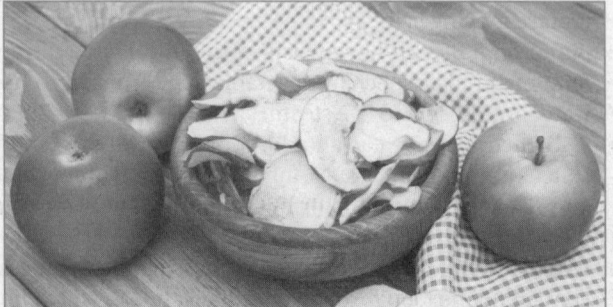

Fig. 11.31: Drying method of preservation.

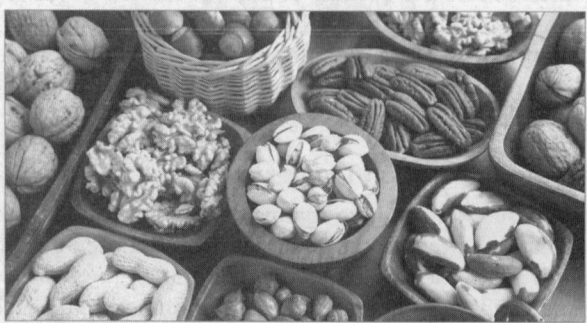

Fig. 11.32: Drying/dehydration of fruits and vegetables.

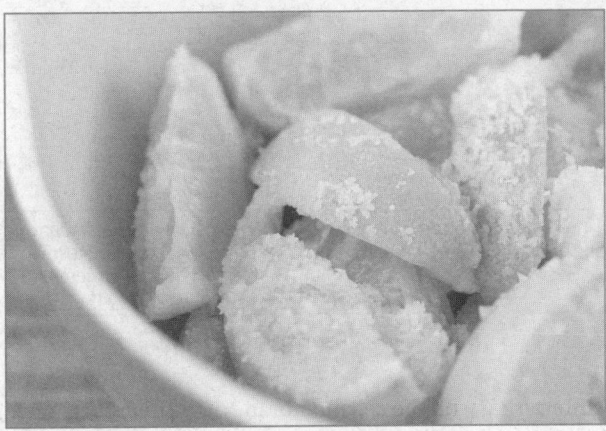

Fig. 11.33: Drying by osmosis.

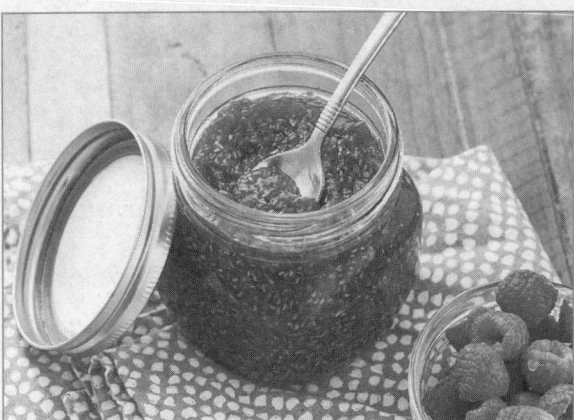

Fig. 11.34: Jam.

5. **Drying by osmosis:** Drying also results when fish is heavily salted. In this case, the moisture is drawn out from all cell tissues. The water is then bound with the solute, making it unavailable to the microorganisms.

   In osmotic dehydration of fruits, the method involves the partial dehydration of fruits by osmosis in a concentrated sugar solution or syrup **(Fig. 11.33)**.

6. **Freeze drying:** Removal of water from a product while it is frozen by sublimations is called freeze drying.

PRESERVATION BY HIGH CONCENTRATION OF SUGAR AND SALT

Sugar and salt aid in the preservation of products in which it is used due to their ability to bind water and make it unavailable for microbial growth. Salt is an effective preservative because it also ionizes to yield chlorine ion, which is harmful to organisms and reduces the solubility of oxygen in moisture, which are essential for the growth, and multiplication of microorganisms.

Jams, jellies and fruit juices are an important class of fruit products preserved using high concentration of sugar. Pickles are preserved using high concentration of salt.

Jam (Fig. 11.34)

1. Jams are prepared by boiling fruit pulp with sufficient amount of sugar to a reasonably thick consistency, firm enough to hold the fruit tissue in position.
2. In preparing jam, the fruit is crushed or finely cut and measured quantity of sugar and preservatives are added so that when cooked, the mass is fairly uniform throughout.
3. Jams can be prepared from all varieties of pulpy fruits, such as grapes, mango, sapota, banana, guava, etc.

Jelly (Fig. 11.35)

- Jellies are prepared by boiling fruits in water. The extract obtained is strained and measured quantity of sugar is added to it.
- The mixture is then boiled to a stage at which it will set to a clear gel. A perfect jelly should be transparent, well

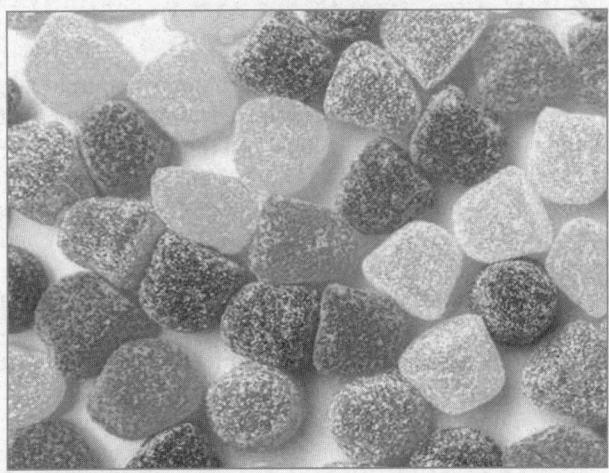

Fig. 11.35: Jelly.

  set, but not too stiff and should have the original flavor of the fruit.
- It should retain its shape when removed from the mould.
- Usually fruits, such as guava, pineapple, apple, grape and a mixture of fruits rich in pectin can be used for the preparation of jellies.

Fruit Juices

- Fruit beverages are prepared from different fruits, such as apple, mango, grapes, lime, pineapple, and sapota and in different forms, such as pure juices, crushes, squashes and cordials **(Fig. 11.36)**.
- The ratio of sugar and fruit juice in the preparation of various beverages is as follows:
  - Crushes: 25% fruit juice and 55% sugar.
  - Squashes: 25% fruit juice and 45% sugar.
  - Cordial: Clarified juice 1 liter and 250 g sugar.

In the preparation of fruit juices, citric acid is usually added to clarify the sugar syrup. Preservatives, such as sodium benzoate are added to tomato and grape juices while potassium meta bisulphite (KMS) is added to all other fruit beverages.

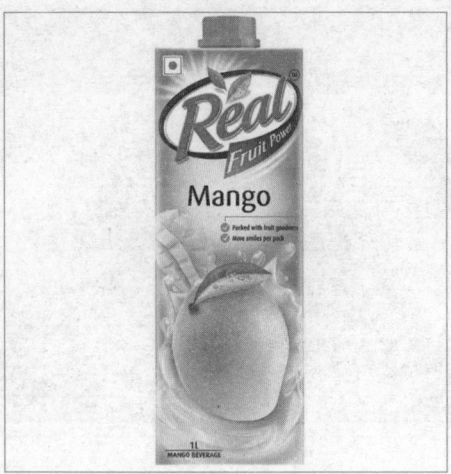

Fig. 11.36: Fruit juice.

Pickling

- The preservation of fruits and vegetables in common salt, vinegar, oil and spices are referred to as pickling. Salt binds the moisture in the food and thereby prevents the growth of microorganisms **(Fig. 11.37)**.
- The layer of oil that floats on the top of pickles prevents the entry and growth of microorganisms like moulds and yeast.
- Spices, like turmeric, pepper, chili powder and asafetida retard the growth of bacteria.
- Vinegar lowers the pH of the product thereby providing an unfavorable acidic environment for microbial growth.
- Mango, lime, ginger, garlic, tomato, chili, mixed vegetables, such as beans, carrot, cauliflower and peas are used widely in the preparation of pickles.

Preservation by Chemical Agents

Preservatives are defined as chemical agents who serve to retard, hinder or mask the undesirable changes in food. These changes may be caused by microorganisms, by enzymes of food or by purely chemical reactions. Certain chemicals when added in small quantities can hinder undesirable chemical reaction in food by **(Fig. 11.38)**:

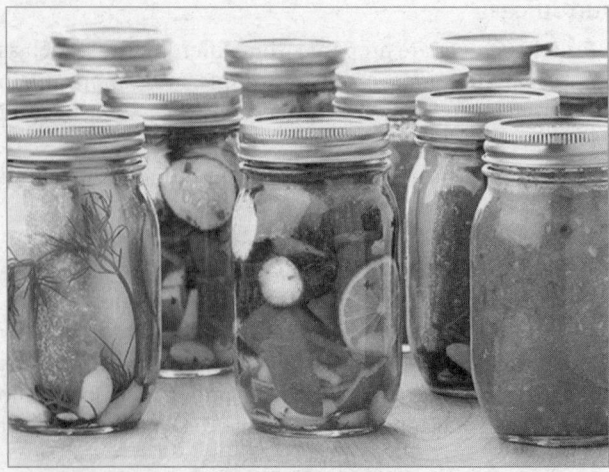

Fig. 11.37: Pickling.

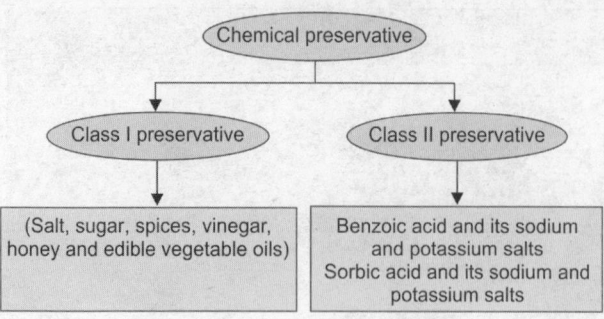

Fig. 11.38: Chemical preservative.

1. Interfering with the cell membrane of the microorganism, their enzyme activity or their genetic mechanism.
2. **Acting as antioxidants:** Maximum amounts allowed to be added to each type of food are regulated by law because higher concentrations can be a health hazard. Benzoic acid in the form of its sodium salt is an effective inhibitor of moulds and is used extensively for the preservation of jams and jellies.

Some of the other chemical preservatives used are:
- Potassium metabisulphite
- Sorbic acid
- Calcium propionate
- Sodium benzoate

The development of off-flavors (rancidity) in edible oils is prevented by the use of Butylated Hydroxy Anisole (BHA), Butylated Hydroxy Toluene (BHT), lecithin which is some of the approved antioxidants.

Figure 11.39 is depicted the preservative agents.

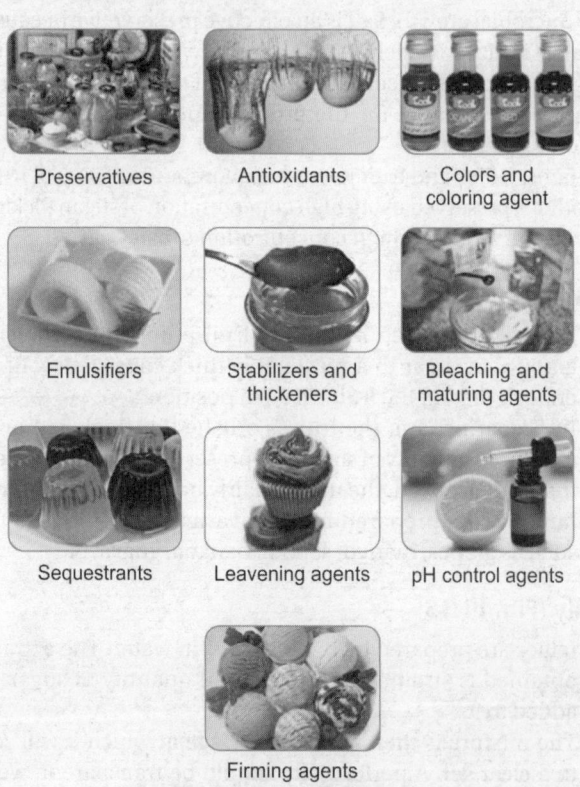

Fig. 11.39: Preservative agents.

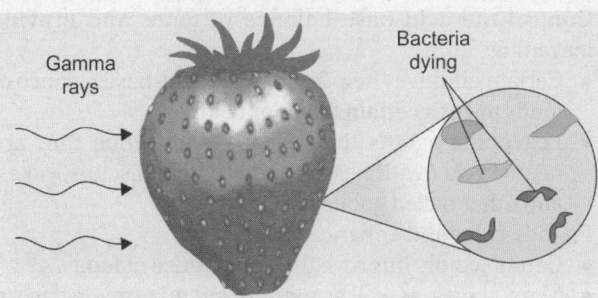

Fig. 11.40: Preservation by radiation.

Preservation by Radiation (Fig. 11.40)

Radiant energy can be used to preserve food. Gamma rays and beta particles produced by special electronic machines are sources of energy used to preserve food.

These waves penetrate throughout the food. As the waves and particles pass through the food, they collide with molecules in the food and in microorganisms. These result in chemical alterations. The goal of irradiation is to kill the microorganism and inactivate the enzymes without altering the food

Changes in the food are minimized if it is done in a vacuum, and if **ascorbic** acid is present. Berries and meat are preserved in this way.

■ FOOD ADDITIVES

Food additives are substances added to food as flavorants, nutrients, preservatives, emulsifiers, or colorants. In addition, foods may contain residues of chemicals used during the production of plant or animal crops, including pesticides, antibiotics, and growth hormones. The use of most food additives is clearly beneficial because it results in improved public health and prevention of spoilage, which enhances the food supply **(Fig. 11.41)**.

❏ Food additives are substances added to food to maintain or improve its safety, freshness, taste, texture, or appearance.
❏ Food additives need to be checked for potential harmful effects on human health before they can be used.
❏ The Joint FAO/WHO Expert Committee on Food Additives (JECFA), is the international body responsible for evaluating the safety of food additives.

Definition

Food additives defined as 'any substance, the intended use of which results or may reasonably be expected to result, directly or indirectly, in its becoming a component or otherwise affecting the characteristics of any food.' In other words, an additive is any substance that is added to food.

Purpose (Fig. 11.42)

Direct additives are those that are intentionally added to foods for a specific purpose. Indirect additives are those to which the food is exposed during processing, packaging, or storing. Preservatives are additives that inhibit the growth of bacteria, yeasts, and molds in foods.

Types of Food Additives

The different types of food additives used in food are **(Fig. 11.43)**:
1. Flavors and sweeteners
2. Antioxidants
3. Preservatives
4. Food colors (dyes)
5. Fat emulsifiers and stabilizing agent
6. Flour improver's antistaling agents and bleaches.
7. Nutritional supplements, such as vitamins, minerals, and amino acids.

Function (Box 11.3)

Food additives serve five main functions. They are:
1. Give the food a smooth and consistent texture:
   - Emulsifiers prevent liquid products from separating.
   - Stabilizers and thickeners provide an even texture.
   - Anticaking agents allow substances to flow freely.

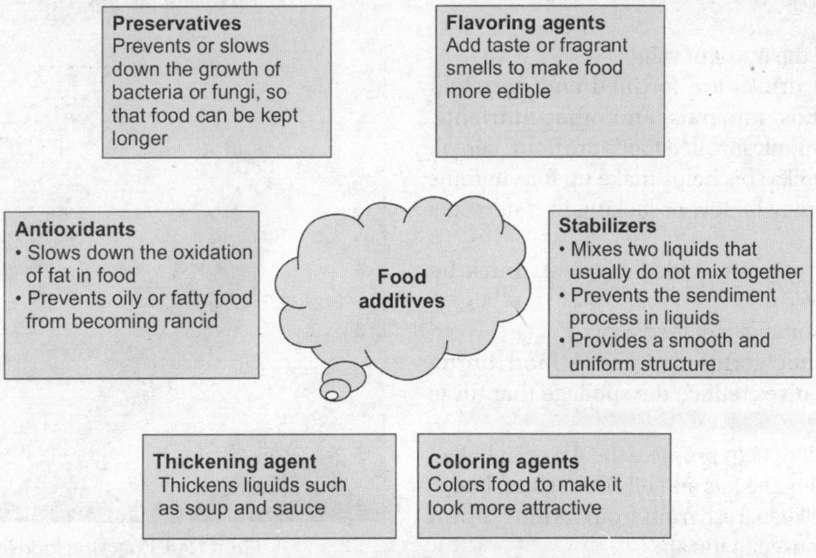

Preservatives
Prevents or slows down the growth of bacteria or fungi, so that food can be kept longer

Flavoring agents
Add taste or fragrant smells to make food more edible

Antioxidants
• Slows down the oxidation of fat in food
• Prevents oily or fatty food from becoming rancid

Food additives

Stabilizers
• Mixes two liquids that usually do not mix together
• Prevents the sendiment process in liquids
• Provides a smooth and uniform structure

Thickening agent
Thickens liquids such as soup and sauce

Coloring agents
Colors food to make it look more attractive

Fig. 11.41: Food additives.

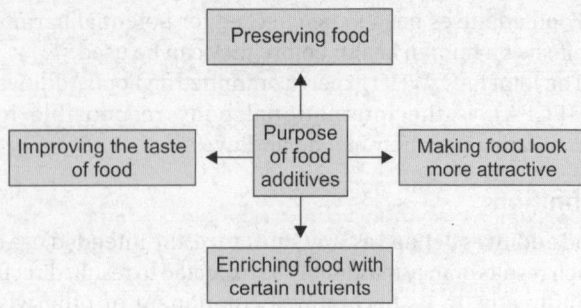

Fig. 11.42: Purpose of food additives.

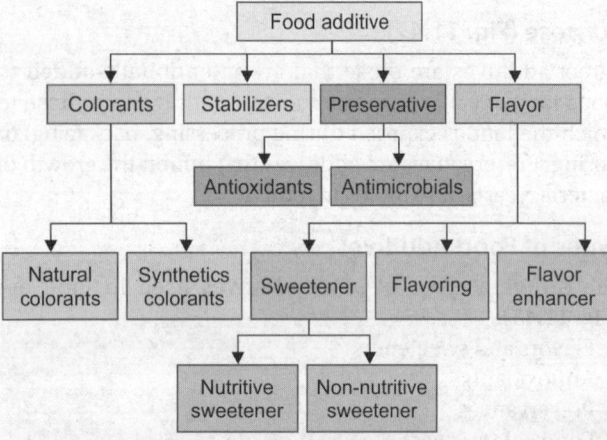

Fig. 11.43: Types of food additives.

> **Box 11.3:** Functions of food additive.
>
> In general, food additives are used to:
> - Preserving foods for survival
> - Decrease the risk of contamination by certain microbes
> - Maintain or improve nutritional quality
> - Enhance appearance, flavor
> - Control the acidity and alkalinity of food and provide leavening
> - Increase shelf-life
> - Reduce waste or
> - Contribute to convenience

2. Improve or preserve the nutrient value:
   - Many foods and drinks are fortified and enriched to provide vitamins, minerals, and other nutrients. Examples of commonly fortified foods are flour, cereal, margarine, and milk. This helps make up for vitamins or minerals that may be low or lacking in a person's diet.
   - All products that contain added nutrients must be labeled.
3. Maintain the wholesomeness of foods:
   - Bacteria and other germs can cause food borne illnesses. Preservatives reduce the spoilage that these germs can cause.
   - Certain preservatives help preserve the flavor in baked goods by preventing the fats and oils from going bad.
   - Preservatives also keep fresh fruits from turning brown when they are exposed to the air.
4. Control the acid-base balance of foods and provide leavening:
   - Certain additives help change the acid-base balance of foods to get a certain flavor or color.
   - Leavening agents that release acids when they are heated react with baking soda to help biscuits, cakes, and other baked goods rise.
5. Provide color and enhance flavor:
   - Certain colors improve the appearance of foods.
   - Many spices, as well as natural and man-made flavors, bring out the taste of food.

Figure 11.44 is depicted the checking food ingredients.

Food Additives Effect on Health

The use of food additives increases the market value, but some of the food additives show the following health problems:
- Usage of food with high food additive may lead to weight gain.
- Artificial colors may cause allergies and hyperactivity in children.
- It shows potential cancer-causing effects.
- Increased use of food additives leads to suppression in the immune response.
- It interferes with hormones, thereby affecting development and growth.
- It causes gastric irritation, diarrhea, asthma, nausea, respiratory irritation, etc.

Food Additives Agents

Food additives can be derived from plants, animals, or minerals or they can be synthetic. They are added intentionally to food to perform certain technological purposes which consumers often take for granted. There are several thousand food additives used, all of which are designed to do a specific job in making food safer or more appealing. WHO, together with FAO, groups food additives into 3 broad categories based on their function.

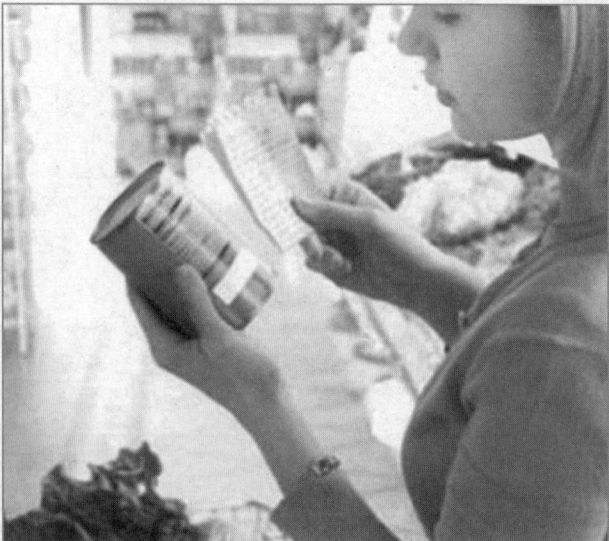

Fig. 11.44: Checking food ingredients.

Flavoring Agents

- Flavoring agents—which are added to food to improve aroma or taste—make up the greatest number of additives used in foods.
- There are hundreds of varieties of flavorings used in a wide variety of foods, from confectionery and soft drinks to cereal, cake, and yoghurt.
- Natural flavoring agents include nut, fruit and spice blends, as well as those derived from vegetables and wine. In addition, there are flavorings that imitate natural flavors.

Figure 11.45 is depicted the types of food additives.

Enzyme Preparations

- Enzyme preparations are a type of additive that may or may not end up in the final food product.
- Enzymes are naturally-occurring proteins that boost biochemical reactions by breaking down larger molecules into their smaller building blocks.
- They can be obtained by extraction from plants or animal products or from microorganisms, such as bacteria and are used as alternatives to chemical-based technology.
- They are mainly used in baking (to improve the dough), for manufacturing fruit juices (to increase yields), in wine making and brewing (to improve fermentation), as well as in cheese manufacturing (to improve curd formation).

Other Additives

- Other food additives are used for a variety of reasons, such as preservation, coloring, and sweetening.
- They are added when food is prepared, packaged, transported, or stored, and they eventually become a component of the food.
- Preservatives can slow decomposition caused by mould, air, bacteria, or yeast. In addition to maintaining the quality of the food, preservatives help control contamination that can cause food borne illness, including life-threatening botulism.
- Coloring is added to food to replace colors lost during preparation, or to make food look more attractive.
- Non-sugar sweeteners are often used as an alternative to sugar because they contribute fewer or no calories when added to food.

Advantages of Food Additives

- Food additives improve the quality, texture, consistency, appearance, and other technical requirements of the food material.
- Food additives are added to increase the shelf-life of the stored food or for cosmetic purposes.
- Antioxidants, preservatives, fat emulsifiers, and stabilizing agents as well as flavor improvers, are used to increase the shelf-life of the stored food. Dyes, flavors,

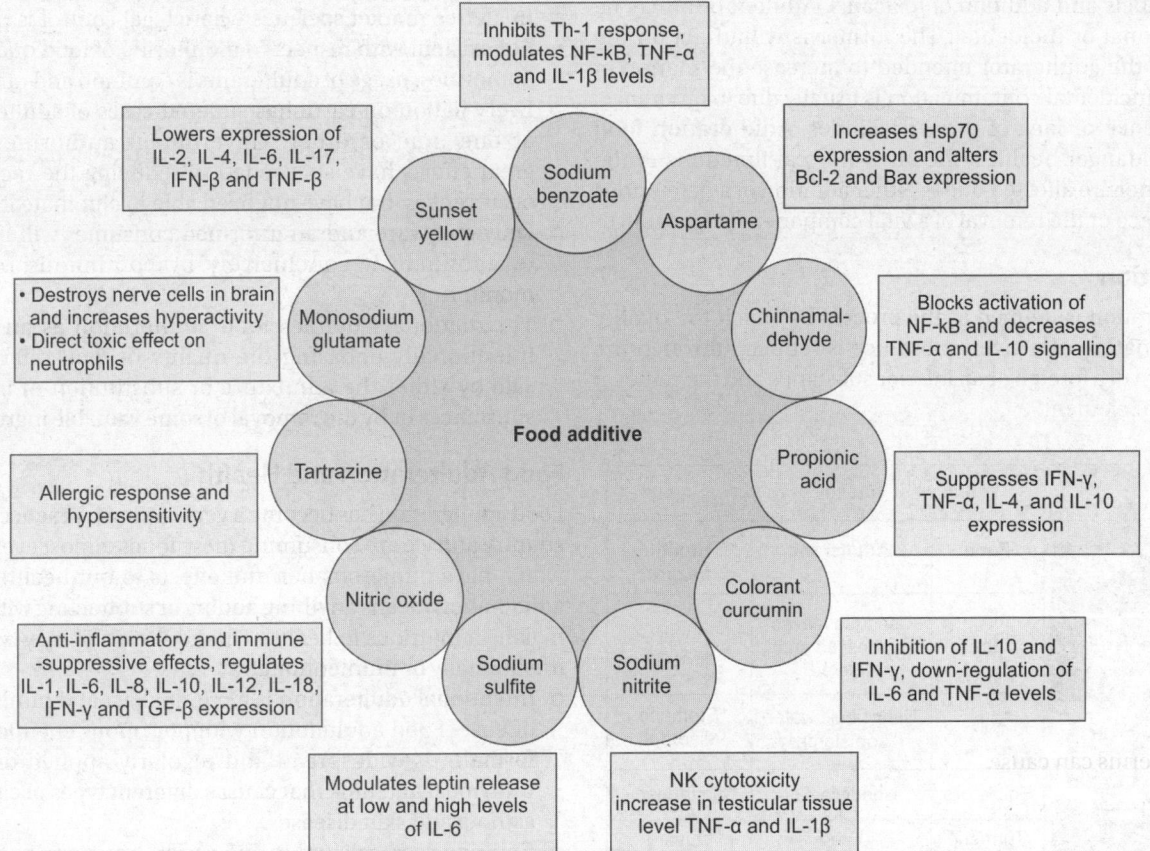

Fig. 11.45: Types of food additives.

and sweetening agents help to improve their cosmetic value.
- Food additives like nutritional supplements, such as vitamins, minerals, and amino acids have unique health benefits.
- With the help of food preservatives, seasonal crops and fruits are available throughout the year.
- Food additives are used to lower the calories.

Disadvantages of Food Additives
- Several additives can cause allergic reactions, gastric irritation, diarrhea, rashes, asthma, nausea, respiratory irritation, risk of cancer, etc.
- It may lead to hyperactivity and affect the nervous system.
- Food additives sometimes destroy vitamins in the food, replacing real ingredients.
- During food preservation, there may be a loss of nutritive value of the food.

FOOD ADULTERATION

Adulteration is defined as the process by which quality or the nature of a given substances is reduced though, the addition of a foreign or an inferior substance and the removal of vital element. A good example of addition of water to milk. Adulteration of food consists of a large number of practice, e.g., mixing, substitution, concealing, the quality, putting up decomposed foods for sale, misbranding or giving false labels and addition of toxicants. Adulteration may be intentional or incidental. The former is willful act on the part of the adulterator intended to increase the margin of profit. Incidental contamination is usually due to ignorance, negligence or lack of proper facilities. Adulteration food may endanger health if the physiological functions of the consumer are affected due to either addition of a deleterious substance or the removal of a vital component **(Fig. 11.46)**.

Definition
Adulteration is defined as the process by which the quality or the nature of a given substance is reduced through the addition of a foreign or an inferior substance and the removal of a vital element.

Watch what you eat		
Food	Adulterant	Health hazard
Tea	Used tea leaves processed and colored	Liver disorder
Milk	Unhygienic water and starch	Stomach disorder
Edible oils	Unedible oils	Carcinogenic
Turmeric powder	Lead chromate	Liver disorder

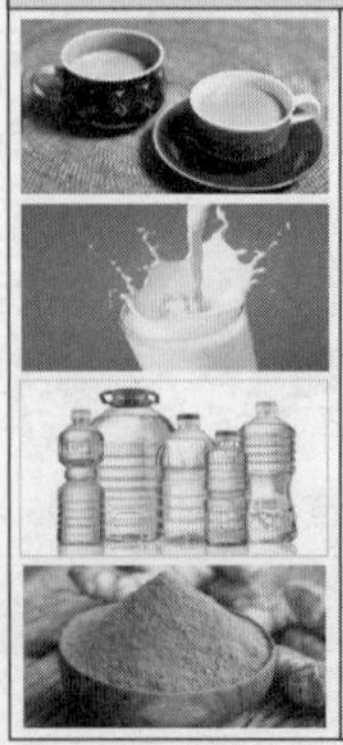

Fig. 11.46: Food adulteration.

- If the product sold by a vendor is not of the nature, substance or quality demanded by the purchaser or which it purports to be.
- If the product offered contains any substance or if it is so processed as to injuriously affect its nature, substance, or quality.
- If any inferior or cheaper substance has been substituted wholly or partly in the product, or any natural constituent has been wholly or partly abstracted from it, to affect its quality.
- If the product had been prepared, packed, or kept under unsanitary conditions, has become contaminated, injurious to health or is unfit for human consumption.
- If the container of the product is composed of any poisonous or deleterious substance which renders its contents injurious to health.
- If the product contains any prohibited coloring matter, preservatives, or contains any permitted coloring matter or preservative in excess of the prescribed limits.
- If the quality or purity of the product falls below the prescribed standard, or its constituents are present in proportions other than those prescribed, whether or not rendering it injurious to health.

Meaning of Food Adulteration
- Food adulteration is a growing menace that unscrupulous traders and manufacture all over the world indulge into exploit gullible consumers to make quick and easy money.
- In all free market societies where legal control is poor or nonexistent with respect to monitoring of food quality by authorities, usage of adulterants is common and rampant.
- Every nation on earth has suffered cases of adulteration at one time or other. Government authorities with great efforts have succeeded in reducing the recurrent occurrences; but have not been able to eliminate it.
- Only an aware and an informed consumer will be able to eliminate it conclusively by continuous routine monitoring.
- The dictionary defines food adulteration as an act of intentionally debasing the quality of food offered for sale by either the admixture or substitution of inferior substances or by the removal of some valuable ingredient.

Food Adulteration and Health
Food adulteration has become a very common practice in our country and we are consuming these foods almost every day, which have numerous harmful effects to our health. Food adulteration means anything adding or subtracting with food making it injurious to health. This adulteration may be done intentionally or unintentionally.
- Intentional adulteration is a criminal act and punishable offense. Food adulteration with poisonous chemical like formalin is widespread and regularly applied on fish, fruit, meat and milk that causes different types of cancers, asthma and skin diseases.
- Coloring dyes, calcium carbide, urea, brunt engine oil and even some permitted preservatives are used in excessive amount that affect multiple organs of human body.

- Mostly it causes cancer like colon, peptic ulcer diseases, and chronic liver diseases including cirrhosis and liver failure, electrolyte imbalance and eventually kidney failure.
- Heart diseases, blood disorders and bone marrow abnormality are also detected.
- Chance of malignancy increases and neurological impairment or brain functions are also often compromised.
- Skin problems are frequently seen including allergic manifestation. We know it is a punishable offence and it creates health hazards and can kill human being, even then we forget everything just for business interest.

Types of Adulterants (Fig. 11.47)

1. **Intentional:** Intentional adulterants are those substances that are added as a deliberate act on the part of the adulterer with the intention to increase the margin of profit, e.g., sand, marble chips, stones, mud, chalk powder, water, dyes, etc. These adulterants cause harmful effects on the body.
2. **Incidental:** These adulterants are found in food substances due to ignorance, negligence or lack of proper facilities. It is not a willful act on the part of the adulterer, e.g., pesticides, droppings of rodents, larvae in food.
3. **Metallic contamination:** Arsenic from pesticides, lead from water, mercury form effluents from chemical industries, tin from cans.

Food Materials and Common Adulterants

- **Cereals (wheat and rice):** Mud, grits and soapstone bits
- **Dals:** Coaltar dyes, khesari dal
- **Black pepper:** Dried seeds of papaya
- **Chilly powder:** Saw dust, brick powder
- **Milk:** Extraction of fat, addition of starch and water
- **Ghee:** Vanaspathi
- **Sweet meats:** Nonpermitted colors
- **Fresh green peas in packing:** Green dye
- **Coffee powder:** Date husk, tamarind husk, chicory
- **Tea dust/leaves:** Black gram husk, tamarind seeds powder, saw dust, used tea dust
- **Butter:** Starch, animal fat.

Table 11.1 is depicted the types of food stuff, adulteration and their harmful effects.

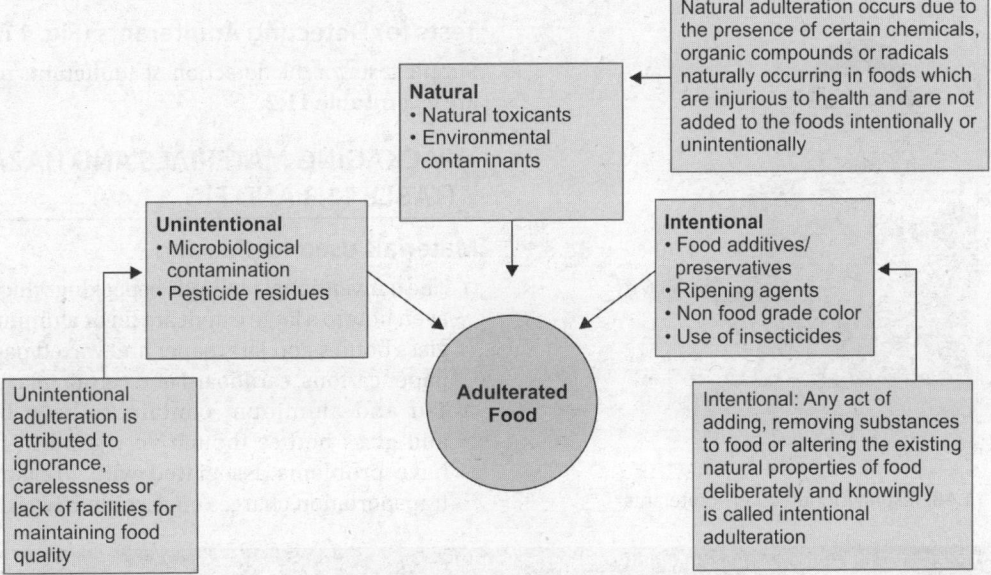

Fig. 11.47: Types of adulteration.

Table 11.1: Types of food stuff, adulteration and their harmful effects.

Food article	Adulterant	Harmful effects
Bengal gram dal and thoor dal	Khesari dal	Lathyrism cancer
Tea	Used tea leaves processed and colored	Liver disorder
Coffee powder	Tamarind seed, date seed powder	Diarrhea
	Chicory powder	Stomach disorder, giddiness and joint pain
Milk	Unhygienic water and starch	Stomach disorder
Khoa	Starch and less fat content	Less-nutritive value
Wheat and other food grains (bajra)	Ergot (a fungus containing poisonous substance)	Poisonous
Sugar	Chalk powder	Stomach-disorder
Black powder	Papaya seeds and light berries	Stomach, liver problems
Mustard powder	Argemone seeds	Epidemic dropsy and glaucoma

Contd...

Contd...

Food article	Adulterant	Harmful effects
Edible oils	Argemone oil	Loss of eyesight, heart diseases, tumors
	Mineral oil	Damage to liver, carcinogenic effects
	Karanja oil	Heart problems, liver damage
	Castor oil	Stomach problem
Asafetida	Foreign resins galbanum, colophony resin	Dysentery
Turmeric powder	Yellow aniline dyes	Carcinogenic
	Nonpermitted colorants like metanil yellow	Highly carcinogenic
	Tapioca starch	Stomach disorder
Chilli powder	Brick powder, saw dust	Stomach problems
	Artificial colors	Cancer
Sweets, juices, jam	Nonpermitted coaltar dye, (metanil yellow)	Metanil yellow is toxic and carcinogenic
Jaggery	Washing soda, chalk powder	Vomiting, diarrhea
Pulses (green peas and dal)	Coaltar dye	Stomach pain, ulcer
Suapari	Color and saccharin	Cancer
Honey	Molasses sugar (sugar plus water)	Stomach disorder
Carbonator water beverages	Aluminum leaves	Stomach disorder
Cloves	Cloves from which volatile oil has been extracted	Cheating, waste of money

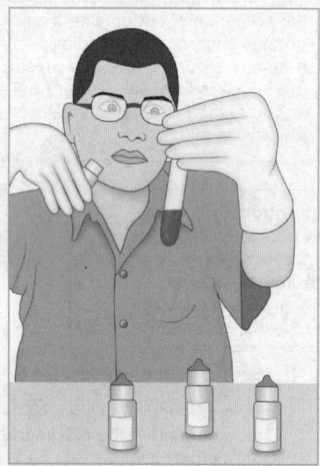

Fig. 11.48: Testing for detecting adulterants.

Tests for Detecting Adulterants (Fig. 11.48)

Simple tests for the detection of adulterants present in foods are given **Table 11.2**.

PACKAGING MATERIALS AND HAZARDS (TABLE 11.3 AND FIG. 11.49)

Materials used for Packing

- The conventional methods of packing which are prevalent even now to a large extent are tin or aluminum containers, glass bottles and jars, paper and waxed paper wrappings, paper cartons, cardboard and certain plastic containers.
- Tin and aluminum containers have become costly and glass bottles though very good in many respects have problems associated with breakage and heavy transportation charges on account of weight.

Table 11.2: Simple tests for the detection of adulterants present in foods.

Sl. No.	Substance	Adulterant	Test
1.	Asafetida (hing)	Resin or gum scented and colored	• Pure asafetida dissolves in water to form a milk white solution • Pure asafetida burns with a bright flame on being ignited (burning)
2.	Sugar	Chalk powder	Dissolve in a glass of water. Chalk will settle down in the bottom
3.	Cardamom	Oil is removed and pods are coated with talcum powder	On rubbing, talcum will stick to the fingers. On testing, if there is hardly any aromatic flavor, it indicates removal of essential oil
4.	Turmeric (haldi)	Metanil yellow coloring	When concentrated hydrochloric acid is added to a solution of turmeric powder, it turns magenta if yellow is present
5.	Chilli powder	Sawdust and color	Sprinkle on the surface of water, sawdust floats. Added color will make the water colored
6.	Coffee	Chicory	Shake a small portion in cold water. Coffee will float while chicory will sink, making the water brown
7.	Coriander powder	Horse dung powdered	Soak in water. Horse dung will float which can be easily detected
8.	Cloves (lavang)	Oil may be removed	If so, cloves may be shrunken in appearance

Contd...

Contd...

Sl. No.	Substance	Adulterant	Test
9.	Cumin seeds (jeera)	May contain grass seeds colored with charcoal dust	If rubbed in hand, fingers will turn black
10.	Ghee	Vanaspathi	Dissolve one teaspoon of sugar in 10 ccs of hydrochloric acid and 10 ccs of the melted ghee and shake thoroughly for one minute. Allow it to stand for 10 minutes. If vanaspathi has been added, the aqueous layer will be red in color
11.	Jaggery	Metanil yellow	Hydrochloric acid added to a solution of jaggery will turn its color to magenta
12.	Rawa	Iron filing to add weight	Pass magnet through the rawa. Iron filings will cling to it
13.	Betelnut powder (*Supari*)	Sawdust and artificial color	Sprinkle in water. Sawdust will float and the added color will dissolve in water.
14.	Milk	• Mashed potato, other starches • Water	Add a drop of tincture of iodine. Iodine, which is brown turns blue if starch is present. Put a drop of milk on a polished vertical surface and allow to flow. Pure milk flows slowly leaving a white trail. Adulterated milk will flow immediately without leaving a mark
15.	Tea dust	Used tea leaves dried, powdered and artificially colored	Sprinkle the dust on a wet white filter paper. Spots of yellow, pink and red appearing on the paper indicates that tea is artificially colored
16.	Edible oil	Argemone	A reddish-brown precipitate is formed when oil and hydrochloric acid are gently mixed with ferric chloride solution, if argemone is present
17.	Saffron	Maizefibers dried, colored and scented	• Genuine saffron is tough. Spurious saffron is brittle and breaks easily • Dissolves easily in water, giving aroma of saffron
18.	Sago	Sand and talcum	Gritty feel in mouth. Pure sago swells on burning and leaves hardly any ash
19.	Black pepper	Dried seeds of papaya fruit	Papaya seeds are shrunken oval in shape and greenish-brown in color and have a repulsive flavor distinct from the bite of black pepper
20.	Coconut oil	Any other oil	Place a small bottle of oil in refrigerator. Coconut oil solidifies leaving the adulterant as a separate layer
21.	Bajra	Fungus (ergot infested)	Immerse in salt water. Fungi will float to the top
22.	Cinnamon (*Dalchini*)	Cassia bark	Added color comes off in water
23.	Common salt	White powdered stone, chalk	Stir a spoonful of simple salt in a glass of water. The presence of chalk will make the solution white
24.	Honey	Molasses (sugar and water)	A cotton wick dipped in pure honey when lighted with a match stick burns, if adulterated it will not burn and will produce a cracking sound
25.	Peanut oil	Cottonseed oil	Mix 2.5 mL of oil or fat with 2.5 mL Halphen's reagent. Lightly screw cap and heat in boiling water for 30 minutes. The test is positive if a rose color is obtained

- Continued use of paper in increased volume dwindles the natural resources.
- Against the conventional materials there has emerged increased usage of newer materials derived synthetically.
- Some polymeric plastic materials are polystyrene, polyvinyls, polyvinydines and derivatives, vinyl acetate, polyethylene, polypropylene and polyesters.
- Folding cartons and paper board boxes are used extensively in the food industry. Tin plate containers-the cylindrical open-top variety are mostly used for processed foods.
- Aluminum is used principally as foil, e.g., chocolates. It is also used as bottle caps and closures and easy open tops for cans.

Table 11.3: Types of packing and their functions.

Rigid packaging	Flexible packaging	Semi-flexible packaging	Function of packaging
• Glass or plastic bottle • Glass, plastic, and metal jar • Plastic and metal pack and can • Cap, tray, tank	• Plastic food bag • Foam packaging • Shrink, bubble, cling plastic wrap • Squeezable tube • Stand-up packet • Vacuum bag	• Caps and closure • Carton box • Tetra pack multi-material	• Protection from oxygen, temperature variation, moisture, light • Biological protection against micro-organisms • Physical protection from damage • Information about the product • Identification of the product

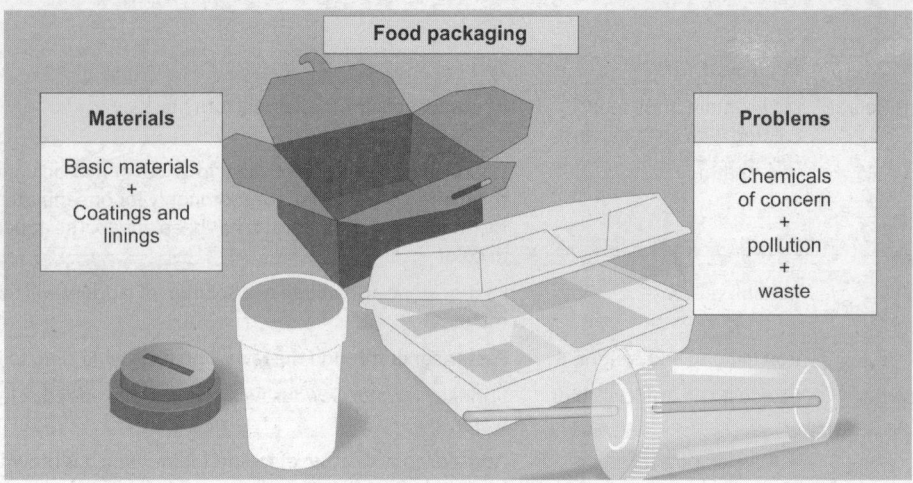

Fig. 11.49: Food packing materials and techniques.

- Polystyrene is principally made into tubs for ice creams, packs for eggs, sausages and small packages for butter, jam and cheese.
- Bags made from the simplest of all plastic polymers, namely, polyethylene or 'polythene' as commonly known have relatively low preserving qualities.
- Material, such as polyesters vinyl acetate derivatives and multilayer films made out of a combination of different materials has good preserving characteristics for food products.
- Timber crates are used extensively for packing weights above 100 kg. Plastic crates are well established in the dairy industry and for the transportation of bottled beer, mineral water and soft drinks. High density polythene is used for milk crates.
- Shrink wrap packaging is a system where heat shrinkable thermoplastic film is wrapped around an article or a group of articles.
- The film is made to shrink around it by the application of heat to achieve a skin light package. Canned food products, bottles and jars of all types can be shrinking wrapped.
- Nowadays it is expected that packaging material be environment friendly or ecofriendly, that is, it should not pose many problems for mankind and hazards to the environment.
- For example, corrugated boxes are ecofriendly and are preferred for exporting. They can be effectively replaced for conventional wooden boxes which need to destroy the trees.

Table 11.4: Chemicals causes hazards.

Source	Why a hazard?
Agricultural chemicals (e.g., pesticides, herbicides)	If improperly applied, some can be acutely toxic or may cause long-term health effects
Cleaning chemicals (e.g., acids, caustics)	Can cause chemical burns if present in the food at high levels
Equipment components (e.g., copper pipe fittings)	Acidic foods can cause leaching of heavy metals from pipes and joints (e.g., copper and lead)
Maintenance chemicals (e.g., lubricants)	Some chemicals that are not approved for food use may be toxic
Packaging materials (e.g., tin)	High nitrite levels in food can cause excessive detinning of uncoated cans resulting in excessive levels of tin in the food

- Recyclability of packaging is desirable so as to preserve the resources of the packaging material for future generations.

Figure 11.50 is depicted the types of chemical hazards, **Table 11.4** is depicted the chemicals causes hazards, and **Figure 11.51** is depicted the packing and preserving the fruits.

Chemical hazards
(Food processing)
- Preservatives
- Colors and dyes
- Flavor enhancers
- Water additives
- Packaging materials
- Processing aids

Fig. 11.50: Types of chemical hazards.

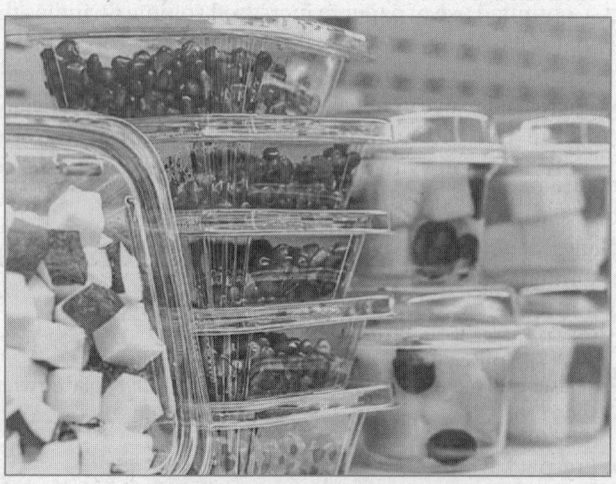

Fig. 11.51: Packing and preserving the fruits.

Packaging Hazards

Plastics, such as cellulose acetate, polyamide polyethylene polypropylene and polyvinyl chloride are often used as packing materials because they are light in weight and are resistant to diffusion due to solvents and high temperatures.

However care should be taken those only food grade plastic packing materials should be used for packaging foods to prevent the following packaging hazards.
- Production of noxious thermal breakdown products which are injurious to health.
- Formation of toxic residues that result when subjected to heat treatment for sterilization of the contents.
- Unfavorable reactions between acid and oil content of the food and the packaging material.

FOOD LAWS

The Government of India is fully aware to the possibilities of food being adulterated. It has therefore, empowered several agencies and promulgated a number of acts and orders to contract the menace. Agencies and institutions have also been created to lay down standards for the quality of foods. The manner in which the food is processed and packaged is also covered by a number of regulations. Following measures have been taken by the government to control the quality of food.

Signage and Customer Notices

It is important to note that though the provisions of FSSAI do not specifically deliver for any statutory and regulatory requirements either for signage or customer notices, but it has certain provisions with regard to advertisement of products by food business operators (FBO's).
- Makes a wrong or misleading representation concerning the need for, or the usefulness.
- Gives to the public any guarantee of the efficacy that is not based on an adequate or scientific justification thereof, provided that where a defense is raised to the effect that such guarantee is based on adequate or scientific justification, the burden and responsibility of proof of such defense shall lie on the person raising such defense.
- Falsely represents that the foods are of a particular quality, quantity, standard, or grade-composition.

Packaging and Labeling

The Packaging and Labeling Regulations provide the general requirements for labeling of food products prescribed under the FSSAI, some of the packaging and labeling rules are as follows:
- Contents on the label shall be clear, prominent, indelible and easily readable by the consumer under normal conditions of buying and use;
- Label in pre-packaged foods products shall be completed in such a way that they will not become separated from the container;
- Pre-packaged food shall not be described or presented on any label or in any manner that is wrong, misleading or illusory or is likely to make an inaccurate impression regarding its character in any respect;
- Where the container is roofed by a wrapper, the wrapper shall carry the necessary information or the label on the container shall be readily readable through the outer wrapper and not obscured by it.
- The particulars of declaration required under these Rules to be mentioned on the label shall be in Hindi or English in Devnagri script: Provided that nothing herein contained shall prevent the use of any other language in addition to the language required under this regulation and regulations.

In addition to above rules and regulations mentioned, every package of food shall also carry the following information on the label:
- Name of the food
- List of ingredients
- Date of manufacturing or packing
- Best before and use by date
- Nutritional information
- Name and complete address of the manufacturer
- Net quantity
- Lot/code/batch identification
- Declaration regarding vegetarian and nonvegetarian
- Declaration regarding food additives
- Country of origin for imported food
- Instructions for use

Prevention of Food Adulteration Act

The Prevention of Food Adulteration Act, (PFA) 1954 operated by the Directorate General of Health Services, Ministry of Health was designed for the following purposes:
- It formulates and monitors the standard of quality and purity of foods with emphasis on prevention of adulteration of foods.
- It is the basic structure intended to protect the common consumer against the supply of adulterated foods.
- It makes provision for prevention of adulteration of food and lays down the rule that no person shall manufacture for sale, store, sell or distribute any adulterated or misbranded food or food which contravenes the provision of act or rules.
- It has set the yardstick to ascertain adulteration. According to this act, a food is deemed to be adulterated—if:
  - It is not of the nature, substance and quality, which the food ought to be.
  - It contains any other substance which affects, or if the article is so processed so as to affect injuriously the nature, substance and quality of the food.
  - It contains added inferior or cheaper substance that affects the nature and quality of the food.
  - Any constituent of the food is removed so as to affect injuriously the nature, quality and substance of the food.
  - It is prepared, packed and stored under unsanitary conditions.
  - It contains any filthy, disgusting, rotten, decomposed substance of a diseased animal or vegetable substance

or is insect-infested or otherwise unfit for human consumption.
- The article is obtained from a diseased animal.
- The article contains a poisonous ingredient or any other ingredient injurious to health.
- The container renders the food injurious to health.
- It contains excessive or prohibited colors.
- It contains excessive or prohibited preservatives.
- It does not satisfy the standards prescribed by the authorities.

Under the provision of the PFA Act, the Government of India has promulgated PFA rules which specify the following details:
- Qualification, duties and functions of food analysts, food inspectors and central food laboratory.
- Procedure for drawing test samples and sending them to the analyst and laboratory.
- Specification for the identity and purity of food.
- Tolerance for contaminants, preservatives, emulsifiers and other additives.

Prevention of Food Adultration

Prevention of Food Adulteration (PFA) Act was amended in 1964, 1976 and lately in 1986 to make the Act more stringent. A minimum imprisonment of 6 months with minimum fine of ₹ 1,000 is envisaged under the act for cases to proven adulteration, where as for the cases of adulteration which may render the food injurious to cause death or such harm which may amount to grievous hurt (within the meaning of section 320 of IPC) the punishment may go up to life imprisonment and fine which shall not less than ₹ 5,000.

CONSUMER PROTECTION

A number of laboratories are authorized by the Central government to collect samples of food suspected to the adulteration and analyze them. They can prosecute the manufacturers of these foods if they find the food to be adulterated. The various laboratories engaged in the collection of samples and analysis of such food.
- Municipal laboratories in big cities
- Food and Drug Administration laboratories of states.
- Central food testing laboratory of the Government of India.
- Laboratories of the export inspection council.
- Central grain analysis laboratory

Food adulteration is a social evil—the general public has lack of awareness of the dangers of adulteration and disinterest it occurs continuously. Unless the public rises up against the trades and unscrupulous food inspectors, the evil cannot be curbed.

PREVENTION OF FOOD ADULTERATION, ACT 1954

Objectives
- To protect the public from poisonous and harmful foods
- To prevent the sale of substandard foods
- To protect the interests of the consumers by eliminating fraudulent practices

Meaning of adulterant: Any material which is or could be employed for the purposes of adulteration.

Definition of food: Any article used as food or drink for human consumption other than drugs and water and includes:
- Any article which ordinarily enters into or is used in the composition or preparation of human food
- Any flavoring matter or condiments and
- Any other article which the Central Government may having regard to its use, nature, substance or quality, declare, by notification in the official gazette as food for the purpose of this Act.

Concept of Adulteration

An article of food shall be deemed to be adulterated:
- If the article sold by vendor is not of the nature, substance or quality demanded by the purchaser.
- If the article contains any other substance which affects the substance or quality thereof.
- If any inferior or cheaper substance has been substituted wholly or in part for the article so as to affect the nature, substance or quality of the product.
- If any constituent of the article has been wholly or in part extracted to affect the quality thereof.
- If the article has been prepared, packed or kept under unsanitary conditions whereby it has become contaminated or injurious to health.
- If the article consists wholly or in part of any filthy, putrefied, rotten decomposed or diseased animal or vegetable substance or is insect-infested or is otherwise unfit for human consumption.
- If the article is obtained from a diseased animal.
- If the article contains any poisonous or other ingredient which renders it injurious to health.
- If the container of the article is composed, whether, wholly or in part of any poisonous or deleterious substance which renders sits contents injurious to health.
- If any coloring matter other than that prescribed in respect thereof is present in the article or if the amounts of the prescribed coloring matter which is present in the article are not within the prescribed limits.
- If the article contains any prohibited preservative or permitted preservative in excess of the prescribed limits.
- If the quality or purity of the Article falls below the prescribed limits of variability which renders it injurious to health
- If the quality or purity of the article falls below the prescribed standard or its constituents are present in quantities not within the prescribed limits of variability which renders it injurious to health.

SALE OF CERTAIN ADMIXTURES PROHIBITED

Sale by himself or by his servant or agent is prohibited in case of:
- Cream which has not been prepared exclusively from milk or which contains less than 25% of milk fat
- Milk which contains added water

- Ghee which contains any added matter not exclusively derived from milk fat
- Selling skimmed milk as whole milk
- Mixture of two or more edible oils as an edible oil
- Vanaspati to which ghee or any other substance has been added
- Any article of food which contains any artificial sweetener beyond the prescribed limit
- Turmeric containing any foreign substance
- Mixture of coffee and other substance except chicory
- Dahi or curd not made out of milk
- Milk or milk products containing constituents other than of milk

PROCEDURE FOR SAMPLING AND ANALYSIS

Any food inspector can enter and inspect any place where any article of food is manufactured or stored for sale or stored for the manufacture of any other article of food for sale or exposed or exhibited for sale or where any adulterant is manufactured or kept and take samples of such article of food or adulterant for analysis.

- Notice will be issued by the Inspector in writing then and there to the seller indicating his intention.
- Three samples are taken and the signature of the seller is affixed to them.
- One sample is sent for analysis to Public Analyst under intimation to the Local Health Authority.
- The other two samples are sent to the local health authority for further reference.

PENALTIES

Guilt will be punished with imprisonment for a term which shall not be less than six months and up to 3 years and with fine up to ₹ 1,000.

IMPORTANT MISCELLANEOUS PROVISIONS

- If any extraneous additions of coloring matter are added, the same should be indicated on the labels.
- From the labels the blending composition of ingredients should be clear to the customer.
- Sale of khesari gram individually or as an admixture is prohibited.
- Prohibition of use of carbide (acetylene) gas in ripening is prohibited.
- Sale of ghee with Reichert value less than the permitted level.
- Sale of admixture of ghee or butter is prohibited.
- Addition of artificial sweetener should be mentioned on the label.
- Sale of food colors without license prohibited.
- Sale of insect damaged dry fruits and nuts prohibited.
- Food prepared in rusted containers, chipped enamel containers and untinned copper/brass utensils are treated as unfit for human consumption.
- Containers not made of plastic material which is not according to the standards are not to be used.
- Selling salseed fat or any other purpose except for bakery and confectionery is prohibited.
- Store of insecticides in the same premises where food articles are stored is prohibited.
- Milk powder or condensed milk can be sold only with ISI mark.
- Use of more than one type of preservative is prohibited.
- Crop contaminants beyond certain specified level is treated as adulterant.
- Naturally occurring toxic substances in the food material beyond certain level is considered as unfit for human consumption.
- No antioxidant, emulsifiers and stabilizing agent is permitted beyond the prescribed level.
- No insecticides should be sprayed on the food items.
- Oils can be manufactured only in factories licensed for such purpose.

FOOD STANDARDS

ISI Standards

Various committees, including representatives from the government, consumers and industry, formulate the Indian Standards Institution (ISI). Standards are laid for vegetable and fruit products, spices and condiments, animal products and processed foods. The products are checked for quality by the ISI in their own network of testing laboratories at Delhi, Mumbai, Kolkata, Madras, Chandigarh and Patna or in a number of public and private laboratories recognized by them.

The AGMARK Standard

The AGMARK standard was set up by the Directorate of Marketing and Inspection of the Government of India by introducing an Agricultural produce Act in 1937. The word 'AGMARK' seal ensures quality and purity. A sample AGMARK seal is as below The word AGMARK is derived from the words 'Agricultural Marketing'. It is a standard of quality based on the physical and chemical characteristics of food, both the natural and those acquired during processing. Products graded under AGMARK include vegetable oils, ghee, butter, rice, groundnut, pulses and spices. These standards ensure accurate weight and correct selling price.

BUREAU OF INDIAN STANDARDS

The Bureau of Indian Standards (BIS) lays down criteria for standardization of vegetables and fruit products, spices and condiments, animal products and processed food. Manufacturers are allowed to use the BIS label on each unit of their product, if their products conform to the standards laid down by BIS. The products are checked for quality by laboratories certified by BIS. BIS is also known as ISI (Indian Standard Institution). Some of the items which require compulsory BIS certification under PFA Act include artificial food colors, natural food colors, food additives, infant formula; milk-cereal based weaning foods, milk powder and condensed milk.

Export Inspection Council

The council has been constituted to check the quality of a number of food materials meant for export. The council has powers to reject any food, which does not measure up to the standards prescribed for the food. Canned food, such as mango juice, pineapple juice, frozen food, such as shrimp, pomfrets are subject to scrutiny by this body before export.

FOOD AND NUTRITION BOARD

The Food and Nutrition Board was formed in 1964 under the Ministry of Agriculture to bring variety in the dietary habits with the dual objective of reducing the demand of food grains and to make the individual diet more nutritious. In April 1993, the board was brought under the women and child development department in accordance with the National Nutrition Policy.

Activities of Food and Nutrition Board

Education and Training in Nutrition

- Nutrition demonstration programs.
- Training in domestic preservation of fruits and vegetables.
- Integrated nutrition education.
- To observe nutrition weeks (1–7 September).
- To observe world food day (16 October).
- To observe world breastfeeding week (1–7 August).

Development and Enhancement of Nutritive Foods

- Assessment of regularity and quality of supplementary food in anganwadi.
- To encourage production of nutritious foods in the community.
- Fortification of food:
  - To fortify milk with vitamin A.
  - To fortify salt with iodine.
- Food analysis.
- Research and development.
- National nutrition policy and implementation.
  - Constitution of a standing committee for implementation of national nutrition program.
  - Activities for control of micro nutritional deficiencies.
  - Nutritional surveillance.
  - Planning of district level diet and nutritional programs and their implementation.

NUTRITION SOCIETY OF INDIA

The Nutrition Society of India (NSI) was established in 1967, is an organization dedicated to keep abreast of the latest developments in the basic and applied aspects of science of Nutrition. The society continues to analyze issues related to the diverse aspects of nutrition. The society activities involve scientists, programmers and policy makers throughout the country and abroad who are working in the field. Through its annual conference, the society provides a forum for new ideas, encourages innovations, recognizes important research findings, increases awareness of the latest survey data and promotes action programs.

FOOD AND AGRICULTURAL ORGANIZATION

Food and Agricultural Organization (FAO) is one of the specialized agencies of the United Nations formally formed in 1945 with headquarter in Rome. It was the first United Nations organization specialized agency created to look after several areas of World cooperation. FAO's primary aim is to increase agriculture production to keep pace with growing population in the world (**Fig. 11.52**).

Chief Aims

- To increase the efficiency of farming, fisheries and forestry.
- To improve the condition of rural people.
- To ensure that the food is consumed by the people who need it in sufficient quantities and in right proportions.
- To develop and maintain a better state of nutrition throughout the world.
- To help nations raise their living standards.

The main functions of FAO are:

- To help nations raise their living standards.
- To improve nutrition level of people of all countries.
- To secure improvement of production and distributions of all food and agricultural products.
- To improve the conditions of rural populations.

The main activity of this agency is to promote production of food to keep pace with the rising world population. The joint WHO/FAO expert committee provides the base for many cooperative activities, such as nutritional surveys, training courses, seminars, and the coordination or related research programs.

Objectives of FAO

The FAO has organized a World Freedom from Hunger Campaign (FFHC) in 1960. The primary objective of FAO is

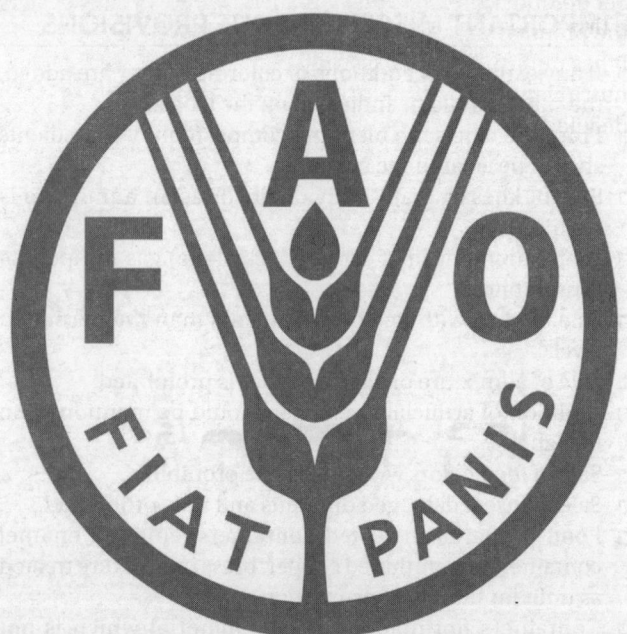

Fig. 11.52: Logo of Food and Agricultural Organization.

towards ensuring that the food is consumed by the people who need it in sufficient quantities and in right proportions to develop and maintain a better state of nutrition throughout the world.

FAO and Other Organizations

- The FAO also collaborating with other international agencies, such as UNICEF, WHO in applied nutritional program.
- The joint WHO/FAO expert committee have provided the basis for many cooperative activities—nutritional surveys training courses, seminars and the coordination of research programs on brucellosis and other zoonoses.

Cooperative for Assistance and Relief Every-Where

Cooperative for assistance and relief everywhere (CARE) was founded in North America in 1945. It is one of the world's largest independent nonprofit, non-sectarian international relief and developmental organization. CARE provides emergency aid and long-term development assistance.

CARE began its operation in India in 1950. Till the end of 1980s, the primary objective of CARE India was to provide food for children in the age group of 6–11 years. From mid 1980s CARE India focused its food support in the ICDS programme and in development programmes in the areas of health and income supplementation.

CARE India has given help in the field of medicine, literacy, vocational training and agriculture. It also helps schools by providing garden tools, pumps and improved seeds to grow more food. It also provides mobile medical vans, X-ray machines, diagnostic equipments, eye glasses and frames, medical books, medicine and vitamins.

NIN (National Institute of Nutrition), Hyderabad

Set up under Indian Council of Medical Research (ICMR) is the premier research institution of the country **(Fig. 11.53)**. It has published many research publications including "The nutritive value of Indian Foods". This handbook provides detailed information on the nutrients composition of a wide range of common Indian foods. Up to date information on nutritional requirement and recommended dietary allowances and guidelines for formulation of nutritionally rich diets are also provided by NIN for the benefit of health professionals and informed public. The data on nutrient composition of foods given are based mainly on Indian research work carried out at the National Institute of Nutrition, Hyderabad itself.

Vision: "To achieve optimal nutrition of vulnerable segments of population, such as women of reproductive age, children, adolescent girls and elderly by 2020." (NIN website)

Mission: "To enable food and nutrition security conducive to good health, growth and development and increase productivity through dedicated research, so as to achieve the national nutrition goals set by the government of India in the national nutrition policy." (NIN website)

Objectives

- To identify various dietary and nutrition problems prevalent among different segments of the population.
- To continuously monitor diet and nutrition situation of the country.
- To evaluate effective methods of management and prevention of nutritional problems.
- To conduct operational research connected with planning and implementation of national nutrition programs.
- To dovetail nutrition research with other health programs of the government.
- Human resource development in the field of nutrition.
- To disseminate nutrition information.
- To advice governments relating to nutrition.

Central Food Technological Research Institute

Central Food Technological Research Institute (CFTRI) is situated in Mysuru. It came into existence during 1950. A network of its founders and inspiring and dedicated scientists had the great vision to pursue in depth research and development in the areas of food science and technology. The Bengal famine of 1943 and the ravages of the Second World War made the Government of India realize that the key to food security was in the right intervention of science and technology to conserve, preserve, process and distribute the available food resources. CFTRI was declared open on 21st October 1950 as the next step **(Fig. 11.54)**.

Through the decades since then, CFTRI has produced and provided scores of technology solutions that have given a powerful thrust to the development of indigenous food industries and played a notable role in the socioeconomic transformation of the nation.

Technology Milestones of CFTRI

- Formation of infant food using buffalos milk.
- Extraction of plant protein for the nutrition base for a new class of food supplements: Energy food, Indian multipurpose food, miltone and several weaning foods.
- Improvement in the efficiency of process for handling, drying and willing of staple cereals.

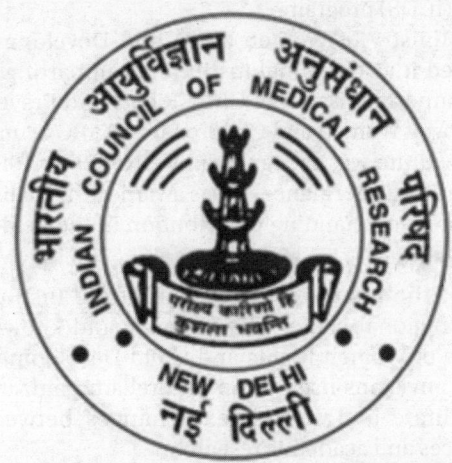

Fig. 11.53: Logo of Indian Council of Medical Research (ICMR).

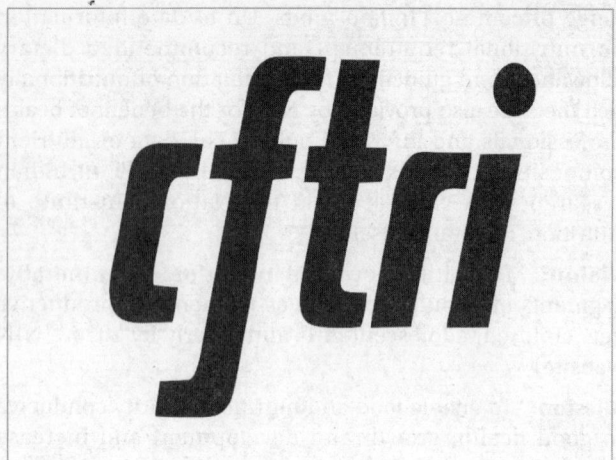

Fig. 11.54: Logo of Central Food Technological Research Institute.

- Design and fabrication of energy efficient and cost effective equipment for milling food grains and pulses.
- Refinement of millets and production of diversified millet products with enhanced nutritive value.
- Efficient methods for parboiling paddy.
- Formulation of products for preparing traditional Indian snacks.
- Production of spice and oil resins by indigenous technology.
- Fermentation and drying of cocoa mass, cocoa butter and cocoa powder by indigenous technology.

Support Area Milestones

- Establishment of the International Food Technology Training Centre (IFTTC) in collaboration with FAO—the nucleus of an internationally referred center of excellence in advanced knowledge in foods.
- Selection by the UNU as an Associated Institution.
- Recognition by the University of Mysore for postgraduate studies and research in food technology, food science and allied disciplines.
- Adoption by the National Information System for Science and Technology (NISSAT) as a sectoral information centre (NICFOS) for food science and technology in India.
- Establishment of a state-of-the-art pilot plant.
- Establishment of the International School of Milling Technology: An Indo-Swiss venture.
- ISO 9001 certification.

Vision

- A model organization for scientific industrial research and a path setter in the new paradigm of self-financed R&D in the country.
- A global platform providing competitive R&D and high quality science-based technical services across the world.
- A vital source of science and technology for national societal mission which provide a human a face to the organization's endeavors.

Mission

- Generate and apply knowledge of food science and food technology for optimal conservation and utilization of the nation's resources.
- Integrate scientific and technological knowledge into conventional and traditional systems and local and regional realities.
- Add value and utility to agro-resources through R&D and contribute to sustain development, food security and food safety.
- Aid and promote the development of food industry through interdisciplinary, innovative and state-of-the-art solutions.
- Set national standards for food quality, and spread food quality consciousness all around.
- Sustain leadership in long-term strategic research and technology development.
- Integrate the food supply chain from the cultivator to the consumer so that cultivators get optimal returns from processing, and consumers get the food that they want, when they want, where they want, in whatever form they want and at affordable cost.
- Build and bolster bonds with nodal agencies from the global to the grassroots level, particularly in the area of multilevel human resources development.
- Develop new knowledge continuously, to address contemporary challenges and answer future emergencies.

National Institute of Public Cooperation and Child Development

National Institute of Public Cooperation and Child Development (NIPCCD) is a premier organization devoted to promotion of voluntary action research, training and documentation in the field of women and child development. It was established in New Delhi in the year 1966 under Societies Registration Act of 1860. It functions under the aegis of the Ministry of Women and Child Development. The Institute has four Regional Centers, at Guwahati (1978), at Bengaluru (1980), at Lucknow (1982), and Indore (2001) to cater to the specific needs of the country. This institute trains the functionaries of the Integrated Child Development Services (ICDS) program.

The Ministry of Women and Child Development has designated it as the nodal institute for imparting training for two important issues of Child Rights and Prevention of Trafficking of Women and Children for SAARC countries.

The institute was recognized by UNICEF in 1985 for its expertise and performance. It was awarded the Maurice Pate Award for its outstanding contribution in the field of child development.

Vision of the institute: The vision of the Institute is to become regional center of excellence and knowledge in the fields of Women Rights and Child Development. This institute envisions itself as an umbrella organization that will facilitate and stimulate exchanges between field experiences and academic research.

Mission of the institute:
The Institute shares the belief that human progress and overall development is fundamentally rooted in the progress of women and children and in the realization of their rights. Working with this conviction the strategic mission of NIPCCD is defined as:

- Developing into an organization with a strong civil society orientation while retaining characteristic advantages of technical institutions.
- Forging strategic alliance with premier training institutes in other countries.
- Intensification of collaborative ventures in the areas of training, research and documentation.
- Acquiring flexibility in offering a broad spectrum of training opportunities that meet the changing demands in the context of issues related to women and children at national, regional and international level.
- Integrating select programs of the Institute into the professional training system, though accreditation of these programs by the AICTE and other accrediting Institutions.

CONCLUSION

Cooking is an art. It is linked with the dietary habits and cultural pattern of people. Almost all foods consumed today need some form of cooking and processing before they are fit for serving and consumptions. The three R's for nutrient preservation are to reduce the amount of water used in cooking, reduce the cooking time and reduce the surface area of the food that is exposed. Waterless cooking, pressure cooking, steaming, stir-frying and microwaving are least destructive of nutrients. Frozen vegetables can be steamed.

BIBLIOGRAPHY

1. Antia FP. Clinical Dietetics and Nutrition, 3rd edition. Oxford University Press, Bombay, 1986.
2. Briggs GM, Doris HC: Nutrition and Physical Fitness, 11th edition. Harcourt College Publishers, New York, USA, 1984.
3. Cataldo CB, Whitney EN, DeBruyne LK. Nutrition and Diet Therapy–Principles and Practice, West Publishing Co St Paul, 2003.
4. Joshi SA. Nutrition and Dietetics, Tata McGraw Hill, New Delhi, India, 1992.
5. Schmidl MK, Labuza TP (Eds). Essentials of Functional Foods. Gaithersburg, MD: Aspen Publishers; 2000.
6. Shils MS, Benjamin CA, Catherine R, Robert J. Cousins: Modern Nutrition in Health and Disease, 10th edition. Lippincott, Williams & Wilkins, Baltimore, USA, 2005.
7. Swaminathan M. Essentials of Food and Nutrition, Volume I and II, 2nd edition. Ganesh, Madras, India, 1985.

REVIEW QUESTIONS

Long Essays
1. Explain the various methods of cooking and its effect on nutrients.
2. Write a note on household methods of preservation of foods. What are the golden rules to prevent vitamin loss?
3. Describe personal hygiene of food handlers. Explain the signs of good meat hygiene and hygiene of slaughter houses.
4. a. What are food additives? Enumerate the classification of food additives.
   b. Write a note on food adulteration.
5. Define cooking; explain the principles of cooking.
6. Discuss the various methods of cooking with examples.
7. What is effect of cooking on food? Explain with examples.
8. Define food hygiene and discuss various methods of food storage.
9. Define food adulteration, types of adulterants and legislature measures to control it.

Short Essays
1. What are purposes of cooking?
2. What are different methods of cooking?
3. What is safe food handling?
4. Explain food hygiene and sanitation.
5. Explain food preservation.
6. Mention various food storage methods.
7. What are different household methods used for preservation of food.
8. What is the different food borne disease?
9. What are various methods to control food adulteration?
10. Explain PFA–1954 Act.

Short Answers
1. Canning and bottling.
2. Principles of food preservation.
3. Solar cooking.
4. Microwave cooking.
5. Dry heat methods.
6. Pressure cooking.
7. Moist heat methods.
8. Objectives of cooking.
9. Central food technological research institute.
10. Food and nutrition board.
11. AGMARK standard.
12. Consumer protection.
13. Food laws.
14. Types of adulterants.
15. Flavoring agents.
16. Food additives.
17. Preservation by chemical agents.
18. Canning procedure.
19. Causes of food spoilage.
20. Measures to prevent loss of nutrients.

CHAPTER 12

Nutrition Assessment and Nutrition Education

CHAPTER OUTLINE

- ❖ Objectives of Nutritional Assessment
- ❖ Methods of Assessment—Clinical Examination, Anthropometry, Laboratory and Biochemical Assessment,
- ❖ Assessment of Dietary Intake Including Food Frequency Questionnaire (FFQ) Method
- ❖ Nutrition Education—Purposes, Principles and Methods

■ TERMINOLOGY

- ▫ **Bitot's spots:** Clinical sign of vitamin A deficiency, characterized by dryness of the eyes accompanied by foamy accumulations on the conjunctiva that often appear near the outer edge of the iris.
- ▫ **Body mass index (BMI):** Defined as an individual's body mass (in kilograms) divided by height (in meters squared)—BMI units = kg/m^2. Acute malnutrition in adults is measured by using BMI.
- ▫ **Early warning system:** An information system designed to monitor indicators that may predict or forewarn of impending food shortages, worsening of the nutritional situation or famine.
- ▫ **Goiter:** Swelling of the thyroid gland in the neck caused by iodine deficiency.
- ▫ **Growth monitoring and promotion:** Individual-level assessment where the growth of infants and young children are monitored over time in order to identify and address growth faltering and growth failure.
- ▫ **Height-for-age nutritional index:** A measure of stunting or chronic malnutrition.
- ▫ **Mid-upper-arm circumference:** The circumference of the mid-upper arm is measured on a straight left arm (in right-handed people) midway between the tip of the shoulder (acromion) and the tip of the elbow (olecranon). It measures acute malnutrition or wasting in children aged 6–59 months. The mid-upper-arm circumference (MUAC) tape is a plastic strip, marked with measurements in millimeters. MUAC <115 mm indicates
- ▫ **Nutritional index:** Different nutritional indices measure different aspects of growth failure (wasting, stunting and underweight) and thus have different uses. The main nutritional indices for children are weight-for-height, MUAC-for-age, sex and height, height-for-age, weight-for-age, all compared to values from a reference population. In emergency situations, weight-for-height (wasting) is commonly used for nutritional assessments.
- ▫ **Nutrition survey:** Survey to assess the severity, extent, distribution and determinants of malnutrition in a population. Nutrition surveys in emergencies assess the extent of undernutrition or estimate the numbers of children who might require supplementary and/or therapeutic feeding or other nutritional support.
- ▫ **Nutritional screening:** Individual-level assessment where each person is measured in order to identify and refer those needing further check-ups or such services as supplementary or therapeutic feeding.
- ▫ **Rickets:** Caused by vitamin D deficiency, rickets affects bone development; severe cases result in bowing of the legs.
- ▫ **Scurvy:** Caused by vitamin C deficiency; typical signs of scurvy include swollen and bleeding gums and the slow healing of wounds or reopening of old wounds.
- ▫ **Wasting:** Technically defined as below minus 2 standard deviations from median weight-for-height of a reference population.
- ▫ **Weight-for-age:** Nutritional index, a measure of underweight (or wasting and stunting combined).
- ▫ **Weight-for-height:** Nutritional index, a measure of acute malnutrition or wasting.

■ INTRODUCTION

Nutritional status is now recognized as a significant indicator of the health of the individuals and/or population. It is important for screening and identification of individuals and populations who are affected/at risk with malnutrition. This, in turn, bears importance in formulating nutritional intervention and awareness programs. Nutritional status can be assessed using a number of methods. The direct methods are anthropometry, biochemical assessment, clinical signs and symptoms, and dietary intake. The indirect methods are based on vital statistics. A nutrition assessment is an in-depth evaluation of both objective and subjective data related to an individual's food and nutrient intake, lifestyle, and medical history. Once the data on an individual is collected and organized, the practitioner can assess and evaluate the nutritional status of that person. The assessment leads to a plan of care, or intervention, designed to help the individual either maintain the assessed status or attain a healthier status.

DEFINITION

- "Nutritional assessment can be defined as the interpretation from dietary, laboratory, anthropometric, and clinical studies. It is used to determine the nutritional status of individual or population groups as influenced by the intake and utilization of nutrients"—**Gibson, 2005**.
- A nutritional assessment can be defined as—a structured way to establish the nutritional status and energy requirements by objective measurements and whereby, accompanied by objective parameters and in relation to specific disease indications, an adequate (nutritional) treatment can be developed for the patient. All this happens preferably in a multidisciplinary setting.
- Nutritional assessment may be defined as a judgment of the quality and quantity of the intake and the subsequent utilization of nutrients. The methods adopted for nutritional assessment can be classified into two groups—Direct Methods and Indirect Methods—**WHO**.

MEANING OF NUTRITION ASSESSMENT

- A nutrition assessment is an in-depth evaluation of both objective and subjective data related to an individual's food and nutrient intake, lifestyle, and medical history. Once the data on an individual is collected and organized, the practitioner can assess and evaluate the nutritional status of that person.
- **An easy way to remember types of nutrition assessment is ABCD:** Anthropometric, biochemical, clinical, and dietary. Anthropometry is the measurement of the size, weight, and proportions of the body.
- Common anthropometric measurements include weight, height, MUAC, head circumference, and skin fold.
- The purpose of nutrition assessment is to obtain, verify, and interpret data needed to identify nutrition-related problems, their causes, and significance.
- It is an ongoing, nonlinear and dynamic process that involves data collection and continual analysis of the patient/client's status compared to specified criteria.
- **The NCP includes four steps:** Nutrition assessment, nutrition diagnosis, nutrition intervention, and nutrition monitoring and evaluation.
- A comprehensive nutritional assessment includes:
  - Anthropometric measurements of body composition
  - Biochemical measurements of serum protein, micronutrients, and metabolic parameters
  - Clinical assessment of altered nutritional requirements and social or psychological issues that may preclude adequate intake.

PURPOSE

- The purpose of nutrition assessment is to obtain, verify, and interpret data needed to identify nutrition-related problems, their causes, and significance.
- It is an ongoing, nonlinear and dynamic process that involves data collection and continual analysis of the patient/client's status compared to specified criteria.
- This contrasts with nutrition monitoring and evaluation where food and nutrition professionals use the same data to determine changes in patient/client behavior, nutritional status, and the efficacy of nutrition intervention.

OBJECTIVES

- To be aware of the methods that is being employed by researchers to document nutritional status
- To know the importance of studying nutritional status in a country, such as India
- Understand that WHO has evaluated the methods that can be used and has also come up with recommendations that needs to be understood
- To realize that each method has its own merits and demerits that need to be understood so as to use a method that is well-suited to the study model and conditions.
- To recognize the symptoms of different deficiency diseases and infections need to be learnt.

GOALS

- Timely identification of malnourished patients or patients at risk, so that the dietician can start her nutritional treatment as soon as possible;
- To determine the quantity of malnutrition, so an adequate assessment of the individual nutritional need is possible
- Collecting data for diagnostic purposes;
- Monitoring changes in the nutritional status during a nutritional intervention;
- Collecting data for scientific research;
- Monitoring the patient's nutritional status during hospitalization;
- Improving the nutritional assessment method.

SYSTEMS OF NUTRITIONAL ASSESSMENT

Three types of nutritional assessment systems have been employed both in population-based studies and in the care of hospitalized patients:

1. **Nutrition surveys:** Cross-sectional evaluations of selected population groups; conducted to generate baseline nutritional data, to learn overall nutrition status, and to identify subgroups at nutritional risk
2. **Nutrition surveillance:** Continuous monitoring of the nutritional status of selected population groups (e.g., at-risk groups) for an extended period of time; conducted to identify possible causes of malnutrition
3. **Nutrition screening:** Comparison of individuals' parameters of nutritional status with predetermined standards; conducted to identify malnourished individuals requiring nutritional intervention (**Fig. 12.1**).

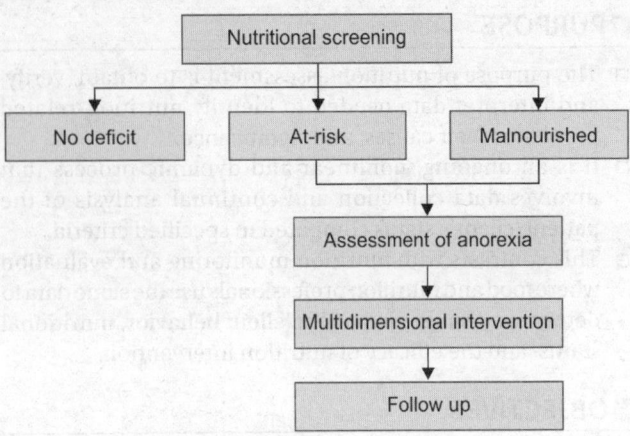

Fig. 12.1: Nutritional screening techniques.

METHODS OF NUTRITIONAL ASSESSMENT (FIG. 12.2)

Systems of nutritional assessment can employ a wide variety of specific methods. In general, however, these methods fall into five categories:

1. **Dietary assessment:** Estimation of nutrient intakes from evaluations of diets, food availability, and food habits (using such instruments as food frequency questionnaires, food recall procedures, diet histories, food records).
2. **Anthropometric assessment:** Estimation of nutritional status on the basis of measurements of the physical dimensions and gross composition of an individual's body.
3. **Clinical assessment:** Estimation of nutritional status on the basis of recording a medical history and conducting a physical examination to detect signs (observations made by a qualified observer) and symptoms (manifestations reported by the patient) associated with malnutrition.
4. **Biochemical assessment:** Estimation of nutritional status on the basis of measurements of nutrient stores, functional forms, excreted forms, and/or metabolic functions.
5. **Sociologic assessment:** Collection of information on non-nutrient-related variables known to affect or be related to nutritional status (e.g., socioeconomic status, food habits and beliefs, food prices and availability, food storage and cooking practices, drinking water quality, immunization records, incidence of low birth-weight infants, breastfeeding and weaning practices, age- and cause-specific mortality rates, birth order, family structure).

Figure 12.3 is depicted the nutritional assessment steps.

TYPES OF ASSESSMENT

Direct Methods

Direct methods are directly related with the individual and the parameters taken are considered to be objective, whereas indirect methods are the methods which rely on various demographic indices that are related to the community. Each method is unique in its advantages and limitations. Ideally, the results of all the methods should be taken together to assess nutritional status and formulate suitable intervention programs to improve the level of nutrition and health.

Figure 12.4 is depicted the direct nutritional assessment.

Types of Direct Methods

1. Anthropometric measurements
2. Biochemical assessments
3. Clinical examinations
4. Dietary assessments

It can be remembered as "ABCD"
A for Anthropometric measurements
B for Biochemical assessments

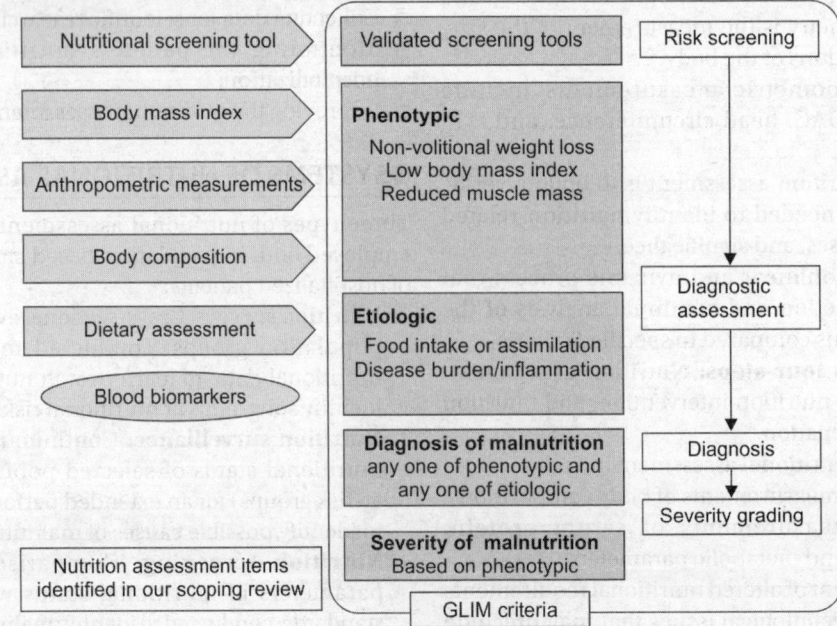

Fig. 12.2: Nutrition assessment methods.

Chapter 12: Nutrition Assessment and Nutrition Education

Nutritional screening:
Use MUST screen system; when the score is 2 or more, there is a high risk

⇩

Refer to dietitian

⇩

Nutritional assessment:
- History (24-hour dietary record, food frequency)
- Activity states (bed rest, light)
- Feeding status (e.g., normal, acceptable, poor appetite, NPO)
- GI function (e.g., normal, vomiting, diarrhea)
- Biochemical tests (blood, urine)

⇩

Nutritional intervention (education):
Registered dietitians can provide nutritional information, care and support for patients and their families who are currently dealing with cancer

⇩

Nutritional monitoring and evaluation:
- Check patient/client/group understanding and compliance with plan
- Measure and compare to patient's previous status, nutrition goals, or reference standards

Fig. 12.3: Nutritional assessment steps.

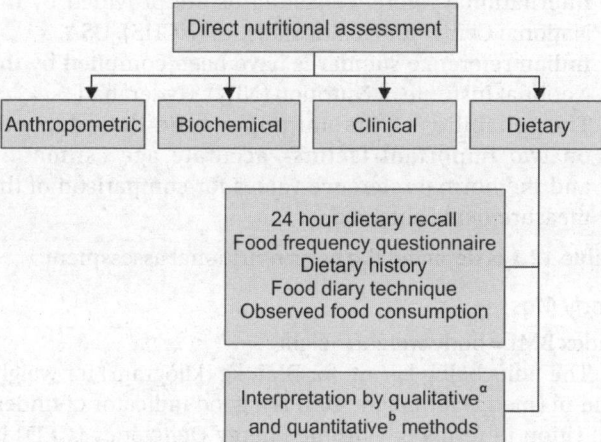

Fig. 12.4: Direct nutritional assessment.

C for Clinical examinations
D for Dietary assessments

Indirect Methods

☐ These are the vital statistics data that are obtained from' the census and demographic data. They also include data from other important sources, such as per capita income and population density.

☐ The World Health Organization (WHO) has played a significant role in formulating and standardizing the methods used to assess nutritional status of individuals and populations.

☐ Very important recommendations were given by the WHO Expert Committee on Medical Assessment of Nutritional Status in 1963.

Anthropometric Methods

Anthropometry is a technique to assess nutritional status and body composition of an individual or population. The most commonly utilized measurements to assess nutritional status are height/length, weight, mid-upper arm circumference, head circumference, chest circumference and waist circumference (**Figs. 12.5A to D**).

☐ The commonly utilized indices are the body mass index, height-for-age, weight-for-age, weight for-height, waist-hip ratio and waist-height ratio.

☐ The method of biochemical assessment estimates the concentrations of essential dietary constituents in the body to evaluate malnutrition.

☐ The important tests are hemoglobin estimation, urine and stool examination. Specific vitamins and micro-nutrients deficiencies can also be documented using this method.

☐ Clinical signs and symptoms are observed in the skin, mouth, gums, nails, lips, eyes and hair of the subjects. The internal signs are in the cardiovascular, gastrointestinal and nervous systems.

☐ The qualitative dietary method uses food pyramids to estimate food requirements, servings and consumption, while the quantitative method calculates the amount of energy and specific nutrients for each food using food consumption tables.

☐ Body composition of an individual or population. Anthropometry is the single most universally applicable,

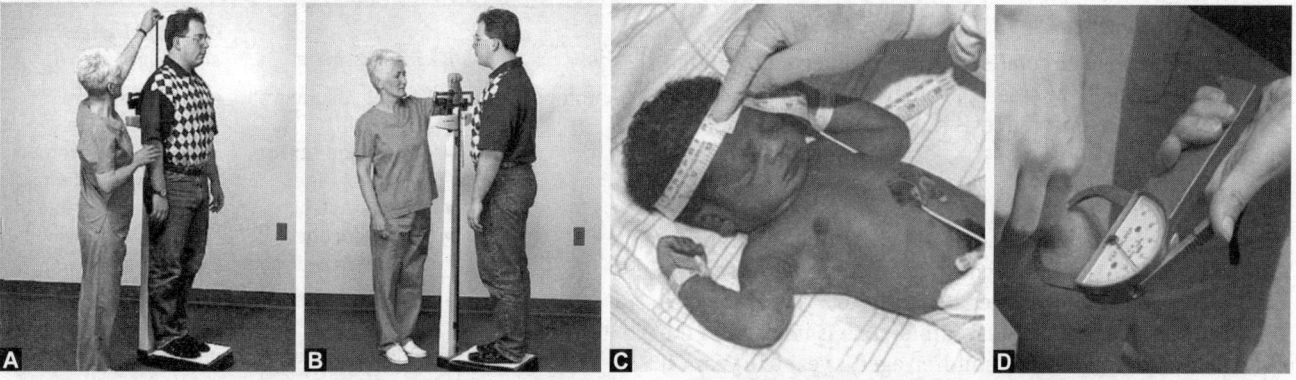

Figs. 12.5A to D: Steps of anthropometric measurements.

inexpensive, and non-invasive technique available to assess the size, proportions and composition of the human body.

The most commonly utilized measurement is as follows:
- Height/length
- Weight
- Mid-upper arm circumference (MUAC)
- Head circumference
- Chest circumference
- Waist circumference

Height
Height is very important for assessing nutritional status—as a normal individual attains a particular height at a particular age and has to be measured in a standardized manner.

Weight
- An individual has to obtain a standard weight for age to attain normal nutritional status.
- Weight increases with the increase in the age of a healthy child. There are standard range of weight of a child given age/height and standard range of height given age.
- If a child falls short of the minimum values of these ranges the child is underweight.
- On the other hand, if the child lies above the maximum values of the ranges then he/she is overweight.

Mid-upper Arm Circumference (MUAC)
- MUAC can be used for screening under-weight. It can be utilized along with BMI to identify the preferential loss of peripheral tissue stores of fat and protein.
- It is very useful to assess the nutritional status of children aged less than 5 years as it does not change much during the age of 1 year till 5 years.
- It is also of great value especially when a large number of children are to be covered and there is confusion regarding their ages.
- MUAC colored tape is being regularly used during emergencies, such as famines.
- MUAC values below 23.0 cm and below 22.0 cm are considered to be undernourished for adult males and females respectively.
- For children the cutoff point is 12.5 cm for both boys and girls. A series of MUAC cut-off points have also now been identified to allow the screening of individual adults under extreme conditions, e.g., during famines.

Head Circumference
Brain size and head circumference can be affected by undernutrition, especially in case of protein energy malnutrition. The greatest circumference is to be measured for head circumference.

Chest Circumference
Chest circumference is a useful indicator of growth in the 2nd and 3rd years of life. A chest/heap circumference ratio of <1 recorded in children aged 6 months to 5 years indicates undernutrition. If the chest circumference is more than the head circumference among children aged 1 year to 5 years, it is an indication of protein energy malnutrition.

Waist Circumference
Waist measurement can be used to assess obesity, and two levels of risk have been identified. These are:
1. **Risk Level I:** Males >94.0 cm, females >80.0 cm
2. **Risk Level II:** Males >102.0 cm, females >88.0 cm

Level I—it is utilized for the maximum acceptable waist circumference, while Level II is significant for the screening of obesity and requires weight reduction management therapy.

Commonly Used Indices to Determine Nutritional Status
- The commonly used indices in this regard are the body mass index (BMI), height-for-age, weight-for-age, weight-for-height, waist-hip ratio and waist height ratio, these indices are expressed in terms of Z-scores or percentiles.
- The WHO recommends a comparison of these indices with an international reference population to determine undernutrition.
- The justification for use of a reference population is the empirical finding that well-nourished children in all communities follow very similar growth patterns.
- If the measurements and indices are compatible with those of the reference standards then the individual is considered to be nutritionally healthy. If lower than the values, then the individual suffers from undernutrition.
- In case the observed values are higher than those of the reference, then it is a case of overnutrition.
- International reference standards are provided by the National Center for Health Statistics (NCHS), USA.
- Indian reference standards have been compiled by the National Institute of Nutrition (NIN), Hyderabad.
- The reliability of the anthropometric data depends on two important factors—accurate age estimation and the normal reference values for comparison of the measurements obtained.

Table 12.1 is depicted the basic nutritional assessment.

Body Mass
Index BMI = body weight/height^2

The units being kg/mt^2 for BMI, kg (kilogram) for weight and m (meter) for height. BMI is a good indicator of undernutrition in terms of Chronic Energy Deficiency (CED) in populations and is non-invasive, inexpensive and can be

Table 12.1: Basic nutritional assessment.

Tool	Basic assessment	Additional assessment and comments
Anthropometry	• Weight, height in all patients • BMI for age/sex in 5–18 years age • BMI in adults • Weight for age z-scores in 0–5 years	• Mid upper arm circumference • In pregnant women, those with edema, and those unable to stand
Biochemical and laboratory assessment	• Hemoglobin in all cases • Peripheral smear in case of anemia	Serum electrolytes required in severe undernutrition

used for large-scale surveys well suited for the assessment of malnutrition because it is.

Height-for-age
Individual height reflects the total increase in size of the person and indicates adequate nutritional status. The height-for-age index is a long-term measure of the duration of malnutrition. Low height for age is also known as stunting, stunting usually occurs before age two.

Weight-for-age
Changes in weight are more pronounced than height, as weight is more sensitive to changes in individual growth patterns. The weight-for-age index is a commonly used indicator of body size and it reflects food intake levels. This index is a good indicator of' short-term and acute under-nutrition.

Weight-for-height
Sometimes, it is difficult to ascertain the correct date of birth and subsequently the age of the individual. Then the relation between weight and height instead of weight for-age can be used. This index provides an indication of thinness of the individual and shows chronic and acute under-nutrition. Wasting refers to low weight-for-height.

Waist-hip Ratio (WHR)
- Waist-hip ratio = Waist circumference in cm/hip circumference in cm.
- WHR values >0.90 in males and >0.80 in females are considered to be high risk for diseases, such as diabetes.

Waist-height Ratio
Waist-height ratio = Waist circumference in cm/height in cm. A cut-off value of 0.5 is suggested for both sexes to assess obesity.

Some New Indices and Cut-offs
- The Composite Index of Anthropometric Failure (CIAF) The conventional indices of stunting, underweight and wasting only allow for the categorization of children into the general categories of undernutrition and do not provide an opportunity to determine the overall prevalence of undernutrition that is associated with multiple failures.
- The number of children suffering from undernutrition was being underestimated primarily due to overlapping of the children into multiple categories of anthropometric failure.
- The conventional anthropometric indices are unable to depict the overall prevalence of undernutrition because a researcher has to 'choose' a certain category of anthropometric failure for assessing nutritional status.
- Hence, while some stunted children may not be affected with wasting and/or underweight, and other similar combinations, others might suffer from all three nutritional failures of stunting, underweight and wasting.
- The CIAF is thus, an aggregated single anthropometric measure providing an overall estimate of under-nourishment in children.

Biochemical Methods
The underlying principle of this method is that any changes in the quantity and composition of the diet is reflected by variations in the concentrations of nutrients or their associated compounds in different body tissues and fluids along with the appearance or disappearance of metabolites.
- The method of biochemical assessment estimates the concentrations of essential dietary constituents in the body to evaluate nutritional status.
- Hemoglobin estimation is the most important test to interpret the overall state of nutrition.
- This indicates prevalence of anemia and deficiencies in proteins and trace elements.
- Stool examination is utilized to test for the presence of ova and or intestinal parasites.
- Urine examination can be used for albumin and sugar tests.

Vitamins and Proteins in Assessing Nutritional Status
- Vitamins promote other metabolic reactions in the body' that produce energy.
- This in turn leads to better maintenance of cells and tissues, along with promoting growth and development. Hence, a determination of the levels of these vitamins of different body tissues (biomarkers) can help to ascertain deficiencies.
- The important vitamins needed by the body are vitamins A, B, C, D, E, and K. Vitamin A deficiency is indicated by plasma B-carotene levels and fasting plasma amino acid pattern, which in turn indicate a deficiency of plasma retino.
- Deficiency in vitamin B1 (thiamine) is determined by thiamine levels in urine. The biomarker for riboflavin or vitamin B2 deficiency is urinary riboflavin and the function of the enzyme red cell glutathione reductase is impaired.
- The biomarker for the determination of vitamin B6 deficiency is urinary 4-pyridoxic acid, indicating plasma pyridoxal 5' phosphate dysfunction.
- Deficiency in vitamin B12 is indicated in plasma holotranscobalamin n levels which in turn show a deficiency in the function of the enzymes plasma vitamin B12 and plasma methylmalonate.
- Analysis of plasma and urinary ascorbate levels is associated with a deficiency in vitamin C. There is a cell depletion of leucocyte ascorbate in the long term.
- Vitamin D deficiency is, documented by the analysis of 25-hydroxy-vitamin D in the plasma.
- The deficiency results in the improper function of the enzyme plasma alkaline phophatase. The ratio of plasma tocopherol to cholesterol plus triglyceride is the biomarker to determine deficiency in vitamin E status.
- Vitamin K deficiency is determined by the plasma analysis of phylloquinone. This deficiency results in the impairment in the function of plasma prothrombin,
- Proteins are responsible for maintaining fluid balance, blood clotting, cell growth and repair, and immunity.
- Proteins also provide fuel for the body and glucose for the synthesis of sugar.

Water	30 mL/kg
Vitamin A	600–700 µg retinol equivalents/day
Vitamin B12	2.5 µg/day either from supplement or foods fortifies
Folate	400 µg/day
Vitamin C	60–100 mg/day
Vitamin D	10–15 µg/day
Vitamin E	100–400 IU/day
Vitamin K	60–90 µg/day
Chromium	50 µg/day
Copper	1.3–1.5 mg/day
Zinc	
High Zn availability (50+%)	Men 4.2 mg/day; Women 3.0 mg/day
Moderate Zn availability (30%)	Men 7.0 mg/day; Women 4.9 mg/day
Low Zn availability (15%)	Men 14.0 mg/day; Women 9.8 mg/day

- These **water needs** may be insufficient for underweight adults
- An alternative approach is: 100 mL/kg for the first 10 kg, 50 mL/kg for the next 10 kg and 15 mL/kg for the remaining weight
- Unless there is a renal failure or some other reason for restriction, even underweight adults, should receive at least 1500 mL of fluid per day

- **Vitamin D, B12, and Ca deficiencies** should be assessed and treated properly
- Daily intake of vitamin B12 should be 10–15 µg
- Vitamin D and calcium requirements are controversial (see Chapter 4: Vitamin D and calcium deficiency in the elderly)

Fig. 12.6: WHO: Food-based guidelines for older adults.

- Diets low in energy and proteins lead to a situation known as protein-energy malnutrition (PEM) and kwashiorkor. Analysis of urinary nitrogen indicates reduced intake of proteins.

Figure 12.6 is depicted the WHO's food-based guidelines for older adults.

Essential Trace Elements in Assessing Nutritional Status

- Trace elements are those elements that are present in the human body in minute quantities. Their concentrations are measured in parts per million.
- Essential trace elements act as catalytic or structural components of larger molecules and they have specific functions which are indispensable for life.
- These trace elements are required by man in amounts ranging from 50 µg to 18 mg per day.
- The main essential trace elements are iron, zinc, selenium, iodine, chromium and copper.
- Iron and transferrin levels in plasma are utilized for determining iron levels and documenting iron deficiency. Plasma zinc is the best biomarker for zinc deficiency.
- Plasma selenium concentrations together with toe nail selenium levels are the established biomarkers of selenium status.
- Iodine deficiency is analyzed from the concentrations of iodine in urine.
- Chromium deficiency can be assessed using urine and plasma chromium levels.
- Serum or plasma copper is the most widely used biomarker for copper deficiency.

Advantages

- The principal advantages of the biochemical method are that it is precise, accurate, reliable and extremely useful in assessing and detecting early cases of malnutrition before the appearance of the clinical signs.
- The biochemical measurements usually reflect the immediate past intake of nutrients or the changes produced by a longstanding deficient intake of a nutrient.
- The main disadvantages are that most of the tests are still quite expensive, time consuming and not routinely done.
- Good laboratory facilities and trained personnel are a prerequisite. Often in the field situation, it becomes difficult to collect and transport tissue samples which are biologically active.

CLINICAL ASSESSMENT (SIGNS AND SYMPTOMS)

Clinical examination is a simple, yet objective method to assess nutritional status. The signs and symptoms can be in the skin, mouth, gums, nails, lips, eyes and hair of the subjects under study. Clinical examination may be defined as the method of assessing the nutritional status of an individual by examining the clinical signs and symptoms.

Classification of the Physical Signs and Symptoms

- The 1963 WHO Expert Committee on Medical Assessment of Nutritional Status provided a classification of the physical signs that can be utilized for nutritional assessment.

- This classification was subsequently updated in the World Health Organization Monograph Series No. 53 entitled "The Assessment of the Nutritional Status of the Community" published in the year 1966.
- The WHO classification is very helpful when a rapid nutritional screening of a population is required within a stipulated time frame and also for specific research studies that needs to evaluate certain signs and symptoms.

Group I: This group constitutes those signs that are of paramount importance in nutritional assessment studies. These signs are sometimes associated with deficiencies in one or more micronutrients and are strongly related to malnutrition. This group is the best suited for individual assessment of nutritional status.

Group II: This group consists of those signs that are unclear and require more precise investigation. The signs mayor may not be related to malnutrition. The signs under this category are usually noticed among populations in the developing countries.

Group III: Signs that are not related to malnutrition are included in this group. But the problem is that these signs can bear similarities to that of malnutrition. So, it really needs a trained eye to differentiate between the two.

Physical Signs of Malnutrition (Table 12.2)

- Physical signs and symptoms need to be recorded in a precise manner. The signs of malnutrition can be multiple.
- An experienced observer should possess the inherent capability of going for a more precise assessment of the body, after the initial findings based on a single sign.
- He/she also has to take into account the physical environment of the subject, along with the cultural features that can contribute to malnutrition.
- The age of the subject also plays an important role as the signs of a particular deficiency.
- The two aspects that are vital for proper and objective diagnosis are the reliability of the signs of symptoms and the experience of the investigator.
- For convenience, the signs and symptoms are being classified into two categories. The categories are:
  - Physical signs and general appearance
  - Internal signs
- The physical signs and symptoms need to be recorded as accurately and possible. This can only be attained by the nutritionist/health worker by constant practice.
- The age of the individual under study is also related to the signs and their interpretation. Any physical finding that is

Table 12.2: Physical signs (appearance) indicative of malnutrition.

Body region	Signs	Possible deficiencies
Skin	Petechiae	Vitamins A, C
	Purpura	Vitamins C, K
	Pigmentation	Niacin
	Edema	Protein, vitamin B1
	Pallor	Folic acid, iron, biotin, vitamins B12, B6
	Decubitus	Protein, energy
	Seborrheic dermatitis	Vitamin B6, biotin, zinc, essential fatty acids
	Unhealed wounds	Vitamin C, protein, zinc
Nails	Pallor or white coloring	Iron, protein, vitamin B12
	Clubbing, spoon-shape, or transverse ridging/banding; excessive dryness, darkness in nails, curved nail ends	
Head/Hair	Dull/lackluster; banding/sparse; alopecia; depigmentation of hair; scaly/flaky scalp	Protein and energy, biotin, copper, essential fatty acid
Eyes	Pallor conjunctiva	Vitamin B12, folic acid, iron
	Night vision impairment	Vitamin A
	Photophobia	Zinc
Oral cavity	Glossitis	Vitamins B2, B6, B12, niacin, iron, folic acid
	Gingivitis	Vitamin C
	Fissures, stomatitis	Vitamin B2, iron, protein
	Cheilosis	Niacin, vitamins B2, 86, protein
	Pale tongue	Iron, vitamin B12
	Atrophied papillae	Vitamin B2, niacin, iron
Nervous system	Mental confusion	Vitamins B1, B2, B12, water
	Depression, lethargy	Biotin, folic acid, vitamin C
	Weakness, leg paralysis	Vitamins B1, B6, B12, pantothenic acid
	Peripheral neuropathy	Vitamins B2, B6, B12
	Ataxia	Vitamin B12
	Hyporeflexia	Vitamin B1
	Muscle cramps	Vitamin B6, calcium, magnesium
	Fatigue	Energy, biotin, magnesium, iron

indicative of malnutrition should be a clue that needs to be pursued more precisely.
- The physical signs and symptoms are strongly related to the ethnic features of the population under study.
- In a diverse country, such as India, this is even more evident. The main advantages of this method are that it is inexpensive, rapid, reliable and easy to perform in any situation.
- It is also non-invasive and do not require the collection, transportation and analysis of any biologically active material.
- No specialized laboratory is required as such. Whereas the main disadvantage of this method is that it is often not possible to detect early cases of malnutrition and that some of the clinical signs may not be specific to a particular nutrient deficiency and often one sign is an indicator of two or more such deficiencies. Moreover, the prevalence of the different clinical signs of malnutrition is quite low.
- There also can be differences in the assessment of the clinical signs by different observers (interobserver error). The physical signs and symptoms can also vary over time periods.
- Physical clinical examination constitutes an inseparable portion in nutritional assessment studies, even though some authorities have opined that it would not be wise to interpret the clinical results alone.
- Used in a cautious manner in conjunction with the other methods of assessing nutritional status, they can provide a comprehensive assessment of the same.

DIETARY HISTORY

The dietary data can be collected from individuals and/or families depending on the need and the model/hypothesis. This method has assumed prime importance as nutritionists have now recognized that nutrition has a major role to play so far as the prevalence of obesity, heart diseases and diabetes are concerned. This prevalence is now termed as "aetiology of common chronic diseases".

- Dietary surveys are nowadays being increasingly used for both population estimates and individual assessments.
- Dietary survey may be defined as the systematic study of the dietary intake of individuals and populations/communities. The dietary methods can be both qualitative and quantitative.
- Qualitative method typically uses food pyramids to estimate food requirements, servings and consumption and quantitative method calculates the amount of energy and specific nutrients for each food using food consumption tables which are subsequently compared with the RDA.
- Dietary surveys are extensively used in the areas of nutritional epidemiology, clinical assessment, population surveillance and experimental research. The dietary surveys have some general advantages.
- They are inexpensive, relatively easy, objective and yet easy to reproduce. No sophisticated laboratory is required.
- It is a non-invasive method and there is no requirement of the collection, transportation and analysis of any human tissue. However, the dietary surveys have certain general disadvantages.
- The assessment of the food amount is usually done by the subjects who may be erroneous.
- There may be variations in the daily diet that may not be accurately reflected. There also could be under-reporting by the respondents and of course, measurement errors.

Types of Dietary Surveys
- Twenty-four hour recall
- Weighed intake
- Food frequency questionnaire
- Food diary
- Dietary history

Twenty-four Hour Recall Method
- All the food items that were consumed during the last 24 hours are recorded in the "24-hour recall method".
- This method is utilized in large-scale nutritional surveys.
- The subject is usually asked to recall and describe in as much detail as possible his/her food intake during the last 24-hours either through an interview or by a questionnaire.
- The most widely preferred subject for this method is the housewife. The investigator asks her to recall the kind and amount of the food used, the preparations actually made and distributed to the family members.
- Standard measuring containers, such as cups, glasses, saucers and spoons are used to help the subject in recalling the information. To get proper information, the investigator may use several stages in which each data obtained are checked and verified.
- The main advantages of this method are that it is inexpensive, quick, easy and relies on short-term memory.
- The 24-hour recall method for a single day is not very suited for correlation with the biochemical or clinical findings. The 24-hour recall method should be repeated for at 'least 2–3 consecutive days.
- Some individuals may find it difficult to vividly recall the details about the last day's diet. The day of the recall may also not be the typical normal day of the individual.
- Lastly, the individual being interviewed may not be always speaking the truth.

Weighed Intake Method
- In this case, the investigator remains actually present when the subject is eating and the food amounts are weighed before serving, during serving and subsequently the left-over (food not consumed).
- The differences between the amounts of food served and not consumed give the amount of food actually consumed by the individual.
- The principal advantage of weighed intake method is that it is a very intensive method.
- The main demerit of the weighed intake method is that it is time consuming.
- Furthermore, there can be cultural taboos in some societies to eat in front of a stranger or grant the investigator entry to the kitchen.

Food Frequency Questionnaire (FFQ)

- The FFQ method tries to obtain long-term dietary habits. The individuals generally complete the FFQ themselves.
- The detailed instructions are sent by post along with the questionnaire.
- However, in the developing countries, such as India, it is advisable for the investigator to fill up the questionnaire after interviewing the subjects.
- In the FFQ method, the individual is asked about how often specific food items are consumed.
- The responses of the subjects are standardized so that the subjects just need to tick mark on the specific responses.
- The frequency is generally calculated as per week/fortnight/month. The list of food items should not generally exceed 150 items. To standardize, categories ranging from never to six times per day are the usual format.
- The FFQ method has been used in large epidemiological studies to assess food patterns associated with inadequate intake of nutrients and descriptive information of the food and diet.
- The FFQ check list has two main parts, namely—a list of different food items and the frequency of consumption of these food items.
- The main advantage is that this method is quick and inexpensive, involving more coverage of the respondents.
- The data obtained can be analyzed in a very short time as the reponses are standardized. However, the FFQ method gives only a qualitative description and frequency of the food items consumed.
- It does not indicate the amounts of food consumed. It also becomes difficult to explain the association between the diet patterns and certain diseases. Sometimes, the questionnaire may be long and may need modifications to keep pace with the changing dietary habits.

Food Diary

- The subject is required to keep a record in written form (diary) and photographs of all the food and beverages consumed over a certain period of time.
- This method generally utilized when interviewing all the members regarding their dietary intakes. is not possible due to some practical constraints.
- A time period of one week can be used in the diary to estimate the dietary intake.
- The subject's arc initially tutored to describe and weigh/estimate the amount food immediately prior to eating and subsequently to record left over's, if any. Standardized bowls and utensils are given to them prior to writing the diary. Even though the subject burden appears to be the highest while using this method, the food diary method has been effectively used in a number of large prospective epidemiological studies and for validating the results obtained from other methods of dietary assessment.
- This method consists of dietary records kept just at the time of eating. So there is no question of any kind of "recall".
- The method is reliable as sufficient number of days is covered by each subject. The subjects also take interest in filling up the diary.
- The main disadvantage is that individuals are sometimes not able to estimate the quantity of food consumed accurately.
- The subject concerned can also be illiterate. Maintaining a diary can also be cumbersome for some individuals.
- Often, individuals modify their diets so that not much information can be noted in the diary and the records are kept to a minimum. The subject may not be writing the correct dietary information and become biased.

Dietary History

- Dietary history records the dietary practices of the respondents over a prolonged period of time.
- The investigator obtains a retrospective estimate of the food intake using this method. The time duration covered is 3 months to one year.
- The information is recorded either through interviews and/or questionnaires addressed to the subject.
- This method is not used in large scale epidemiological surveys. The main advantage is that it can be used for individual assessment.
- This method is now used increasingly by dieticians in the clinical context. Since the time period covered by this method is large, the individuals often cannot remember what they had consumed during the last one year. Moreover, each interview takes a very long time, often up to 90 minutes. The method is also not cost effective.

NUTRITIONAL EDUCATION

Nutrition education is essential to the community because a number of factors influence the food habits, such as sociocultural practices, educational and economic level of community, and availability of food in a geographical area. Once the food habits are established they are handed down from generation to generation and such habits are based on false idea and ignorance. Educating people regarding nutrition is important. In nutrition education the primary aim is to remove prejudices and to import good dietary habits people are ignorant about balanced diets they should be educated about the nutritive value of food, storage, preparation, cooking, serving and eating of food. Traditional belief religious beliefs, food fads and geographic, changing food habits.

MEANING

- Nutrition education means a planned sequential instructional program that provides knowledge and teaches skills to help students adopt and maintain lifelong healthy eating habits.
- Nutrition education means a program to promote better health by providing accurate and culturally sensitive nutrition, physical fitness, or health (as it relates to nutrition) information and instruction to participants, caregivers, or participants and caregivers in a group or individual setting overseen by a dietitian or individual of comparable expertise.

Box 12.1: Aspects of nutrition education.
- Helps community in providing information.
- Nutritional need of individuals
- Functions and sources of nutrients
- Food items that are nutritious, cheap and locally available
- Importance and composition of balanced diet
- Correct method of cooking to minimize nutrient loss
- Correct food habit
- Meeting nutritional requirement with the help of kitchen garden
- Hygiene and sanitation and immunization

☐ Nutrition education means individual or group education sessions and the provision of information and educational materials designed to improve health status, achieve positive change in dietary habits, and emphasize relationships between nutrition and health, all in keeping with the individual's personal, cultural, and socioeconomic preferences.

Box 12.1 is depicted the aspects of nutrition education.

AIMS

☐ The natural resources of food.
☐ Assessment of their nutritional behaviors and beliefs.
☐ Appreciating the importance of the standard of living improving programs.

Importance of Nutrition Education

It is an important tool to improve the nutrition of the community in the developing countries.
☐ Nutrition education gives the knowledge in right direction and corrects faulty practices.
☐ It educates people to make best use of their limited income.
☐ It educates people to make wise food choices for health and well-being of the family members.
☐ It tells about the appropriate eating habits.
☐ If the whole family is given nutrition education the nutritional status of the whole family will improve with the result the coming generation will be born with good nutritional status and the problem of malnutrition can be decreased to a great extent.

Traditional Belief

☐ Consumption of papaya fruit by pregnant woman is believed to lead to abortion.
☐ Dhal is not given to mother which will produce flatus to mother and indigestion to baby.
☐ **Religions belief:** Muslims are for bidden from eating pork and while Hindus are for bidden from eating beef.

Geographic

☐ Soil climate water resources local agricultural practice. The type of food that can be grown in the locality the food that can be practiced in that locality is the staple food. Because of all these reasons nutrition education is important.
☐ Nutrition education on good nutrition is necessary in improving dietary habits, helps them to select right food stuff within their economy.

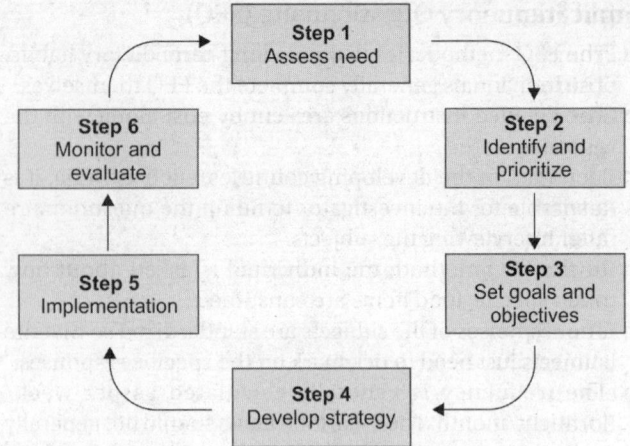

Fig. 12.7: Steps of nutrition assessment and interventions.

☐ Nutrition education must be given in simple words and in a language which is easily understood by people.
☐ Success of nutrition education will depend on whether people have understood the importance of it and have started practicing on the new ideas given to them.

Figure 12.7 is depicted the steps of nutrition assessment and interventions.

Approaches to Nutritional Education

Food is one of the important and basic biological needs of man. Food is the foundation for good health. It is essential for life, growth and repair of human body, regulation of body mechanism and production of energy for work. Nutritional education is essential part in community development.

Objectives and Need of Nutritional Education

☐ To educate the individual, the family and community about the food sources, food and their nutritive values, proper methods of cooking, balanced diet and requirements of energy.
☐ To educate the individual, the family and community about food selection, preparation, purchase and storage.
☐ To provide information about food substitutes, changes and modification in diet.
☐ To educate the effects of various cooking methods on the nutrients.
☐ To provide information about the importance of various nutrients and their required amount.
☐ To inform about various signs and symptoms of nutritional deficiencies and early detection of disease condition.
☐ To explain about the importance of food hygiene.
☐ To underline the nutritional requirements of the vulnerable group (children, pregnancy, location, and old age).
☐ To provide health education to avoid bad habits, prejudices, idiosyncrasies and wrong motions regarding diet.
☐ To educated various methods and techniques of prevention and control of nutritional deficiencies.

Implications for Nutrition Education

- Promote traditional diets and eating patterns with their positive aspects.
- Encourage the use of easily and locally available fruits and vegetables.
- Encourage cooking methods that require less fat.
- Respect and observe the religious and cultural food restrictions.
- Promote healthy eating habits for the whole family rather than an individual.
- Identify the target groups that are vulnerable, such as young children, pregnant and lactating women and the elderly.
- Local members of the community, such as health workers, mothers may be involved.
- The health workers need to have thorough knowledge of nutrition and health issues.
- Nutrition education material, such as leaflets, posters or audio video must be prepared in local language.
- The health workers must be fluent in local language to communicate effectively.

Methods of Nutritional Education

- **Individual nutrition education:** During pregnancy, lactation and to the mothers of malnourished children, nutrition education in their homes, is more effective.
- **Group nutritional education:** Community program for the entire families in the community are collected in particular place and cooking demonstration is more useful in information's are given.
- The following techniques can be used to make nutrition education more effective, e.g., role playing nutrition drama, puppet show, music and folk dance, posters, pictures, tape recorder, computer, television, films about nutrition.

Nutrition education can be organized during

- Home visit
- School health programs
- During organization of special clinics, e.g., antenatal clinic, postnatal clinic, and preschool clinic, etc.
- Special community health programs and health camps
- Indoor and outdoor clinics with patients and their attendants.

Opportunities for Nutrition Education

- During home visits.
- During conduction of special clinics, e.g., antenatal clinic, postnatal clinic, well baby clinic, under five-clinics, preschool clinic, etc.
- While conducting School Health Programme.
- With patients and their attendants in outdoor and indoor clinics.
- In ladies clubs meetings, during nutrition demonstration.

Principles of Nutrition Education

It is difficult to change the dietary habits of person. Hence, the nurse should be aware about her role and responsibilities while imparting nutrition education. For this, nurse should observe the following principles:

- The following factors are important in nutrition education:
  - The educational level of the individual or the community.
  - Culture, religion, dietary habits and idiosyncrasies.
  - Local availability of foodstuff.
  - Cleanliness of house and surroundings.
- The individual should be given sufficient time to adopt new ideas and habits.
- Any changes or suggestions regarding diet should be made according to the individual's practices, religion and culture.
- The individuals/patients should be made familiar with the importance and objectives of nutrition education.
- The local names should be used for the foodstuff and the education should be imparted in day-to-day language.
- The persons should be encouraged to ask question to satisfy their queries regarding nutrition.
- Nutrition education should be combined with reproductive and child health.
- The food articles which are not within the purchasing power of the individual or which are not consumed by him should not be advised to be included in the diet.

Responsibilities of Nurse in Nutrition Education/Teaching

- Assessing the health status of the individual/the family/the community.
- Making an early diagnosis of nutritional diseases and deficiencies and their treatment.
- Paying special attention to nutrition of the vulnerable groups, e.g., children, pregnant and lactating women and poor class people and to check adulteration.
- Telling the importance of kitchen garden/village shak vaatika.
- Imparting applied nutrition education using modem and attractive techniques.

CONCLUSION

Nutritional assessment can be defined as the interpretation from dietary, laboratory, anthropometric, and clinical studies. It is used to determine the nutritional status of individual or population groups as influenced by the intake and utilization of nutrients. Nutritional status represents meeting of human body needs for nutritive and protective substances and the reflection of these in physical, physiological, and biochemical characteristics, functional capability, and health status. Information about nutritional status, i.e., nutritional assessments, is essential for identification of potential critical nutrients (at population groups at risk of deficiency); formulation of recommendations for nutrient intake; development of effective public health nutrition (PHN) program for nutrition-related diseases prevention; and monitoring the efficiency of such interventions.

BIBLIOGRAPHY

1. Tobin KJ. Fast-food consumption and educational test scores in the USA. Child Care Health Dev. 2013;39(1): p. 118-24.
2. Hooper C, Fisher B, Munoz K. Physical Activity and Nutrition for Health. Champaign, IL: Human Kinetics, 2008.
3. Lutz CA, Karen RP. Nutrition and Diet Therapy, 4th edition. Davis FA, Philadelphia, USA, 1995.
4. Patwardhan VN. Nutrition in India, 2nd edition. Indian Journal of Medical Sciences, New Delhi, 1961.
5. Leverton RM. Food Becomes You: Better Health through Better Nutrition, Doubleday Publishing, Boston, USA, 1980.
6. Martin EA, Ardath AC. Nutrition in Action 4th edition, Holt Rinehart and Winston, New York, 1978.

REVIEW QUESTIONS

Long Essays

1. Describe in detail about nutrition assessment.
2. Explain clinical assessment.
3. Discuss methods of nutritional assessment.
4. Enumerate responsibilities of nurse in nutrition education/teaching.

Short Essays

1. Principles of nutrition education.
2. Systems of nutritional assessment.
3. Nutritional education.
4. Anthropometric methods.
5. Food frequency questionnaire.

Short Answers

1. Nutrition surveillance.
2. Body mass.
3. Importance of nutrition education.
4. Biochemical assessment.
5. Nutritional index.
6. Mid-upper-arm circumference.
7. Bitot's spots.
8. Body mass index (BMI).
9. Weight-for-age.
10. Weight-for-height.
11. Nutritional screening.
12. Nutrition survey.

CHAPTER 13

National Nutritional Programmes and Role of Nurse

CHAPTER OUTLINE

- Nutritional Problems in India
- National Nutritional Policy
- National Nutritional Programmes—Vitamin A Supplementation, Anemia Mukt Bharat Programme, Integrated Child Development Services (ICDS), Mid-day Meal Scheme (MDMS), National Iodine Deficiency Disorders Control Programme (NIDDCP), Weekly Iron Folic Acid Supplementation (WIFS) and Others as Introduced
- Role of Nurse in Every Program

INTRODUCTION

Every day 799 million people in developing countries—about 18% of the world's population—go hungry. In South Asia one person in four goes hungry, and in sub-Saharan Africa the share is as high as one in three. Around 175 million children under five are estimated to be underweight, a third of preschool children are stunted, 16% of newborn babies weigh less than 2.5 kg and 243 million adults are severely malnourished. Two billion women and children are anemic, 250 million children suffer from vitamin A deficiency and two billion people are at risk from iodine deficiency (Micronutrient Initiative, 1998). Malnutrition has different levels of causation. It is strongly linked with poverty—poor children are more likely to be underweight at birth and less likely to receive energy-rich complementary food (Brown et al. 1998) and iodized salt (UNICEF 1998). In India, nutrition affects growth and development of a person. That is why, food security has been a major goal of development policy in India since the beginning of planning. There was acute starvation and shortage of food at the time of independence of the country. The major public health problems were chronic energy malnutrition, kwashiorkor, marasmus and micronutrient deficiencies, such as goiter, beriberi, blindness due to vitamin-A deficiency and anemia.

NATIONAL NUTRITIONAL PROGRAMMES

The Government of India has launched various nutritional programs to benefit mostly for mothers and children and to tackle major problems of malnutrition prevailing in India. Lack of nutrients will lead to decrease in work output, physical intolerance and increase in mortality and morbidity particularly among the pregnant women, lactating mothers and children up to 5 years forming the vulnerable group of the population.

- **Vertical nutritional programs:** Programs operating at national levels are called vertical programs, such as ICDS, vitamin 'A' prophylaxis programs, iodine deficiency disorder control programs, etc.
- **Horizontal nutritional programs:** Programs operating at state level and integrated with primary health centers are horizontal programs, e.g., Balwadi Nutrition Programme and Tamil Nadu Integrated Nutritional Programmes, etc.

Most of the nutritional programs do not have much impact, particularly on the mortality of the vulnerable group. The reasons are as follows:

1. Poor community participation
2. Negligence of the nutrition
3. Poor implementation of the programs
4. Old stock supplies
5. Unaware of the program by the people.

The Government of India have initiated several large scale supplementary feeding programs, and programs aimed at overcoming specific deficiency diseases through various ministries to combat malnutrition including Ministry of Health and Family Welfare, Ministry of Social Welfare and Ministry of Education. The major factors leading to malnutrition in India include inadequate intake of calories and proteins, deficiency of certain micronutrients (such as iron, vitamin A, calcium or iodine). Maldistribution of essential food commodities, low purchasing power, lack of knowledge about balanced nutrition and limited access to healthcare facilities. The vicious cycle of poverty, malnutrition and ill-health has to be combated through the integrated efforts of socioeconomic development, better nutrition is widely lacking, especially amongst those who live below. They are direct and indirect interventions programs as described below:

Direct

I. Department of Women and Child Development
- Integrated Child Development Services (ICDS) Scheme
- Nutrition Programme for Adolescent Girls
- Nutrition Advocacy and Awareness General Programmes for Food and Nutrition Board (FNB)
- Follow-up action on National Nutrition Policy 1993

II. Ministry of Health and Family Welfare
- Iron and Folic Acid Supplementation of Pregnant Women.
- Vitamin A supplementation of children of 9–36 months age groups.
- National Iodine Deficiency Disorder Control Programme

III. Department of Elementary Education and Literacy
- Mid-day Meal for Primary School Children
- Indirect

IV. Department of Agriculture and Cooperation
- Increased Food Production
- Horticulture Interventions

V. Food and Public Distribution
- Targeted Public Distribution System
- Antyodaya Anna Yojana
- Annapurna Scheme

VI. Rural and Urban Development
- Food for Work Program
- Poverty Alleviation Program
- Safe Drinking Water and Sanitation Program
- National Rural Employment Guarantee Scheme

VII. Ministry of Health
- National Rural Health Mission (NRHM)
- Integrated Management of Neonatal and Childhood Illnesses (IMNCI)
- Various Public Health Measures

VIII. Department of Elementary Education and Literacy
- Sarva Shiksha Abhiyan
- Adult Literacy Program

IX. Department of Women and Child Development
Various women's welfare and support programs.

HISTORY OF NUTRITIONAL PROGRAMS

A number of programs were implemented in the past from time to time with minor successes or failures. Some of these are mentioned:

- **Special Nutrition Programme (SNP):** The program was launched in the country in 1970–71. It provided supplementary feeding of about 300 calories and 10 grams of protein to preschool children and about 500 calories and 25 grams of protein to expectant and nursing mothers for six days a week. This program was operated under Minimum Need Programme. The program was taken up in rural areas inhabited predominantly by lower socioeconomic groups in tribal and urban slums. Fund for nutrition component of ICDS Programme was shared with SNP budget.
- **Balwadi Nutrition Programme:** Fund for the supplementary feeding of Balwadi Nutrition Programme was given by the Central Government which was launched in 1970–71 through voluntary organizations. It had provided 300 calories and 10 grams of protein per child (3–5 years) per day for 270 days a year.
- **Applied Nutrition Programme (APN):** The Applied Nutrition Programme (ANP) was introduced as a pilot scheme in Odisha in 1963 which later on extended to Tamil Nadu and Uttar Pradesh with the objectives of:
  - Promoting production of protective food, such as vegetables and fruits and ensures their consumption by pregnant and nursing mothers and children. During 1973, it was extended to all the state of the country.
  - The nutritional education was the main focus and efforts were directed to teach rural communities through demonstration how to produce food for their consumption through their own efforts.
  - The beneficiaries were children between 2–6 years and pregnant and lactating mothers. Nutrition worth 25 paisa per child per day and 50 paisa per woman per day was provided for 52 days in a year.
  - No definite nutrient content had been specified. The idea was to provide better seeds and encourage kitchen gardens, poultry farming, beehive keeping, etc., but this program did not produce any impact.
  - The community kitchens and school gardens could not function properly due to lack of suitable land, irrigation facilities, and low financial investment.
- **The Tamil Nadu Integrated Nutrition Program (TINP):** The Tamil Nadu Integrated Nutrition Project was started in 1980 targeting 6–36 months old children, and pregnant and lactating women.

The objective of TINP was:
- To reduce malnutrition up to 50% among children under 4 years of age;
- To reduce infant mortality by 25%;
- To reduce vitamin-A deficiency in the under 5 year from about 27% to 5%; and
- To reduce anemia in pregnant and nursing women from about 55% to about 20%.

The project had four major components:
1. Nutrition services,
2. Health services,
3. Communication, and
4. Monitoring and evaluation.

The projects were assisted by World Bank and with the goal of universalization of ICDS. All the TINP blocks were converted into ICDS blocks.

- **Wheat-based supplementary nutrition programme:** A centrally sponsored program was introduced in 1986 but now transferred to the State Sector. This program follows the norms of SNP or of the nutrition component of the ICDS. Central assistance for the program consists of supply of free wheat and supportive costs for other ingredients, cooking, transport, etc.

GUIDING PRINCIPLES

The implementation of the National Nutrition Strategy will be guided by the following key principles of action.

- **A life cycle approach:** A life cycle approach will be adopted, with a focus on critical periods of nutritional vulnerability and opportunity for enhancing human development potential.
- **Early preventive action:** Emphasis on preventing under nutrition, as early as possible, across the life cycle.
- **Inclusive and gender sensitive:** It will be rooted in a rights based framework that seeks to promote the rights of women and children to survival, development, protection and participation—without discrimination.
- **Community empowerment and ownership:** Families and communities will be enabled for improved care behaviors and nutrition of children and women, to demand quality services, to contribute to increased service utilization and to participate in community-based monitoring.
- Valuing, recognizing and enhancing contribution of Anganwadi workers, helpers and ASHAs
- **Decentralization and flexibility:** Contextually relevant, decentralized approaches will be promoted, with greater flexibility at state, district and local levels for greater and sustained program effectiveness and impact, in harmony with the approach of cooperative federalism.
- Ownership of Panchayati Raj institutions and urban local bodies
- Foster innovation
- Informed by science and evidence
- Ensure that there is no conflict of interest

CURRENT NUTRITIONAL DEFICIENCY STATUS

There is a wide gap in food production and food consumption. The achievement of macro-food grain security at the national level did not percolate own to household and the level of chronic food insecurity in India is still high. Many aspects of life and development are reflected in this one statistic—including the income and education of parents, the prevalence of disease, the availability of clean water, efficacy of health services, infant feeding practices, access to food and care, food and dietary habits, the health and nutritional status of mothers, and more broadly, the position of women in society.

- According to NFHS -3 in 2005–06, 46% of children below three years of age were underweight, 38% were stunted and 19% were wasted that are lower than sub-Saharan Africa.
- Approximately 26.1% of the population is still living below poverty line. Undernourishment is higher among rural than urban children. The proportion of underweight children in urban areas was 36% as against 49% in rural areas.
- Similarly, levels of stunting and wasting are higher in rural than in urban areas
- It is estimated that 2.2 million children are afflicted with cretinism and about 6.6 million are mildly retarded and suffer from motor handicaps. It is also estimated that iodine deficiency accounts for 90,000 still births and neonatal deaths.
- Nutritional blindness affects 7 million children in India per year resulting mainly from the deficiency of vitamin A, couples with PEM. Prevalence of conjunctival xerosis and Bitot's spot was observed to be as high as 7.8% among slum children, followed by industrial labor (6.3%).
- Prevalence of Low Birth Weight babies in India ranged between 26% and 57% in the urban slums and 35% and 41% in rural areas. 40% of the adults in rural area and 50% of the tribal adults are suffering from chronic energy deficiency.
- There is a problem of over nutrition in certain areas and certain groups of people in the country which have serious health effects.

FIVE YEAR PLANS ON NUTRITIONAL ASPECTS

I. **10th FYP:** Initiatives of 10th five year plan (FYP) to have paradigm shift
   1. Household food security to nutritional security for family and individuals.
   2. Untargeted food supplementation in vulnerable group to screening of all persons to identify various grade of undernutrition and appropriate management.
   3. Lack of focused interventions on prevention of overnutrition to promotion of appropriate lifestyle and dietary intakes for prevention and management of over nutrition and obesity.
   4. Integration of various sectors to support the nutritional program for better output.

II. **11th FYP:** National nutrition goals for 11th five year plan
   1. Reduce the prevalence of underweight in children under 5 years to 20%.
   2. Eradicate the prevalence of severe undernutrition in children under five years.
   3. First hour breastfeeding rates to increase to 80%
   4. Exclusive breastfeeding rates to increase to 90%
   5. Complementary feeding rate at six months to increase to 90%
   6. Reduce prevalence of anemia in high-risk groups (infants, preschool children, adolescent girls, pregnant and lactating women) to 25%.
   7. Eliminate vitamin A deficiency in children under 5 years as a public health problem and reduce sub-clinical deficiency of vitamin A in children by 50%.
   8. Reduce prevalence of iodine deficiency disorders to less than 5%.

NUTRITION INTERVENTIONS

Infant and Young Child Care and Nutrition

These interventions will focus on children under 3 years, through the promotion of:

- Universal early initiation (within 1 hour of birth) and exclusive breastfeeding for the first six months of life.
- Universal timely and appropriate complementary feeding after six months, along with continued breastfeeding for two years or beyond.
- Universal growth monitoring and promotion of young children-using WHO CGS with counseling of mothers/families using the Mother Child Protection Card.
- Universal access to infant and young child care (including ICDS, crèches, linkages with MGNREGA), with improved supplementary nutritional support/THR through ICDS.
- Enhanced care, improved feeding during and after illness, nutritional support, referrals and management of severely and acutely undernourished and/or sick children.

Infant and Young Child Health

- Improved newborn care and care of low birth weight babies.
- Bi-annual vitamin A supplementation for children 9-59 months
- Universal, timely and complete immunization of infants against vaccine preventable diseases (and subsequent booster doses) with quality assurance.
- Ensuring that young children receive micronutrient supplementation and bi-annual deworming as per MHFW guidelines. This includes—IFA supplementation for children 6-59 months and Bi-annual deworming for children over 12-59 months (linked to bi-annual VAS rounds).
- Prevention and management of common neonatal and childhood illnesses, such as diarrhea (with ORS and zinc supplementation) and acute respiratory infections (ARI) and severe acute malnutrition, at community and facility level.

Maternal Care, Nutrition and Health

- Improved supplementary nutritional support during pregnancy and lactation (ICDS).
- Improved antenatal care—including health and nutrition counseling (also family support for extra diet and rest to ensure adequate weight gain), IFA supplementation, consumption of adequately iodized salt and screening/management of severe anemia.
- Enhanced maternity protection (through the effective implementation of PMMVY)
- Institutional deliveries, lactation management, improved post-natal and newborn care.
- Promoting marriage at the right age, first pregnancy at the right age, inter pregnancy recoupment/birth spacing and shared care/parenting responsibilities.
- Promoting Women's Literacy and Empowerment

Adolescent Care, Nutrition and Health

- Equal care of the girl child at different stages of the life cycle—linked to the Beti Bachao Beti Padhao initiative.
- Improved access to health care, counseling support through school health programs, ARSH and deworming as per MHFW National Deworming Initiative.
- Improved access to nutritional support through Mid-day Meals in schools (MHRD) and through SABLA for out of school girls.
- Universal access of girls in school and girls out of school to IFA supplementation.
- Girls' education, skill development and female literacy.
- Changing gender constructs—gender sensitization and life skills for adolescents.
- No child marriage—marriage of young women after the age of 18 years.
- Addressing micronutrient deficiencies—including anemia

Community Nutrition (Interventions Addressing the Community)

- Ensuring universal access to safe drinking water, sanitation and hygiene, in an open defecation free environment, through Swachh Bharat.
- Prevention and treatment for malaria through the Use of bed-nets and/or intermittent preventive therapy for malaria (as per MHFW protocols) in malaria-endemic areas; facilitating mosquito control measures; other relevant health/disease control measures specific for the state/district, relevant for improving nutrition at community levels, such as JE, kala azar, etc.
- Ensuring access to household food security, social protection systems and safety nets.
- Nutrition education to ensure that optimal feeding and caring practices, dietary diversity nutritious foods; sanitation and hygiene and healthy lifestyles are promoted-addressing undernutrition and also the dual burden of malnutrition. (This includes nutrition education in the school curriculum and in colleges).
- Focused interventions to reaching the most nutritionally vulnerable community groups (such as SC, STs, minorities, others) and address multiple nutritional vulnerabilities, such as those related to seasonal distress, disease outbreaks, natural disasters (such as floods, drought, earthquakes) and other situations.
- Flexible responses to other state/district specific needs for improving nutrition at community levels.

NUTRITIONAL PROBLEMS IN INDIA

The common nutritional deficiencies in India are protein energy malnutrition (PEM), anemia, iodine deficiency disorder, vitamin A deficiency and vitamin D deficiency.

Protein Energy Malnutrition

Protein energy malnutrition is a syndrome synonymous with undernutrition. In PEM, there is a low intake of food containing sufficient energy and protein and involves deficiency of other nutrients. PEM occurs because the diet is inadequate in both quantity and quality nutrition, and is insufficient to satisfy the physiological requirements. It commonly occurs in infants and children. It can adversely affect their physical and mental development. It also occurs in adults and extreme forms of PEM are referred as Kwashiorkor and Marasmus.

Several interventions have been found helpful to tackle this condition, such as reducing low birth weight by ensuring better maternal nutrition, encouraging breastfeeding, use of clean purified water, better hygiene, introducing nutrient dense foods, ensuring sufficient amount of protein and use of therapeutic food. Protein-rich foods are lean chicken, fish, turkey, eggs, milk and milk products, such as curd should be the part of the diet. For vegetarians, paneer, cheese and plant proteins, such as pulses, legumes, nuts and seeds are a good choice.

Vitamin A Deficiency

Vitamin A deficiency is a lack of vitamin A in blood and tissues. Vitamin A deficiency is defined as—tissue concentration of vitamin A low enough to have adverse health consequences. Depletion of body stores of vitamin A impairs normal physiology functions. It adversely affects visual function, integrity of epithelial lining and immunity. Few causes are inadequate breastfeeding, inadequate consumption of vitamin A-rich foods, general malnutrition and inflammatory conditions. Prevention and management involve food-based approach and vitamin A supplementation. Vitamin A food sources are dairy products, eggs, and orange and yellow vegetables and fruits.

Anemia—Iron Deficiency

The most common encountered anemia is caused by the deficiency of iron, wherein there is insufficient iron in the body to maintain normal physiological functions of the tissues. The causes include low dietary intake of iron-rich foods, frequent consumption of tea and coffee which contain polyphenols that reduce the absorption of iron, and low intake of vitamin C-rich foods with iron-rich foods which can help improve the absorption of iron.

Prevention and treatment would include promoting iron-rich foods, fortification, using lemon and other sources of vitamin C along with iron rich foods. Use of iron utensils for cooking also tends to increase the iron content. Iron-rich foods are such as green leafy veggies, nuts, seeds, millets, meat, egg and liver.

Vitamin D Deficiency

Vitamin D deficiency affects bone health, cardiovascular health, immunity, hormone health and inflammation. Prevention and management include consumption of vitamin D foods, such as beef liver, eggs, fortified milk, and cheese, getting adequate sunshine and supplementation.

Food is information to the body and plays an important role in managing the common nutritional deficiencies in India and hence must be consumed wisely. If you are concerned about having any of these nutritional deficiencies, do approach your health care provider for advice.

■ NATIONAL NUTRITIONAL POLICY

National Nutrition Policy (NNP) has been adopted by the Government in 1993. The National Nutrition Policy (NNP) identified key action in various areas having impact on nutrition, such as agriculture, food production, food supply, education, information, health care, social justice, tribal welfare, urban development, rural development, labour, women and child development, people with special needs and monitoring and surveillance. The core strategy envisaged under NNP is to tackle the problem of nutrition through direct nutrition interventions for vulnerable groups as well as through various development policy instruments which will improve access and create conditions for improved nutrition.

Figure 13.1 is depicted the national nutritional programmes.

Direct Short-term Nutrition Intervention

The direct short-term nutrition intervention suggested by NNP includes:
- Nutrition interventions for specially vulnerable group, such as children below 6 years, adolescent girls and pregnant and lactating women, expanding the safety nets, facilitating behavior change among mothers, reaching the adolescent girls and ensuring better coverage of expectant women;
- Fortification of essential food items with appropriate nutrients;
- Popularization of low cost nutritious foods prepared from indigenous and locally available raw materials;
- Control of micronutrient deficiencies among vulnerable groups.

Indirect Long-term Nutrition Interventions

The indirect long-term nutrition interventions leading to institutional and structural changes including:
- Food security for improved availability of food grains;
- Improvement of dietary patterns through production and demonstration;
- Policies for effecting income transfers so as to improve the entitlement package of the rural and urban poor

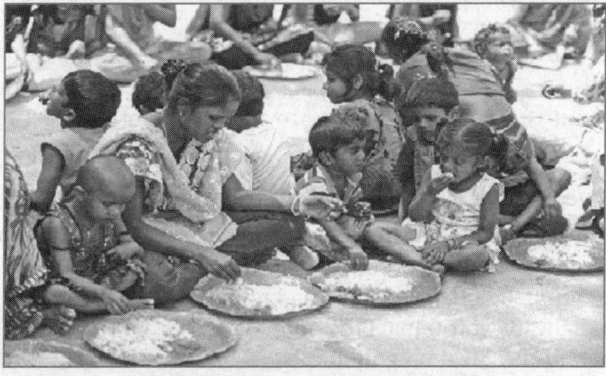

Fig. 13.1: National nutritional programmes.

improving the purchasing power and strengthening public distribution system;
- Land reforms measures for reducing vulnerabilities of landless and landed poor;
- Strengthen health and family welfare program;
- Imparting basis health and nutrition knowledge;
- Prevention of food adulteration;
- Improvement in nutrition surveillance;
- Monitoring of nutrition programs;
- Research into various aspects of nutrition;
- Equal remuneration for women;
- Communication through established media
- Minimum wage administration to ensure its strict enforcement and timely revision and linking it with price rise through a suitable nutrition formula a special legislation for providing agricultural women laborers the minimum support, and at least 60 days leave by the employer in the last trimester of her pregnancy;
- Community participation for generating awareness on NNP active participation of community members in management nutrition programs and related interventions through beneficiaries committees, participation of women in food production and processing, promoting kitchen gardens, food preservation, preparation of weaning food, generating demand of nutrition services;
- Education and literacy;
- Improvement in status of women.

SPECIAL NUTRITIONAL PROGRAMME

This is primarily a Food Distribution Programme, initiated 1970 in India as a crash program. Diet surveys conducted among preschool children in several regions had clearly indicated that the primary factor in the home diets of a majority of Indian children suffering from various grades of protein calorie malnutrition.

The Government of India in 1970 initiated, on a priority basis, the special nutrition program for tribal and urban slum children in different parts of the country.

Objectives

- The program is operated through the Ministry of Social Welfare and Community.
- It was suggested that the supplement should provide approximately a minimum of 300 calories and 9 g of protein per day per child.
- The supplement actually consisted of cereal, pulse, oil seed and jaggery (wheat 60 g, Bengal gram 10 g, ground nut 10 g and jaggery 30 g, provides 400 calories and 12 g protein).

Types of Special Nutritional Programme

The Government of India has launched several nutritional programs for the prevention of nutritional diseases.
- Supplementary Feeding Programme.
- Balwadi Nutritional Programme
- Mid-day Meal Programme
- Integrated Child Development Services Scheme (ICDS)
- Anemia Control Programme
- Vitamin A prophylaxis
- National Goitre Control Programme.
- **The Supplementary Feeding Programme:** This program was started in 1970 for nutritional benefit of preschool children (6 months to 6 years) pregnant women and nursing mothers. The supplementary food supplies 300 calories of energy and 10 to 12 g of protein per child per day. The beneficiary mother receives daily 500 calories and 25 g of protein. This supplement is provided to them for about 300 days in a year.
- **Balwadi Nutrition Programme:** This program is being organized by the Central Social Welfare Board from the year 1970–71. National level organizations give active support in Balwadi Nutrition Programme and provide help to the voluntary agencies for implementation of the same. These organizations are Indian Tribal Caste Association, Indian Council for Child Welfare, Kasturba Gandhi National Memorial Trust and Harijan Sevak Sangh.
  Balwadi were established in rural areas for providing preparatory education to children in the age group of 3 to 6 years. The supplement provided to the beneficiaries supplies 300 calories and 10 g of protein per child per day.
- **Mid-day Meal Programme:** Mid-day Meal Programme has an important role in providing balanced diet to school children. This is an effort taken by Government of India. Since 1960's to provide at least one nutritious meal and diet supplements to children in primary and middle schools. It was first organized in 1957 in Tamilnadu successfully
  In this program, one-third of the child's daily requirement can be fulfilled. CARE, UNICEF and many international, governmental voluntary agencies give their contribution in this. The primary objective of mid-day meal program is to improve the nutritional status of children and imparting nutritional education and to ensure universal primary education.
- **Integrated Child Development Service Scheme (ICDS):** This project was started in the year 1975 in pursuance of the national policy for children. The beneficiaries are preschool children below 6 years, pregnant and lactating mothers.
- **Vitamin A Prophylaxis Programme:** This Programme was launched by Ministry of Health and Family Welfare in 1970. For the success of the National Programme for Control of Blindness, it is necessary to prevent disease due to deficiency of vitamin A. For these children under 5 years of age are given vitamin A containing 2,00,000 IU orally, every 6 months through this program in India every year. The primary responsibility of implementation of this program rests on the maternal and child health using of the health and family welfare department. Integrated Child Development Services (ICDS) have an important role in the implementation of this program.
- **Anemia Control Programme:** This program consists of distribution of iron and folic acid tablets to pregnant women and young children (1–12 years). Mother and child health (MCH) centers in urban areas, primary health

centers in rural areas and ICDS projects are engaged in the implementation of this program.
- **National Goitre Control Programme:** The National Goitre Control Programme was launched by the Government of India in 1962 in the conventional goiter belt in the Himalayan region with objectives of identification of goiter endemic areas to supply iodized salt.
- **Tamil Nadu Integrated Nutrition Project:** This program was started in 1980. This provides a package of health and nutrition services to the rural pregnant and lactating mothers and their children in the rural blocks of Tamil Nadu. The second phase the targets were revised and expanded with the implementation of ICDS everywhere, the blocks will be converted into ICDS blocks.

INTEGRATED CHILD DEVELOPMENT SERVICES SCHEME (FIG. 13.2)

Integrated Child Development Services (ICDS) scheme was launched on 2nd October, 1975 (5th Five Year Plan) in pursuance of the National Policy for Children in 33 experimental blocks. The network consists of 5659 projects in rural and urban slum pockets. Now the goal is universalization of ICDS throughout the country.

The primary responsibility for the implementation of the program is with the Department of Women and Child Development, Ministry of Human Resources Development at the center and the nodal departments at the state which may be Social Welfare, Rural Development, Tribal Welfare, Health and Family Welfare or Women and Child Development.

Beneficiaries

- Children below 6 years,
- Pregnant and lactating women,
- Women in the age group of 15–45 years,
- Adolescent girls in selected blocks.

Objectives of ICDS

- To improve the nutritional and health status of preschool children in the age-group of 0–6 years;
- To lay the foundation of proper psychological development of the child;
- To reduce the incidence of mortality, morbidity, malnutrition and school dropout;
- To achieve effective coordination of policy and implementation amongst the various departments to promote child development; and
- To enhance the capability of the mother to look after the normal health and nutritional needs of the child through proper nutrition and health education

Tenth Five Year Plan

10th Five Year Plan has emphasized on:
1. Strengthening the nutrition and health component so that there is appropriate intra-familial distribution of food;

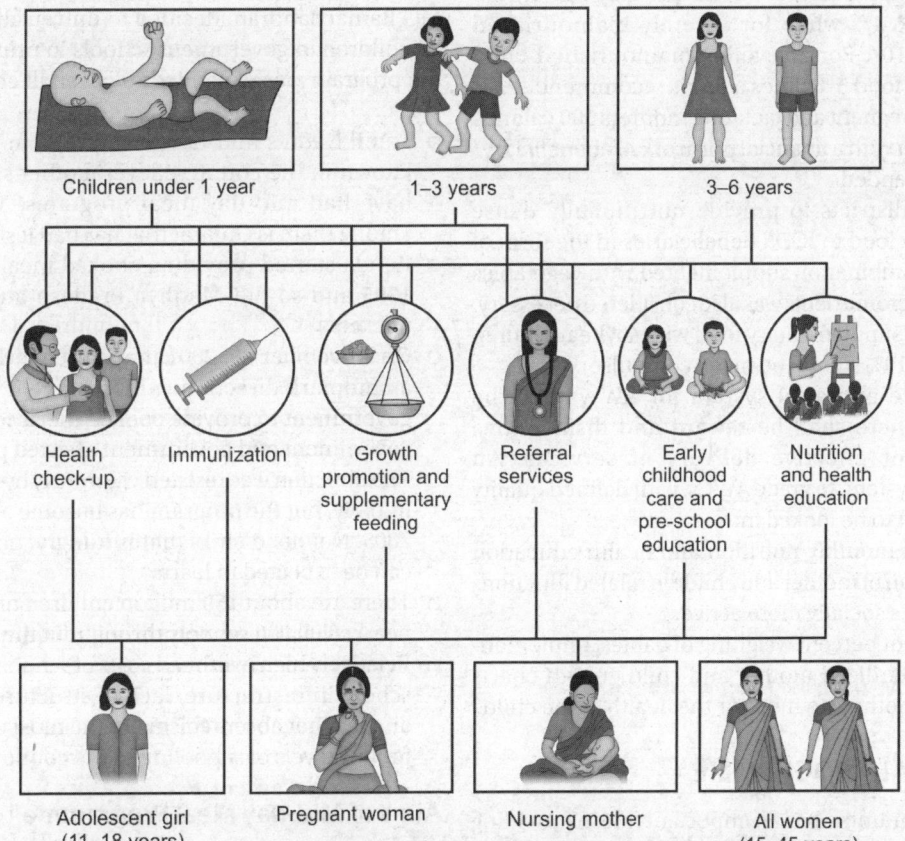

Fig. 13.2: ICDS scheme.

2. Reaching children in 6–36 months age group, pregnant and lactating women;
3. Weighing all vulnerable population and put on treatment with follow-up in 3 months;
4. Ensuring universal screening of all children at least once a quarter to identify growth falters.
5. Focus on intervention including take home supplements, to ensure conversion of Grade III and IV to Grade II in next quarter;
6. Looking for and treating health problems associated with severe undernutrition;
7. Enhancing the quality and impact of ICDS through training and supervision;
8. Intersectoral coordination for nutrition action;
9. Creating nutrition awareness; and
10. Establishing reliable monitoring and evaluation.

Eleventh Five Year Plan

1. Overall objective is to reduce child malnutrition through strengthening of ICDS services.
2. Wheat flour fortified with iron, vitamin A, folic acid should be supplied.
3. The calories and protein norms for children in age group of six months to six years need to be enhanced to 500 calories and 10 g protein child/day from the existing 300 calories and 8–10 g protein. Severely malnourished children in this age group need to be given 600 calories and 20 g protein/child/day. Financial norms for normal children for supplementary food per day should be enhanced to ₹ 4/- while for severely malnourished children to ₹ 10/. For a severely malnourished child nutrient dense food 5–6 times a day is recommended.
4. Similarly, for pregnant and lactating mothers 500 calories and 20 g protein with a financial norm of ₹ 4/- beneficiary/day is recommended.
5. Flexibility to districts to provide nutritionally dense supplementary food to ICDS beneficiaries in the form of cereal-pulse combination supplemented with vegetables and fruits or micronutrients was also considered necessary. Fortification of supplementary food with soybean flour in the range of 5–10% should be made compulsory.
6. A performance appraisal system for AWWs may be introduced. There shall be reward and disincentive mechanism for effective delivery of services. An accreditation system, to grade AWCs, with defined quality standards need to be looked into.
7. Observation of monthly nutrition and health education days, celebration of mother and children related functions will make AWCs socially more active.
8. Regular and cent percent weighing of babies, implementation of standardized mother and child growth charts will facilitate mothers to monitor the health of the child.

MID-DAY MEAL PROGRAMME

Mid-day Meal Programme has an important role in providing balanced diet to school children. This is an effort taken by Government of India. Since 1960's to provide at least one nutritious meal and diet supplements to children in primary and middle schools. It was first organized in 1957 in Tamilnadu successfully.

In this program, one-third of the child's daily requirement can be fulfilled. CARE, UNICEF and many international, governmental voluntary agencies give their contribution in this. The primary objective of midday meal program is to improve the nutritional status of children and imparting nutritional education and to ensure universal primary education.

Concept of Mid-day Meal Programme

- In India, the Mid-day Meal Programme was first started at Madras (Chennai) city in 1961.
- The Mid-day Meal Programme was launched in the country as a whole in 1962–1963.
- Nearly 12 million children benefited by this program in 1947 and 16 million children in 1979.
- Food material consisting of corn, soymilks and salad oil supplied by CARE has been the sheet anchor of the School Lunch Programme in a majority of places.

History of Mid-day Meal Programme

One of the pioneers of the scheme is the Madras Presidency that started providing cooked meals to children in corporation schools in the Madras city in 1923. The program was introduced in a large scale in 1960s under the Chief Ministership of K Kamaraj Nadar. But the first major thrust came in 1982 when the then Chief Minister of Tamil Nadu, Dr MG Ramachandran, decided to universalize the scheme for all children in government schools in primary classes. Later the program was expanded to cover all children up to class 10.

- Tamil Nadu's mid-day meal program is among the best known in the country. Several other states of India also have had mid-day meal programs. The most notable among them is Gujarat that has had it since the late 1980s.
- Kerala started providing cooked meals in schools since 1995 and so did Madhya Pradesh and Orissa in small pockets.
- On November 28, 2001 the Supreme Court of India gave a landmark direction, which made it obligatory for the government to provide cooked meals to all children in all government and government assisted primary schools.
- The direction was resisted vigorously by state governments initially, but the program has become almost universal by 2005. Neither a child that is hungry, nor a child that is ill can be expected to learn.
- There are about 150 million children officially enrolled in nearly 8,00,000 schools throughout the country.
- Relatively high overhead costs of school coupled with poor school infrastructure, lack of structure, lack of teachers and teacher absenteeism are the most often cited reasons for low levels of schooling in the country.

Aims of Mid-day Meal Programme

Realizing this need the National Programme of Nutritional Support to Primary Education, popularly known as Mid-Day

Meal (MDM) Scheme was formally launched on 15 August 1995 with the aim of improving in three areas:
- School attendance,
- Reduced dropouts,
- A beneficial impact on children's nutrition

Beside these, MDM could be a valuable means of imparting health and nutrition education not only to children but also to the parents and the community. MDM could also create employment opportunities for poor women of the village. Majority of cooks engaged in the programs could be women, most of them coming from underprivileged backgrounds. Mid-day meal has been effective in improving enrolment rates particularly of girls (Dreze and Goyal 2003). From October 2002, the program has been extended to children studying in government supported schools.

Nursing Foundation of India Recommendations

Following recommendations are made in a report by Nutrition Foundation of India:
- The children in classes 1–8th could be included as beneficiaries of the program, as being practiced in the states of Gujarat and Tamil Nadu.
- Each MDM should provide roughly a third of the daily nutrient requirement (350–500 kcal depending on the age of the child). The meal should contain apart from cereals, a good quality of vegetables, particularly, dark green leafy vegetables to combat micronutrient deficiencies.
- Meal should be of hygienic quality that demands monitoring of the raw material and cooked preparation by trained personal.
- In urban areas a centralized kitchen should be set up and meal should be prepared, transported, and served hygienically. This model was adopted by Chennai and Naandi Foundation in Hyderabad and ISKON group in Bengaluru. In rural areas, self-help groups and Panchayat should be involved.
- Mobilization of funds and ₹ 2.50–2.75 per child per meal should be allocated through various existing schemes.
- **Convergence of synergistic activities:** School health services, environmental sanitation and safe water supply, sensitization of teachers, involvement and networking of professional bodies and communities.

NATIONAL NUTRITIONAL ANEMIA PROGRAM

Anemia among children: Anemia is a serious concern for young children as it can adversely affect cognitive performance, behavioral and motor development, coordination language development and scholastic achievement as well increase morbidity from infectious deceases.

Hemoglobin levels are classified into three categories: Mild (10.0–10.9 g/dL), moderate (8.0–9.9 g/dL) and severe (less than 8.0 g/dL). The proportion of anemic children of 6–35 months has risen from 74% in 1998–99 to 79% in 2005–06. The increases is noticed in both rural and urban areas though the increase is higher in rural than in urban areas.

The level of anemia among children of 6–35 months varies from 56% in Kerala and 59% in Himachal Pradesh, 85% in Uttar Pradesh and 88% in Bihar. The levels of anemia are also higher among rural than urban children. And the rural-urban differential has widened from 4 percentage points in 1998–99 to 8 percentage points in 2005–06.

Available studies on prevalence of nutritional anemia in India show that 65% infant and toddlers, 60% 1–6 years of age, 88% adolescent girls (3.3% have hemoglobin <7 g/dL; severe anemia) and 85% pregnant women (9.9% severe anemia) having anemia.

Anemia in adult: The prevalence of anemia was marginally higher in lactating women as compared to pregnancy. The commonest is iron deficiency anemia.

The program was launched in 1970 to prevent nutritional anemia in mothers and children. Under this program, the expected and nursing mothers as well as acceptors of family planning are given one tablet of iron and folic acid containing 60 mg elementary iron which was raised to 100 mg elementary iron, however folic acid content remained same (0.5 mg of folic acid) and children in the age group of 1–5 years are given one tablet of iron containing 20 mg elementary iron (60 mg of ferrous sulfate and 0.1 mg of folic acid) daily for a period of 100 days.

This program is being taken up by Maternal and Child Health (MCH) Division of Ministry of Health and Family Welfare. Now it is a part of RCH Program. But this program has failed to make any impact in India. Experiences from other countries in controlling moderately-severe anemia have suggested that long-term measures, such as fortification of food items, such as milk, cereal, sugar and salt with iron are beneficial interventions. India has also identified fortification of salt with iron as a useful measure to control anemia. Pilot project of salt fortification with iron has been started in Tamil Nadu. Nutrition education to improve dietary intakes in family for receiving needed macro- and micro-nutrients as protein, iron and vitamins, such as folic acid, 12 C, etc., for hemoglobin synthesis is important. Nutritional Anemia Control Programme should be comprehensive and incorporate nutrition education through school health and ICDS infrastructure to promote regular intake of iron folic acid-rich foods, to promote intake of food which helps in absorption of iron and folic acid and adequate intake of food.

Iron supplementation can be risky for children living with high malarial areas and can lead to severe illness and death. As India has many high malarial states where prophylactic iron may be risky. An alternative policy is required in such areas. According to another research study conducted in Teheran revealed that the expectant mothers should not unnecessarily be given iron ills unless anemic, as it may cause development of high blood pressure and hence small gestation age babies.

Table 13.1 is depicted the iron deficiency anemia for various age group.

SPECIAL NUTRITION PROGRAMME (SNP)

The Special Nutrition Program was launched in 1970, as a crash program to provide supplementary nutrition to children below 6 years of age, and pregnant and lactating

Table 13.1: Iron deficiency anemia for various age group.

Iron deficiency anemia	Percentage
Children (6–35 months)	79 (NFHS-3)
• 6–11 months	71.7–80
• 12–23 months	77.7–78
• 24–35 months	72
• <6 month–6 years (<11 g/dL)	70
• 5–1 years	73
Adolescent girls <12 g/dL)	52–88
• Mild anemia	34
• Moderate anemia	15.7
• Severe anemia	1.8
Adolescent girls in urban slum of Delhi	46.6
Pregnant and lactating women (<11 g/dL)	58 (NFHS-3)
	81.7 (ICMR)
Women 15–49 years ever married	56 (NFHS-3)
Adult male (<13 g/dL)	24 (NFHS-3)

mothers. The socially and economically handicapped are to be reached through this program, as well as those in slums, drought prone and flood affected areas. It is now envisaged that the special nutrition program should include some of the components of the ICDS, in order to render it more effective, properly selected target groups of mothers and children are to be supported with basic health inputs, including nutrition and health education.

The objectives of the program are to improve the nutritional status of pregnant and lactating mothers and children below 6 years of age in the weakest sections and most vulnerable areas. The objectives are now to include a reduction in mortality and morbidity in children below 6 years, enhance the capacity of mothers to look after the daily health and nutritional needs of children and to strengthen the supportive services.

The main activities of the program are:
1. To provide supplementary nutrition's.
2. To provide health services including supply of vitamin A solution and iron and folic acid tablets (since 1976).

This program is for the nutritional benefit of children below 6 years of age, pregnant and nursing mothers and is in operation in urban slums, tribal areas and backward rural areas. The supplementary good supplies about 30 kcal and 10–12 g of protein child per day. The beneficiary mothers receive daily 500 kcal and 25 g of proteins, this supplement is provided to them for about 300 days in a year. This program is gradually merged into ICDS.

The major objective of the program is to prevent anemia. The specific objectives as identified from general description of the program are as follows:
- To assess the baseline prevalence of nutritional anemia in mothers and young children through estimation of Hb levels.
- To put the mothers and children with low Hb levels (less than 10 g% and less than 8 g%) on antianemic treatment.
- To put the mothers with Hb levels more than 10 g/dL and children with more than 8 g/dL on the prophylaxis program.
- To monitor continuously the quality of the tablets, distributions and consumption, and to assess periodically the Hb levels of the beneficiaries.
- To negative mothers, through relevant education, to consume the WA tablets and to give the same to their children.

NATIONAL GOITRE CONTROL PROGRAMME (NGCP)

The Government of India realizing the magnitude of endemic goiter launched the NGCP in 1962. It aimed at replacement of ordinary salt by iodized salt, particularly in goiter endemic regions. Surveys indicated that the problem of the goiter and iodine deficiency disorders was more widespread than it was thought earlier, with nearly 145 million people estimated to be living in known endemic areas of the country. As a result, the program started in 1986 with objective to replace the entire edible salt by iodized salt in a phased manner by 1992.

The objectives of NGCP are
- Initial survey to assess the magnitude of the iodine deficiency disorders.
- Supply of iodized salt in place of common salt to the entire country by 1992.
- Repeat surveys to assess the importance of iodized salt after 5 years.

Accordingly the program has been implemented and shown some progress. But reveals strengthening of NGCP. Areas requiring strengthening of the NGCP related to:
- Irregular distribution of iodized salt for varying periods.
- Lack of supportive supervision for the quality of iodized salt distributed.
- Failure of lifting of the allotted quotas of iodized salt by wholesale agents for further distribution to retailers.
- Poor interpersonal relationship between salt dealers and food inspectors, the implementation of PFA act.
- Coordination between department of food and civil supply. Health and wholesale dealers.

NATIONAL PROGRAMME FOR PROPHYLAXIS AGAINST BLINDNESS DUE TO VITAMIN-D DEFICIENCY

The National Program for Prophylaxis against Blindness Due to Vitamin 'A' Deficiency was launched in 1970 under Ministry of Health as a part of MCH program. Studies have shown that in the southern and eastern parts of the country, about 30–50% preschool children have eye problems as a result of vitamin 'A' deficiency. It is estimated that 2% of the total blindness in India is caused by vitamin 'A' deficiencies.

The specific objective of the program is reduction of diseases and prevention of blindness due to vitamin "deficiency. An evaluation of the program has shown that in areas where it has been implemented well there was significant reduction in the prevalence of signs of vitamin 'A' deficiency. The reason for coverage have been inadequate supplies of vitamin 'A' and adoption of clinic approach instead of house to house visit for the distribution. As a part of RCH program (earlier (CS SM)) attention now focused upon children up to 3 years of age.

BALWADI NUTRITION PROGRAMME

The Balawadi Nutrition Programme was started in 1970–71, or the preschool child as it is operated through balawadis and day care centers, and is under the charge of the social welfare department.

- The objective of the program is to supply one-fourth of the calorie requirements and half of the protein requirements of the preschool child as a measure to improve the nutritional status.
- It is to be a supplement to what the child receives at home. As far as possible, locally available food stuff is to be utilized.
- Children belonging to the lower socioeconomic group would be selected. Community involvement would be encouraged.
- The nutrition supplement providing 300 calories and 10 g of protein per day for 270 days a year is provided in balawadis or day care centers where some non-formal education of the preschool child is given.
- It is envisaged that package including basic health components are to be included as in the ICDS.
- This program is directed by the Ministry of Social Welfare through several voluntary organizations.
- Balawadi is managed by balsevikas assisted by helper, coordination committees at the center, state, district, block along with the community, are to ensure regular supply of resources and effective management.

WORLD FOOD PROGRAMME (WFP)

World Food Programme is the world's largest international food aid organization, serving in 84 countries working with the goal of achieving "A world in which every man, woman and child has access at all times to the food needed for an active and healthy life. Without food, there can be no sustainable peace, no democracy and no development". Founded in 1963 as the food aid arm of the United Nation after the Rome Declaration on World Food Security in 1996, WFP is committed to achieve the goal of reducing half the number who are without adequate access to food by 2015.

World Food Programme in India

Nearly half of the world's hungry reside in India. Despite a substantial increase in food grain production since her independence in 1947, India is still classified as low-income and food deficit country. Around 35% of India's population is considered food insecure, consuming less than 80% of minimum energy requirements. However, National Sample Survey organization claimed it has reduced to 27%. Without adequate nutrition, a person may be unable to perform work productively, or a child may be unable to learn school lessons to his/her capacity, or a mother may give birth to a child with permanent impaired brain development.

WFP's Goal and Objectives in India

- Improve nutrition and quality of life for the most vulnerable population at critical times in their lives;
- Make sustainable improvements in household food security for the poorest, especially for women and child, and invest funds in development for long-term security;
- Strengthen channels for locally-produced food grains and support local entrepreneurship; and
- Advocate for eco-restoration through participatory methods and development.

Beneficiaries

- Poor women, particularly mothers, and children at risk;
- Poor forest-dependent population;

Over the years, more than 70 development projects of WFP have included supplementary feeding, and supported forestry, livestock and dairy development, irrigation, and rural development activities. A blend of precooked maize and soya fortified with micronutrients called CSB (Corn-soya blend) has been developed in India in the name of Indiamix, distributed through existing infrastructure of the ICDS projects. The Indiamix project is operational in Rajasthan, Uttar Pradesh, Odisha, Madhya Pradesh, Gujarat, Kerala, Assam, and Bihar.

Nutritive Value of Indiamix (Table 13.2)

Indiamix is precooked, nutritious commodity, appropriate for both on the spot feeding and take home rations made from wheat (75%) and full-fat soybean (25%) or alternatively, maize (40%), and wheat (40%) and full-fat soya bean (20%) and has the nutritive values providing 80–90% of Recommended Dietary Allowance (RDA) of a child for iron and vitamin A.

Activities under WFPs: Helping women to gain better access to food, education, and involvement in community decisions. It works in many directions: access to maternal and child health care, improving child survival, "food for work" program in collaboration with forest department, providing food in emergencies, access to health services, potable water and sanitation, proper caring practices for young children, education particularly girls and women, supporting generation of biogas, protection of forest through mass awareness and active participation, irrigations, income generating projects, creating market by local manufacturing of Indiamix, and effective program implementation.

Table 13.2: Nutritive value of Indiamix.

Nutrients	Amount per 100 g
Protein (g)	20
Fat (g)	6
Crude fiber (g)	2
Carbohydrate (g)	60
Energy (kcal)	390
Calcium (mg)	191
Iron (mg)	15
Vitamin A (µg)	1454

APPLIED NUTRITION PROGRAMME

The concept and philosophy of the Applied Nutrition Programme arose early in the 1950s, out of the realization that the problem of improving nutritional condition and preventing malnutrition could not be solved by scattered, uncoordinated activities mainly of a relief nature, such as the free distribution of food to the vulnerable segments of the population.

Applied Nutritional Programmes (ANP) has been defined as co-coordinated educational activities among health, agricultural and educational departments and other interested agencies, with the active participation of the people to help them. Emphasis is placed on community action and the production of low cost productive foods.

Their utilization for vulnerable groups in the family, especially infants and toddlers is emphasized, sometimes through community supplementary feeding programs, with/without externally provided foods. The implementation should be continuously adapted to changing conditions.

Objectives

- To increase the production of protective foods, e.g., milk fruits, vegetables eggs and fish, etc.
- To ensure effective utilization of these protective foods by pregnant and nursing women, preschool and school children.
- Nutritional education of Applied Nutrition Programme in community development blocks.
- To assist in the extension of Applied Nutrition Programme in community development blocks.
- To promote sound and hygienic practices for production, preservation and use of protective foods through demonstration and education among village communities.

The main objectives of the program are:
- To make people conscious of their nutritional needs and
- To increase production of nutritious foods and their consumptions.
- To provide supplementary nutrition to vulnerable groups through locally produced foods.

The main components of the ANP are:
- Production of protective foods.
- Training of functionaries involved in the production of these foods.
- Nutrition education and demonstration (demonstration of improved technique of cooking and feeding were also used).

The program is coordinated by the Ministry of Rural Reconstruction.

At the state level, the panchayati raj and community development is generally in-charge of the program. In the field, block development officer is in charge of the program.

Activities of Applied Nutritional Programme

- **Training of personnel:** As a first phase facilities for conducting practical courses in poultry management, dairying, fisheries (inland and marine) horticulture and home science, and in the teaching of applied human nutrition are being strengthened in selected training institutions, such as rural extension training centers.
- **Program at the state level:** As soon as the subsidiary plan of operation is signed for a state government a coordination committee is established at the state, district and block levels. The state nutrition officer, in consultation with the officer-in-charge of the Applied Nutritional Programme in the state, formulates a training program for different categories of persons employed in the implementation of this program.
- **Production of productive foods:** It is being achieved at the village level by (a) establishing school gardens and orchard (b) setting up poultry units (c) production of fish in local tanks (d) inshore fishery in selected centers in coastal areas. The medical officer and their staffs in the primary health center will help impart nutrition to the people who come to the center and sub-center for medical care.

Role of Other Agencies

- **Women's organization:** Women's organization has an important role to play as they are being entrusted with the feeding of preschool and school children. These organizations are being supplied utensils. For cooking and serving balanced diets. Training program and cooking demonstrations have been organized by this women's organization.
- **Balwadi:** Under this program, a certain number of Balwadis have to be organized in each block where the preschool children can gather for reaction and lunch.
- **Youth clubs:** These clubs are encouraged to take plots of land for cultivation of vegetables, so that the youth team practices farming. This system also establishes a spirit of competition among the youths. Youth clubs are also encouraged to take up poultry units.
- **School teachers:** The success of the program for school gardens will depend upon the interest and leadership of the teacher. Therefore, the subject of nutrition has been included in the syllabus of teacher training courses.
- **Role of international agencies:** The international agencies responsible for this program are UNICEF, FAQ and WHO. The UNICEF also provides assistance for the production of text books, literature and visual education aids. The FAQ provides technical assistance for all the components of the program. WHO through its regional offices provides technical assistance in the field of health.

INTEGRATED CHILD DEVELOPMENT SERVICES

Integrated Child Development Scheme (ICDS), services was initiated by the Government of India under the Ministry of Social and Women's Welfare on October 2nd in 1975, in pursuance of the National Policy for Children which was recommended by the Shrivastav Committee during the 5th-five year plan (1974–1979). At present, the most important scheme in the field of child welfare is the ICDS scheme. The integrated child development services scheme has been implemented in India since 1975. There are about 100 such workers in each ICDS project. According to the available statistics, there are over 5320 ICDS blocks are functioning in India and 185 ICDS blocks are functioning in Kamataka, Karnataka.

Figure 13.3 is depicted the structure of Ministry of Women and Child Welfare.

The selection criteria of an Anganwadi worker are as follows:

- Educational qualification—SSLC pass or fail.
- Willing to serve for the community.
- Belongs to the same community/culture.
- In case of more volunteers from the same community.
- Village committee will select the candidate.

Objectives of ICDS

- To improve the nutritional and health status of children in the age group of 0–5 years.
- To lay the foundation for proper psychological, physical and social development of the child.
- To achieve effective coordination and implementation among the various departments working for the promotion of child development.
- To reduce morbidity, mortality and malnutrition among 0–5 years children and reproductive age mothers.
- To enhance the capability of the mother and nutritional needs of the child through proper nutrition and health education.

Packages of ICDS Scheme

- Supplementary nutrition.
- Immunization.
- Health check-up.
- Medical referral services.
- Nutrition and health education for women.
- Nonformal education for 3–5 years children.

The primary health centers of the ICDS blocks have been strengthened by the following additional inputs:

- One medical officer
- Two lady health visitors
- Eight ANM's in rural blocks and four ANM's in urban and tribal projects.

Anganwadis were established as focal points for the delivery of ICDS services. Each village with a population of 1000 has one anganwadi.

The anganwadi worker is the key person for the delivery of services at the anganwadis. An anganwadi worker has the following functions:

- Organizing supplementary nutrition feeding at the center.
- Non-formal preschool education
- Primary medical care
- Health and nutrition education to women
- Assisting the PHC staff in the implementation of the health components of one ICDS, eliciting community support and maintaining records.

MINIMUM NEED PROGRAMME

Launched at the very outset of the 5th five year plans (1975–80), the main aim of the program is to meet certain minimum needs of the people, and thus raise their living standards.

The minimum needs identified under this program are:

- Nutrition
- Rural health
- Elementary education
- Rural water supply
- Adult education
- Rural roads
- Rural electrification
- Rural housing
- Environmental improvement of urban slums.

The modes of meeting the nutritional needs of the people-children are:

- By extending nutritional support to 11 million eligible individuals.
- By expanding the Special Nutrition Programme for all the ICDS projects and
- By consolidating the Mid-day Meal Programmes and links it with health, portable water and sanitation.

20-POINTS PROGRAMME

The 20-Points Programme was launched in 1975 as a agenda for national action for promoting social justice and economic growth. In 1986, the program was modified.

The modified 20-Points Programme has at least eight points concerning health in some way or the others as indicated below:

- Point 1 relates to rural poverty
- Point 7 relates to clean drinking water
- Point 8 relates to "Health for all"
- Point 9 relates to "Two-child" norm
- Point 10 relates to expansion of education
- Point 14 relates to housing
- Point 15 relates to improvement in slums
- Point 17 relates to protection of environments

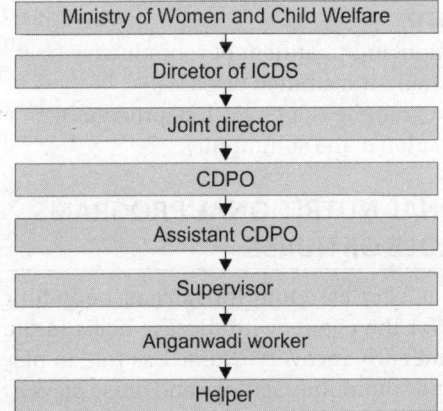

Fig. 13.3: Ministry of women and child welfare.
(CDPO: Child Development Project Officer; ICDS: Integrated Child Development Scheme)

CHILD SURVIVAL AND SAFE MOTHERHOOD PROGRAMMES

Every year over 27 million pregnancies take place in the country. All women need additional care during pregnancy. They need to eat and rest more than they did when they were not pregnant. All women need to be advised on the preparations they must make for delivery. These women must be given periodic health check-ups so that maternal complications or risk factors are identified in time and treatment started early and the women are counseled to deliver in a hospital.

The program is introduced as part of the overall strategy for reduction of:
- IMR to below 60 per 1000 live births.
- Child mortality to below 10 per 1000 child population.
- Reduction of percentage of LBW babies to less than 10%.
- Maternal mortality to below 2 per 1000 live births by 2000.
- Perinatal mortality should be less than 35 per 1000 live births.
- Immunization coverage should be 100%.
- Deliveries by trained personnel by 100%.
- Antenatal care should be 100%.
- Control of blindness should be less than 0.3. The CSSM came in to force in August 1992 and this is implemented with financial assistance from World Bank and UNICEF.

Objectives
- Sustaining and strengthening the ongoing Universal Immunization Programme.
- Continuing ORT program for children below the age of 5 years
- Introducing and expanding the program for control of acute respiratory infection for children below 5 years of age.
- Universalizing the Vitamin 'A' prophylaxis program from 6 months to 5 years.
- Iron and folic acid administration program to pregnant mother and children up to 5 years.
- Improving newborn care and maternal care at the community level.

Components
- Package consisting of UIP, ORT, prophylaxis, schemes and ART in all states and Union Territories.
- Safe motherhood programs for six high MMR states of Assam, Bihar, Madhya Pradesh, Odisha, Rajasthan and Uttar Pradesh.

Two districts of Tamil Nadu had been taken up earlier under UNICEF-assisted pilot project. The CSSM project will be implemented in a phased manner.

REPRODUCTIVE AND CHILD HEALTH PROGRAMME

This program followed revisions in the CSSM Programme as per recommendation made at the International Conference on Population and Development in Cairo in 1994 and was born in 1997.

The package of services offered by RCH Programme is: Program addresses the needs that have emerged over years of implementing the Family Welfare Programme. Unification of many women and child health areas will now enable health workers to move easily and completely understand service needs and deliver services accordingly. As opposed to the Family Welfare Programme, the RCH Programme aims to be more in tune with the ground realities concerning the:
- Overall health needs of women and children
- Implementation needs of health workers
- Local demographic needs and conditions.

Program Components: The Reproductive and Child Health Programme will build on the success of the UIP and the CSSM Programme. In addition, it will cover all aspects of women's reproductive health across their reproductive cycle, from puberty to menopause. In a nutshell, Reproductive and Child Health Programme will cover the services offered under the CSSM and the Family Welfare Programme as well as two new interventions, namely management of reproductive tract infections and adolescent reproductive health.

For the children:
- Essential newborn care
- Exclusive breastfeeding
- Immunization
- Appropriate management of ARI
- Vitamin A prophylaxis
- Treatment of anemia.

For the mother:
- Tetanus toxoid immunization
- Prevention and treatment of anemia
- Antenatal care and early identification of maternal complications.
- Deliveries conducted by trained personnel
- Promotion of institutional deliveries
- Management of obstetrical emergencies
- Birth spacing

For the eligible couples:
- Prevention of unwanted pregnancy
- Safe abortion

For RTI/STD:
- Prevention and treatment of reproductive tract infection and sexually-transmitted diseases.
- RCH Programme is a target-free program with voluntary participation of the community.

NATIONAL NUTRITIONAL PROGRAMS AND ROLE OF NURSE

Nutrition is very essential for normal body functioning. Nutrition for the clients with disease helps in the prompt healing and early recovery. Nurse has role to play in both hospital and community settings and nurse plays a dramatic role in different levels of health care. Broadly categorizing nurse has different roles at different levels.

Health Education

Health education being an extremely powerful component in achieving the adequate healthy life, nurse uses health education component as a tool in every setting and where ever needed, such as hospitals, clinics, community, schools, etc.

- Nurse educates about healthy and balanced diet to the peoples.
- Gives knowledge about recommendations required by different age and gender groups.
- Educated about best and easy ways to achieve good nutritious diet.
- Managing easy nutrients from locally available foods
- Education about the menu planning.

Hospitals

Nurse working in different wards of hospital are very vigilant in maintaining adequate nutrition levels for the client admitted.

- In hospital, nurse has to take care of nutritional aspects of the admitted client in ward.
- Educates the client as well as family members regarding the importance of the healthy and nutritious diet.
- Nurse maintains the adequate diet plans for the client.
- Helps in monitoring the conditions of the client, such as vomiting, input-output, electrolyte monitoring, in order to add different components in the diet.
- Maintaining parental nutrition for the client.
- Maintenance of adequate hydration.

Community

In community, nurse focuses on the prevention aspect, i.e., helps in giving the basic education regarding prevention of certain nutritional deficiency disease. At the community level the nurse can act as:

- Community health nurse.
- School health nurse.

And work in different sectors where she mainly works at grass root levels to correct the nutritional deficiencies in the client.

- Nurse rectifies the different patterns of the nutrition opted by the people.
- Nurse collaborates with government and non-government. agencies working for nutritional betterment of public sectors.
- Nurse plays a role in school health programs as school health nurse, helps in identification of malnourished children and maintains growth charts.
- Involvement of family.

CONCLUSION

Malnutrition is a major health problem in India. The efforts of the Government to combat and reduce under nutrition have been threefold—increasing food production, increasing purchasing capacity and organizing nutrition programmes. Supplementary feeding and nutrient deficiency control programmes are considered to be a short-term strategy and curative in their approach. There are essentially helpful for immediate child protection instead of sustained child development. Planned community nutrition education with community participation is an appropriate strategy for achieving and sustaining positive changes in food choices and utilization.

BIBLIOGRAPHY

1. Abrams SA, et al. A micronutrient-fortified beverage enhances the nutritional status of children in Botswana. Journal of Nutrition. 2003; 133:1834-40.
2. Antia FP. Clinical Dietetics and Nutrition, 3rd edition. Oxford University Press, Bombay, 1986.
3. Briggs GM, Doris HC. Nutrition and Physical Fitness, 11th edition. Harcourt College Publishers, New York, USA, 1984.
4. Garrow JSS, James WPT, Ralph A. Human Nutrition & Dietetics, 10th edition. WB Saunders, Philadelphia, USA, 1999.
5. Joshi SA. Nutrition and Dietetics, Tata McGraw Hill, New Delhi, India, 1992.
6. Joshi SA. Nutrition and Dietetics, Tata McGraw Hill, New Delhi, India, 1992.
7. Latham MC, et al. Micronutrient dietary supplements—a new fourth approach. Archivos Latinoamericanos de Nutricion. 2001;51(1 Suppl 1):37-41.
8. Martin EA, Ardath AC. Nutrition in Action, 4th edition, Holt Rinehart and Winston, New York, 1978.
9. McDivitt ME, Sumati RM. Human Nutrition—Principles and Applications in India, Revised Edition, Prentice Hall, New Delhi, 1973.
10. Nutrition Advisory Committee of the Indian Research Fund Association (IRFA). A report of the twelfth meeting. New Delhi, India; 1944.
11. Rao BSN. Nutrient requirement and safe dietary intake for Indians. Bull Nutr Foundation India. 2010;31:1-5.
12. Swaminathan M. Essentials of Food and Nutrition, Volume I and II, 2nd edition. Ganesh, Madras, India, 1985.

REVIEW QUESTIONS

Long Essays

1. Discuss in detail about nutritional problems in India.
2. Enumerate five year plans on nutritional aspects.
3. Explain National Nutritional Policy.
4. Describe about National Nutritional Programmes.

Short Essays

1. Enumerate various National Nutritional Programmes of India.
2. List various agencies working towards food and nutrition.
3. What are the various ways to assess the nutritional status?
4. Define nutrition education. Explain in detail the methods of imparting nutrition education.
5. Discuss the role of nurse in nutritional education.
6. Explain National Nutritional Programmes (NNP).
7. Explain Mid day Meal Programme.
8. Explain Vitamin A Deficiency Prophylaxis Programme.
9. Explain National Iodine Deficiency Disorders Programme.
10. How can nutritional anemia be prevented?
11. Explain ICDS Programme.
12. What is the role of FAO to improve nutrition of people of all countries?
13. Explain nutritional assessment.

Short Answers

1. Integrated Child Development Services (ICDS) Scheme.
2. Anemia Control Programme.
3. Vitamin A Prophylaxis Programme.
4. Community nutrition.
5. Infant and young child care and nutrition.
6. National Nutritional Programmes and role of nurse.
7. 20-points Programme.
8. Minimum Need Programme.
9. WFP's goal and objectives in India.
10. National Goitre Control Programme.
11. Aims of Mid Day Meal Programme.
12. Applied Nutrition Programme.
13. Balwadi Nutrition Programme.
14. Special Nutrition Programme.
15. Horizontal Nutritional Programmes.
16. Vertical Nutritional Programmes.

CHAPTER 14

Food Safety

CHAPTER OUTLINE

- ❖ Definition, Food Safety Considerations and Measures
- ❖ Food Safety Regulatory Measures in India—Relevant Acts
- ❖ Five Keys to Safer Food
- ❖ Food Storage, Food Handling and Cooking
- ❖ General Principles of Food Storage of Food Items (e.g., Milk, Meat)
- ❖ Role of Food Handlers in Foodborne Diseases
- ❖ Essential Steps in Safe Cooking Practices

TERMINOLOGY

- **Bacteria:** Bacteria are found in all foods. Most are killed by high temperatures, but some form toxins which may or may not be killed by heat.
- **Calibration:** the process of standardizing a temperature monitoring instrument to ensure that it will measure within a specific temperature range in which the instrument is designed to operate.
- **Chemicals:** Chemical foodborne illnesses are among the most deadly. Chemicals and other "natural" toxins formed in food include agents, such as scombrotoxin and ciguatoxin. Store cleaning supplies in a different area away from stored food.
- **Control (verb):** To take all necessary actions to ensure and maintain compliance with criteria established in the Hazard Analysis Critical Control Points (HACCP) Plan.
- **Control (noun):** The state wherein correct procedures are being followed and criteria are being met.
- **Control measures:** Actions and activities that can be used to prevent or eliminate a food safety hazard or reduce it to an acceptable level.
- **Corrective actions:** Actions to be taken when the results of monitoring at the CCP indicate a loss of control.
- **Critical control point (CCP):** A step at which control can be applied and is essential to prevent or eliminate a food safety hazard or reduce it to an acceptable level.
- **Critical limit:** A criterion which separates acceptability from unacceptability.
- **Cross-contamination:** Cross-contamination is when bacteria spread between food, surfaces or equipment.
- **Detergent:** A chemical used to remove grease, dirt and food, such as washing-up liquid.
- **Disinfectant:** A chemical that kills bacteria. Check that surfaces are clean of grease, dirt and food before you use a disinfectant. Chemicals that kill bacteria are sometimes called germicides, bactericides or biocides.
- **Contaminant:** Something that shouldn't be in food and can make the food unsafe to eat. Examples are harmful chemicals, physical objects (e.g., glass, metal fragments) and microorganisms ('germs', bacteria, viruses, parasites–see definition below).
- **Cross contamination:** When harmful microorganisms or chemicals spread between food, surfaces, hands or equipment. For example, if a cutting board used to prepare raw chicken is then used to prepare salad vegetables, microorganisms from the chicken juice on the board will spread to the salad. Because the salad won't be cooked, the microorganisms will not be killed before it is eaten.
- **Environmental sample:** A small amount of soil, water, food or other material taken (e.g., from a restaurant, factory or farm) to test in a lab to see if it contains harmful microorganisms.
- **Employee:** Any person working in or for a food service establishment who engages in food preparation or service, who transports food or Food containers, or who comes in contact with any food utensils or equipment.
- **Equipment:** All stoves, ranges, hoods, meat blocks, tables, counters, Refrigerators, freezers, sinks, dishwashing machines, steam tables and similar items, other than utensils, used in the operation of a food service establishments.
- **Fixed food establishment:** A food service establishment which operates at a specific location and is connected to electric utilities, water, and a sewage disposal system.
- **Foodborne illness:** A general term often used to describe any disease or illness caused by eating contaminated food or drink.
- **Foodborne infections:** These occur when "enough" of the live bacterial cells that have reproduced in the food, small intestine, or both are consumed. The severity of the infection depends on the virulence of the bacteria, resistance of the victim, and the number of cells that survive digestion.

- **Foodborne intoxications:** These result from a poison or toxin produced by reproductive bacterial cells in food or in the human body. Bacterial toxins have varying resistance to heat; some can even survive boiling. Other toxins can be a natural part of the food, for example, certain types of mushrooms.
- **Foodborne illness outbreak:** The Centers for Disease Control define an outbreak of foodborne illness as illness that involves two or more persons who eat a common food, with the food confirmed as the source of the illness by a laboratory analysis. The only exception is that a single case of botulism qualifies as an outbreak.
- **Food contact surfaces:** Surfaces of equipment and utensils with which normally comes in contact, and those surfaces from which food may drain, drip, or splash back onto surfaces normally in contact with Food.
- **Food poisoning:** An illness that occurs when people eat food that has been contaminated with harmful germs (particularly bacteria and viruses) or toxins (poisonous substances).
- **Food preparation:** The manipulation of foods intended for human consumption by such means as washing, slicing, peeling, chipping, shucking, scooping and/or portioning.
- **Food service establishment:** Any facility, where food is prepared and intended for individual portion service, and includes the site at which individual portions are provided.
- **HACCP:** A system which identifies, evaluates, and controls hazards which are significant for food safety.
- **HACCP plan:** A document prepared in accordance with the principles of HACCP to ensure control of hazards which are significant for food safety in the segment of the food chain under consideration.
- **Hazard:** A biological, chemical or physical agent or factor with the potential to cause an adverse health effect.
- **Hazard analysis:** The process of collecting and evaluating information on hazards and conditions leading to their presence to decide which are significant for food safety and therefore should be addressed in the HACCP plan.
- **Kitchenware:** All multi-use utensils, other than tableware (such as pots, pans).
- **Limited food service establishment:** Any establishment with a food operation, so limited by the type and quantity of foods prepared and the equipment utilized, that poses a lesser degree of risk to the public's health, and, for the purpose of fees, requires less time to monitor.
- **Monitor:** The act of conducting a planned sequence of observations or measurements of control parameters to assess whether a CCP is under control.
- **Parasites:** These tiny organisms can cause severe illness. Parasites need nutrients from their host to complete their life cycle. They are always associated with raw or undercooked meat and fish, including pork, bear meat and others.
- **Pathogen:** Any disease producing agent, microorganism or germ.
- **Perishable foods:** Any food of such type or in such condition as may spoil; provided, that foods which are in hermetically sealed containers processed by heat or other means to prevent spoilage and properly packaged, dehydrated, dry or powered foods so low in moisture content as to retard development of microorganism are not considered readily perishable.
- **Potentially hazardous food:** Any perishable food that is capable of supporting rapid and progressive growth of infectious or toxigenic microorganisms.
- **Safe temperatures:** As applies to potentially hazardous foods, means Temperatures of 41°F or below, or 140°F or above.
- **Sanitizer:** A two-in-one product that acts as a detergent and a disinfectant.
- **Single-service articles:** Any cups, containers, closures, plates, straws, place mats, napkins, doilies, spoons, stirrers, paddles, knives, forks, wrapping materials, and all similar articles, which are constructed wholly or in part from paper or paper material, foil, wood, plastic, synthetic or other readily destructible materials, for one time and one person use and then discarded.
- **Step:** A point, procedure, operation or stage in the food chain including raw materials, from primary production to final consumption.
- **Tableware:** Multi-use eating and drinking items, including flatware, knives, forks, spoons, glasses, cups, etc.
- **Temperature:** A critical measurement for ensuring the safety and quality of many food products.
- **Utensil:** Implements, such as pots, pans, ladles or food containers used in the preparation, storage, transportation or serving of food.
- **Verification:** The application of methods, procedures, and tests, in addition to those used in monitoring to determine compliance with the HACCP plan, and/or whether the HACCP plan needs modification.
- **Viruses:** Viruses grow or reproduce only on living cells. They are often found in untreated water or sewage-contaminated water, and viruses from human feces on unwashed hands can infect others by passing the virus to food.

INTRODUCTION

Food safety is about handling, storing and preparing food to prevent infection and help to make sure that our food keeps enough nutrients for us to have a healthy diet. Unsafe food and water means that it has been exposed to dirt and germs, or may even be rotten, which can cause infections or diseases, such as diarrhea, meningitis, etc. These diseases can make people very sick or even be life threatening. When people are sick, they are weak and would have difficulty working or concentrating at school. Some of these infections also make it difficult for our bodies to absorb the nutrients they need to get healthy. Unsafe or stale foods also deteriorate and are of poor quality, which means they lose nutrients and so we do not get enough of what we need for a healthy diet.

CONCEPT OF FOOD SAFETY

- Unsafe food-containing harmful bacteria, viruses, parasites or chemical substances, causes more than 200 diseases—ranging from diarrhea to cancers.

- An estimated 600 million—almost 1 in 10 people in the world—fall ill after eating contaminated food and 420,000 die every year, resulting in the loss of 33 million healthy life years (DALYs).
- US$ 110 billion is lost each year in productivity and medical expenses resulting from unsafe food in low- and middle-income countries.
- Children under 5 years of age carry 40% of the foodborne disease burden, with 125,000 deaths every year.
- Diarrheal diseases are the most common illnesses resulting from the consumption of contaminated food, causing 550 million people to fall ill and 230,000 deaths every year.
- Food safety, nutrition and food security are inextricably linked. Unsafe food creates a vicious cycle of disease and malnutrition, particularly affecting infants, young children, elderly and the sick.
- Foodborne diseases impede socioeconomic development by straining healthcare systems, and harming national economies, tourism and trade.
- Food supply chains now cross multiple national borders. Good collaboration between governments, producers and consumers helps ensure food safety.

FOUR STEPS TO FOOD SAFETY (FIG. 14.1)

Following four simple steps at home—clean, separate, cook, and chill—can help protect you and your loved ones from food poisoning.

Clean

Wash your hands and surfaces often:
- Germs that cause food poisoning can survive in many places and spread around your kitchen.
- Wash hands for 20 seconds with soap and water before, during, and after preparing food and before eating.
- Wash your utensils, cutting boards, and countertops with hot, soapy water.
- Rinse fresh fruits and vegetables under running water.

Separate

Do not cross-contaminate:
- Raw meat, poultry, seafood, and eggs can spread germs to ready-to-eat foods—unless you keep them separate.
- Use separate cutting boards and plates for raw meat, poultry, and seafood.
- When grocery shopping, keep raw meat, poultry, seafood, and their juices away from other foods.
- Keep raw meat, poultry, seafood, and eggs separate from all other foods in the refrigerator.

Cook to the Right Temperature

- Food is safely cooked when the internal temperature gets high enough to kill germs that can make you sick. The only way to tell if food is safely cooked is to use a food thermometer. You cannot tell if food is safely cooked by checking its color and texture.
- Use a food thermometer to ensure foods are cooked to a safe internal temperature. Check this chart for a detailed list of temperatures and foods external icon, including shellfish and precooked ham.
- **Whole cuts of beef, veal, lamb, and pork, including fresh ham (raw):** 145°F (then allow the meat to rest for 3 minutes before carving or eating)
- **Fish with fins:** 145°F or cook until flesh is opaque
- **Ground meats, such as beef and pork:** 160°F
- **All poultry, including ground chicken and turkey:** 165°F
- **Leftovers and casseroles:** 165°F

Chill: Refrigerate Promptly

Bacteria can multiply rapidly if left at room temperature or in the "Danger Zone" between 40°F and 140°F. Never leave perishable food out for more than 2 hours (or 1 hour if exposed to temperatures above 90°F).
- Keep your refrigerator at 40°F or below and know when to throw food out external icon.
- Refrigerate perishable food within 2 hours. If the food is exposed to temperatures above 90°F (such as a hot car or picnic), refrigerate it within 1 hour.
- Thaw frozen food safely in the refrigerator, in cold water, or in the microwave. Never thaw foods on the counter because bacteria multiply quickly in the parts of the food that reach room temperature.

MAJOR FOODBORNE ILLNESSES AND CAUSES (FIG. 14.2)

Foodborne illnesses are usually infectious or toxic in nature and caused by bacteria, viruses, parasites or chemical substances entering the body through contaminated food or water. Foodborne pathogens can cause severe diarrhea or debilitating infections including meningitis. Chemical contamination can lead to acute poisoning or long-term diseases, such as cancer. Foodborne diseases may lead to long-lasting disability and death. Examples of unsafe food include uncooked foods of animal origin, fruits and vegetables contaminated with feces, and raw shellfish containing marine biotoxins.

Bacteria

- ***Salmonella, Campylobacter,* and *Enterohaemorrhagic Escherichia coli*** are among the most common foodborne pathogens that affect millions of people annually—sometimes with severe and fatal outcomes. Symptoms are fever, headache, nausea, vomiting, abdominal pain and diarrhea. Examples of foods

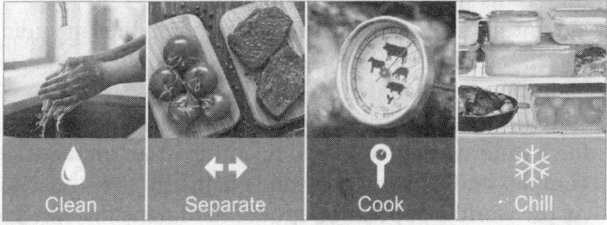

Fig. 14.1: Four steps to food safety.

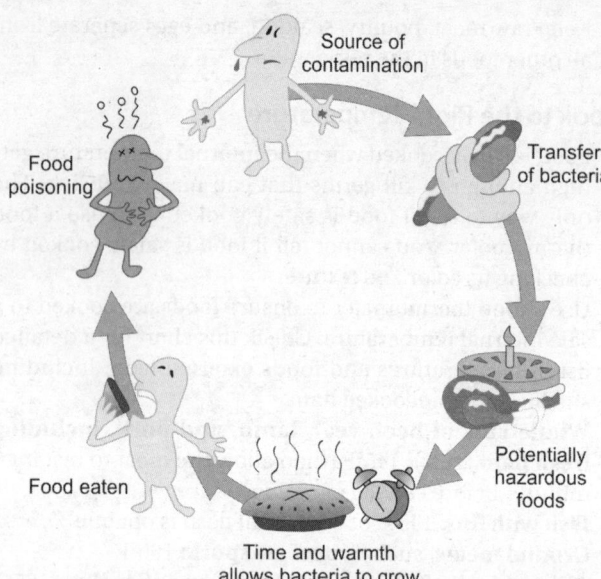

Fig. 14.2: Major foodborne illnesses and causes.

involved in outbreaks of salmonellosis are eggs, poultry and other products of animal origin. Foodborne cases with *Campylobacter* are mainly caused by raw milk, raw or undercooked poultry and drinking water. *Enterohaemorrhagic Escherichia coli* is associated with unpasteurized milk, undercooked meat and fresh fruits and vegetables.

- *Listeria* infection leads to miscarriage in pregnant women or death of newborn babies. Although disease occurrence is relatively low, *Listeria's* severe and sometimes fatal health consequences, particularly among infants, children and the elderly, count them among the most serious foodborne infections. *Listeria* is found in unpasteurized dairy products and various ready-to-eat foods and can grow at refrigeration temperatures.
- *Vibrio cholerae* infects people through contaminated water or food. Symptoms include abdominal pain, vomiting and profuse watery diarrhea, which may lead to severe dehydration and possibly death. Rice, vegetables, millet gruel and various types of seafood have been implicated in cholera outbreaks.

Antimicrobials, such as antibiotics, are essential to treat infections caused by bacteria. However, their overuse and misuse in veterinary and human medicine has been linked to the emergence and spread of resistant bacteria, rendering the treatment of infectious diseases ineffective in animals and humans. Resistant bacteria enter the food chain through the animals (e.g., *Salmonella* through chickens). Antimicrobial resistance is one of the main threats to modern medicine.

Viruses

Norovirus infections are characterized by nausea, explosive vomiting, watery diarrhea and abdominal pain. Hepatitis A virus can cause long-lasting liver disease and spreads typically through raw or undercooked seafood or contaminated raw produce. Infected food handlers are often the source of food contamination.

Parasites

Some parasites, such as fish-borne trematodes, are only transmitted through food. Others, for example, tapeworms, such as *Echinococcus* species, or *Taenia solium*, may infect people through food or direct contact with animals. Other parasites, such as *Ascaris*, *Cryptosporidium*, *Entamoeba histolytica* or *Giardia*, enter the food chain via water or soil and can contaminate fresh produce.

Prions

Prions, infectious agents composed of protein, are unique in that they are associated with specific forms of neurodegenerative disease. Bovine spongiform encephalopathy (BSE, or "mad cow disease") is a prion disease in cattle, associated with the variant Creutzfeldt-Jakob disease (vCJD) in humans. Consuming bovine products containing specified risk material, e.g., brain tissue, is the most likely route of transmission of the prion agent to humans.

Chemicals

Of most concern for health are naturally occurring toxins and environmental pollutants.
- **Naturally occurring toxins** include mycotoxins, marine biotoxins, cyanogenic glycosides and toxins occurring in poisonous mushrooms. Staple foods, such as corn or cereals can contain high levels of mycotoxins, such as aflatoxin and ochratoxin, produced by mould on grain. A long-term exposure can affect the immune system and normal development, or cause cancer.
- **Persistent organic pollutants (POPs)** are compounds that accumulate in the environment and human body. Known examples are dioxins and polychlorinated biphenyls (PCBs), which are unwanted by-products of industrial processes and waste incineration. They are found worldwide in the environment and accumulate in animal food chains. Dioxins are highly toxic and can cause reproductive and developmental problems, damage the immune system, interfere with hormones and cause cancer.
- **Heavy metals,** such as lead, cadmium and mercury cause neurological and kidney damage. Contamination by heavy metal in food occurs mainly through pollution of air, water and soil.

THE EVOLVING WORLD AND FOOD SAFETY

- Safe food supplies support national economies, trade and tourism, contributes to food and nutrition security, and underpins sustainable development.
- Urbanization and changes in consumer habits, including travel, have increased the number of people buying and eating food prepared in public places.
- Globalization has triggered growing consumer demand for a wider variety of foods, resulting in an increasingly complex and longer global food chain.
- As the world's population grows, the intensification and industrialization of agriculture and animal production

to meet increasing demand for food creates both opportunities and challenges for food safety. Climate change is also predicted to impact food safety.
- These challenges put greater responsibility on food producers and handlers to ensure food safety.
- Local incidents can quickly evolve into international emergencies due to the speed and range of product distribution.
- Serious foodborne disease outbreaks have occurred on every continent in the past decade, often amplified by globalized trade.

FOOD SAFETY: A PUBLIC HEALTH PRIORITY

Unsafe food poses global health threats, endangering everyone. Infants, young children, pregnant women, the elderly and those with an underlying illness are particularly vulnerable. Every year 220 million children contract diarrheal diseases and 96,000 die. Unsafe food creates a vicious cycle of diarrhea and malnutrition, threatening the nutritional status of the most vulnerable.
- The International Conference on Food Safety held in Addis Ababa in February 2019, and the International Forum on Food Safety and Trade held in Geneva in 2019, reiterated the importance of food safety in achieving the Sustainable Development Goals.
- Governments should make food safety a public health priority, as they play a pivotal role in developing policies and regulatory frameworks, and establishing and implementing effective food safety systems.
- Food can become contaminated at any point of production and distribution, and the primary responsibility lies with food producers. Yet a large proportion of foodborne disease incidents are caused by foods improperly prepared or mishandled at home, in food service establishments or at markets.
- Not all food handlers and consumers understand the roles they must play, such as adopting basic hygienic practices when buying, selling and preparing food to protect their health and that of the wider community.
- Everyone can contribute to making food safe. Here are some examples of effective actions:

Role of Policy Maker
- Build and maintain adequate food systems and infrastructures (e.g., laboratories) to respond to and manage food safety risks along the entire food chain, including during emergencies;
- Foster multisectoral collaboration among public health, animal health, agriculture and other sectors for better communication and joint action;
- Integrate food safety into broader food policies and programmes (e.g., nutrition and food security);
- Think globally and act locally to ensure that food produced domestically remains safe when imported internationally.

FOOD SAFETY CONSIDERATIONS AND MEASURES

Clean and safe food is very important to prevent germs from getting into foods and water. Such germs not only cause diseases, but they also destroy valuable nutrients in the food.
- Wash hands with soap and clean water after going to the toilet, changing babies' nappies and working with animals. Also wash hands before working with food and before eating.
- Wash all fruit and vegetables in clean water before eating and cooking. Add a teaspoon of salt to this water.
- Wash the udder of the cow or goat well before milking.
- Wash dishes and utensils (knives, spoons, etc.) immediately after use and store them in a clean place where flies or dust cannot get on them.
- Choose fruit and vegetables that are fresh and healthy-looking.
- Boil water and milk for at least 5 minutes. (A small glass bottle, or china cup or saucer placed in the pot will stop the milk from boiling over).
- Do not eat cracked eggs. Wipe eggs clean with a clean, damp cloth before use, cook eggs until they are no longer runny.
- Avoid buying or eating food which is old. Check the sell-by dates on food products.
- Cook or reheat food properly, but avoid overcooking, because this can destroy nutrients. Also avoid cooking food in too much water, because the nutrients get lost when they go into the water.
- Keep cooked and raw foods apart when preparing or storing them. This helps to prevent germs from moving from one to the other.
- If you do not have a fridge, do not keep cooked food for more than a few hours in cool weather. In warm weather, eat it as soon as possible. To avoid waste, rather cook smaller amounts than cooking too much food which has to then be kept too long or thrown away.
- Keep food warm only as long as really needed; otherwise let if cool as soon and fast as possible. Warmth will encourage germs to breed.
- If you have a fridge, avoid keeping cooked food or raw meat for more than 24 hours unless it is in the freezer.
- Water and food should be stored in clean, covered containers in a cool, dark place. Covered containers protect food from dust, insects or rats and coolness helps food to last longer.
- Do not keep food in open tins, which can get rusty. Rather keep the food in clean plastic containers with lids.
- Keep food storage and preparation places clean and tidy.
- Prevent human and animal feces from getting into water.
- Keep chickens away from the home. Chicken feces carry germs and attract flies.
- Avoid or prevent littering. This attracts flies, rats and other organisms which spread disease.

TIPS FOR MAINTAINING FOOD SAFETY

- Keep the refrigerator temperature at 4°C. This temperature is intended to prevent the development of most pathogenic bacteria that may be in food.
- Cool food down within a short time after cooking or consuming it to 4°C. Avoid keeping food outside of the refrigerator for more than an hour. Cooked food should be cooled down by various means, such as by immersing in a container with cold water, within two hours of cooking it, to the temperature of the refrigerator.
- It is recommended to use disposable paper towels in the kitchen. If non-disposable tea towels are used, they should be washed frequently. Towels that are used to clean working surfaces that have been in contact with food could become contaminated with bacteria, some of which are pathogenic bacteria that convey diseases.
- Cutting boards that come into contact with raw meat, fish and poultry should be cleaned with soap and hot water after each use. The cutting board should be rubbed with a scrubber sponge or brush with dishwashing liquid, rinsed well with hot water and air-dried. The scrubber sponge should be replaced frequently. These measures are in order to prevent the development of bacteria that remain on the cutting board. Do not use the same board to cut cooked meat.
- Raw food, especially red meat, poultry and fish products, should be cooked thoroughly. Cooking of food, including meat, must reach a minimum temperature at the center of the product of 72°C. Meat products that have undergone cooking change their color. It is recommended to use a special kitchen thermometer, a special thermometer probe for checking food to measure the temperature at the center of the food and ensure thorough cooking. Do not use a mercury thermometer made of glass.
- Do not consume raw eggs or eggs that have been treated with mild heat (soft boiled egg, fried egg). Do not prepare foods at home that to not undergo heat treatment and are based on fresh eggs, e.g., ice cream, mayonnaise, etc. Foods prepared with fresh eggs that are not destined to undergo heat treatment could be contaminated with *Salmonella enterica* bacteria (a bacteria that causes food poisoning).
- Clean kitchen utensils (cutlery, plates, pots) with a scrubbing sponge or brush, hot water and dishwashing fluid; and air-dry them after rinsing in water. Avoid wiping kitchen utensils with a tea towel which could be contaminated with bacteria and re-contaminate the clean food utensils.
- Wash your hands with hot water and soap immediately after handling raw food—vegetables, fruit, raw meat, poultry, fresh eggs or fish.
- Defrosting of frozen food should be done in the refrigerator or microwave oven in a suitable container that prevents direct contact with other food products. Defrosting of uncooked meat, fish and poultry shall be done in the refrigerator only, on the lowest shelf.
- Do not purchase perishable foods (meat, poultry, fish, dairy and egg products) at places that are not organized, air-conditioned, and have appropriate equipment, such as refrigerators and freezers.
- When purchasing fruits and vegetables, avoid their direct contact with other food products. Do not eat fruits or vegetables before cleaning them.
- **Cleaning fruits and vegetables:**
  - Wash the fruit/vegetable well with tap water, until the gross debris is removed
  - Soak the fruit/vegetable in water with liquid soap, and rinse using a brush
  - Dry the fruit/vegetable in air or with a clean paper towel.

FOOD HYGIENE/SANITATION

Food sanitation implies cleanliness in the producing preparing storing and servicing of food and water. Food sanitation is essential aspect of food preparation. It needs to emphasize at every stage of food handling and preparation. Some of the items which need particular attention to ensure that food is safe for consumption are a safe and portable water supply.

Selection of wholesome ingredients and hygienic handling to prevent the entry of spoilage and pathogenic organisms, both during preparation and serving. In addition, all equipment during coming in contact with food supply be scrupulously clean, the surrounding should be clean and there should be a proper and safe method for the disposal of waste. Inculcation of hygienic habits would help in preventing foods from being contaminated during handling.

Definition

The WHO has defined **food safety/food hygiene** as all conditions and measures that are necessary during the production, processing, storage, distribution and preparation of food to ensure that it is safe, sound wholesome and fit for human consumption.

According to WHO "as all conditions and measures that are necessary during the production, processing storage, distribution and preparation of food, to ensure that it is safe, sound, wholesome and fit for human consumption.

Food hygiene: Food is a potential source of infection and is liable to contamination by microorganisms, and any point during its journey from the production to the consumer. Food hygiene, in its widest sense, implies hygiene in the production, handling, distribution and serving of all types of food.

The primary aim of food hygiene is to prevent food poisoning and other foodborne illnesses, which can be grouped under the following headings.

Milk hygiene: Milk is an efficient vehicle for a great variety of disease agents, the source of infection or contamination of milk may be the diary animal, human handler or the environment. For example, a contaminated vessel, polluted water, flies, dusts, etc.

Table 14.1 is depicted the terms used in food safety measures.

Table 14.1: Terms used in food safety measures.

Sl. No.	Term	Description
1.	Clean	Free from dirt, dust, grease, waste, food residues and all other foreign visible materials as well as objectionable odor
2.	Contamination	Foods exposed to conditions which permit: • Introduction of foreign matters including dust, dirt, chemicals and pests, or • Introduction or multiplication of disease—causing microorganisms or parasites, or • Introduction or production of toxins
3.	Cross-contamination	Transfer of microorganisms or contaminants from one food (usually raw) to another food either directly when one food touches another, or indirectly through hands or equipment
4.	Equipment	Apparatus, vessels, containers, utensils, machines, instruments or appliances used for storing, handling, cooking and cleaning of food
5.	Food contact surfaces	Surfaces that will come into contact with food in a food premises
6.	Food handler	Any person who engages in the handling of food, equipment or utensils that will come into contact with food for a food business
7.	Food premises	Any place where food is supplied, prepared, processed, handled, stored, packaged, displayed, served or offered for sale for human consumption
8.	Open food	Uncooked perishable food and food not contained in containers as to exclude risks of contamination.
9.	Pathogen	A disease-causing microorganism
10.	Pest	Any animal or insect that may contaminate food or a food contact surface. This includes rats, mice, cockroaches and flies
11.	Potable	Suitable for human to drink or ingest
12.	Potentially hazardous food	Food that requires temperature control to minimize the growth of any pathogenic microorganisms that may be present or to prevent the formation of toxin
13.	Poultry	Any domesticated bird whether live or dead (chickens, ducks, geese, quails, etc.) commonly used for human consumption
14.	Ready-to-eat food	Food that is ready for immediate consumption at the point of sale. It could be raw or cooked, hot or chilled, and can be consumed without further heat-treatment
15.	Utensils	Articles, vessels, containers or equipment used in the handling, preparation, processing, packaging, displaying, serving, dispensing, storing, containing or consumption of food

Principles of Food Sanitation

- The food handlers are free from any communicable diseases.
- Human air, nasal, discharge, skin can also be source of microorganisms therefore persons handling food, must wash hands with soap before starting preparation and refrain from touching hair or wiping nose during food preparation.
- **Personal hygiene:** A high standard of personal hygiene among individuals engaged in the handling, preparation and cooking of food is needed.
- **Food handling techniques:** The handling of ready to eat food with bare hands should be reduced to a minimum.
- **Sanitary conditions:** Sanitation of all work surfaces, utensils and equipment must be ensured. Food premises should be kept free from rats, mice, flies and dust.

Sources of Food Contamination (Fig. 14.3)

- Water used for washing or cleaning is not potable.
- Soil adhering to foods grown close to ground in not completely removed.
- Container or utensils used for storage and preparation are not clean.
- Personnel handling food have unhygienic habits.
- Personnel handling food suffer from communicable diseases.

Hygienic Practices of Food Handlers (Fig. 14.4)

- Hand should be washed properly and should be clean always.
- Fingernails should be kept short and free from dirt.
- Head covering should be used to prevent loose hair falling into the food.
- Aprons should be worn.
- Coughing, sneezing, smoking in vicinity of food should be avoided.

FOOD POISONING

Food poisoning is caused by the consumption of food or drinks contaminated with pathogens (including bacteria, viruses and parasites), bacterial or biochemical toxins or toxic chemicals. Patients usually show gastrointestinal symptoms, such as nausea, abdominal pain, diarrhea and vomiting, although other symptoms, such as fever may also develop. The incubation period varies from hours to days depending on the causative agent.

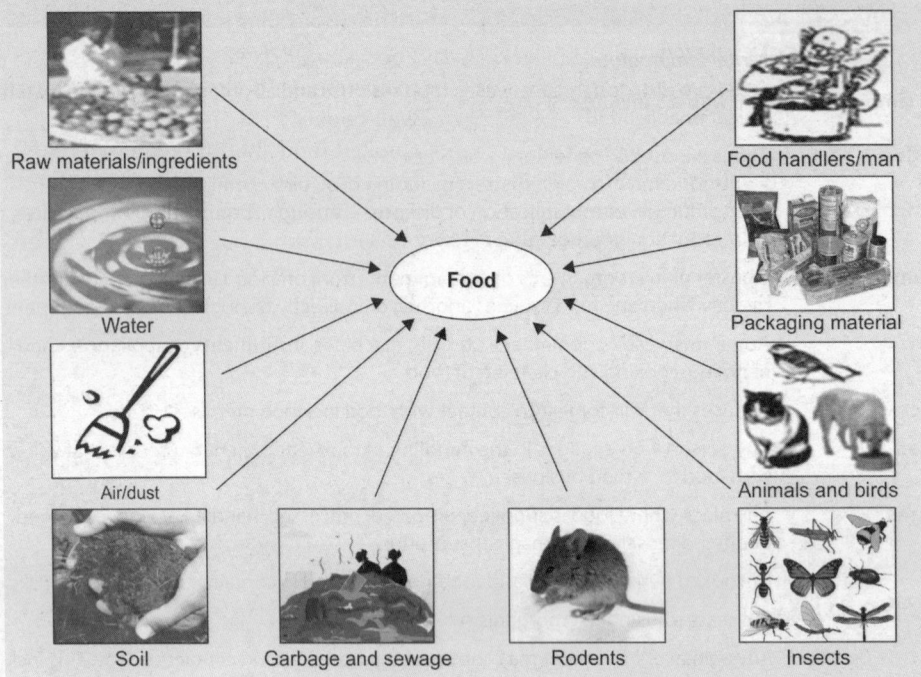

Fig. 14.3: Sources of food contamination.

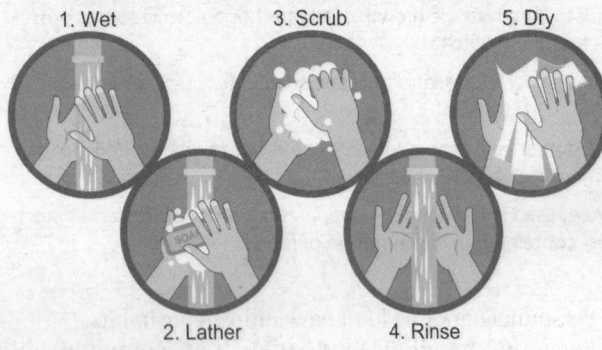

Fig. 14.4: Hygienic practices of food handlers.

Foodborne Disease

- **Bacterial:** Typhoid and paratyphoid, diarrhea and dysentery
- **Viral:** Viral hepatitis, poliomyelitis,
- **Protozoa:** Amoebas
- **Intestinal worms:** Tapeworm and round worm
- **Others:** Food poisoning

Common Types of Bacterial Food Poisoning (Table 14.2)

In Hong Kong, bacterial food poisoning caused by pathogenic bacteria is the commonest type of food poisoning. There are various kinds of bacterial food poisoning, but the following are the most prevalent:

Common Contributing Factors to Bacterial Food Poisoning

- **Contamination of cooked food:** Cooked food has been contaminated by food handlers, raw food, food contact surfaces or pests.

Table 14.2: Common types of bacterial food poisoning.

Sl. No.	Name of bacteria	Common foods involved
1.	Salmonella species	Raw or undercooked egg and egg products (e.g., Tiramisu); undercooked meat, poultry and their products (e.g., barbecued and preserved meat, goose intestines, etc.)
2.	Staphylococcus aureus	Foods which have been subject to a large amount of handling with no subsequent cooking or reheating (e.g., lunch boxes, cakes, pastries, sandwiches, etc.)
3.	Vibrio parahaemolyticus	Raw or undercooked seafood, shellfish, marine products and salted food (e.g., jellyfish, cuttlefish, salted vegetables and smoked knuckles, etc.)
4.	Bacillus cereus	Leftover cooked rice, fried rice, meat products and vegetables
5.	Clostridium perfringens	Cross-contaminated and inadequately cooked meat and meat products (e.g., stew and meat pies, etc.).

- **Improper storage of cooked food:** Cooked food has been stored between 4°C and 60°C for a prolonged period.
- **Inadequate cooking of food:** Raw food has not been cooked thoroughly to reduce any pathogen present.
- **Inadequate reheating of cooked food:** Cooked food has not been reheated to 75°C.
- **Inadequate thawing of food before cooking:** Insufficiently thawed food, which still has a high bacterial count or pathogen content and which needs a longer time to reach the temperature that kills the bacteria and pathogens in cooking, has not been cooked for sufficiently long time.

Table 14.3: Food thermometer.

Food type	Internal temperature
Beef, pork, veal, and lamb (chops, roasts, steaks)	145°F with a 3 minute rest time
Ground meat	160°F
Ham, uncooked (fresh or smoked)	145°F with a 3 minute rest time
Ham, fully cooked (to reheat)	140°F
Poultry (ground, parts, whole, and stuffing)	165°F
Eggs	Cook until yolk and white are firm
Egg dishes	160°F
Fin fish	145°F or flesh is opaque and separates easily with fork
Shrimp, lobster, and crabs	Flesh pearly and opaque
Clams, oysters, and mussels	Shells open during cooking
Scallops	Flesh is milky white or opaque and firm
Leftovers and casseroles	165°F

- **Preparation of food too early in advance:** Food has been prepared too early in advance but has not been stored under proper temperature control.
- **Infected food handlers:** Food handlers infected with communicable diseases have engaged in handling food.
- **Consumption of raw food:** Food (e.g., shrimps) that usually has a high bacterial count or pathogen content has been eaten in a raw state without cooking.
- **Use of unsafe food source:** Food has been purchased from an unapproved or unreliable source, such as hawkers.
- **Use of leftovers:** Use of food leftovers (e.g., cooked rice) that have been stored between 4°C to 60°C for a prolonged period.

Table 14.3 is depicted the food thermometer.

Prevention of Bacterial Food Poisoning

In principle, the best way to avoid bacterial food poisoning is to ensure safe food production. Essential measures include:

Purchase of Food

- Do not buy foods that are not properly protected (e.g., siu mei and lo mei that has been exposed to the open air during transportation, or cooked food that has not been covered properly).
- Do not purchase food from unlicensed sources, especially for cooked or cold food (because the place and ways in which they cook their foods are usually not hygienic).
- Do not buy any food which looks abnormal (e.g., swollen or dented canned foods).
- Food to be eaten raw, such as sashimi and rock oysters, should be obtained from a reliable and reputable source to ensure their quality.

Handling of Food

- Food should be thoroughly cooked before being served to customers (both meat and marine products should be well-cooked).
- Cooked food should be prepared and stored separately from raw food (to avoid cross-contamination).
- Food handlers should thoroughly wash their hands after going to the toilet and before handling food (to prevent the soiled hands from contaminating the food). In any case, do not touch cooked food with bare hands.
- Anybody suffering from diarrhea, vomiting, sore throat or inflamed wounds (unless properly bandaged with waterproof plastic tapes) should not handle or touch any food so as to prevent the food from being contaminated by food poisoning bacteria.

Storage of Food

- Food should be served once it is prepared (that means food should be served either hot or cold. Food that is neither hot nor cold is conducive to the growth of bacteria).
- Leftovers should best be discarded. Otherwise, it should be properly stored in refrigerators (4°C or below) and thoroughly reheated to 75°C or above before being served to customers.
- Any food that is not to be served immediately should be stored at a temperature below 4°C or above 60°C. Do not store food at room temperature which is favorable to bacterial growth or production of toxins.

Practical Rules for Good Sanitation

- Tie hair neatly before starting food preparation, use hair net or cap if necessary. Wash hands thoroughly with soap and water before starting preparation.
- Wash fruits, vegetables, cereals and beans thoroughly before preparation with portable water. Boil milk in a clean container as soon as possible after receipt and keep covered.
- Use portable water in food preparation.
- Boil water used for drinking or for preparation of cold beverages, if the purity of water is not guaranteed.
- Utensils and equipments used for preparation should be scrupulously cleaned.
- Cooked food should be stored covered, preferably in the container in which it is cooked.
- Left over foods, such as rice, vegetables should be stored either in a refrigerator kept in a pan of cold water. Reheating before use is advisable.

HYGIENE CONTROL

Control of hygiene when working with food is essential. This is because food must be kept safe. This is done by:
- Protecting food from contamination by harmful bacteria
- Preventing bacteria from multiplying to dangerous levels
- Destroying harmful bacteria in or on food by thorough cooking
- Disposing of harmful food safely.

The basic rules of food hygiene are outlined below:
Always wash your hands before touching food, particularly after visiting the toilet, after touching animals, your own skin and hair, and after touching raw food.

- Always cover any break in the skin of your hands, or sores or spots, with a waterproof adhesive dressing (preferably a highly colored one so you notice it if it comes off).
- No smoking during the preparation of food.
- Avoid preparing food if you have any illness (particularly skin, nose or throat infections and sickness and diarrhea).
- Do not allow animals into the food preparation area.
- Cover food to protect it from flies and other insects.
- Wrap all food waste and dispose of it in a covered waste bin.
- Clean as you go. Wash surfaces with hot water and detergent.
- Wipe spills up immediately with kitchen tissue and place this in a covered bin.
- Serve food as soon as possible after preparing it.
- Never allow raw food to come in contact with cooked food; common ways in which cooked food is contaminated from raw food are through the hands, knives and working surfaces.
- Wear clean clothing and be clean yourself.
- Do not cough or sneeze over food.

Temperature Control

Control of temperature is very important in the cooking and storage of food. The Food Safety (Temperature Control) Regulations 1995 sets out the safe temperatures for the storage, heating and chilling of food, as shown in the table below.

Method Temperature

- Freezer −18°C to −22°C
- Refrigerator legal requirement 8°C; good practice 5–6°C
- Hot holding food, hot food must be maintained at a temperature of 63°C
- Reheating commercially manufactured food that has been cooked once during manufacture
- Temperature of reheated food must reach a minimum of 82°C.

Pest Control

A food pest is any animal that can live on or in food, causing damage or contamination. The main types of pests are:
1. Insects, such as flies, cockroaches and weevils
2. Birds
3. Rodents, such as rats and mice.

Flies land on food and carry bacteria on their bodies. In addition, they defecate on food and regurgitate half-digested food from a previous meal onto the food. They can also lay eggs and their dead bodies can be found in food.

Cockroaches can deposit feces on food and spread bacteria, and small insects, such as weevils live in stored foods and food products, such as flour and cereals.

Rodents, such as mice and rats carry bacteria and pass these on by either walking on the food or on work surfaces. Mice particularly have a tendency to urinate on food.

Some birds can also carry bacteria. Food can be contaminated by droppings and feathers and by insects that they carry on their bodies.

Some birds will contaminate milk by pecking through the foil tops of bottles left on the doorstep.

Protecting premises where food is stored or manufactured is the most important way of preventing possible infection of or damage to food.

The owner of the premises must ensure that the building is kept in good repair with no obvious points of entry for pests. Food pests tend to, such as warm, dark, damp undisturbed places, so it is important for food storage and preparation areas to be cool, clean and dry

EFFECTS OF UNSAFE PRACTICES

Food can be contaminated in a variety of ways—both physical and chemical. Physical contaminants include bones, shells or pips and stalks from food, food packaging, nuts or bolts from equipment, jewellery, hair, fingernails, plasters, dust and dirt, and insects and their droppings and eggs.

Chemical contamination can be caused by cleaning chemicals, if they are not kept separate from food and food preparation areas, and agricultural chemicals, for example, on fruit and vegetables if they have been sprayed. They must be cleaned thoroughly or peeled before eating.

Leftover food or drink from metal containers should always be transferred to a non-metallic container and stored covered in a refrigerator. Acidic and salty food can attack the metal once a can is opened, which then affects the food.

Biological contamination is contamination by bacteria or viruses where they multiply on the food to dangerous levels, or by moulds which cause toxins on food. When they are eaten, they cause illness.

Legislation, Regulations and Codes of Practice

Food safety legislation requires that establishments preparing and serving food ensure that food is safe to eat. Three of the main laws and regulations are:

Food Safety Act 1990

The Food Safety Act is the main piece of legislation that governs the safety of food. The Act says that it is illegal to sell or keep for sale food that is unfit for people to eat or causes food to be dangerous to health, or is not of acceptable content or quality, or is labeled or advertised in any way that misleads the consumer. If prosecuted, people who work with food must show that they have taken all reasonable steps to avoid causing any of the above.

Food Safety (General Food Hygiene) Regulations 1995

These regulations cover the basic hygiene principles that businesses must follow and relate to staff, premises and food handling. They affect anyone who owns manages or works in

a food business, whether it is a caravan in a lay-by selling tea, coffee and snacks, or a five-star hotel. The regulations cover the following:
- The supply and selling of food in a hygienic way.
- Identification of possible food hazards.
- Control of identified hazards to prevent harm to customers.
- The establishment of effective control and monitoring procedures to ensure that harm does not come to customers.

Food Safety (Temperature Control) Regulations 1995

These regulations cover the following aspects of food hygiene:
- The stages of the food chain that is subject to temperature controls.
- The temperatures at which certain foods must be kept.
- Which foods are exempt from specific temperature controls?
- When the temperature controls allow flexibility.

The safe temperatures are set out in the **Table 14.3**.

Hazard Analysis Critical Control Point (HACCP)

HACCP is a universal food safety system. It aims to protect food from contamination by:
- Identifying critical points in the food handling process that might cause contamination
- Putting controls in place to prevent microbiological, chemical and physical contamination of food
- Monitoring the critical points to ensure that contamination does not occur.

This means that all potential hazards at each stage of food handling, from delivery of raw products to the serving of fully prepared food, must be identified. The whole process is designed to ensure that any problems can be dealt with before they cause any problems or illness.

ROLE OF FOOD HANDLERS IN FOODBORNE DISEASES

A food handler is anyone who works in a food business and who either handles food or surfaces that are likely to be in contact with food, such as cutlery, plates and bowls. A food handler may do many different things for a food business. Examples include making, cooking, preparing, serving, packing, displaying and storing food. Food handlers can also be involved in manufacturing, producing, collecting, extracting, processing, transporting, delivering, thawing or preserving food.

If a food handler has a foodborne illness:
- Food handlers must tell their work supervisor if they have any of the following symptoms while they are at work—vomiting, diarrhea, a fever or a sore throat with a fever.
- The only exception to this is if the food handler knows that he/she has these symptoms for a different reason. For example, a food handler may be vomiting at work because of pregnancy.
- Food handlers must also tell their supervisor if they have been diagnosed as having or carrying a foodborne illness. As well as reporting the foodborne illness, the food handler must not handle any food where there is a chance they might make the food unsafe or unsuitable because of their illness.
- Also, if a food handler stays on at work to do other work, he/she must do everything reasonable to make sure that they do not contaminate any food.
- **Note:** Illnesses that can be passed on through food include hepatitis A and those caused by giardia, *Salmonella* and *Campylobacter*.

If a food handler has skin injuries or sores or is otherwise unwell:
- Food handlers must tell their supervisor about any infections or conditions, such as a cold or other problem that may result in discharges from their ears or nose or eyes if there is any chance that they might make food unsafe or unsuitable for people to eat as a result of their condition.
- Also, if they continue to handle food with such a condition, food handlers must do whatever is reasonable to make sure that they do not contaminate any food.
- For example, an infected sore could be completely covered by a bandage and clothing or by a waterproof covering if on an area of bare skin, and medication can be used to dry up discharges.
- If a food handler knows or suspects he/she might have contaminated some food
- Food handlers must tell their supervisor if they know or think they may have made any food unsafe or unsuitable to eat. For example, jewellery worn by a food handler may have fallen into food.

Personal Hygiene

Food handlers' personal hygiene practices and cleanliness must minimise the risk of food contamination. The most important things they need to know are that they must:
- Do whatever is reasonable to prevent their body, anything from their body or anything they are wearing, coming into contact with food or food contact surfaces;
- Do whatever is reasonable to stop unnecessary contact with ready-to-eat food;
- Wear clean outer clothing, depending on the type of work they do;
- Make sure bandages or dressings on any exposed parts of the body are covered with a waterproof covering;
- Not eat over unprotected food or surfaces likely to come in contact with food;
- Not sneeze, blow or cough over unprotected food or surfaces likely to come into contact with food;
- Not spit, smoke or use tobacco or similar preparations where food is handled; and
- Not urinate or defecate except in a toilet.

Some Special Hand Washing Rules for Food Handlers

Food handlers are expected to wash their hands whenever their hands are likely to contaminate food. This includes washing their hands:

- Immediately before working with ready-to-eat food after handling raw food;
- Immediately after using the toilet;
- Before they start handling food or go back to handling food after other work;
- Immediately after smoking, coughing, sneezing, using a handkerchief or disposable tissue, eating, drinking or using tobacco or similar substances; and
- After touching their hair, scalp or a body opening

ESSENTIAL STEPS IN SAFE COOKING PRACTICES

The way we cook our food is as important as the way we prepare and store it. Inadequate cooking is a common cause of food poisoning. Cross-contamination from raw to cooked foods, such as from hands, chopping boards or utensils, can also cause food poisoning. Most foods, especially meat, poultry, fish and eggs, should be cooked thoroughly to kill most types of food poisoning bacteria. In general, food should be cooked to a temperature of at least 75°C or hotter. When food is cooked, it should be eaten promptly, kept hotter than 60°C, or cooled, covered and stored in the fridge or freezer.

Safety when Cooking High-risk Foods

Food poisoning bacteria grow more easily on some foods than others. High-risk foods include:
- Raw and cooked meat—such as chicken and minced meat, and foods containing them, such as casseroles, curries and lasagne
- Dairy products—such as custard and dairy-based desserts, such as custard tarts and cheesecake
- Eggs and egg products—such as mousse
- Small goods—such as ham and salami
- Seafood—such as seafood salad, patties, fish balls, stews containing seafood and fish stock
- Cooked rice and pasta
- Prepared salads—such as coleslaws, pasta salads and rice salads
- Prepared fruit salads
- Ready-to-eat foods—such as sandwiches, rolls, and pizza that contain any of the food above.

High-risk Foods and the Temperature Danger Zone

Take care with high-risk foods. You should remember to:
- Keep high-risk foods out of the temperature danger zone of between 5°C and 60°C.
- If high-risk foods have been left in the temperature danger zone for up to 2 hours the food should be reheated, refrigerated or consumed.
- If high-risk foods have been left in the temperature danger zone for longer than 2 hours, but less than 4 hours, they should be consumed immediately.
- Throw out any high-risk foods that have been left in the temperature danger zone for more than 4 hours.

Cook all Food to a Temperature of 75°C

How you cook food is very important. Different foods need a different approach:

- Aim for an internal temperature of 75°C or hotter when you cook food. Heating foods to this temperature kills most food poisoning bacteria. Use a thermometer to check the internal temperature of foods during the cooking process.
- Cook mince, sausages, whole chickens or stuffed meats right through to the centre. You should not be able to see any pink meat and the juices should be clear.
- Cook steak, chops and whole cuts of red meat to your preference as food poisoning bacteria are mostly on the surface.
- Cook fish until it flakes easily with a fork.
- Cook foods made from eggs, such as omelettes and baked egg custards thoroughly.

Food Safety with Raw Eggs

- Take extra care when preparing foods that contain raw egg, such as homemade mayonnaise, sauces, such as hollandaise, and desserts, such as tiramisu and mousse.
- Bacteria present on eggshells and inside the egg can contaminate these types of food and cause food poisoning.
- Avoid giving food containing raw eggs to pregnant women, young children, elderly people and anyone with a chronic illness.

Food Safety and Microwave Cooking

Microwaves are a quick and convenient way to cook food. However, if they are not used correctly, they can cook food unevenly. This may leave food partially cooked or not reaching a uniform temperature of 75°C. When you cook food in the microwave:
- Cut food into evenly sized pieces if possible or put larger or thicker items towards the outside edge of the dish.
- Cover the food with a microwave-safe lid or microwave plastic wrap. This will trap the steam and promote more even cooking.
- Rotate and stir food during cooking.
- Wait until the standing time is over before you check that the cooking is complete. Food continues to cook even after the microwave is turned off.

Cooling and Storing Food

- If you need to store food for later use, wait until the steam stops rising, cover the food and put it in the fridge. This helps keep the food out of the temperature danger zone as fast as possible.
- Large portions of food cool faster when you put them into shallow trays or divide them into smaller portions.
- If you need to keep food warm, keep it hotter than 60°C and out of the temperature danger zone.
- Under ideal conditions, cooked food can be stored in the fridge for a few days. If you want to keep cooked food longer, freeze the food immediately after cooling in the fridge.
- Always store cooked food separately from raw food, especially raw meats, poultry and fish.
- Keep raw meats and poultry at the bottom of the fridge to avoid raw juices dripping onto other food. Ensure that all food is covered or sealed.

Reheat Food to Steaming Hot

- Reheat food until it is steaming hot-above 75°C or, preferably, boiling. Food should steam throughout, not just on the edges.
- Take care when reheating food in a microwave oven. Follow the same actions as when cooking with a microwave to ensure all the food is heated to above 75°C.

CONSUMER CONTROL POINTS FOR FOOD SAFETY

Purchasing

- Keep your food safe from the moment you put it in your grocery cart.
  - Purchase meat and poultry products last.
  - Keep packages of raw meat and poultry separate from other foods.
  - Consider using plastic bags to enclose individual packages of raw meat and poultry.
  - Make sure meat and poultry products are refrigerated as soon as possible after purchase.
  - Canned goods should be free of dents, cracks or bulging lids. (Botulism is a concern.)
- When buying food and taking it home, remember to keep raw meat and poultry away from other foods, especially fresh foods, such as fruits and vegetables. Place raw meat and poultry at the lowest level of the cart, so it cannot drip on other foods
  - Make sure foods are kept cold between the store and your home
  - Take into account the outside temperature and adjust your trip home so that food you purchase at the grocery store will not reach the DANGER ZONE, between 40° and 140°F (5°–60°C).
  - Check package sell-by or pull-by dates to make sure they are current make sure you have enough storage space in the refrigerator or on your shelves
- When purchasing food from a vendor or having it catered, remember to:
  - Consider our Brown First Policy
  - Use only Brown Dining Services approved vendors. These vendors have provided the necessary documentation of their RI Department of Health Food licensing, certifications and liability insurances.

Storing

- Proper storage maintains quality and prevents contamination.
- At home, refrigerate or re-wrap and freeze meat, fish and poultry immediately.
- To prevent raw juices from dripping on other foods, store meat, fish and poultry in plastic bags or on a plate.
- Wash hands with soap and water for 20 seconds before and after handling raw meat, poultry or seafood products.
- Store canned goods in a cool, clean, dry place. Avoid extreme heat or cold.

Preparing

Food can cause foodborne illness when conditions in the environment encourage bacterial growth.

- The importance of hand-washing cannot be overemphasized.
- Do not let juices from raw meat, poultry or seafood come in contact with cooked foods or foods that will be eaten raw, such as fruits or salad ingredients.
- Wash hands, counters, equipment, utensils and cutting boards with soap and water immediately after use.
- Thaw foods in the refrigerator, never at room temperature.
- When using a microwave oven to thaw food, cook it immediately after thawing. Always wash and rinse your cutting board between uses, especially after cutting up raw meat.
- Wash and rinse using hot, soapy water. Sanitize and air dry.
- Use the 10 steps to a safe kitchen to ensure your food is prepared in a safe manner.

Cooking

Thorough cooking destroys harmful bacteria.

- **Cook food thoroughly:** If harmful bacteria are present, only thorough cooking will destroy them.
- Use a meat thermometer to determine if your meat, poultry or casserole has reached a safe internal temperature.
- Avoid interrupted cooking. Never partially cook products to later finish them on the grill or in the oven.
- When microwaving foods, use microwave-safe containers.
- Cover, rotate, and allow for standing time of at least two minutes, which contributes to thorough cooking.

Serving

Choose a serving style which will allow food to be served as quickly as possible, while maintaining desirable temperatures below 40° (4°C) or above 140°F (60°C).

- Wash hands with soap and water before serving or eating food. Never leave potentially hazardous foods, raw or cooked, at room temperature any longer than necessary—never longer than 2 hours.
- Keep hot foods above 140°F (60°C) and cold foods below 40°F (4°C).
- RI Law states that consumers under the age of twelve may not be served raw or partially cooked comminuted foods of animal origin.
- Provide information regarding ingredients to alert persons with food allergies.
- Cross contamination during preparation is also dangerous for persons with allergies. Some of the most common food allergens are—milk, fish, shellfish, wheat, eggs, nuts, citrus, melons, strawberries and soy.
- When serving food, wear non-latex rubber or plastic gloves, such as vinyl, nitrile and synthetics.
- The state of RI has banned latex gloves in food establishments to protect the public from the increasing problem of latex allergies.

Handling Leftovers

Follow these steps to ensure safe handling of leftovers:
- Wash hands before and after handling leftovers.
- Use clean utensils and surfaces.
- Divide leftovers into small units and store in shallow containers for quick cooling.
- Refrigerate within 2 hours of cooking. Reheat leftovers thoroughly to a temperature of 165°.
- Bring soups, sauces and gravies to a rolling boil.
- The most common food handling mistake is cooling food too slowly!

CONCLUSION

Food safety (or food hygiene) is used as a scientific method/discipline describing handling, preparation, and storage of food in ways that prevent foodborne illness. The occurrence of two or more cases of a similar illnesses resulting from the ingestion of a common food is known as a foodborne disease outbreak. This includes a number of routines that should be followed to avoid potential health hazards. In this way, food safety often overlaps with food defense to prevent harm to consumers. The tracks within this line of thought are safety between industry and the market and then between the market and the consumer. In considering industry to market practices, food safety considerations include the origins of food including the practices relating to food labeling, food hygiene, food additives and pesticide residues, as well as policies on biotechnology and food and guidelines for the management of governmental import and export inspection and certification systems for foods. In considering market to consumer practices, the usual thought is that food ought to be safe in the market and the concern is safe delivery and preparation of the food for the consumer.

BIBLIOGRAPHY

1. Akil L, Ahmad HA, Reddy RS. Effects of climate change on Salmonella infections. Food borne Pathogens and Disease. 2014;11:974-80.
2. Bhaskaram P. Micronutrient malnutrition, infection, and immunity: An overview. Nutrition Reviews. 2002;60:S40-S45.
3. Charlton KE, et al. Fish, food security and health in Pacific Island countries and territories: a systematic literature review. BMC public health. 2016;16(1): p. 285.
4. Forman J, Silverstein J. Organic foods: Health and environmental advantages and disadvantages. Pediatrics. 2012; 130, e1406-e1415.
5. Joshi SA. Nutrition and Dietetics, Tata McGraw Hill, New Delhi, India, 1992.
6. Lutz CA, Karen RP. Nutrition and Diet Therapy, 4th edition. Davis FA, Philadelphia, USA, 1995.
7. Puckett RP. "Food Service Manual for Health Care Institutions, Third Edition". American Hospital Association, Jossey-Bass, Wiley Imprint, San Francisco, USA. 2004:371-3.
8. Truswell AS. "ABC of Nutrition, Fourth Edition", BMJ Books, London, UK. 2003:32-40.
9. Williams P. "Food Toxicity and Safety". In: Mann J, Truswell AS (Eds). "Essentials of Human Nutrition, Second Edition. Oxford University Press, Oxford, UK. 2002:415-6.

REVIEW QUESTIONS

Long Essays
1. Explain in detail about food poisoning.
2. Discuss the major foodborne illnesses and causes.
3. Describe food safety considerations and measures.

Short Essays
1. Four steps to food safety.
2. Safety when cooking high-risk foods.
3. Role of food handlers in foodborne diseases.
4. Food safety act 1990.
5. Hygiene control.
6. Prevention of bacterial food poisoning.
7. Contributing factors to bacterial food poisoning.
8. Common types of bacterial food poisoning.
9. Principles of food sanitation.
10. Food hygiene/sanitation.
11. Food safety: A public health priority.

Short Answers
1. Foodborne intoxications.
2. Food contact surfaces.
3. Food poisoning.
4. Cross contamination.
5. Contaminant.
6. Foodborne illness.
7. Foodborne infections.
8. Cross-contamination.
9. Disinfectant.
10. Hazard analysis critical control point (HACCP).
11. Milk hygiene.

SECTION 2

Applied Biochemistry

SECTION OUTLINE

15. Introduction to Biochemistry
16. Carbohydrates
17. Lipids
18. Proteins
19. Clinical Enzymology
20. Acid Base Maintenance
21. Heme Catabolism
22. Organ Function Tests
23. Immunochemistry

CHAPTER 15

Introduction to Biochemistry

CHAPTER OUTLINE

- Definition, Meaning and Concept of Bio-chemistry
- History of Bio-chemistry
- Importance of Biochemistry in Nursing
- Review of Structure, Composition and Functions of Cell
- Microscope: Parts and Types

TERMINOLOGY

- **Cell:** The cell is the basic structural and functional unit of the life as the life starts form a single cell. The living body is made up of innumerable cells.
- **Biomolecules:** The living matter is composed of mainly six elements—carbon, hydrogen, oxygen, nitrogen, phosphorus and sulfur. These elements constitute about 90% of the dry weight of human body. Several other functionally important element are also found, e.g., sodium, potassium, chloride, calcium, magnesium, ferrous, and copper, etc. Carbon is the most predominant and versatile element of life.
- **Microscope:** The microscope is the standard instrument for magnification in the clinical laboratory. It is used to largely for morphological identification of cells, microorganism and tissues. Microscopes are used in pathology, microbiology, cytology and genetics. microscope is an instrument used to observe minute objects, such as bacteria and is a combination of a variety of lens system which can magnify the object by 1000 times.
- **Biochemistry:** Biochemistry is the science concerned with the chemical basis of life. It is the chemistry of the living matter in its different phases of activity, from the smallest microorganism, such as viruses to the most complex and highly evolved ones as human beings.
- **Anabolism:** All metabolisms in which complex biomolecules are built up from simpler ones. These processes usually require cellular energy.
- **Joule (J):** A unit for energy (or work), defined as the work done by a force of 1 Newton when the object it acts on moves 1 meter.
- **Ketone bodies:** The chemicals acetoacetate, beta-hydroxybutyrate, and acetone, which are produced from excess acetyl-CoA (during starvation).

INTRODUCTION

Biochemistry is the study of the chemistry of, and relating to, biological organisms. It forms a bridge between biology and chemistry by studying how complex chemical reactions and chemical structures give rise to life and life's processes. Biochemistry is sometimes viewed as a hybrid branch of organic chemistry which specializes in the chemical processes and chemical transformations that take place inside of living organisms, but the truth is that the study of biochemistry should generally be considered neither fully "biology" nor fully "chemistry" in nature. Biochemistry incorporates everything in size between a molecule and a cell and all the interactions between them.

Biochemistry essentially remains the study of the structure and function of cellular components (such as enzymes and cellular organelles) and the processes carried out both on and by organic macromolecules—especially proteins, but also carbohydrates, lipids, nucleic acids, and other biomolecules. All life forms alive today are generally believed to have descended from a single protobiotic ancestor, which could explain why all known living things naturally have similar biochemistries. Even when it comes to matters which could appear to be arbitrary, such as the genetic code and meanings of codons, or the "handedness" of various biomolecules—it is irrefutable fact that all marine and terrestrial living things demonstrate certain unchanging patterns throughout every level of organization, from family and phylum to kingdom and clade.

DEFINITION AND SIGNIFICANCE IN NURSING

Definitions

- Biochemistry is defined as the chemistry of biology. The science of biochemistry has also been called physiological chemistry and biological chemistry. Biochemistry is concerned chiefly with the chemistry of biological processes; it attempts to utilize the tools and concepts of chemistry particularly organic and physical chemistry, for elucidation of the living system.

- Biochemistry can also define as the study of the molecular basis of cellular function. It has evolved into the common language for translating the advances of molecular genetics into cellular and chemical terms. Biochemists study a broad range of cellular functions from gene transcription to the structure and function of macromolecules.

MEANING AND CONCEPT OF BIOCHEMISTRY

- Biochemistry is used to learn about the biological processes which take place in cells and organisms.
- Biochemistry may be used to study the properties of biological molecules, for a variety of purposes. For example, a biochemist may study the characteristics of the keratin in hair so that a shampoo may be developed that enhances curliness or softness.
- Biochemists find uses for biomolecules. For example, a biochemist may use a certain lipid as a food additive.
- Alternatively, a biochemist might find a substitute for a usual biomolecule. For example, biochemists help to develop artificial sweeteners.
- Biochemists can help cells to produce new products. Gene therapy is within the realm of biochemistry. The development of biological machinery falls within the realm of biochemistry.

HISTORY OF BIOCHEMISTRY

Sl. No.	Year	Description
1.	1835	Jons Berzelius writes a paper on chemical catalysis, uses amylase as an example.
2.	1859	Charles Darwin publishes On the Origin of Species.
3.	1860	Recognized fermentation
4.	1865	Gregor Mendel publishes his theory of genetics.
5.	1869	Fredrick Meischer discoverse DNA in cell nuclei.
6.	1897	Eduard and Hans Buchner extracts materiel from yeast that catalyzes the conversion of glucose to alcohol.
7.	1900	Gregor Mendel's work on genetics is rediscovered.
8.	1914	Fritz Lipmann elucidates the role of ATP in energy metabolism.
9.	1926	James Sumner obtains crystalline jack bean urease and demonstrates that it is a protein.
10.	1926	Thomas Hunt Morgan writes The Theory of the Gene.
11.	1934	Arnold Beckman develops the first pH meter.
12.	1937	Hans Krebs discovers the citric acid cycle (TCA cycle).

Contd...

Contd...

Sl. No.	Year	Description
13.	1941	George Beadle and Edward Tatum propose the one-gene, one-enzyme hypothesis.
14.	1944	Oswald Avery, Colin MacLeod, and Maclyn McCarthy use chemical methods to establish that DNA is the genetic material.
15.	1950	Edwin Chargaff publishes observation that A=T, G=C (Chargaff's rules).
16.	1952	Linus Pauling and Robert Corey propose the **a**-helix and the **b**-pleated sheet structures for proteins.
17.	1952	Alfred Hershey and Martha Chase provide additional support for DNA as genetic material.
18.	1953	James Watson and Frances Crick put forth the double helix model DNA.
19.	1953	Fredrick Sanger determines the first amino acid sequence of a protein (insulin).
20.	1956	Earl Sutherland isolates cyclic AMP.
21.	1957	Matthew Meselson and Franklin Stahl carry out experiment to demonstrate semiconservative DNA replication.
22.	1960	John Kendrew and Max Pertuz obtain the first three dimensional structure of proteins (hemoglobin and myoglobin).
23.	1960	Jerald Huritz and Samuel Weiss discover RNA polymerase.
24.	1961	Francois Jacob and Jaques Monod propound the operon model of gene control.
25.	1963	Allosteric model for inhibition of enzymes (Jean-pierrre Changuex, F Jacob, and J Monod).
26.	1964	Acrylamide gel electrophoresis of proteins is developed.
27.	1965	Marshal Nirenberg, H Gobind Khorana, and severo Ochoa complete the elucidation of the genetic code.
28.	1965	3-D model of first enzyme (lysozyme by David Phillips.
29.	1965	Robert Holley determines the structure of a transfer-RNA.
30.	1965	Jerome Vinograd discovers superhelical twisting.
31.	1968	Mark Ptashne and Walter Gilbert identify the first repressor genes.
32.	1969	Paula DeLucia and John Cairns isolate a mutant of *E. coli* called pol A1.
33.	1969	First synthesis of an enzyme (ribonuclease).
34.	1970	Hamilton Smith discovers restriction endonucleases.
35.	1970	Howard Temin and David Baltimore discover reverse transcriptase.

Contd...

Contd...

Sl. No.	Year	Description
36.	1973	Stanley Cohen and Herbert Boyer prepare recombinant DNA.
37.	1974	Sung-Hou Kim, et al. produces the first X-ray structure of transfer RNA.
38.	1977	Cesar Milstein discovers how to produce monoclonal antibodies.
39.	1977	Allan Maxam and Walter gibert develop chemistry for sequencing DNA.
40.	1977	Fredrick Sanger, S Nicklen and AR Coulson develop chemistry for sequencing DNA.
41.	1977	Phillip Sharp and Richard Roberts discover intron (intervening sequences).
42.	1982	First X-ray structure of a membrane protein.

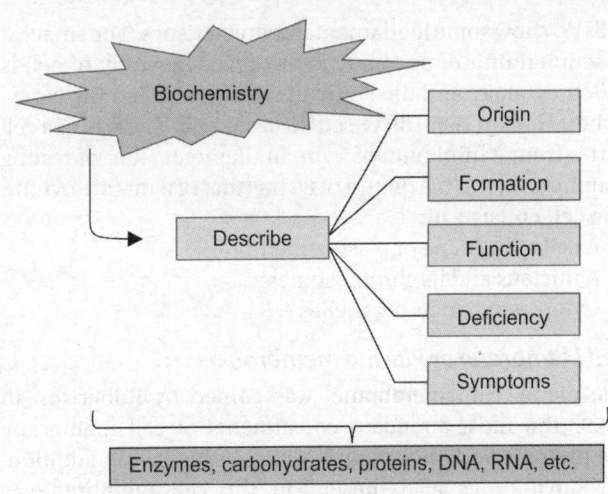

Fig. 15.1: Need of studying biochemistry.

NEED OF STUDYING BIOCHEMISTY (FIG. 15.1)

Biochemical approaches to the simplification and understanding of biological systems require two types of background. First, biochemists must be thoroughly skilled in the basic principles and techniques of chemistry, such as stoichiometry, photometry, organic chemistry, oxidation and reduction, chromatography, and kinetics. Second, biochemists must be familiar with the theories and principles of a wide variety of biological and physical disciplines often used in biochemical studies, such as genetics, radioisotope tracing, bacteriology, and electronics. This need reflects the biochemists' ready acceptance and use of theories and techniques from allied areas and disciplines. Today, the findings of biochemistry are used in many areas, from genetics to molecular biology and from agriculture to medicine. The first application of biochemistry was probably the making of bread using yeast, about 5000 years ago.

Importance of Biochemistry in Nursing

Applications of the basic principles of biochemistry are essential to the nursing profession. The correct diagnosis, nursing care plans, treatment, prevention and control of infectious diseases depend on a sound knowledge of medical biochemistry. Biochemistry is perhaps the most rapidly developing branch of medicine. No wonder, the major share of Nobel prizes in medicine has gone to research workers engaged in biochemistry.

- Biochemistry is of great use within the field of nursing, with many practical applications that can assist you in becoming a better nurse.
- Biochemistry is the study of how chemical reactions occur within living things and refers generally to medicine and nutrition, where practical applications are concerned.
- Another avenue that is related to biochemistry is the environment, such as how life forms react to greenhouse gases and other studies. These studies allow us to gain more insight upon what we put into our bodies, through either medicine or food, ensuring that we do not harm ourselves with either poison or excessive doses.
- Biochemistry is sometimes referred to as biological chemistry, governing all life forms and life processes. It controls the flow of information by biochemical signaling and the chemical energy flow through metabolism, revealing the huge complexity of life.
- Biochemistry is generally concerned with things, such as proteins, lipids and carbohydrates, focusing more on the processes rather than individual molecules.
- In recent times, over the past 40 years, biochemistry has become increasingly successful in terms of helping us understand the chemical processes within living organisms, to the extent that practically every area of life science from medicine to botany now interlinks with biochemistry.
- The current main focus where biochemistry is concerned surrounds the process within which biological molecules give rise to processes that occur in living cells, helping us understand and study whole organisms to a much deeper level.
- Using biochemistry can be helpful in the nursing profession, allowing nurses to determine how much medicine should be prescribed or given to each patient they encounter. It ensures that nobody gets too high of a dose for their body and that people recover in as little time as is possible.

REVIEW OF STRUCTURE, COMPOSITION AND FUNCTIONS OF CELL

Cell and its Various Components

All living organisms are composed of cells which are minute compartments within which various processes of life occur. Microscopic organisms, such as bacteria, some algae and recomposed of single cells. Human body starts from a single cell but contains about 1013 cells at maturity. Our body contains about 200 distinct type of cells. They are muscle cells, bone and cartilage cells, nerve cells, skin cells, visual cells in the eye and many others. Although each cell may show distinct characteristics for the particular functions performed, cells do show some fundamental characteristics. The smallest functional unit of our body is the cell. The study of cell is called cytology and the study of tissues is called histology. Robert Hooke (1665) first used the term 'cell'. The size of a cell varies from a minimum of 6 um in diameter (that of resting lymphocyte) to a maximum of 80 tm (that of a mature ovum).

The cell consists of:
1. A cell membrane or plasma membrane
2. A nucleus and its chromosomes
3. Cytoplasm and its organelles

Cell Membrane or Plasma Membrane

The name 'Unit membrane' was coined by Robertson in 1959. The most abundant constituents of cell membrane are proteins and phospholipids in the ratio 3:2. In addition, carbohydrate is also present in the cell membrane as lipopolysaccharides or glycoproteins. The phospholipid layer is a bilayer with the hydrophobic ends of each lipid molecule pointing towards the interior of the membrane and hydrophilic ends pointing towards the exterior.

The cell membrane is a permeability barrier. If a cell is placed n hypotonic solution and if it contains molecules, which cannot penetrate its outer membrane, it will swell; conversely, it will shrink if placed in a hypertonic medium. In both instances water moves down its concentration gradient. Thus, the cell behaves is an osmometer. Nonpolar molecules (gases, lipids) move freely across the membrane; polar molecules penetrate the membrane much less readily and indeed it is the selective permeability of the plasma membrane to certain ions, which determines the excitability characteristics of nerve and muscle cells.

STRUCTURE AND COMPOSITION OF CELL

Although the general chemical nature of the membrane found it the cell boundary was predicted on the basis of physiological data, the detailed molecular structure is not yet known. Models of cell membranes prepared by combining their lipid and protein constituents (partly known from chemical analysis of purified cell membrane preparations) exhibit some physiological characteristics similar to those of natural membranes. The role of lipid—lipid interactions in membrane structure have been at the center of attention because such interactions can explain much of the presently known phenomena of membrane transport. Quantitative studies of isolated cell membranes revealed that enough lipids are present to be arranged as a bilayer coating the cell. Artificial mixtures of extracted cellular polar lipids (lecithin, phospholipid, and steroids) under appropriate conditions will form a bimolecular layer spontaneously. Presumably the polar (hydrophilic) ends of the lipids form the two outer borders, making them available for interaction with other polar molecules such as proteins. On a weight basis, membranes contain a significantly larger amount of protein than lipid (ratio up to 4:1); however, due to the high molecular weight of proteins, this relationship is reversed on a molar basis (protein to lipid ratio ranging from 1:100 to 10:100). Some proteins are associated peripherally with one of the polar surfaces of the lipid bilayer. Other proteins, the integral membrane proteins, are not restricted to the surfaces of the plasma membranes but extend into the bimolecular lipid layer.

Figure 15.2 is depicted the structure and parts of cell.

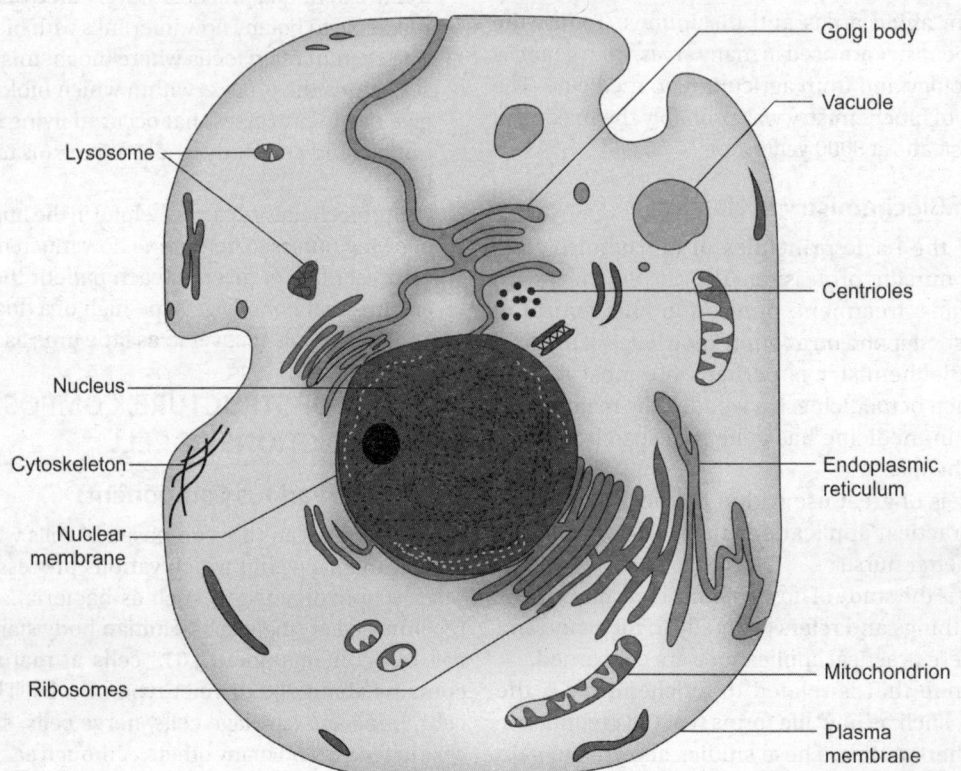

Fig. 15.2: Structure and parts of cell.

In addition to lipid and protein, carbohydrate is associated with the cell membrane as lipopolysaccharide and as protein polysaccharide. The carbohydrate moieties of the membrane serve to modify the electric charge at its surface and provide specific surface binding sites. Cytochemically demonstrable polysaccharide protein complex is associated with many cell surfaces as an extracellular layer. In some places, particularly at luminal surfaces, this layer forms a fuzzy coat—often referred to as a glycocalyx, which may act as a crude filter and/or facilitate the attachment of molecules for endocytic transport across the cell membrane.

STRUCTURE OF THE UNIT MEMBRANE

A pattern generally found in almost all cellular membranes prepared for microscopy by conventional techniques consists of three layers, i.e., two electron dense layers on either side of a single electron lucent layer. This has been termed a unit membrane, or a three layered membrane. Electron microscopic examination of osmium tetroxide fixed sectioned tissue shows the cell membrane to be 7-10 nm wide. The electron lucent line in the unit membrane is thought to represent the lipid layer. Hydrophobic bonding in the lipid bilayer region may make it inaccessible to osmium deposition. Thus, the two electron dense lines would result from deposition of osmium at the surfaces of this bilayer. There is much physiological evidence to suggest that the lipid bilayer is interrupted by proteins which, as hydrophilic molecules, connect the two outer surfaces of the membrane and provide transmembrane channels for transfer of water molecules and ions. The protein components of the plasma membrane are either tightly associated with it or more readily dissociated from it.

Additional electron microscopic structural information comes from unfixed membranes studied by the freeze—etching technique. When rapidly frozen tissue is fractured by a sharp knife, the membranes tend to fracture along the middle layer of their bimolecular lipid leaflets. The evaporation of a thin layer of carbon or platinum into the exposed surface produces a replica, which is viewed in the electron microscope. Intramembrane particles are seen mainly in replicas of membranes having integral proteins (and also in various lipids—cholesterol mixtures).

Figure 15.3 is depicted the cell membrane.

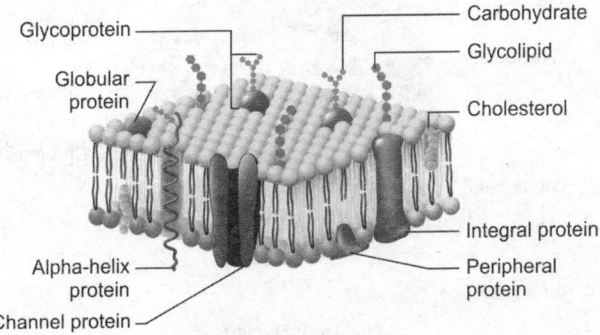

Fig. 15.3: Cell membrane.

In most metabolically active membranes, repeating structures are visible at various intervals within the layer. These structures may represent proteins that extend through much of the thickness of the membrane. This interpretation is supported by evidence from other techniques, which label the outer portions of integral proteins at either the outside, or inside surface. The positions of the intramembranous particles may be more or less stable. With varying physiological conditions the distribution pattern of these particles may shift within a membrane. This lateral mobility of components, e.g., proteins, within the membrane is seen if cells of different origins are caused to fuse. Rather than a patchwork of the two original membrane particle patterns the result is an intermixture of both characteristics. Hormone effects resulting in transmembrane signaling may depend on this mobility.

For example, formation of a receptor dimer may be required for activation and receptor and integral membrane proteins may need to associate in order to activate adenylate cyclase and thereby increase the level of the intracellular second messenger.

The lipid bilayer serves as a transport medium for lipid-soluble molecules to gain entry into the cell membrane. The lipid bilayer serves as a transport medium for lipid soluble molecules to gain entry into the cell, whereas protein lined hydrophilic "pores" probably provide channels for diffusion of polar entities, such as water and ions. Surprisingly, certain lipid bilayer show rates of movement sufficient to account for osmosis. The permeability to water, however, seems to be inversely related to the proportion of cholesterol in the phospholipid membranes.

Cell Membrane

Membrane components are subject to continual turnover. In certain cell types, portions of the membrane invaginate into the cell and pinch off to form the boundary of an intracellular vesicle, vacuole, or tubule. External material is carried into the cell by this process, referred to as Endocytosis. This material and its enclosing membrane may fuse with lysosomes, or after delivering endocytosed material to an intracellular endosome, the specialized endocytic vesicle membrane may return to the plasma membrane.

Endocytosis	*Exocytosis*
It is the process of ingestion of substances by the cell through plasma membrane	It the process of expel molecules outside the cell
It involves the formation of vesicles containing the substances	In exocytosis, the vesicles containing the waste substances fuse with the plasma membrane
Endocytosis helps to bring molecules inside the cells	Release enzymes, hormones, proteins and glucose to be used in other parts of the body

The fusion to the plasma membrane with membranes of intracellular origin is termed exocytosis. When secretary granules exocytose at the cell membranes they release their internal material to the outside of the cell but their membrane are retrieved as endocytic vesicles.

These vesicles may, in fact, return to their intracellular origin, the Golgi area. As a result, there is a flow of membrane and of material enclosed in membrane-delimited spaces between the surface and intracellular compartments. Similar exchanges seem to occur between certain intracellular organelles, notably the endoplasmic reticulum and the Golgi apparatus. In the various processes involving formation of vesicles (e.g., pinocytic endocytosis) there is often a "bristle" coating, presumably clathrin or a related protein, on the cytoplasmic side of the vesicle membrane. Exocytosis and incorporation into the surface of intracellular membrane containing transport units (e.g., channels or transporters) may be the structural basis for rapid changes of cell permeability by increasing the numbers of cell membrane transporters in response to hormonal stimulation.

Figure 15.4 is depicted the endocytosis and exocytosis.

Structure of Cell Surface

Stable imaginations and invaginations of the cell membrane are important elements in providing a dramatic increase in surface areas contact between cell and environment. Microvilli, finger- like envaginations, are generally associated with cell surfaces involved in absorption processes, such as in the intestine and kidney. Conversely, in striated muscle, one finds and invagination of the cell membrane, the transverse tubule, associated with each sarcomere. Since the transverse tubules are continuous with the surface membrane they provide a direct route for the communication of alterations at the cell surface to the contractile system deep within the muscle fiber.

The Nucleus (Fig. 15.5)

The nucleus has two principal functions—replication of deoxyribonucleic acid (DNA) and synthesis of ribosomal, messenger, and transfer ribonucleic acids (RNAs). Because it is best understood, we shall discuss in some detail ribosomal RNA synthesis, which occurs in the nucleolus. Each nucleus possesses one or more nucleoli not delimited by membranes. Each nucleolus consists of a roughly spherical dense array of fibrils and granules rich in RNA. Often the nucleolus is found in intimate association with special regions of DNA (known as nucleolus organizer regions), which is presumed to carry the information for ribosomal RNA.

Nucleolar RNA (45S predominantly) is almost certainly a precursor form of ribosomal RNA found in the cytoplasm; if one labels RNA synthesized in the nucleolus with radioactive nucleotides, labeled RNA molecules are subsequently detected in the cytoplasm. These RNA molecules complex with protein and form respectively a 30S and a 60S sub-cytoplasm to form a ribosome (15–25 nm in diameter). There may be several million ribosomes in a given cell.

The specific function of ribosomal RNA is not well understood; generally speaking, however, all three types of RNA are involved in the translation of genetic information constrained in the DNA molecule into specific proteins that are synthesized in the cytoplasm. The ribosomes interact in the process of protein synthesis with two other types of RNA. Large messenger RNA molecules (mRNAs) determine the sequence of amino acids in proteins by specifying the order of attachment of the small transfer RNAs carrying the appropriate amino acids. Our belief that DNA is the template for these RNAs is derived largely from experiments with prokaryotic (bacterial) cells.

As the information in a messenger RNA molecule is being read, several ribosome attach via their smaller subunits to the mRNA. The combination of an mRNA and its attached ribosomes is referred to as a polysome. Each ribosome of a polysome synthesizes a polypeptide chain, so that several chains will be produced simultaneously by a polysome. The nascent peptide seems to be attached to the larger ribosomal subunit; completed protein is released to the cytoplasm. An average polypeptide may be synthesized in 10–20 s.

Morphology of the Nucleus

The interphase nucleus is readily seen in the light microscope as a spheroidal body with a "suggestion" of internal organization. The DNA-containing material can be specifically stained. The nuclear chromatin can be resolved into two types—euchromatin (loosely coiled) and heterochromatin (Compact). It seems likely that the euchromatic regions are more active in the transcription process than the heterochromatic regions, i.e., there is little demonstrable RNA synthesis in chromosomes that are largely or entirely composed of heterochromatin, as in the

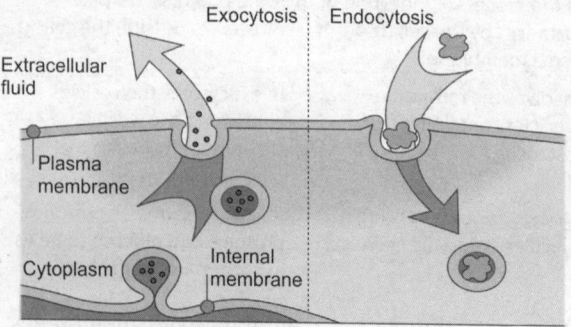

Fig. 15.4: Endocytosis and exocytosis.

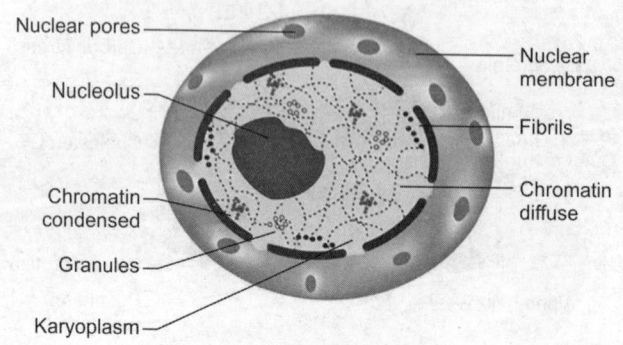

Fig. 15.5: Nucleus.

case of sperm cells, polymorphonuclear leukocytes, and the Barr body (one of the X chromosomes of female cells). The association of euchromatin with active transcription may account for some of the selective genetic expression associated with characteristic chromosomal uncoiling patterns found in different tissues within the same organism or at different developmental stages in the same tissue.

Chemical analysis has shown that the chromosome consists of DNA associated with basic proteins (histones) and with other (nonhistone) protein. It has been speculated that the complexing of histone with DNA may have a protective or structural function (preventing alternation or denaturation of the DNA, controlling coiling, etc.), or the histone may have a repressor function (interfering with the template activity of DNA). The amounts of RNA and nonbasic nuclear protein seem to vary in parallel with the metabolic activity of the cell, e.g., sperm cell nuclei have essentially neither RNA nor non basic protein.

Isolated chromosomes studied by electron microscopy appear as masses of fibers around 25 nm in diameter, or may have a beaded look with periodic DNA coiling around histone groups (nucleosomes). An individual DNA double helix coated with protein measures less than 5 nm, and while it is known that the fibers of chromosomes are coiled, the nature of the packaging of nucleic acid and proteins is yet to be described. Nevertheless, there are theories, consistent with current evidence, suggesting that a single chromosome contains one, or at most a very few, extremely elongated DNA molecules complexed with protein and coiled into a fiber structure which is seen in the electron microscope.

Cytoplasm

It consists of various organelles, which are suspended, in the cytoplasm. The organelles include ribosomes, endoplasmic reticulum, mitochondria, microtubules and microfilaments, golgi complex and centrioles.

- **Mitochondria:** Mitos-granule, chondrium-rod. The mitochondria is bounded by outer membrane and inner-folded membrane called cristae. Both walls are separated by intermembranous space. All mitochondria is said to be of maternal origin. They are called the powerhouse of cells. The enzymes for the Kreb's cycle are located in the matrix. The mitochondria, also called as the power house of the cell, are the major intracellular components of a eukaryotic cell. Mitochondrial membrane is a double layered structure. Its two layers are separated from each other by intra membrane space **(Fig. 15.6)**.

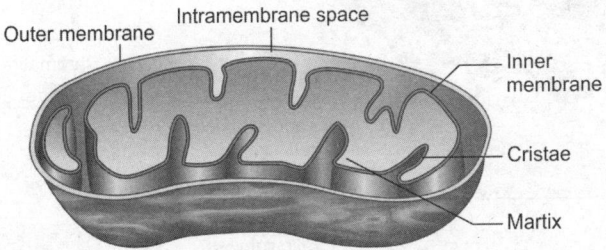

Fig. 15.6: Structure of mitochondria.

- **Golgi apparatus:** It is made up of anastomosing tubules of membranes and vesicles. It helps in formation of secretary products of carbohydrates.
- **Endoplasmic reticulum:** It consists of membranes which are arranged in the form of flattened sacs. The network of membrane enclosed spaces that extends throughout the cytoplasm constitutes endoplasmic reticulum (ER).

Some of these thread-like structures extend from the nuclear pores to the plasma membrane. A large portion of the ER is studded with ribosomes to give a granular appearance which is referred to as rough endoplasmic reticulum. Ribosomes are the factories of protein biosynthesis. During the process of cell fractionation, rough ER is disrupted to form small vesicles known as microsomes. It may be noted that microsomes as such do not occur in the cell.

The smooth endoplasmic reticulum does not contain ribosomes. It is involved in the synthesis of lipids (triacylglycerols, phospholipids, sterols) and metabolism of drugs, besides supplying O_2 for the cellular functions.

It is of two types:
a. Smooth endoplasmic retinaculum without ribosomes.
b. Rough endoplasmic retinaculum with ribosomes.

Smooth endoplasmic retinaculum is involved in lipid synthesis and rough endoplasmic retinaculum is involved in synthesis of proteins.

- **Ribosomes:** It has two subunits—40s and 60s. Few are attached to endoplasmic retinaculum and few are free. They play important role in protein synthesis.
- **Lysosomes:** They are vesicle, such as structure, which contain enzymes, which include proteases, carbohydrates, lipases, hydrolytic enzymes, etc. Lysosomal enzymes help in destruction of bacteria. All cells contain lysosomes except mature erythrocytes.
- **Microtubules and microfilaments:** The cytoplasms of cells contain elements, which are tubular called microtubules and some solid fibers called microfilaments. The microtubules are composed of protein tubulin and they form the cytoskeleton of the cell. Microfilaments are composed of G actin sub-units. They form actin and myosin filaments of muscles.
- **Centriole:** There is pair of centrioles in each cell. Each centriole has two cylindrical bodies placed at right angles to each other. Transverse section of the centriole shows three tubules in single group and thus 9 groups of tubules. They help in synthesis of microtubules during cell division.

Projections, which arise from cell surface, include:
- **Cilia:** They are hair like projection from the cell. For example, cilia in uterine tube
- **Flagella:** They resemble cilia. They are larger in size compared to cilia. For example, tail of spermatozoan
- **Microvilli:** They are finger like extension of cell surface. For example, small intestine

Junctional complex: There are three types of junctions—(a) Zonula Occludens, (b) Zonula Adherens, (c) Macula adherens

Figure 15.7 is depicted the structure of cytoplasm and nucleus.

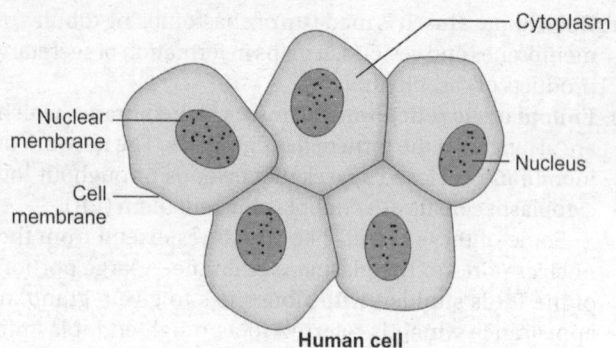

Fig. 15.7: Structure of cytoplasm and nucleus.

Intracellular Membrane Systems of Nuclear Envelope

The boundary of the nucleus, the nuclear envelope, is a double membrane complex. Each membrane is approximately 7–8 nm thick. The envelope, a flattened sac with an enclosed perinuclear space, resembles the rough endoplasmic reticulum (ER)—(1) the cytoplasmic surface of the outer (cytoplasmic) nuclear membrane has granules which appear to be ribosomes; (2) direct continuities are seen between the cytoplasmic portion of the nuclear membrane and the ER; and (3) the presence of certain enzymes can be demonstrated cytochemically in both the perinuclear space and the cisternae of the ER.

The inner surface often nuclear membrane is often associated with chromatin an "internal dense lamella", the latter may provide some rigidity to the structure. The inner and outer membranes of the envelope join at intervals to form "pores" tens of nanometers in diameter.

How does a "directive" of the nucleus reach the cytoplasm or, conversely, how do cytoplasmic and other external feedback messages reach the nucleus? Non-nuclear substances can act as inducers or repressors of the synthesis of specific proteins in the cytoplasm. This almost certainly requires interaction with genes. Furthermore, most gene products (e.g., mRNA) must leave the nucleus and enter the cytoplasm to express their effects. Permeability properties of the nucleus are too complex to be explained by simple holes. The morphology of the nuclear boundary provides for two alternative routes for the transfer of information either across membranes of the perinuclear sac or through "pores." The pores are often referred to as "annuli" to emphasize that they are not simple holes but rather organized regions—often pores are seen which contain a diaphragm or plug. In addition, the membrane adjacent to the pore may show morphological traces of special organization.

To date, the morphological evidence in support of the physiological and biochemical data on transnuclear transport through pores rests mainly on a few observations, such as the movement of electron dense material (thought to be RNA-containing granules) through the nuclear pores in the insect salivary gland and some other tissues, and the movement of a marker (colloidal gold) into the nucleus when it is injected into the cytoplasm of Ameba. Clear morphological evidence on passage of material across the nuclear membranes as distinct from the pores, is not available.

Endoplasmic Reticulum

Often an integrated biochemical and ultrastructural investigation (involving cell disruption, isolation, and analysis of a homogeneous organelle population) leads to the clearest understanding of organelle function in situ. From such studies, in a variety of cell types, a fraction of membrane—delimited vesicles, referred to as microsomes, is recovered.

Figure 15.8 is depicted the three-dimensional endoplasmic reticulum.

The microsomes perform several functions, including the provision of a base for the attachment of ribosomes, the

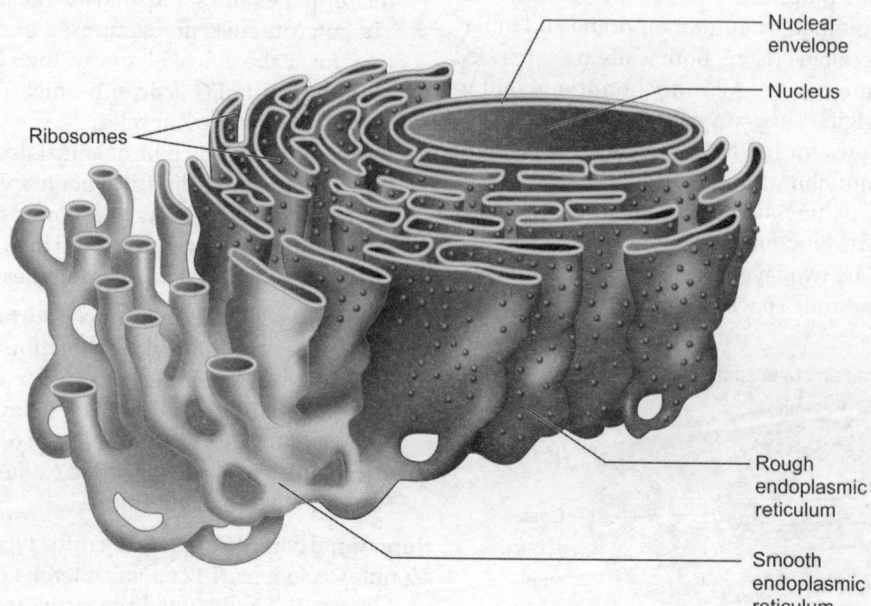

Fig. 15.8: Three-dimensional endoplasmic reticulum..

biosynthesis of lipids, and in the case of striated muscle, the accumulation and release of calcium. In the intact cell, microsomal vesicles are not found as such; rather, one observes a tubular network known as the ER. It is assumed that the majority of microsomal vesicles represent a reproducible, preparative artifact arising during cell disruption by the shearing into fragments and closing up of the tubules and sacs of the ER.

Rough ER: As noted above, the ER (and/or the microsomes derived from the ER) can provide a base for the attachment of ribosomes. Such ribosome carrying ER is referred to as rough ER. Microsomal vesicles derived from this rough ER were found to be capable of protein synthesis, the newly synthesized protein appearing in the vesicle lumen. In the rough ER in situ, the nascent protein likewise can be demonstrated within the reticulum lumen. This unidirectional passage into the lumen is thought to result from the folding of the original 0.5 to 1.0 nm wide protein into a three-dimensional structure which is large enough to be retained. The rough ER seems to grow by synthesizing more of it. The newly made rough ER may lose its ribosomes and thus become converted to smooth ER. The relative proportions of rough and smooth ER vary within different cells; for example, the rough ER is extensive in cells which specialize in synthesizing protein for export, while the smooth ER is extensive in steroid secreting cells.

Figure 15.9 is depicted the differences between rough and smooth endoplasmic reticulum.

Smooth ER: As noted above, the ER, which lacks ribosomes, is referred to as the smooth ER. The membrane of the ER carries enzymes, which are important in several biosynthetic pathways. For example, the enzymes required for the synthesis of steroid are found in microsomal fractions of steroid secreting cells.

Figure 15.10 is depicted the rough endoplasmic reticulum and smooth endoplasmic reticulum.

Enzymes involved in triglyceride synthesis as well as phospholipid synthesis are also found in this fraction the phospholipid sometimes appearing in the ER as small fat droplets. In liver cells, important drug degrading enzymes are associated with the smooth ER. Also, in the hepatocytes, the close spatial relationship of the smooth ER with glycogen, the major storage form of glucose, suggests that the smooth ER may function in glycogen metabolism. In muscle, the smooth ER (sarcoplasmic reticulum) controls the local concentration of calcium ions near the contractile machinery and thereby influences the contraction and relaxation process.

Golgi Apparatus (Fig. 15.11)

The Golgi apparatus is believed to be a site for the concentration of protein and polysaccharide. It is also a site for completion of the synthesis of the carbohydrate moiety of glycoprotein, e.g., the synthesis of the carbohydrate moieties of thyroglobulin and immunoglobulin begins in the ER, but the terminal sugars are added in the Golgi apparatus. In the case of synthesis of polysaccharides destined for secretion,

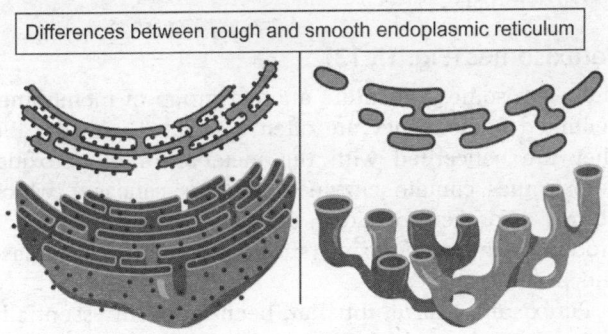

Fig. 15.9: Differences between rough and smooth endoplasmic reticulum.

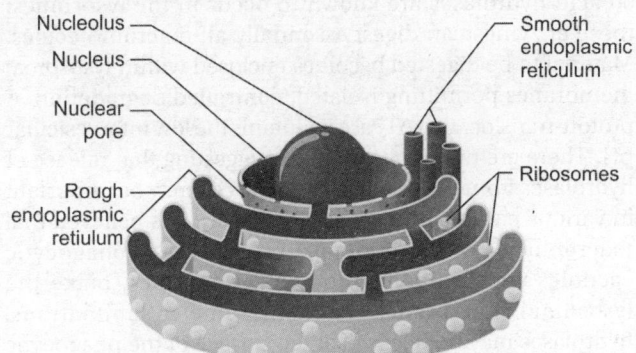

Fig. 15.10: Rough endoplasmic retiulum and smooth endoplasmic reticulum.

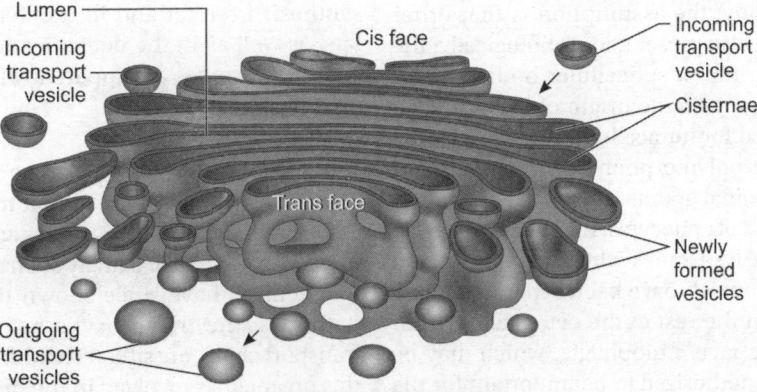

Fig. 15.11: Golgi apparatus.

the precursors are first seen in the Golgi apparatus. Therefore, the apparatus is believed to be the site of synthesis and packaging of polysaccharides for secretion. These products are usually packaged as "granules" within Golgi derived vacuoles or vesicles, which then migrate away from the Golgi apparatus. The enzymes involved in the polymerization of polysaccharide or addition of carbohydrate to protein, glycosyltransferases, have recently been used as marker enzymes for the biochemical isolation of the Golgi apparatus.

The Golgi apparatus consists of stack of several membranous saccules with associated vacuoles and vesicles. The ER in some cell types is assumed to contribute to the "forming face" or "outer" surface of the Golgi apparatus. Within the stacked membranes of the Golgi apparatus materials are concentrated as they pass from the saccules on the "outer" surface to those forming the "inner" surface of the apparatus. In addition while passing through the Golgi cisternae, these luminal proteins are modified covalently by removal and addition of specific sugars. In exocrine and endocrine cells the mature secretary granules are generally found in association with the "inner" saccules.

Lysosomes

Lysosomes have been found in virtually all-animal cells, which have been studied. As organelles they are best defined by biochemical and cytochemical criteria—a lysosome is a membrane-delimited body containing demonstrable acid hydrolase activity and an intervesicular pH of 5-6. Over 30 acid hydrolases are known to occur in the lysosomes; these enzymes can digest essentially all macromolecules. Material to be digested becomes enclosed within lysosomal membranes permitting isolated, controlled degradation. A proton-translocating ATPase maintains the low intervesicular pH. There are numerous findings suggesting that release of hydrolases from the lysosome into the cell may be important in various pathological states. In silicosis, it is believed that macrophages of the lung take up silica into phagocytic vacuoles which, upon fusion with lysosomes, make the lysosomal membranes leaky. In some inflammations, hydrolases may be released at the surface of the phagocytic cells and affect the adjacent tissues. In many cases, these findings are yet to be fully evaluated.

Microscopic identification of lysosomes often consists of demonstration of acid phosphatase activity within a membrane-delimited body; the assumption is that other lysosomal hydrolases are also present. Morphologically, the Lysosomes are mostly group of subcellular bodies. Their appearance depends largely on the origin of the enclosed material which is destined for intracellular digestion by the lysosomal hydrolases. In polymorphonuclear white blood cells, Golgi-derived lysosomal granules fuse with phagocyte vacuoles formed as a result of endocytosis of foreign material. Autophagic vacuoles are lysosomes which contain bits of the cell's own substance which have been separated along with the hydrolases from the rest of the cytoplasm within a membrane-delimited space. Autophagia, which may be enhanced by stress, is hypothesized to be important for the turnover of some cell constituents **(Fig. 15.12)**.

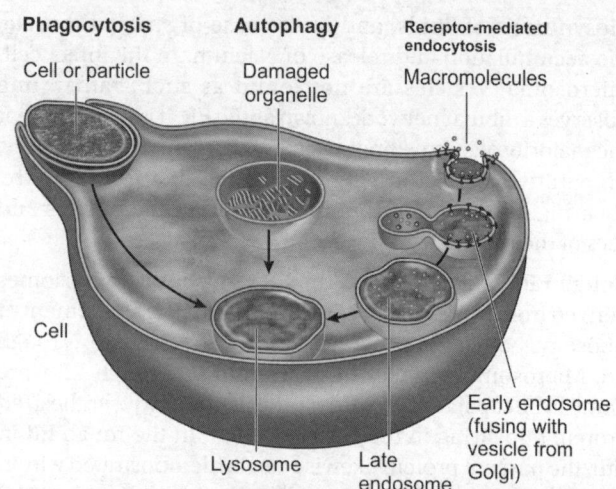

Fig. 15.12: Microscopic identification of lysosomes.

The degraded soluble products of lysosomal hydrolysis can either enter the anabolic pool to reused in biosynthesis or to be secreted. An example of the latter is the secretion of thyroid hormone. Thyroid colloid travels from the follicle lumbar within endocytic vacuoles which then fuse with the lysosomes; the colloid is hydrolyzed and thyroxin is released. It is also noteworthy that indigestible residues accumulate within lysosomes, a phenomenon which accompanies the aging process in neural and other cells. The accumulation of lipid deposits in blood vessels may be one factor contributing to the development of arteriosclerosis.

Peroxisomes (Fig. 15.13)

The peroxisomes constitute another group of membrane-delimited bodies. They are often associated with the ER. They are concerned with the metabolism of peroxide: peroxisomes contain enzymes (such as catalase), which destroy hydrogen peroxide and other enzymes, which produce hydrogen peroxide (such as D-amino acid oxidase and, in some species).

Peroxisomes have, thus far, been found in essentially all cell types, of which liver and kidney are among the best-established examples. The function of peroxisomes is currently under active investigation, and there is evidence that, in some species, they are involved in carbohydrate synthesis from fat and in the degradation of purines and fats, as well as in the detoxification of hydrogen peroxide. New peroxisomes are apparently formed by division of pre-existing peroxisomes.

Mitochondria

The early cytologists noted that mitochondria were closely associated with motile processes and were situated in regions of intense metabolic activity such as sites of active transport. Biochemists have since shown that two major metabolic pathways, the tricarboxylic acid cycle and the electron transport chain, are situated within the mitochondrion; thus, this organelle is involved in the metabolism of lipids, amino acids, and carbohydrates.

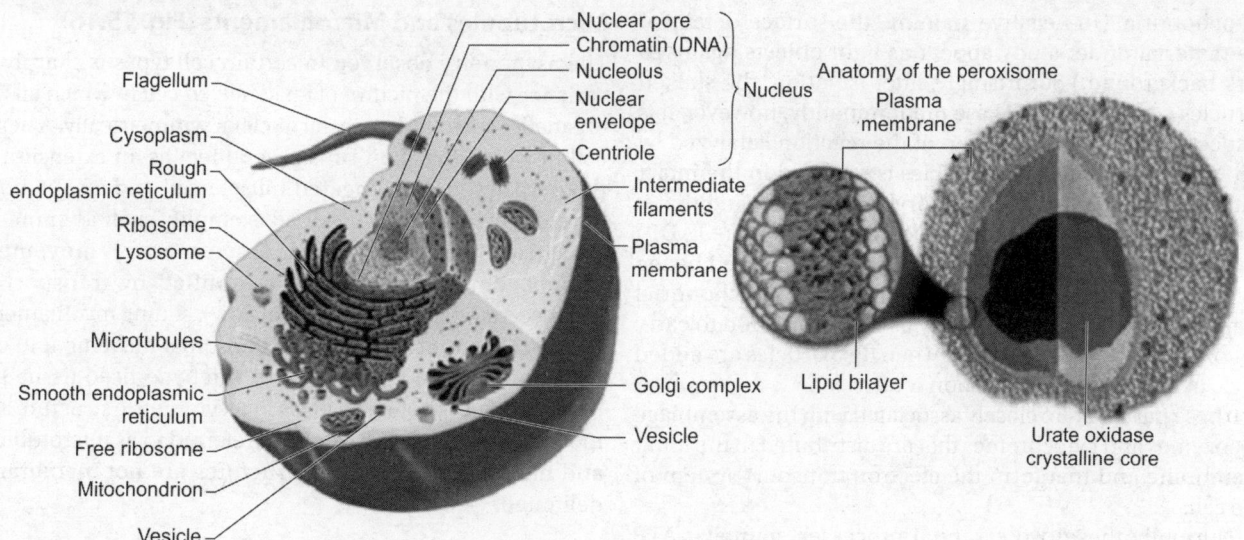

Fig. 15.13: Peroxisomes.

Mitochondrion has a length of 5-10 nm and a diameter of 0.5-1.0 nm. It is bounded externally by two lipoprotein membranes (each about 7 nm thick), the inner one of which is thrown into folds termed cristae or tubules. Within the inner membrane is a matrix containing granules, RNA and DNA. The DNA is a small circular molecule and is thought to provide some, but not all, of the necessary information for replication of the mitochondria.

Figure 15.14 is depicted the structure of a mitochondrion.

The RNA is responsible for synthesis of a few of the proteins of the mitochondrion; the majority of the mitochondria enzymes are synthesized on cytoplasmic ribosomes under the direction of the nuclear DNA. From physiological and biochemical evidence, it is generally believed that the respiratory enzymes and the components of oxidative phosphorylation are associated in an ordered array on the inner membrane. The order is thought to promote the sequential interaction of substrates and enzymes in these multienzyme systems with concomitant conservation of energy. Therefore, much effort has been directed toward isolation of modular physiological units from inner membrane fraction. The fact that multienzyme assemblies can be obtained from mitochondria has been encouraging. Moreover, morphological studies support the multienzyme assembly can be obtained from mitochondria has been encouraging.

Moreover, morphological studies support the multienzyme assembly hypothesis. First, the respiratory activity or mitochondria is roughly proportional to the amount of inner membrane a finding which could be explained by presuming an increased number of repeating units or respiratory assemblies associated with the increased membrane area. Second, a repetitive array of particles found in certain preparations suggests a similarly repetitive assemblage of inner membrane enzyme systems. These regularly space particles are attached by small stalks to the inner membrane of unfixed and negatively stained isolated

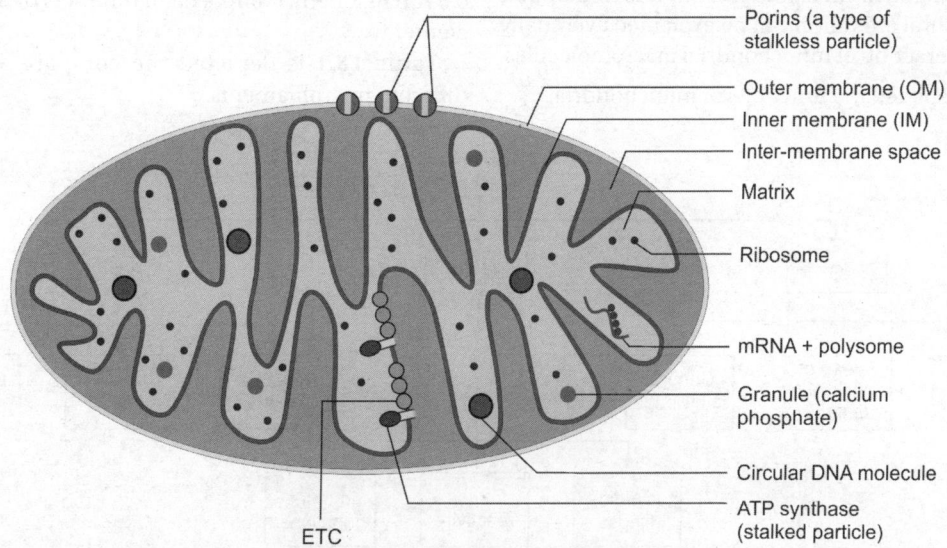

Fig. 15.14: Structure of a mitochondrion.

mitochondria. (In negative staining, the surface details of the material under study appear as light objects against a dark background.) Surprisingly, after isolation, the stalked particles contained an ATPase predominantly; however, it is suspected that the equilibrium of the reaction catalyzed by the ATPase in the stalked particles is reversed in the intact mitochondrial oxidative phosphorylation system and that it couples phosphorylation of adenosine diphosphate (ADP) with electron transport. This suggestion is supported by the fact that dissociation of the particle from submitochondrial preparations abolishes the ability of the preparation to carry out oxidative phosphorylation; when the particles are added back, oxidative phosphorylation returns too.

These particles are closely associated with the assemblage of enzymes and cytochromes that are distributed in the inner membrane and that form the electron transport system of the cell.

Normally these two essential processes, namely—ATP formation and electron transport, are tightly coupled. The morphology of the inner membrane enzyme system remains a matter of current dispute.

The outer membrane of the mitochondrion has different enzyme content, a larger percentage of lipids, and is more permeable to simple sugars than the inner membrane. In addition to the demonstrable membrane-anchored enzymes of both inner and outer membranes, certain enzymes (such as those of the tricarboxylic acid cycle) are solubilized after disruption of the mitochondria. These enzymes are presumed to be situated in the matrix or possibly loosely attached to a mitochondrial membrane.

Physiologists can clearly define the metabolic state of the mitochondria in terms of electron transport and oxidative phosphorylation. Careful electron microscopic study of isolated mitochondria, in situ, has related states—(1) the condensed state in which the matrix appears dense and the space between the inner and outer membrane is enlarged; this state is seen when oxidative phosphorylation is proceeding at a rapid rate under conditions of excess ADP and inorganic phosphate, and (2) the orthodox state. When ADP and P. are rate-limiting in oxidative phosphorylation. It is hoped that this kind of structural alteration can be explained eventually in terms of the interaction of mitochondrial macromolecules.

Figure 15.15 is depicted the functions of mitochondria.

Microtubules and Microfilaments (Fig. 15.16)

The asymmetry observed in certain cell types is sharply at variance with the picture of an idealized cell in which all the organelles surround a central nucleus symmetrically. A nerve cell in which the axon runs several feet as an extension of the perikaryon an elongated muscle cell and a squamous (or columnar) epithelial cell all exemplify such asymmetry. Likewise, the nonrandom (asymmetric) movement of subcellular elements is exemplified by transport of neurosecretory products (axonal flow), sliding myofilaments in muscle contraction, and chromosomal movement in cell division. Electron microscopy of aldehyde-fixed tissue has revealed a morphological basis for asymmetric structure and movement in the form of entities referred to as microtubules and microfilaments; these structures are not membrane-delimited.

Microtubules and Centrioles

In cross-section, microtubules are 20–30 nm in diameter and may be followed for several microns in longitudinal sections. They are found in many regions in which phase contrast and polarizing microscopy had previously demonstrated the presence of formed oriented, elongated elements. Microtubules are often associated with oriented movement, e.g., axonal transport of neurotransmitter from the nerve cell body (where synthesis occurs) to the synaptic terminal where transmitter is released. In nerve cells, microtubule subunits are also synthesized in the cell body but assembled in the axon.

One of the best-established examples of microtubule association with movement in all cells is chromosomal movement in the mitotic spindle. The mitotic poles—toward which the microtubules of the spindle orient and toward which the chromosomes move—have centrioles, usually two per cell. In the interphase cell, the pair of centrioles is generally found with long axes at right angles to each other. Each centriole is a cylinder 0.15 nm in diameter had 0.5 nm in length, composed of nine sets of microtubule like elements.

Table 15.1 is depicted the compare and contrast of different microfilaments.

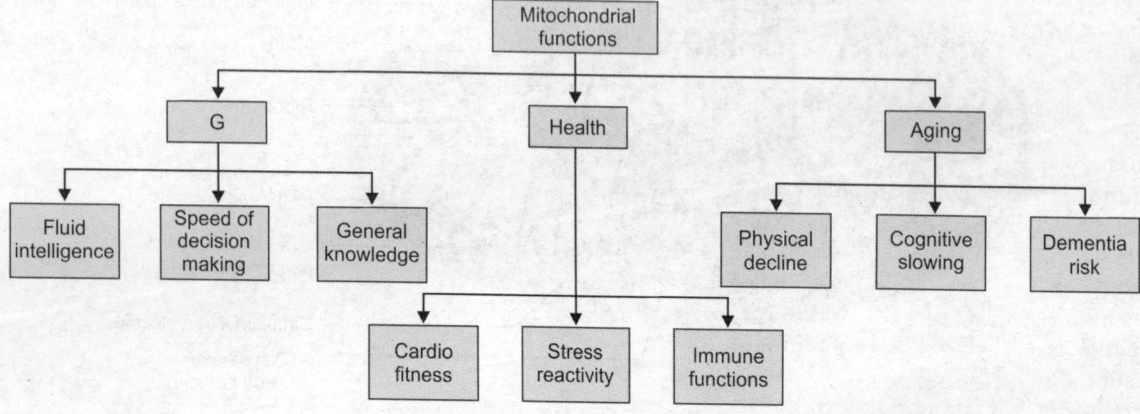

Fig. 15.15: Functions of mitochondria.

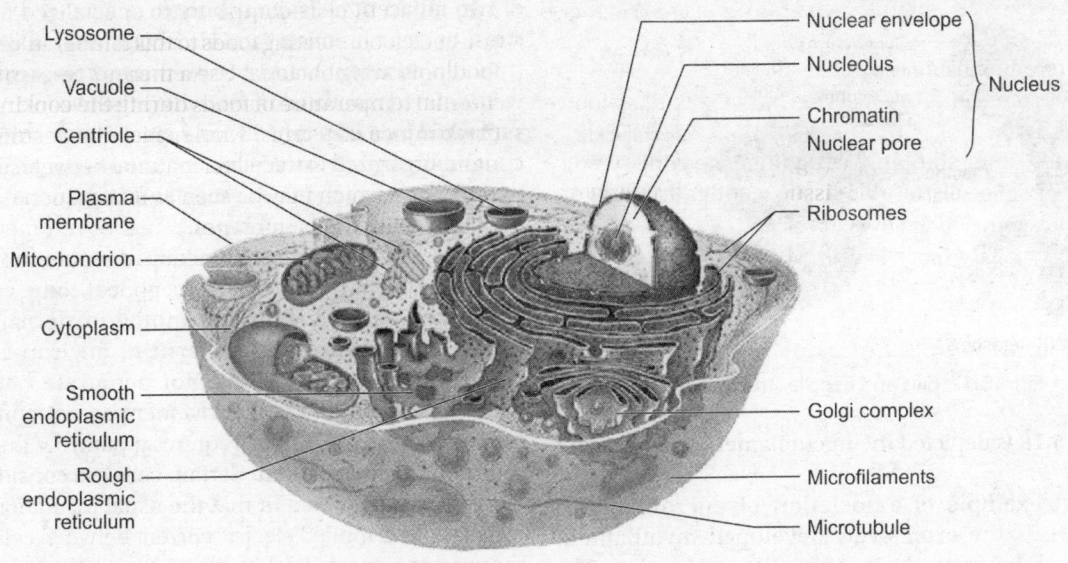

Fig. 15.16: Microtubules and microfilaments: Structural components of the cell (cytoskeleton) in eukaryotes.

helical fashion to form the microtubules. In normal cells, the microtubular protein appears to be present in a form, which is assembled into tubules (e.g., for the formation of the mitotic spindle) under appropriates but as yet not understood, stimulation.

Cilia and Flagella

Microtubule-like structures may also be organized into organelles. Cilia and flagella are rapidly beating cell processes, which extend 10–200 nm from the cell and are surrounded by a membrane, which is continuous with the plasma membrane. The intracellular basal bodies of cilia and flagella are also composed of microtubular structures arranged in the pattern of nine basic units (often referred to as "9+0"); they are widely assumed to be an alternate form of the centrioles.

Cilia and flagella generally have, in addition to the basic nine outer sets, a central pair of microtubules ("9+2"). Good evidence suggests that the sliding of tubules within a doublet is the motile force. The process of beating requires cellular energy as indicated by the findings that exogenous ATP can cause beating in isolated cilia and flagella and that the "arms" of the nine sets of microtubules contain and ATPase. The tubules of the cilia are composed of molecules similar to those of the other cellular microtubules.

Figure 15.17 is depicted the cilia and flagella structure.

Microfilaments

Microfilaments are heterogeneous classes of long, thin and non-tubular structures. Thin microfilaments, 5–7 nm in diameter, are made of actin. Among the most commonly seen microfilaments are those, which appear to serve as the structural core of microvilli. Also frequently encountered are tonofilaments on the intracellular side of desmosomes.

Table 15.1: Compare and contrast of different microfilaments.

	Microfilament	Intermediate filaments	Microtubule
Subunit	Actin monomers	Diverse	Tubulin dimers
Relative size (largest, midsize, or smallest)		Largest	
Dynamic or static			
Major function	• Cell shape and support • Cell movement • Cell division • Vesicle transport • Muscle contraction	Cell shape and support	Cell shape and support Cell movement Cell division Vesicle transport Muscle contradiction
Associates with which cell junction (if any)	Adherens junction	• Desmosomes • Hemidesmosome	

The organization of microtubules can be disrupted by physical mean (freezing or high pressure) or by chemical treatment especially with colchicines. When this is done motion is inhibited and some of the structure collapses. Therefore, the affinity of microtubular protein for colchicines serves as a means of identifying microtubular protein in a cell fraction. Isolated and disrupted microtubules yield protein subunits of approximately 6×10^4 daltons. These appear to be globular subunits, which may be arranged in

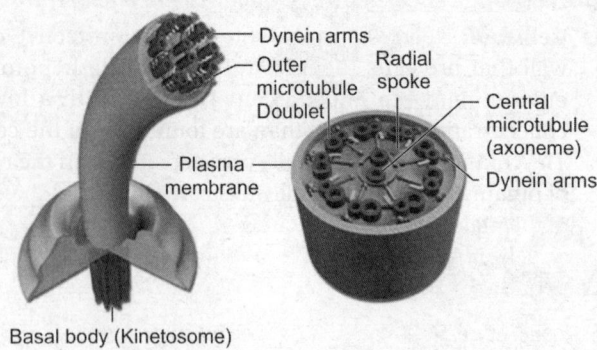

Fig. 15.17: Cilia and flagella structure.

Figure 15.18 is depicted the microfilament structure and assembly.

The best example of association of microfilaments with motion is the extensively developed myofilament system, which forms the basis of muscle contraction. The myofilament proteins, actin and myosin, have now been localized in many other cell types as result of improved techniques for the cellular localization of specific proteins. Results of the application of antibody to actin have implicated some of this protein as a constant component of thin (5 nm diameter) microfilaments. Likewise a myosin like protein associated with transiently formed thick microfilaments (10 run), is found in virtually all cells.

Junctional Complex

We have thus far limited our view of the cell to those entities circumscribed by and including its boundary, the plasma membrane. Cells rarely are continuous with one another; usually a space of 10–20 them. Cells are associated in tissues by various means; the best described is the junctional complex in epithelial cell. In this complex then plasma membranes of two adjacent cells contribute to specialized attachment sites: at tight junction (zonula occludens), a desmosome (macula adherens), and between these two usually a less well-defined zonula adherens where the two membranes are separated by a constant 20 nm space. The desmosome may contain organized extracellula material between the two cell membranes, which may be seen as an additional dense line in parallel with the membranes.

In the region of the tight junction, the outermost layers of the two cellular unit membranes appear to be very closely associated or fused with one another; externally applied tracer molecules (such as ferritin, an iron-containing electron dense protein) cannot penetrate between the cells at the tight junction. Movement across epithelial cell layers with tight junctions requires a pathway through cells rather than around them. Certain cells are considered to be electronically coupled in that the usual insulation effect on passage of an applied electric current between cells is greatly reduced at a specialized junctional area. This area has been called a gap junction because in a thin section it appears to have many small regions of contact between the plasma membranes with obliteration of (gaps in) the adjacent dense lines. Communication between and coordination of the individual cells of cardiac muscle may be effected via such gap junctions.

Prokaryote and Eukaryote Cell Organization (Fig. 15.19)

During the 1950s, scientists developed the concept that all organisms may be classified as prokaryotes or eukaryotes. The cells of all prokaryotes and eukaryotes possess two basic features—a plasma membrane and cytoplasm. However, the cells of prokaryotes are simpler than those of eukaryotes. For example, prokaryotic cells lack a nucleus, while eukaryotic cells have a nucleus. Prokaryotic cells lack internal cellular bodies (organelles), while eukaryotic cells possess them. Examples of prokaryotes are bacteria and cyanobacteria (formerly known as blue-green algae). Examples of eukaryotes are protozoa, fungi, plants, and animals.

Prokaryote

Prokaryotes are single-cell organisms, including bacteria and their bacteria-like cousins Archaea. Prokaryotic cells are much simpler than the more evolutionarily advanced eukaryotic

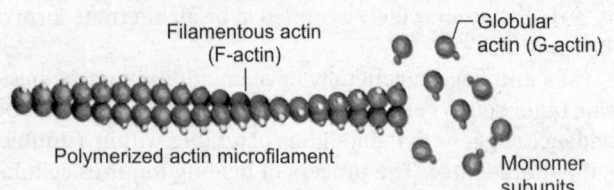

Fig. 15.18: Microfilament structure and assembly.

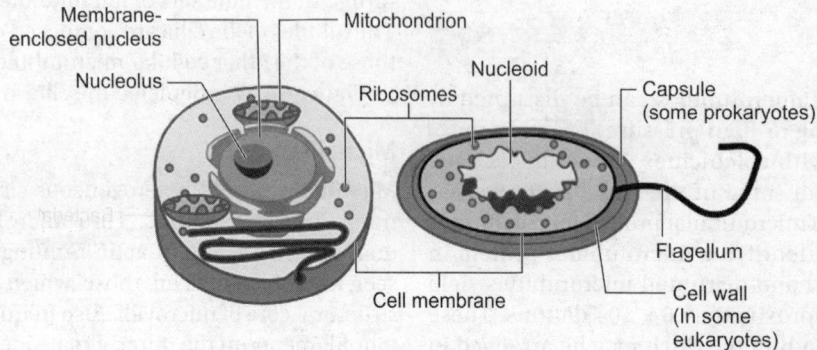

Fig. 15.19: Prokaryote and eukaryote cell organization.

cell. Whereas eukaryotic cells have many different functional compartments, divided by membranes, prokaryotes only have one membrane, the plasma membrane, which encloses all of the cell's internal contents. If a eukaryotic cell is analogous to a big house with many different rooms, a prokaryotic cell is like a one-room, studio apartment. Here is a list and description of the main cellular components of prokaryotes. Labeled diagrams of a prokaryotic cell and a related assignment appear below.

Internal Structures of Prokaryotic Cells

- **Plasma membrane:** The plasma membrane is a double-layer of phospholipids with associated proteins and other molecules. It is essentially the "bag" that holds all of the intracellular material and regulates the movement of materials into and out of the cell.
- **Cytoplasm:** This is the gel-like fluid that the cell is filled with, inside the plasma membrane—liquid with all of the cellular organelles suspended within.
- **Cytoskeleton:** It is only recently been discovered that rod-shaped bacteria and Archaea possess cytoskeletal proteins that function in a similar way to the cytoskeleton of eukaryotic cells. This scaffolding provides structural support to the cell and plays a role in cell-division.
- **Ribosomes:** All cells, both prokaryotic and eukaryotic, have multiple ribosomes within. Ribosomes are the protein-making machinery of the cell.

Genetic Material of Prokaryotes

- **Nucleoid:** The nucleoid is the region of the prokaryotic cytoplasm that contains the genome—the main genetic material (DNA) of the cell. Bacteria and Archaeans typically have a single, circular chromosome.
- **Plasmids:** In addition to the bacterial chromosome, bacteria may also contain one or more plasmids. A plasmid is a non-essential piece of DNA that confers an advantage to the bacteria, such as antibiotic resistance, virulence (the ability to cause disease) and conjugation (a bacterium's ability to share its plasmids with other bacteria). Plasmids are also found in some eukaryotic microbes, such as yeasts.

Prokaryotic Cell Structures Outside of Plasma Membrane

- **Cell wall:** Nearly all prokaryotes have a protective cell wall that prevents them from bursting in a hypotonic environment (an aqueous environment with a lower concentration of solutes than are found within the cell). The composition of cell walls vary depending on the type of organisms, but most cell walls contain a combination of the major organic molecules—proteins, carbohydrates and lipids. Bacteria have a unique molecule called peptidoglycan in their cell wall. Archaean cell walls do not contain this molecule. Cell wall composition of bacteria allows scientists to classify them as either Gram-positive or Gram-negative.
- **Glycocalyx:** The glycocalyx is a layer present in some bacteria, and located outside of the cell wall. There are two types of glycocalyces—slime layers and capsules. Slime layers help bacteria stick to things and protect them from drying out, particularly in hypertonic environments. Capsules also allow bacteria to stick to things, but have the added benefit of helping encapsulated bacteria hide from the host's immune system.
- **Cell extensions:** There are several different types of cell extensions associated with bacteria, all a made of delicate protein strands. Bacterial cell extensions include:
  1. *Flagella:* Long whip-like extensions that help bacteria move about the environment.
  2. *Fimbriae:* Allow bacteria to adhere to target host cells, so play a major role in bacterial virulent.
  3. *Conjugation pili:* The tubes used to transfer plasmids from donor to recipient Bacteria.

Figure 15.20 is depicted the structures of prokaryotic cells.

Eukaryote

Prokaryotic cells are fundamentally different in their internal organization from eukaryotic cells. Notably, prokaryotic cells lack a nucleus and membranous organelles. The nucleus is bounded by the nuclear envelope, a double membrane with many nuclear pores through which material enters and leaves. Animals, plants, fungi, and protists are all eukaryotes.

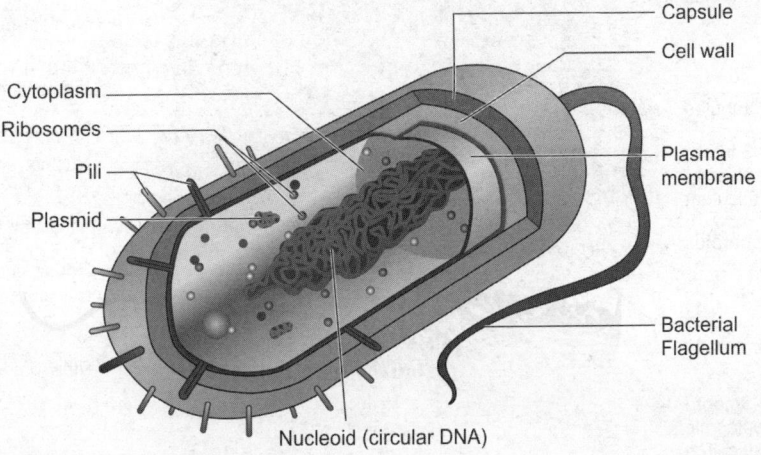

Fig. 15.20: Structures of prokaryotic cells.

Eukaryotic cells are more complex than prokaryotic cells and are found in a great many different forms as mentioned above, animals are not the only kind of creature to have eukaryotic cells. Plants, fungi and protists are also eukaryotic organisms. There are several important differences between plant and animal cells. The description of the animal cell above points out that at least higher plants have no centrioles in their cells. There are also three kinds of structures found in plant cells and not in animal cells.

1. **Plant cells have cell walls:** Animal cells do not. As noted in the description of the prokaryotic cell wall, the cell must also have a plasma membrane. Plant cells have cell walls in addition to plasma membranes, not instead of plasma membranes. Plant cell walls are composed all or partially of a carbohydrate called cellulose, which is quite different from the peptidoglycan of prokaryotic cell walls. The primary function of the cell wall is support, and inconjunction with the central vacuole, to create turgor (stiffness) in plant structures like leaves.

2. **Plant cells contain a specialized vacuole called the central vacuole:** This is a large, membrane bound structure filling most of the interior of the cell. The central vacuole is filled mostly with water, but always with some impurities—mineral or protein—so that the water concentration is always less than 100%. When the cell is surrounded by sufficient water, osmosis causes the central vacuole to swell, and thus causes the cell to press against the inside of the cell wall. This phenomenon in all of the cells of a leave causes the leaf's tissues to be stiff, and keeps this delicate structure spread out so it can serve its vital function as a solar panel.

3. **Plant cells contain a family of organelles called plastids:** There are several kinds of plastids, all related to each other and, under appropriate conditions, capable of modifying from one type to another. The best known of these plastids is the chloroplast, which performs the function of photosynthesis. Chloroplasts are double-membrane-bound, like mitochondria. Also like mitochondria, their inner membrane is very complicated. In fact, it is formed into many thylakoid structures which perform the same function performed by the thylakoids in prokaryotic cells. Despite common beliefs, Fungi are not plants. Biologically speaking, they are more animal-like than plant-like. They just look like plants to us. They do no photosynthesis and have no plastids. They have cell walls, but they are different from plant cell walls, and are clearly a separate evolutionary development. The cell walls of Fungi are typically composed of a material called chitin. Strangely enough, we also find chitin in one of the most successful of all animal phyla, the Arthropoda (which includes spiders, insects, crabs and lobsters). Arthropods have endoskeletons made of chitin. Again, a separate evolutionary invention.

Another odd aspect of cell structure in many Fungi is that, in some groups, the concept of a "cell" is only very loosely applicable. There are Fungi which are largely composed of a single, huge structure with many, many nuclei and no subdivisions into cellular chambers. And there are Fungi whose bodies are divided by incomplete subdivision, with continuous cytoplasm connecting all of the "cells" into one giant super-cell. Protists are very diverse—typical of a more primitive (meaning evolutionarily older) group of organisms. This group contains animal-like cells, plant-like cells, and fungus-like cells, as well as a dizzying assortment of in-betweens and oddities. The task of classifying protists is dreadfully difficult.

Figure 15.21 is depicted the structures of eukaryotic cells.

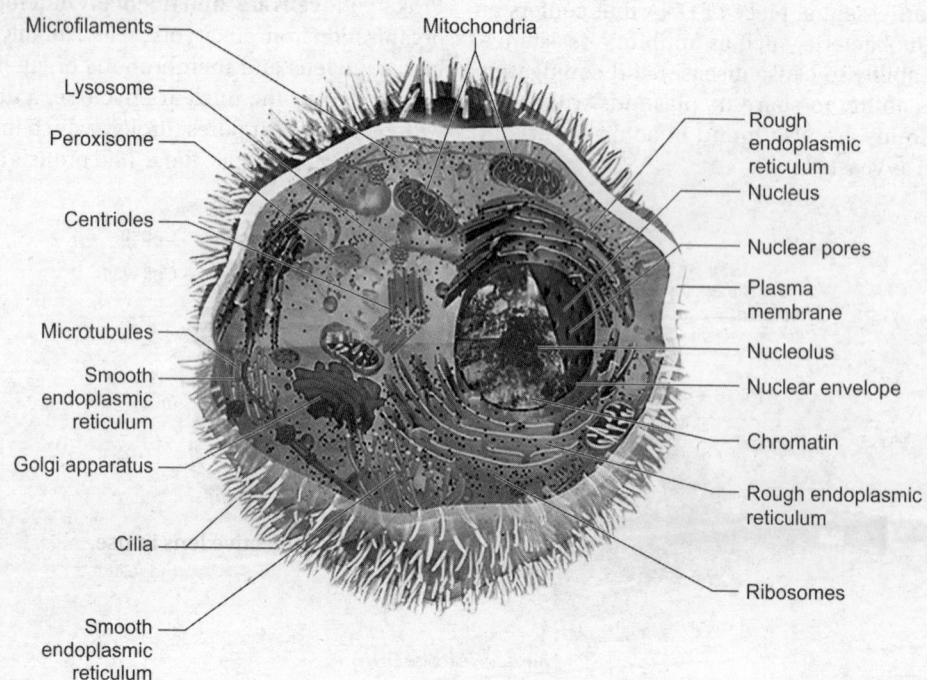

Fig. 15.21: Structures of eukaryotic cells.

Microscope (Fig. 15.22)

Historians credit the invention of the compound microscope to the Dutch spectacle maker, Zacharias Janssen, around the year 1590. The compound microscope uses lenses and light to enlarge the image and is also called an optical or light microscope. The simplest optical microscope is the magnifying glass and is good to about ten times (10X) magnification.

The **compound** microscope has two systems of lenses for greater magnification—(1) the ocular, or eyepiece lens that one looks into and (2) the objective lens, or the lens closest to the object. Before purchasing or using a microscope, it is important to know the functions of each part. Microscopes can be classified based on the physical principle that is used to generate an image. Different microscopes visualize different physical characteristics of the sample (e.g., elasticity can be visualized with acoustic microscopes). Image contrast, resolution (which determines magnification) and destructiveness of the sample are other relevant parameters.

- **Eyepiece lens:** The lens at the top that you look through. They are usually 10X or 15X power.
- **Tube:** Connects the eyepiece to the objective lenses
- **Arm:** Supports the tube and connects it to the base
- **Base:** The bottom of the microscope, used for support
- **Illuminator:** A steady light source (110 volts) used in place of a mirror. If your microscope has a mirror, it is used to reflect light from an external light source up through the bottom of the stage.
- **Stage:** The flat platform where you place your slides. Stage clips hold the slides in place. If your microscope has a mechanical stage, you will be able to move the slide around by turning two knobs. One moves it left and right, the other moves it up and down.
- **Revolving nosepiece or turret:** This is the part that holds two or more objective lenses and can be rotated to easily change power.
- **Objective lenses:** Usually you will find 3 or 4 objective lenses on a microscope. They almost always consist of 4X, 10X, 40X and 100X powers. When coupled with a 10X (most common) eyepiece lens, we get total magnifications of 40X (4X times 10X), 100X, 400X and 1000X. To have good resolution at 1000X, you will need a relatively sophisticated microscope with an Abbe condenser. The shortest lens is the lowest power, the longest one is the lens with the greatest power. Lenses are color coded and if built to DIN standards are interchangeable between microscopes. The high power objective lenses are retractable (i.e., 40XR). This means that if they hit a slide, the end of the lens will push in (spring loaded) thereby protecting the lens and the slide. All quality microscopes have achromatic, parcentered, parfocal lenses.
- **Rack stop**: This is an adjustment that determines how close the objective lens can get to the slide. It is set at the factory and keeps students from cranking the high power objective lens down into the slide and breaking things. You would only need to adjust this if you were using very thin slides and you were not able to focus on the specimen at high power. (Tip: If you are using thin slides and cannot focus, rather than adjust the rack stop, place a clear glass slide under the original slide to raise it a bit higher).
- **Condenser lens**: The purpose of the condenser lens is to focus the light onto the specimen. Condenser lenses are most useful at the highest powers (400X and above). Microscopes with in stage condenser lenses render a sharper image than those with no lens (at 400X). If your microscope has a maximum power of 400X, you will get the maximum benefit by using a condenser lenses rated at 0.65 NA or greater. 0.65 NA condenser lenses may be mounted in the stage and work quite well. A big advantage to a stage mounted lens is that there is one less focusing item to deal with. If you go to 1000X then you should have a focusable condenser lens with an NA of 1.25 or greater. Most 1000X microscopes use 1.25 Abbe condenser lens systems. The Abbe condenser lens can be moved up and down. It is set very close to the slide at 1000X and moved further away at the lower powers.
- **Diaphragm or iris:** Many microscopes have a rotating disk under the stage. This diaphragm has different sized holes and is used to vary the intensity and size of the cone of light that is projected upward into the slide. There is no set rule regarding which setting to use for a particular power. Rather, the setting is a function of the transparency of the specimen, the degree of contrast you desire and the particular objective lens in use.
- **Method of focusing microscope:** The proper way to focus a microscope is to start with the lowest power objective lens first and while looking from the side, crank the lens down as close to the specimen as possible without touching it. Now, look through the eyepiece lens and **focus upward**

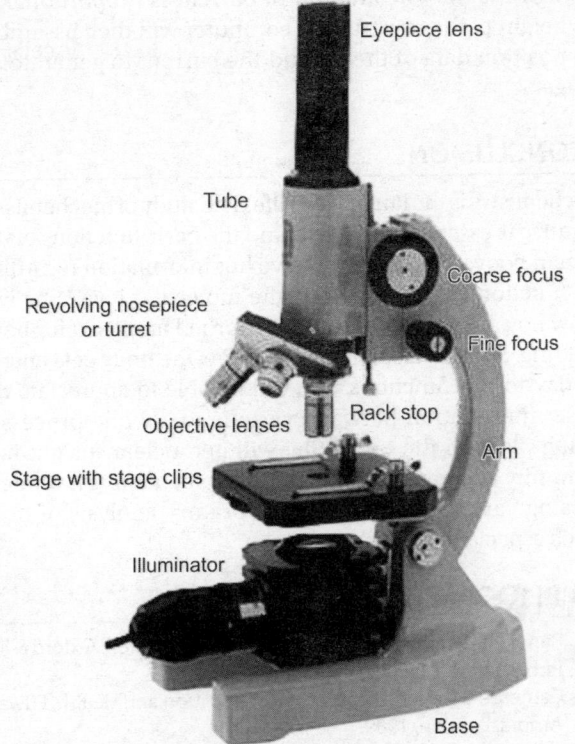

Fig. 15.22: Microscope.

only until the image is sharp. If you cannot get it in focus, repeat the process again. Once the image is sharp with the low power lens, you should be able to simply click in the next power lens and do minor adjustments with the focus knob. If your microscope has a fine focus adjustment, turning it a bit should be all that is necessary. Continue with subsequent objective lenses and fine focus each time.

Types of Microscope

How many different types of microscopes are there? More than you probably thought. I tried to research a list of different types, based on the physical principle used to make an image. Of course, one could also classify the microscopes based on their area of application, their cost, their versatility or any other aspect. These classification systems do have a problem: In this case, one type of microscope can be allocated to several groups, and the system becomes "messy".

Optical microscopes

These microscopes use visible light (or UV light in the case of fluorescence microscopy) to make an image. The light is refracted with optical lenses. The first microscopes that were invented belong to this category. The price of optical microscopes varies from very cheap to nearly unfordable (for the private person, at least). Optical microscopes can be further subdivided into several categories:

1. **Compound microscope:** These microscopes are composed of two lens systems, an objective and an ocular (eye piece). The maximum useful magnification of a compound microscope is about 1000x.
2. **Stereo microscope (dissecting microscope):** These microscopes magnify up to about maximum 100x and supply a 3-dimensional view of the specimen. They are useful for observing opaque objects.
3. **Confocal laser scanning microscope:** Unlike compound and stereo microscopes, these devices are reserved for research organizations. They are able to scan a sample also in depth. A computer is then able to assemble the data to make a 3D image.

X-ray microscope

As the name suggests, these microscopes use a beam of X-rays to create an image. Due to the small wavelength, the image resolution is higher than in optical microscopes. The maximum useful magnification is therefore also higher and is between the optical microscopes and electron microscopes. One advantage of X-ray microscopes over electron microscopes is, that it is possible to observe living cells.

Scanning acoustic microscope (SAM)

These devices use focused sound waves to generate an image. They are used in materials science to detect small cracks or tensions in materials. SAMs can also be used in biology where they help to uncover tensions, stress and elasticity inside biological structure.

Scanning helium ion microscope (SHIM or HeIM)

As the name suggests, these devices use a beam of Helium ions to generate an image. There are several advantages to electron microscopes, one being that the sample is left mostly intact (due to the low energy requirements) and that it provides a high resolution. It is a relatively new technology and the first commercial systems were released in 2007.

Neutron microscope

These microscopes are still in an experimental stage. They have a high resolution and may offer better contrast than other forms of microscopy.

Electron microscopes

Modern electron microscopes can magnify up to 2 million times. This is possible, because the wavelength of high energy electrons is very small. At the same time, the high energy electrons are pretty tough on the sample being observed. It may take a long time to completely dehydrate and prepare the specimen. Some biological specimens also need to be coated with a very thin layer of a metal before they can be observed.

- **Transmission electron microscopy (TEM):** In this case, the electron beam is passed through the sample. The result is a two dimensional image.
- **Scanning electron microscopy (SEM):** Here the electron beam is projected on the sample. The electrons do not go through the sample but bounce off. This way it is possible to visualize the surface structure of the specimen. The image appears 3-dimensional.

Scanning probe microscopes

It is possible to visualize individual atoms with these microscopes. The image of the atom is computer-generated, however. A small tip measures the surface structure of the sample by rastering over the surface. If an atom projects out of the surface, then a higher electrical current will flow through the tip. The amount of current is proportional to the height of the structure. A computer will then assemble the position data of the tip and the current to generate an image.

CONCLUSION

Biochemistry is the language of life. The study of biochemistry by nurse is essential to understand the basic functions of the human body. This study will give her information regarding the functioning of the cells at the molecular level. She will know how the food is digested, absorbed and used for body building. She will also understand how the body gets energy for day-to-day functions. She will be able to appreciate the close interrelation between various metabolic processes taking place in the body. She will get a clear insight into immunity and genes from a study of biochemistry. Modern nursing care depends on the laboratory analysis of body fluids especially the blood.

BIBLIOGRAPHY

1. Bamji MS, et al. (Ed). Textbook of Human Nutrition, Oxford & IBH Publishing Co. Pvt. Ltd. New Delhi, 1998.
2. Cameron GA, Fox B. Food Science, Nutrition and Health, Edward Arnold, London, 1989.

3. Frazier WC, West Hoff DC. Food Microbiology, Tata McGraw Hill Publishing Co, Ltd, New Delhi, 1986.
4. Garrow JS, James WPT. Human Nutrition and Dietetics, Churchill Living Stone, 1993.
5. Gopalan C, Rama Sastic BV, Balsosubramaniam SC. Reprinted Nutritive Value of Indian Foods. NIN, Hyderabad, 1996.
6. Gopalan C, Rama Sastri BV, Balasubramanian SC. Nutritive Value of Indian Foods, National Institute of Nutrition, ICMR, Hyderabad, 1989.
7. Lehninger AL, Nelson DL, Cox MM. Lehninger principles of biochemistry. New York: Worth Publishers, 2000.
8. Madigan MT, Martinko JM, Bender KS, Buckley DH, Stahl DA. Brock biology of microorganisms (Fourteenth edition.). Boston: Pearson, 2015.
9. Park K. Park's Text Book of Preventive and Social Medicine. Banarsidas Bhanot Publishers, Jabalpur, 1995.
10. Rodwell VW, Botham KM, Kennelly PJ, Weil PA, Bender DA. Harper's illustrated biochemistry, 30th edition. New York, NY: McGraw-Hill Education LLC, 2015.

REVIEW QUESTIONS

Long Essays
1. Define biochemistry; explain in detail about the importance of biochemistry in nursing.
2. Define cell, explain the of structure, composition and functions of cell.
3. Define microscope, explain different types, and explain in detail about.

Short Essays
1. Definition, meaning and concept of biochemistry.
2. History of biochemistry.
3. Chemical composition of cell.
4. Difference between endocytosis and exocytosis.
5. Golgi apparatus: structure and functions.
6. Microtubules and microfilaments.
7. Microscope: parts and types.
8. Difference between diffusion and osmosis?
9. Difference between prokaryotic and eukaryotic cell?
10. Explain the composition and functions of cell?
11. Describe fluid mosaic model of cell structure?
12. Explain active and passive transport mechanism with labelled diagram?
13. Describe transport mechanism of cell based on solubility of lipid?
14. Define diffusion. Enumerate the factors influencing diffusion?
15. Classify and describe about types of diffusion?

Short Answers
1. Enlist four functions cell wall.
2. Enlist four functions of golgi bodies.
3. Enlist four functions of endoplasmic reticulum.
4. Enlist four functions of mitochondria.
5. Enlist four functions of peroxisome.
6. Enlist four functions of ribosome.
7. Enlist four functions of lysosome.
8. Enlist four functions of centrosome.
9. Enlist four functions of plasma membrane.
10. Enlist four functions of nucleolus.

CHAPTER 16

Carbohydrates

CHAPTER OUTLINE

- Digestion, Absorption and Metabolism of Carbohydrates and Related Disorders
- Regulation of Blood Glucose
- Diabetes Mellitus—Type 1 and Type 2, Symptoms, Complications and Management in Brief
- Investigations of Diabetes Mellitus
- OGTT—Indications, Procedure, Interpretation and Types of GTT Curve
- Mini GTT, Extended GTT, GCT, IV GTT
- HbA1c (Only Definition)
- Hypoglycemia—Definition and Causes

TERMINOLOGY

- **Carbohydrate:** Carbohydrates are defined as polyhydroxy aldehydes or ketones or compounds which produce them on hydrolysis. For example, glucose, fructose, sucrose, starch, lactose, glycogen, etc. The term sugar is applied to carbohydrates which are soluble in water, crystalline in nature and are sweet in taste.
- **Uric acid pathway:** The process of oxidation of glucose to pyruvate or lactate under aerobic or anaerobic conditions respectively, along with the formation of ATP.
- **Citric acid cycle:** A cycle system of enzymatic reactions for oxidation of acetyl residues to carbon dioxide, in which formation of citrate is the first step; also known as the Krebs cycles or tricarboxylic acid cycle.
- **Diabetes mellitus:** A metabolic disease resulting from insulin deficiency; characterized by a failure in glucose transport from the blood into cells at normal glucose concentration.
- **Furanose:** A sugar that contains a five-membered ring as a result of intramolecular hemiacetal formation.
- **Gluconeogenesis:** The production of sugars from non-sugar precursors, such as lactate or amino acids. Applies more specifically to the production of free glucose by vertebrate livers.
- **Glycogen:** A polymer of glucose residue in 1, 4 linked, with 1.6 linkages at branch points.
- **Glycosidic bond:** The bond between a sugar and an alcohol, also the bond that links two sugars in disaccharides, oligosaccharides and polysaccharides.
- **Hexose monophosphate pathway:** An oxidative pathway beginning with glucose 6-phosphatase and leading, via 6-phosphogluconate, to pentose phosphates and yielding NADPH. It also called the pentose.
- **Krebs cycle:** A cycle system of enzymatic reactions for the oxidation of acetyl residues to carbon dioxide, in which formation of citrate is the first step; also known as the Krebs cycles or tri-carboxylic acid cycle.
- **Polysaccharide:** A liner or branched chain structure containing many sugar molecules linked by glycosidic bonds.
- **Reducing sugar:** A sugar in which the carbonyl (anomeric) carbon is not involved in a glycosidic bond and that can therefore undergoing oxidation.
- **Glycogenolysis:** The breakdown of glycogen is called glycogenolysis.
- **Glycogenesis:** When surplus amount of carbohydrate is present in the body, it is stored as glycogen. Synthesis of glycogen is called glycogenesis. If the blood glucose level is decreased, the stored glycogen is broken down and glucose is released to maintain the blood glucose level.
- **Glycans:** Polysaccharides that on hydrolysis yield many monosaccharides bound by oxygen bridge. They are non-sugars and from colloids with water.
- **Carbohydrates:** Polyhydroxy aldehydes or polyhydroxy ketones or substances that yield such compounds on hydrolysis.
- **Monosaccharide:** A carbohydrate consisting of a single sugar unit.
- **Hexose:** A simple sugar with a backbone containing 6 carbon atoms.
- **Pentose:** A simple sugar with a backbone containing 5 carbon atoms.
- **Disaccharide:** A carbohydrate consisting of two sugar units.
- **Oligosaccharides:** A carbohydrate consisting of 3–10 monosaccharides.

- **Polysaccharide:** A linear or branched polymer of more than 10 monosaccharide units linked by glycosidic bonds.
- **Diabetes mellitus:** If the glucose level exceeds 180 mg% (renal threshold level), it is excreted in the urine and this condition is called diabetes mellitus.

INTRODUCTION

Carbohydrates include a large group of compounds commonly known as starches or sugars, widely distributed in plants and animals. Chemically, they are described as polyhydric alcohols,' having potentially active aldehyde and ketone groups. In general, carbohydrates are white solids, freely soluble in water with the exception of certain polysaccharides. Carbohydrates of lower molecular weight have a sweet taste.

Types, Structure, Composition and Uses of Carbohydrate

Carbohydrates are polyhydroxy aldehydes or polyhydroxy ketones or substances that yield such compounds on hydrolysis. Carbohydrates are organic compounds made up of carbon, hydrogen and oxygen.

Structure of Carbohydrate

Carbohydrates are important macromolecules that consist of carbon, hydrogen, and oxygen in a 1:2:1 ratio (can be written as $C_n(H_2O)_n$). Carbohydrates are organic compounds organized in the form of aldehydes or ketones with multiple hydroxyl groups coming off the carbon chain. Carbohydrates are the most abundant organic compounds in living organisms and account for one of the four major biomolecular classes including proteins, lipids, and nucleic acids. They originate as products from carbon dioxide and water by **photosynthesis**,

$nCO_2 + nH_2O$ (+ reducing agents and energy from photon [sunlight]) $\rightarrow$ **ADP** + $C_nH_{2n}O_n + nO_2$

Chemically, carbohydrates contain carbon, hydrogen and oxygen. Generally, the composition in carbohydrates is in the proportion of two of hydrogen and one of oxygen atoms as in water (H_2O). Glucose which is a simple carbohydrate has a molecular formula of $C_6H_{12}O_6$. All simple sugars contain a potential aldehyde or ketone group. All the compound sugars which are made up of simple sugar molecules also contain the potential aldehyde group either in the free form or in the combined form. The importance of potential aldehyde or ketone group is that they are associated with reducing properties.

Types of Carbohydrates

Carbohydrates are classified into four major groups—there are a variety of interrelated classification schemes. The most useful classification scheme divides the carbohydrates into groups according to the number of individual simple sugar units. **Monosaccharides** contain a single unit; **disaccharides** contain two sugar units; and **polysaccharides** contain many sugar units as in polymers-most contain glucose as the monosaccharide unit.

Figure 16.1 is depicted the classifications of carbohydrate.

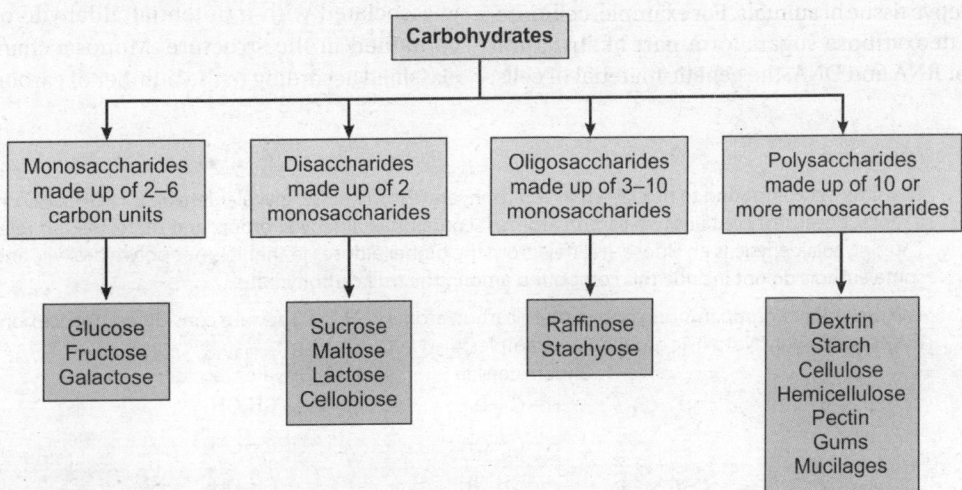

Fig. 16.1: Classifications of carbohydrate.

Classifications

Sl. No.	Classification	Description
1.	Monosaccharide	Monosaccharide contains only one molecule of sugar and they cannot be broken into simpler substances by hydrolysis. They are further subdivided according to the number of carbon atoms contained in their structure as indicated below: • Diose has tow carbon atoms. Molecular formula, $C_2H_4O_2$, e.g., glycolaldehyde • Triose has three carbon atoms. Molecular formula, $C_3H_6O_3$, e.g., glyceraldehyde, dihydroxyacetone • Tetrose has four carbon atoms. Molecular formula, C4H8O4, e.g., erythrose, threose • Pentose has five carbon atoms. Molecular formula, $C_5H_{10}O_5$, e.g., ribose, deoxyribose, xylose • Hexose has six carbon atoms. Molecular formula, $C_6H_{12}O_6$, e.g., glucose, fructose, galactose, mannose • Heptose has seven carbon atoms. Molecular formula, $C_7H_{14}O_7$, e.g., sedoheptulose, glucoheptose
2.	Oligosaccharides	Oligosaccharides yield two to ten monosaccharide units on hydrolysis. Strictly speaking disaccharides also come under this group. Examples of oligosaccharides other than disaccharides are, (a) Raffinose: Trisaccharide, (b) Stachyose: Tetrasaccharide, (c) Verbascose: Pentasaccharide
3.	Disaccharides	Disaccharides yield two molecules of monosaccharides on hydrolysis. They have a molecular formula of C12H22O11, e.g., (a) Sucrose, (b) Lactose, (c) Maltose
4.	Polysaccharides	Polysaccharides yield more than ten molecules of onosacdiarides on hydrolysis. They have a molecular formula of (C6 H10 O5), e.g., (a) Starch, (b) Glycogen, (c) Dextrins, (d) Cellulose, (e) Dextran, (f) Insulin

Functions of Carbohydrate

The chief function of carbohydrates in the body is that of a fuel. When carbohydrates are oxidized in the body they liberate carbon dioxide, water and energy. They supply the major portion of energy required by living cells. Certain carbohydrates can be used as the starting material for the biological synthesis of compounds such as fatty acids and amino acids.

❒ Carbohydrates serve as energy stores, fuels and metabolic intermediates.
  • Glycogen and starch are storage of polysaccharides found in animals and
  • **Plants respectively:** These are broken down to generate glucose molecules.
  • Glucose is utilized for production of energy.
❒ Carbohydrates serve as structural and protective elements in the cell wall of bacteria and plants. They are also present in the connective tissue of animals. For example, cellulose.
❒ Ribose and deoxyribose sugars form part of structural framework or RNA and DNA, the genetic material of cells;

❒ Carbohydrates are attached to many proteins and lipids. Such carbohydrates (glycoproteins and glycolipids) play important role in the cell—cell communication and in interaction between cells and other elements. These form part of the cell membrane.
❒ Carbohydrates serve as precursors for compounds, such as fats and amino acids.

Monosaccharides, Disaccharides, Polysaccharides, and Oligosaccharides

Monosacchraides

Monosaccharides are called simple sugars because they are the simplest units of carbohydrate and contain only one molecule of the sugar which cannot be split further into simpler molecules. Monosaccharides are regarded as polyhydric alcohols having reducing property which is associated with a potential aldehyde or ketone group, contained in the structure. Monosaccharides are further classified according to the number of carbon atoms.

Sl. No.	Types	Description
1.	Diose	The simplest compound to be classed as a carbohydrate is the diose, glycolaldehyde ($CH_2OH \cdot CHO$). It is classified as a 'diose', because it contains two carbon atoms. It contains an aldehyde group, and therefore, it is referred as aldose. Thus, glycolaldehyde is an aldose. It differs from the higher aldoses in that it is not polyhydroxylic and for this reason, some authors do not include this compound among the true carbohydrate.
2.	Triose	The next higher group. Trioses contain three carbon atoms ($C_3H_6O_3$). They are considered true carbohydrates because they contain polyhydroxylic groups. For examples: 1. Glyceraldehyde 2. Dihydroxyacetone $\begin{array}{c} H-C=O \\ \mid \\ H-C-OH \\ \mid \\ CH_2OH \end{array}$ $\begin{array}{c} CH_2OH \\ \mid \\ C=O \\ \mid \\ CH_2OH \end{array}$ Glyceraldehyde, which can be considered as the simplest monosaccharide is an aldotriose because it is a triose and contains an aldehyde group. Dihydroxyacetone is a ketotriose because it is a triose and contains a ketone group. The phosphate esters of glyceraldehyde and dihydroxyacetone occur as intermediates in the glycolysis of carbohydrates.

Contd...

Contd...

Sl. No.	Types	Description
3.	Tetroses	They contain four carbon atoms ($C_4H_8O_4$), e.g., (1) Erythrose, (2) Threose, (3) Erythrulose. Erythrose and threose are aldotetroses while erythrulose is a ketotetrose. D-Threose, D-Erythrose, D-Erythrulose
4.	Pentose	They contain five carbon atoms ($C_5H_{10}O_5$), e.g., (1) Ribose, (2) Deoxyribose, (3) Xylulose, (4) Arabinose Pentoses are physiologically important because ribose and deoxyribose are constituents of nucleic acids. Ribose is also a constituent of the vitamin riboflavin. Xylulose is a metabolite of glucuronic acid and is excreted in the urine of individuals suffering from Pentosuria, which is an inborn error of pentose metabolism. Arabinose is found in plants. D-Ribose, D-Deoxyribose, D-Xylulose
5.	Hexoses	These are physiologically important compounds. They contain six carbon atoms. Molecular formula-C6H 1206. The common hexoses are: (1) Glucose, (2) Fructose, (3) Galactose, (4) Mannose. Glucose, galactose and niannose are aldohexoses, each having an aldehyde group. Fructose is a ketohexose having a ketone group. Of the hexoses, glucose is most important, because it is the sugar contained in blood. Glucose and fructose occur freely in plants and fruits. Galactose is a component of lactose which is the disaccharide of milk. Polysaccharides containing mannose are found in ivory nuts, orchid tubers and yeast. D-Fructose, D-Galactose, D-Mannose Hexoses are as a class optically active. It will be seen that the various aldohexoses differ in their structures mainly in the spatial arrangement of hydrogen and hydroxyl groups, around each carbon atom of the molecule. But this little difference is enough to produce marked variation in the physical properties of the different hexoses.
6.	Heptose	A heptose is a monosaccharide with seven carbon atoms. Heptose is an obligatory component of the LPS core domain; its absence results in a truncated LPS structure resulting in susceptibility to hydrophobic antibiotics. The core heptose trisaccharide consists of L-glycero-D-manno-heptose, but analysis of the peracetylated sugars indicated that the 1,4-linked heptose is likely D-glycero-D-manno-heptose. D-glycero-D-manno-heptose is a constituent of lipopolysaccharide (LPS) cores of Gram-negative bacteria, and also a component of the S-layer glycoprotein of the Gram-positive bacterium *Aneurinibacillus thermoaerophilus*.

Disaccharides

Two monosaccharides connected by a glycoside link form a disaccharide. The disaccharide lactose found in milk is a disaccharide composed of one glucose and one galactose unit with the glycosidic link between carbon 4 of glucose and carbon 1 of galactose in the p-configuration. Since the anomeric carbon of galactose is involved in the glycosidic bond, lactose is a galactoside. The full chemical name of lactose is (beta-D-galacto pyranosyl-D-glucopyranose. The anomeric carbon of the glucose component remains free and has therefore reducing properties and exhibits mutarotation and 3-lactose are distinguished by the configuration around the free anomerie carbon of the glucose portion but they are both 3-galactosides. The enzyme galactosidase can be induced in *E.coli* by growing it on lactose which is hydrolyzed to galactose and glucose before being metabolized.

Sl. No.	Classification	Description
1.	Lactose	(4β-D-Galactopyranosyl-α-D-Glucopyranose) α-Lactose Latin word for milk "lact"; a disaccharide found in milk containing **glucose and galactose**.
2.	Sucrose	(α-D-Galactopyranosyl-β-D-Fructofuranose) Sucrose French word for sugar—"sucre", a disaccharide containing **glucose and fructose**; table sugar, cane sugar, beet sugar. Sucrose the common table sugar, is obtained from sugarcane and sugar beets. It is readily hydrolyzed through the action of acid or of a specific enzyme named sucrose into glucose and fructose. The anomeric carbons of both sugars are involved in the linkage and it is therefore non-reducing and does not display mutarotation. Sucrose can be looked upon, therefore, either as a glucoside or a fructoside. It has been shown that in the hydrolysis of sucrose with sucrase in the presence of O^{18}-labeled water the point of cleavage lies between the C2 of fructose and the bridge oxygen.
3.	Maltose:	4α-D-Galactopyranosyl-β-D-Glucopyranose β-maltose French word for "malt"; a disaccharide containing **two units of glucose**; found in germinating grains, used to make beer. Maltose is 4O-(O-D-glucopyranosyl)- D-glucopyranose while cellobiose is 4–0-(3-D-glucopyranosyl)- D-glucopyranose. Though the only chemical defference between the two lies in the orientation about the connecting oxygen atom, this leads to a great difference in their nutritional value.
4.	Cellobiose	4β-D-Galactopyranosyl-D-Glucopyranose Cellobiose Both maltose and cellobiose are reducing sugars capable of mutarotation and participate in the formation of further glycosidic links leading to the formation of starches and celluloses respectively.

Oligosaccharides

They are composed of three to ten monosaccharide units linked to each other by the removal of water molecules. They are formed during break down of starch into simpler sugars, e.g., raffinose and stachyose. They are not as common in food as the mono, di and polysaccharides.

Polysaccharides

Polysaccharides consist of straight or branched chains of many monosaccharid units joined together by means of glycosidic bonds. They may be subdivided into two broad groups, the homopolysaccharides and the heteropolysaccharides. The homopolysaccharides yield on hydrolysis a single type of sugar unit, such as a hexose, a pentose, a sugar acid or an amino sugar. The most abundant polysaccharides are of this type. The sugar units present are hexoses, such as D-glucose, D-mannose, D-galactose and to a small extent L-galactose, D-idose and L-altrose, pentoses, such as D-xylose, L-arabinose and D-arabinose, the amino sugars D-glucosamine and D-galactosamine, the sugar acids D-glucuronic acid, D-galacturonic acid, D-manfluronic acid, L-iduronic acid and the deoxy sugars L-fucose and L-rhamflose. The heteropolysaccharides yield a mixture of building units, including monosaccharides and their derivatives, the amino sugars and sugar acids. In terms of their function, the polysaccharides can be considered under two classes, the 'skeletal or structural' polysaccharides which provide the framework for a rigid structure in plants and animals and 'nutrient' polysaccharides, such as starch and glycogen which serve as a food reserve of monosaccharides in plants and aminals.

Classifications: 1. Homopolysaccharides, 2. Heteropolysaccharides

1. Homopolysaccharides

Sl. No.	Classification	Description
1.	**Starch**	It is the reserve carbohydrate of plant kingdom. They are present abundantly in potatoes, tapioca, rice, wheat and other food grains. Starch consists of 2 polysaccharide components—water soluble amylose and a water insoluble amylopectin. Amylose is a long un-branched chain with 200–1000 D-glucose units held by alpha (1–4) glycosidic linkages. Amylopectin is a branched chain with (1–6) glycosidic bonds at the branching points and (1–4) linkages everywhere else. Starch $\xrightarrow{\text{Amylase}}$ Dextrins $\xrightarrow{\text{Hydrolysis}}$ Maltose and glucose
2.	Dextrins	They are breakdown products of starch by the enzyme amylase or dilute
3.	Inulin	It is a long chain homoglycan composed of D-fructose. It occurs in dahlia, onion, garlic, etc. It is clinically used to find renal clearance value and glomerular filtration rate (GFR).
4.	Glycogen	It is the reserve carbohydrate in animals and often referred to as "animal starch". It is stored in liver and muscle. Glycogen is composed of glucose units joined by glycosidic linkages. Its structure is similar to amylopectin with more number of branches.
5.	Cellulose	It is the chief carbohydrate in plants. It is the predominant constituent of plant cell wall. It is made up of —D-glucose units linked by (1–4) glycosidic bonds. Cellulose is not digested by human enzyme. It is a major constituent of dietary fiber.

2. **Heteropolysaccharides:** Mucopolysaccharides are negatively charged heteropolysaccharides. Mucopolysaccharides or glycosaminoglycans (GAG) are mainly made up of amino sugars and uronic acids. Functions: (i) Essential components of tissue structure, (ii) Collagen and elastin fibers embedded in a matrix or ground substance which is predominantly composed of GAG. For example, hyaluronic acid, heparin, chondroitin sulfate, dermatan sulfate, keratin sulfate, etc.

Sl. No.	Classification	Description
1.	Hyaluronic acid	It is present in vitreous humor, skin, synovial fluid, umbilical cord and ovum. It is composed of N-acetylglucosamine and glucuronic acid held together by I (1–3) glycosidic bond. It acts as a lubricant and a shock absorbant in joints and it further acts as a cementing substance and contributes semi-permeability to membrane.
2.	Heparin	It occurs in liver, lungs, thymus, blood, etc., and consists of sulfated glucosamine and glucuronic acid (or iduronic acid). It acts as an anticoagulant and also as an enzyme.
3.	Chondroitin sulfate	It occurs in skin, heart, valves, b6nes, tendons, cartilages, etc. It is composed of glucuronic acid and N-acetylglucosamine sulfate. It is required for synthesis of osteocytes and cartilages. It is a constituent of basement membrane and cell surface.
4.	Dermatan sulfate	Mostly, it occurs in the skin, blood vessels, etc., and composed of iduronic acid and N-acetylglucosamine sulfate.
5.	Keratan sulfate	It is the only GAG which does not contain any uronic acid. It is present in cornea and tendon. It is composed of galactose and N-acetylglucosamine sulfate.

Digestion and Absorption of Carbohydrates (Fig. 16.2)

Digestion of carbohydrates is necessary because only monosaccharides can be absorbed into the blood stream. Food is chewed in the mouth and it mixes with saliva. The enzyme ptyaun splits starch into dextrin and maltose.

In the stomach, it mixes with gastric juice but it contains no enzyme of carbohydrate digestion.

There are two pathways for the transport of materials absorbed by the intestine:
1. Hepatic portal system—leads directly to the liver transporting water soluble nutrients.
2. Lymphatic vessels—lead to the blood by way of the thoracic duct and transport lipid soluble nutrients.

Based on sites, digestion is of 3 types: Extracellular, surface and intracellular digestion.

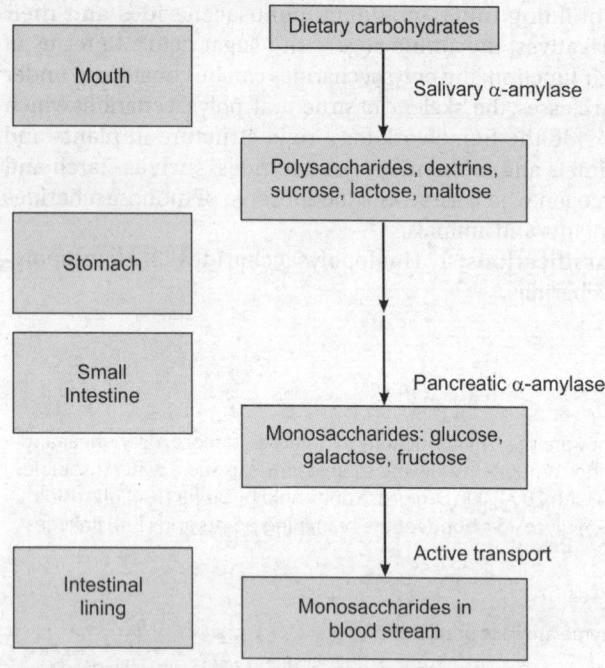

Fig. 16.2: Digestion and absorption of carbohydrate.

Absorbed digestive products are carried to liver via portal circulation where a part of glucose and the entire fructose and galactose are converted into glycogen. A part of glucose passes into general circulation, where it is used by various tissues as a fuel for energy (ATP). A small remaining part is converted to glycogen by muscles and into fat and stored in adipose tissue. Waste products of carbohydrate metabolism are CO_2 and H_2O, excreted by the body.

Transport of glucose: Glucose is an essential substrate for the metabolism of most cells. Because glucose is a polar molecule, transport through biological membranes requires specific transport proteins.

Active transport-cotransporters: Transport of glucose through the apical membrane of intestinal and kidney epithelial cells depends on the presence of secondary active Na^+/glucose symporters, SGLT-1 and SGLT-2, which concentrate glucose inside the cells, using the energy provided by cotransport of Na^+ ions down their electrochemical gradient.

Passive transport-GLUTs: Facilitated diffusion of glucose through the cellular membrane is otherwise catalyzed by glucose carriers (protein symbol GLUT, gene symbol SLC2 for solute carrier family 2) that belong to a superfamily of transport facilitators (major facilitator superfamily) including organic anion and cation transporters, yeast hexose transporter, plant hexose/proton symporters, and bacterial sugar/proton symporters. Molecule movement by such transporter proteins occurs by facilitated diffusion. This makes them energy-independent, unlike active transporters, which often require the presence of ATP to drive their translocation mechanism, and stall if the ATP/ADP ratio drops too low.

Digestion and absorption from GI tract:

Sl. No.	Organ	Major functions
1.	Stomach	Saliva containing o-amylase is produced and polysaccharides are partially digested.
2.	Stomach	Gastric juice with HC1 and proteases is produced and proteins are partially digested.
3.	Pancreas	Many enzymes and $NaHCO_3$ required for intestinal digestion are released.
4.	Liver	Bile acids are synthesized.
5.	Gallbladder	Bile is stored
6.	Small intestine	Food stuffs are finally digested and digested products are absorbed.
7.	Large intestine	Electrolytes are absorbed and bacterial utilization of certain undigested and or unabsorbed foods.

Digestion occurs in the small intestine by pancreatic amylase, intestinal amylase, sucrose, lactose, and maltase and iso-maltase enzymes. The ultimate digestive products are glucose, fructose and glactose. Non-digestible carbohydrates (cellulose, hemicelluloses, pentosans and galactans) add bulk to the intestinal contents and are excreted in the feces.

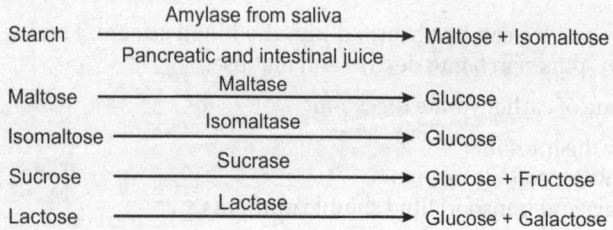

Absorption of monosaccharides occurs in small intestine.

Carbohydrate Metabolism

Carbohydrate metabolism begins with digestion in the small intestine where monosaccharides are absorbed into the blood stream. Blood sugar concentrations are controlled by three hormones—insulin, glucagon, and epinephrine. If the concentration of glucose in the blood is too high, insulin is secreted by the pancreas. Insulin stimulates the transfer of glucose into the cells, especially in the liver and muscles, although other organs are also able to metabolize glucose. In the liver and muscles, most of the glucose is changed into glycogen by the process of **glycogenesis** (anabolism). Glycogen is stored in the liver and muscles until needed at some later time when glucose levels are low. If blood glucose levels are low, then eqinephrine and glucogon hormones are secreted to stimulate the conversion of glycogen to glucose. This process is called **glycogenolysis** (catabolism).

If glucose is needed immediately upon entering the cells to supply energy, it begins the metabolic process called **glycoysis** (catabolism). The end products of glycolysis are **pyruvic acid and ATP**. Since glycolysis releases relatively little ATP, further reactions continue to convert pyruvic acid to acetyl CoA and then citric acid in the citric acid cycle. The majority of the ATP is made from oxidations in the citric acid cycle in connection with the electron transport chain.

Figure 16.3 is depicted the mechanism of digestion and **Figure 16.4** is depicted the carbohydrate metabolism.

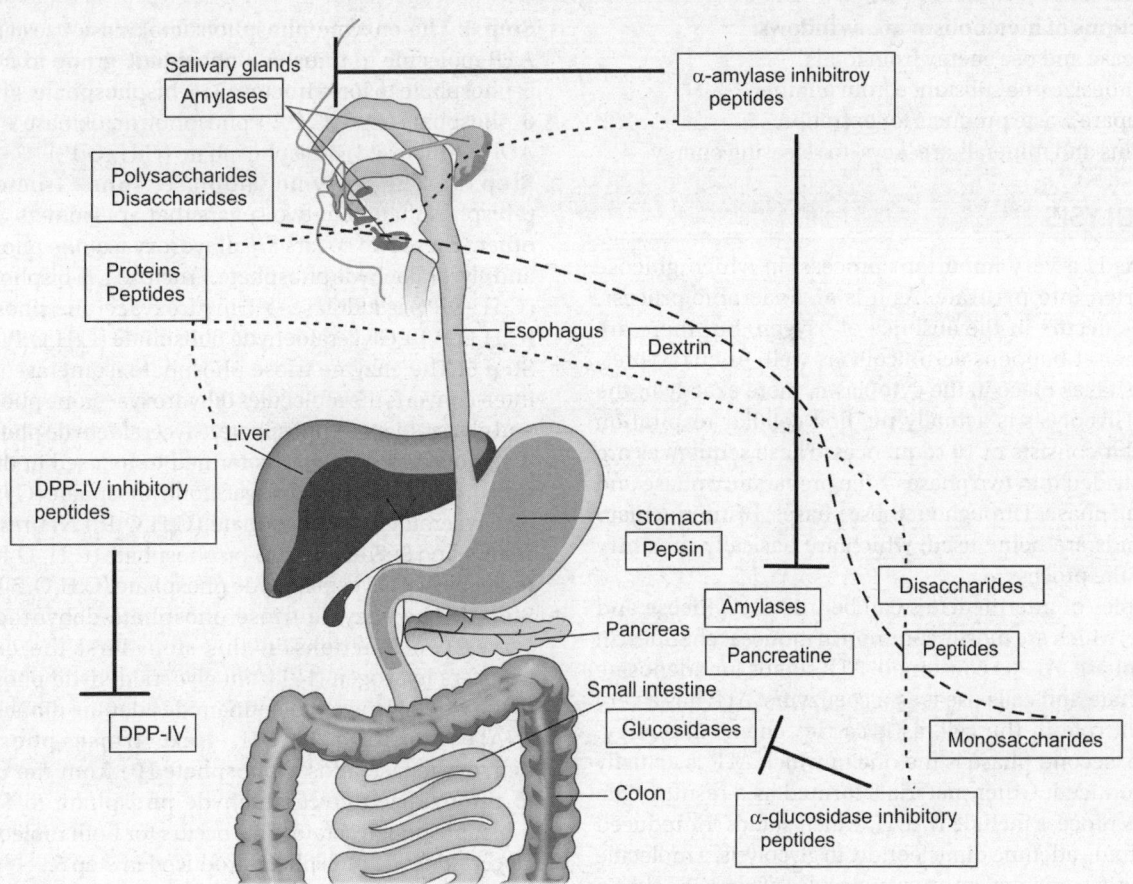

Fig. 16.3: Mechanism of digestion.

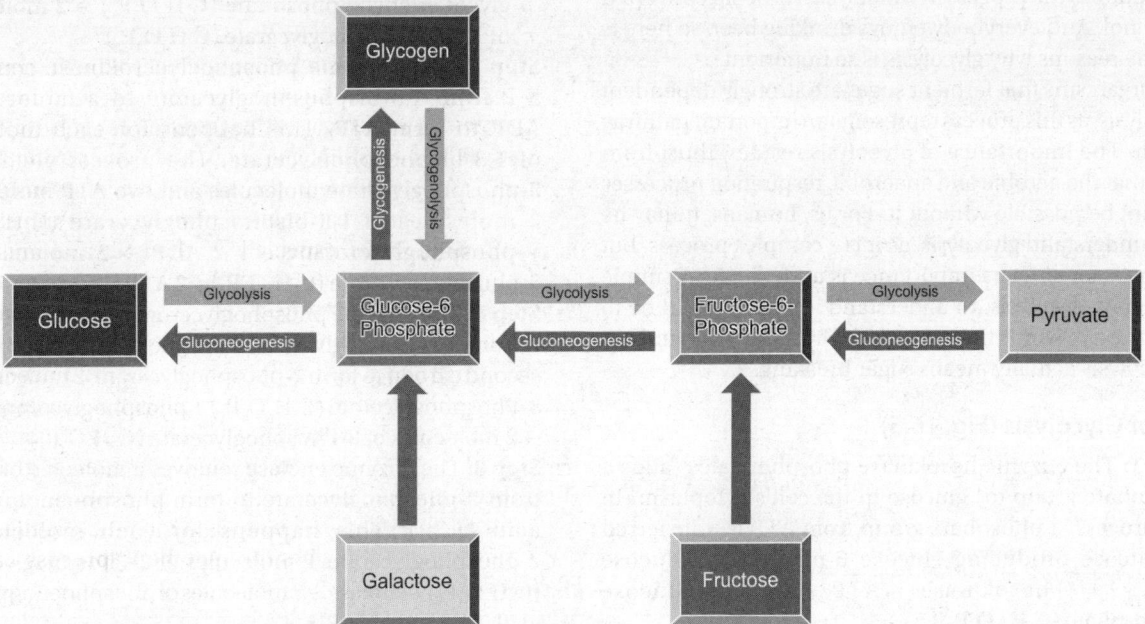

Fig. 16.4: Carbohydrate metabolism.

During strenuous muscular activity, pyruvic acid is converted into lactic acid rather that acetyl CoA. During the resting period, the lactic acid is converted back to pyruvic acid. The pyruvic acid in turn is converted back to glucose by the process called **gluconeogenesis** (anabolism). If the glucose is not needed at that moment, it is converted into glycogen by glycogenesis. You can remember those terms if you think of "genesis" as the formation-beginning.

The functions of metabolism are as follows:
- To release and use energy from foods.
- To synthesize one substance from another.
- To prepare waste products for excretion.
- Vitamins and minerals are 'keys' to releasing energy.

GLYCOLYSIS

Glycolysis is a very important process, in which glucose is converted into pyruvate. As it is an anaerobic process, glycolysis occurs in the absence of oxygen, but there are times when it happens aerobically as well. In eukaryotes, glycolysis takes place in the cytoplasm, more exactly in the cytosol. Glycolysis is actually the first cellular respiration step, and it consists of 10 sequences. These sequences are further divided into two phases—the preparatory phase and the pay-off phase. Throughout these phases, 10 intermediary compounds are being used, which are basically the entry points of the process.

Examples of intermediates can be fructose, glucose and galactose, which are mostly common in monosaccharides. In the first phase, ATP is consumed. ATP stands for adenosine triphosphate and cells use it as a coenzyme. ATP has a very important role in the cell, as it carries chemical energy. Then, the second phase is the one in which ATP is actually being produced. Other materials formed as a result of the glycolysis process include NADH, which stands for reduced nicotinamide adenine dinucleotide. In glycolysis, a molecule of glucose in converted into two molecules of pyruvic acid. So glycolysis is basically the starting point for other respiration processes, such as fermentation. Everybody knows that fermentation is the process in which yeast is being converted into alcohol. And everybody enjoys drinking beer, so here is one of the reasons why glycolysis is so important.

The organisms that ferment sugar are strongly dependent on glycolysis, as this process represents an important pathway for them. The importance of glycolysis resides, thus, from the fact that the aerobic and anaerobic respiration processes would not be possible without it. For us, humans, it may be hard to understand glycolysis, as it is a complex process, but one thing is for sure: its importance is undeniable. A simple definition of glycolysis, to understand it better, would be to think of the two words that it is formed from. You will find out that glycolysis actually means sugar breaking.

Steps of Glycolysis (Fig. 16.5)

- **Step 1:** The enzyme hexokinase phosphorylates (adds a phosphate group to) glucose in the cell's cytoplasm. In the process, a phosphate group from ATP is transferred to glucose producing glucose 6-phosphate. Glucose ($C_6H_{12}O_6$) + hexokinase + ATP → ADP + Glucose 6-phosphate ($C_6H_{11}O_6P_1$).
- **Step 2:** The enzyme phosphoglucoisomerase converts glucose 6-phosphate into its isomer fructose 6-phosphate. Isomers have the same molecular formula, but the atoms of each molecule are arranged differently. Glucose 6-phosphate ($C_6H_{11}O_6P_1$) + Phosphoglucoisomerase → Fructose 6-phosphate ($C_6H_{11}O_6P_1$).
- **Step 3:** The enzyme phosphofructokinase uses another ATP molecule to transfer a phosphate group to fructose 6-phosphate to form fructose 1, 6-bisphosphate. Fructose 6-phosphate ($C_6H_{11}O_6P_1$) + phosphofructokinase + ATP → ADP + Fructose 1, 6-bisphosphate ($C_6H_{10}O_6P_2$).
- **Step 4:** The enzyme aldolase splits fructose 1, 6-bisphosphate into two sugars that are isomers of each other. These two sugars are dihydroxyacetone phosphate and glyceraldehyde phosphate. Fructose 1, 6-bisphosphate ($C_6H_{10}O_6P_2$) + aldolase → Dihydroxyacetone phosphate ($C_3H_5O_3P_1$) + Glyceraldehyde phosphate ($C_3H_5O_3P_1$).
- **Step 5:** The enzyme triose phosphate isomerase rapidly inter-converts the molecules dihydroxyacetone phosphate and glyceraldehyde phosphate. Glyceraldehyde phosphate is removed as soon as it is formed to be used in the next step of glycolysis. Dihydroxyacetone phosphate ($C_3H_5O_3P_1$) → Glyceraldehyde phosphate ($C_3H_5O_3P_1$) Net result for steps 4 and 5: Fructose 1, 6-bisphosphate ($C_6H_{10}O_6P_2$) ↔ 2 molecules of Glyceraldehyde phosphate ($C_3H_5O_3P_1$).
- **Step 6:** The enzyme triose phosphate dehydrogenase serves two functions in this step. First the enzyme transfers hydrogen (H^-) from glyceraldehyde phosphate to the oxidizing agent nicotinamide adenine dinucleotide (NAD^+) to form NADH. Next triose phosphate dehydrogenase adds a phosphate (P) from the cytosol to the oxidized glyceraldehyde phosphate to form 1, 3-bisphosphoglycerate. This occurs for both molecules of glyceraldehyde phosphate produced in step 5.
  - Triose phosphate dehydrogenase + 2 H^- + 2 NAD^+ → 2 NADH + 2 H^+
  - Triose phosphate dehydrogenase + 2 P + 2 glyceraldehyde phosphate ($C_3H_5O_3P_1$) → 2 molecules of 1,3-bisphosphoglycerate ($C_3H_4O_4P_2$)
- **Step 7:** The enzyme phosphoglycerokinase transfers a P from 1,3-bisphosphoglycerate to a molecule of ADP to form ATP. This happens for each molecule of 1,3-bisphosphoglycerate. The process yields two 3-phosphoglycerate molecules and two ATP molecules. 2 molecules of 1,3-bisphosphoglycerate ($C_3H_4O_4P_2$) + phosphoglycerokinase + 2 ADP → 2 molecules of 3-phosphoglycerate ($C_3H_5O_4P_1$) + 2 ATP
- **Step 8:** The enzyme phosphoglyceromutase relocates the P from 3-phosphoglycerate from the third carbon to the second carbon to form 2-phosphoglycerate. 2 molecules of 3-Phosphoglycerate ($C_3H_5O_4P_1$) + phosphoglyceromutase → 2 molecules of 2-Phosphoglycerate ($C_3H_5O_4P_1$)
- **Step 9:** The enzyme enolase removes a molecule of water from 2-phosphoglycerate to form phosphoenolpyruvic acid (PEP). This happens for each molecule of 2-phosphoglycerate. 2 molecules of 2-Phosphoglycerate ($C_3H_5O_4P_1$) + enolase → 2 molecules of phosphoenolpyruvic acid (PEP) ($C_3H_3O_3P_1$)
- **Step 10:** The enzyme pyruvate kinase transfers a P from PEP to ADP to form pyruvic acid and ATP. This happens for each molecule of PEP. This reaction yields 2 molecules of pyruvic acid and 2 ATP molecules. 2 molecules of PEP ($C_3H_3O_3P_1$) + pyruvate kinase + 2 ADP → 2 molecules of pyruvic acid ($C_3H_4O_3$) + 2 ATP.

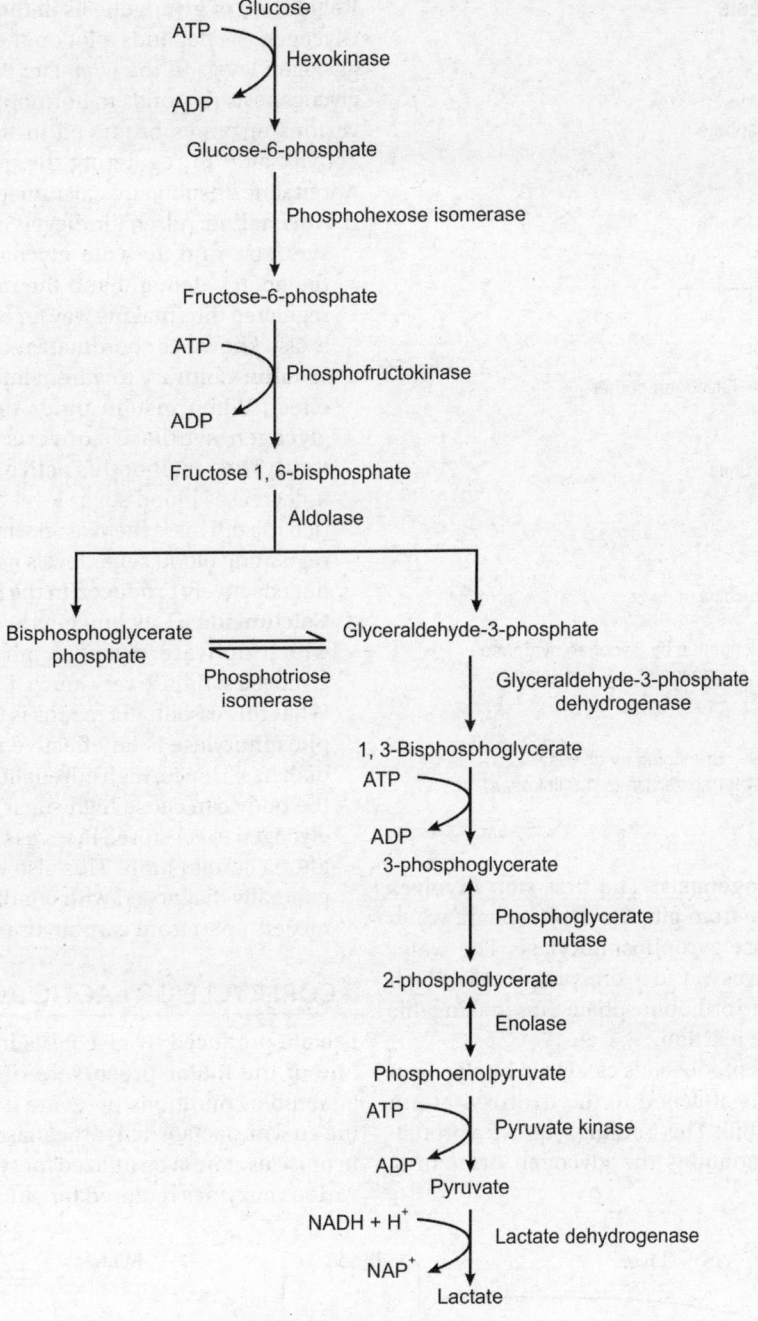

Fig. 16.5: Steps of glycolysis.

GLYCOGENESIS

Glycogenesis is an important metabolic activity in which molecules of glucose in the body is converted to glycogen in order to be stored in the liver, etc. In theory, it is defined as a process in which glucose molecules are added to glycogen chains. Glycogenesis is activated when the body is in a state of rest or during high glucose level in the blood (due to high carbohydrate diet or due to diabetes) thus making insulin activate this process to reduce blood sugar level. However, the synthesis of glycogen largely depends on the energy and glucose levels in the body.

There are 2 steps in glycogenesis. Glucose is first converted into glucose-6-phosphate by the action of glucokinase. This glucose-6-phosphate is converted into glucose-1,6-bisphosphate by phosphoglucomutase and later into glucose-1-phosphate.

Definition: The synthesis of glucose from noncarbohydrate precursors is called gluconeogenesis. This metabolic pathway is very important because glucose is the primary energy source for the brain. Erythrocytes do not have mitochondria and derive all of their energy by glycolysis converting glucose into two molecules of lactate.

Pathway of Glycogenesis

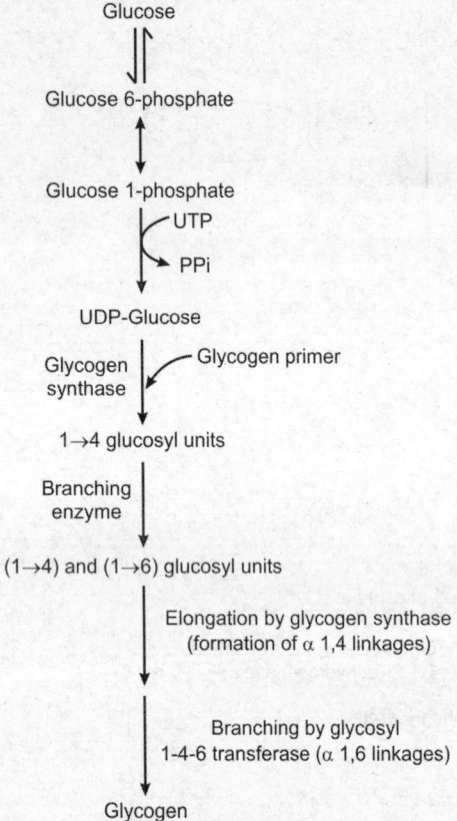

Steps involved in glycogenesis: The first step involves synthesis of UDP-glucose from glucose-1-phosphate when catalyzed by UDP-glucose pyrophosphorylase. The water present in this reaction gives way to hydrolysis process which converts pyrophosphate to orthophosphate thus making this first step a non-reversible reaction.

The UDP-glucose thus produced is catalyzed by glycogen synthase in which it gets attached to the hydroxyl group forming α-1,4-glycosidic link. This binding requires a protein like glycogenin which contains the glycogen branching enzyme.

Regulation of glycogenesis in the body:
Glycogenesis depends a lot on the blood glucose levels and glycogen levels in the liver, etc. But it should be noted that glycogenesis responds to hormonal activity in the body. The various enzymes produced in the body under hormonal activity aide in regulating the glycogen levels. These are Adrenaline, insulin and calcium ions.

- **Adrenaline:** Adrenaline levels in the body inhibit glycogen synthase and activate glycogen phosphorylase. Thus the energy demand and the rate of energy burn out are regulated thus making way for optimized glycogenesis and is also known as coordinate reciprocal control.
- **Insulin:** Contrary to adrenaline, Insulin has an opposite effect. When insulin binds to the protein primer, the glycogen synthase converts to non-phosphorylated form. The result of this active glycogen synthase is that it decreases blood sugar level even after a carbohydrate-rich meal. This is the reason why insulin is so important in regulating blood sugar levels in our body. When insulin is not effectively produced in the body, it results in diabetes.
- **Calcium ions:** Calcium ions act as secondary messengers which activate glycogen phosphorylase and inhibit glycogen synthase very much like the effects of Adrenaline. What this essentially means is that inhibition of glycogen phosphorylase is an effective method of treating type-2 diabetes. Hence, high adrenaline rush or calcium levels in the body can cause high sugar levels in the body leading glycogen to get stored in excess in the liver. This is harmful after a certain limit. This also explains why diabetics are generally diagnosed with conditions of hypertension and anxiety apart from carbohydrate and sugar-rich diet.

CORI CYCLE OR LACTIC ACID CYCLE (FIG. 16.6)

Lactate produced by glycolysis in active skeletal muscle is one of the major precursors of gluconeogenesis. Under anaerobic conditions pyruvate is converted into lactate by the enzyme lactate dehydrogenase (LDH). Lactate produced in muscles cannot be utilized for synthesis of glucose because various enzymes required for gluconeogenesis are absent in

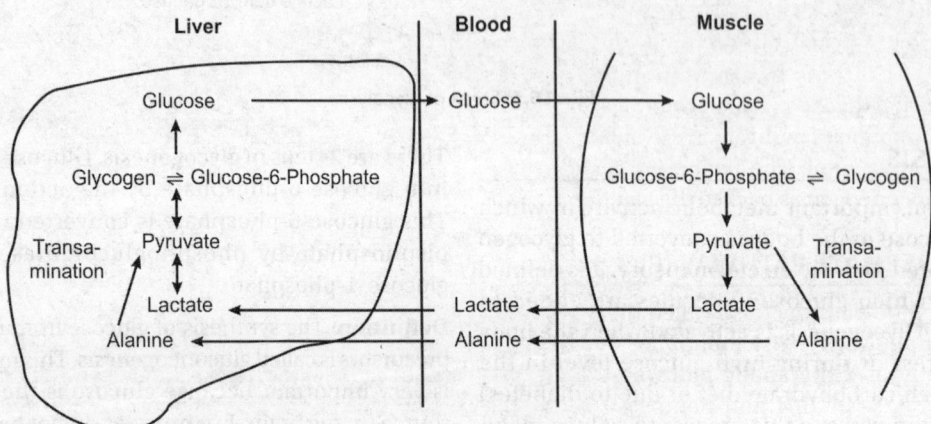

Fig. 16.6: Coricycle or lactic acid cycle.

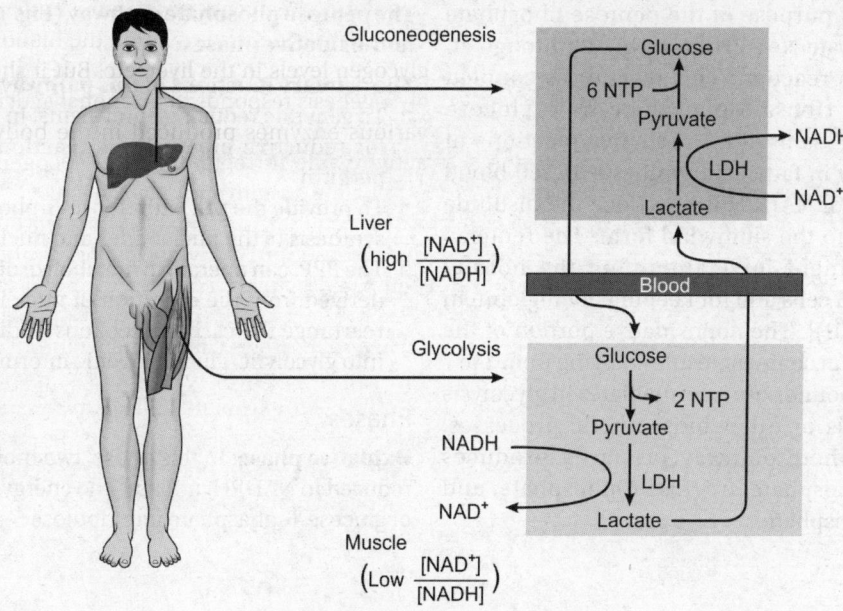

Fig. 16.7: Glucose-alanine cycle.

muscles. Lactate formed in skeletal muscles is transported to the liver with the help of blood, In liver lactate is oxidized into pyruvate which is converted into glucose by gluconeogenesis. The glucose formed at the end is again transported to the muscles.

Vigorous exercise leads to an oxygen shortage producing anaerobic conditions in the muscle cells. In order to regenerate NAD⁺ to keep glycolysis going pyruvate is reduced to lactate. The lactate produced by the muscles is released into the blood where it is carried to the liver. In the liver, lactate is reoxidized into pyruvate which is then converted to glucose via gluconeogenesis. In this way, the liver shares in the metabolic stress produced by vigorous exercise.

During exercise the liver releases glucose into the blood stream to fuel the muscles. The muscles produce lactate which is carried back to the liver where by gluconeogenesis it is converted back into glucose. This cycle is called cor cycle.

Glucose-alanine cycle (Fig. 16.7): During starvation amino acids are transported from muscles to the liver. Alanine is the major amino acid in this transportation process. In glucose alanine cycle glucose is transported from liver to the muscles with formation of pyruvate. Pyruvate undergoes transamination to form alanine. The alanine is transported to liver, followed by gluconeogensis back to the glucose.

PENTOSE PHOSPHATE PATHWAY (FIG. 16.8)

The pentose phosphate pathway (also called the phosphogluconate pathway and the hexose monophosphate shunt and the HMP shunt) is a metabolic pathway parallel to glycolysis. It generates NADPH and pentoses (5-carbon sugars) as well as ribose 5-phosphate, a precursor for the synthesis of nucleotides.

The pentose phosphate pathway starts with G6P

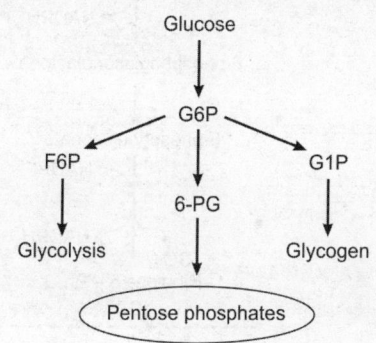

Fig. 16.8: Pentose phosphate pathway: Oxidative and non-oxidative phases.

Definition

- The pentose phosphate pathway is primarily an anabolic pathway that utilizes 6 carbons of glucose to generate 5 carbon sugars and reducing equivalents. However, this pathway oxidizes glucose and under certain conditions can completely oxidize glucose to CO_2 and water.
- The pentose phosphate pathway (also called phosphogluconate pathway or hexose monophosphate shunt [HMP shunt]) is a cytosolic process that serves to generate NADPH and the synthesis of pentose (5-carbon) sugars. There are two distinct phases in the pathway. The first is the oxidative phase, in which NADPH is generated, and the second is the non-oxidative synthesis of 5-carbon sugars. This pathway is an alternative to glycolysis. While it does involve oxidation of glucose, its primary role is anabolic rather than catabolic.

Purposes: The main purpose of the pentose phosphate pathway is to regenerate NADPH from NADP$^+$ through an oxidation/ reduction reaction. This reaction is coupled to the formation of ribose 5-phosphate from glucose 6-phosphate. NADPH is used for reductive reactions in anabolism, especially in fatty acid synthesis. In red blood cells, the major role of NADPH is to reduce the disulfide form of glutathione to the sulfhydryl form. The reduced glutathione is pertinent for maintaining the normal structure of red blood cells and for keeping hemoglobin in the ferrous state [Fe(II)]. The nonoxidative portion of the pathway creates carbon chain molecules ranging from 3 to 7 carbons. These compounds are intermediates in glycolysis and gluconeogenesis or other biosynthetic processes. The pentose phosphate pathway primarily produces NADPH, ribose 5-phosphate, fructose 6-phosphate, and glyceraldehyde 3-phosphate.

The pentose phosphate pathway (Fig. 16.9): Oxidative and non-oxidative phases:

The primary functions of this pathway are as follows:
- To generate reducing equivalents, in the form of NADPH, for reductive biosynthesis reactions that cell need to perform.
- To provide the cell with ribose-5-phosphate (R5P) for the synthesis of the nucleotides and nucleic acids.
- The PPP, can operate to metabolize dietary pentose sugars derived from the digestion of nucleic acids as well as to rearrange the carbon skeletons of dietary carbohydrates into glycolytic/gluconeogenic intermediates.

Phases

Oxidative phase: In this phase, two molecules of NADP$^+$ are reduced to NADPH, utilizing the energy from the conversion of glucose-6-phasphate into ribulose 5-phosphate.

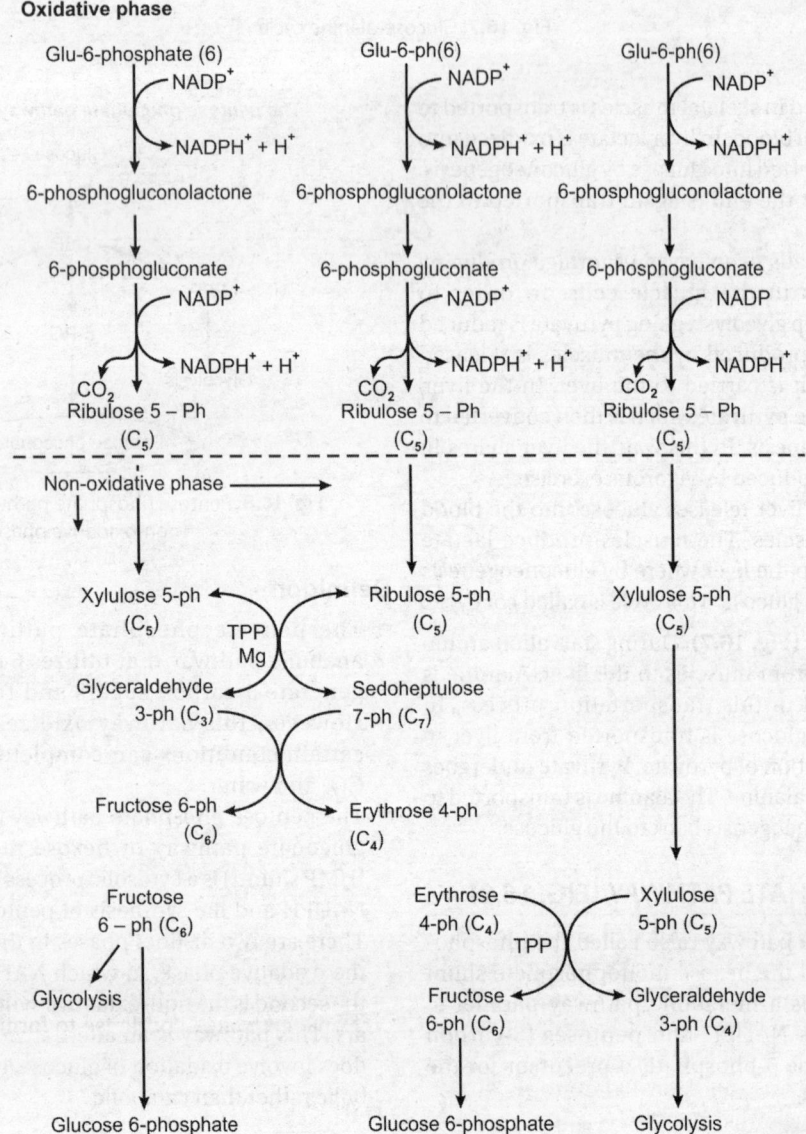

Fig. 16.9: Pentose phosphate pathway.

Sl. No.	Reactants	Products	Enzyme	Description
1.	Glucose 6-phosphate + $NADP^+$	→ 6-phosphogluco-nolactone + **NADPH**	Glucose 6-phosphate dehydrogenase	Dehydrogenation. The hemiacetal hydroxyl group located on carbon 1 of glucose 6-phosphate is converted into a carbonyl group, generating a lactone, and, in the process, NADPH is generated
2.	6-phosphogluconolactone + H_2O	→ 6-phosphogluconate + H^+	6-phosphogluconolactonase	Hydrolysis
3.	6-phosphogluconate + $NADP^+$	$NADP^+$ → ribulose 5-phosphate + **NADPH** + CO_2	**NADPH** + CO_2 6-phosphogluconate dehydrogenase	Oxidative decarboxylation. $NADP^+$ is the electron acceptor, generating another molecule of NADPH, a CO_2, and ribulose 5-phosphate
4.	Ribulose 5-phosphate	Ribose 5-phosphate	Phosphopentose isomerase	Isomerization. (Can also be considered part of nonoxidative phase)

The overall reaction for this process is: Glucose 6-phosphate + 2 $NADP^+$ + H_2O → ribulose 5-phosphate + 2 NADPH + 2 H^+ + CO_2

Non-oxidative phase

Sl. No.	Reactants	Products	Enzyme
1.	Ribulose 5-phosphate	→ ribose 5-phosphate	Phosphopentose isomerase
2.	Ribulose 5-phosphate	→ xylulose 5-phosphate	Phosphopentose epimerase
3.	Xylulose 5-phosphate + ribose 5-phosphate	→ glyceraldehyde 3-phosphate + sedoheptulose 7-phosphate	Transaldolase
4.	Sedoheptulose 7-phosphate + glyceraldehyde 3-phosphate	→ erythrose 4-phosphate + fructose 6-phosphate	Transaldolase
5.	Xylulose 5-phosphate + erythrose 4-phosphate	→ glyceraldehyde 3-phosphate + fructose 6-phosphate	Transaldolase

Regulation: Glucose-6-phosphate dehydrogenase is the rate-controlling enzyme of this pathway. It is allosterically stimulated by $NADP^+$. The ratio of NADPH: $NADP^+$ is normally about 100:1 in liver cytosol. This makes the cytosol a highly-reducing environment. Formation of $NADP^+$ by a NADPH-utilizing pathway, thus, stimulates production of more NADPH.

CITRIC ACID CYCLE

History of citric acid cycle: The citric acid cycle is a series of enzyme catalyzed chemical reactions that takes place in the mitochondria. In 1937, this first stage of cellular respiration was first identified by Albert Szent-Gyorgyi and Hans Krebs, hence the name Krebs cycle (officially referred to as the Svent-Gyorgyi-Krebs Cycle). Szent-Gyorgyi was awarded the Nobel Prize in 1937 for his discoveries of a biological combustion process and Krebs was awarded the Nobel Prize in 1953 for the discovery of the citric acid cycle.
Description: Under aerobic conditions the end product of glycolysis is pyruvic acid. The next step is the formation of **acetyl coenzyme A** (acetyl CoA)—this step is technically not a part of the citric acid cycle.

Acetyl CoA, whether from glycolysis or the fatty acid spiral, is the initiator of the citric acid cycle. In carbohydrate metabolism, acetyl-CoA is the link between glycolysis and the citric acid cycle. The initiating step of the citric acid cycle occurs when a four carbon compound (oxaloacetic acid) condenses with acetyl-CoA (2 carbons) to form citric acid (6 carbons).

The whole purpose of a "turn" of the citric acid cycle is to produce two carbon dioxide molecules. This general oxidation reaction is accompanied by the loss of hydrogen and electrons at four specific places. These oxidations are connected to the electron transport chain where many ATP are produced.

The reactions for the citric acid cycle are shown in the graphic on the left. These reactions are more familiar than those from glycolysis. Unless the instructor states otherwise, you should study these reactions so that you can—tabulate the ATP and CO_2 generated; name the type of reaction at each step; and write the structure of any compound which has been blanked out. You should not memorize these structures but derive them from knowledge of reaction principles.

Definition: The citric acid cycle is the first stage of a two tier process called cellular respiration. It is also known as the tricarboxylic acid cycle (TCA) and, more commonly, as the Krebs cycle. Cellular respiration is the process by which glucose is transformed into ATP (adenosine triphosphate) or a useful form of chemical energy.

Citric Acid Cycle Reaction Steps (Fig. 16.10)

- **Reaction 1 (Synthesis of citric acid):** Acetyl CoA and oxaloacetic acid condense to form citric acid. The acetyl group CH_3COO is transferred from CoA to oxaloacetic acid at the ketone carbon, which is then changed to an alcohol. The net effect is to join a 2 carbon piece with a 4 carbon piece to make citric acid which is 6 carbons. This is just called the synthesis of citric acid.

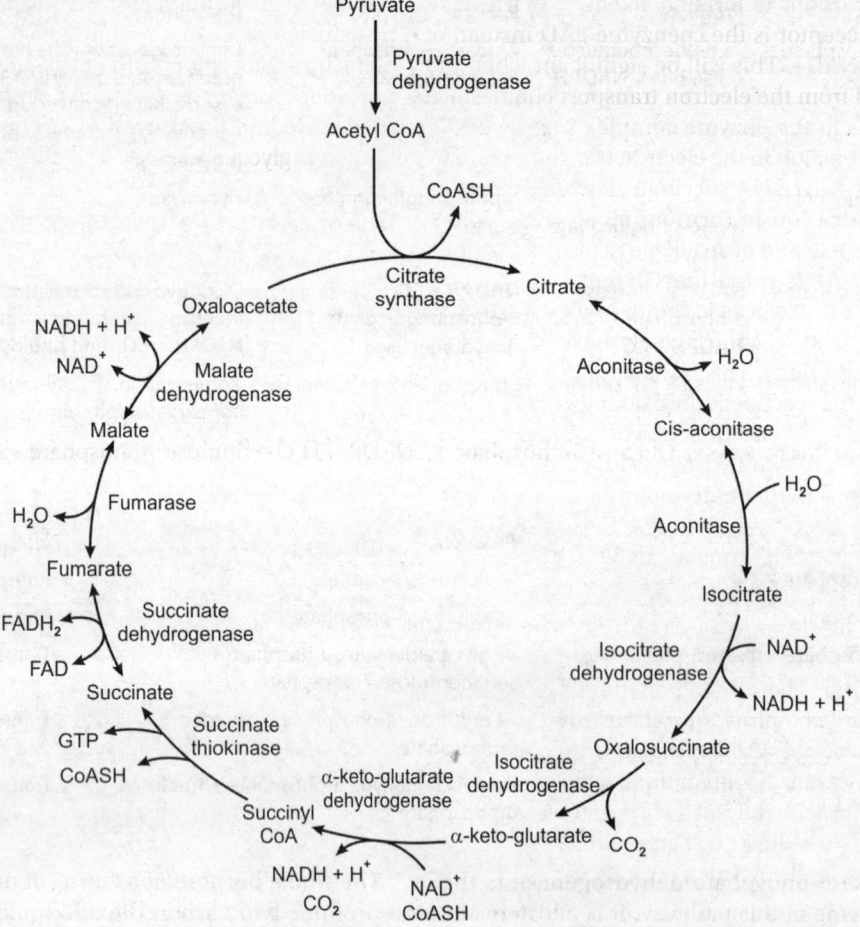

Fig. 16.10: Citric acid cycle reaction steps.

- **Reaction 2 (Dehydration of an alcohol):** Two steps (Rx. 2 and 3) are required to isomerize the position of the -OH group on citric acid. This first step is a dehydration of an alcohol to make an alkene. The cis-aconitic acid remains bound to the enzyme aconitase in readiness for the next step.
- **Reaction 3 (Hydration to make alcohol):** This reaction is a hydration reaction of an alkene to make an alcohol. This hydration does not follow Markovnikov's Rule. The net effect of reactions 2 and 3 has been to move the -OH group from C-3 to C-2, which is isocitric acid.
- **Reaction 4 (Oxidation):** This is the first oxidation reaction in which an alcohol is converted to a ketone. Two hydrogens and 2 electrons are transferred to NAD⁺ to NADH + H⁺. This is the entry point into the electron transport chain. The product of this reaction, oxalosuccinic acid, remains attached to the isocitrate dehydrogenase for the next step.
- **Reaction 5 (Decarboxylation):** This is the first step where a carbon group is lost as carbon dioxide in a decarboxylation reaction. The remaining compound now has 5 carbons and is called alpha-ketoglutaric acid. This reaction is also catalyzed by isocitrate dehydrogenase.
- **Reaction 6 (Oxidation, decarboxylation, thiol ester synthesis):** This complex oxidative decarboxylation is guided by three enzymes in much the same fashion as the formation of acetyl CoA from pyruvic acid. This is actually the only non-reversible step in the entire cycle and

prevents the cycle from operating in the reverse direction. This is the second oxidation reaction in which an alcohol is converted to a ketone. Two hydrogens and 2 electrons are transferred to NAD⁺ to NADH + H⁺. This another entry point into the electron transport chain.

This is the second step where a carbon group is lost as carbon dioxide in a decarboxylation reaction. Essentially, although not the exact same carbons, the two carbons from the acetyl CoA have been converted to carbon dioxide at the end this step. The remaining 4 carbon group is attached to the CoA through a thiol ester high energy bond. Notice that the final product, succinyl CoA, has 4 carbons in the succinate group at one end of the CoA molecule.

This reaction is catalyzed by alpha-ketoglutarate dehydrogenase complex.
- **Reaction 7 (Hydrolysis of Succinyl CoA):** Synthesis of ATP

The hydrolysis of the thioester bond (exothermic) is coupled with the formation of ATP (Actually guanosine triphosphate is formed first but is further coupled with the ADP to make ATP). This is the only "visible" ATP formed in the entire cycle. Succinic acid, a 4 carbon acid, is the product of this reaction. This is the start of the return to the beginning of the cycle.

This reaction is catalyzed by succinyl CoA.
- **Reaction 8 (Oxidation):** This slightly unusual oxidation reaction results in the removal of the hydrogens from

saturated alkyl carbons to form an alkene, fumaric acid. The hydrogen acceptor is the coenzyme FAD instead of the more usual NAD+. This will be significant when the ATP is tabulated from the electron transport chain, since this coenzyme is in the enzyme complex 2. Only 2 ATP result from this reaction in the electron transport chain. This reaction is catalyzed by succinate dehydrogenase.

- **Reaction 9 (Hydration to form an alcohol):** This is a simple hydration reaction of an alkene to form an alcohol. Take your pick where you place the -OH group since it must be adjacent to a carboxylic acid group in either case and forms malic acid. This reaction is catalyzed by fumarase.
- **Reaction 10 (Oxidation):** This is the final reaction in the citric acid cycle. The reaction is the oxidation of an alcohol to a ketone to make oxaloacetic acid. The coenzyme NAD⁺ causes the transfer of two hydrogens and 2 electrons to NADH + H⁺. This is a final entry point into the electron transport chain.

This reaction is catalyzed by malate dehydrogenase.

Function: The citric acid cycle takes certain compounds that donate protons and electrons to the electron transport chain, according to "Citric Acid (Krebs) Cycle" at ccbcmd.edu. The electron transport chain then generates ATP through the process of oxidative phosphorylation. Furthermore, Krebs cycle also produces 2 ATP through the process of substrate phosphorylation. Through the supply of precursor metabolites, the citric acid cycle also plays an important role in the flow of carbon through the cell. In general, it is made up of eight distinct steps (each of which is catalyzed by a unique enzyme).

Features: The citric acid cycle begins when coenzyme A transfers its 2-carbon acetyl group to the 4-carbon compound oxaloacetate. This step results in a 6-carbon molecule citrate. In step 2, the citrate is rearranged to form isocitrate (an isometric form of the molecule), according to ccbcmd.edu. In step 3, the isocitrate is oxidized and a carbon dioxide molecule is removed. The removal produces a 5-carbon molecule called alpha-ketoglutarate. In step 4, alpha-ketoglutarate is oxidized, the carbon dioxide molecules are removed and coenzyme A is added to form succinyl-CoA (a 4-carbon compound). In step 5 of the citric acid cycle, CoA is removed from succinyl-CoA to produce succinate. Energy is released and is used to make GTP (guanosine triphosphate) and, in turn, to make ATP. In step 6, succinate is oxidized to create fumarate and, in step 7, water is added to fumarate to form malate. In step 8, malate is oxidized to produce oxaloacetate (the beginning compound of the citric acid cycle).

GLYCOGENOLYSIS

Glycogenolysis is the process of converting the food storage carbohydrate polymer glycogen into glucose for the body to use as energy. Glycogen is a polysaccharide—a long sugar chain—of glucose molecules with side branches. It is a way for animal cells to store excess carbohydrates until needed. Glycogen is found in the liver and in muscle tissue.

The process of glycogenolysis can be triggered by low blood sugars, through the action of the hormone glucogon, which is released by the pancreas and travels to the liver. It can also be actuated as a stress response by the action of the adrenal gland hormone epinephrine, also known as adrenaline. Both hormones trigger the catabolism of glycogen, its breakdown to glucose and the release of energy. This process is also known as glycogenolysis.

Glycogenolysis Pathway (Fig. 16.11)

Glycogenolysis begins with the removal of individual glucose molecules from the glycogen chain. A molecule of inorganic phosphate is then added to the glucose molecule to make glucose-1-phosphate. This reaction is carried out by the enzyme glycogen phosphorylase. It is the key regulatory step of the process. If it adds a phosphate group, the reaction proceeds. If it removes one, the process stops.

Function: Glycogenolysis transpires in the muscle and liver tissue, where glycogen is stored, as a hormonal response to epinephrine (e.g., adrenergic stimulation) and/or glucagon, a pancreatic peptide triggered by low blood glucose concentrations.

Liver (hepatic) cells can consume the glucose-6-phosphate in glycolysis, or remove the phosphate group using the enzyme glucose 6-phasphatase and release the free glucose into the bloodstream for uptake by other cells.

Muscle cells will not release glucose, but instead use the glucose-6-phosphate in glycolysis.

Reaction of Glycogenolysis

- **First step:** The overall reaction for the 1st step is: Glycogen (n-residues) + Pi ⟷ Glycogen (n-1 residues) + G1P. Here, glycogen phosphorylase cleaves the bond at the 1 position by substitution of a phosphoryl group. It breaks down glucose polymer at α-1-4 linkages until 4 linked glucoses are left on the branch. [Furthermore, glycogen phosphorylase (EC 2.4.1.1) can be used as a marker enzyme to determine glycogen breakdown].

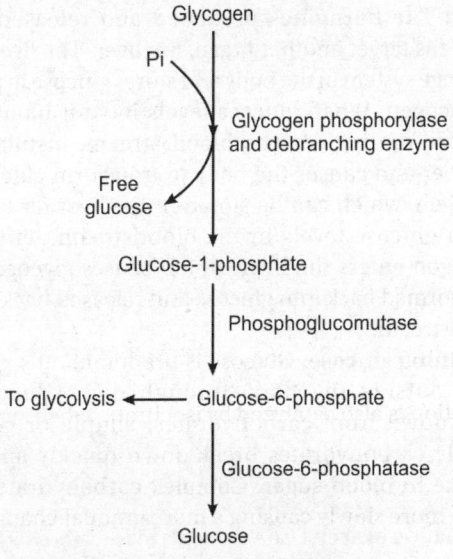

Fig. 16.11: Glycogenolysis pathway.

- **Second step:** The second step involves the enzyme glucan transferase]/debranching enzyme, which transfers the three remaining glucose units to another 1, 4 terminal of glycogen, which exposes the branching point. Another enzyme, α-1,6 glucosidase, then removes the final glucose residue of the branch, thereby destroying the branch. It is removed by hydrolysis and produces a glucose molecule. This is the only case in which a glycogen metabolite is not glucose-1-phosphate.
- **Third step:** The third and last stage converts G1P (glucose-1-phosphate) to G6P (glucose-6-phosphate) through the enzyme phosphoglucomutase.

REGULATION OF BLOOD SUGAR LEVEL

The normal blood sugar level is 80–100 mg/dL (RBS), in fasting it is 70–90 mg/dL, in postprandial 80–110 mg/dL. The regulation of glucose is an important system inside the human body. Glucose is the primary fuel for the brain and a secondary fuel for muscle function and red blood cell production. Thus insuring that enough glucose is available is imperative. However, an excess of glucose brings about its own problems. The best known disease caused by a glucose imbalance is diabetes.

- **Regulation of blood sugar:** For the body to survive, it must constantly receive energy in the form of adenosine triphosphate (ATP). To create ATP, the body needs adequate levels of a substance called glucose. Since the amount of energy you need varies depending on the activity being performed, the amount of glucose needed throughout the day must also vary.
- **Pancreas:** Blood glucose regulation starts with the pancreas. The pancreas is an integral part of this process because of its ability to produce two different types of hormones called insulin and glucagon. When glucose levels get too high, the body activates the pancreas to produce more insulin. When glucose levels are too low, the body activates the pancreas to produce more glucagon.
- **Liver:** The hormones produced and released by the pancreas target another organ, are liver. The liver acts as a storage system in the body and stores glucose in the form of glycogen. When glucose levels in your bloodstream become too high in the blood stream, insulin enters the liver and causes the body to transform glucose into glycogen, which can be stored in the liver for later use. When glucose levels in the bloodstream get too low, glucagon enters the liver, which causes glycogen to be transformed back into glucose and released back into the bloodstream.
- **Obtaining glucose:** Glucose is predominantly garnered from outside the body through diet. Glucose is a breakdown from carbohydrates, simple or complex. Simple carbohydrates break down quickly and cause a spike in blood sugar. Complex carbohydrates break down more slowly causing a more gradual change to the body's blood sugar. Once the glucose is brought into the body, it takes one of three pathways toward use. The most direct route is from the small intestine to the bloodstream where it is immediately converted into ATP (adenosine tri-phosphate). This goes directly to the brain. The secondary route is through the musculoskeletal system where the glucose is stored inside the muscles. Once this route is taken, the glucose cannot return back into the bloodstream and is used to power the muscle itself. The third route is to reusable storage in the liver. The liver holds onto glucose in the form of glycogen to release later, as well as playing a vital role in regulating the amount of glucose available in the blood, in conjunction with the pancreas.
- **Glucose and the liver:** The liver is the primary storehouse for glucose in the body in the form of glycogen. It is capable of holding 10% of its total volume this way. While it is the liver that stores the glycogen, it is the pancreas that regulates when it releases the stores out into the body.
- **Glucose and the pancreas:** The pancreas is an organ primarily responsible for sending out regulatory hormones. The regulatory hormones involved in the regulation of glucose are insulin and glucagon. Insulin is released when glucose levels in the blood rise too high. It tells the liver to take up glucose from the blood and store it for later. Glucagon, the opposite of insulin, is produced when glucose levels in the blood fall too low and causes the liver to let go of its stores in order to keep everything running smoothly. Diabetes is caused by a problem with the body's reaction to insulin.
- **Glucose and the brain:** The brain uses 75% of the stores of glucose in the body. According to the Franklin Institute (2009), "brain cells need two times more energy than the other cells in the body." This is because unlike most cells, brain cells are constantly in a state of metabolic activity. Even when a person is sleeping, brain cells are busy fixing things upstairs to keep the body running smoothly. This high demand is the reason that the glucose regulation in the body is so important.
- **Glucose and diabetes:** Diabetes is the best known disease of abnormal glucose regulation. In its primary form, the pancreas does not produce enough insulin to keep the regulatory system running correctly, so insulin has to be introduced from the outside as well as careful control of the patient's diet. The secondary form is insulin resistant; the body does not use the available insulin well and, once again, careful control of the diet is imperative.
- **Hyperglycemia** is the condition of having too much glucose in the blood. Hypoglycemia means there is too little. While both of these can occur without the presence of diabetes, they are strongly linked with diabetes due to the problems with insulin.

Figure 16.12 is depicted the hormonal regulation of blood glucose and **Figure 16.13** is depicted the glucose regulation in the pancreas.

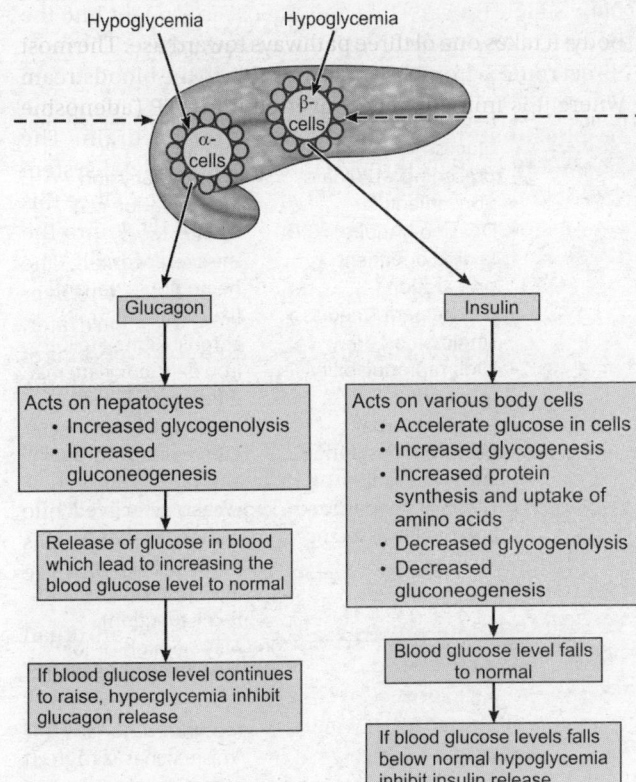

Fig. 16.12: Hormonal regulation of blood glucose.

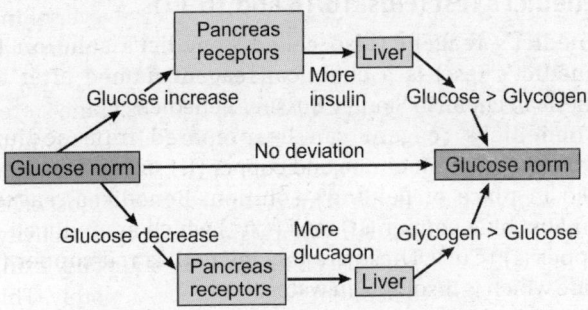

Fig. 16.13: Glucose regulation in the pancreas.

Blood Glucose Monitoring (Fig. 16.14)

A blood glucose meter is an electronic device for measuring the blood glucose level. A relatively small drop of blood is placed on a disposable test strip which interfaces with a digital meter. Within several seconds, the level of blood glucose will be shown on the digital display.

Needing only a small drop of blood for the meter means that the time and effort required for testing is reduced and the compliance of diabetic people to their testing regimens is improved. Although the cost of using blood glucose meters seems high, it is believed to be a cost benefit relative to the avoided medical costs of the complications of diabetes.

Blood glucose monitoring is a way of testing the concentration of glucose in the blood (glycemia). Particularly important in the care of diabetes mellitus, a blood glucose

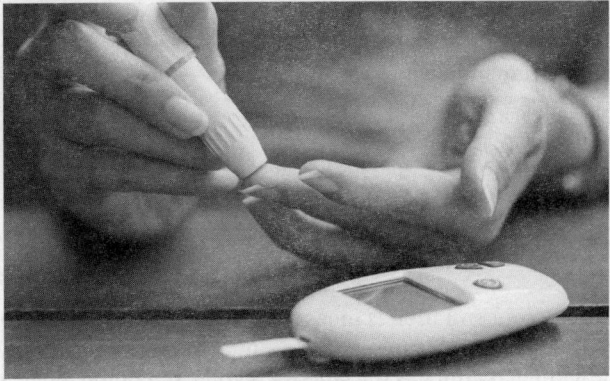

Fig. 16.14: Blood glucose monitoring.

test is performed by piercing the skin (typically, on the finger) to draw blood, then applying the blood to a chemically active disposable 'test-strip'. Different manufacturers use different technology, but most systems measure an electrical characteristic, and use this to determine the glucose level in the blood. The test is usually referred to as capillary blood glucose and sometimes incorrectly called BM Stix (after one of the companies that makes the test kit).

Recent Advances Include

- 'Alternate site testing', the use of blood drops from places other than the finger, usually the palm or forearm. This alternate site testing uses the same test strips and meter, is practically pain free, and gives the real estate on the finger tips a needed break if they become sore. The disadvantage of this technique is that there is usually less blood flow to alternate sites, which prevents the reading from being accurate when the blood sugar level is changing.
- **'No coding' systems:** Older systems required 'coding' of the strips to the meter. This carried a risk of 'miscoding', which can lead to inaccurate results. Two approaches have resulted in systems that no longer require coding. Some systems are 'autocoded', where technology is used to code each strip to the meter. And some are manufactured to a 'single code', thereby avoiding the risk of miscoding.
- **'Multi-test' systems:** Some systems use a cartridge or a disc containing multiple test strips. This has the advantage that the user does not have to load individual strips each time, which is convenient and can enable quicker testing.
- **'Downloadable' meters:** Most new systems come with software that allows the user to download meter results to a computer. This information can then be used, together with healthcare professional guidance, to enhance and improve diabetes management. The meters usually require a connection cable, unless they are designed to work wirelessly with an insulin pump, or are designed to plug directly into the computer.

Glucose Tolerance Test (GTT)

After a night without food, the patient drinks a test dose of 100 g of glucose dissolved in a glass of water. The blood

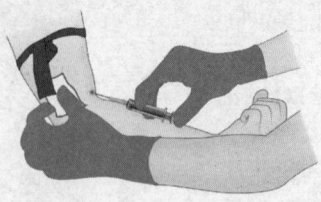

Glucose tolerance test Normal persons	
Fasting	60–100 mg/dL
After 1 hour	200 mg/dL
After 2 hours	140 mg/dL

Fig. 16.15: Glucose tolerance test and their normal values.

glucose concentration is measured before the test dose and at 30 min intervals for several hours thereafter. A normal individual assimilates the glucose readily, the blood glucose rising to no more than about 80 to 120 mg/100 mL; little or no glucose appears in the urine. Diabetic individuals assimilate the test dose of glucose poorly; their blood glucose level far exceeds the kidney threshold (about 180 mg/100 mL), causing glucose to appear in their urine (**Fig. 16.15**).

Barfoed's Test

A biochemical test to detect monosaccharide (reducing) sugars in solution, devised by the Swedish physician CT Barfoed (1815–99).

$$R\text{—}CHO + 2Cu^{2+} + 2H_2O \longrightarrow R\text{—}COOH + Cu_2O + 4H$$

Reducing saccharide → Carboxylic (red) acid

Barfoed's reagent, a mixture of ethanoic (acetic) acid and copper (II) acetate, is added to the test solution and boiled. If any reducing sugars are present a red precipitate of copper (II) oxide is formed. The reaction will be negative in the presence of disaccharide sugars as they are weaker reducing agents.

Test	Advantages	Disadvantages
FPG	• Can be performed as a single blood draw • Most commonly used test • Majority of the global diabetes prevalence epidemiology studies were based on the FPG criteria	• Requires overnight fast (at least 8–12 h) • Less sensitive than the OGTT
Oral glucose tolerance test (OGTT)	• Includes assessment of both FPG and the 2-h PG after the oral glucose load • Allows assessment of the glucose response after an oral glucose challenge • Identifies more individuals with dysglycemia than the FPG or HbA1c	• Requires overnight fast • Administration of glucose causes nausea and vomiting in a subset of the population (~2–5%) • 2-h test duration • Sensitive to day-to-day variations due to diet or exercise • The values vary according to the time of day of testing • Reproducibility is not as good as the FPG or HbA1c

Contd...

Contd...

Test	Advantages	Disadvantages
HbA1c	• Reflects integrated glucose levels over preceding ~180 days • Convenient • Does not require fasting or patient preparation • Can be performed as a single blood draw • High reproducibility (precision) • Less day-to-day perturbations during stress and illness • Globally standardized and quality assurance in place	• Less sensitive than the FPG and 2-h PG • The accuracy and interpretation can be affected by the presence of hemoglobin variants (i.e., sickle cell trait), chronic kidney failure, iron deficiency anemia, differences in red blood cell lifespan, and differences with age and race • Weakly associated with the diabetes pathophysiology (e.g., insulin sensitivity, and B-cell function) • May be high or low relative to underlying average glucose levels (accuracy –HbA1c "mismatches" as a reflection of average glucose levels)

Benedict's Test (Figs. 16.16 and 16.17)

Benedict's reagent (also called Benedict's solution or Benedict's test) is a chemical reagent named after an American chemist, Stanley Rossiter Benedict.

Benedict's reagent can be prepared from sodium carbonate, sodium citrate and copper (II) sulfate. It is often used in place of Fehling's solution. Benedict's reagent contains blue copper (II) ions (Cu^{2+}) which are reduced to copper (I) (Cu^+). These are precipitated as red copper (I) oxide which is insoluble in water.

Benedict's reagent is used as a test for the presence of all monosaccharides, and generally also reducing sugars. These include glucose, galactose, mannose, lactose and maltose. Even more generally, Benedict's test will detect the presence of aldehydes (except aromatic ones), and alpha-hydroxy-ketones, including those that occur in certain ketoses.

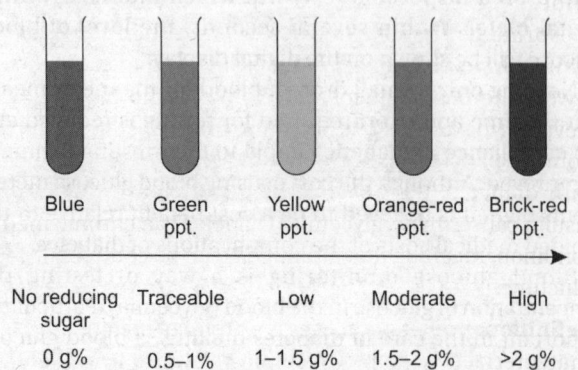

Fig. 16.16: Benedict's test results (for levels of reducing sugar).

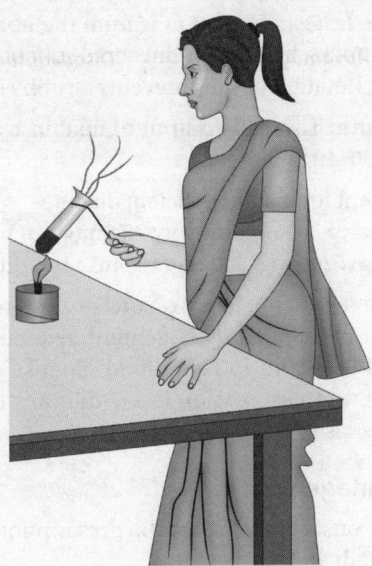

Fig. 16.17: Benedict's test.

Thus, although the ketose fructose is not strictly a reducing sugar, it is an alpha-hydroxy-ketone, and gives a positive test because it is converted to the aldoses glucose and mannose by the base in the reagent.

$$R\text{—}CHO + 2CU^{2+} + 5\, OH \longrightarrow R\text{—}CO + 2CUO + 3H_2O$$

Reducing carbohydrate — Carbohydrate (red ppt) Ion

Benedict's test is used to identify reducing sugars, such as monosaccharides. When a reducing sugar is heated with the Benedict's reagent the blue solution turns to a brick red color. The biuret test is used to identify proteins. If there is protein present a pale purple layer is formed, if not it remains light blue.

Diabetes Mellitus

Diabetes mellitus is a group of metabolic diseases characterized by high blood sugar (glucose) levels that result from defects in insulin secretion, or action, or both. Diabetes mellitus, commonly referred to as diabetes (as it will be in this article) was first identified as a disease associated with "sweet urine," and excessive muscle loss in the ancient world. Elevated levels of blood glucose (hyperglycemia) lead to spillage of glucose into the urine, hence the term sweet urine.

Normally, blood glucose levels are tightly controlled by insulin, a hormone produced by the pancreas. Insulin lowers the blood glucose level. When the blood glucose elevates (for example, after eating food), insulin is released from the pancreas to normalize the glucose level. In patients with diabetes, the absence or insufficient production of insulin causes hyperglycemia. Diabetes is a chronic medical condition, meaning that although it can be controlled, it lasts a lifetime.

Definition: Diabetes mellitus is a group of metabolic disease characterized by hyperglycemia resulting from defect in insulin secretion, insulin action or both

Diabetic mellitus result in long time damage dysfunction and failure of various organs especially the heart, kidney and eyes.

Classification of Diabetes Mellitus

1. Type 1 or insulin dependent
2. Type 2 or non-insulin dependent
3. Juvenile diabetes mellitus
4. Pregnancy-induced diabetes mellitus

- **Type 1 or insulin dependent (IDDM):** It is characterized by autoimmune beta cell, destruction, which is attributing to a genetic predisposition coupled with one or more viral agents and possible chemical agents. It depends on exogenous insulin to sustain life. Onset generally before age of 30 years but may occur at any age, Persons body built is generally leaning rarely obese.
- **Type 2 (non-insulin dependent) (NIDDM):** Majority of (90%) people with diabetes mellitus are type 2, has strong genetic influences but has no connection with HLAC (human leukocyte antigen).

The absolute requirement of exogenous insulin is episodic no requirement for exogenous insulin to sustain life. Onset usually after 40 years of age but may occur at any age

Etiology

- Insufficiency of insulin
- A failure in production of insulin
- The use of insulin by the cells may be prohibited by some antagonistic factors, such as the growth hormone from anterior pituitary gland or adrenocortico-glucocorticoids
- The need for insulin may be greater than the available supply.
- Destruction of insulin by liver or other tissues
- In children diabetes mellitus develops because of primary derangement in the insulin producing cells.
- Hereditary predisposition.
- Congenital rubella and cytomegalovirus.
- Endocrinopathies, e.g., acromegaly, Cushing's syndrome.
- Impaired glucose tolerance.
- Drug induced, i.e., IV pentamidine.

Clinical features: Type one requires insulin therapy and careful, lifelong control of the balance between glucose intake and insulin dose. The decreased or defective production of insulin is characterized by the following symptoms:

1. **Decreased permeability of the cell membrane** for glucose resulting in the accumulation of glucose in the blood. This condition is known as hyperglycemia. Glucose concentration increases as high as 500 mg/100 mL of blood.
2. **Polyuria:**
   - This means excretion of increased quantity of urine.
   - This is to excrete the additional quantity of glucose in urine (glucosuria).
3. **Polydipsia:**
   - The excessive thirst which leads to increased consumption of water. This condition is known as polydipsia.

- This is to replace the volume of water excreted due to polyuria.
4. **Polyphagia:** Excessive appetite leads to polyphagia and increased intake of food. This is to replace the lost nourishment. The diabetic has voracious appetite, but in spite of over eating; they lose weight and become lean and emaciated.
5. As glucose is not enough for energy production, increased mobilization of fat from adipose tissue occurs. But the metabolism of fat is incomplete resulting in the production of large amounts of the intermediary products of fat metabolism, namely—ketone bodies (e.g., acetoacetate and β-hydroxybutyrate). This condition is known as 'ketosis' and excess ketone bodies cause severe acidosis, ultimately resulting in 'coma'.
6. Deposition of lipids in the walls of the blood vessels resulting atherosclerosis".

Diagnostic Evaluation
- Complete history and physical examination
- Blood tests including fasting blood sugar (FBS) post postprandial blood sugar (PPBS) glycosylated, hemoglobin, cholesterol
- Triglyceride levels, blood urea nitrogen and serum creatinine
- Urine for complete urine analysis, microalbuminuria, culture and sensitivity glucose and acetone
- Fundoscopic examination
- Neurological examination
- Blood pressure monitoring
- Monitoring of weight
- Doppler scan

Medial Management
- Dietary management
- Oral hypoglycemic drugs
- Insulin
- Exercise

Dietary Management
- **Low energy weight reducing diet:** Dietary prescription which causes a daily deficit of 500 kcal provides realistic diet and reduces weekly weight loss of 0.5 kg.
- Weight maintenance diet
- The diet should be high in carbohydrates and low in fat.

Types of insulin: There are 3 types of insulin—
1. **Short-acting insulin:** It is regular insulin. It is rapid acting and it is a zinc suspension.
2. **Intermediate-acting insulin:** It is semilente suspension and composed of neutral protamine hagedorn.
3. **Long-acting insulin:** It is extended insulin of zinc suspension and having a long action, composed of ultralente protamine insulin.

Rotation of site: The speed with which peak serum concentration are reached various with anatomic sites for injection. The fastest absorption is from the abdomen arm, thigh, and buttocks. Insulin administered subcutaneously for better action. Rotation of sites prevents atrophy of muscles.

Dose of insulin: The daily output of insulin by pancreatic islets cells is 30–40 units.

Initial treatment for insulin deficient diabetes
- **Blood sugar:** >300 mg/100 mL: 20 units
- **Blood sugar:** 200 mg–300 mg/100 mL: 10 units

Exercise: Regular consistent exercise is considered an essential part of diabetic management. Exercise improves insulin sensitivity and lowers blood glucose during and after exercise. Exercise session is 5–7 minutes of warm up, stretching exercise.

Nursing Management
- The nurse must clarify the insulin prescription in terms of type, strength and species.
- Observe for the symptoms of hyperglycemia
- Reduce overall blood glucose and minimize fluctuation
- Achieve weight reduction in obese patients to reduce insulin resistance
- Avoid weight gain associated with therapeutic agents
- Avoid atherogenic diets which may aggravate diabetic complication
- Advice the patient not to skip meals. The body requires food at regularly spaced intervals throughout the day
- Educate the patient about benefits of exercise

Acute complications: Hypoglycemia, diabetic ketoacidosis, hyperglycemic coma

Chronic Complications
- **Microvascular:** Diabetic retinopathy, nephropathy, neuropathy, radiculopathy
- **Macrovascular:** Dyslipidemia, hypertension, coronary artery disease

Hypoglycemia: Definition and Causes
Hypoglycemia is a condition in which your blood sugar (glucose) level is lower than normal. Glucose is your body's main energy source. Hypoglycemia is often related to diabetes treatment. But other drugs and a variety of conditions—many rare—can cause low blood sugar in people who do not have diabetes. Hypoglycemia needs immediate treatment when blood sugar levels are low. For many people, a fasting blood sugar of 70 milligrams per deciliter (mg/dL), or 3.9 millimoles per liter (mmol/L), or below should serve as an alert for hypoglycemia. But your numbers might be different.

Figure 16.18 is depicted the signs and symptoms of hypoglycemia.

Causes of Hypoglycemia
- **Too few carbohydrates:** As carbohydrates are your body's main source of glucose, not having enough of them can cause a drop in blood sugar.

Dizziness
This may be the case after experiencing continual disorientation and a light-headed feeling.

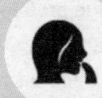

Unceasing hunger
Comparable to being unsatisfied after you have eaten a full and balanced meal over and over.

Irritability
Certain symptoms, such as hypoglycemia may cause confusion and anxiety that make you feel testy.

Clammy skin
Moderate hypoglycemia often makes people feel clammy with sweaty, cold hands and feet.

Mood swings
Fluctuations in blood glucose can result in rapid mood changes, including depression.

Fig. 16.18: Signs and symptoms of hypoglycemia.

- **Skipping meals:** Just like consuming too few carbohydrates, skipping meals can prevent your body from receiving the energy it needs from glucose.
- **Strenuous physical activity:** Exercising more than usual, especially if you have not eaten enough carbohydrates at a meal, can cause a hypoglycemic episode.
- **Excessive drinking:** Alcohol can interfere with your body's ability to metabolize glucose.
- **Not eating soon enough after insulin treatment:** If you take insulin as prescribed during mealtimes, but delay eating, this can cause hypoglycemia.
- **Too much insulin:** If you take too much insulin, this can cause your blood sugar to crash.

Signs and Symptoms

Each person's reaction to low blood sugar is different. From milder, more common indicators to most severe, signs and symptoms of low blood sugar include:
- Feeling shaky
- Being nervous or anxious
- Sweating, chills and clamminess
- Irritability or impatience
- Confusion
- Fast heartbeat
- Feeling lightheaded or dizzy
- Hunger
- Nausea
- Color draining from the skin (pallor)
- Feeling sleepy
- Feeling weak or having no energy
- Blurred/impaired vision
- Tingling or numbness in the lips, tongue or cheeks
- Headaches
- Coordination problems, clumsiness
- Nightmares or crying out during sleep
- Seizures

Treatments for Hypoglycemia

- **Adjusting your medications:** You may need to change how often you take insulin or other medications, which medications you are on, how much you take, and when you take them.
- **Working with a registered dietitian on a personalized meal plan that stabilizes blood sugar levels:** There is no one-size-fits-all hypoglycemia diet, but a nutritionist can help you figure out a consistent meal plan tailored to you, and teach you how to count carbohydrate grams to go along with your health and routine.
- **Increasing and improving self-monitoring of your blood glucose levels:** Knowing your blood glucose level throughout the day—when you get up, before meals, and after meals, etc.—can help you keep it from getting too low.
- **Limiting consumption of alcoholic beverages:** Alcohol interferes with the way your body metabolizes glucose. If you are prone to hypoglycemia, consider decreasing how much alcohol you consume.
- **Glucose tablets (dextrose):** Make sure you always have glucose tablets on hand, whether at home, school, the office, or the gym. After taking the tablet, check your blood sugar. If it is still low, take another tablet. If that does not help, check with your doctor.

Glycogen Storages Diseases

In 1929, von Gierke provided the initial description of glycogen-storage disease type I (GSD I) from autopsy reports of 2 children whose large livers contained excessive glycogen. He also reported similar findings in the kidneys. Both children had frequent nosebleeds before their deaths, consistent with histories documented in current patients.

In 1952, Cori and Cori reported 6 similar patients. Two of the patients had almost total deficiency of hepatic glucose-6-phosphatase, whereas the remaining 4 had normal enzyme activity. These authors recognized that defects in the enzymology of hepatic glycogen-storage disease may cause a heterogeneous group of disorders. However, the mystery of patients with these clinical symptoms (despite normal phosphatase activity) remained unsolved until 1978, when Narisawa et al identified a defect in intracellular transport of the enzyme substrate.

Table 16.1 is depicted the types of glycogen storage diseases.

Section 2: Applied Biochemistry

Table 16.1: Types of glycogen storage diseases.

Type/doctor	Enzyme/Gene	Organs	Frequency	Potential signs	Treatment
Oa	Glycogen synthase/GYS2	Liver	Unknown	Hypoglycemia, potential increase in ketones, morning fatigue, convulsions, variable signs and symptoms	Symptomatic, e.g., frequent meals and uncooked starch to avoid episodes of hypoglycemia, a high protein diet
Ob	Glycogen synthase/GYS1	Muscle	Unknown	Exercise intolerance, cardiomyopathy, fainting, muscle biopsy lacks glycogen	Symptomatic, e.g., frequent meals and uncooked starch to avoid episodes of hypoglycemia, a high protein diet
Ia/von Gierke	Glucose-6-phosphatase/G6PC	Liver, kidney, small intestine	1/125,000	Hypoglycemia, lactic acidosis, hyperuricemia, hyperlipidemia, hepatomegaly, osteoporosis	Symptomatic, e.g., physically modified corn starch, allopurinol, statins
Ib	Glucose-6-phosphate transporter/SLC37A4	Liver, kidney, small intestine	1/500,000	Same as type Ia but with neutropenia, inflammatory bowel disease, dental diseases	Symptomatic, e.g., physically modified corn starch, allopurinol, statins
II/Pompe	Lysosome acid alpha-glucosidase/GAA	Skeletal and cardiac muscle	1/40,000	Myopathy, hypotonia, hepatomegaly, heart defects	Enzyme replacement therapy
III/Cori or Forbes	Glycogen debranching enzyme/AGL	Liver, skeletal and cardiac muscle	1/100,000	Hypoglycemia hepatomegaly, myopathy, cirrhosis	Symptomatic, e.g., physically modified corn starch, allopurinol, statins
IV/Anderson	Glycogen branching enzyme/GBE1	Heart, liver	1/600,000	Hepatomegaly, liver dysfunction, cirrhosis, myopathy	Symptomatic, e.g., liver transplantation

Types of Glycogen Storage Diseases

Sl. No.	Types	Description
1.	**Von gierke's diseases** (Glycogen storage disease type I)	Glycogen storage disease (GSD) type I is also known as von Gierke disease or hepatorenal glycogenosis. Von Gierke described the first patient with GSD type I in 1929 under the name hepatonephromegalia glycogenica. In 1952, Cori and Cori demonstrated that glucose-6-phosphatase (G6Pase) deficiency was a cause of GSD type I. In 1978, Narisawa et al. proposed that a transport defect of glucose-6-phosphate (G6P) into the microsomal compartment may be present in some patients with GSD type I. Thus, GSD type I is divided into GSD type Ia caused by G6Pase deficiency and GSD type Ib resulting from deficiency of a specific translocase T1. Apart from the substrate translocation defect, patients with GSD type I have altered neutrophil functions predisposing them to Gram-positive bacterial infections. Later, other translocases were discovered, adding 2 more subtypes of GSD to the disease spectrum. GSD type Ic is deficiency of translocase T2 that carries inorganic phosphates from microsomes into the cytosol and pyrophosphates from the cytosol into microsomes. GSD type Id is deficiency in a transporter that translocates free glucose molecules from microsomes into the cytosol.
2.	**Pompe disease** (Glycogen storage disease type II)	GSD type II, also known as acid maltase deficiency or Pompe disease, is a prototypic lysosomal disease. Its clinical presentation clearly differs from other forms of GSD. Deficiency of a lysosomal enzyme, alpha-1,4-glucosidase, causes GSD type II. Pompe initially described the disease in 1932. An essential pathologic finding is the accumulation of normally structured glycogen in most tissues. Three forms of the disease exist—infantile, juvenile, and adult. In the classic infantile form, the main clinical signs are cardiomyopathy and muscular hypotonia. In the juvenile and adult forms, the involvement of skeletal muscles dominates the clinical presentation. The images below illustrate histologic findings of GSD type II.
3.	**Forbes diseases** (Glycogen storage disease type III)	GSD type III is also known as Forbes-Cori disease or limit dextrinosis. In contrast to GSD type I, liver and skeletal muscles are involved in GSD type III. Glycogen deposited in these organs has an abnormal structure. Differentiating patients with GSD type III from those with GSD type I solely on the basis of physical findings is not easy.

Contd...

Contd...

Sl. No.	Types	Description
4.	**Anderson's disease** (Glycogen storage disease type IV)	GSD type IV, also known as amylopectinosis or Andersen disease, is a rare disease that leads to early death. In 1956, Andersen reported the first patient with progressive hepatosplenomegaly and accumulation of abnormal polysaccharides. The main clinical features are liver insufficiency and abnormalities of the heart and nervous system.
5.	**McArdle disease** (Glycogen storage disease type V)	GSD type V, also known as McArdle disease, affects the skeletal muscles. McArdle reported the first patient in 1951. Initial signs of the disease usually develop in adolescents or adults. Muscle phosphorylase deficiency adversely affecting the glycolytic pathway in skeletal musculature causes GSD type V. Like other forms of GSD, McArdle disease is heterogeneous.
6.	**Hers disease** (Glycogen storage disease type VI)	GSD type VI, also known as Hers disease, belongs to the group of hepatic glycogenoses and represents a heterogenous disease. Hepatic phosphorylase deficiency or deficiencies of other enzymes that form a cascade necessary for liver phosphorylase activation cause the disease. In 1959, Hers described the first patients with proven phosphorylase deficiency.
7.	**Tarui's disease** (Glycogen storage disease type VII)	SD type VII, also known as Tarui disease, arises as a result of phosphofructokinase (PFK) deficiency. The enzyme is located in skeletal muscles and erythrocytes. Tarui reported the first patients in 1965. The clinical and laboratory features are similar to those of GSD type V.

Galactosemia

Galactosemia is a disorder that affects how the body processes a simple sugar called galactose. A small amount of galactose is present in many foods. It is primarily part of a larger sugar called lactose, which is found in all dairy products and many baby formulas.

Causes

Galactosemia is an inherited enzyme disorder (transmitted as an autosomal recessive trait). It occurs in approximately 1 out of every 60,000 births among Caucasians, while the rate is different for other groups. There are 3 forms of the disease—galactose-1 phosphate uridyl transferase deficiency (classic galactosemia, the most common and most severe form), deficiency of galactose kinase, and deficiency of galactose-6-phosphate epimerase.

People with galactosemia are unable to fully break down the simple sugar galactose. Galactose makes up half of lactose, the sugar found in milk. Lactose is called a disaccharide (meaning 2 and saccharide meaning sugar) because it is made up of two sugars, galactose and glucose, bound together. If an infant with galactosemia is given milk, derivatives of galactose build up in the infant's system, causing damage to the liver, brain, kidneys, and eyes. Individuals with galactosemia cannot tolerate any form of milk (human or animal) and must carefully watch intake of other galactose-containing foods. Exposure to milk products may result in liver damage, mental retardation, cataract formation, and kidney failure.

After drinking milk for a few days, a newborn with galactosemia will refuse to eat and develop jaundice, vomiting, lethargy, irritability, and convulsions. The liver will be enlarged and the blood sugar may be low. Continued feeding of milk products to the infant leads to cirrhosis of the liver, cataract formation in the eye (which may result in partial blindness), and mental retardation.

Symptoms

- Jaundice (yellowish discoloration of the skin and the whites of the eyes)
- Vomiting
- Poor feeding (baby refusing to drink milk-containing formula)
- Poor weight gain
- Lethargy
- Irritability
- Convulsions
- Exams and tests
- Hepatomegaly (enlarged liver)
- Hypoglycemia (low blood sugar)
- Aminoaciduria (amino acids are present in the urine and/or blood plasma)
- Cirrhosis
- Ascites (fluid collects in the abdomen)
- Mental retardation
- Cataract formation

Diagnostic investigations: Prenatal diagnosis by direct measurement of the enzyme galactose-1-phosphate uridyl transferase.

The presence of "reducing substances" in the infant's urine with normal or low blood sugar while the infant is being fed breast milk or a formula containing lactose. A simple test on the urine indicates the presence of a reducing substance, and a specific enzymatic study on the urine can prove the substance to be galactose.

- Presence of chemicals, called ketones, in the urine
- Measurement of enzyme activity in the red blood cells
- Blood culture for bacterial infection (*E. coli* sepsis)

Treatment

- Once the disease is recognized, treatment consists of strictly avoiding all milk, milk-containing products, and other foods that contain galactose. The infant can be fed with soy formula, meat-base formula, or Nutramigen (a protein hydrolysate formula), or other lactose-free formula.
- The condition is lifelong and requires abstinence from milk, milk products, and galactose-containing foods for life.

- Calcium supplements are recommended.
- Parents need to take care and educate the child to avoid not only milk and milk products, but also those foods that contain dry milk products. For this reason, it is essential to read product labels and be an informed consumer.

Prevention

A personal knowledge of family history is helpful. If there is a family history of galactosemia, genetic counseling will help prospective parents make decisions about pregnancy and prenatal testing. Once the diagnosis of galactosemia is made, genetic counseling is recommended for other members of the family.

Many states have mandatory screening of newborns for galactosemia. Parents may receive a call from a health care provider that says the screening test indicates possible galactosemia. At that time, the parents should promptly stop milk products and have a blood test done for galactosemia through their doctor.

HEREDITARY FRUCTOSE INTOLERANCE

Hereditary fructose intolerance is a disorder in which a person lacks the protein needed to break down fructose. Fructose is a fruit sugar that naturally occurs in the body. Man-made fructose is used as a sweetener in many foods, including baby food and drinks.

Causes, Incidence, and Risk Factors

- This condition occurs when the body is missing an enzyme called aldolase B.
- This substance is needed to break down fructose.
- If a person without this substance eats fructose and sucrose (cane or beet sugar, table sugar), complicated chemical changes occur in the body. The body cannot change its energy storage material, glycogen, into glucose. As a result, the blood sugar falls and dangerous substances build up in the liver.
- Hereditary fructose intolerance is inherited, which means it is passed down through families. If both parents carry an abnormal gene, each of their children has a 25% chance of being affected. The condition may be as common as 1 in 20,000 people in some European countries.

Symptoms (Fig. 16.19)

Symptoms can be seen after a baby starts eating food or formula.

The early symptoms of fructose intolerance are similar to those of galactosemia. Later symptoms relate more to liver disease.

Symptoms may include:
- Convulsions
- Excessive sleepiness
- Irritability
- Jaundice
- Poor feeding as a baby
- Problems after eating fruits and fructose/sucrose-containing foods
- Vomiting

Diagnostic evaluation:
- Physical examination may show:
  - Enlarged liver and spleen (hepatosplenomegaly)
  - Yellow skin or eyes
- Tests that confirm the diagnosis include:
  - Blood clotting tests
  - Blood sugar test
  - Enzyme studies
  - Genetic testing
  - Kidney function test
  - Liver function test
  - Liver biopsy
  - Uric acid blood test
  - Urinalysis

Blood sugar will be low, especially after receiving fructose or sucrose. Uric acid levels will be high.

Treatment: Removing fructose and sucrose from the diet is an effective treatment for most patients. Complications are treated. For example, some patients can take medication to lower the level of uric acid in their blood and decrease their risk for gout.

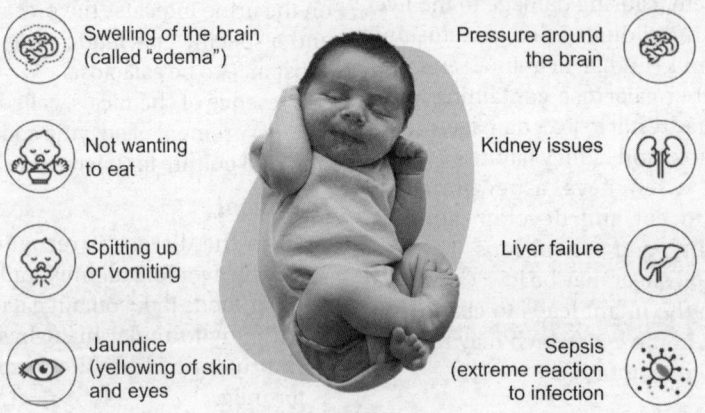

Fig. 16.19: Hereditary fructose intolerance symptoms.

Complications

- Avoidance of fructose-containing foods due to their effects
- Bleeding
- Death
- Gout
- Illness from eating foods containing fructose or sucrose
- Liver failure
- Low blood sugar (hypoglycemia)
- Seizures

Disorders of Pyruvate Metabolism

Hereditary disorders of pyruvate metabolism. They are difficult to diagnose and describe because pyruvate is a key intermediate in glycolysis, gluconeogenesis, and the tricarboxylic acid cycle. Some inherited metabolic disorders may alter pyruvate metabolism indirectly. Disorders in pyruvate metabolism appear to lead to deficiencies in neurotransmitter synthesis and, consequently, to nervous system disorders.

Inherited disorders of liver metabolism are in general due to single enzyme defects that result in abnormalities in the synthesis or catabolism of proteins, carbohydrates, or lipids. This group of diseases comprises disorders of the amino acid, iron, bilirubin and sphingolipid metabolism as well as disorders of the coagulation cascade, the urea cycle and diverse transport processes. These diseases either lead to structural liver damage or, if the defective enzyme is produced predominantly in the liver, to injury to other organ systems. In this review article, we discuss the pathogenesis, clinical presentation, diagnosis and therapy of hereditary hemochromatosis, Wilson's disease and alpha 1-antitrypsin deficiency which represent the most common hereditary liver diseases.

CONCLUSION

A carbohydrate is a large biological molecule, or macromolecule, consisting only of carbon (C), hydrogen (H), and oxygen (O), usually with hydrogen: oxygen atom ratio of 2:1. Carbohydrates are technically hydrates of carbon; structurally it is more accurate to view them as polyhydroxy aldehydes and ketones. Carbohydrates are a group of naturally occurring carbonyl compounds (aldehydes or ketones) that also contain several hydroxyl groups. It may also include their derivatives which produce such compounds on hydrolysis. They are the most abundant organic molecules in nature and are also referred to as "saccharides". The carbohydrates which are soluble in water and sweet in taste are called "sugars" Carbohydrates absorbed in the small intestine and are hydrolyzed to monosaccharides prior to absorption. The digestion of starch begins with the action of salivary alpha-amylase/ptyalin, although its activity is slight in comparison with that of pancreatic amylase in the small intestine

BIBLIOGRAPHY

1. Lehninger AL, Nelson DL, Cox MM. Lehninger principles of biochemistry. New York: Worth Publishers, 2000.
2. Madigan MT, Martinko JM, Bender KS, Buckley DH, Stahl DA. Brock biology of microorganisms, Fourteenth edition. Boston: Pearson, 2015.
3. Robert K, Murray RK, Granner DK, Mayes PA, Rodwell VW. Harpers Biochemistry, 23rd edition. Prentice-Hall International Inc, 1993.
4. Rodwell VW, Botham KM, Kennelly PJ, Weil PA, Bender DA. Harper's illustrated biochemistry, 30th edition. New York, NY. McGraw-Hill Education LLC, 2015.

REVIEW QUESTIONS

Long Essays

1. Define carbohydrates. List down the classification of carbohydrates. Explain monosaccharide in detail.
2. Explain in detail about digestion and absorption of carbohydrate.
3. Describe about glycogen storage diseases.
4. Describe in detail steps, regulation, and energetics and amphibolic nature of tricarboxylic acid cycle.
5. Define gluconeogenesis. Describe in detail about the pathway of gluconeogenesis.
6. Describe briefly about the disorders of carbohydrate metabolism, regulation of blood sugar and significance of glucose tolerance test.

Short Essays

1. Classify monosaccharides with examples.
2. Classify polysaccharides with examples.
3. Write short note on absorption of carbohydrates.
4. Describe the composition and functions of cell.
5. Enumerate the functions and structure of mitochondria.
6. Types, structure, composition and uses of carbohydrate.
7. Carbohydrate metabolism.
8. Steps of glycolysis.
9. Cori cycle (con cycle or lactic acid cycle).
10. Pentose phosphate pathway.
11. Citric acid cycle: Citric acid cycle reaction steps.
12. Glycogenolysis pathway.
13. Regulation of blood sugar level.

Short Answers

1. Diabetes mellitus.
2. Gluconeogenesis.
3. Hexose monophosphate pathway.
4. Krebs cycle.
5. Morphology of nucleus.
6. Glycogenesis.
7. Blood glucose monitoring.
8. Glucose tolerance test (GTT).
9. Barfoed's test.
10. Benedict's reagent.
11. Hypoglycemia.
12. Galactosemia.
13. Hereditary fructose intolerance.
14. Disorders of pyruvate metabolism.

CHAPTER 17

Lipids

CHAPTER OUTLINE

- Fatty Acids—Definition, Classification
- Definition and Clinical Significance of MUFA and PUFA, Essential Fatty Acids, Trans Fatty Acids
- Digestion, Absorption and Metabolism of Lipids and Related Disorders
- Compounds Formed from Cholesterol
- Ketone Bodies (Name, Types and Significance Only)
- Lipoproteins—Types and Functions (Metabolism not Required)
- Lipid Profile
- Atherosclerosis (in Brief)

TERMINOLOGY

- **Lipids:** These are the greasy materials which may be extracted from animal and plant tissue. Lipids are extracted out from tissues by hot alcohol, ether and benzene. Lipids are soluble in organic solvents such as chloroform.
- **Essential fatty acids:** The group of polyunsaturated fatty acids produced by plants, but not by humans-required in human diet.
- **Ether:** A molecule containing two carbon linked by an oxygen atom.
- **Fatty acid:** A long chain hydrocarbon containing a carboxyl group at one end. Saturated fatty acids have completely saturated hydrocarbon chain. Unsaturated fatty acids have one or more carbon-carbon double bonds in their hydrocarbon chains.
- **Steroids:** Compounds that are derivatives of a tetracyclic structure composed of a cyclopentane ring fused to a substituted phenanthrene nucleus.
- **Sterols:** A class of lipids containing the steroid nucleus.
- **Triacylglycerides:** Also called triglycerides, these are fats and oils that comprise the major energy source for the body. Triacylglycerides are composed of a glycerol backbone to which 3 fatty acids are esterified.
- **Phospholipids** Phospholipids are similar to fats but one of the fatty acid groups is replaced by a phosphate group. Amphiphilic nature (hydrophilic heads and hydrophobic tails) form a bilayer arrangement essential in cell membrane structure Lecithin present in brain, nervous tissue, sperm and egg yolk Cephalins present in brain and erythrocytes
- **Glycolipids:** They contain a fatty acid, sphingosine (amino alcohol-contains both an amine functional group and an alcohol functional group), carbohydrate or carbohydrate derivative. Is an essential part of cell.
- **Lipoproteins:** A lipoprotein contains both proteins and lipids water-bound to the proteins. It is structure consists of—a core consisting of droplets of triacylglycerols and/ or cholesteryl esters a surface monolayer of phospholipid, cholesterol and specific proteins (apolipoproteins, e.g., apoprotein B-100 in low density lipoprotein). Many enzymes, transporters, structural proteins, antigens and toxins are lipoproteins.
- **Emulsification** is the dispersion of one phase into another in fine particles. The emulsification of fats into dispersion allows high surface area for the fatty particles and increases the rate of any chemical reaction. One familiar emulsion is milk in which finely-divided fat particles are dispersed in water containing proteins.
- **Hydrolysis** means a reaction of a substance with water. Thus, the reaction of fats with water is called hydrolysis of the fat.
- **Enzymes** are catalysts. Catalysts, you recall, reduce the activation energy for a process, lowering the temperature at which it can take place. You cannot hydrolyze a fat in water at any appreciable rate. The molecule is stable. Yet in the body, hydrolysis takes place quickly under the influence of an enzyme.

INTRODUCTION

Lipids are organic compounds of biological nature that includes fats, oils and waxes. They are insoluble in water but soluble in nonpolar solvents, such as ether, chloroform and benzene. Lipids are utilizable by living organisms. In the normal mammal at least 10% to 20% of the body weight is lipid. They form important dietary constituent on account of their high calorific value and fat soluble vitamins (vitamins A, D, E and K) along with the essential fatty acids. Lipids are distributed in all organs, particularly in adipose tissues in which lipids represent more than 90% of the cytoplasm of a cell.

Definition

- Chemically lipids are defined as esters of glycerol and fatty acids or as the triglycerides of fatty acids, general formula of lipid = Glycerol + Fatty acid = Triglycerides
- Lipids are a heterogeneous group of compounds, including fats, oils, steroids, wax and related compounds, which are related more by their physical than by their chemical properties. Lipids may be regarded as organic substances relatively insoluble in water, soluble in organic solvents (alcohol, ether, etc.), actually or potentially related to fatty acids and utilized by the living cells.

Biological Functions of Lipids

Lipids are stored in a relatively water-free state in the tissues in contrast to carbohydrates which are heavily hydrated to perform a wide variety of functions.

- Body lipids are reservoir of potential chemical energy. Lipids can be stored in the body in almost unlimited amount in contrast to carbohydrates. Furthermore, lipids have a high calorific value (9.3 calories per gram) which is twice as great as carbohydrate. Large amount of energy is stored as lipid than as carbohydrates.
- Lipids which forms the major constituent of biomembranes are responsible for membrane integrity and regulation of membrane permeability.
- The subcutaneous lipids serve as insulating materials against atmospheric heat and cold and protect internal organs.
- They serve as a source of fat soluble vitamins (vitamin A, D, E and K) and essential fatty acids. (linoleic, linolenic and arachidonic acid).
- Lipids serve as metabolic regulators of steroid hormones and prostaglandins.
- Lipids present in inner mitochondrial membrane actively participate in electron transport chain.
- Polyunsaturated fatty acids help in lowering blood cholesterol.
- Squalamine, a steroid, is an potential antibiotic and antifungal agent.

FATTY ACIDS

The fatty acids are the basic units of lipid molecules. Fatty acids are derivatives of aliphatic hydrocarbon chain that contains a carboxylic acid group. Over 200 fatty acids have been isolated from various lipids.

They differ among themselves in hydrocarbon chain length, number and position of double bonds as well as in the nature of substituents, such as oxy, keto, epoxy groups and cyclic structure. Depending on the absence, or presence of double bonds, they are classified into saturated and unsaturated fatty acids.

Saturated fatty acids do not contain double bonds. The hydrocarbon chain may contain 12 to 18 carbon atoms., e.g., palmitic and stearic acids.

- $CH_3(CH_2)_{14}COOH$ - Palmitic acid (C-16)
- $CH_3(CH_2)_{16}COOH$ - Stearic acid (C-18)

Unsaturated fatty acids are classified into different types depending on the number of double bonds present in the hydrocarbon chain. These fatty acids are mainly found in plant lipids.

Unsaturated Fatty Acid

Sl. No.	Name of fatty acid	No. of double bonds
1.	Oleic acid	1
2.	Linoleic acid	2
3.	Linolenic acid	3
4.	Arachidonic acid	4

ESSENTIAL FATTY ACIDS

Fatty acids required in the diet are called essential fatty acids (EFA). They are not synthesized by the body and are mainly polyunsaturated fatty acids (PUFA).

For example, linoleic acid, linolenic acid, arachidonic acid

Functions of Essential Fatty Acids

They are required for membrane structure and function, transport of cholesterol, formation of lipoproteins and prevention of fatty liver.

Deficiency of Essential Fatty Acids

The deficiency of essential fatty acid results in phrynoderma or toad skin.

Biosynthesis of Fatty Acids

- Biosynthesis of fatty acids occurs in all organisms and in mammals it occurs mainly in adipose tissue, mammary glands, and liver.
- Fatty acid synthesis takes place in the cytosol in two steps:
  a. Formation of medium chain fatty acid of chain length 16 carbon atoms.
  b. Lengthening of this carbon chain in microsomes for larger fatty acids.
- Acetyl-CoA serves as a source of carbon atoms for saturated as well as unsaturated fatty acids.

Acetyl-CoA can be formed from excessive dietary glucose and glucogenic amino acids (amino acids which can be converted to glucose). Carbohydrates and amino acids in the presence of oxygen is converted to pyruvate which in turn can be converted to acetyl-CoA.

Synthesis of Fatty Acids

Reactions of fatty acid syntheses complex (Fig. 17.1): The remaining reactions of fatty acid synthesis are catalyzed by a multifunctional enzyme known as fatty acid synthase complex and it has 2 subunits. Each subunit contains 6 enzymes and an acyl carrier protein (ACP). The sequence of reactions for the extra mitochondrial synthesis of fatty acids:

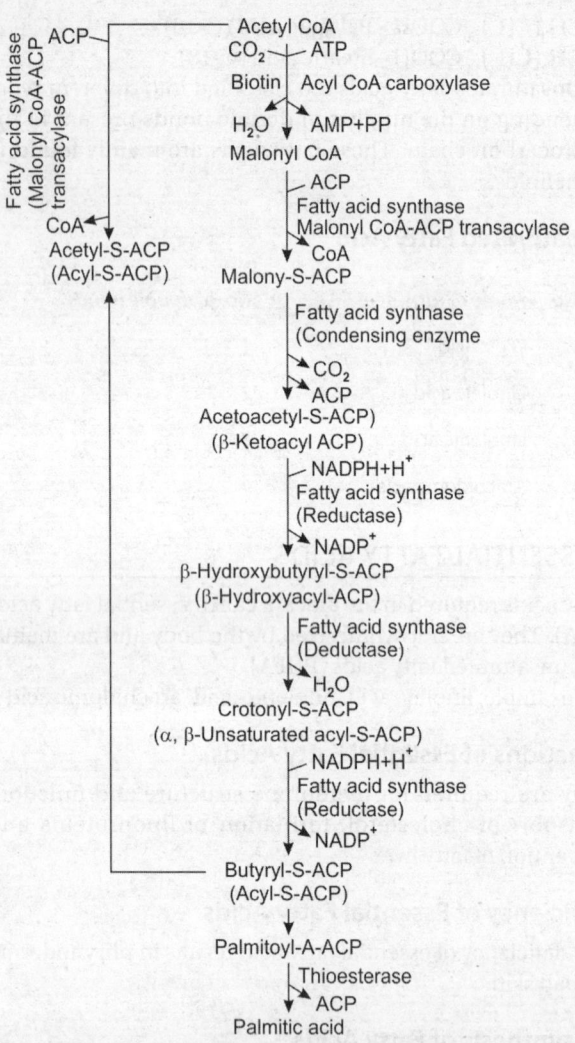

Fig. 17.1: Reactions of fatty acid syntheses.

1. The two carbon fragment of acetyl COA is transferred to ACP of fatty acid synthesis catalyzed by the enzyme acetyl COA ACP transacylase.
2. The enzyme malonyl COA-ACP transacylase transfers malonate from malonyl COA to bind to ACP
3. The acetyl unit attached to cysteine is transferred to malonyl group (bound to ACP). The malonyl moiety loses CO_2 which was added by acetyl COA carboxylase. The reaction is catalyzed by 3-ketoacyl ACP synthase.
4. 3-keto acyl ACP reductase reduces ketoacyl group to hydroxy acyl group. The reducing equivalents are supplied by NADPH.
5. 3-hydroxy acyl ACP undergoes dehydration. A molecule of water is eliminated and a double bond is introduced between a and 3 carbons.
6. A second NADPH dependent reduction catalyzed by enoyl-ACP reductase occurs to produce acyl—ACP

The carbon chain attached to ACP is transferred to cysteine residue and the reactions 2 to 6 are repeated 6 more times. At the end of 7 cycles the fatty acid synthesis is complete. The enzyme palmitoyl thioesterase separates palmitate from fatty acid synthase.

This completes the synthesis of palmitate.
- Regulation of biosynthesis of fatty acids
- Conversion of acetyl COA to malonyl COA is the rate limiting step in fatty acid biosynthesis.
- Hormones regulate acetyl COA carboxylase by a separate mechanism.
  - **Phosphorylation and dephosphorylation:** Insulin promotes fatty acid synthesis. Consumption of high carbohydrate or fat free diet increases the synthesis of acetyl COA carboxylase and fatty acid synthase which promote fatty acid synthesis.

Lipids Classification

Lipids are broadly classified into simple, complex and derived, which are further subdivided into different groups.
- **Simple lipid:** these are esters of fatty acids with various alcohols.
  - **Fats and oils:** esters of fatty acids with glycerol. The difference between fat and oil is only physical. Thus, oil is a liquid while fat is a solid at room temperature.
  - **Waxes:** esters of fatty acids (usually long chain) with alcohols other than glycerol. These alcohols may be aliphatic is most commonly found in waxes.
- **Compound/complex lipid:** Esters of fatty acids containing groups in addition to an alcohol and a fatty acid.
  - **Phospholipids:** Lipids containing, in addition to fatty acids and an alcohol, a phosphoric acid residue. They frequently have nitrogen containing bases and other constituents, e.g., in 'glycerophopholipids' the alcohol is glycerol and in 'sphingo -phospholipids' the alcohol is sphingosine.
  - **Glycolipids:** Lipids containing a fatty acid, sphingosine, carbohydrate and nitrogenous base glycerol and phosphate are absent, e.g., cerebrosides, gangliosides.
  - **Lipoproteins:** Macromolecular complexes of lipids with protein.
  - **Other complex lipids:** Lipids, such as sulfolipids, and amino lipids.
- **Precursor and derived lipids:** These include fatty acids, glycerol, steroids, other alcohols, fatty aldehydes, and ketone bodies, hydrocarbons, lipid-soluble vitamins and hormones.

PROPERTIES OF LIPIDS

Lipids consist of a broad group of compounds that are generally soluble in organic solvents but only sparingly soluble in water. Lipids in food exhibit unique physical and chemical properties. Their composition, crystalline structure, melting properties and ability to associate with water and other non-lipid molecules are especially important to their functional properties in many foods. During the processing, storage and handling of foods, lipids undergo complex chemical changes and react with other food constituents, producing numerous compounds both desirable and deleterious to food quality. Cooking oil includes the well-known olive, sunflower, and canola oils and the not so well-known coconut, soy, and palm oils. Palm oil is similar to coconut. Because of its highly saturated, it issued to make shortening and frying oil. The oil palm fruits produce two types of oil, palm oil which is extracted from the per carp of the fruit and palm kernel oil from the seeds, both of which are important in the world trade. Edible palm oil shall have the following characteristics:

- Density at 50° relative to the density of water at 25°C, ranging from 0.8910 to 0.9030.
- Refractive index, at 50°C, ranging from 1.449 to 1.455.
- Saponification value ranging from 190 to 209 milligrams of potassium hydroxide pergram of oil.
- Iodine value (Wij's) ranging from 50 to 55.
- An acid value of—not more than 10 milligrams of potassium hydroxide per gram of virgin oil; or not more than 0.6 milligrams of potassium hydroxide per gram of non-virgin oil.
- Peroxide value not more than 10 milliequivalents peroxide oxygen per kilogram of oil..
- Unsaponifiable matter of not more than 12 grams per kilogram of oil.
- Total carotenoids of the oil of the red palm of—not less than 500 milligrams per kilogram; and not more than 2000 milligrams per kilogram calculated as beta-carotene.

LIPID METABOLISM

Digestion converts the foods we eat to a form that the body can use for energy or store for future needs as fat. Digestion is a catalyzed process—chemical reactions take place in the body that would not occur without the presence of catalysts called enzymes. The specific enzymes that operate to catalyze fat digestion are called lipases.

When we enjoy a typical Western diet for a day we may consume on the order of 30% to 40% fat. These dietary lipids often include as much as 100 g of triglycerides such as tristearin a much smaller amount (4–8 g) of phospholipids, 0.4–0.5 g of cholesterol, the fat soluble vitamins A, D, E, and K, and small amounts of waxes from plant and animal cell walls. As we consume these wonderful foods the digestion process begins in the stomach and can be thought of as four major events:

- The secretion of bile and the various lipases into the stomach (lipid breaking enzymes),
- The emulsification or mixing of the lipids and the water soluble lipases and bile phases,
- The enzymatic hydrolysis of the ester linkages in the triglycerides,
- The formation of lipid containing bile salt micelles which transport the lipids to the cells for resynthesis or oxidation.

Biosynthesis of Fatty Acids

- Biosynthesis of fatty acids occurs in all organisms and in mammals it occurs mainly in adipose tissue, mammary glands, and liver.
- Fatty acid synthesis takes place in the cytosol in two steps.
  a. Formation of medium chain fatty acid of chain length 16 carbon atoms.
  b. Lengthening of this carbon chain in microsomes for larger fatty acids.

- Acetyl CoA serves as a source of carbon atoms for saturated as well as unsaturated fatty acids. Acetyl CoA can be formed from excessive dietary glucose and glucogenic amino acids (amino acids which can be converted to glucose). Carbohydrates and aminoacids in the presence of oxygen is converted to pyruvate which inturn can be converted to acetyl CoA.

Oxidation of Fatty Acids

The digestion of fats starts in the small intestine. Fats are emulsified by the bile salts and hydrolyzed by the pancreatic lipases to form free fatty acids. These free fatty acids combine with glycerol (produced by the glycolytic process) to form triglycerides. They combine with proteins to form lipoproteins and enter into circulation to perform various biological functions such as oxidation, storage and formation of new lipids. Thus the various fatty acids may exist in the free form as well as in the esterified form (Triglyceride) in blood.

Fatty acids are the immediate source for oxidation of fats in various tissues viz. liver, adipose tissue, muscles, heart, kidney, brain, lungs and testes.

B-Oxidation: Fatty acids are oxidized to CO_2 and water with the liberation of large amount of energy. Oxidation is brought about in the mitochondria because all the enzymes required for oxidation are present in the mitochondria. Oxidation of fatty acids is of three types, based on the position of the carbon atom which gets oxidized.

However beta-oxidation of fatty acids is predominant and widely prevalent and it provides large amount of energy than and oxidation. Beta-oxidation of fatty acids can be conveniently studied under different stages as detailed below.

Activation of Fatty Acids

Fatty acids are relatively inert chemical molecules and hence they must be converted to an active intermediate for the initiation of B-oxidation. The activation of fatty acids takes place in the cytosol in the presence of ATP, coenzyme A and acyl CoA synthetase. The activated fatty acid then enters into mitochondria with the help of a carrier protein, carnitine in the presence of an enzyme carnitine acyltransferase.

Oxidation of acyl CoA (fatty acid) takes place through several steps leading to the formation of acetyl CoA (C2) and an acyl CoA having two carbon atoms less than the original fatty acid with which the β-oxidation cycle originally started. Acyl CoA then enters into a similar oxidation cycle until all the carbon atoms are released as acetyl CoA. These reactions require cofactors, such as flavin adenine dinucleotide (FAD) and nicotinamide adenine dinucleotide (NAD^+).

Structural Biochemistry/Lipid Droplets and Cellular Lipid Metabolism

Lipid droplets are the lipid storage organelles of all organisms. Their important roles include cellular and organismic energy storage Lipid droplets could be found nearly in every cell. They are cytoplasmic organelles that store lipids; some examples are triglycerides and cholesterol. Under nutrient deprivation, droplet triglycerides are hydrolyzed to create free fatty acids, which are then oxidized and used to provide energy.

Lipid droplets in a cellular organism are typically composed of nonpolar, hydrophobic lipids, also known as neutral lipids. The droplets contain a hydrophobic center that is encircled by a phospholipid monolayer. There are two major types of lipid droplets; sterol esters and triacylglycerols. As the lipid droplets form there can be a variety of lipid droplet proteins along the monolayer. The amount of lipid droplets in each cell can vary and currently scientists are unable create an algorithm to predict the lipid droplet concentration.

Lipid droplets are formed on or in close proximity of endoplasmic reticulum. Through the use of the electron microscope, it was possible to see that lipid droplets and cisternae have a close relationship but the mechanism of formation has yet to be discovered. There are over 800 genes that affect lipid droplet accumulation. When testing to see how these multitudes of genes affect lipid droplet formation, knockdown of genes led to differing lipid droplet formation changes. Depending on the gene that was knocked-down, some of the lipid droplets decreased in concentration, increased in size, or increased in size and were more dispersed. Proteins were also found to affect lipid droplet formation. For example, with the over-expression of fat-inducing transcript-2 (FIT2) proteins, there are more lipid droplets. Consequently, knockdown of FIT2 leads to fewer lipid droplets.

Lipid droplets are capable of interacting with other cellular organelles. They interact with the endoplasmic reticulum, endosomes, mitochondria, and peroxisomes. These interactions can sometimes mediate some cellular mechanisms, such as lipid trafficking, neutral lipid metabolism, and synthesis/catabolism of steroid hormones. A majority of these interactions occur at the endoplasmic reticulum.

Properties of Lipid Droplets

- Almost every cell has lipid droplets or has the capacity to produce them
- Some bacteria use lipid droplets to store lipids themselves
- Lipid droplets' abundance varies greatly in cells.
- Lipid droplets' size also varies greatly depending on cell types. Many cells are known to contain small LDs (100–200 nm). On the other hand, in white adipocytes, for instance, have diameters up to 100 micrometers, occupying most of the cytoplasm.

Functions of Lipid Droplets

- Generally they are intracellular lipid reservoirs that become useful as they provide building blocks for cell membranes or substrates for energy metabolism
- Lipid droplets may be used as places for synthesizing some lipids. For instance, TGs are produced in the Er and lipid droplets.
- Lipids droplets may be used to store some proteins.
- Lipid droplets are involved in hepatitis C virus assembly

Lipid Droplets and Tissues

- **Adipose tissue:** In mammals and birds, adipose tissues is located in specific areas in the body and are regulated by hormones. They are more prominently used as insulation for endotherms. There are two types of adipocytes—white adipocytes and brown adipocytes. Adipocytes are the cells that are utilized by the body to store lipids in lipid droplets. White adipocytes store lipids in a single large lipid droplet in the cytoplasm. They are also known to store cholesterol esters and fat-soluble vitamins. The white adipocytes utilize leptin to regulate the lipid storage. Brown adipocytes catabolize lipids in order to generate heat. They store lipids in smaller and more numerous lipid droplets in the cytoplasm.
- **Liver:** The liver has the second greatest lipid in LD form storage capacity. They store the lipid droplets in hepatocytes. In humans, a high amount of lipid droplets can lead to an illness called fatty liver.
- **Small intestine:** The small intestine is where a majority of nutrient absorption occurs. By utilizing its microvilli, the small intestine is able to absorb 95% of a meal's fat content. The lipid droplets are stored in intestinal enterocytes. The enterocytes have a large surface area and are able to store and synthesize triacylglycerols (TGs).
- **Yolk sac:** The yolk sac stores lipids in a similar manner to intestinal enterocytes and liver hepatocytes. They are able to store lipid droplets and export via apoB-containing lipoproteins.
- **Skeletal muscle:** Muscle is not known to be a large lipid storage unit. When humans store lipids in their skeletal muscles it is usually a side effect of obesity because of insulin resistance. There is an exception with this in highly-trained athletes. Athletes use a high volume of ATP when they are training so the body needed a way to keep a lipid reserve for when the muscles need more energy. This compensation occurs with the lipid droplets being stored in skeletal muscle cells near the mitochondria. This is considered the athlete's paradox because lipid droplet storage in skeletal muscles is usually a bad sign.
- **Adrenal cortex:** The adrenal cortex is able to store large amounts of sterol esters (SEs). The SEs are most likely stored in the form of cholesterols for steroid hormone synthesis. Also the yellow coloring of the tissue can be credited to the lipids

Disorders of Lipid Metabolism

Certain genetic disorders or medical conditions, such as diabetes, hypothyroidism, kidney disease and liver disease can cause dysfunction of your lipid metabolism (your body's use of lipids). A poor diet, sedentary lifestyle and/or certain medications also can influence your lipid levels. The major lipids in the blood stream are cholesterol and triglycerides.

- **Cholesterol** is carried through the body in lipoproteins (compounds that move cholesterol and triglycerides through your blood). Cholesterol helps to form and repair cells in your body. There are two types of cholesterol.
- **LDL**, or low density cholesterol, is considered "bad" cholesterol because when it is too high it causes coronary artery (heart) disease that can lead to heart attack.
- **HDL**, or high density cholesterol, is considered "good" because it protects against coronary artery disease.

- **Triglycerides** supply energy for your body. When triglycerides are very high they cause severe inflammation of the pancreas, called pancreatitis. In some patients, high triglycerides also increase the risk for coronary heart disease.

Common Treatments for Lipid Metabolism Disorders

- **Diet:** Following a healthy diet that is free of trans fat and reduced in saturated fats is the most important way you can lower your bad cholesterol. Lowering triglycerides also may require decreasing your weight, alcohol intake, and variably simple sugars.
- **Exercise:** Regular aerobic exercise will help raise your HDL (good) cholesterol level and reduce your risk of coronary artery (heart) disease and heart attack.
- **Medication:** Your doctor may prescribe a variety of medications when diet and exercise are not effective in lowering cholesterol and/or triglyceride levels. These medications must be used in combination with a healthy diet and exercise plan.
- **LDL apheresis:** A new therapy that is used with patients whose high cholesterol levels do not respond to diet, exercise and medication. The LDL apheresis procedure involves two intravenous (IV) lines, one inserted into each arm.

Ketone Bodies

Ketone bodies are three different water soluble, biochemical that are produced by the liver from fatty acids during periods of low food intake (fasting) and starvation for cells of the body to use as energy instead of glucose. Two of the three are used as a source of energy in the heart and brain while the third (acetone) is a degradation breakdown product of acetoacetic acid. Radioactive tracing of acetone determines that between 2% and 30% is excreted from the body. Ketone bodies are picked up by cells and converted back into acetyl CoA which then enters the citric acid cycle and electron transport chain for energy. In the brain, ketone bodies are also used to make acetyl CoA into long chain fatty acids because long chain fatty acids cannot pass through the blood brain barrier. The liver breaks down protein to produce glucose during starvation for the very few glucose obligate cells that cannot use ketone bodies. In the brain, ketone bodies are a vital source of energy during fasting or strenuous exercise. Although termed "bodies", they are molecules, not particles.

The three endogenous ketone bodies are acetone, acetoacetic acid, and beta-hydroxybutric acid Other ketone bodies, such as beta-ketopentanoate and beta-hydroxypentanoate may be created as a result of the metabolism of synthetic triglycerides such as triheptanoin.

Ketone bodies become major body fuels during fasting and consumption of a high-fat, low-carbohydrate (ketogenic) diet. Hyperketonemia is associated with potential health benefits. Ketone body synthesis (ketogenesis) is the last recognizable step of lipid energy metabolism, a pathway that links dietary lipids and adipose triglycerides to the Krebs cycle and respiratory chain and has three highly regulated control points: (1) adipocyte lipolysis, (2) mitochondrial fatty acids entry, controlled by the inhibition of carnitine palmitoyltransferase I by malonyl coenzyme A (CoA) and (3) mitochondrial 3-hydroxy-3-methylglutaryl CoA synthase, which catalyzes the irreversible first step of ketone body synthesis. Each step is suppressed by an elevated circulating insulin level or insulin/glucagon ratio. The utilization of ketone bodies (ketolysis) also determines circulating ketone body levels. Consideration of ketone body metabolism reveals the mechanisms underlying the extreme fragility of dietary ketosis to carbohydrate intake and highlights areas for further study.

Metabolism of Ketone Bodies

Acetoacetic acid, 3-hydroxybutyric acid and acetone are classified as ketone bodies, acetone bodies or ketones. The process of their formation is known as ketogenesis. Ketone bodies are produced in the liver. They are acidic and detected by Rothera's test.

Ketogenesis

In a diabetic patient, in starvation, or in any situation in which carbohydrate metabolism is restricted, the body utilizes oxaloacetate to produce glucose for brain and muscles. This reduces the amount of oxaloacetate available for Krebs cycle and acetyl CoA cannot be properly metabolized. When this occurs, acetyl CoA is changed into acetoacetyl-C0A which is converted into acetoacetic acid in the liver by the enzyme deacylase. Acetoacetic acid may be changed into acetone and beta- hydroxybutyric acid:

The ketone bodies pass into the blood stream in very small amounts under the normal circumstances. The total ketone bodies concentration in blood is normally, below 1 mg per 100 mL of blood and the average excretion in urine in 24 hours is less than 125 mg. Normally the ketone bodies are carried in the blood stream, mainly to the kidneys and muscles, where acetoacetic acid is oxidized after conversion to acetoacetyl CoA. The latter is then cleaved by thiolase when 2 moles of acetyl CoA are formed. They then enter the (citric acid) tricarboxylic acid cycle. This process of oxidation of ketone bodies is called ketolysis and is an alternate source of energy for the peripheral tissues.

Ketosis

When the rate of ketogenesis in the liver exceeds the rate of ketolysis in the periphery, the concentration of ketone bodies in the blood increases resulting in ketonemia. At this stage, ketone bodies are excreted in detectable quantity in the urine. This is ketonuria—when ketonuria and ketonemia are marked, acetone which is volatile escapes in the exhaled air giving rise to acetone smell in the breath. Ketonemia, ketonuria and the acetone odor of the breath together is ketosis. If ketosis is severe, acidosis will set in and this is accompanied by excretion of large amounts of water to carry the ketone bodies. At this stage, the patient becomes profoundly acidotic and passes into comatose stage.

Two main causes of ketosis are starvation and diabetes mellitus. In starvation there is deprivation of carbohydrates and in diabetes, carbohydrates are not efficiently utilized. The person survives on his own stores of glycogen in the liver for energy. When this is depleted, energy is derived by the breakdown of fats in the body. The accelerated fat metabolism leads to the formation of large amounts of acetyl CoA and ketone bodies giving rise to ketosis and ketonuria.

Diabetic Ketoacidosis

Ketosis is more common in type 1 diabetes mellitus. Deficiency of insulin promotes lipolysis. There is accelerated rate of fatty acid oxidation and acetyl CoA is increased in the mitochondria. As oxaloacetate is diverted for gluconeogenesis, the TCA cycle cannot consume all the acetyl CoA. Hence, more acetyl CoA is converted to ketone bodies. This leads to accumulation of ketone bodies in blood. The ketonemia leads to ketonuria. The presence of ketone bodies in urine is assessed by Rothera's test. The accumulation of acidic ketone bodies lowers the plasma pH. So, metabolic acidosis occurs. The condition is called diabetic ketoacidosis. Smell of acetone in the breath is noticed.

Ketosis also leads to dehydration. The hyperglycemia and glycosuria produce osmotic diuresis. Since ketone bodies are excreted as their sodium or potassium salts, there is loss of fixed bases from the body. The typical acidotic breathing or Kussmaul respiration is due to compensatory hyperventilation. Adolf Kussmaul described the peculiar pattern of breathing in diabetic coma in 1874. If not treated promptly and properly, the condition may be fatal. Patient may become unconscious, comatose and die.

The major lines of management are parenteral administration of insulin along with glucose to control the diabetes, bicarbonate and water to correct the acidosis and electrolytes to maintain the electrolyte balance.

Gout

The word **gout** comes from Latin gutta and old French *gote* meaning "a drop". Several hundred years ago gout was thought to be caused by drops of viscous humors that seeped from blood into the joints. In fact, this supposition was not that far from the truth. When a patient experiences the symptoms of a gout attack uric acid has been accumulating in his blood, and uric acid deposits have been forming in the joints. "A disorder of purine metabolism, occurring especially in men, characterized by a raised but variable blood uric acid level and severe recurrent acute arthritis of sudden onset resulting from deposition of crystals of sodium urate in connective tissues and articular cartilage; most cases are inherited, resulting from a variety of abnormalities of purine metabolism. The familial aggregation is for the most part galtonian with a threshold of expression determined by the solubility of uric acid. However, gout is also a feature of the Lesch-Nyhan syndrome, an X-linked disorder."

Gout causes attacks of pain and swelling in one or more joints. An anti-inflammatory painkiller usually eases an attack quickly. Lifestyle factors may reduce the risk of having gout attacks. These include losing weight (if overweight), eating a healthy diet, and not drinking much alcohol or sugar-sweetened soft drinks. If gout attacks recur, then taking vitamin C supplements and/or allopurinol each day can prevent them.

- **Signs and symptoms of gout are generally acute:** They come on suddenly without warning. A significant proportion of patients experience them at night.
- **Severe pain in the joints:** The patient may experience pain in his ankles, hands, wrists, knees or feet. More commonly the big toe is affected (podagra). Many patients describe the affected areas as warm/hot. The fluid sacs that cushion tissue (bursae) may become inflamed (bursitis)—when this happens in the elbow it is called olcranon bursitis, while in the knee prepatellar bursitis.
- **Gradually goes away:** A bout can last for over a week if left untreated—and then gradually goes away during the following week or two.
- **Itchy and peeling skin later:** As the gout subsides the skin around the affected area may be itchy and peel. By the end of it the patient feels fine.
- **Redness and inflammation:** The sufferer will most likely have tender, red and swollen joint(s) in the areas that experienced the most pain.
- **Red/purplish skin:** The affected area may become red or purplish, making the patient think he has an infection.
- **Fever:** Some patients have an elevated temperature.
- **Less flexibility:** The affected joint may be harder to use, the patient has limited movement.
- **No symptoms:** Some patients experience no symptoms. In these cases it may develop into chronic gout.
- **Nodules:** The gout may first appear as tophi (nodules) in the elbows, hands, or ears.

Gout usually occurs in attacks. An attack typically develops quickly over a few hours. It usually causes severe pain in one joint. The base of the big toe is the most commonly affected joint. Walking can be very painful and even the weight of bedclothes can hurt.

However, any joint can be affected. Sometimes two or more joints are affected. Affected joints usually swell and the nearby skin may look red and inflamed. If left untreated, a gout attack may last several days but usually goes completely within 7-10 days. Less severe attacks can occur which may be mistaken at first for other forms of arthritis. Weeks, months or even years may go by between attacks. Some people only ever have one attack.

Diagnosis: Gout is usually diagnosed if you have the typical gout symptoms and a raised blood level of uric acid. If there is doubt as to the cause of the pain and swelling, your doctor may take some fluid out of a swollen joint. This is done with a needle and syringe. The fluid is looked at under the microscope. Crystals of uric acid (urate) can be seen in the fluid to confirm the diagnosis of gout. After examining you, your doctor may carry our either or both these tests:

- **Blood test:** To measure your levels of uric acid. This test is not definitive as some people with high uric acid levels never have gout symptoms; while others who have gout symptoms do not have high levels of uric acid in their blood.
- **Joint fluid test:** A needle is used to collect fluid from the affected joint. The liquid is then examined under a microscope to see whether urate crystals are present.

Complications: Gout does not commonly cause any further problems. However, some are possible:

- **Recurrent gout:** While some people just get one attack, and never experience another one again, others may have recurrent attacks. There are drugs which help reduce the number of recurrent attacks, or even eliminate them.
- **Advanced gout:** If the gout is not treated urate crystals may form under the skin in nodules, they are known as tophi. They may become swollen and tender whenever the patient has a gout attack, but are not painful otherwise.
- **Kidney stones:** Urate crystals can accumulate in the urinary tract of a patient who suffers from gout. This causes kidneys stones. There are drugs which can lower the chances of developing kidney stones.
- **Damage to joints:** If the tophi (nodules) become inflamed the joints could become damaged.
- **Gout might spread:** The gout could spread to other joints.
- **Medication:** Gout is usually treated with medications, these include:
  - **NSAIDs (nonsteroidal anti-inflammatory drugs):** These help combat inflammation and pain. Ibuprofen and naproxen are NSAIDs. There is an increased risk of stomach pain, ulcers and bleeding for some patients who take this drug - the higher the dosage, the higher the risk.
  - **Colchicine:** An effective drug for gout. However, a number of patients might experience diarrhea, vomiting and/or nausea. Colchicine is often given to patients who are unable to take NSAIDs.
  - **Steroids:** These may help combat inflammation and relieve pain. The patient may receive the medication orally or it could be injected right into the joint. Some patients who take steroids may experience a thinning of bones, poor wound healing, while others find that their immune systems become weaker and it is harder to fight off infections. Steroids are usually given to patients who are unable to take either colchicines or NSAIDs.

CHOLESTEROL

Cholesterol is a lipid with a unique structure consisting of four linked hydrocarbon rings forming the bulky steroid structure. There is a hydrocarbon tail linked to one end of the steroid and a hydroxyl group linked to the other end. The hydroxyl group is able to form hydrogen bonds with nearby carbonyl oxygen of phospholipid and sphingolipid head groups. Cholesterol is known as a "sterol" because it is made out of a alcohol and steroid. Cholesterol is present in most animal membranes with varying amounts but is absent in prokaryotes and intracellular membranes.

Steroid, as cholesterol, is one of the most basic lipids and consists of multiple rings of connected atoms, such as hexagons and pentagon. Some examples of steroids are vitamin D, estrogen, and cortison, which are molecules that are critical for keeping the body running smoothly. All steroids are made in cells either from the sterols lanosterol in animals and fungi, or from cycloartenol in plants. Steroids are important in the reproductive system in the body and in the structure and function of membranes. In addition, they can affect the nervous system as they are active in the brain. For example, steroids can be used in medicine such as anesthetics where they slow down the brain function before surgery.

Cholesterol is also a key regulator of membrane fluidity in animals. It is able to insert itself into bilayers perpendicular to the membrane plane. The hydroxyl group forms hydrogen bonds with the carbonyl oxygen of a phopholipid head group while the hydrocarbon tail positions itself in the non-polar core of the bilayer. Since the structure of cholesterol differs from phospholipids, it disrupts the normal reactions between fatty acid chains. Cholesterol is also able to form lipid rafts when it forms specific complexes with certain phospholipids which results in membranes that are less fluid and less subject to phase transitions. This also increases the permeability of the cell membrane to hydrogen and sodium ions. Cholesterol is usually synthesized in animals and smaller cholesterol can be generated in plants. They are important in the composition of cell membranes and also steroid hormones.

Functions of Cholesterol

Cholesterol serves a variety of functions in human body. This includes:

- The manufacture of steroids, or cortisone-like hormones, including vitamin D and the sex hormones testosterone,

estrogen and cortisone. This in turn controls a myriad of bodily functions.
- Assisting the liver in the manufacture of bile acids, this is essential for digestion and absorption of fat-soluble vitamins such as vitamin A, D, E and K.
- Formation of the myelin sheath, a neuron consisting of fat-containing cells that insulate the axon from electrical activity. This ensures proper function of our brains by aiding route of electrical impulses. The absence of cholesterol might lead to loss of memory and difficulty in focusing.
- As a cell to interconnect "lipid molecules", which are needed to stabilize our cell membranes.
- As a source of energy
- Maintenance of our body temperature
- Protection of internal organs
- Modulation the fluidity of cell membranes

Cholesterol Metabolism
- LDL binds to a specific receptor, the LDL receptor (integral membrane protein)
- Segment of the plasma membrane containing the LDL-LDL-receptor complex then invaginates and buds off from the membrane to form an internal vesicle.
- The LDL separates from the receptor and is recycled back to the membrane in a separate vesicle. Vesicle containing LDL fuses with a lysosome leading to the degradation of the LDL and the release of cholesterol.

This process can be beneficial because hormones and antibodies can transport proteins use this method. However, on the downside the pathway is also available to viruses and toxins as a means of entry into the cell.

Biosynthesis of Cholesterol
Important intermediates of cholesterol biosynthesis and enzymes involved.
- **Formation of acetyl CoA:** A molecule of acetic acid combines with coenzyme A (CoA) to produce Acetyl CoA in the presence of an enzyme Acetyl CoA synthetase.
- **Formation of acetoacetyl CoA** Two molecules of acetyl-CoA condense to form an acetoacetyl-CoA molecule, catalyzed by the enzyme "thiolase".
- **Formation of HMG CoA:** The acetoacetyl-CoA further undergoes condensation with one more molecule of acetyl-CoA to form HMG-CoA (3-hydroxy-3-methylglutaryl-CoA). The enzyme which mediates this reaction is called HMG-CoA synthetase.

Health Significance of Cholesterol
Cholesterol and triglycerides cannot dissolve in the blood. They have to be transported within the cells by carriers called lipoproteins. Low-density lipoprotein (LDL) and very low-density lipoprotein (VLDL) are known as the "bad" cholesterols while high-density Lipoprotein (HDL) is known as "good" cholesterol.

Hypercholesterolemia is a condition when there is an extremely high level of cholesterol in the body. Usually, this means that there is a high concentration of LDL and low concentration of HDL. When too much LDL circulates the blood cell, it can built up the inner walls of arteries that feed the heart and brain, therefore, cause the clogging of the arteries. The health significance is that they are prone to cardiovascular diseases. If a clot forms and blocks the narrowed artery, a series of cardiovascular diseases, such as hypertension, myocardial infarction, arteriosclerosis, angina pectoris, heart attack or stroke can result. High levels of cholesterol are also closely associated to diabetes.

HDL is known as "good" cholesterol in that it removes excess cholesterol in the arteries and transport it back to the liver for excretion or re-utilization, and thus preventing the arteries from clogging.

Hypocholesterolemia is a condition when there is an extremely low level of cholesterol in the body. This condition is usually rare, but if they do occur, it might be because of other illness that has caused the body to generate low or no cholesterols.

Important Derivatives of Cholesterol
- **Bile salts:** As polar derivatives of cholesterol, bile salts are highly effective detergents because they contain both polar and nonpolar regions. Bile salts are synthesized in the liver, stored and concentrated in the gallbladder, and then released into the small intestine. Bile salts, the major constituent of bile, solubilize dietary lipids. Solubilization increases in the effective surface area of lipids with two consequences—more surface area is exposed to the digestive action of lipases and lipids are more readily absorbed by the intestine. Bile salts are also the major breakdown products of cholesterol.
- **Synthesis of bile salts from bile acids:** Bile acids are of two types, namely—primary and secondary bile acids. Primary bile acids include cholic acid and chenodeoxycholic acid and secondary bile acids include deoxycholic acid and lithocholic acid.
- **Importance:** Bile acids are C24 steroids, detergent like compounds that are responsible for the emulsification and absorption of lipids in the intestine.
- **Bile salts:** Cholic acid is conjugated in the liver with either glycine or taurine through peptide linkages forming the bile salts glycocholic acid and taurocholic acid respectively. They combine with sodium and potassium present in the bile and form water soluble alkaline bile salts, namely sodium glycocholate and sodium taurocholate respectively.

Importance
- Bile salts are the digestion promoting constituents of bile.
- They lower surface tension and thus can emulsify fats.
- They also activate lipases.

STEROID HORMONES
Cholesterol is the precursor of the five major classes of steroid hormones—progestagens, glucocorticoids, mineralocorticoids, androgens, and estrogens. These

hormones are powerful signal molecules that regulate a host of organismal functions. Progesterone, a progestagen, prepares the lining of the uterus for implantation of an ovum. Progesterone is also essential for the maintenance of pregnancy. Androgens of male secondary sex characteristics, whereas estrogens (such as estrone) are required for the development of female secondary sex characteristics. Estrogens, along with progesterone, also participate in the ovarian cycle. Glucocorticoids (such as cortisol) promote gluconeogenesis and the formation of glycogen, enhance the degradation of fat and protein, and inhibit the inflammatory response. They enable animals to respond to stress-indeed, the absence of glucocorticoids can be fatal. Mineralocorticoids (primarily aldosterone) act on the distal tubules of the kidney to increase the reabsorption of Na^+ and the excretion of K^+ and H^+, which leads to an increase in blood volume and blood pressure. The major sites of synthesis of these classes of hormones are the corpus luteum, for progestagens; the ovaries, for estrogens; the testes, for androgens; and the adrenal cortex, for glucocorticoids and mineralocorticoids

ATHEROSCLEROSIS

Atherosclerosis refers to the fatty deposits block the arteries. Healthy arteries are smooth inner lining and blood can flow though them easily. However, if arteries are damaged, the infection can roughen the lining and cause inflammation. White blood cells go to the damaged arteries and begin to take up lipids, including cholesterol. Fatty acids start to grow at this affected area. This makes the artery become stiff and obstructs the blood flow. If unrecognized and treated, atherosclerosis can lead to heart attack due to the death of cardiac muscle tissue. Drugs called statins which lover LDL (low-density lipoprotein (LDL), "bad cholesterol") can be used to treat atherosclerosis. Aspirin is also know to help the recurrence of heart attacks.

Causes: High blood cholesterol can result from a variety of factors. For instance,
- Genetic factors
- **Age:** usually over age 45 in men and age 55 in women
- Gender: Before menopause, women tend to have lower total cholesterol levels than men of the same age. After menopause, women's LDL (bad) cholesterol levels tend to increase.
- Lack of physical activity
- Certain medications, e.g., some diuretics, immunosuppressants, and corticosteroids
- Diseases, such as diabetes, hypothyroidism
- Cigarette smoking
- High dietary intake of cholesterol
- Obesity

Cholesterol content in food: The American Heart Association recommends a daily intake of less than 300 mg of cholesterol. Moreover, people with high LDL (bad) blood cholesterol levels or people who are taking cholesterol medication should limit themselves to a consumption of less than 200 mg of cholesterol per day.

Clinical manifestations: The symptoms of atherosclerosis vary widely. Patients with mild atherosclerosis may present with clinically important symptoms and signs of disease and MI, or sudden cardiac death may be the first symptom of coronary heart disease. However, many patients with anatomically advanced disease may have no symptoms and experience no functional impairment. The spectrum of presentation includes symptoms and signs consistent with the following conditions—asymptomatic state (subclinical phase), Stable Angina Pectoris, unstable angina (i.e., ACS), AMI, chronic ischemic cardiomyopathy, congestive heart failure, sudden cardiac arrest.

History may include the following—chest pain, shortness of breath, weakness, tiredness, reduced exertional capacity, dizziness, palpitations, leg swelling, weight gain.

Symptoms related to risk factors: Progressive luminal narrowing of an artery due to expansion of a fibrous plaque results in impairment of flow once at least 50–70% of the lumen diameter is obstructed. This impairment in flow results in symptoms of inadequate blood supply to the target organ in the event of increased metabolic activity and oxygen demand. Stable angina pectoris, intermittent claudication, and mesenteric angina are examples of the clinical consequences of this mismatch.

Rupture of a plaque or denudation of the endothelium overlying a fibrous plaque may result in exposure of the highly thrombogenic subendothelium and lipid core. This exposure may result in thrombus formation, which may partially or completely occlude flow in the involved artery. Unstable angina pectoris, MI, transient ischemic attack, and stroke are examples of the clinical sequelae of partial or complete acute occlusion of an artery. Atheroembolism is a distinct clinical entity that may occur spontaneously or as a complication of aortic surgery, angiography, or thrombolytic therapy in patients with advanced and diffuse atherosclerosis.

Angina pectoris is characterized by retrosternal chest discomfort that typically radiates to the left arm and may be associated with dyspnea. Angina pectoris is exacerbated by exertion and relieved by rest or nitrate therapy. Unstable angina pectoris describes a pattern of increasing frequency or intensity of episodes of angina pectoris and includes pain at rest. A prolonged episode of angina pectoris that may be associated with diaphoresis is suggestive of MI.

LIPOPROTEINS

A **lipoprotein** is a biochemical assembly that contains both proteins and lipids. The lipids or their derivatives may be covalently or non-covalently bound to the proteins. Many enzymes, transporters, structural proteins, antigens, adhesins and toxins are lipoproteins. Examples include the high density (HDL) and low density (LDL) lipoproteins which enable fats to be carried in the blood stream, the transmembrane proteins of the mitochondrion and the chloroplast, and bacterial lipoproteins function of lipoprotein particles is to transport water-insoluble lipids (fats) and cholesterol around the body in the blood.

Lipoprotein class	Density (g/mL)	Diameter (nm)	Protein % of dry wt	Phospholipid %	Triacylglycerol % of dry wt
HDL	1.063–1.21	5–15	33	29	8
LDL	1.019–1.063	18–28	25	21	4
IDL	1.006–1.019	25–50	18	22	31
VLDL	0.95–1.006	30–80	10	18	50
Chylomicrons	<0.95	100–500	1–2	7	84

Lipids are transported in blood as large macromolecules; these are complexes with proteins. Free fatty acids are the exception, mainly binding to albumin. Hydrophobic lipids, triglycerides and phospholipids are within the lipoprotein core, with the polar portions of phospholipids and the water-soluble alcohol portion of free cholesterol projecting into the aqueous environment, causing solubilization of the lipoprotein. Types of lipoproteins are chylomicrons, very-low-density lipoprotein (VLDL), intermediate-density lipoprotein (IDL), Low-density lipoprotein (LDL) and High-density lipoprotein (HDL). Lipoprotein classes can be separated physicochemically, either by electrophoresis witch uses surface charge or by ultracentrifugation which uses relative density.

Lipoproteins differ in the ratio of protein to lipids, and in the particular apoproteins and lipids that they contain. They are classified based on their density:

- Chylomicron (largest; lowest in density due to high lipid/protein ratio; highest in triacylglycerols as % of weight)
- VLDL (very low density lipoprotein; 2nd highest in triacylglycerols as % of weight)
- IDL (intermediate density lipoprotein)
- LDL (low density lipoprotein, highest in cholesteryl esters as % of weight)
- HDL (high density lipoprotein, highest in density due to high protein/lipid ratio).

Chylomicrons are the largest, lightest lipoproteins; they carry dietary triglycerides to be hydrolyzed by peripheral tissues lipoprotein lipase (LPL). Fatty acids either provide energy or are stored as triglycerides. Whereas VLDL carry triglycerides synthesized in the liver also to the periphery. LDL are the main cholesterol carriers, delivering cholesterol to peripheral tissues, or back to the liver, through LDL receptors. IDL normally undergo rapid conversion to LDL or are removed by the liver.

As triglycerides are removed, chylomicrons and VLDL shrink in size, and are further catabolized as remnants. Chylomicron remnants are removed by a liver chylomicron remnant receptor, known as LRP (LDL receptor-related protein) or the α2-macroglobulin receptor, VLDL remnants, intermediate-density lipoproteins (IDL), are acted on by hepatic lipase, removed by the liver or converted to low-density lipoproteins (LDL).

PHOSPHOLIPIDS

Phospholipids are so designated because they contain phosphoric acid. They are present in all cells, plants as well as animals. They are present both in cytoplasm as well as in the cell membranes and serve important functions in both cell activity and cell permeability.

The most common phospholipid is the glycerol phospholipids. They contain glycerol phosphate, two fatty acids and a nitrogen compound that may be choline, ethanol amine, or serine. Lecithins and cephalins are examples of phospholipids. Any lipid containing phosphorus is called phospholipids. Phospholipids are good emulsifying agents. They are found in cell membranes and in subcellular structures where lipids and water soluble materials interact Phospholipids are made up of fatty acids, nitrogenous base, phosphoric acid and glycerol or other alcohol. Phospholipids can be classified based on the alcohol moiety of the phospholipid as follows:

- **Glycerophosphatides:** Glycerol is the alcohol moiety in this group. This includes lecithins, cephalins, phosphatidylserine, plasmalogens and diphosphatidylglycerols.
- **Phosphoinositides:** In this, the cyclic hexahydric alcohol "inositol" replaces the nitrogenous base.
- **Sphingolipids:** In this group of substances, glycerol is replaced by a complex amino alcohol "Sphingosine". These are clinically important phospholipids in human.

Biosynthesis of phospholipids: All tissues synthesize phospholipids, but at different rates. In all tissues except liver, phospholipids are synthesized, utilized and degraded in situ; while in liver large proportion of the phospholipids after synthesis is transferred to the plasma and as a matter of fact, liver is practically the sole source of plasma phospholipids.

CONCLUSION

The lipids are a heterogeneous group of compounds, including fats, oils, steroids, waxes, and related compounds, which are related more by their physical than by their chemical properties. Lipids are a class of compounds distinguished by their insolubility in water and solubility in nonpolar solvents. Lipids are important in biological systems because they form the cell membrane, a mechanical barrier that divides a cell from the external environment. Lipids also provide energy for life and several essential vitamins are lipids. Lipids can be divided in two major classes, nonsaponifiable lipids and saponifiable lipids. A nonsaponifiable lipid cannot be broken up into smaller molecules by hydrolysis, which includes triglycerides, waxes, phospholipids, and sphingolipids. A saponifiable lipid contains one or more ester groups allowing it to undergo hydrolysis in the presence of an acid, base, or enzyme. Nonsaponifiable lipids include steroids, prostaglandins, and terpenes. Within these two major classes of lipids, there are several specific types of lipids important to life, including fatty acids, triglycerides, glycerophospholipids, sphingolipids, and steroids.

BIBLIOGRAPHY

1. Eric EC, Stumpf PK, Brueins G, Ray HD. Outlines of Biochemistry. John Wiley & Sons, NY, 1987.
2. Garrette, Grisham. Principles of Biochemistry. Saunders College Publishing, 1994.
3. Lieberman M, Marks AD. Marks 'Basic Medical Biochemistry: A Clinical Approach, 3rd edition. Baltimore: Lippincott Williams & Wilkins, 2009.
4. Thomas MD, Wiley AJ. Text Book of Biochemistry, 4th edition. Inc publication, New York, 1997.
5. Zubay GL. Biochemistry, 4th edition (1988) WMC Brown Publishers, 1994.

REVIEW QUESTIONS

Long Essays

1. Define lipids; explain the biological functions of lipids.
2. Define fatty acids; explain in detail about essential fatty acids.
3. Describe lipid metabolism in detail.
4. Define ketones bodies; explain in detail about diabetic ketoacidosis.
5. Define cholesterol. Explain in detail about metabolism of cholesterol.

Short Essays

1. Properties of lipids.
2. Classify lipids with suitable examples.
3. What are essential and nonessential fatty acids?
4. Write short on importance of cholesterol.
5. Write short note on digestion and absorption of lipids.
6. Functions of essential fatty acids.
7. Lipoproteins.
8. Health significance of cholesterol.
9. Disorders of lipid metabolism.
10. Phospholipids.
11. Steroid hormones.
12. Atherosclerosis.
13. Important derivatives of cholesterol.

Short Answers

1. Enlist four functions of bilirubin.
2. Enlist four functions of lipids.
3. Enlist four functions of bile salts.
4. Enlist four functions of steroid hormones.
5. Enzymes.
6. Emulsification.
7. Lipoproteins.
8. Triacylglycerides.
9. Essential fatty acids.
10. Functions of cholesterol.
11. Gout.
12. Functions of lipid droplets.
13. Oxidation of fatty acids.
14. Biosynthesis of fatty acids.

CHAPTER 18

Proteins

CHAPTER OUTLINE

- Classification of Amino Acids Based on Nutrition, Metabolic Rate with Examples
- Digestion, Absorption and Metabolism of Protein and Related Disorders
- Biologically Important Compounds Synthesized from Various Amino Acids
- In Born Errors of Amino Acid Metabolism—Only Aromatic Amino Acids (in Brief)
- Plasma Protein—Types, Function and Normal Values
- Causes of Proteinuria, Hypoproteinemia, Hypergammaglobulinemia
- Principle of Electrophoresis, Normal and Abnormal Electrophoretic Patterns (in Brief)

TERMINOLOGY

- **Amino acids:** Alpha-amino substituted carboxylic acid, the building blocks of proteins.
- **Aminotransferases:** Enzymes that catalyze the transfer of amino acid groups from alpha-amino to alpha-keto acids, also called transaminases.
- **Transamination:** The transfer of an amino (-NH2) group from an amino acid to keto acid is known as transamination. This reaction involves reversible transfer of an amino group from amino acid to keto acid.
- **Deamination:** Deamination involves removal of amino group from amino acid in the form of NH3. The ammonia liberated is diverted for urea synthesis. The remaining carbon skeleton of amino acid is catabolized to keto acid.
- **Ammonia toxicity:** Brain is very vulnerable to marginal concentration of ammonia. Elevated blood ammonia levels cause blurring of vision and slurring of speech. If nor corrected in time, it may lead to coma or death.
- **Essential amino acids:** Amino acids that cannot by synthesized by humans (and other vertebrates) and must be obtained from the diet.
- **G proteins:** A family of heterotrimeric GTP-binding proteins that act in intracellular signaling pathways. Commonly, ligand binding to a serpentine receptor induces the exchange of GTP for bound GDP, enabling the G protein to activate a downstream enzyme in a signaling pathway. G proteins have intrinsic GTPase activity and therefore can self-inactivate.
- **Urea cycle:** A metabolic pathway in the liver that leads to the syntheses of urea from amino groups and CO_2. The function of the pathway is to convert the ammonia resulting from catabolism to a nontoxic form, which is then secreted.
- **Polypeptide:** A linear polymer of amino acids held together by peptide linkages. The polypeptide has a directional sense, with an amino- and a carboxy-terminal end.
- **Protein kinases:** Enzymes that transfer the terminal phosphoryl group of ATP or another nucleoside triphosphate to a Ser, Thr, Tyr, Asp, or in a target protein, thereby regulating the activity or other properties of that protein.
- **Peptide bond:** A substituted amide linkage between the alpha amino group of one amino acid and the alpha-carboxyl group of another, with the elimination of the elements of water.
- **Peptide:** An organic molecule in which a covalent amide bond is formed between the os-amino group of one amino acid and the a-carboxyl group of another amino acid, with the elimination of a water molecule. The resulting connection is called a peptide bond.

INTRODUCTION

Proteins contain carbon, hydrogen, nitrogen and sulfur as major constituents. Some proteins also contain phosphorus as the chief constituent. Proteins are present as the main constituent of all living matter. Proteins are among the central molecules of biology. In fact, along with nucleic acids, they are the most essential as virtually all the chemical functions of the living cell are performed by protein enzymes (there are minority of RNA-based enzymes also). In addition, most of the scaffoldings that hold cells, chromosomes and other molecules together are made up of proteins. Proteins transmit and commute signals from the external environment to cell interior, duplicate genetic information, transform the energy in light, carryout chemical reactions with tremendous efficiency, transport molecules between cell compartments, etc. In a way proteins constitute the most complex, precise and minute example of nanotechnology known by humans. Proteins are the most perfect nanomachines.

STRUCTURAL ORGANIZATION OF PROTEIN

Sl. No.	Classification	Description
1.	Primary structure of proteins	Primary structure of a protein refers to the order and sequence of amino acid residues $H_2N-CH-CO-NH-CH-CO-NH-CH-CO-NH-CH-$ $\quad\;\; |\qquad\qquad |\qquad\qquad\quad |\qquad\qquad\quad |$ $COOH\;\; R_1\qquad\quad R_2\qquad\qquad R_3\qquad\qquad R_n$
2.	Secondary structure of proteins	Secondary level of protein structure includes folding and twisting patterns of a polypeptide chain. Secondary structure includes a-helix and n-sheet structure. • **Alpha-helix:** Alpha-helix refers to the right handed folding of the protein chain. A coil or helix is formed by twisting the back bone of a polypeptide chain. It is the must stable confirmation of a polypeptide chain, e.g., a keratin. There are 3 to 6 amino acids in one turn. • **Beta structure:** The second regular conformation present in a protein is referred to as 13 structures. This conformation has a pleated edge. Therefore, this conformation is also called as B-pleated sheet structure. 13-sheet orientation is formed due to stretching of the polypeptide chain and forming interchain peptide linkages.
3.	Tertiary structure of proteins	Tertiary structure involves intramolecular folding of the polypeptide chain forming a compact three-dimensional structure which has a specific shape.
4.	Quaternary structure of protein	Multi subunit proteins contain several identical and or different chains where each polypeptide is referred to as a subunit. These polypeptides are associated with a specific geometry. Spatial arrangement of these subunits is referred to as quaternary structure of a protein.

IMPORTANCE OF PROTEIN

Biological Importance

- Some proteins form essential part of a particular structure in the body, e.g., collagen (bone and cartilage) keratins (hair and nail), etc.
- Proteins catalyze biological reactions and act as enzymes such as pepsin
- Protein act as hormones and regulate metabolic processes within the body, e.g., insulin
- Proteins serve as carriers for the transport of substances within the body, e.g., hemoglobin for oxygen (O_2), ceruloplasmin for copper.
- Proteins act as receptors, such as hormone receptors.
- Storage proteins bind a substance for storage in different tissues, e.g., Ferritin stores Fe^{3+}
- Proteins such as X-globulins act as antibodies and provide immunity to the body.

Biochemical Importance

- Proteins are basic constituents of cytoplasm of the cell.
- Proteins are fundamental constituents of the structural and functional organization of the cell.
- Chemically enzymes are proteins.
- Many of the hormones are proteins.
- Proteins play major part in the transport of the O_2 and CO_2 by hemoglobin and special enzymes in red blood cells.
- Proteins, such as thrombin, fibrinogen, etc., participate in the blood clotting as clotting factor.
- Antibodies are proteins by nature, which act as defense against infections.
- Some proteins, such as actin and myosin carry out mechanical work in the muscle.
- A protein rhodopsin of retina carry out function of sensing the light.
- Plasma proteins function in the homeostatic control of the volume of the circulating blood and that of the interstitial fluid.

General Properties of Protein

- Proteins are complex substances of high molecular weight, consisting largely of chains of alpha amino acids, united in peptide linkage. The constituent amino acids may be obtained by hydrolysis of the proteins.
- They contain C, H, O, N and sometimes P and S. Elements, such as Fe: Cu, I and Zn are occasionally present.
- The molecular weight of the proteins varies from 6000 to many millions. Because of the high molecular weight, most proteins are not diffusible through membranes, such as cellophane.
- Proteins are generally soluble in water, weak salt solution, dilute acids and alkalies. Owing to their large size, they form colloidal solution and exhibit the properties associated with the colloidal state of the matter; the number of the molecules occupying a given volume of the solution is lesser. Consequently, properties, such as osmotic pressure, surface tension, viscosity, lowering of the freezing point, rising of the boiling point, become less.
- Proteins possess free ionic or electrically charged groups, so that they can migrate in an electrical field. Owing to their charges, they combine with ionic reagents giving rise to insoluble compounds.
- Proteins are precipitated by salts of heavy metals, such as silver, mercury and lead in an alkaline medium. Here, the metals combine with the carboxyl groups to form metal proteinate. One important application of this property is the use of proteins as antidote in metallic poisoning. Egg white and milk are commonly used, when the metal is precipitated along with the proteins of egg and milk.
- Proteins are precipitated by certain alkaloidal reagents. These are picric acid, trichloroacetic acid, phosphotungstic acid, phosphomolybdic acid and sulfosalicylic acid. Here the proteins react with the NH2 groups.
- Proteins are amphoteric substances because they contain both NH_2 and COOH groups. They can react with acids and bases.
- Some proteins in solution coagulate on heating. They are called heat coagulable proteins; examples are, albumin and globulin.
- **Color reaction:** All proteins give color reaction, when treated with certain reagents. Certain reactive chemical groups, situated in the amino acids and the peptide linkages possessed by all proteins are responsible for the production of the colors.
- Proteins are hydrolyzed to their constituent amino acids by boiling with acids and alkali, and by the action of appropriate proteolytic enzymes.

CLASSIFICATIONS OF PROTEIN

Sl. No.	Classifications	Description
I.	Simple proteins	1. **Albumins:** Blood (serum albumin); milk (lactalbumin); egg white (ovalbumin); lentils (legumelin); kidney beans (phaseolin); wheat (leucosin). Globular protein; soluble in water and dilute salt solution; precipitated by saturation with ammonium sulfate solution; coagulated by heat; found in plant and animal tissues. 2. **Globulins:** Blood (serum globulins); muscle (myosin); potato (tuberin); Brazil nuts (excelsin); hemp (edestin); lentils (legumin). Globular protein; sparingly soluble in water; soluble in neutral solutions; precipitated by dilute ammonium sulfate and coagulated by heat; distributed in both plant and animal tissues.

Contd...

Contd...

Sl. No.	Classifications	Description

		3. **Glutelins:** Wheat (glutenin); rice (oryzenin). Insoluble in water and dilute salt solutions; soluble in dilute acids; found in grains and cereals.
		4. **Prolamins:** Wheat and rye (gliadin); corn (zein); rye (secaline); barley (hordein). Insoluble in water and absolute alcohol; soluble in 70% alcohol; high in amide nitrogen and proline; occurs in grain seeds.
		5. **Protamines:** Sturgeon (sturine); mackerel (scombrine); salmon (salmine); herring. Soluble in water; not coagulated by heat; strongly basic; high in arginine; associate with DNA; occurs in sperm cells.
		7. **Histones:** Thymus gland; pancreas; nucleoproteins (nucleohistone). Soluble in water, salt solutions, and dilute acids; insoluble in ammonium hydroxide; yields large amounts of lysine and arginine; combined with nucleic acids within cells.
		8. **Scleroproteins:** Connective tissues and hard tissues. Fibrous protein; insoluble in all solvents and resistant to digestion.
		   ■ **Collagen:** Connective tissues, bones, cartilage, and gelatin. Resistant to digestive enzymes but altered to digest gelatin by boiling water, acid, or alkali; high in hydroxylamine.
		   ■ **Elastin:** Ligaments, tendons, and arteries. Similar to collagen but cannot be converted to gelatin.
		   ■ **Keratin:** Hair, nails, hooves, horns, and feathers. Partially resistant to digestive enzymes; contains large amounts of sulfur, as cystine.

II.	Conjugated proteins	1. **Nucleoproteins:** Cytoplasm of cells (ribonucleoprotein); nucleus of chromosomes (deoxyribonucleoprotein) viruses, and bacteriophages. Contains nucleic acids, nitrogen, and phosphorus. Present in chromosomes and in all living forms as a combination of protein with either RNA or DNA. 2. **Mucoprotein:** Saliva (mucin); egg white (ovomucoid). Proteins combined with amino sugars, sugar acids, and sulfates. 3. **Glycoprotein:** Bone (osseomucoid); tendons (tendomucoid); cartilage (chondromucoid). Containing more than 4% hexosamine, mucoproteins; if less than 4%, then glycoproteins. 4. **Phosphoproteins:** Milk (casein); egg yolk (ovovitellin). Phosphoric acid joined in ester linkage to protein. 5. **Chromoproteins:** Hemoglobin; myoglobin; flavoproteins; respiratory pigments; cytochromes. Protein compounds with such nonprotein pigments as heme; colored proteins. 6. **Lipoproteins:** Serum lipoprotein; brain, nerve tissues, milk, and eggs. Water-soluble protein conjugated with lipids; found dispersed widely in all cells and all living forms. 7. **Metalloproteins:** Ferritin; carbonic anhydrase; ceruloplasmin. Proteins combined with metallic atoms that are not parts of a nonprotein prosthetic group.
III.	Derived proteins	1. **Proteans:** Edestan (from elastin) and myosan (from myosin). Results from short action of acids or enzymes; insolvent in water. 2. **Proteases:** Intermediate products of protein digestion. Soluble in water; uncoagulated by heat; and precipitated by saturated ammonium sulfate; result from partial digestion of protein by pepsin or trypsin. 3. **Peptones:** Intermediate products of protein digestion. Same properties as proteases except that they cannot be salted out; of smaller molecular weight those proteases. 4. **Peptides:** Intermediate products of protein digestion. Two or more amino acids joined by a peptide linkage; hydrolyzed to individual amino acids.

Color Reaction of Proteins

Proteins give a number of color reactions with reagents because of amino acids present in them.

1. **Biuret test:** When protein solution is made alkaline with NaOH and a drop of dilute $CuSO_4$ is added to it, pink or violet colored complex is formed.
2. **Millon's reactions:** Phenolic compounds, when heated with, mercuric nitrate in nitric acid and traces of nitrous acid, develop a red color. The tyrosine present in protein is responsible for the test.
3. **Sakaguchi reaction:** Guanidines present in arginine in alkaline solution give a red color with α-naphthol and sodium hypochlorite.
4. **Nitroprusside test:** Cysteine gives a red color with sodium nitroprusside in dilute ammoniacal solution.
5. **Folin's reaction:** Amino acids give a red color with sodium 1,2-naphthoquinone-4-sulfonate in alkaline solution.

Amino Acid

Proteins and peptides represent the polymers of alpha-amino acids, which can exist in either dextro (D) or levo (L) form, also known as stereoisomers. Dextro and levo refer to the absolute confirmation of optically active components. Aside from glycine, all other amino acids can be described as mirror images not able to be superimposed.

Amino acid structure

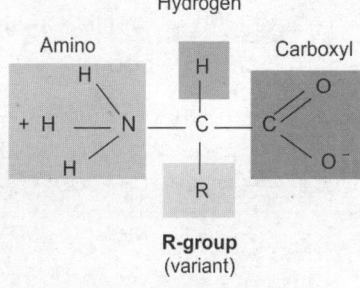

Major part of them, which are found in nature, appear to be of the L-type. That is why eukaryotic proteins turn out to be always composed of levo amino acids, despite the fact that dextro ones can be found in bacterial cell walls and a number of peptide antibiotics. Thus far, more than three hundred kinds of amino acids have been discovered in nature. However, only 20 of them are usually found as compounds of human peptides and proteins. Molecule of an amino acid contains carboxyl (COOH) and amino (NH_2) functional groups, and each molecule features a different side chain, also known as R group, which vary greatly in properties.

$$\text{pK (amino group)} = 9.4 \; H_3N^+ - \underset{\underset{H}{|}}{\overset{\overset{R}{|}}{C}H} - COO^- \; \text{pK (COO}^- \text{group)} = 2.2$$

Classifications of Aminoacids

Experts classify amino acids based on lots of different features. One of them is whether or not people can acquire them through the diet. According to this factor, scientists recognize 3 types—the nonessential, essential, and conditionally essential amino acids. However, the classification as essential or nonessential does not actually reflect their importance, as all twenty of them are necessary for human health. Those 8 called essential (or indispensable) cannot be produced by the body and therefore should be supplied by food—leucine, isoleucine, lysine, threonine, methionine, phenylalanine, valine, and tryptophan. One more amino acid, histidine, can be considered semi-essential, as the human body does not always need dietary sources of it. Meanwhile, conditionally essential amino acids are not usually required in the human diet, but are able to become essential under some circumstances. Finally, nonessential ones are produced by the human body either out of the essential ones or from normal proteins breakdown. These include asparagine, alanine, arginine, aspartic acid, cysteine, glutamic acid, glutamine, praline, glycine, tyrosine, and serine.

One more classification depends on the side chain structure, and experts recognize 5 types in this classification:

1. Containing sulfur (cysteine and methionine)
2. Neutral (asparagine, serine, threonine, and glutamine)
3. Acidic (glutamic acid and aspartic acid) and basic (arginine and lysine)
4. Aliphatic (these include leucine, isoleucine, glycine, valine, and alanine)
5. Aromatic (these include phenylalanine, tryptophan, and tyrosine)

There is another classification based on structure of the side chain that divides the list of twenty into 4 groups, two of which are main groups and two are subgroups—nonpolar, polar, acidic and polar, basic and polar. For example, side chains having pure hydrocarbon alkyl or aromatic groups are considered non-polar, and their list includes phenylalanine, glycine, valine, leucine, alanine, isoleucine, proline, methionine, and tryptophan. Meanwhile, if the side chain contains different polar groups, such as amides, acids, and alcohols, they are classified as polar. Their list includes tyrosine, serine, asparagine, threonine, glutamine, and cysteine. Further classification goes for acidic-polar (includes aspartic acid and glutamic acid), if the side chain has a carboxylic acid, and basic-polar (includes lysine, arginine, and histidine), if the side chain contains an amino group. They are over 300 amino acids occur in nature but 20 amino acid occur only in protein, they classified according to the synthesis by the body into:

- **1-Non-essential amino acids:** Which the body can synthesized alanine, proline, asparagine, aspartic acid, cysteine, tyrosine, serine, glycine, glutamine and glutamic acid.
- **2-Essential amino acids:** Which the body cannot synthesize it. Isoleucine, leucine, lysine, methionine, valine, phenyl alanine, threonine, tryptophan, histidne and arginine.

Physical classification of amino acids:

1. **Hydrophobic:** Alanine, isoleucine, methionine, phenylalanine, proline, tryptophan, tyrosine and valine.
2. **Hydrophilic:** Arginine, asparagine, aspartic acid, cysteine, glutamic acid, glutamine, glycine, histidine, lysine, serine and threonine.

Chemical Structure of Aminoacides

Sl. No.	Types	Description
I.	Aliphatic side chain	**Amino acids with aliphatic side chains:** Structurally simplest amino acids, glycine, alanine, valine, leucine, isoleucine belong to this class. They contain monoamino, monocarboxylic groups. The valine, leucine, isoleucine have branched chains in their structure. Alanine, glycine, isoleucine, leucine, proline and valine
1.	Glycine	$H-CH(NH_3^+)-COO^-$
2.	Alanine	$CH_3-CH(NH_3^+)-COO^-$
3.	Valine	$(H_3C)_2CH-CH(NH_3^+)-COO^-$

Contd...

Contd...

Sl. No.	Types	Description
4.	Leucine	$\begin{array}{c}CH_3\\ \diagdown\\ CH-CH_2-CH-COO^-\\ CH_3\diagup|\\ NH_3^+\end{array}$
5.	Isoleucine	$\begin{array}{c}CH_3\\ |\\ CH_3\\ \diagdown\\ CH-CH-COO^-\\ H_3C\diagup|\\ NH_3^+\end{array}$
II.	**Hydroxy amino acids**	**Hydroxyl group containing amino acids:** Serine, threonine and tyrosine are hydroxyl groups containing amino acids of which tyrosine is also classified under aromatic amino acids.
1.	Serine	$\begin{array}{c}CH_2-CH-COO^-\\ ||\\ OHNH_3^+\end{array}$
2.	Threonine	$\begin{array}{c}H_2C-CH-CH-COO^-\\ ||\\ OHNH_3^+\end{array}$
III.	**Sulfur-containing amino acid:**	**Sulfur-containing amino acids:** Cysteine, cystine and methionine are members of this class. They are characterized by the presence of sulfhydryl, disulfide and thioether group respectively. Amino acid cystine is formed by condensation of two molecules of cistern. Cysteine and methionine
1.	Cysteine	$\begin{array}{c}CH_2-CH-COO^-\\ ||\\ SHNH_3^+\end{array}$
2.	Cystine	$\begin{array}{c}H_2C-CH-COO^-\\ ||\\ SNH_3^+\\ |\\ S\\ |\\ CH_2-CH-COO^-\\ |\\ NH_3^+\end{array}$
3.	Methionine	$\begin{array}{c}CH_2-CH_2-CH-COO^-\\ ||\\ S-CH_3NH_3^+\end{array}$
IV.	**Acidic amino acids**	**Acidic amino acids and their amides:** Aspartic acid and glutamic acid are dicarboxylic monoamino acids. While asparagine and glutamine are respective amines of these dicarboxylic acids. They are acidic amino acids. Aspartic acid and glutamic acid
1.	Aspartic acid	$\begin{array}{c}^-OOC-CH_2-CH-COO^-\\ |\\ NH_3^+\end{array}$
2.	Glutamic acid	$\begin{array}{c}^-OOC-CH_2-CH_2-CH-COO^-\\ |\\ NH_3^+\end{array}$
3.	Glutamine	$\begin{array}{c}H_2N-C-CH_2-CH_2-CH-COO^-\\ \||\\ ONH_3^+\end{array}$
4.	Asparagine	$\begin{array}{c}H_2N-C-CH_2-CH-COO^-\\ \||\\ ONH_3^+\end{array}$
V.	**Basic amino acids**	**Basic amino acids:** Lysine, arginine, histidine are dibasic, monocarboxylic amino acids. Presence of one more amino group makes them basic in nature. Histidine contains imidazole ring. Arginine, histidine and lysine
1.	Lysine	$\begin{array}{c}CH_2-CH_2-CH_2-CH_2-CH-COO^-\\ ||\\ NH_3^+NH_3^+\end{array}$

Contd...

Contd...

Sl. No.	Types	Description
2.	Arginine	NH—CH$_2$—CH$_2$—CH$_2$—CH—COO$^-$ | | O=NH$_2^+$ NH$_3^+$ | NH$_2$
3.	Histidine	(imidazole ring)—CH$_2$—CH—COO$^-$ | NH$_3^+$
VI.	**Aromatic amino acids**	Aromatic amino acids, amino acids phenylalanine, tyrosine and tryptophan are characterized by the presence of aromatic ring. The phenylalanine and tyrosine contain benzene ring and tryptophan contain indole ring. Histidine can be grouped in here. But owing to basic nature, it is also considered under basic amino acids. Phenyl alanine, tryptophan and tyrosine
1.	Phenylalanine	(benzene)—CH$_2$—CH—COO$^-$ | NH$_3^+$
2.	Tyrosine	HO—(benzene)—CH$_2$—CH—COO$^-$ | NH$_3^+$
3.	Tryptophan	(indole)—CH$_2$—CH—COO$^-$ | NH$_3^+$
VII.	**Imino acid**	Imino acids presence of secondary amino group in proline makes it imino acid. Hydroxylation of proline converts it into hydroxyproline. Hydroxyproline is the active component of cross linking of collagen.
1.	Proline	Pro: H$_2$C—CH$_2$ / H$_2$C—N—C—H / COO$^-$ or (pyrrolidine ring)—COO$^-$

Classification of Amino Acids based on Polarity (Chemical Nature)

The nature of R group attached to amino acids determines the polar nature of amino adds. The amino acids may be divided into two broad groups on the basis of polar nature of R groups

- **Non-polar amino acids:** They are also known as hydrophobic or water hating amino acids. The absence of charge on the R groups of these amino acids makes them non-polar amino acids. The amino acids—alanine, leucine, isoleucine, valine, methionine, phenylalanine, tryptophan and proline are members of this group.
- **Polar amino acids:** They are also referred to as hydrophilic amino acids. The amino acids, such as arginine, asparagine, aspartic acid, cysteine, glutamic acid, glutamine, glycine, histidine, lysine, serine, and threonine are in this class of amino acids. These amino acids may contain no-charge on their R groups, e.g., glycine, threonine, etc., or they may contain positive side chains of R groups, e.g., lysine, arginine and histidine. Amino acids, such as aspartic acid and glutamic acids are characterized by negatively charged R side chains.

Propertites of Amino Acids

Amino acids are crystalline solids able to dissolve in water. Meanwhile, they only dissolve sparingly in organic solvents, and the extent of their solubility depends on the size and nature of the side chain. Amino acids feature very high melting points-up to 200–300°C, and other properties vary for each particular amino acid.

I. Physical Properties

- **Solubility:** Most of the amino acids are soluble in water.
- **Melting point:** Amino acids generally melt at higher temperatures, often above 200°C
- **Taste:** Amino acids may be sweet (glycine, alanine, valine) or bitter (argentine, isoleucine)
- **Optical properties:** All the amino acids except glycine possess optical isomers due to the presence of asymmetric carbon atom
- **Amino acids as ampholytes:** Amino acids contain both acidic (-COOH) and basic (-NH2) groups. They can donate a proton or accept a proton; hence amino acids are regarded as ampholytes.

- **Formation of zwitter ions:** On account of the presence of both acidic and basic groups which are readily ionizable, the amino acids behave as 'amphoteric electrolytes' and give both anion and cations in solution (zwitter ions).

Amino acids thus may have either a positive charge or a negative charge. In low pH (acidic) amino acid exists in cationic form (positively charged) while at high pH (strongly alkaline) it exists in anionic form (negatively charged).

$$\text{R-CH-COOH} \underset{}{\overset{H^+}{\longleftrightarrow}} \text{R-CH-COO}^- \underset{}{\overset{H^-}{\longleftrightarrow}} \text{R-CH-COO}^-$$
$$\quad\ \ |\qquad\qquad\qquad\quad |\qquad\qquad\qquad\ \ |$$
$$\quad NH_3^+\qquad\qquad\quad\ \ NH_3\qquad\qquad\quad\ \ NH_2$$
$$\quad \text{Cation}\qquad\qquad\quad \text{Zwitterion}\qquad\qquad\ \text{Anion}$$

II. Chemical Properties Due to Carboxyl

- They can form esters with alcohols or salts with bases.
- With ammonia, they form the corresponding amides, e.g.,
  - Aspartic acid + NH_3 — Asparagine
  - Glutamic acid ± NH_3 — glutamine
- Amino acids undergo decarboxylation to produce corresponding amines, e.g.,
  - Histidine—histamine
  - Tyrosine—tyramine

Due to Amino Group

- They can form salts with acids
- The amino group can be methylated or benzylated.
- Amino acids react with Sanger's reagent [Fluro-2, 4-dinitrobenzene (FDNB)] in an alkaline medium to give colored complex
- Amino acids react with Edman's reagent (phenyliso-thiocyanate) which enables the identification of the N-terminal amino acid.
- **Reaction with ninhydrin:** The α-amino acids react with ninhydrin to form a purple blue or pink color complex
  - Amino acid+ninhydrin— Keto acid + NH_3 + Co_2 + Hydrindantin
  - Hydrindantin + NH_3 + Ninhydrin—Ruhemann's purple
- **Oxidative deamination:** The amino acids undergo oxidative deamination to liberate free ammonia, e.g., glutamate→α-Ketoglutarate + NH_3
- Formation of a peptide bond

Functions of Amino Acids

Most amino acids are available in a balanced diet. But an imbalanced diet can lead to a deficiency in one of these essential nutrients. Vegetarians must make an extra effort to consume the necessary balance of grains and legumes to avoid a deficiency. Each essential amino acid must be consumed every day. Unlike other nutrients and fats, the body does not store amino acids. If one of the essential amino acids is missing, then proteins do not function properly.

Amino acid is the building unit of protein, which have important role in our body because—1-Amino acids used to compose antibodies which have role in immune system against microbial infection, 2-Amino acids used to regulate cell growth and bio-synthesis of purine and pyrimidine (this compounds have role in DNA synthesis)

I. Functions served by intact amino acid

- *Synthesis of cell protoplasm:* Amino acids are necessary to build up living cells, since proteins are main and essential constituents of them.
- *Taking up wear and tear:* Amino acids repair the damaged parts when tissue proteins break down during metabolism.
- *Storage of protein:* In adult/elderly people, protein breakdown exceeds protein synthesis; proteins cannot be stored when nitrogen equilibrium is established. But they can be stored in active/growing age, when protein synthesis exceeds protein breakdowns.
- *Essential amino acids:* There are some amino acids, which cannot be synthesized in the body, but are essential for growth and maintenance of life.
- *Other synthesis process:* Amino acids help in synthesis of bile acids, plasma proteins, hemoglobin, hormones, enzymes, milk proteins in lactating mothers, glutathione and cytochrome, purine and pyrimidine, melanin, antibodies, and formation of rhodypsin and urea. When the above functions are served by the amino acids in tact form, to the required stage, the surplus amounts of amino acids break down and undergo the following next group of functions.

II. Functions of amino acids while breaking down

- *Supply of energy:* Amino acids liberate energy on break down at the rate of 4.3 Calories per gram of protein.
- *Dynamic action:* Amino Acids while breaking down, excret a specific stimulating action to the extent of about 30% on tissue metabolism.
- *Deamination:* During deamination under the influence of certain enzymes, the amino acid losses its radicle, into nitrogenous part and non-nitrogenous part, each of which perform separate function.

The nitrogenous part, ammonia, a large part (80%) of it is converted to urea, and the smaller part combines with acids to form ammonium salts. It is also utilized for the synthesis of simple amino acids, such as glycine, alanine, glutamic acid; and some nitrogenous substances, such as creation, purine, uric acid, pyrimidine, lecithin, etc. The non-nitrogenous residues are utilized as carbohydrates, and some also get broken down as fatty acids in the body. It sulfur and phosphorus components get converted into their compounds before excretion.

Digestion and Absorption of Proteins

Protein digestion begins in the stomach. Gastric juice produced by stomach contains Hcl and protease proenzyme pepsinogen. I-Id—the pH of the stomach is less than 2.0 due to the presence of Hcl, secreted by parietal cells of gastric gland. The acid performs 2 important functions—denaturation of proteins and killing of certain micro organisms. The denatured proteins are more susceptible to proteases for digestion. Pepsin is produced by the serous cells of the stomach as pepsinogen. Pepsinogen is converted to active pepsin by gastric Hcl. Pepsin is an acid-stable endopeptidase optimally active at a very low pH (2.0) acids. Pepsin digestion of proteins results in peptides and a few amino.

- **Digestion of proteins by pancreatic protease:** The proteases of pancreatic juice are secreted as zyogens and then converted to active forms. The processes are initiated by the release of 2 polypeptide hormones cholecystokinin and secretin from the intestine. The key enzyme for the activation of zymogen is enteropeptidase produced by intestinal mucosal epithelial cells. Enteropeptidase converts trypsinogen to trypsin. Trypsin is a common activator of all other pancreatic zymogens to produce active proteases, namely—chymotrypsin, elastase and carboxypeptidases. Specificity of pancreatic proteases trypsin, chymotrypsin and elastase are endopeptidases active at neutral pH. Gastric Hcl is neutralized by pancreatic $NaHCO_3$ in the intestine and this creates favorable pH for the action of proteases.
- **Action of carboxypeptidases:** The pancreatic carboxypeptidase's are metalloenzymes that are dependent on Zn 2+ for their catalytic activity. The combined action of pancreatic proteases results in the formation of free amino acids and small peptides (2–8 amino acids)
- **Digestion of proteins by small intestinal enzymes:** The luminal surface of intestinal epithelial cells contains aminopeptidases and dipeptidases. Aminopeptidases repeatedly cleaves N-terminal amino acid one by one to produce free amino acid and smaller peptides. The dipeptidases act on different dipeptides to liberate amino acids.

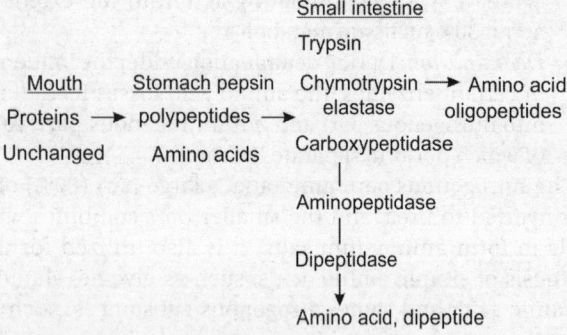

- **Absorption of amino acids and dipeptides:** The free amino acids, dipeptides and to some extent tripeptides are absorbed by intestinal epithelial cells. The di and tripeptides after being absorbed are hydrolysed into free amino acids in the cytosol of epithelial cells. The small intestine possesses an efficient system to absorb free amino acids. L-amino acids are more rapidly absorbed than D-amino acids.

Mechanism of Amino Acid Absorption

Amino acids are primarily absorbed by a similar mechanism as for the transport of glucose. It is basically a Na^{2+} dependent active process linked with the transport of Na^{2+}. As the Na^+ diffuses along with the concentration gradient amino acid also enters the intestinal cell. Both Na^+ and amino acids share a common carrier and transported together. The energy is supplie1 individually by ATP.

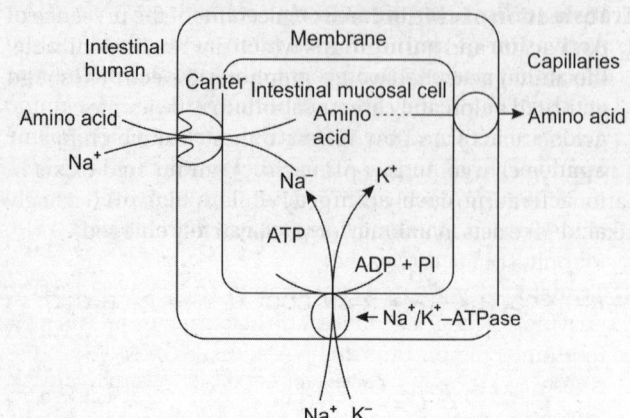

Absorption of intact proteins and polypeptides: For a short period, immediately after birth, the small intestine of infants can absorb intact proteins and polypeptides. The uptake of proteins occurs by a process called as endocytosis or pinocytosis. The direct absorption of intact proteins is very important for the transfer of maternal immunoglobulins to the off spring. The intact proteins and polypeptides are not absorbed by the adult intestine.

Biosynthesis of Protein

The biosynthesis of protein molecules in the cell by sequential addition of various amino acids using peptide bond is called protein synthesis.

The amino acids are linked together in succession to produce a linear polypeptide chain. The polypeptide chain is a unit of a protein molecule.

- **Protein biosynthesis:** In a protein molecule amino acids are joined together by peptide bonds. In the process of protein synthesis also known as translation of mRNA, the amino acids are added sequentially in a specific number. The protein synthesizing mechanism involves the following steps:
  a. **Transcription:** The formation of RNA complementary to a DNA strand is called transcription. In this process, the RNAs required for protein synthesis are synthesized on DNA strands. This reaction is catalyzed by the enzyme RNA polymerase. The enzyme, RNA polymerase I, II, III are involved in the synthesis of rRNA (ribosomal RNA) mRNA (messenger RNA) and tRNA (transfer RNA) respectively in the eukaryotes. In prokaryotes only one type of:
  RNA polymerase is present to synthesize all the three classes of RNA. In the DNA double helix, one of the strands serves as a template to produce RNA. The RNA produced by transcription is inactive and is called pre-RNA. They become active after further processing. All these RNA are processed through chemical reactions and structural modifications.
  b. **Translation:** Translation is a process by which the base sequence of DNA transcribed to the mRNA is interpreted into amino acid sequence of a polypeptide chain.

Translation involves the following steps:
1. **Activation of amino acid:** Amino acids, the building blocks of proteins, are present in the cytoplasm. They are activated before they are transported by tRNA. The amino acids are activated by ATP with the help of the enzyme amino acyl synthetase. Amino acyl synthetase is specific in activating each amino acid. The activated amino acid is called amino acyl adenylate or amino acyl AMP. Pyrophosphate is released.
2. **Transfer of activated amino acid to tRNA:** The same enzyme that activates the amino acid catalyses its transfer to a molecule of transfer RNA at the 3' hydroxyl of the ribose, an ester with a high potential for group transfer. In this reaction, AMP and the enzyme amino acyl synthetase are released.
3. **Initiation of polypeptide chain:** Protein synthesis is initiated by the selection and transfer of the first amino acid into ribosomes. This process requires ribosome subunits, amino acyl tRNA complex, mRNA and initiation factors (IF). Initiation of polypeptide chain involves the following steps.
   a. The 30s ribosomal subunit attaches to the 5¢ end of the mRNA to form an mRNA 30s complex. This process requires the initiation factor IF-3 and Mg2+ ions. The attachment is made at the first codon of the mRNA.
   b. The first codon of mRNA will be always AUG. This codon specifies the amino acid methionine. So the first amino acid in the synthesis of any polypeptide chain is methionine.
   c. The tRNA having the anticodon UAC (complementary to AUG) transports methionine to the 30s ribosome and attaches itself to the initiation codon on mRNA. The tRNA, mRNA and 30s ribosome subunit form a complex called 30s-preinitiation complex. This process requires initiation factors and GTP.
   d. 30s-preinitiation complex joins with 50s ribosomal subunit to form initiation complex. The initiation complex is formed of 70s ribosome, mRNA and met-RNA (methionine RNA).
   e. The 70s ribosome has two slots for the entry of amino acyl tRNA, namely—P site (peptidyl site) and A site (amino acid site). The first tRNA, i.e., met RNA is attached to the P site of 70s ribosome.
4. **Elongation of polypeptide chain:** Elongation refers to sequential addition of amino acids to methionine, as per the sequence of codon in the mRNA. It involves the following steps:
   a. The second codon in the mRNA is recognized and as per the recognition, the Aminoacyl-tRNA containing the corresponding anticodon moves to the 70s ribosome and fits into the A-site. Here the anticodon of tRNA base pairs with the second codon of mRNA.
   b. A peptide bond is formed between the carboxyl group of first amino acid of site P and the amino group of second amino acid of A-site. The peptide bond links two amino acids to form a dipeptide. The bonding is catalyzed by the enzyme peptidyl transferase, which is present in 50s ribosomal subunit.
   c. After the formation of peptide bond, the methionine and tRNA are separated by an enzyme called tRNA deacylase.
   d. The dissociated tRNA is then released from P-site into the cytoplasm for further amino acylation.
   e. Now the ribosome moves on the mRNA in the 5'®3' direction so that the first codon goes out of ribosome, the second codon comes to lie in the P-site from A-site and the third codon comes to lie in the A-site. Simultaneously, the second tRNA is shifted from A-site to P-site. All these events, the movement of ribosome, the release of first tRNA from P-site and shifting of second tRNA from A-site to P-site constitute **translocation**. Translocation is catalyzed by the enzyme **translocase**.
   f. The third codon is recognized and the aminoacyl-tRNA containing the corresponding anticodon moves to the 70s ribosome and fits into the A-site. The anticodon base pairs with the codon. A peptide bond is formed between the third amino acid of site-A and the second amino acid of the dipeptide present in the P-site. Thus a tripeptide is formed.
   g. The amino acids are added one by one as per the codon in the mRNA and hence the tripeptide is converted into polypeptide chain.
   The polypeptide chain elongates by the addition of more and more amino acids.
   h. The elongation of polypeptide chain is brought about by a number of protein factors called elongation factors.
5. **Termination of polypeptide chain:** Termination is the completion of polypeptide chain. By termination, a polypeptide chain is finished and released. The polypeptide chain is **completed, when the ribosome reaches the 3¢ end of mRNA.**
   - The 3' end contains stop codons or termination codons. They are UAG or UAA or UGA. Termination is helped by the terminating protein factors. The terminated polypeptide chain is released from the ribosome.
   - After the release of polypeptide chain, the 70s unit dissociates into 50s and 30s subunits. These subunits are again used in the formation of another initiation complex.
   - The polypeptide chain released after translation is inactive. It is processed to make it active. In the processing, the initiating amino acid methionine is removed. Along with methionine a few more amino acids are removed from the N-terminal of the polypeptide. The processing is carried out by deformylase and amino peptidase. This processing is called as post translational modifications.

Protein Metabolism

The ingested proteins are metabolized to amino acids by peptide bond cleaving enzymes known as proteinases.

General reactions of amino acids: The general reactions of amino acids include deamination, transamination and decarboxylation. The reactions of deamination and transamination bring about the formation of keto acids which can undergo a further series of changes. Inter-conversion between keto acids and amino acids results in the synthesis of many nutritionally non-essential amino acids. These provide for the synthesis of protein and important non-protein nitrogenous materials. During protein synthesis, the amino acids are absorbed from the blood, as the liver does not store them.

Catabolism of amino acids: Although each amino acid follows its own specific metabolic pathway, a few general reactions are found to be common in the catabolism of nearly all the amino acids. Most of the amino acids are converted to a-keto acids by the removal of nitrogen in the form of ammonia which is quickly transformed into urea or it gets incorporated into some other amino acids.

- **Oxidative deamination:** Deamination means removal of the amino groups from amino acids. This is the mechanism where in the amino acids lose two hydrogen atoms (dehydrogenation) to form keto acids and ammonia.

  Oxidative deamination is accompanied by oxidation and is catalyzed by specific amino acid oxidases or more appropriately, dehydrogenases present in liver and kidneys. The process of oxidative deamination takes place in two steps.

  The first step is oxidation (dehydrogenation) of amino acid resulting in the formation of imino acid. The imino acid then undergoes the second step, namely hydrolysis which results in a keto acid and ammonia.

  The first reaction is catalyzed by amino acid oxidase (also called dehydrogenase) and the coenzyme FAD or FMN takes up the hydrogen.

  There are two types of amino acid oxidases depending upon the substrate, on which they act, namely,
  a. L-amino acid oxidases which act on L-amino acids (FMN acts as coenzyme).
  b. D-amino acid oxidases which act on D-amino acids (FAD acts as coenzyme).

  FMN occurs only in the liver and kidney and FAD occurs in all animal tissues. The major site of oxidative deamination is liver but kidney and other tissues also have a role.

  The oxidative deamination of L-glutamic acid is an exceptional case where the deamination needs not only the zinc-containing enzyme L-glutamic acid dehydrogenase but also NAD^+ or $NADP^+$ as coenzymes.

- **Transamination:** The process of transfer of an amino group from an amino acid to an α-keto acid, resulting in the formation of a new amino acid and keto acid is known as transamination. In other words, it is deamination of an amino acid, coupled with amination of a keto acid.

  Transamination is catalyzed by transaminases or aminotransferases with pyridoxal phosphate functioning as coenzyme. There are two active transaminases in tissues, catalyzing interconversions. They are:
  a. Aspartate aminotransferase (AST) is also known as glutamate-oxaloacetate transaminase (GOT)
  b. Alanine aminotransferase (ALT) is also known as Glutamate-pyruvate transaminase (GPT)

- **Decarboxylation:** This refers to the removal of CO_2 from the carboxyl group of amino acids. The removal of CO_2 needs the catalytic action of enzymes decarboxylases and the pyridoxal phosphate coenzyme. The enzymes act on amino acids resulting in the formation of the corresponding amines with the liberation of CO_2.

  There are several amino acid decarboxylases found in various tissues, such as liver, kidney, intestine, spleen, lung and brain. They convert the amino acids into the respective amines and liberate CO_2. For example, histidine is converted to histamine by the action of histidine decarboxylase.

  The amino acid tryptophan is converted to tryptamine, tyrosine to tyramine, etc. Such amines are called biogenic amines which are physiologically important.

- **Transmethylation:** The transfer of methyl group from one compound to another is called transmethylation and the enzymes involved in the transfer are known as transmethylases.

  Transfer of methyl group usually involves methionine (amino acid containing methyl group). By this process various important, physiologically active compounds, such as epinephrine, creatine, thymine and choline are synthesized in the body. Detoxification of certain toxic substances are also carried out by this process (e.g., nicotinic acid is detoxified by methionine into a nontoxic methyl derivative namely N-methyl nicotinamide). Methionine is a principal methyl donor. It has to be activated by ATP which requires a methionineactivation enzyme of liver, known as methionine glutamate-oxaloacetate adenosyltransferase. By the action of this enzyme, methionine is converted to active methionine.

  The active methionine thus formed is known as S-adenosyl methionine and in the activation reaction, ATP transfers its adenosine moiety to methionine and loses three molecules of phosphate, one as orthophosphate (Pi) and two as pyrophosphate (PPi).
  - Active Methionine + Norepinephrine—Epinephrine
  - Active Methionine + Nictoinamide—N-methyl nicotinamide
  - Active Methionine + Uracil—Thymine
  - Active Methionine + Guanidinoacetate—Creatine
  - (Methyl group donor) (Methyl group acceptor)
  - Active methionine contains S-methyl bond which is a high energy bond and hence methyl group is liable and can be easily transferred to a methyl group acceptor

- **Catabolism of the carbon skeleton of amino acids:** The carbon skeletons left behind after deamination are identified as a-keto acids. They may take any one of the following pathways:
  - **Synthesis of amino acids:** They may get reductively aminated by reversal of transdeamination or undergo transamination to form once again the original amino acids.
  - **Glucogenic pathway:** The keto acids of some amino acids may get converted to the intermediates of carbohydrate metabolism, such as α-keto glutarate, oxaloacetate, pyruvate, fumarate and succinyl CoA and hence could be converted to glucose and glycogen

and these amino acids are said to by glucogenic amino acids.

The pathways of three important glucogenic amino acids are shown below. Though the routes vary with each amino acid, they all converge at the stage of pyruvic acid.

Glucogenic amino acids constitute more than 50% of the amino acids, derived from animal protein. The process of conversion of the keto acids of glucogenic amino acids to carbohydrate metabolites is known as gluconeogenesis.

- **Ketogenic pathway:** The keto acids formed from the deamination of certain amino acids are closely related to fats rather than carbohydrates. They metabolise to form acetyl CoA or acetoacetyl CoA or acetoacetate (ketone bodies) which are the intermediates of fatty acid metabolism and not glucose and this amino acid are said to be ketogenic amino acids.

Ketogenic amino acids constitute only a minority and follow specialized and complex pathways. Examples are leucine, isoleucine, phenylalanine and tyrosine. Among these, leucine is purely ketogenic, whereas the other three amino acids are both ketogenic and glucogenic.

Urea Cycle

Living organisms excrete the excess nitrogen resulting from the metabolic breakdown of amino acids in one of three ways. Many aquatic animals simply excrete ammonia. Where water is less, plentiful processes have evolved that convert ammonia to less toxic waste products which require less water for excretion. One such product is urea, which is excreted by most terrestrial vertebrates; another is uric acid, which is excreted by birds and terrestrial reptiles.

Accordingly, living organisms are classified as being ammonotelic (ammonia excreting), urotelic (urea excreting) and uricotelic (uric acid excreting). Some animals can shift from ammonotelism to ureotelism or uricotelism if their water supply becomes restricted.

Urea is synthesized in the liver by the enzymes of the urea cycle. It is then secreted into the blood stream and sequestered by the kidneys for excretion in the urine.

The urea cycle reactions were elucidated by Hans Krebs and Kurt Henseleit. This cycle starts with the amino acid ornithine. The cycle is confined only to the mitochondria and cytoplasm of the cells of liver and it is found that the enzyme, arginase which is required in the final step of urea formation is present only in the liver and absent in all the other tissues. Urea cycle occurs partially in the mitochondria and partially in the cytosol with ornithine and citrulline being transported across the mitochondrial membrane by specific membrane systems. The following are the various reactions in the process of urea formation

- **Carbamoyl phosphate formation:** Carbamoyl phosphate synthetase catalyses the condensation and activation of NH^{4+} and HCO_3^- to form carbamoyl phosphate.
- **Citrulline formation from ornithine:** Ornithine transcarbamylase transfers the carbamoyl group of carbamoyl phosphate to ornithine, yielding citrulline the reaction occurs in the mitochondria so that ornithine, which is produced in the cytosol, must enter the mitochondria via a specific transport system. Likewise, since the remaining urea cycle reactions occur in the cytosol, citrulline must be transported from the mitochondria Citrulline undergoes condensation with amino group of aspartate to form arigininosuccinate this reaction requires ATP, Mg^{2+} and the enzyme argininosuccinate synthetase.
- **Formation of arginine and fumarate:** The enzyme argininosuccinase catalyses the elimination of arginine from the aspartate carbon skeleton forming fumarate.
- **Formation of urea:** The fifth and the final reaction in the urea cycle is the hydrolysis of arginine by the enzyme arginase to yield urea and ornithine. Ornithine is then returned to the mitochondria for another round of the cycle.

Formation of Nicin

Niacin is pyridine 3-carboxylic acid. Nicotinamide or niacinamide is the amide of nicotinic acid. It derives its name from nicotine, from which it can be prepared by oxidation. In tissues, it is present as nicotinamide which is the physiologically active form. Nicotinamide, the active component in NAD^+ and $NADP^+$. Niacin is synthesized in the body from tryptophan, an essential amino acid. Administration of tryptophan or proteins rich in tryptophan is followed by increased excretion of niacin metabolites. Diets deficient in tryptophan produce a deficiency of niacin in the body. The following scheme has been proposed by Hayaishi and others for the conversion of tryptophan into niacin in liver.

Formation of Melanin

The melanins, the pigments of skin and hair are complex polymers in which a major constituent is formed from tyrosine via dihydroxyphenylalanine (DOPA). The formation of melanins from tyrosine, which occurs in animals, plants and certain bacteria (*B. niger*), is due to the action of polyphenol oxidases or tyrosinases. Tyrosinase, is a copper containing mixed function oxidase that carries out a tricky sequence.

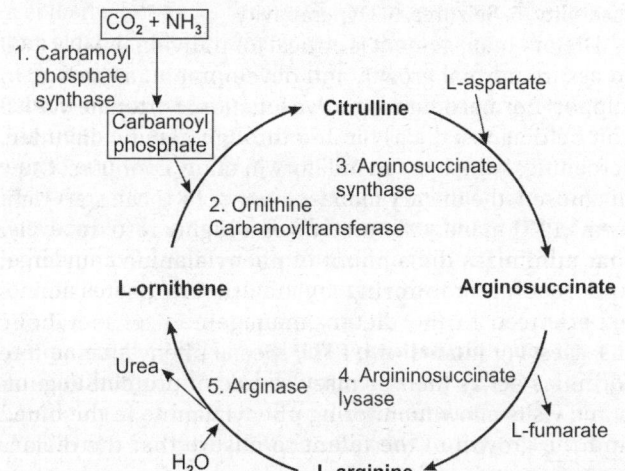

While the melanins of human beings are derived from tyrosine through DOPA, most polyhydroxy phenyl and aminophenyl compounds having ortho or para groups can be oxidized to pigmented polymers and the type of melanin is best shown by indicating the substance from which the melanin is formed. Thus, we may have dopa-melanin, adrenaline-melanin, homogentisic acid—melanin, p-phenylenediamine melanin, etc.

Melanin forms a reversible oxidation—reduction system, in which the reduced and the oxidized form is black. Melanins appear in tissues as regular, spheroid granules and represent formed elements rather than precipitated aggregates. Melanins are produced in pigment—forming cells, the melanocytes, and their formation is stimulated by adrenal cortical and especially pituitary hormones.

Formation of Thyroid Hormone

The thyroid gland is a bilobed organ in the anterior portion of the neck. Thyroid gland in normal adult weighs 20–25 g. Thyroxine the hormone is secreted by this gland. Thyroxine is stored in the colloid of the thyroid follicles, a form of glycoprotein called thyroglobulin. Hydrolysis of thyoglobulin yields monoiodotyrosine, diiodotyrosine, triiodotyrosine and thyroxine. Of these, triiodothyroxine is considered to possess a biological potency greater than thyroxine.

Thyroxine is synthesized in thyroid gland from tyrosine. First inorganic iodide is oxidized to organic iodide (2I I2). Tyrosine is iodinated in the third position to form 3-monoiodotyrosine. The next iodination occurs in the fifth position to form 3,5-diiodotyrosine. Two molecules of diiodotyrosine couple to form a mole of tetra iodotyrosine which is thyroxine. Alanine is liberated.

Synthesis of thyroxine is accelerated by thyroid stimulating hormone (TSH) and inhibited by antithyroid drugs, such as thiocarbamides and amino benzenes. Thyroid has the capacity of trapping inorganic iodine from circulation and storing it for utilization in the synthesis of thyroxine and its precursors. Depending upon the need for thyroxine and its iodinated derivatives, a proteolytic enzyme hydrolyses thyroglobulin, under the stimulating influence of TSH.

Formation of Catecolamines

The adrenal glands in the human adult are situated close to the upper pole of the kidneys and average 45 x 26 x 6 mm in size and weighs about 10 g each. The adrenal gland is divided into two distinct portions—the medulla and cortex. Catecholamines are secreted from the medullary portion of the adrenal gland.

These two hormones, belonging to the catecholamine class of organic compounds, have potent biological activity in both metabolic and physiologic regulations. Epinephrine regulates carbohydrate metabolism, it has the effect of causing liver and muscle glycogenolysis, hyperglycemia and glucosuria. The hormone causes increased oxygen consumption, its effect being more rapid from that of thyroxine. Nor epinephrine causes increase in blood pressure by causing an increase in peripheral resistance. The hormone has, however, little effect on carbohydrate metabolism. Tyrosinegets converted to form norepinephrine and epinephrine.

- Tyrosine is first hydroxylated to 3, 4-dihydroxyphenylalanine (DOPA) by a specific enzyme. DOPA is an intermediate which is common to the synthesis of both epinephrine and melanin.
- DOPA is next decarboxylated to dopamine by a decarboxylase in the presence of pyridoxal phosphate.
- Next dopamine isoxidised toyield norepinephrine. There action is catalyzed by dopamine hydroxylase and ascorbic acid
- Methylation of norepinephrine in the medulla gives rise to epinephrine. The methyl group is derived from S-adenosylmethionine.

Protein Metabolism Disorders

Protein is a key constituent of most foods we eat, including meat, beans, milk products and grains. Infants with protein metabolism disorders cannot drink human milk because it also contains proteins and amino acids that cannot be metabolized. Infants with protein metabolism disorders are unable to metabolize certain amino acids and require specialized formulas without the offending amino acid, allowing the baby to receive essential nutrients for growth. Examples of protein metabolism disorders include:

- Phenylketonuria (PKU)
- Maple syrup urine disease (MSUD)
- Tyrosinemia
- Homocystinuria

Phenylketonuria (PKU)

Phenylketonuria, often referred to as PKU, is one of the most common protein metabolism disorders. Normally, the human body metabolizes the essential amino acid phenylalanine into tyrosine. Infants with PKU do not have the enzyme needed to make this conversion. Consequently, their bodies have excess amounts of phenylalanine and low tyrosine levels. The following symptoms may result from untreated PKU:

1. Lethargy, 2. Light pigment, 3. Eczema, 4. Intellectual disability, 5. Seizures, 6. Hyperactivity

Dietary management is critical for individuals with PKU to assure normal growth and development, as well as to support normal neurocognitive function. Fortunately, PKU can be diagnosed early in life through genetic disorders screenings, which are mandatory in many countries. Once diagnosed, the dietary management of PKU can start right away. PKU management involves a highly restrictive diet that minimizes the amount of phenylalanine consumed and regular monitoring by healthcare professionals experienced in the dietary management of metabolic diseases. For infants with PKU, special phenylalanine-free formulas act as their primary source of protein. Regular clinic visits allow monitoring phenylalanine in the blood and the growth of the infant to ensure that the dietary management is successful.

Maple Syrup Urine Disease (MSUD)

MSUD is a potentially deadly disorder that affects the way the body breaks down three amino acids, leucine, isoleucine, and valine. When they are not being used to build a protein, these three amino acids can be either be recycled or broken down and used for energy. They are normally broken down by six proteins that act as a team and form a complex called BCKD (branched-chain alpha-ketoacid dehydrogenase).

People with MSUD have a mutation that results in a deficiency for one of the 6 proteins that make up this complex. Therefore, they cannot break down leucine, isoleucine, and valine. They end up with dangerously high levels of these amino acids in their blood, causing the rapid degeneration of brain cells and death if left untreated. Defects in any of the six subunits that make up the BCKD protein complex can cause the development of MSUD. The most common defect is caused by a mutation in a gene on chromosome 19 that encodes the alpha subunit of the BCKD complex (BCKDHA). There is a classic form of MSUD and several less common forms. Each form varies in its severity and characteristic features. However, all subtypes of the disorder can be caused by mutations in any of the 6 genes used to build the BCKD protein complex.

A baby who has the disorder may appear normal at birth. But within three to four days, the symptoms appear. These may include—loss of appetite, fussiness, and sweet-smelling urine. The elevated levels of amino acids in the urine generate the smell, which is reminiscent of maple syrup. This is how MSUD got its name. If left untreated, the condition usually worsens. The baby will have seizures, go into a coma, and die within the first few months of life.

Treatment involved dietary restriction of the amino acids leucine, isoleucine, and valine. This treatment must begin very early to prevent brain damage. Babies with the disease must eat a special formula that does not contain the amino acids leucine, isoleucine, and valine. As the person grows to adulthood, he/she must always watch their diet, avoiding high protein foods, such as meat, eggs, and nuts. If levels of the three amino acids still get too high, patients can be treated with an intravenous (given through a vein) solution that helps the body use up excess leucine, isoleucine, and valine for protein synthesis. Gene therapy is also a potential future treatment for patients with MSUD. This would involve replacing the mutated gene with a good copy, allowing the patient's cells to generate a functional BCKD protein complex and break down the excess amino acids.

Tyrosinemia

Elevated blood tyrosine levels are associated with several clinical entities. The term tyrosinemia was first given to a clinical entity based on observations (e.g., elevated blood tyrosine levels) that have proven to be common to various disorders, including transient tyrosinemia of the newborn (TTN), hereditary infantile tyrosinemia (tyrosinemia I), Richner-Hanhart syndrome (tyrosinemia II), and tyrosinemia III. In addition, a mysterious entity called tyrosinosis has been described once in the literature. This designation was chosen at a time when specific enzymatic diagnosis was unavailable; leaving a clinical description that has not been duplicated in the 50 years since its publication. Transient tyrosinemia is believed to result from delayed enzyme maturation in the tyrosine catabolic pathway. This condition is essentially benign and spontaneously disappears with no sequelae. Transient tyrosinemia is not categorized as an inborn error of metabolism because it is not caused by a genetic mutation. Hereditary infantile tyrosinemia, or tyrosinemia I, is a completely different disease. Patients have a peculiar (cabbage-like) odor, renal tubular dysfunction (Fanconi syndrome), and survival of less than 12 months of life if untreated. Fulminant onset of liver failure occurs in the first few months of life.

For many years, the diagnosis was based on the observation that plasma tyrosine and methionine levels were significantly elevated. Postmortem examination revealed that both the liver and the kidney had a highly unusual pattern of nodular cirrhosis, the histopathologic hallmark of the disease. In the early 1970s, researchers discovered that most severe liver diseases caused such findings regardless of etiology, and, in the late 1970s, the biochemical and enzymatic causes of the disease were reported. Tyrosinemia II is a disease with a clinical presentation distinctly different from that described above. This presentation includes herpetiform corneal ulcers and hyperkeratotic lesions of the digits, palms, and soles, as well as mental retardation. Tyrosinemia III is an extremely rare cause of intermittent ataxia, without hepatorenal involvement or skin lesions, and is also not discussed further in this article.

Homocystinuria

Homocystinuria is an inherited disorder that affects the metabolism of the amino acid methionine. Homocystinuria is inherited in families as an autosomal recessive trait. This means that the child must inherit the non-working gene from both parents to be seriously affected. Homocystinuria has several features in common with Marfan syndrome. Unlike Marfan syndrome, in which the joints tend to be "loose," in homocystinuria the joints tend to be "tight." Newborn infants appear healthy. Early symptoms, if present at all, are not obvious. Symptoms may occur as mildly delayed development or failure to thrive. Increasing visual problems may lead to diagnosis of this condition. Other symptoms include—chest deformities, flush across the cheeks, intellectual disability, long limbs, mental disorders, nearsightedness, spidery fingers, tall, thin build There is no cure for homocystinuria. However, just under half of people respond to high doses of vitamin B6 (also known as pyridoxine). Those who do respond will need to take vitamin B6 supplements for the rest of their lives. Those who do not respond will need to eat a low-methionine diet. Most will need to be treated with trimethylglycine (a medication also known as betaine). Neither a low-methionine diet nor medication will improve existing intellectual disability. Medication and diet should be closely supervised by a physician who has experience treating homocystinuria. Taking a folic acid supplement and adding cysteine (an amino acid) to the diet are helpful

Non-protein Nitrogenous Substances

NPN: Nonprotein nitrogen is nitrogen in the blood that is not a constituent of protein, e.g., nitrogen associated with urea, uric acid, creatine, creatinine and polypeptides. NPN substances in urine are urea, creatine, creatinine, uric acid, amino acids, allantoin and hippuric acid.

- **Urea:** About 25 to 30 g of urea is excreted daily in urine. As urea is the end product of protein metabolism, urea excretion in urine is an index of protein intake in diet. Urea in urine is increased in exaggerated protein metabolism, fevers and increased adrenocortical activity. It is decreased in the last stages of severe hepatic diseases and in acidosis. Urea can be detected by sodium hypobromide test, where it undergoes decomposition to nitrogen on being exposed to the reagent and a brisk effervescence ensues.
- **Sodium hypobromide test:** Add about 5 drops of sodium hypobromide solution to a test tube containing about 5 mL of the sample urine and note the brisk effervescence of the liberated nitrogen gas. Urease test—the enzyme urease converts the urea into ammonia and carbonic acid both of which react with each other to form ammonium carbonate under experimental conditions. This results in an alkaline solution that can be detected by the addition of phenolphthalein indicator when a pink color is produced.
- **Procedure:** Label two test tubes as "test' and "control" containing 5 mL of urine in each. Add 2 mL of urease suspension to the test tube marked as "test" and 2 mL of inactivated urease suspensions to the test tube marked "control".

Incubate both the test tubes at room temperature for 15 minutes and then add 2 drops of phenolphthalein indicator solution to each test tube. Pink color will be produced in the test tube having active enzyme.

Uric acid: It is derived as an end product of the breakdown of cellular nucleoproteins. The daily excretion is 0.6 to 1 g. An increase in the excretion of uric acid is observed in leukemia, in severe liver disease and in various stages of gout. Deposits of urates and uric acid in the joints and tissues are also characteristics of gout, so that this disease appears to be a form of arthritis.

CONCLUSION

Twenty percent of the human body is made up of proteins. Proteins are the large, complex molecules that are critical for normal functioning of cells. They are essential for the structure, function, and regulation of the body's tissues and organs. Proteins are made up of smaller units called amino acids, which are building blocks of proteins. They are attached to one another by peptide bonds forming a long chain of proteins. Proteins are the agents of biological functions, virtually occurring in every cellular activity in the form of enzymes, regulatory proteins, transport proteins, storage proteins, contractile and motile proteins, structural proteins, adapter proteins, and protective and exploitive proteins. Proteins are digested at the intestinal region by several groups of proteolytic digestive enzymes (proteases), with different specificities for the amino acids forming the peptide bond to be hydrolyzed.

BIBLIOGRAPHY

1. Concepts in Experimental Biochemistry, Brooks/Cole Publishing company, 1999.
2. Jain JL. Fundamentals of Biochemistry, S Chand publications, 2004.
3. Stryer L. Biochemistry, 4th edition. WH Freeman & Co, 1995.
4. Zubay GL. Principles of Biochemistry, 3rd edition. In: William WP, Dennis EV (Eds). WC Brown Publishers, 1995.

REVIEW QUESTIONS

Long Essays
1. Define protein; explain the structural organization of proteins.
2. Explain the classifications of protein.
3. Define aminoacid, explain the classifications of aminoacid.
4. Define urea cycle; explain the steps of urea cycle.

Short Essays
1. Biological importance of proteins.
2. General properties of protein.
3. Chemical structure of aminoacid.
4. Functions of amino acids.
5. Digestion and absorption of proteins.
6. Biosynthesis of protein.
7. Protein metabolism.
8. Formation of catecolamines.
9. Formation of thyroid hormone.
10. Protein metabolism disorders.
11. Phenylketonuria (PKU).
12. Maple syrup urine disease (MSUD).

Short Answers
1. Aminotransferase.
2. Transamination.
3. Deamination.
4. Essential amino acids.
5. Albumins.
6. Protein kinases.
7. Urea cycle.
8. Globulins.
9. Non-polar amino acids.
10. Catabolism of amino acids.
11. Tyrosinemia.
12. Uric acid.
13. Sodium hypobromide test.
14. Homocystinuria.

CHAPTER 19

Clinical Enzymology

CHAPTER OUTLINE

- Isoenzymes—Definition and Properties
- Enzymes of Diagnostic Importance in:
  - Liver Diseases—ALT, AST, ALP, GGT
  - Myocardial Infarction—CK, Cardiac Troponins, AST, LDH
- Muscle Diseases—CK, Aldolase
- Bone Diseases—ALP
- Prostate Cancer—PSA, ACP

TERMINOLOGY

- **Enzymes:** A molecule, most often a protein that contains a catalytic site for a biochemical reaction.
- **Phenylketonuria:** A human disease caused by a genetic deficiency in the enzyme that converts phenylalanine to tyrosine. The immediate cause of the disease is an excess of phenylalanine, which can be alleviated by a diet low in phenylalanine.
- **Substrate:** The substances changed or acted on by enzymes called substrate.
- **Catabolism:** Catabolic pathway involves the breakdown or digestion of large, complex molecules.
- **Anabolism:** Anabolic pathway involves the synthesis of large molecules, generally it joining smaller molecules to getter.
- **Co-enzymes:** There are other groups that contribute to the reactivity of enzymes besides amino acid residues.

INTRODUCTION

There are about 2700 enzymes in the human body, which are divided into three major groupings; metabolic enzymes, food enzymes and digestive enzymes. Depending on their functions, the enzymes are usually located in different parts of the body, such as the stomach or the mouth. Any of numerous proteins produced in living cells that accelerate or catalyze the metabolic processes of an organism. Enzymes are usually very selective in the molecules that they act upon, called **substrates**, often reacting with only a single substrate. The substrate binds to the enzyme at a location called the **active site** just before the reaction catalyzed by the enzyme takes place. Enzymes can speed up chemical reactions by up to a million fold, but only function within a narrow temperature and pH range, outside of which they can lose their structure and become **denatured**. Enzymes are involved in such processes as the breaking down of the large protein, starch, and fat molecules in food into smaller molecules during digestion, the joining together of nucleotides into strands of DNA, and the addition of a phosphate group to ADP to form ATP.

Definition

- Enzymes are defined as the chemical reactions in all cells of living things operate in the presence of biological catalysts.
- An enzyme is a protein formed by the body that acts as a catalyst to cause a certain desired reaction. Enzymes are very specific. Each enzyme is designed to initiate a specific response with a specific result.
- There are many enzymes in the human body. In cystic fibrosis, the term enzyme generally refers to the enzymes created by the pancreas that are intended to initiate a reaction that digests food.

Characteristics of Enzymes

Enzymes, the biochemical catalysts posses the following important characteristics:

- They increase the rate of reaction without themselves being used-up.
- Their presence does not affect the nature or properties of end products.
- Small amount of an enzyme can accelerate chemical reaction.
- They are very specific in their action; a single enzyme catalyzes only a single chemical reaction of a group of related reactions.
- They are sensitive to even a minor change in Ph, temperature and substrate concentration. Some enzymes require a co-factor for their proper functioning.
- They lower the activation energy of the reaction.

Classifactions of Enzymes (Table 19.1)

Enzymes are biocatalysts—the catalyst of life. A catalyst is defined as substance that increases the velocity or rate of a chemical reaction without itself undergoing any change in the overall process. All enzymes are protein in nature but all proteins are not necessarily enzymes.

Classifications: Enzymes are sometimes considered under two broad categories

- **Intracellular enzymes:** They are functional within the cells where they are synthesized
- **Extracellular enzymes:** These enzymes are active outside the cell, all the digestive enzymes belong to this group.

International Union of Biochemistry (IUB) has set a system of enzyme classification in 1964. Accordingly enzymes are classified in to 6 major classes:

(1) Oxidoreductases, (2) Transferases, (3) Hydrolases, (4) Lyases, (5) Isomerases, and (6) Ligases.

1. **Oxidoreductases:** Enzymes involved in the oxidation reduction reactions, i.e., they catalyze the addition of oxygen or removal of hydrogen, e.g., alcohol dehydrogenase, cytochrome oxidase, etc.
2. **Transferases:** Enzymes that catalyze the transfer of functional groups from one substrate to another, e.g., hexokinase, phosphorylase, transaminase.
3. **Hydrolases:** Enzymes that bring about hydrolysis of various compounds with the addition of a molecule of water, e.g., lipase, amylase, pepsin, alkaline phosphatase.
4. **Lyases:** Enzymes specialized in the addition or removal of water, ammonia, CO_2, aldolase, fumarase.
5. **Isomerases:** These are involved in the isomerization of a substrate and in turn catalyze the interconversion of one isomeric form to the other, e.g., phosphohexose isomerase, retinol isomerase, etc.
6. **Ligases:** Enzymes catalyzing the synthetic reactions where two molecules are joined together and ATP is used, e.g., glutathione synthetase, acetyl-coA carboxylase, etc.

Functions of Enzymes

Enzymes are biological compounds that increase the rate of a chemical reaction within the body. Almost all enzymes in the human body are proteins. These enzyme proteins than cause something to happen faster than it normally would. The body controls the rate at which many things happen by controlling the amount of individual enzymes it produces. If the body wants to slow down the rate at which something happens, it stops making a certain enzyme, or even creates a different enzyme to destroy the first enzyme. By using enzymes, the body is able to micromanage the rates of many different activities inside the body. There are literally thousands of different enzymes in the body that regulate nearly every activity. Below is a brief outline of some of the major systems involved and some sample enzymes from that system.

- **Digestion:** Nearly every type of food we consume has an enzyme that has a singular job of breaking that food down into a smaller compound. For instance, our saliva contains an enzyme called Amylase that breaks starches down into a simpler carbohydrate called maltose. When the maltose gets into your small intestines, another enzyme called maltase, then breaks the maltose down further into glucose, which is absorbed by the small intestines and enters the bloodstream. Similarly, there is an enzyme called lipase that breaks down fats, and another enzyme called pepsin that breaks down proteins so they can be absorbed by the digestive tract.
- **Detoxification:** Another common use for enzymes is the destruction of harmful things within the body. These enzymes are found in many different places including the bloodstream and liver. For instance, in the liver is an enzyme called catalase, whose sole purpose is to breakdown hydrogen peroxide, which is toxic to the body. Catalase takes the harmful hydrogen peroxide and converts it into oxygen and water. Besides the liver, enzymes are also an important part of our immune response.
- **Movement:** Enzymes are important part of the neuromuscular system that controls movement. Not only are enzymes an integral part of information transportation between neurons, but enzymes are also critical the actual contraction of muscles, controlling the rate at which ATP (energy) is provided for the cells.

While and enzyme is simply a biological catalyst whose function is to speed up a chemical reaction. In most situations that rates of these reactions without the enzyme is so slow as to result in death. For instance, without enzymes, a person would absorb only an insignificant fraction of the nutrients that is eaten. Starvation would begin almost immediately. Toxic chemicals in the body gradually degrade, but the rate at which they do so is so slow that a person would die from their effects long before the toxin falls apart on its own.

Table 19.1: Classification of enzymes.

Group of enzyme	Reaction catalyzed	Examples
Oxidoreductase	Transfer of hydrogen and oxygen atoms or electrons from one substrate to another	Dehydrogenases Oxidases
Transferases	Transfer of a specific group (a phosphate or methyl, etc.) from one substrate to another	Transaminase Kinases
Hydrolases	Hydrolysis of a substrate	Estrases Digestive enzymes
Isomerases	Change of the molecular form of the substrate	Phospho-hexo-isomerase, fumarase
Lyases	Nonhydrolytic removal of a group or addition of a group to a substrate	Decarboxylases Aldolases
Ligases (synthetases)	Joining of two molecules by the formation of new bonds	Citric acid synthetase

MECHANISM OF ENZYME ACTIVITY (FIG. 19.1)

Enzymes are proteins that allow certain chemical reactions to take place much quicker than the reactions would occur on their own. Enzymes function as catalysts, which mean that they speed up the rate at which metabolic processes and reactions occur in living organisms. Usually, the processes or reactions are part of a cycle or pathway, with separate reactions at each step. Each step of a pathway or cycle usually requires a specific enzyme. Without the specific enzyme to catalyze a reaction, the cycle or pathway cannot be completed. The result of an uncompleted cycle or pathway is the lack of a product of that cycle or pathway. And, without a needed product, a function cannot be performed, which negatively affects the organism.

Catalysts and activation energy: Reactions are not impossible without enzymes. Enzymes do not change during reactions, nor do they change the other contents of the reaction. They just speed up the rate at which all parts of the reaction react. In a chemical reaction, the reaction is said to be completed when equilibrium is reached. Chemical reactions have forward directions and backward directions, and reactions tend to move in both directions until no more products are created from the reactants, and products are no longer converted back into reactants.

$$A + B \longleftrightarrow C + D$$
$$(\text{reactants}) \longleftrightarrow (\text{products})$$

That is the point of equilibrium. The equilibrium constant is written as: Reactions will occur with the free energy available in the system (*system* is referring to the area where the reaction is occurring). There is always some energy in the system before a reaction begins, and this free energy is called G. The amount of change in the free energy of a reaction is labeled ΔG (the Greek letter delta, Δ, is used to represent change).

- **Exergonic reactions** give off energy, so they represent a negative change in free energy ($-\Delta G$) — that is, the free energy is given off, so there is a "loss" of free energy. In actuality, the energy is just transferred. Exergonic reactions will continue until equilibrium is reached, because they yield energy.
- **Endergonic reactions** absorb energy into the system, so the free energy in the system increases ($+\Delta G$). This increase appears to be a "gain" in energy, when really it is just another energy transfer. Endergonic reactions kind of quit while they are ahead. Because endergonic reactions take in energy, the reactions peter out so that less energy is taken in. They usually do not reach equilibrium.

There are two theories as to how reactions occur:
In the collision theory, it is thought that reactions occur because molecules collide; the faster they collide, the faster the reaction occurs. The energy level that must be reached for the molecules to collide is called the *activation energy*. The activation energy is affected by heat, because a higher temperature increases the energy of each molecule.

In the transition state theory, reactants are thought to form bonds and then break bonds until they form products. As this forming and breaking happens, free energy increases until it reaches a transition state (also called activated complex), which is viewed as the midpoint between reactants and products. Reactions proceed faster if there is a higher concentration of activated complex.

If the free energy of activation is high, the transition state is low, and the reaction is slow. The reaction rate is proportional to the concentration of the activated complex. If the activation energy is lower, the reaction occurs faster because more activated complexes can form.

In living organisms, the reactions that need to occur have high activation energies. So, to get reactions to occur, either the temperature must be increased, or the activation energy must be decreased. But the internal temperature of a living thing cannot be raised too high like chemicals in a laboratory can be. Instead, living organisms rely on enzymes to lower the activation energies so that reactions can occur quickly.

Cofactors and Coenzymes: Coexisting with Enzymes

Enzymes are made mostly of proteins, but they also have some nonprotein components. When these nonprotein components must be included in order for the enzyme to act as a catalyst, then the nonprotein component is called a cofactor. Examples of cofactors are potassium, magnesium, or zinc ions.

A coenzyme is a type of cofactor. Coenzymes are small molecules that can separate from the protein component of the enzyme and react directly in the catalytic reaction. An important function of coenzymes is that they transfer electrons, atoms, or molecules from one enzyme to another.

Vitamins are closely connected to coenzymes. The function of vitamins is that they help to make coenzymes. Niacin, which is one of the B vitamins, helps to make nicotinamide adenine dinucleotide (NAD), which is one of the coenzymes that carries electrons from Krebs cycle through the electron transport chain to produce ATP. Without NAD, very little ATP would be produced, and the organism would be low in energy.

Factors Affecting Enzymes Activity

All enzymes exhibit maximum activity under optimal conditions. Enzyme activity is markedly, affected by several factors. The important factors that influence the velocity of enzyme reaction are

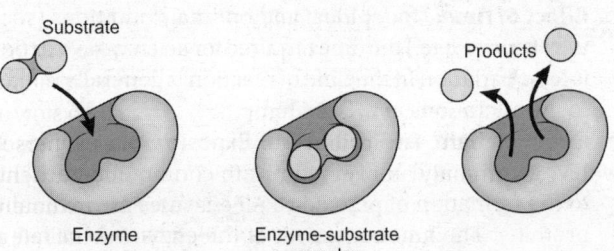

Fig. 19.1: Mechanism of enzyme of activity.

- Concentration of enzyme
- Concentration of substrate
- Effect of temperature
- Effect of pH
- Effect of product concentration
- Effect of activators
- Effect of time
- Effect of light and radiation
- **Concentration of enzyme:** As the concentration of enzyme is increased, the velocity of reaction proportionately increases.

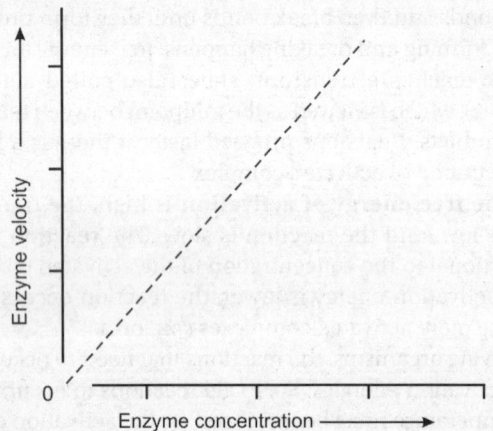

- **Concentration of substrate:** Increased in the substrate concentration gradually increases the velocity of enzyme reaction within a limited range of substrate levels. Further increase in substrate concentration thereafter does not increase the rate of reaction

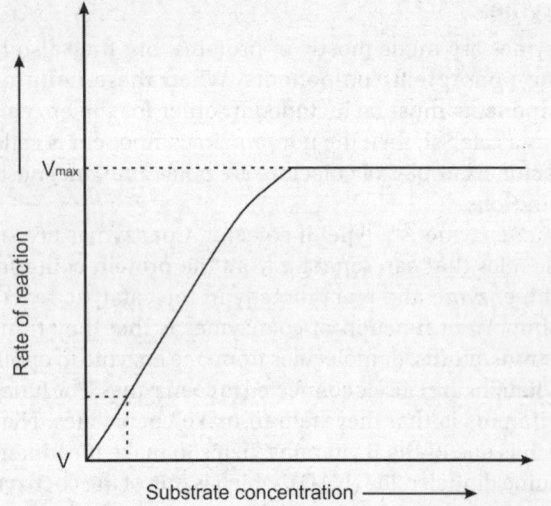

- Effect of substrate concentration on enzyme activity
- Three distinct phases of the reaction are observed. In the first phase, at low substrate concentration velocity is directly proportional to substration concentrate. In the second phase, the substrate concentration is not directly proportional to the enzyme activity. In the third and final phase, the reaction is independent of substrate concentration. Km or the michelis menten constant is defined as the substrate concentration at half of the maximal velocity in the enzyme catalyzed reaction.

- **Effect of temperature:** Velocity of an enzyme reaction increases with increase in temperature up to a maximum and then declines. Effect of temperature on Enzyme activity. In general, when enzymes are exposed to temperature above 5°C, denaturation occurs.

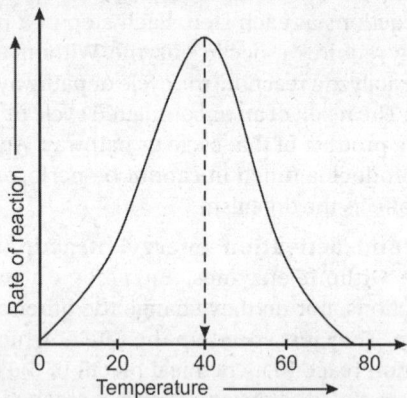

- **Effect of pH:** Every enzyme has an optimum pH at which the velocity of reaction is maximum.
Effect of pH on enzyme activity

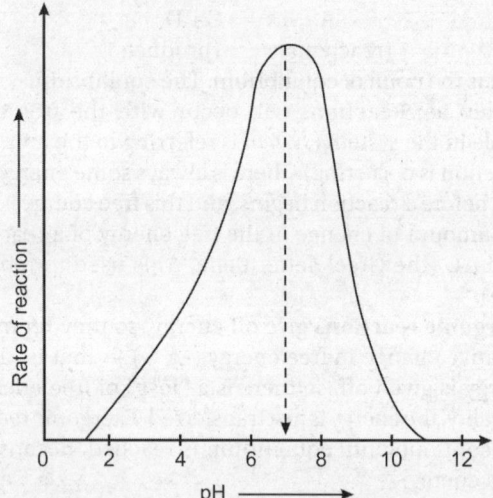

Effect of product concentration: The accumulation of reaction products generally decreases the enzyme activity
- **Effect of activators:** Some of the enzymes require certain inorganic metallic cations (Mg^2, Mn^2, Mn^{2+} CO^2, Cu^2, NA^+, K^+ for their optimum activity. Metals function as activators of enzyme velocity.
- **Effect of time:** Under ideal and optimal conditions (such as pH, temp., etc.) the time required for an enzyme reaction is less. Variation in the time of reaction is generally related to the alterations in pH and temp.
- **Effect of light and radiation:** Exposure of enzymes to UV, gamma and X-rays inactivate certain enzymes due to the formation of peroxides. All enzymes are invariably proteins. The functional unit of the enzyme is called as holoenzyme which is often made up of apoenzyme (the protein part) and a coenzyme (non-protein organic part)

Holoenzyme-Apoenzyme + coenzyme (active enzyme) (Protein part) (Non-protein part).

ISO-Enzymes

Isozymes were first described by RL Hunter and Clement Markert (1957) who defined them as different variants of the same enzyme having identical functions and present in the same individual.

Definitions:
- Enzyme variants that are the product of different genes and thus represent different loci (described as isozymes) and
- Enzymes that are the product of different alleles of the same gene (described as allozymes).

Isozymes (also known as **isoenzymes** or more generally as **multiple forms of enzymes**) are enzymes that differ in amino acid sequence but catalyze the same chemical reaction. These enzymes usually display different kinetic parameters (e.g., different Km values), or different regulatory properties. The existence of isozymes permits the fine-tuning of metabolism to meet the particular needs of a given tissue or developmental stage (for example lactate dehydrogenase (LDH)). In biochemistry, isozymes (or isoenzymes) are isoforms (closely related variants) of enzymes. In many cases, they are coded for by homologous genes that have diverged over time. Although, strictly speaking, allozymes represent enzymes from different alleles of the same gene, and isozymes represent enzymes from different genes that process or catalyze the same reaction, the two words are usually used interchangeably.

- LDH is found in many body tissues, such as the heart, liver, kidney, skeletal muscle, brain, blood cells, and lungs.
- LDH exists in 5 forms, which differ slightly in structure.
- LDH-1 is found primarily in heart muscle and red blood cells.
- LDH-2 is concentrated in white blood cells.
- LDH-3 is highest in the lung.
- LDH-4 is highest in the kidney, placenta, and pancreas.
- LDH-5 is highest in the liver and skeletal muscle.

LD is a tetrameric cytoplasmic enzyme, composed of H and M subunits. The most usual designation of the isoenzyme is LD-I (H4), LD-II (H3M), LD-III (H2M2), LD-IV (HM3), and LD-V (M4). Tissue specificity is derived from the fact that there is tissue-specific synthesis of subunits in well-defined ratios. Most notably, heart muscle cells preferentially synthesize H subunits, while liver cells synthesize M subunits nearly exclusively. Skeletal muscle also synthesizes largely M subunits so that LD-V is both a liver and skeletal muscle form of LD. The LD-I and LD-V forms are most often used to indicate heart or liver pathology, respectively.

LD-I appear elevated in the serum about 24 to 48 hours after a myocardial infarction (MI), but is generally not as useful as troponin or creatine kinase-MB (CK-MB) for detection of MI, unless the MI occurred at least 24 hours prior to testing. Normally, LD-II is greater than LD-I; however, when a MI has occurred, there is a "flip" in the usual ratio of LD-I/LD-II from <1 to >1 (or at least >0.9). Use of the ratio for evaluation of patients with possible cardiovascular injury has largely been replaced by TPNT/82428 Troponin T, Serum.

The LD-V form is pronounced in patients with either primary liver disease or liver hypoxia secondary to decreased perfusion, such as occurs following an MI. However, LD-V is usually not as reliable as the transaminases (e.g., aspartate aminotransferase, alanine aminotransferase) for evaluating liver function. LD-V also may be elevated in muscular damage and diseases of the skin.

Coenzymes

Coenzyme, any of a number of freely diffusing organic compounds that function as cofactors with enzymes in promoting a variety of metabolic reactions. Coenzymes participate in enzyme-mediated catalysis in stoichiometric (mole-for-mole) amounts, are modified during the reaction, and may require another enzyme-catalyzed reaction to restore them to their original state.

Definition: A coenzyme is a substance that works with an enzyme to initiate or aid the function of the enzyme.

Examples: The B vitamins serve as coenzymes essential for enzymes to form fats, carbohydrates and proteins. Examples include nicotinamide adenine dinucleotide (NAD), which accepts hydrogen (and gives it up in another reaction), and ATP, which gives up phosphate groups while transferring chemical energy (and reacquires phosphate in another reaction). Most of the B vitamins are coenzymes and are essential in facilitating the transfer of atoms or groups of atoms between molecules in the formation of carbohydrates, fats, and proteins. Many enzymes require certain non-protein small additional factors. The cofactors may be organic or inorganic.

- The non-protein organic, low mol.wt and dialyzable substance associated with enzyme function is known as coenzyme. The term prosthetic group is used when a non-protein moiety is tightly bound to enzyme.
- Coenzymes are second substrates or cosubstrates since they have affinity with the same enzyme comparable with that of substrates. Coenzymes undergo alterations during the enzymatic reactions.
- Coenzymes from B-Complex vitamins—derivatives of B-Complex vitamins, e.g., tpp FMN, FAD, NAD, NADI PU COA, FH4 biotin, coenzymes, methylcobalamin
- Non-vitamin coenzymes these are some organic substances which function as coenzymes. They are called as non-vitamin coenzymes. For example, ATI UDI S-adenosyl methionine, etc.
- Nucleotide coenzymes contains nitrogenous base, sugar and PO_4, e.g., NAD, NADP FMN, FAD, COA, etc.
- Coenzymes do not decide the enzyme specificity. The specificity of enzymes is mostly dependent on the apoenzyme and not on the coenzyme.

Clinically Important Enzymes

Certain tissue cells contain characteristic enzymes which enter the blood only when the cells to which they are confined are damaged or destroyed. The presence in the blood of significant quantities of these specific enzymes indicates the probable site of tissue damage gives a listing of a few enzymes of diagnostic importance and their relationship to the overall metabolic scheme.

Common enzymes used for clinical diagnosis include:
- Acid phosphatase
- Alanine aminotransferase
- Alkaline phosphatase
- Amylase
- Angiotensin converting enzyme
- Aspartate aminotransferase
- Cholinesterase
- Creatinine kinase
- Gamma-glutamyl transferase
- Lactate dehydrogenase
- Renin

Aldolase

Aldolase is present most significantly in skeletal and heart muscle. Damage to skeletal muscle produces high serum levels of aldolase, particularly in the case of progressive muscular dystrophy. Aldolase may also be slightly increased in early stages of viral hepatitis and advanced cancer of the prostate.

Creatine Phophokinase (CPK or CK)

CPK catalyzes the reversible transfer of phosphate groups between creatine and phosphocreatine as well as between ATP and ADP. Most of the CPK resides in skeletal muscle, heart muscle, and in the gastrointestinal tract. CPK enters the blood rapidly following damage to muscle cells. At first CPK seemed to be an excellent marker for acute myocardial infarction (heart damage) or skeletal muscle damage. Unfortunately, the CPK levels rise and fall rapidly and coincide with a variety of other circumstances including surgical procedures, vigorous exercise, a fall, or a deep intramuscular injection. The measurement of CPK levels still provides valuable differentiating diagnostic information.

Lipase

Lipase is an enzyme secreted by the pancreas into the duodenum. Damage to the pancreas as in acute pancreatitis results in lipase in the blood from the secretory cells.

LDH

This enzyme catalyzes the reversible reaction between pyruvic and lactic acids. LDH is present in nearly all types of metabolizing cells, but different cells have different forms of the enzyme which can be distinguished. The enzyme is especially concentrated in the heart, liver, red blood cells, kidneys, muscles, brain, and lungs. Normal value of LDH in serum is 100–200 U/L. Values in the upper range are generally seen in children. Strenuous exercise will slightly increase the value. LDH level is 100 times more inside the RBC than in plasma, and therefore minor amount of hemolysis will result in a false-positive test.

- **LDH and, heart attack:** In myocardial infarction, total LDH activity is increased, while H4 iso-enzyme is increased 5–10 times more. The magnitude of the peak value as well as the area under the graph will be roughly proportional to the size of the myocardial infarct.
  - Differential diagnosis: Increase in total LDH level is seen in hemolytic anemia's, hepatocellular damage, muscular dystrophy, carcinomas, leukemias, and any condition which causes necrosis of body cells. Since total LDH is increased in many conditions, the study of iso- enzymes of LDH is of great importance.
- **Iso-enzymes of LDH:** LDH enzyme is a tetramer with four subunits. But the subunit may be either H (heart) or M (muscle) polypeptide chains. These two are the products of two different genes. Although both of them have the same molecular weight (32 kD), there are minor amino acid variations. So five combinations of H and M chains are possible; H4, H3M, H2M2, M3H and M4 varieties, forming five iso-enzymes. All these five forms are seen in all persons. M4 form is seen in skeletal muscles; it is not inhibited by pyruvate. But H4 form is seen in heart and is inhibited by pyruvate. Normally LDH-2 (H3M1) concentration in blood is greater than LDH-1 (H4); but this pattern is reversed in myocardial infarction; this is called flipped pattern. The iso-enzymes are usually separated by cellulose acetate electrophoresis at pH 8.6. They are then identified by adding the reactants finally producing a color reaction. (Another 6th isoenzyme, called LDH-X, composed of 4 X subunits is present in post pubertal human testes).

The total LDH can be further separated into five components or fractions labeled by number—LDH-1, LDH-2, LDH-3, LDH-4, and LDH-5. Each of these fractions, called isoenzymes, is used mainly by a different set of cells or tissues in the body. The LDH isoenzymes test assists in differentiating heart attack, anemia, lung injury, or liver disease from other conditions that may cause the same symptoms. LDH-1 is found mainly in the heart. LDH-2 is primarily associated with the system in the body that defends against infection. LDH-3 is found in the lungs and other tissues, LDH-4 in the kidney, placenta, and pancreas, and LDH-5 in liver and skeletal muscle. Normally, levels of LDH-2 are higher than those of the other isoenzymes.

Certain diseases have classic patterns of elevated LDH isoenzyme levels. For example, an LDH-1 level higher than that of LDH-2 is indicative of a heart attack or injury; elevations of LDH-2 and LDH-3 indicate lung injury or disease; elevations of LDH-4 and LDH-5 indicate liver or muscle disease or both. A rise of all LDH isoenzymes at the same time is diagnostic of injury to multiple organs.

One of the most important diagnostic uses for the LDH isoenzymes test is in the differential diagnosis of myocardial infarction or heart attack. The total LDH level rises within 24–48 hours after a heart attack, peaks in two to three days, and returns to normal in approximately five to ten days. This pattern is a useful tool for a delayed diagnosis of heart attack. The LDH-1 isoenzyme level, however, is more sensitive and specific than the total LDH. Normally, the level of LDH-2 is higher than the level of LDH-1. An LDH-1 level higher than that of LDH-2, a phenomenon known as "flipped LDH," is strongly indicative of a heart attack.

Creatine Kinase (CK)

It was called as creatine phosphokinase in old literature. Normal serum value for CK is 15–100 U/L for males and 10–80 U/L for females.

- **CK and heart attack:** CK value in serum is increased in myocardial infarction. The CK level starts to rise within three hours of infarction. Therefore, CK estimation is very useful to detect early cases, where ECG changes may be ambiguous. The CK level is not increased in hemolysis or in congestive cardiac failure; and therefore CK has an advantage over LDH. The area under the peak and slope of initial rise are proportional to the size of infarct.
- **CK and muscle diseases:** The level of CK in serum is very much elevated in muscular dystrophies (500–1500 iu/L). The level is very high in the early phases of the disease. In such patients a fall in CK level is indicative of deteriorating condition, because by that time, all muscle mass is destroyed. In female, carriers of this X-linked disease (genotypically heterozygous), CK is seen to be moderately raised. CK level is highly elevated in crush injury, fracture and acute cerebrovascular accidents. Estimation of total CK is employed in muscular dystrophies and MB iso-enzyme is estimated in myocardial infarction.

Cardiac Troponins (CTI/CTT)

They are not enzymes. However, it is now increasingly being employed as a marker for myocardial infarction, and hence it is described here. The troponin complex consists of three components; troponin C (calcium binding), troponin-I (actomyosin ATPase inhibitory element), and troponin T (tropomyosin binding element). Troponin I (TnI) is encoded by three different genes, giving rise to three is forms; the 'slow' and "fast" moving forms are skeletal variety. Cardiac is form is specific for cardiac muscle. It has molecular weight of 24 kD. Troponin I is released into the blood within four hours after the onset of cardiac symptoms, peaks at 12–16 hours and remains elevated for 5–9 days post-infarction. Therefore, CTI is very useful as a marker at anytime interval after the heart attacks. It is 75% sensitive index for myocardial infarction. It is not increased in muscle injury; whereas CK2 may be elevated in some muscle injury. CTI level greater than 1.5 mg/L is indicative of myocardial damage. It is usually assayed by ELISA or RIA techniques. Two isoforms of cardiac Troponin T (TnT1 and TnT2) are present in adult cardiac tissues. Serum level of TnT2 increases within four hrs of myocardial infarction, and remains high up to 14 days. The TnT2 estimation is 100% sensitive index for myocardial infarction.

Aspartate Aminotransferase (AST)

It is also called as serum glutamate-oxaloacetate transaminase (SGOT). AST needs pyridoxal phosphate as co-enzyme. AST is estimated by taking aspartate, ct-ketoglutarate, pyridoxal phosphate (vitamin B6) and patient's serum as the source of AST. The oxaloacetate formed may be allowed to react with dinitrophenyl hydrazine to produce a color which is estimated colorimetrically at 520 nm.

Normal serum level of AST is 8–20 U/L. It is significantly elevated in myocardial infarction. It is moderately elevated in liver diseases. However, a marked increase in AST may be seen in primary hepatoma. AST has two iso-enzymes; cytoplasmic and mitochondrial. In mild degree of tissue injury, cytoplasmic form is seen in serum. Mitochondrial type is seen in severe injury.

Transaminase (GOT and GPT)

Glutamic-oxaloacetic transaminase (GOT) occurs in large concentrations in the heart and liver with moderate amounts in skeletal muscle, kidneys, and pancreas. GOT levels can be used to diagnose myocardial infarction within 10–48 hours. Other conditions with elevated GOT include arrhythmias and severe angina of the heart, and liver damage.

Glutamic-pyruvic transaminase (GPT) is found in significant quantities in liver, kidney, and skeletal muscle, in decreasing order. When liver cells are damaged, GOT and GPT levels rise especially early in the disease. In hepatitis, transaminase levels rise several days before jaundice begins. The enzyme levels are especially useful in assessing subtle and early changes in biliary obstruction and active cirrhosis.

Gamma-glutamyl Transferase

The old name was gamma-glutamyl transpeptidase. It can transfer 'γ-glutamyl residues to substrate. In the body, it is used in the synthesis of glutathione. GGT has 11 iso-enzymes. It is seen in liver, kidney, pancreas, intestinal cells and prostate gland. It is estimated at pH 8.5 using the following reaction: γ-glutamyl-nitroanilide > nitroaniline + glycinyl glycine + glutamyl glycyl glycine.

The nitroaniline thus produced is quantitated colorimetrically at 405 nm.

Normal serum value of GGT is 10–30 U/L. It is slightly higher in normal males, due to the presence of prostate gland. This value is moderately increased in infective hepatitis and prostate cancers. The GGT level is highly elevated in alcoholism, obstructive jaundice and neoplasms of liver. GGT-2 is positive for 90% of hepatocellular carcinomas. It is not elevated in cardiac or skeletal diseases.

GGT is a microsomal enzyme. Its activity is induced by alcohol, phenobarbitone and rifampicin. GGT is clinically important because of its sensitivity to detect alcohol abuse. GGT is increased in alcoholics even when other liver function tests are within normal limits. GGT level is rapidly decreased within a few days when the person stops to take alcohol. Increase in GGT level is generally proportional to the amount of alcohol intake.

Enzyme profile for liver diseases: Enzymes commonly studied by diagnosis of liver diseases are ALT, ALP, NTP and GGT.

Acid Phosphatase (ACP)

It hydrolyses phosphoric acid ester at pH between 4 and 6.

Methods for assay are the same as described for ALP; but the pH of the medium is kept at 5 to 5.4. Normal serum value for ACP is 2.5–12 U/L. ACP is secreted by prostate cells, RBC, platelets and WBC. Iso-enzymes of ACP are described. Erythrocyte ACP gene is located in chromosome 2; osteoclast ACP gene is on chromosome 19; lysosomal gene is on 11 and prostate ACP gene is on 13. The prostate iso-enzyme is inactivated by tartaric acid. Cupric ions inhibit erythrocyte ACP. Normal level of tartrate labile fraction of ACP is 1 U/L.

ACP total value is increased in prostate cancer and highly elevated in bone metastasis of prostate cancer. In these conditions, the tartrate labile iso-enzyme is elevated. This assay is very helpful in follow up of treatment of prostate cancers. ACP is therefore an important tumor marker. Since blood cells contain excess quantity of ACP, care must be taken to prevent hemolysis while taking blood from the patient. Prostate massage may also increase the value. So blood may be collected for ACP estimation before per rectal examination of patient. ACP is present in high concentration in semen, a finding which is used in forensic medicine in investigation of rape.

Prostate-specific Antigen (PSA)

It is produced from the secretory epithelium of prostate gland. It is normally secreted into seminal fluid, where it is necessary for the liquefaction of seminal coagulum. It is a serine protease, and is a 32 kD glycoprotein; encoded in chromosome number 1 9. In blood, it is bound to alpha-2-macroglobulin and alpha-1-antitryp-sin; a very small fraction is in the free from also. Normal value is 1–5 ug/L. It is very specific for prostate activity. Values between 4–10 ug/L is seen in benign prostate enlargement; but values above 10 ug/L are indicative of prostate cancer.

Gamma-glutamyl Transpeptidase (GGT)

GGT catalyzes the transfer of the glutamyl groups among different polypeptides and amino acids. Clinically significant GGT found in the blood comes from cells that line the biliary tract. GGT levels rise dramatically with obstructive diseases of the biliary tract and liver cancers. GGT is especially useful in assessing liver function associated with alcohol-induced liver disease.

Enzymes and Disease Conditions

Liver Diseases

Some of the many enzymes found in hepatocytes can be measured in the serum and are used as tests of liver function. We now review the current knowledge of their physiology and pathophysiology and outline their clinical usefulness. We divide them into two categories—enzymes that primarily reflect cholestasis, such as the alkaline phosphatase, the 5-nucleotidase, and the gamma-glutamyl transpeptidase, and those that primarily reflect hepatocellular necrosis, such as the aminotransferases.

Renal Diseaes

The serum enzymes of patients with end-stage renal disease (ESRD) are commonly abnormal. This is due in part to the absence of renal excretion and to the frequent presence of multiple comorbid conditions. Since the diagnosis of many diseases is based upon the detection of elevated levels of these enzymes, the accurate clinical assessment of the patient with ESRD is hampered by a paucity of knowledge concerning the serum concentrations of different enzymes in various disease states. The use and significance of variations in the concentrations of serum enzymes in dialysis patients will be reviewed here. A discussion of serum cardiac enzymes in patients with renal failure is presented separately. The serum enzymes most commonly used to help assess the diagnosis of hepatobiliary disease include the aminotransferases, alkaline phosphatase, and gamma glutamyl transpeptidase.

Aminotransferases-serum concentrations of aspartate and alanine aminotransferase [AST (SGOT) and ALT (SGPT)] are routinely measured to assess liver function in patients with and without renal failure. The aminotransferases are normally present in the circulation in low concentrations, usually <40 international units/L. the concentrations of serum aminotransferases in both chronic dialysis and chronic renal failure patients most commonly fall within the lower end of the range of normal values (1–4). Although the exact cause is unknown, possible underlying reasons may be related to pyridoxine deficiency (pyridoxal phosphate is a necessary coenzyme for ALT and AST) (5–7) and/or the presence of an inhibitory substance in the uremic milieu

Cardiac Diseases

Levels of cardiac enzymes are principally utilized to help assess the presence or absence of acute myocardial injury. Abnormal elevations in the serum concentrations of these enzymes may be the key diagnostic element in determining admission to the hospital and/or coronary care units. They are also increasingly being used as predictive markers for short- and long-term adverse outcomes, particularly among those presenting with acute coronary syndromes. The principal cardiac enzymes are cardiac troponin T (cTnT), cardiac troponin I (cTnI), and the MB isoenzyme of creatine kinase (CK-MB).

CONCLUSION

Enzymes are biological molecules that catalyze (i.e., increase the rates of) chemical reactions. In enzymatic reactions, the molecules at the beginning of the process, called substrates, are converted into different molecules, called products. Almost all chemical reactions in a biological cell need enzymes in order to occur at rates sufficient for life. Their functionality depends on how proteins are folded, what they bind to, and what they react with. For protein-based catalysts, amino acid polarization lies at the core of catalytic activity. Since enzymes are selective for their substrates and speed up only a few reactions from among many possibilities, the set of enzymes made in a cell determines which metabolic pathways occur in that cell.

BIBLIOGRAPHY

1. Bais R, Panteghini M. Principles of clinical enzymology. In: Burtis CA, Ashwood ER, Bruns DE (Eds). Tietz Textbook of Clinical Chemistry and Molecular Diagnostics, 4th edition. Philadelphia, PA: Elsevier Saunders, 2006:191-218.
2. Boyd JW. The rates of disappearance of L-lactate dehydrogenase isoenzymes from plasma. Biochim Biophys Acta. 1967 Mar 15;132(2):221–31.
3. Konttinen A, Somer H. Determination of serum creatine kinase isoenzymes in myocardial infarction. Am J Cardiol. 1972 Jun; 29(6):817–820
4. Posen S. Turnover of circulating enzymes. Clin Chem. 1970 Feb;16(2):71–84.
5. Price CP, Hill PG, Sammons HG. The nature of the alkaline phosphatase of bile. J Clin Pathol. 1972 Feb; 25(2):149–54.
6. Sweetin JC, Thomson WH. Enzyme efflux and clearance. Clin Chim Acta. 1973 Nov 15; 48(4):403–11.
7. Wilkinson JH. Clinical significance of enzyme activity measurements. Clin Chem. 1970 Nov;16(11):882–90.

REVIEW QUESTIONS

Long Essays
1. Define enzyme, explain the properties of enzyme.
2. Describe the mechanism of enzyme activity.
3. Explain the factors affecting enzymes activity.

Short Essays
1. Classifications of enzymes.
2. Functions of enzymes.
3. Cofactors and coenzymes.
4. ISO-enzymes.
5. Enzymes and disease conditions.
6. Clinically important enzymes.
7. ISO-enzymes of LDH.

Short Answers
1. Co-enzymes.
2. Anabolism.
3. Catabolism.
4. Phenylketonuria.
5. Enzymes.
6. Creatine phophokinase.
7. Aldolase.
8. Creatine kinase (CK).
9. Acid phosphatase (ACP).
10. Gamma-glutamyl transferase.
11. Transaminase (GOT and GPT).

CHAPTER 20

Acid Base Maintenance

CHAPTER OUTLINE

- ❖ pH—Definition, Normal Value
- ❖ Regulation of Blood pH—Blood Buffer, Respiratory and Renal
- ❖ ABG—Normal Values
- ❖ Acid Base Disorders—Types, Definition and Causes

INTRODUCTION

Acid–base balance refers to the balance between input (intake and production) and output (elimination) of hydrogen ion. The body is an open system in equilibrium with the alveolar air where the partial pressure of carbon dioxide PCO_2 is identical to the carbon dioxide tension in the blood. Maintenance of acid–base balance is fundamental for the normal functioning of biological processes, mainly due to the pH dependence of enzyme function. This article reviews definitions of acid–base balance and describes normal physiology of acid–base metabolism in the extracellular fluid and blood. The individual roles of the kidney, liver, bone, and lungs in maintenance of acid–base balance are outlined in detail in both health and disease. The pathogenesis of common conditions (diabetes, renal failure, drug intoxication) affecting acid–base balance are assessed as well as potential treatment strategies.

Figure 20.1 is depicted the pH scale.

CONCEPT AND MEANING OF ACID BASE MAINTENANCE

❑ To maintain homeostasis, the human body employs many physiological adaptations. One of these is maintaining an acid-base balance. In the absence of pathological states, the pH of the human body ranges between 7.35 to 7.45, with the average at 7.40.

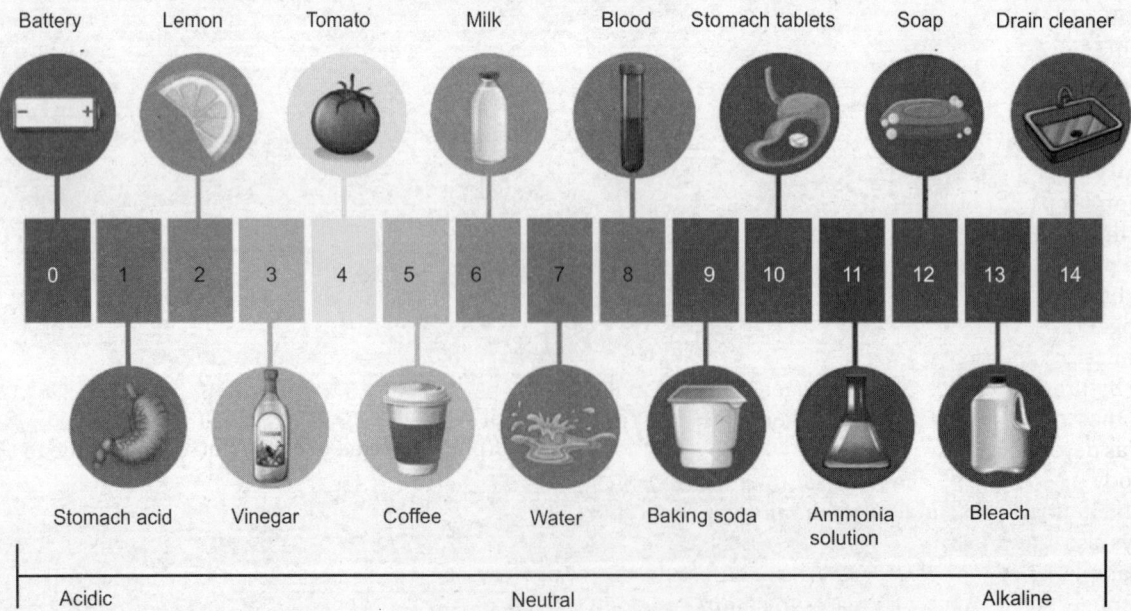

Fig. 20.1: The pH scale.

- A pH at this level is ideal for many biological processes, one of the most important being the oxygenation of blood. Also, many of the intermediates of biochemical reactions in the body become ionized at a neutral pH, which causes the utilization of these intermediates to be more difficult.
- A pH below 7.35 is an acidemia, and a pH above 7.45 is an alkalemia. Due to the importance of sustaining a pH level in the needed narrow range, the human body contains compensatory mechanisms.
- The human body experiences four main types of acid-based disorders—metabolic acidosis, metabolic alkalosis, respiratory acidosis, and respiratory alkalosis.
- If one of these conditions occurs, the human body should induce a counterbalance in the form of an opposite condition. For example, if a person is experiencing a metabolic acidemia, their body will attempt to induce a respiratory alkalosis to compensate. It is rare for the compensation to make the pH completely normal at 7.4.
- When using the term acidemia or alkalemia, one is denoting that overall the pH is acidic or alkalotic, respectively. While not necessary, it can be useful to employ this terminology to distinguish between individual processes and the overall pH status of the patient since multiple imbalances can happen at the same time.

- Conversely, when the pH is too high (i.e., during alkalosis), the respiratory rate decreases to retain acid in the form of CO_2. The kidneys excrete bicarbonate (base) in the urine and retain hydrogen ions (acid).

pH	Examples of solutions
0	Battery acid, strong hydrofluoric acid
1	Hydrochloric acid secreted by stomach lining
2	Lemon juice, gastric acid, vinegar
3	Grapefruit juice, orange juice, soda
4	Tomato juice, acid rain
5	Soft drinking water, black coffee
6	Urine, saliva
7	"Pure" water
8	Sea water
9	Baking soda
10	Great salt Lake, milk of magnesia
11	Ammonia solution
12	Soapy water
13	Bleach, oven cleaner
14	Liquid drain cleaner

DEFINITION

Acid-base balance refers to the mechanisms the body uses to keep its fluids close to neutral pH (that is, neither basic nor acidic) so that the body can function normally.

BLOOD GASES

pH

- pH is a scale from 0–14 used to determine the acidity or alkalinity of a substance. A neutral pH is 7, which is the same pH as water.
- Normally, the blood has a pH between 7.35 and 7.45. A blood pH of less than 7.35 is considered acidic, and a blood pH of more than 7.45 is considered alkaline.
- The pH of blood is a measure of hydrogen ion concentration. A low pH, less than 3.5, occurs in acidosis when the blood has a high hydrogen ion concentration.
- A high pH, greater than 7.45, occurs in alkalosis when the blood has a low hydrogen ion concentration.
- Hydrogen ions are by-products of the metabolism of substances, such as proteins, fats, and carbohydrates. These by-products create extra hydrogen ions (H^+) in the blood that need to be balanced and kept within normal range as described earlier.
- The body has several mechanisms for maintaining blood pH. The lungs are essential for maintaining pH and the kidneys also play a role.
- For example, when the pH is too low (i.e., during acidosis), the respiratory rate quickly increases to eliminate acid in the form of carbon dioxide (CO_2).
- The kidneys excrete additional hydrogen ions (acid) in the urine and retain bicarbonate (base).

PaCO$_2$

- $PaCO_2$ is the partial pressure of arterial carbon dioxide in the blood. The normal $PaCO_2$ level is 35–45 mm Hg. CO_2 forms an acid in the blood that is regulated by the lungs by changing the rate or depth of respirations.
- As the respiratory rate increases or becomes deeper, additional CO_2 is removed causing decreased acid (H^+) levels in the blood and increased pH (so the blood becomes more alkaline). As the respiratory rate decreases or becomes more shallow, less CO_2 is removed causing increased acid (H^+) levels in the blood and decreased pH (so the blood becomes more acidic).
- Generally, the lungs work quickly to regulate the $PaCO_2$ levels and cause a quick change in the pH. Therefore, an acid-base problem caused by hypoventilation can be quickly corrected by increasing ventilation, and a problem caused by hyperventilation can be quickly corrected by decreasing ventilation.
- For example, if an anxious patient is hyperventilating, they may be asked to breathe into a paper bag to rebreathe some of the CO_2 they are blowing off.
- Conversely, a postoperative patient who is experiencing hypoventilation due to the sedative effects of receiving morphine is asked to cough and deep breathe to blow off more CO_2.

HCO$_3$

- HCO_3 is the bicarbonate level of the blood and the normal range is 22–26. HCO_3 is a base managed by the kidneys and helps to make the blood more alkaline.
- The kidneys take longer than the lungs to adjust the acidity or alkalinity of the blood, and the response is not visible

upon assessment. As the kidneys sense an alteration in pH, they begin to retain or excrete HCO_3, depending on what is needed.
- If the pH becomes acidic, the kidneys retain HCO_3 to increase the amount of bases present in the blood to increase the pH.
- Conversely, if the pH becomes alkalotic, the kidneys excrete more HCO_3, causing the pH to decrease.

PaO_2

PaO_2 is the partial pressure of arterial oxygen in the blood. It more accurately measures a patient's oxygenation status than SaO_2 (the measurement of hemoglobin saturation with oxygen). Therefore, ABG results are also used to manage patients in respiratory distress.

Function of pH

The physiological pH of the human body is essential for many processes necessary to life including oxygen delivery to tissues, correct protein structure, and innumerable biochemical reactions that rely on the normal pH to be in equilibrium and complete.

Oxygen Delivery to Tissues

- The oxygen dissociation curve is a graph depicting the relationship of the partial pressure of oxygen to the saturation of hemoglobin.
- This curve relates to the ability of hemoglobin to deliver oxygen to tissues. If the curve is shifted to the left, there is a decreased p50, meaning that the amount of oxygen needed to saturate hemoglobin 50% is lessened and that there is an increased affinity of hemoglobin for oxygen.
- A pH in the alkalotic range induces this left shift. When there is a decrease in pH, the curve is shifted to the right, denoting a decreased affinity of hemoglobin for oxygen.

Protein Structure

- It would be hard to overstate the importance of proteins in the human body. They makeup ion channels, carry necessary lipophilic substances throughout our mostly lipophobic body, and participate in innumerable biological processes.
- For proteins to complete necessary functions, they must be in the proper configuration. The charges on proteins are what allow their proper shape to exist.
- When pH is altered outside of the physiological range, these charges are altered. The proteins are denatured leading to detrimental changes in architecture that cause a loss of proper function.

Biochemical Processes

- Throughout the human body, many chemical reactions are in equilibrium. One of the most important was previously mentioned with the equation:

$$H_2O + CO_2 <-> H_2CO_3 <-> H^+ + HCO_3^-$$

- The Le Chatelier Principle states that when the variables of concentration, pressure, or temperature are changed, a system in equilibrium will react accordingly to restore a new steady state. For the reaction above, this states that if more hydrogen ions are produced, the equation will shift to the left so that more reactants are formed, and the system can remain in equilibrium.
- This is how compensatory pH mechanisms work; if there is a metabolic acidosis present, the kidneys are not excreting enough hydrogen ions and/or not reabsorbing enough bicarbonate.
- The respiratory system reacts by increasing minute ventilation (often by increasing respiratory rate) and expiring more CO_2 to restore equilibrium.

ORGAN SYSTEMS INVOLVED IN pH BALANCE

- Every organ system of the human body relies on pH balance; however, the renal system and the pulmonary system are the two main modulators. The pulmonary system adjusts pH using carbon dioxide; upon expiration, carbon dioxide is projected into the environment.
- Due to carbon dioxide forming carbonic acid in the body when combining with water, the amount of carbon dioxide expired can cause pH to increase or decrease.
- When the respiratory system is utilized to compensate for metabolic pH disturbances, the effect occurs in minutes to hours.
- The renal system affects pH by reabsorbing bicarbonate and excreting fixed acids. Whether due to pathology or necessary compensation, the kidney excretes or reabsorbs these substances which affect pH.
- The nephron is the functional unit of the kidney. Blood vessels called glomeruli transport substances found in the blood to the renal tubules so that some can be filtered out while others are reabsorbed into the blood and recycled.
- This is true for hydrogen ions and bicarbonate. If bicarbonate is reabsorbed and/or acid is secreted into the urine, the pH becomes more alkaline (increases).
- When bicarbonate is not reabsorbed or acid is not excreted into the urine, pH becomes more acidic (decreases).
- The metabolic compensation from the renal system takes longer to occur—days rather than minutes or hours.

Buffer Systems in the Body

The buffer systems in the human body are extremely efficient, and different systems work at different rates. It takes only seconds for the chemical buffers in the blood to make adjustments to pH. The respiratory tract can adjust the blood pH upward in minutes by exhaling CO_2 from the body.
- The renal system can also adjust blood pH through the excretion of hydrogen ions (H^+) and the conservation of bicarbonate, but this process takes hours to days to have an effect.
- The buffer systems functioning in blood plasma include plasma proteins, phosphate, and bicarbonate and carbonic acid buffers.
- The kidneys help control acid-base balance by excreting hydrogen ions and generating bicarbonate that helps maintain blood plasma pH within a normal range. Protein buffer systems work predominantly inside cells.

Protein Buffers in Blood Plasma and Cells

- Nearly all proteins can function as buffers. Proteins are made up of amino acids, which contain positively charged amino groups and negatively charged carboxyl groups.
- The charged regions of these molecules can bind hydrogen and hydroxyl ions, and thus function as buffers.
- Buffering by proteins accounts for two-thirds of the buffering power of the blood and most of the buffering within cells.

Hemoglobin as a Buffer

- Hemoglobin is the principal protein inside of red blood cells and accounts for one-third of the mass of the cell.
- During the conversion of CO_2 into bicarbonate, hydrogen ions liberated in the reaction are buffered by hemoglobin, which is reduced by the dissociation of oxygen. This buffering helps maintain normal pH.
- The process is reversed in the pulmonary capillaries to re-form CO_2, which then can diffuse into the air sacs to be exhaled into the atmosphere. This process is discussed in detail in the chapter on the respiratory system.

Phosphate Buffer

- Phosphates are found in the blood in two forms: sodium dihydrogen phosphate (NaH_2PO_4–NaH_2PO_4-), which is a weak acid, and sodium monohydrogen phosphate ($Na_2HPO_4 Na_2HPO_4$), which is a weak base.
- When $Na_2HPO_4 Na_2HPO_4$ comes into contact with a strong acid, such as HCl, the base picks up a second hydrogen ion to form the weak acid $Na_2H_2PO_4 Na_2HPO_4$ and sodium chloride, NaCl.
- When $NaHPO_4 NaHPO_4$ (the weak acid) comes into contact with a strong base, such as sodium hydroxide (NaOH), the weak acid reverts back to the weak base and produces water. Acids and bases are still present, but they hold onto the ions.

Bicarbonate—carbonic Acid Buffer

- The bicarbonate-carbonic acid buffer works in a fashion similar to phosphate buffers. The bicarbonate is regulated in the blood by sodium, as are the phosphate ions.
- When sodium bicarbonate ($NaHCO_3$), comes into contact with a strong acid, such as HCl, carbonic acid (H_2CO_3), which is a weak acid and NaCl are formed. When carbonic acid comes into contact with a strong base, such as NaOH, bicarbonate and water are formed.
- As with the phosphate buffer, a weak acid or weak base captures the free ions, and a significant change in pH is prevented.
- Bicarbonate ions and carbonic acid are present in the blood in a 20:1 ratio if the blood pH is within the normal range. With 20 times more bicarbonate than carbonic acid, this capture system is most efficient at buffering changes that would make the blood more acidic.
- This is useful because most of the body's metabolic wastes, such as lactic acid and ketone bodies, are acids. Carbonic acid levels in the blood are controlled by the expiration of CO_2 through the lungs.
- In red blood cells, carbonic anhydrase forces the dissociation of the acid, rendering the blood less acidic. Because of this acid dissociation, CO_2 is exhaled (see equations above).
- The level of bicarbonate in the blood is controlled through the renal system, where bicarbonate ions in the renal filtrate are conserved and passed back into the blood. However, the bicarbonate buffer is the primary buffering system of the IF surrounding the cells in tissues throughout the body.

Respiratory Regulation of Acid-base Balance

The respiratory system contributes to the balance of acids and bases in the body by regulating the blood levels of carbonic acid. CO_2 in the blood readily reacts with water to form carbonic acid, and the levels of CO_2 and carbonic acid in the blood are in equilibrium.

Figure 20.2 is depicted the respiratory regulation of blood pH. The respiratory system can reduce blood pH by removing CO_2 from the blood.

- When the CO_2 level in the blood rises (as it does when you hold your breath), the excess CO_2 reacts with water to form additional carbonic acid, lowering blood pH.
- Increasing the rate and/or depth of respiration (which you might feel the "urge" to do after holding your breath) allows you to exhale more CO_2. The loss of CO_2 from the body reduces blood levels of carbonic acid and thereby adjusts the pH upward, toward normal levels.

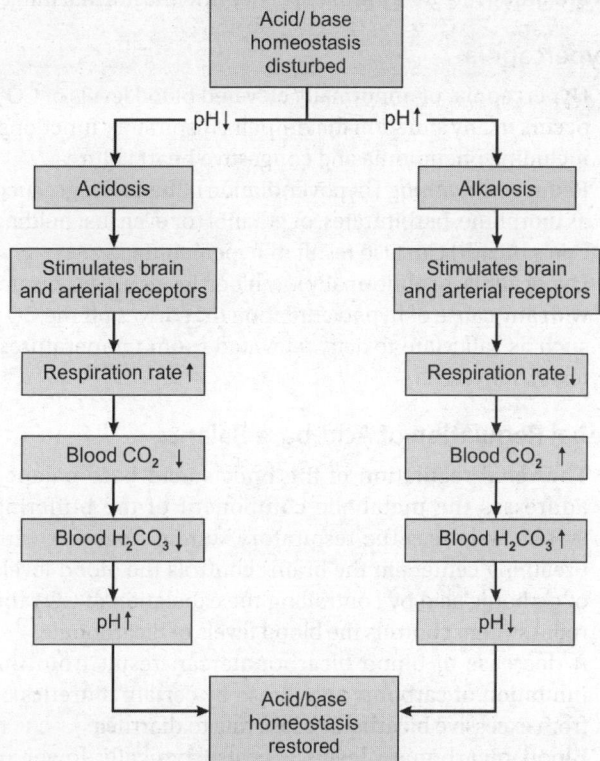

Fig. 20.2: Respiratory regulation of blood pH. The respiratory system can reduce blood pH by removing CO_2 from the blood.

- Excessive deep and rapid breathing (as in hyperventilation) rids the blood of CO_2 and reduces the level of carbonic acid, making the blood too alkaline.
- This brief alkalosis can be remedied by rebreathing air that has been exhaled into a paper bag. Rebreathing exhaled air will rapidly bring blood pH down toward normal.
- The chemical reactions that regulate the levels of CO_2 and carbonic acid occur in the lungs when blood travels through the lung's pulmonary capillaries.
- Minor adjustments in breathing are usually sufficient to adjust the pH of the blood by changing how much CO_2 is exhaled.
- In fact, doubling the respiratory rate for less than 1 minute, removing "extra" CO_2, would increase the blood pH by 0.2. This situation is common if you are exercising strenuously over a period of time.
- To keep up the necessary energy production, you would produce excess CO_2 (and lactic acid if exercising beyond your aerobic threshold). In order to balance the increased acid production, the respiration rate goes up to remove the CO_2. This helps to keep you from developing acidosis.
- The body regulates the respiratory rate by the use of chemoreceptors, which primarily use CO_2 as a signal. Peripheral blood sensors are found in the walls of the aorta and carotid arteries.
- These sensors signal the brain to provide immediate adjustments to the respiratory rate if CO_2 levels rise or fall. Yet other sensors are found in the brain itself.
- Changes in the pH of CSF affect the respiratory center in the medulla oblongata, which can directly modulate breathing rate to bring the pH back into the normal range.

Hypercapnia

- Hypercapnia, or abnormally elevated blood levels of CO_2, occurs in any situation that impairs respiratory functions, including pneumonia and congestive heart failure.
- Reduced breathing (hypoventilation) due to drugs, such as morphine, barbiturates, or ethanol (or even just holding one's breath) can also result in hypercapnia.
- Hypocapnia, or abnormally low blood levels of CO_2, occurs with any cause of hyperventilation that drives off the CO_2, such as salicylate toxicity, elevated room temperatures, fever, or hysteria.

Renal Regulation of Acid-base Balance

- The renal regulation of the body's acid-base balance addresses the metabolic component of the buffering system. Whereas the respiratory system (together with breathing centers in the brain) controls the blood levels of carbonic acid by controlling the exhalation of CO_2, the renal system controls the blood levels of bicarbonate.
- A decrease of blood bicarbonate can result from the inhibition of carbonic anhydrase by certain diuretics or from excessive bicarbonate loss due to diarrhea.
- Blood bicarbonate levels are also typically lower in people who have Addison's disease (chronic adrenal insufficiency), in which aldosterone levels are reduced, and in people who have renal damage, such as chronic nephritis.
- Finally, low bicarbonate blood levels can result from elevated levels of ketones (common in unmanaged diabetes mellitus), which bind bicarbonate in the filtrate and prevent its conservation.
- Bicarbonate ions, HCO_3^-, found in the filtrate, are essential to the bicarbonate buffer system, yet the cells of the tubule are not permeable to bicarbonate ions.

The steps involved in supplying bicarbonate ions

The steps involved in supplying bicarbonate ions to the system and are summarized below:
- **Step 1:** Sodium ions are reabsorbed from the filtrate in exchange for H^+ by an antiport mechanism in the apical membranes of cells lining the renal tubule.
- **Step 2:** The cells produce bicarbonate ions that can be shunted to peritubular capillaries.
- **Step 3:** When CO_2 is available, the reaction is driven to the formation of carbonic acid, which dissociates to form a bicarbonate ion and a hydrogen ion.
- **Step 4:** The bicarbonate ion passes into the peritubular capillaries and returns to the blood. The hydrogen ion is secreted into the filtrate, where it can become part of new water molecules and be reabsorbed as such, or removed in the urine.

It is also possible that salts in the filtrate, such as sulfates, phosphates, or ammonia, will capture hydrogen ions. If this occurs, the hydrogen ions will not be available to combine with bicarbonate ions and produce CO_2. In such cases, bicarbonate ions are not conserved from the filtrate to the blood, which will also contribute to a pH imbalance and acidosis.

The hydrogen ions also compete with potassium to exchange with sodium in the renal tubules. If more potassium is present than normal, potassium, rather than the hydrogen ions, will be exchanged, and increased potassium enters the filtrate. When this occurs, fewer hydrogen ions in the filtrate participate in the conversion of bicarbonate into CO_2 and less bicarbonate is conserved. If there is less potassium, more hydrogen ions enter the filtrate to be exchanged with sodium and more bicarbonate is conserved.

Chloride ions are important in neutralizing positive ion charges in the body. If chloride is lost, the body uses bicarbonate ions in place of the lost chloride ions. Thus, lost chloride results in an increased reabsorption of bicarbonate by the renal system.

Arterial Blood Gas

Arterial blood gas (ABG) sampling is a test often performed in an inpatient setting to assess the acid-base status of a patient. A needle is used to draw blood from an artery, often the radial, and the blood is analyzed to determine parameters such as the pH, pCO_2, pO_2, HCO_3, oxygen saturation, and more. This allows the physician to understand the status of the patient better. ABGs are especially important in the critically ill. They are the main tool utilized in adjusting to the needs of a patient on a ventilator.

Definition

Arterial blood gases (ABG) are measured by collecting blood from an artery, rather than a vein, and are most commonly collected via the radial artery. ABGs measure the pH level of the blood, the partial pressure of arterial oxygen (PaO_2), the partial pressure of arterial carbon dioxide ($PaCO_2$), the bicarbonate level (HCO_3), and the oxygen saturation level (SaO_2).

Normal Values on an ABG

The following are the most important normal values on an ABG:
- pH = 7.35 to 7.45
- pCO_2 = 35 to 45 mm Hg
- pO_2 = 75 to 100 mm Hg
- HCO_3^- = 22 to 26 mEq/L
- O_2 Sat = greater than 95%

Interpretation

The ability to quickly and efficiently read an ABG, especially in reference to inpatient medicine, is paramount to quality patient care.
- Look at the pH
- Decide whether it is acidotic, alkalotic, or within the physiological range
- $PaCO_2$ level determines respiratory contribution; a high level means the respiratory system is lowering the pH and vice versa.
- HCO_3^- level denotes metabolic/kidney effect. An elevated HCO_3^- is raising the pH and vice versa.
- If the pH is acidotic, look for the number that corresponds with a lower pH. If it is a respiratory acidosis, the CO_2 should be high. If the patient is compensating metabolically, the HCO_3^- should be high as well. A metabolic acidosis will be depicted with an HCO_3^- that is low.
- If the pH is alkalotic, again, determine which value is causing this. A respiratory alkalosis will mean the CO_2 is low; a metabolic alkalosis should lend an HCO_3^- that is high. Compensation with either system will be reflected oppositely; for a respiratory alkalosis the metabolic response should be a low HCO_3^- and for metabolic alkalosis, the respiratory response should be a high CO_2.
- If the pH level is in the physiological range but the $PaCO_2$ and/or bicarb are not within normal limits, there is likely a mixed disorder. Also, compensation does not always occur; this is when clinical information becomes paramount.
- Sometimes, it is difficult to ascertain whether a patient has a mixed disorder.

Table 20.1 is depicted the ABG components, descriptions, adult normal values, and critical values.

Other tests that are important to perform when analyzing the acid-base status of a patient include those that measure electrolyte levels and renal function. This helps the clinician gather information that can be used to determine the exact mechanism of the acid-base imbalance as well as the factors contributing to the disorders.

Figure 20.3 is depicted the symptoms of acidosis and alkalosis.

RESPIRATORY ACIDOSIS

Respiratory acidosis develops when carbon dioxide (CO_2) builds up in the body (referred to as hypercapnia), causing the blood to become increasingly acidic. Respiratory acidosis is identified when reviewing ABGs and the pH level is below 7.35 and the $PaCO_2$ level is above 45, indicating the cause of the acidosis is respiratory. Note that in respiratory acidosis, as the $PaCO_2$ level increases, the pH level decreases.

- Respiratory acidosis is typically caused by a medical condition that decreases the exchange of oxygen and carbon dioxide at the alveolar level, such as an acute asthma exacerbation, chronic obstructive pulmonary disease (COPD), or an acute heart failure exacerbation causing pulmonary edema.
- It can also be caused by decreased ventilation from anesthesia, alcohol, or administration of medications, such as opioids and sedatives.
- Chronic respiratory diseases, such as COPD, often cause chronic respiratory acidosis that is fully compensated by the kidneys retaining HCO_3.
- Because the carbon dioxide levels build up over time, the body adapts to elevated $PaCO_2$ levels so they are better

Table 20.1: ABG components, descriptions, adult normal values, and critical values.

Abg component	Description	Adult normal value	Critical value
pH	• Acidity (<7.35) or alkalinity (>7.45) of blood • Measure of H^+ ions (acids) • Affected by the lungs via hypo- or hyperventilation or the kidneys through bicarbonate retention	7.35–7.45	<7.25 >7.60
PaO_2	• Pressure of oxygen in the blood	80–100 mm Hg	<60 mm Hg
$PaCO_2$	• Pressure of carbon dioxide in the blood • CO_2 is an acid managed by the lungs • As $PaCO_2$ increases, the blood becomes more acidic and the pH decreases • As $PaCO_2$ decreases, the blood becomes less acidic and the pH increases	35–45 mm Hg	<25 mm Hg >60 mm Hg
HCO_3	• Bicarbonate level in the blood • HCO_3 is a base managed by the kidneys • As HCO_3 increases, the blood becomes more alkaline and the pH increases • As HCO_3 decreases, the blood becomes more acidic and the pH decreases	22–26 mEq/L	<10 mEq/L >40 mEq/L
SaO_2	Oxygen saturation in the blood	95–100%	<88%

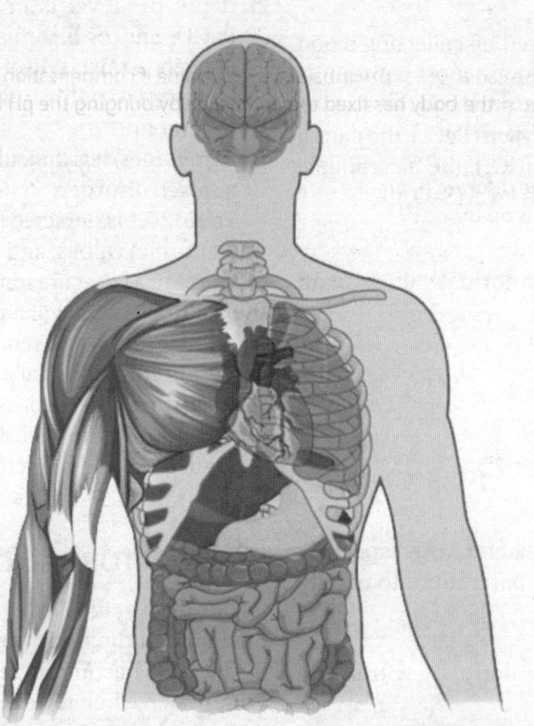

Symptoms of acidosis

Central nervous system
Headache
Sleepiness
Confusion
Loss of consciousness
Coma

Respiratory system
Shortness of breath
coughing

Heart
Arrhythmia
Increased heart rate

Muscular system
Seizures
Weakness

Digestive system
Nausea
Vomiting
Diarrhea

Symptoms of alkalosis

Central nervous system
Confusion
Light-headedness
Stupor
Coma

Peripheral nervous system
Hand tremor
Numbness or tingling in the face, hands, or feet

Muscular system
Twitching
Prolonged spasms

Digestive system
Nausea
Vomiting

Fig. 20.3: Symptoms of acidosis and alkalosis.

tolerated. However, in acute respiratory acidosis, the body has not had time to adapt to elevated carbon dioxide levels, causing mental status changes associated with hypercapnia.
- Acute respiratory acidosis is caused by acute respiratory conditions, such as an asthma attack or heart failure exacerbation with pulmonary edema when the lungs suddenly are not able to ventilate adequately.
- As breathing slows and respirations become shallow, less CO_2 is excreted by the lungs and $PaCO_2$ levels quickly rise.

Table 20.2 is depicted the analyzing ABG results.

Signs of Symptoms of Hypercapnia

Signs of symptoms of hypercapnia vary depending upon the level and rate of CO_2 accumulation in arterial blood:
1. Patients with mild to moderate hypercapnia may be anxious and/or complain of mild dyspnea, daytime sluggishness, headaches, or hypersomnolence.
2. Patients with higher levels of CO_2 or rapidly developing hypercapnia develop delirium, paranoia, depression, and confusion that can progress to seizures and coma as levels continue to rise.

Table 20.2: Analyzing ABG results.

Step	Action
Step 1: pH (normal 7.35–7.45)	If pH is out of range, determine if it is acidosis or alkalosis: • pH <7.35 is acidosis • pH >7.45 is alkalosis

Step 2: $PaCO_2$ (normal 35–45 mm Hg)	• Is the $PaCO_2$ normal?
	  ▪ $PaCO_2$ <35 is considered alkalotic
	  ▪ $PaCO_2$ >45 is considered acidotic
	• If the $PaCO_2$ is abnormal, determine if this is caused by a respiratory problem. Recall that if the imbalance is caused by a respiratory problem, the $PaCO_2$ moves in the opposite direction of the pH:
	  ▪ If the pH is <7.35 (acidosis) and the $PaCO_2$ is >45 (acidotic), this is respiratory acidosis
	  ▪ If the pH is >7.45 (alkalosis) and the $PaCO_2$ is <35 (alkalotic), this is respiratory alkalosis
	**If the imbalance does not appear to be caused by a respiratory problem, move on to evaluate the HCO_3

Step 3: HCO_3 (normal 22–26)	• Is the HCO_3 normal?
	  ▪ HCO_3 <22 is considered acidotic
	  ▪ HCO_3 >26 is considered alkalotic
	• If the HCO_3 is abnormal, determine if this caused by a metabolic problem. Recall that the HCO_3 moves in the same direction as the pH if the imbalance is caused by a metabolic problem:
	  ▪ If pH is <7.35 (acidosis) and the HCO_3 is <22 (acidotic), this is metabolic acidosis
	  ▪ If the pH is >7.45 (alkalosis) and the HCO_3 is >26 (alkalotic), this is metabolic alkalosis

Contd...

Contd...

Step	Action

Step 4: Determine level of compensation	After determining the cause of the pH imbalance, determine if compensation is occurring.
	• Fully compensated = the body has fixed the imbalance by bringing the pH back to normal:
	    ▪ pH is normal (7.35–7.45)
	    ▪ $PaCO_2$ and HCO_3 are both out of range
	    ▪ The cause of the disorder is out of range, and the other value is significantly out of range indicating compensation is occurring
	    ▪ Recall the respiratory rate quickly compensates for metabolic disorders, and the kidneys take longer to compensate for respiratory disorders

	• Partially compensated = the body is working to fix the imbalance but hasn't yet brought the pH back to normal:
	    ▪ pH is abnormal (<7.35 or >7.45).
	    ▪ $PaCO_2$ and HCO_3 are abnormal.
	    ▪ The cause of the disorder is out of range and the other value is moving out of range, indicating compensation is occurring.
	• Uncompensated = the body is not yet working to bring the pH back to normal:
	    ▪ pH is abnormal (<7.35 or >7.45)
	    ▪ $PaCO_2$ or HCO_3 is abnormal, but not both.
	    ▪ The CAUSE of the disorder is out of range but the other value is not yet out of range, indicating compensation is not yet occurring.

Management

Individuals with normal lung function typically exhibit a depressed level of consciousness when the $PaCO_2$ is greater than 75 to 80 mm Hg, whereas patients with chronic hypercapnia may not develop symptoms until the $PaCO_2$ rises above 90 to 100 mm Hg.

Figures 20.4A and B are depicted the metabolic acidosis and respiratory acidosis.
- When a patient demonstrates signs of potential hypercapnia, the nurse should assess airway, breathing, and circulation. Urgent assistance should be sought, especially if the patient is in respiratory distress.
- The provider will order an ABG and prescribe treatments based on assessment findings and potential causes.
- Treatment for respiratory acidosis typically involves improving ventilation and respiration by removing airway restrictions, reversing over sedation, administering nebulizer treatments, or increasing the rate and depth of respiration by using a BiPAP or CPAP devices.
- BiPAP and CPAP devices provide noninvasive positive pressure ventilation to increase the depth of respirations, remove carbon dioxide, and oxygenate the patient.
- If these noninvasive interventions are not successful, the patient is intubated and placed on mechanical ventilation.

Respiratory Alkalosis

Respiratory alkalosis develops when the body removes too much carbon dioxide through respiration, resulting in increased pH and an alkalotic state. When reviewing ABGs, respiratory alkalosis is identified when pH levels are above 7.45 and the $PaCO_2$ level is below 35. With respiratory alkalosis, notice that as the $PaCO_2$ level decreases, the pH level increases.

Figure 20.5 is depicted the respiratory alkalosis.
- Respiratory alkalosis is caused by hyperventilation that can occur due to anxiety, panic attacks, pain, fear, head injuries, or mechanical ventilation. Overdoses of salicylates and other toxins can also cause respiratory alkalosis initially and then often progress to metabolic acidosis in later stages.

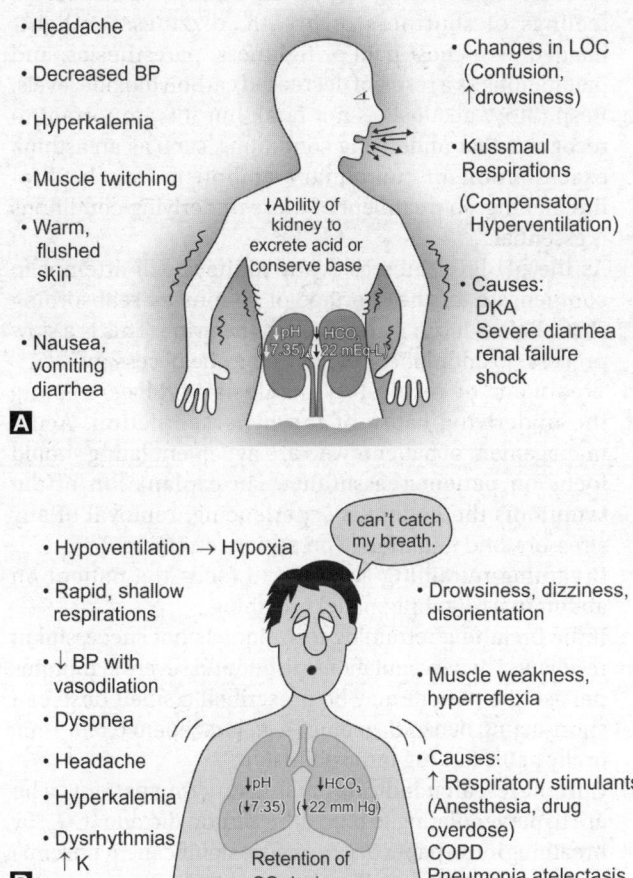

Figs. 20.4A and B: (A) Metabolic acidosis; (B) Respiratory acidosis.

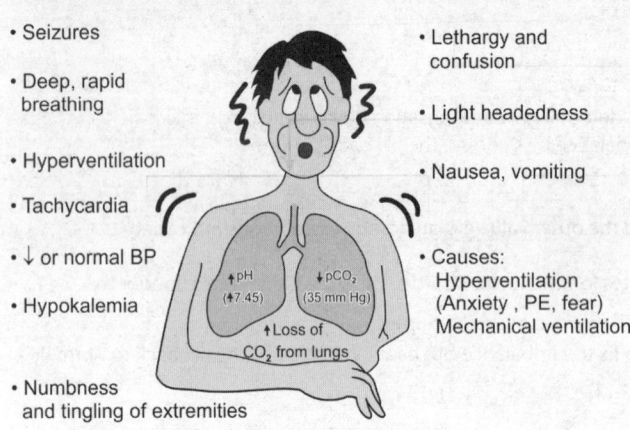

Fig. 20.5: Respiratory alkalosis.

- Acute asthma exacerbations, pulmonary embolisms, or other respiratory disorders can initially cause respiratory alkalosis as the lungs breath faster in an attempt to increase oxygenation, which decreases the $PaCO_2$.
- After a while, however, these hypoxic disorders cause respiratory acidosis as respiratory muscles tire, breathing slows, and CO_2 builds up in the blood.
- Patients experiencing respiratory alkalosis often report feelings of shortness of breath, dizziness or lightheadedness, chest pain or tightness, paresthesias, and palpitations as a result of decreased carbon dioxide levels.
- Respiratory alkalosis is not fatal, but it is important to recognize that underlying conditions, such as an asthma exacerbation or pulmonary embolism can be life-threatening, so treatment of these underlying conditions is essential.
- As the pH level increases, the kidneys will attempt to compensate for the shortage of H^+ ions by reabsorbing HCO_3 before it can be excreted in the urine. This is a slow process, so additional treatment may be necessary.
- Treatment of respiratory alkalosis involves treating the underlying cause of the hyperventilation. Acute management of patients who are hyperventilating should focus on patient reassurance, an explanation of the symptoms the patient is experiencing, removal of any stressors, and initiation of breathing retraining.
- Breathing retraining attempts to focus the patient on abdominal (diaphragmatic) breathing.
- If the breathing retraining technique is not successful in resolving a hyperventilation episode and severe symptoms persist, the patient may be prescribed a small dose of a short-acting benzodiazepine (e.g., lorazepam 0.5 to 1 mg orally or 0.5 to 1 mg intravenously).
- Current research indicates that instructing patients who are hyperventilating to rebreathe carbon dioxide (CO_2) by breathing into a paper bag can cause significant hypoxemia with significant complications, so this intervention is no longer recommended. If rebreathing is used, oxygen saturation levels should be continuously monitored.

Metabolic Acidosis

Metabolic acidosis occurs when there is an accumulation of acids (hydrogen ions) and not enough bases (HCO_3) in the body. Under normal conditions, the kidneys work to excrete acids through urine and neutralize excess acids by increasing bicarbonate (HCO_3) reabsorption from the urine to maintain a normal pH. When the kidneys are not able to perform this buffering function to the level required excreting and neutralizing the excess acid, metabolic acidosis results.

- Metabolic acidosis is characterized by a pH level below 7.35 and an HCO_3 level below 22 when reviewing ABGs.
- It is important to notice that both the pH and HCO_3 decrease with metabolic acidosis (i.e., the pH and HCO_3 move in the same downward direction).
- A common cause of metabolic acidosis is diabetic ketoacidosis, where acids called ketones build up in the blood when blood sugar is extremely elevated.
- Another common cause of metabolic acidosis in hospitalized patients is lactic acidosis, which can be caused by impaired tissue oxygenation.
- Metabolic acidosis can also be caused by increased loss of bicarbonate due to severe diarrhea or from renal disease that causes decreased acid elimination. Additionally, toxins such as salicylate excess can cause metabolic acidosis.
- Nurses may first suspect that a patient has metabolic acidosis due to rapid breathing that occurs as the lungs try to remove excess CO_2 in an attempt to resolve the acidosis.
- Other symptoms of metabolic acidosis include confusion, decreased level of consciousness, hypotension, and electrolyte disturbances that can progress to circulatory collapse and death if not treated promptly.
- It is important to quickly notify the provider of suspected metabolic acidosis so that an ABG can be drawn and treatment prescribed (based on the cause of the metabolic acidosis) to allow acid levels to improve.
- Treatment includes IV fluids to improve hydration status, glucose management, and circulatory support. When pH drops below 7.1, IV sodium bicarbonate is often prescribed to help neutralize the acids in the blood.

Figure 20.6 is depicted the mechanism of metabolic acidosis.

METABOLIC ALKALOSIS (FIG. 20.7)

Metabolic alkalosis occurs when there is too much bicarbonate (HCO_3) in the body or an excessive loss of acid (H^+ ions). Metabolic alkalosis is defined by a pH above 7.45 and an HCO_3 level above 26 on ABG results. Note that both pH and HCO_3 are elevated in metabolic alkalosis.

- Metabolic alkalosis can be caused by gastrointestinal loss of hydrogen ions, excessive urine loss, excessive levels of bicarbonate, or a shift of hydrogen ions from the bloodstream into cells.
- Prolonged vomiting or nasogastric suctioning can also cause metabolic alkalosis. Gastric secretions have high levels of hydrogen ions (H^+), so as acid is lost, the pH level of the bloodstream increases.
- Excessive urinary loss (due to diuretics or excessive mineralocorticoids) can cause metabolic alkalosis due to loss of hydrogen ions in the urine. Intravenous administration

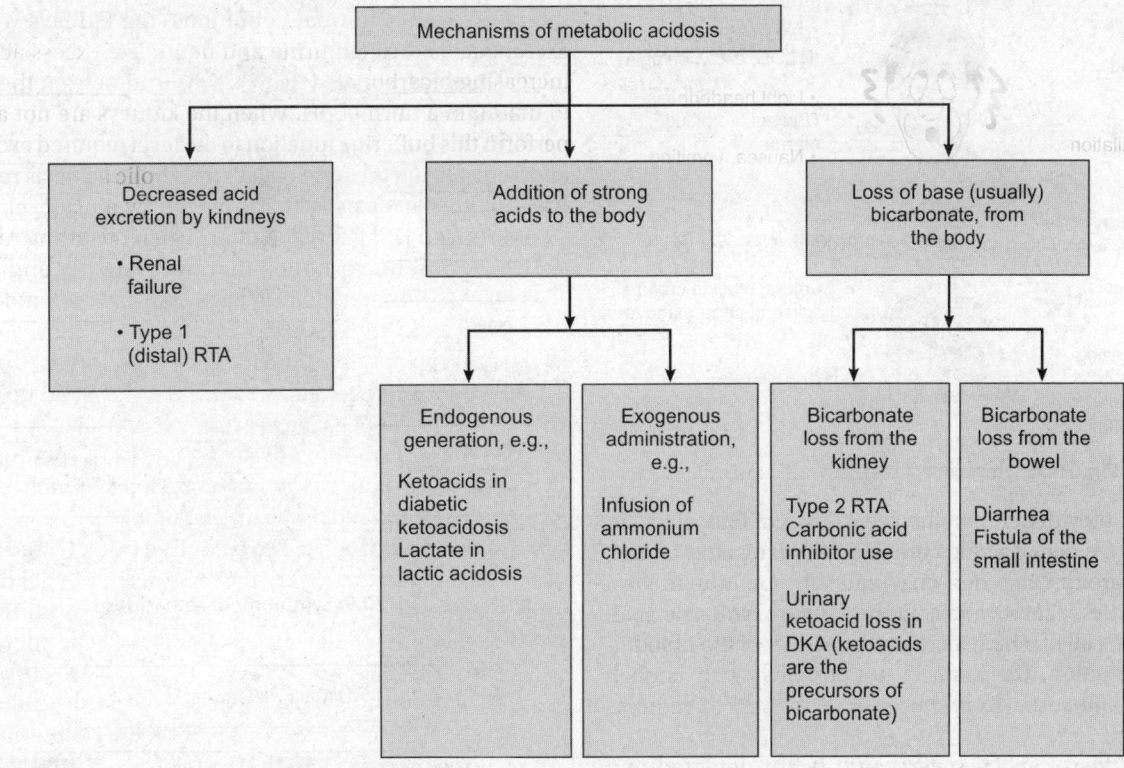

Fig. 20.6: Mechanism of metabolic acidosis.

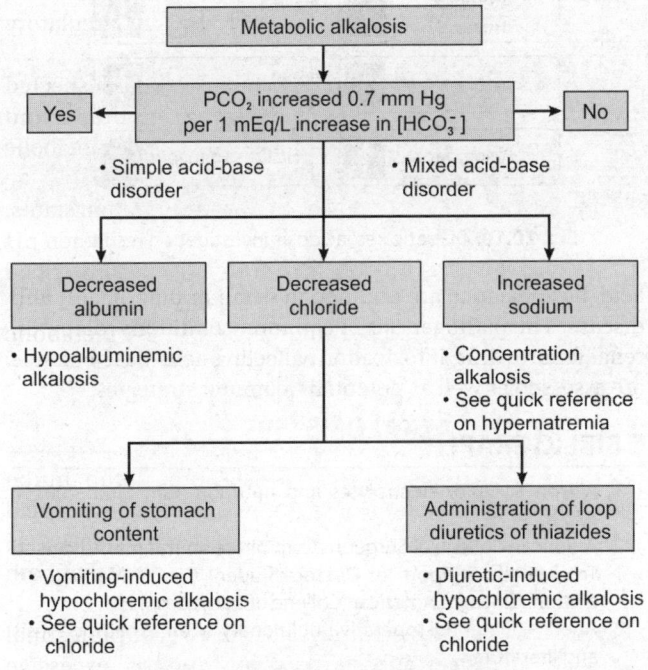

Fig. 20.7: Mechanism of metabolic alkalosis.

of sodium bicarbonate can also cause metabolic alkalosis due to increased levels of bases introduced into the body. Although it was once thought that excessive intake of calcium antacids could cause metabolic alkalosis, it has been found that this only occurs if they are administered concurrently with kayexalate.

- Hydrogen ions may shift into cells due to hypokalemia, causing metabolic alkalosis. When hypokalemia occurs (i.e., low levels of potassium in the bloodstream), potassium shifts out of cells and into the bloodstream in an attempt to maintain a normal level of serum potassium for optimal cardiac function.
- However, as the potassium (K^+) molecules move out of the cells, hydrogen (H^+) ions then move into the cells from the bloodstream to maintain electrical neutrality. This transfer of ions causes the pH in the bloodstream to drop, causing metabolic alkalosis.
- A nurse may first suspect that a patient has metabolic alkalosis due to a decreased respiratory rate (as the lungs try to retain additional CO_2 to increase the acidity of the blood and resolve the alkalosis).
- The patient may also be confused due to the altered pH level. The nurse should report signs of suspected metabolic alkalosis because uncorrected metabolic alkalosis can result in hypotension and cardiac dysfunction.
- Treatment is prescribed based on the ABG results and the suspected cause.
- For example, treat the cause of the vomiting, stop the gastrointestinal suctioning, or stop the administration of diuretics. If hypokalemia is present, it should be treated. If bicarbonate is being administered, it should be stopped. Patients with kidney disease may require dialysis

Figure 20.8 is depicted the symptoms of metabolic alkalosis.

ACID-BASE BALANCE: KETOACIDOSIS

Diabetic acidosis, or ketoacidosis, occurs most frequently in people with poorly controlled diabetes mellitus. When certain tissues in the body cannot get adequate amounts

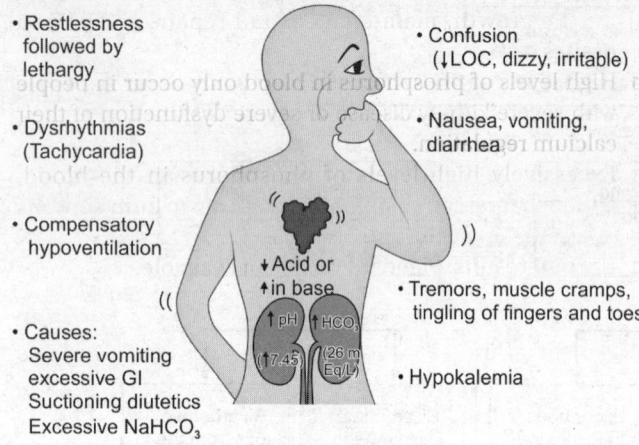

Fig. 20.8: Symptoms of metabolic alkalosis.

of glucose, they depend on the breakdown of fatty acids for energy. When acetyl groups break off the fatty acid chains, the acetyl groups then non-enzymatically combine to form ketone bodies, acetoacetic acid, beta-hydroxybutyric acid, and acetone, all of which increase the acidity of the blood.

In this condition, the brain is not supplied with enough of its fuel—glucose—to produce all of the ATP it requires functioning.

- Ketoacidosis can be severe and, if not detected and treated properly, can lead to diabetic coma, which can be fatal. A common early symptom of ketoacidosis is deep, rapid breathing as the body attempts to drive off CO_2 and compensate for the acidosis.
- Another common symptom is fruity-smelling breath, due to the exhalation of acetone. Other symptoms include dry skin and mouth, a flushed face, nausea, vomiting, and stomach pain.
- Treatment for diabetic coma is ingestion or injection of sugar; its prevention is the proper daily administration of insulin.
- A person who is diabetic and uses insulin can initiate ketoacidosis if a dose of insulin is missed. Among people with type 2 diabetes, those of Hispanic and African-American descent are more likely to go into ketoacidosis than those of other ethnic backgrounds, although the reason for this is unknown.

Figure 20.9 is depicted the symptoms of ketoacidosis and **Figure 20.10** is depicted the diabetic ketoacidosis investigation results.

CONCLUSION

Maintenance of acid–base balance is fundamental for the normal functioning of biological processes, mainly due to the pH dependence of enzyme function. Normal acid–base balance is maintained by the lungs and kidneys. Carbon dioxide, a by-product of normal metabolism, is a weak acid. The lungs are able to prevent an increase in the partial pressure of carbon dioxide (PCO_2) in the blood by excreting the carbon dioxide (CO_2) produced by the body. The individual roles of the kidney, liver, bone, and lungs in maintenance of

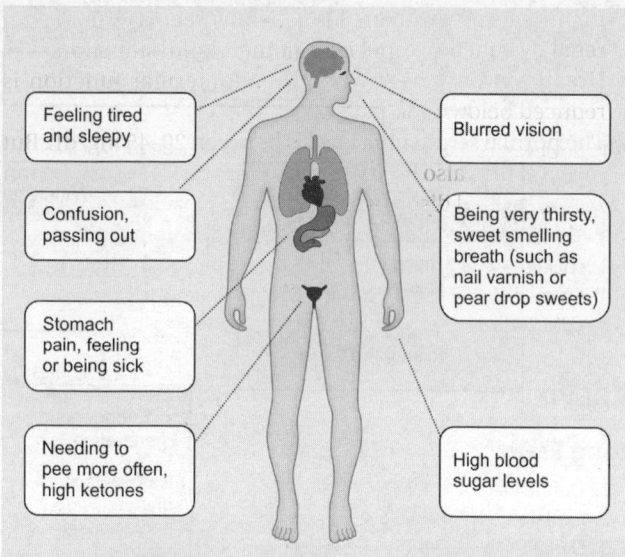

Fig. 20.9: Symptoms of ketoacidosis.

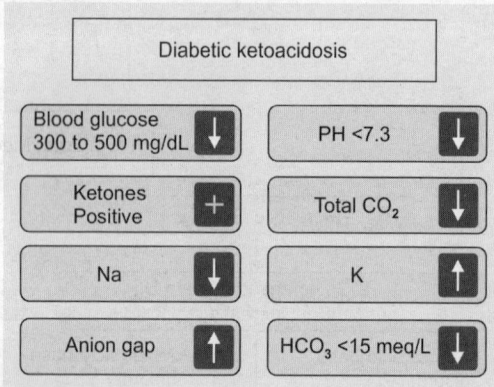

Fig. 20.10: Diabetic ketoacidosis investigation results.

acid–base balance are outlined in detail in both health and disease. The pathogenesis of common conditions (diabetes, renal failure, drug intoxication) affecting acid–base balance are assessed as well as potential treatment strategies.

BIBLIOGRAPHY

1. Allison S. Fluid, electrolytes and nutrition. Clin Med. 2004;4: 573-8.
2. American College of Surgeons Committee on Trauma. Advanced Trauma Life Support for Doctors Student Course Manual, 6th edition. Chicago: American College of Surgeons, 1997.
3. Arieff AI. Fatal postoperative pulmonary edema: pathogenesis and literature
4. Aukland K, Nicolaysen G. Interstitial fluid volume: local regulatory mechanisms. Physiol Rev. 1981;61:556-643.
5. Care of the Critically Ill. 1999;15:11-6.
6. Clinical outcomes in adults. Anesthesia Analg. 2005;100:1093-106.
7. Cuthbertson DP. Effect of injury on metabolism. Biochem J. 1930;2:1244.
8. Gosling P. Fluid balance in the critically ill: the sodium and water audit.

9. Grocott MPW, Mythen MG, Gan TJ. Perioperative fluid management and
10. Guidet B, Soni N, Della RG, et al. A balanced view of balanced solutions. Crit Care. 2010;14:325.
11. Review. Chest. 1999;115:1371-7.
12. Starker PM, Lasala PA, Askanazi J, et al. The response to TPN. A form of nutritional assessment. Ann Surg. 1983;198:720-4.
13. Starling EH. On the absorption of fluids from connective tissue spaces. J Physiol. 1896;19:312-26.
14. Sterns RH, Silver SM. Salt and water: read the package insert. QJM 2003;96:549.

REVIEW QUESTIONS

Long Essays
1. Define acid bases, explain the concept of acid-base balance.
2. Explain the respiratory regulation of acid-base balance.
3. Describe in detail about arterial blood gas analysis.

Short Essays
1. Buffer systems in the body.
2. Organ systems involved in pH balance.
3. Blood gases.
4. Hypercapnia.
5. Renal regulation of acid-base balance.
6. Respiratory acidosis.
7. Metabolic acidosis.
8. Metabolic alkalosis.
9. Ketoacidosis.

Short Answers
1. Function of pH.
2. Protein buffers in blood plasma and cells.
3. Hemoglobin as a buffer.
4. Phosphate buffer.
5. Bicarbonate—carbonic acid buffer.
6. Normal values on an ABG.
7. Signs and symptoms of hypercapnia.

CHAPTER 21

Heme Catabolism

CHAPTER OUTLINE

- Heme Degradation Pathway
- Jaundice—Type, Causes, Urine and Blood Investigations (Van Den Berg Test)

TERMINOLOGY

- **Heme:** The iron-containing prosthetic group found in a number of proteins, such as hemoglobin, myoglobin, and cytochrome P-450.
- **Regulation:** Heme synthesis is regulated precisely to meet the needs of heme-containing proteins (globins).
- **Feedback regulation by heme:** Heme itself inhibits d-ALA synthetase via repression (genetic) along with diminished transport of coproporphyrinogen III from the cytosol to mitochondria and stimulates the synthesis of the protein part of hemoglobin/myoglobin (the globins).
- **Bilirubin:** is yellow, water insoluble and highly toxic.
- **The Van den Bergh test**—measures levels of conjugated and unconjugated bilirubin via coupling of bilirubin with diazonium salts to produce colored azo dyes.
- **Jaundice:** Term used clinically to describe the yellow color seen in hyperbilirubinemia and is due to deposits of bilirubin in the skin and conjunctiva.

INTRODUCTION

One of the many important functions of heme is to serve as the oxygen-carrying moiety in hemoglobin (Hb) that is expressed in cells along the erythroid lineage. Erythropoiesis requires the proper biosynthesis of heme and as erythroblasts mature, their demand for iron and heme increase dramatically. While all the enzymes involved in heme production have been well-characterized, precisely how proto-porphyrin intermediates cross the mitochondrial inner and outer membranes and are shuttled from one enzyme to another remains largely unknown. In addition, the mechanisms of how iron may be subsequently delivered from endosomes to the mitochondria and traverse the mitochondrial outer membrane remain unresolved. A great deal of recent work has, thus, focused on identifying these intracellular heme transport pathways. There is also accumulating evidence that heme can be transported among various tissues in multi-cellular organisms.

The bile goes through the gallbladder into the intestines where the bilirubin is changed into a variety of pigments. The most important ones are stercobilin, which is excreted in the feces, and urobilinogen, which is reabsorbed back into the blood. The blood transports the urobilinogen back to the liver where it is either re-excreted into the bile or into the blood for transport to the kidneys. Urobilinogen is finally excreted as a normal component of the urine.

Figure 21.1 is depicted the heme catabolism.

The catabolism of hemoglobin is outlined in the graphic on the left. Red blood cells are continuously undergoing a hemolysis (breaking apart) process. The average lifetime of a red blood cell is 120 days. As the red blood cells disintegrate, the hemoglobin is degraded or broken into globin, the protein part, iron (conserved for later use), and heme (see middle graphic). The heme initially breaks apart into biliverdin, a green pigment which is rapidly reduced to bilirubin, an orange-yellow pigment (see bottom graphic). These processes all occur in the reticuloendothelial cells of the liver, spleen, and bone marrow. The bilirubin is then

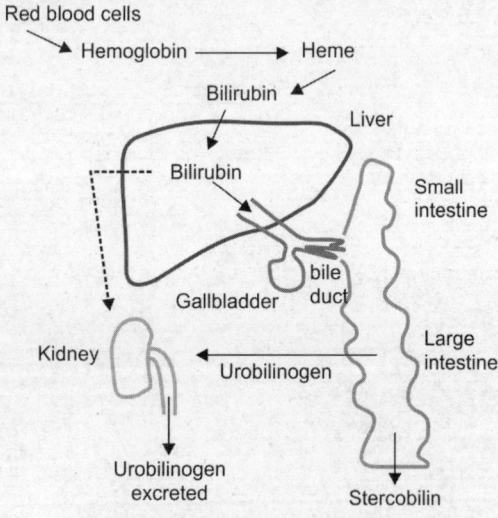

Fig. 21.1: Heme catabolism.

transported to the liver where it reacts with a solubilizing sugar called glucuronic acid. This more soluble form of bilirubin (conjugated) is excreted into the bile.

FUNCTION OF HEME (FIG. 21.2)

Heme has a variety of functions. As a cofactor, it allows for the following:
- Oxygen transport in hemoglobin
- Storage in myoglobin
- A prosthetic group for cytochrome p450 enzymes
- A reservoir of iron
- Electron shuttle of enzymes in the electron transport chain
- Cellular respiration
- Signal transduction-heme regulates the antioxidant response to circadian rhythms, microRNA processing
- Cellular differentiation and proliferation

MECHANISM

Heme Synthesis in Erythroid Cells (Fig. 21.3)

- Heme is synthesized for incorporation into hemoglobin. In immature erythrocytes (reticulocytes), heme stimulates protein synthesis of the globin chains and erythropoietin stimulates heme.
- The kidney releases erythropoietin hormone at low oxygen levels in tissues and stimulates RBC and hemoglobin synthesis.
- Accumulation of heme in erythroid cells is desired as it leads to more globin chain synthesis and required in erythroblast maturation. When red cells mature both heme and hemoglobin synthesis ceases.
- Additionally, control of heme biosynthesis in erythrocytes is controlled by the availability of intracellular iron.

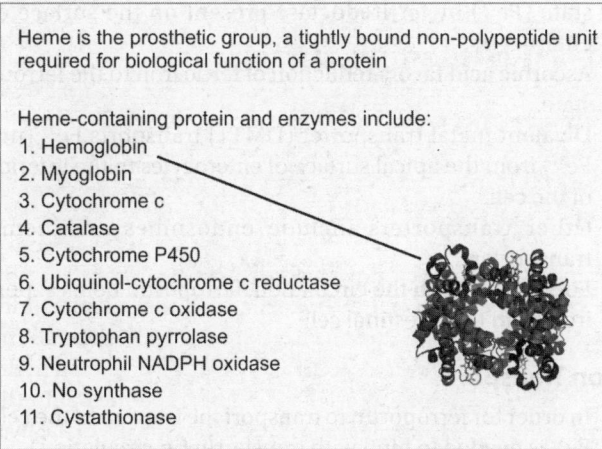

Heme is the prosthetic group, a tightly bound non-polypeptide unit required for biological function of a protein

Heme-containing protein and enzymes include:
1. Hemoglobin
2. Myoglobin
3. Cytochrome c
4. Catalase
5. Cytochrome P450
6. Ubiquinol-cytochrome c reductase
7. Cytochrome c oxidase
8. Tryptophan pyrrolase
9. Neutrophil NADPH oxidase
10. No synthase
11. Cystathionase

Fig. 21.2: Function of heme.

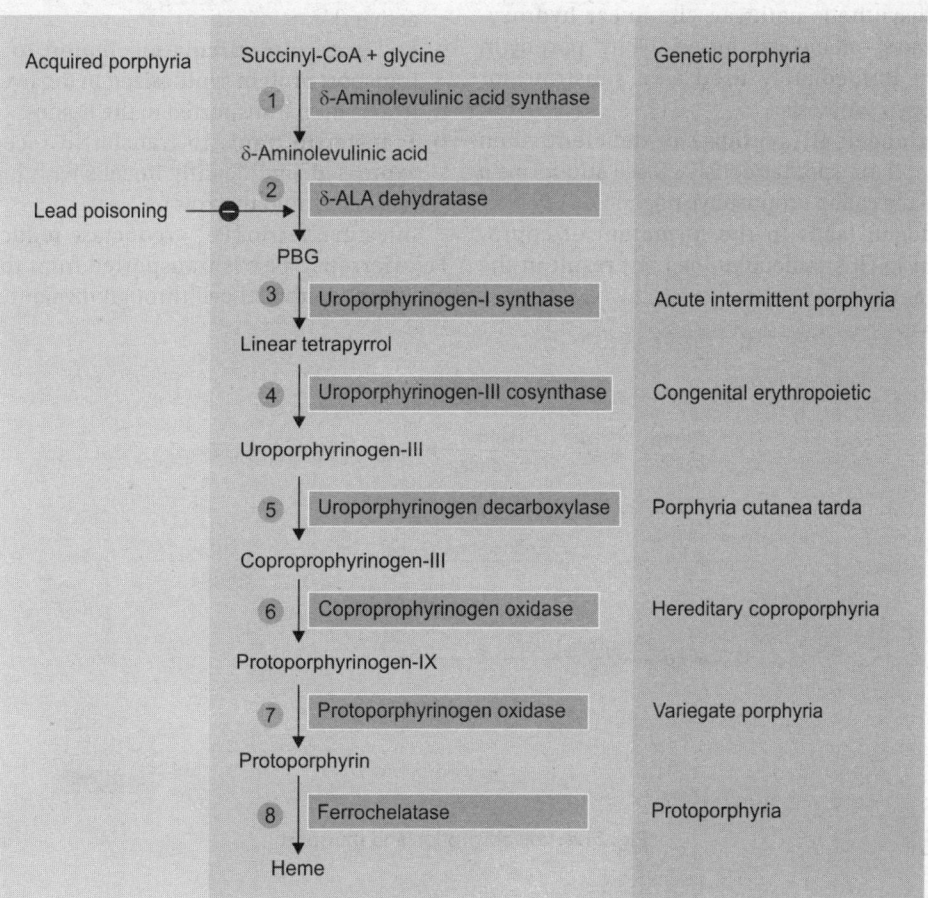

Fig. 21.3: Heme synthesis in erythroid cells.

Heme Synthesis in the Liver

- Heme synthesis in the liver is highly variable and tightly regulated as heme outside proteins causes' damage to hepatocytes at high concentration.
- In the liver, cytochrome P450 (CYP 450) requires heme. Liver contains the isoform ALAS1 which is expressed in most cells.
- Drugs increase ALAS1 activity as they lead to CYP 450 synthesis which needs heme.
- Low intracellular heme concentration stimulates synthesis of ALAS1. Heme synthesis stops when heme is not incorporated into proteins and when heme and hemin accumulate.
- Hemin decreases the synthesis of ALA synthase 1 in three ways: Hemin reduces the synthesis of ALAS1 mRNA, destabilizes ALAS1 mRNA, and inhibits import of the enzyme ALAS1 from the cytosol into mitochondria.

PATHOPHYSIOLOGY

- A defect or mutation in 5'-aminolevulinic acid synthase 2 (ALAS2) leads to a disorder called X-linked sideroblastic anemia.
- It reduces protoporphyrin production and decreases heme. However, iron continues to enter the erythroblast leading to an accumulation in the mitochondria and therefore a manifestation of the disease.
- During the biosynthetic pathway, the linear hydroxymethylbilane can spontaneously form a "faulty" porphyrin ring when not immediately used as a substrate for uroporphyrinogen synthesis.
- If uroporphyrinogen III synthase is deficient, then hydroxymethylbilane spontaneously closes and forms a different molecule called uroporphyrinogen I.
- Uroporphyrinogen leads to the formation of coproporphyrinogen I. This molecule does not result in the formation of heme.

IRON ABSORPTION AND TRANSPORT (FIG. 21.4)

Iron Absorption

Sources of iron:
- Food/diet
- Breakdown of iron-containing products (e.g., hemoglobin)
- Release from reticuloendothelial stores

Dietary iron is absorbed by the enterocytes of the duodenum and proximal jejunum:
- Iron in the ferric state (Fe^{3+}) is reduced to the ferrous state (Fe^{2+}) by ferrireductase present on the surface of enterocytes.
- Ascorbic acid favors reduction of ferric iron to the ferrous state.
- Divalent metal transporter (DMT1) transports Fe^{2+} (not Fe^{3+}) from the apical surface of enterocytes to the interior of the cell.
- Other transporters include endosomes and heme transporter.
- For iron to reach the circulation, ferroportin helps export iron from the intestinal cell.

Iron Transport

- In order for ferroportin to transport the iron out of the cell, Fe^{3+} is needed to bind with transferrin (in circulation).
- Fe^{2+} is oxidized to Fe^{3+} with the aid of hephaestin (a copper-containing membrane protein that has ferroxidase activity).
- Fe^{3+} goes into circulation bound to transferrin (iron transport protein synthesized in the liver).
- Iron is then transported to the tissues.
- Transferrin binds to transferrin receptors, which are expressed significantly in cells with high iron demands (e.g., erythroid marrow).

Intestinal ferric (Fe^{3+}) reductase reduces Fe^{3+} (ferric) to Fe^{2+} (ferrous). Fe^{2+} is transported from the lumen into the intestinal epithelial cell through divalent metal transporter

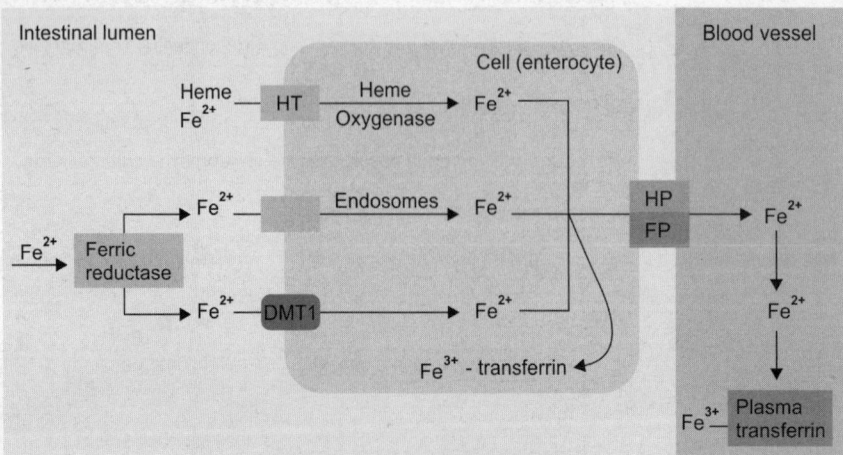

Fig. 21.4: Iron absorption and transport.

1 (DMT1), heme transporter (HT) and/or endosomes. Fe^{2+} can be converted back to Fe^{3+} and bound to transferrin within the intestinal cell or can be transported into the blood by ferroportin (FP) and hephaestin (HP). Oxidized iron (Fe^{3+}), which binds to plasma transferrin, is carried through the circulation to the tissues.

Iron Storage

- **Transferrin carries iron for:**
  - Hematopoiesis in the bone marrow
  - Iron storage in the liver (primary storage site) and other organs
  - Cellular processes requiring iron
- **Storage forms of iron:**
  Ferritin:
  - Main iron storage protein
  - 4500 atoms of iron (when fully loaded)
- **Hemosiderin:** ↑ iron → ferritin forms hemosiderin granules (hemosiderin pigment = aggregates of ferritin micelles)
- **Storage of iron:** Transferrin carries iron for hematopoiesis in the bone marrow, iron storage in the liver (primary storage site) and other organs, and cellular processes requiring iron.

Iron Regulation (Fig. 21.5)

Regulation at the molecular level via the iron response element (IRE) and IRE binding proteins (IRBPs) or iron regulatory proteins (IRPs):

- Involved in posttranscriptional regulation of iron-related genes
- Controls cellular iron uptake, storage and release
- **IRE:** part of the untranslated region (UTR) of the mRNA of the target genes (e.g., ferritin, transferrin receptor, and other iron-metabolizing proteins)
  - Ferritin and ferroportin have the IREs in the 5′ UTR.
  - Transferrin receptor (TfR) has IREs in the 3′ UTR (where binding of IRBP protects from nuclease degradation).
- **IRBPs:** Either a translational enhancer or a translational inhibitor, binding to iron or IRE depending on the required regulation

In Iron Deficiency (Low Iron)

Ferritin

- Ferritin or iron for storage is not needed, as there is low iron for cell usage.
- IRBPs bind ferritin IREs at the 5′ UTR, and interrupt initiation of translation.
- Less ferritin frees up iron for the cells.

TfR

- Since transferrin is needed, IRBPs bind IREs of TfR and produce a different effect.
- IRBP binding to IREs on the 3′ UTR stabilizes the mRNA (protecting from endonucleases).
- This biding allows increased translation of TfR, enhancing iron absorption.

In Iron Abundance (High Iron)

Ferritin

- Ferritin is needed to bind excess iron.
- Iron binds the IRBPs (preventing IREs to be bound), allowing translation of ferritin.

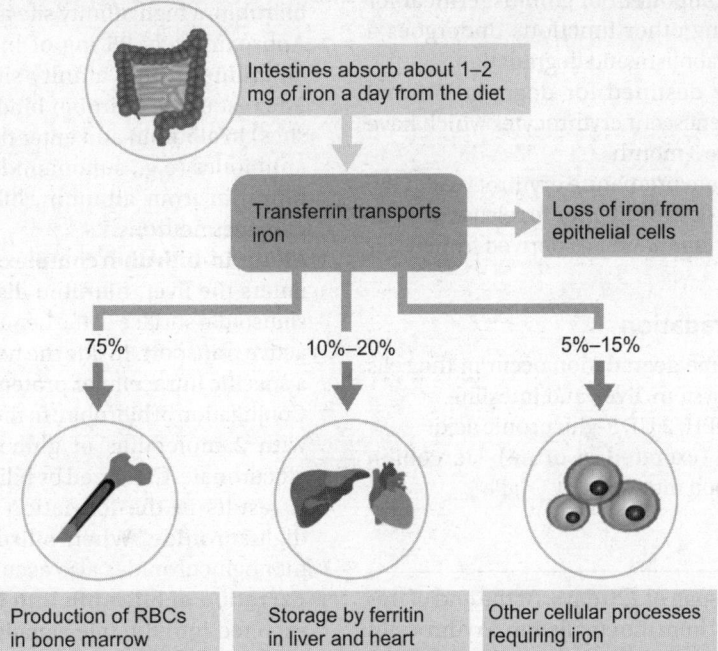

Fig. 21.5: Iron regulation.

TfR

- Increased iron binds the IRBPs.
- Dissociation of IRBPs from the IREs at the 3' UTR exposes the transcripts to endonucleases, increasing mRNA degradation.
- Thus, iron absorption will be inhibited.

Regulation of Iron Availability

Certain conditions require a decrease or increase in iron absorption and circulating iron, a pathway regulated by hepcidin:

- Liver-derived peptide regulating the plasma iron concentration
- Actions (through binding ferroportin):
  - Inhibits intestinal iron uptake
  - Inhibits release of iron from macrophages with old RBCs
- Iron sensing mediated by different proteins:
  - HFE (hereditary iron) protein
  - TfR2
  - Hemojuvelin
- Affected by:
  - ↑ Iron: ↑ hepcidin to reduce iron
  - ↑ Inflammation: ↑ hepcidin to limit iron availability to microorganisms
  - ↑ Erythropoietin: ↓ hepcidin to increase iron for hematopoiesis

HEME DEGRADATION

- Hemes are cyclic tetrapyrroles that contain iron and are commonly found as the prosthetic group of hemoglobin, myoglobin and the cytochromes.
- This small-molecule component of globins, critical for oxygen transport among other functions undergoes a complex process of metabolism and degradation.
- Roughly 80% of heme destined for degradation and excretion comes from senescent erythrocytes which have circulated for on average 3 months.
- The other 20% comes from premature erythrocytes in the bone marrow which are destroyed prior to release into the circulation and a minor component is derived from other cell types.

Location of Heme Degradation

Various components of heme degradation occur in the cells of the reticuloendothelial system, liver, and intestine.

- Substrates: Heme; NADPH; 2 UDP-glucuronic acid.
- Product: Urobilinogen (excreted in urine); stercobilin (excreted in feces); carbon monoxide (CO); Fe^{2+}.

HEME CATABOLISM

- Erythrocytes have a life span of 120 days. At the end of this period, they are removed from the circulation. Erythrocytes are taken up and degraded by the macrophages of the reticuloendothelial (RE) system in the spleen and liver. About 6 g of hemoglobin per day is broken down, and resynthesized in an adult man (70 kg).
- **Fate of globin:** The globin may be reutilized as such for the formation of hemoglobin or degraded to the individual amino acids. The amino acids undergo their own metabolism, including participation in fresh globin synthesis.
- **Sources of heme:** It is estimated that about 80% of the heme that is subjected for degradation comes from the erythrocytes and the rest (20%) comes from immature RBC, myoglobin and cytochromes
- **Heme oxygenase:** A complex microsomal enzyme, heme oxygenase utilizes NADPH and O_2 and cleaves the methenyl bridges between the two pyrrole rings (A and B) to form biliverdin. Simultaneously, ferrous iron (Fe^{2+}) is oxidized to ferric form (Fe^{3+}) and released.
- The products of heme oxygenase reaction are biliverdin (a green pigment), Fe^{3+} and carbon monoxide (CO). Heme promotes the activity of this enzyme. Biliverdin is excreted in birds and amphibia while in mammals it is further degraded
- **Biliverdin Reductase:** Biliverdin's methenyl bridges (between the pyrrole rings C and D) are reduced to methylene group to form bilirubin yellow pigment). Catalyzed by an NADPH dependent soluble enzyme, biliverdin reductase.
- One gram of hemoglobin on degradation finally yields about 35 mg bilirubin. Approximately 250–350 mg of bilirubin is daily produced in human adults. The term bile pigments are used to collectively represent bilirubin and its derivatives.

Table 21.1 is depicted the steps of heme synthesis.

- Transport of bilirubin to liver Bilirubin is lipophilic and therefore insoluble in aqueous solution. Bilirubin is transported in the plasma in a bound (non-covalently) form to albumin. Albumin has two binding sites for bilirubin-a high affinity site and a low affinity site.
- Approximately 25 mg of bilirubin can bind tightly to albumin (at high affinity sites) per 100 mL of plasma. The rest of the bilirubin binds loosely (at the low affinity sites) to albumin and enter the tissues. Certain drugs and antibiotics (e.g., sulfonamides, salicylates) can displace bilirubin from albumin, bilirubin enter the CNS and damages neurons.
- **Albumin-bilirubin complex:** Albumin-bilirubin complex enters the liver, bilirubin dissociates and is taken up by sinusoidal surface of the hepatocytes by a carrier mediated active transport. Inside the hepatocytes, bilirubin binds to a specific intracellular protein namely ligandin.
- Conjugation of bilirubin: In the liver, bilirubin is conjugated with 2 molecules of glucuronate supplied by UDP-glucuronate. Catalyzed by bilirubin glucuronyltransferase. It results in the formation of water soluble bilirubin diglucuronide. When bilirubin is in excess, bilirubin monoglucuronides also accumulated in body.
- **Excretion of bilirubin into bile:** Conjugated bilirubin is excreted into the bile canaliculi against a concentration gradient which then enters the bile. The transport of bilirubin diglucuronide is an active, energy-dependent and rate limiting process. This step is easily susceptible to any impairment in liver function.

Table 21.1: Steps of heme synthesis.

Step	Site of process	Enzyme	Disease associated with enzyme gene mutations
1. Synthesis of aminolevulinic acid	Mitochondria	Aminolevulinic acid synthase	• X-linked sideroblastic anemia (associated with aminolevulinic acid synthase 2 loss-of-function mutations) • X-linked protoporphyria (associated with aminolevulinic acid synthase 2 gain-of function mutations)
2. Formation of porphobilinogen (PBG)	Cytosol	Aminolevulinic acid dehydratase or PBG synthase	Aminolevulinic acid dehydratase porphyria
3. Formation of hydroxymethylbilane (HMB)		PBG deaminase/ HMB synthase	Acute intermittent porphyria
4. Formation of uroporphyrinogen (UPG)		UPG III synthase	Congenital erythropoietic porphyria
5. Synthesis of coproporphyrinogen (CPG) III		UPG decarboxylase	Porphyria cutanea tarda and hepatoerythropoietic porphyria
6. Synthesis of protoporphyrinogen (PPG)	Mitochondria	CPG oxidase	Hereditary coproporphyria
7. Generation of protoporphyrin (PP)		Protoporphyrinogen oxidase	Variegate porphyria
8. Generation of heme		Ferrochelatase/ heme synthase	Erythropoietic protoporphyria

- Fate of bilirubin: Bilirubin glucuronides are hydrolyzed in the intestine by specific bacterial enzymes, namely—β-glucuronidases to liberate bilirubin. And then converted to urobilinogen (colorless compound) A small part of it reabsorbed into circulation. Urobilinogen is converted into urobilin (yellow) in kidney and excreted.
- The color of urine is due to urobilinogen: A major part of urobilinogen is converted bacteria to stercobilin which is excreted along with feces. The characteristic brown color of feces is due to stercobilin.

HEME DEGRADATION PATHWAY (FIG. 21.6)

- Degradation begins inside macrophages of the spleen, which remove old and damaged (senescent) erythrocytes from the circulation.
- RBCs are engulfed by cells of the reticuloendothelial system. The globin is recycled into amino acids, which in turn are catabolized into intermediates of the citric acid cycle and fatty acid oxidation.
- Heme is oxidized; the heme ring is opened by heme oxygenase. The oxidation occurs on a specific carbon, producing the linear tetrapyrrole biliverdin, ferric iron (Fe^{3+}), and CO.
- In the next reaction, second bridging methylene is reduced by biliverdin reductase, producing bilirubin. The green pigment is thus converted to the red-orange bilirubin.
- Bilirubin is then transported in the serum by albumin to the liver, where it is conjugated with glucuronate by bilirubin glucuronyl transferase and excreted in the bile.
- In the intestine, bilirubin is deconjugated and converted to urobilinogen and stercobilin.
- Some urobilinogen is reabsorbed and excreted as urobilin in the urine. Most urobilinogen is oxidized in the feces to stercobilin which gives feces its color.

Significance of Heme Degradation

- Free heme concentration greater than 1 micro M can be toxic because it catalyzes the production of reactive oxygen species. To cope with this problem, heme degradation is very crucial for the body.
- In animals, this pathway is an excretory system by which the heme from the hemoglobin of aging red blood cells, and other hemoproteins, is removed from the body.
- Products of degradation such as CO acts as a cellular messenger and functions in vasodilation. Other metabolites of heme also have additional important functions and are involved in various critical cellular events.
- Heme degradation is believed to be an evolutionarily-conserved response to oxidative stress.
- In higher plants, heme is broken down to the phycobiliprotein phytochrome which is involved in coordinating light responses.
- In algae, it is metabolized to the light-harvesting pigments phycocyanin and phycoerythrin.

Associated diseases: In patients with abnormally high red cell lysis or obstructive liver damage, bilirubin can accumulate, leading to the clinical manifestation of jaundice.

Clinical Relevance

Hereditary Hemochromatosis

- Autosomal recessive disorder most often associated with *HFE* gene mutations. There is increased iron intestinal absorption and iron deposition in several organs, such as the liver, heart, skin and pancreas.
- Clinical presentation includes the triad of cirrhosis, diabetes, and skin bronzing.

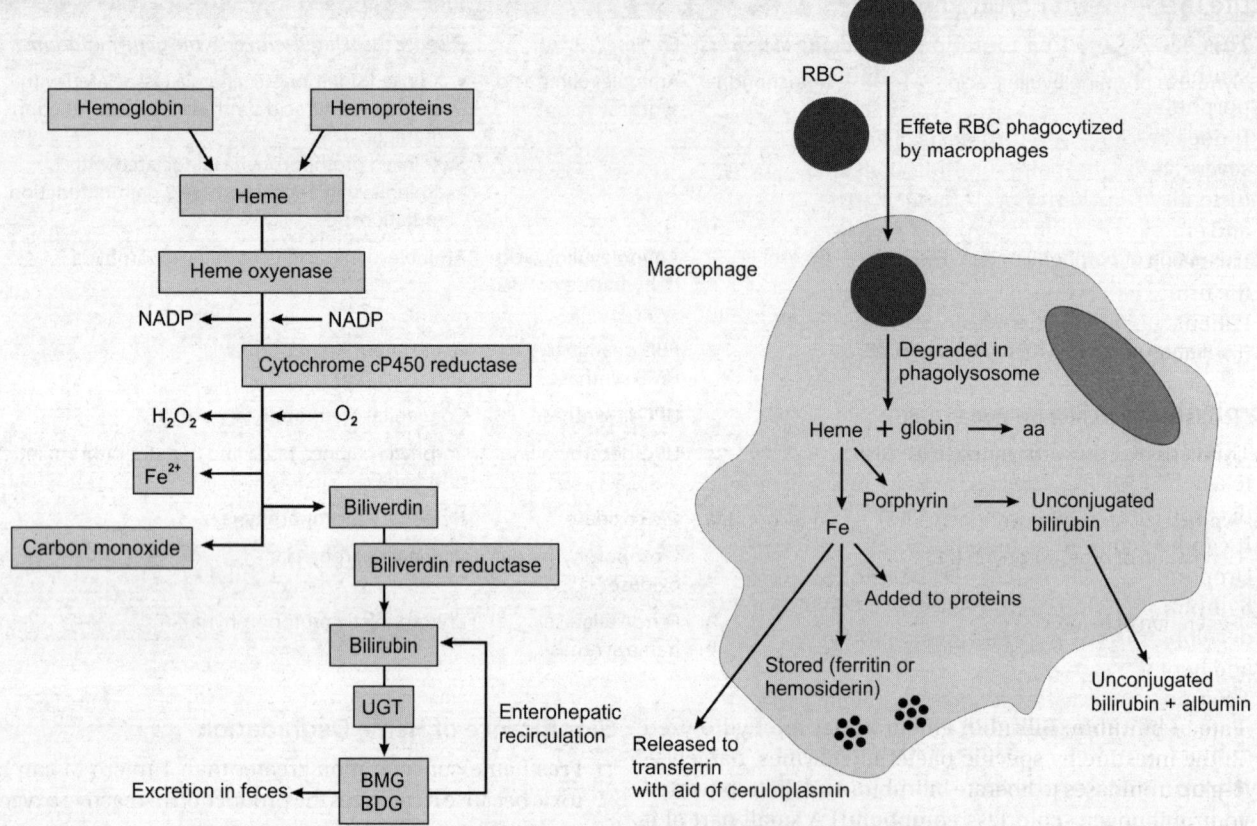

Fig. 21.6: Heme degradation.

- Diagnosis consists of iron studies showing transferrin and ferritin elevation. Genetic screening is recommended for family members.
- Management requires phlebotomy (or iron chelation therapy in some cases) to prevent disease progression. The presence of hepatic fibrosis is a poor prognostic factor.

Porphyrias

- Group of metabolic disorders caused by a disturbance in the synthesis of heme. In most cases, porphyria is caused by a hereditary enzyme defect.
- The disease patterns differ depending on the affected enzyme, and the variants of porphyria can be clinically differentiated between acute and nonacute forms.
- Individuals with porphyria present with photosensitive skin eruptions and sometimes systemic symptoms such as abdominal pain and neuropathy.
- Porphyrias are managed by avoiding triggers, such as sun exposure and consumption of alcohol. When flares occur, therapy is targeted toward symptom relief.

Jaundice

- Abnormal yellowing of the skin and/or sclera caused by the accumulation of bilirubin.
- Hyperbilirubinemia is caused by either an increase in bilirubin production or a decrease in the hepatic uptake, conjugation, or excretion of bilirubin.
- Etiologies often involve the liver and can be prehepatic, intrahepatic, or posthepatic.
- Other symptoms of hyperbilirubinemia include pruritus, pale stools, and darkened urine.
- The diagnosis is made on the basis of liver function tests and imaging. Management is focused on treatment of the underlying condition.

Clinical Significance

Heme synthesis is a biochemical pathway which requires a number of steps, substrates, and enzymes. A deficiency in an enzyme or substrate leads to accumulation of intermediates of heme synthesis in blood, tissues, and urine leading to a clinically significant outcome of a group of disorders called porphyrias. Porphyrias are hepatic or erythropoietic. They can be acute or chronic, lead to neurologic dysfunction, mental disturbance or photosensitivity. Defects of heme synthesis after formation of hydroxymethylbilane leads to photosensitivity of patients. Other symptoms include a change in urine color, abdominal pain, abdominal colic, highly agitated state, tachycardia, respiratory problems, nausea, confusion, weakness of lower extremities.

Porphyrias are acute intermittent, congenital erythropoietic porphyria, porphyria cutanea tarda, hereditary coproporphyria.

Acute Intermittent Porphyria

- This occurs due to a mutation in hydroxymethylbilane synthase, which leads to an accumulation of ALA and porphobilinogen.
- It does not affect erythroblasts. The disease presents as severe abdominal pain, vomiting, constipation, abdominal distention, and behavioral changes (irritability, insomnia, and emotional lability), hypertension and tachycardia.
- Lab results show elevated urinary porphobilinogen and the urine darkens on exposure to air and sunlight.
- Patients presenting with acute intermittent porphyria are not photosensitive.

Porphyria Cutanea Tarda

- This variant is the most common type of porphyria. It is due to a deficiency or decreased activity in uroporphyrinogen decarboxylase (UROD).
- It can be acquired or hereditary (autosomal dominant). Uroporphyrin accumulates in the urine.
- Symptoms include photosensitivity leading to blisters developing in sun-exposed areas and hyperpigmentation, and hepatic injury.
- Treatment includes avoidance of sunlight, hydroxychloroquine, and phlebotomy.

Erythropoietic Porphyria

- This occurs due to a deficiency in ferrochelatase, the enzyme responsible for the final formation of heme in the biosynthesis pathway by combining protoporphyrin IX and ferrous iron.
- Deficiency leads to an accumulation of protoporphyrin IX in erythrocytes.
- Symptoms include painful photosensitivity—swelling burning and itching in sun-exposed areas; sometimes hepatic dysfunction.

Lead Poisoning

- Lead interacts with zinc cofactors for ALA dehydratase and ferrochelatase leading to inhibition of these two enzymes in the biochemical biosynthetic pathway of heme.
- This inhibition leads to mostly ALA and some protoporphyrin IX accumulating in urine.
- Symptoms include abdominal pain, vomiting, fatigue irritability and developmental disability in children.

■ JAUNDICE

Jaundice is a term that is used to describe a yellow colored tinge to the skin, and a yellowing of the whites of the eyes. The body fluids of someone who is affected by jaundice can also become yellow in color.

Bilirubin

- Jaundice is caused by the buildup of bilirubin in the blood. Bilirubin is a yellow colored substance that is produced when red blood cells are broken down.
- Normally, the liver 'picks up' bilirubin and it is filtered by the kidneys, before being excreted (passed out) of the body in urine. However, if there is something wrong with the liver, or the biliary system (which produces a waste substance called bile), an excess amount of bilirubin is produced.

Neonatal Jaundice

Jaundice is very common in newborn babies. It occurs as a result of the liver being underdeveloped and not fully functional. In most cases, neonatal jaundice is nothing to worry about, it requires no treatment, and usually disappears after a week or so.

Jaundice in Adults and Older Children

Jaundice that occurs in adults and older children is usually a sign of an underlying health problem. There are three types of jaundice which are described below.

Hepatocellular Jaundice

Hepatocellular jaundice is the most common type of jaundice. It occurs when bilirubin is unable to leave the liver cells and cannot be removed from the body by the kidneys. Hepatocellular jaundice is usually caused by liver failure, liver disease (cirrhosis), hepatitis (inflammation of the liver), or by taking certain types of medication.

Hemolytic Jaundice

Hemolytic jaundice is where too much bilirubin is produced as a result of a large number of red blood cells being broken down. This can be due to a number of conditions, such as anemia, or a problem with the metabolism (the way that the body produces and uses energy).

Obstructive Jaundice

Obstructive jaundice occurs when there is an obstruction (blockage) in the bile duct, which prevents bilirubin from leaving the liver. This type of jaundice is usually caused by a gallstone, a tumor, or a cyst in the bile duct, or pancreas.

Causes of Jaundice

The liver is a very important organ. One of the functions of the liver is to 'pick up' and remove bilirubin (a yellow colored substance) from the body.

Jaundice is Caused by Excess Bilirubin

Bilirubin is produced when red, oxygen-carrying, blood cells are broken down. The bilirubin is transported in the bloodstream to the liver which usually removes it from the blood so that it can be excreted (passed) from the body in urine.

However, if there is too much bilirubin in the blood, or if, for some reason, the liver cannot get rid of it, the excess will cause jaundice.

Jaundice usually occurs as a result of a separate health condition which causes a buildup of bilirubin, or prevents the liver from functioning properly and disposing of bilirubin.

Some common conditions that can cause jaundice are outlined below.

Acute Hepatitis

Acute hepatitis is a condition that causes inflammation (swelling) of the liver, usually as a result of the hepatitis A, B, C, D, or E viruses.

Acute hepatitis can also develop as a result of drinking excess amounts of alcohol over a long period of time, or taking certain types of medication.

Obstruction of the Bile Ducts

If the bile ducts (tiny tubes in the liver that remove bile) become blocked—for example, by a gallstone—or if they are damaged—for example, by a condition such as cirrhosis (a serious condition that destroys healthy liver tissue)—the obstruction, or damage, can result in a buildup of bilirubin.

Hemolytic Anemia

Hemolytic anemia can occur when a large number of red blood cells are destroyed, leading to an increase in the production of bilirubin.

Hemolytic anemia may be caused by a blood-borne disease, such as malaria, or an autoimmune disease (where the body's immune system, which helps prevent infection, attacks healthy cells and tissue).

Gilbert's Syndrome

Gilbert's syndrome is a condition that affects approximately 3% of the UK population. It is an inherited condition (it runs in families) that adversely affects the ability of enzymes (proteins that cause chemical reactions between other substances) to function properly, and process the excretion of bile. People with Gilbert's syndrome will sometimes experience mild jaundice.

See the 'useful links' section for more information about Gilbert's syndrome.

Neonatal Jaundice

Neonatal jaundice is very common with around 50% of all newborn babies being affected. It often occurs as a result of the baby's liver not being fully developed, which means that it is unable to deal with bilirubin.

Neonatal jaundice often occurs 2–4 days after birth, and usually clears up without treatment, around 7–10 days. However, if jaundice lasts for longer than this, further investigations to find out whether there is another underlying cause will be needed.

Other, Rarer Conditions

As well as the conditions outlined above, there are also a number of other, rarer conditions that can cause jaundice. These are listed below.

- **Crigler-Najjar syndrome**—an inherited condition that adversely affects the enzyme responsible for processing bilirubin, leading to an excess build up of bilirubin.
- **Dubin-Johnson syndrome**—an inherited condition that prevents bilirubin from being secreted (passed out) of the liver's cells.
- **Rotor's syndrome**—an inherited condition that is similar to Dubin-Johnson syndrome, but does not involve the retention of bilirubin in the liver's cells.
- **Pseudojaundice**—a harmless type of jaundice that is unrelated to bilirubin, where the skin turns a yellowish color due an excess amount of beta-carotene in the blood (carotenemia), usually from eating large quantities of carrots, pumpkin, or melon.

Risk Factors

Jaundice most often happens as a result of an underlying disorder that either causes the production of too much bilirubin or prevents the liver from getting rid of it. Both of these result in bilirubin being deposited in tissues.

Underlying conditions that may cause jaundice include:

- **Acute inflammation of the liver:** This may impair the ability of the liver to conjugate and secrete bilirubin, resulting in a buildup.
- **Inflammation of the bile duct:** This can prevent the secretion of bile and removal of bilirubin, causing jaundice.
- **Obstruction of the bile duct:** This prevents the liver from disposing of bilirubin.
- **Hemolytic anemia:** The production of bilirubin increases when large quantities of red blood cells are broken down.
- **Gilbert's syndrome:** This is an inherited condition that impairs the ability of enzymes to process the excretion of bile.
- **Cholestasis:** This interrupts the flow of bile from the liver. The bile containing conjugated bilirubin remains in the liver instead of being excreted.

Types of Jaundice

Various conditions of jaundice result from the accumulation of bilirubin in the blood. A **jaundice** condition is characterized by yellow colored skin due to the presence of bilirubin.

Hemolytic Jaundice

Excessive hemolysis or breakdown of red blood cells causes the formation of higher than normal amounts of bilirubin. Bilirubin made in the liver goes into bile and then into the gall bladder and into the intestines where most is excreted. The liver works normally, but could eventually be damaged from overwork. Usually the liver can handle the excess and the bilirubin is excreted via intestines and does not usually spill over into the kidneys. Urobilinogen levels are likely to be elevated in the blood and urine.

Hepatic Jaundice

Hepatic jaundice is caused by damage or disease in the liver. Heme enters the liver but it does not take out as much bilirubin as is normal. Bilirubin builds up in the blood and spills over into the kidneys which filter it out into the urine. The amount of urobilinogen in the urine will be either normal or low if not enough bilirubin is being removed by the liver into bile and the intestines.

Biliary Obstruction

If bilirubin cannot reach the intestinal area because of a blockage in the bile duct, than bilirubin builds up in the blood because it cannot get out of the liver. Bilirubin is then removed by the kidneys into the urine. Little if any, urobilinogen will be found in the urine since little or no bilirubin is reaching the intestines.

Symptoms of Jaundice (Fig. 21.7)

Yellow skin is the main symptom of jaundice

The most obvious sign of jaundice is a yellow tinge to the skin and the whites of the eyes.

The yellowing of the skin is usually first noticeable on the head and face, before spreading down the body. In people with dark skin, yellowing of the whites of the eyes is often more noticeable.

Figure 21.8 is depicted the complications of jaundice.

Other Symptoms

Depending on the cause of your jaundice, as well as a yellowing of the skin, you may also have other symptoms including:
- Tiredness
- Abdominal pain
- Weight loss
- Vomiting
- Fever—a temperature of 38°C (100.4°F), or above.

If you have obstructive jaundice, your skin may be very itchy. Your urine will also probably be darker than usual, and your stools may be paler.

Figure 21.9 is depicted the Van Den Bergh reaction.

Diagnosing Jaundice

If you have jaundice, you will have a number of tests in order to find out how severe it is, and to determine the underlying cause.

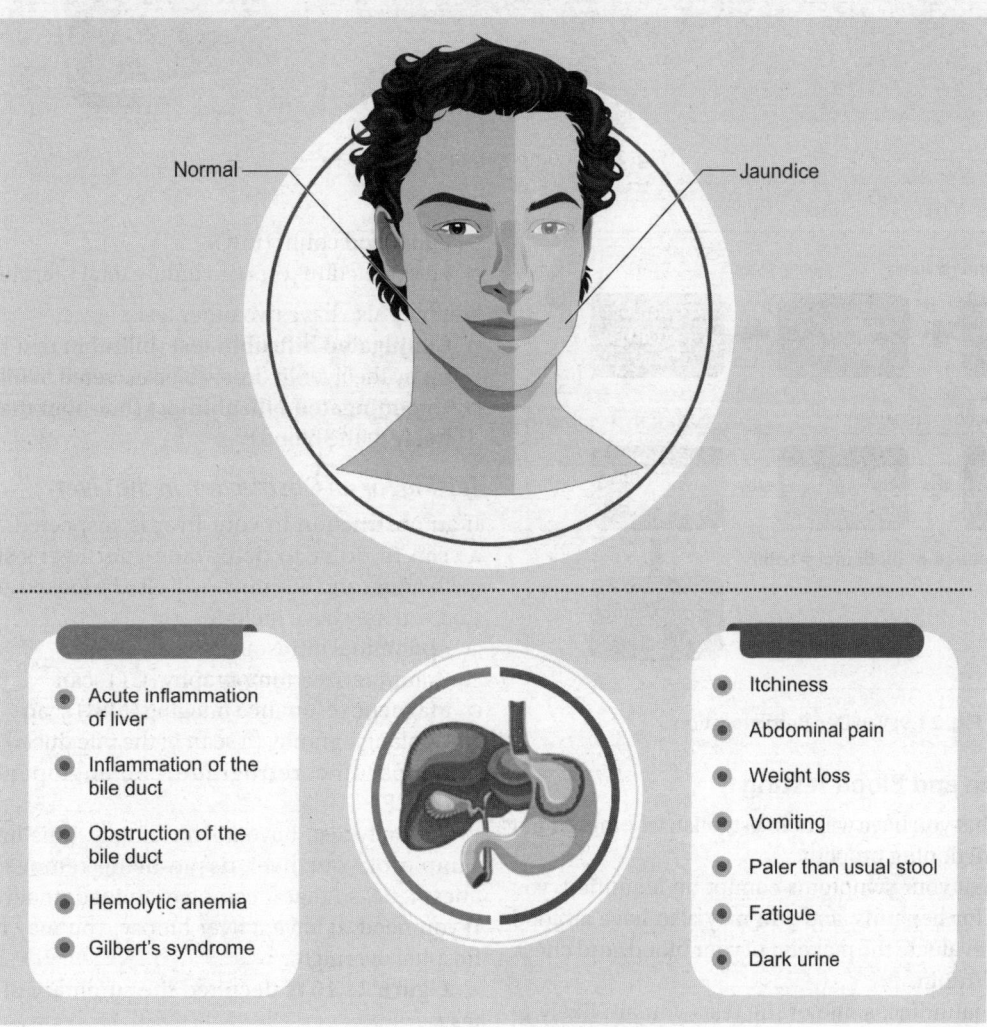

Fig. 21.7: Symptoms of jaundice.

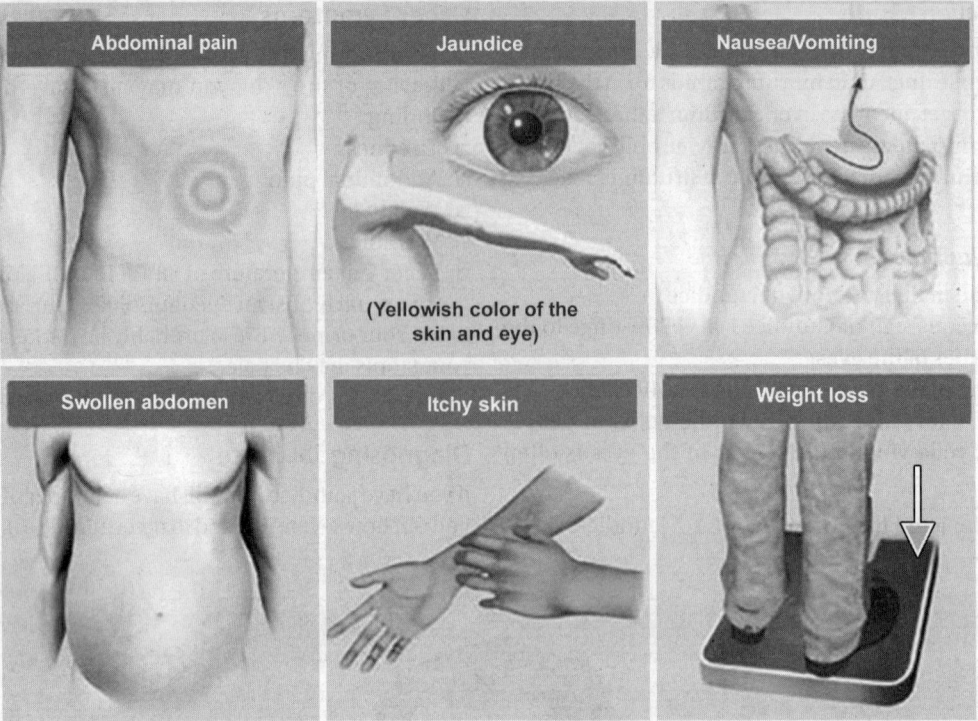

Fig. 21.8: Complications of jaundice.

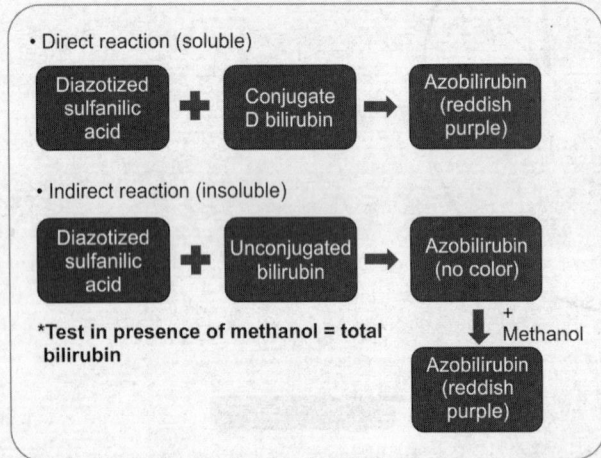

Fig. 21.9: Van Den Bergh reaction.

Liver Function and Blood Testing

The first tests that you have will help establish whether or not your liver is functioning properly.

If the cause of your symptoms cannot be identified, you may be tested for hepatitis, and you may also have a blood test in order to evaluate the makeup of your blood, and check the levels of bilirubin.

If you have jaundice, some of the tests you are likely to have included:
- Hepatitis A
- Hepatitis B
- Hepatitis C
- Full blood count (FBC)
- Liver function tests (including total bilirubin)

You may also have two other tests:
- **Conjugated bilirubin test** (bilirubin that has been taken up by the liver in order to be excreted in bile), and
- **Unconjugated bilirubintest** (bilirubin that is circulating freely in the blood).

Testing for an Obstruction in the Liver

If an obstruction in your liver is suspected, you may have a scan in order to determine your liver's structure. Your gallbladder and bile ducts will also be looked at. Imaging tests that you may have include:
- Abdominal ultrasound
- Computerized tomography (CT) scan
- Magnetic resonance imaging (MRI) scan
- Cholangiography (a scan of the bile ducts)
- Endoscopic retrograde cholangiopancreatography (ERCP)

You may also have a liver biopsy. This involves a small sample of your liver tissue being removed under local anesthetic, so that it can be examined under a microscope. If you need to have a liver biopsy, you may need to stay in hospital overnight.

Figure 21.10 is decpited the summary of liver function tests.

Treating Jaundice

The treatment of jaundice in adults and older children will depend on the underlying condition that is causing it.

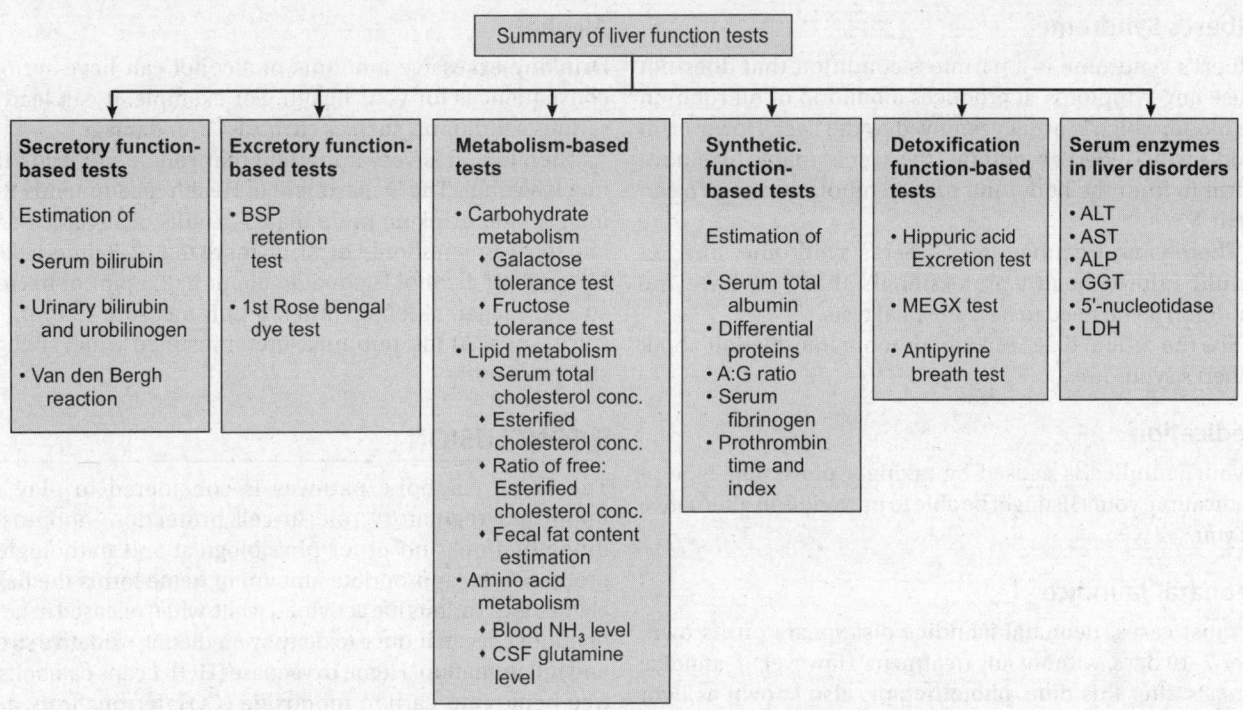

Fig. 21.10: Summary of liver function tests.

After having a number of different tests (see the 'diagnosis' section) to determine the cause of your jaundice, the appropriate treatment will be recommended.

Anemia

Anemia is a condition that occurs when there is a reduced number of red blood cells, or a reduced concentration of hemoglobin (a substance that stores and carries oxygen in red blood cells). There are a number of different types of anemia and each type has a different cause.

If your jaundice is being caused by anemia, you may need to increase the amount of iron in your blood by taking iron supplements, or by including more iron-rich foods in your diet.

See the 'useful links' section for further information about anemia.

In cases of autoimmune hemolytic anemia (where the body's immune system attacks healthy red blood cells), treatment with corticosteroids may be required. However, if corticosteroids fail to successfully control the condition, immunoglobulin (IgG) may be recommended.

Immunoglobulin is a type of protein that functions as an antibody (a substance that fights infection).

Hepatitis

Hepatitis is a condition that is caused by a virus, and results in inflammation of the liver. There are several types of hepatitis virus that can infect the liver. Hepatitis A and B are the most common types.

If your jaundice is caused by hepatitis, you might need to take anti-viral, or steroid, medication. However, not all types of hepatitis can be treated.

See the 'useful links' section for further information about hepatitis.

Cirrhosis

Cirrhosis (liver damage) is a serious condition that destroys healthy liver tissue, leaving scar tissue that can block the flow of blood through the liver. Cirrhosis progresses slowly, gradually causing the liver to stop functioning.

Cirrhosis cannot be cured, but treatment can slow the condition's progress. Treatment also aims to reverse any liver damage that has already occurred. If you have cirrhosis, depending on the underlying cause, you may be prescribed medication, and/or advised to cut down on your consumption of alcohol.

See the 'useful links' section for more information about cirrhosis.

Obstruction

If your jaundice is caused by an obstruction, such as a gallstone, or a tumor, you may need surgery in order to remove it.

Gallstones are usually treated by surgically removing your gallbladder, using a procedure called a cholecystectomy. A cholecystectomy is minimally invasive surgery ('keyhole' surgery), where a small incision is made.

However, in about 10% of cases, keyhole surgery is not possible and an open cholecystectomy is required, where the gallbladder is removed through a larger incision in the abdomen.

See the 'useful links' section for more information about gallstone removal.

Gilbert's Syndrome

Gilbert's syndrome is a harmless condition that does not cause any symptoms. It produces a buildup of bilirubin in the blood, which is usually removed by the liver. However, in people with Gilbert's syndrome, the liver is unable to remove bilirubin from the body, and mild, temporary jaundice can occur.

There is no treatment for Gilbert's syndrome, but you should inform health professionals that you have the condition if you need to have hospital tests.

See the 'useful links' section for more information about Gilbert's syndrome.

Medication

If your jaundice is caused by taking a particular type of medication, your GP might be able to prescribe an alternative for you.

Neonatal Jaundice

In most cases, neonatal jaundice disappears on its own, after 7–10 days, without any treatment. However, if jaundice persists after this time, phototherapy, also known as light therapy, may be needed.

During phototherapy, the baby is exposed to ultraviolet (UV) light, usually for a period of 1–2 days. The UV light breaks down the bilirubin, making it easier for the baby's liver to get rid of. If phototherapy does not work, and the levels of bilirubin are very high, a blood transfusion may be needed.

Preventing Jaundice

Jaundice often develops as a result of an underlying health condition and can therefore be difficult to prevent.

However, jaundice is related to the functioning of the liver, so it is very important that you take steps to keep this vital organ healthy and working properly.

In order to do this, you should ensure that you lead a healthy lifestyle by eating healthily, exercising regularly, and not drinking more than the recommended daily amounts of alcohol.

Diet

Make sure that you eat a healthy, balanced diet that is low in saturated fat, and contains at least five portions a day of a variety of fruit and vegetables.

It is also very important to drink plenty of fluids. You should drink a minimum of 1.2 liters (eight glasses) of water a day, plus more in hot weather and when exercising.

Exercise

In order to remain fit and healthy, you should exercise at least five times a week, for a minimum of 30 minutes each session.

The exercise that you do should raise your heart and breathing rates, and leave you slightly sweaty and out of breath afterwards. Visit your GP for a health check if you have not exercised before, or for a long period of time.

Alcohol

Drinking excessive amounts of alcohol can have serious consequences for your health. For example, it can lead to serious conditions, such as cirrhosis (liver damage).

Therefore, it is very important that you do not drink too much alcohol. The Department of Health recommends that men should drink no more than 3-4 units of alcohol a day, and that women should drink no more than 2-3 units a day.

A unit of alcohol is equal to about half a pint of normal strength lager, cider, or bitter, a pub measure (25 mL) of spirits, or a 50 mL pub measure of fortified wine, such as sherry, or port.

CONCLUSION

The heme catabolic pathway is considered to play an important regulatory role in cell protection, apoptosis, inflammation, and other physiological and pathological processes. An appropriate amount of heme forms the basic elements of various life activities, while when released in large quantities, it can induce toxicity by mediating oxidative stress and inflammation. Heme oxygenase (HO)-1 cans catabolism free heme into carbon monoxide (CO), ferrous iron, and biliverdin (BV)/bilirubin (BR). The diverse functions of these metabolites in immune systems are fascinating. Decades work shows that administration of degradation products of heme, such as CO and BV/BR exerts protective activities in systemic lupus erythematosus (SLE), rheumatoid arthritis (RA), multiple sclerosis (MS) and other immune disorders.

BIBLIOGRAPHY

1. Abraham NG, Asija A, Drummond G, Peterson S. Heme oxygenase -1 gene therapy: recent advances and therapeutic applications. Curr. Gene Ther. 2007;7 (2):89–108.
2. Bloomer JR. "Liver metabolism of porphyrins and haem". Journal of Gastroenterology and Hepatology. 1998;13(3):324–9.
3. Hames D, Hooper N. Biochemistry, Third edition. Taylor & Francis Group: New York, 2005.
4. Pelley JW, Goljan EF. Biochemistry. Third edition. Philadelphia: USA, 2011.
5. Poulos TL. "Heme Enzyme Structure and Function". Chemical Reviews. 2014, 9th April;114(7):3919–62.
6. Smith CM, Marks AD, Lieberman MA, Marks DB, Marks DB. Marks' basic medical biochemistry: A clinical approach. Philadelphia: Lippincott Williams & Wilkins, 2005.

REVIEW QUESTIONS

Long Essays

1. Define heme, explain the functions of heme.
2. Describe in detail about iron absorption and transport.
3. Explain detail about heme degradation pathway.
4. Define jaundice, explain types of jaundice.

Short Essays

1. Heme synthesis in erythroid cells.
2. Heme synthesis in the liver.
3. Iron storage and iron regulation.

4. Heme degradation.
5. Heme catabolism.

Short Answers
1. Albumin-bilirubin complex.
2. Hereditary hemochromatosis.
3. Porphyrias.
4. Jaundice.
5. Van den bergh test.
6. Feedback regulation by heme.
7. Gilbert's syndrome.
8. Hemolytic anemia.
9. Jaundice in adults and older children.
10. Neonatal jaundice.
11. Lead poisoning.
12. Erythropoietic porphyria.
13. Acute intermittent porphyria.
14. Porphyria cutanea tarda.

CHAPTER 22

Organ Function Tests

CHAPTER OUTLINE

- Renal
- Liver
- Thyroid

KIDNEY FUNCTION TEST

The main function of the kidney is excretion of water soluble waste products from our body. The kidney has various filtration, excretion and secretary functions. Derangement of any of these function would result in either decreased excretion of waste products and hence their accumulation in the body or loss of some vital nutrient from the body. Based on the level of these excretory products and nutrients in the urine as well as in blood we can make an accurate calculation to decipher the efficiency of the kidney to undertake its various functions.

Functional Components of a Kidney

- The functional unit of the kidney is called a nephron. It consists of two main parts, the glomerulus and the tubular system.
- The glomerulus is composed of a bowman's capsule and a tuft of leaky blood vessels encapsulated by the Bowman's capsule. The primary purpose of the glomerulus is filtrations.
- The leaky vessels filter into the glomerulus almost all the water, electrolytes, small proteins, nutrients such as sugar, etc., and excretory products such as urea, etc.
- The filtrations are dependent on the size and charge of the particles. The average pore size is 8 nm hence particles of only smaller size will pass through.
- Also the basement membrane carries a negative charge hence preventing negatively charged particles from passing through.
- The tubular system is responsible for reabsorption of most of the water, electrolytes, nutrients as well as excretion of the remaining nutrients by means of secretion into the tubules. These tubules are responsible for the concentration of urine.

Components of Kidney Function Test

The components of the kidney function test can be broadly divided into two categories. The tests that are part of the Kidney function test panel are: (a) Urine examination, (b) Serum urea, (c) Serum creatinine, (d) Blood urea nitrogen (BUN), (e) Calcium, (f) Phosphorus, (g) Protein, (h) Albumin, (i) Creatinine clearance, (j) Urea clearance, (k) Inulin clearance, (l) Dilution and concentration test, and (m) Serum electrolyte levels.

Urine Examination

Before we do a quantitative examination of urine a qualitative examination is necessary as it can provide excellent clues to the nature and location of the lesion in the renal system. This examination consists of a physical examination where the color, odor, quantity, specific gravity, etc., of the urine is noted. Microscopic examination of urine is done to rule out any pus cells, RBC casts, crystals.

Kidney function test items	Reference		Units
Blood urea nitrogen	BUN	5–25	mg/dL
Creatinine	CRE	0.3–1.4	mg/dL
Uric acid	UA	2.5–7.0	mg/dL
Albumin-globulin in ratio	A/G ratio	1.0–1.8	
Creatinine clearance/ 24 hours urine	CC	M: 71–135 F: 78–116	mL/min
Renin	Penin	0.15–3.95	pg/mL/h
Creatinine urine	Creatinine urine	60–250	mg/dL
Natrium	Na	135–145	meq/L
Potassium	K	3.4–4.5	meq/L
Calcium	Ca	8.4–10.6	mg/dL
Phosphorus	IP	2.1–4.7	mg/dL
Alkaline phosphatase	ALP	27–110	U/L

Serum Urea

Urea is the end product of protein catabolism. The urea is produced from the amino group of the amino acids and is produced in the liver by means of the urea cycle.

- Urea undergoes filtrations at the glomerulus as well as secretion and reabsorption at the tubular level. The rise

in the level of serum urea is generally seen as a marker of renal dysfunction especially glomerular dysfunction.
- Urea level only rises when the glomerular function is reduced below 50%.
- The normal serum urea level is between 20–45 mg/dL. But the level may also be affected by diet as well as certain non kidney related disorders.
- A high protein diet may increase the blood urea level. Similarly a low protein diet may decrease blood urea level. Other causes of protein catabolism such as any hyper metabolic conditions, starvation, etc., also causes increased blood urea levels.
- Similarly the level of urea may also be decreased in case of hepatic injury. So even though blood urea is not an excellent marker of renal dysfunction as it rises quite late in the dysfunction and its rise is also not exclusive to kidney dysfunction, but for practical purposes serum urea level is still one of the most ordered test and forms an important part of the kidney function test.
- Urea is measured in diagnostic labs either by UV kinetic method using alpha-ketoglutarate as an NH^{3+} acceptor in presence of enzyme glutamate dehydrogenase.
- It is also measured calorimetrically by Berthelot's end point method and is read in visible range using a calorimeter

Blood Urea Nitrogen (BUN)
- Sometimes the serum urea level is expressed as blood urea nitrogen. BUN can be easily calculated from the serum urea level.
- The molecular weight of urea is 60 and it contains two nitrogen atoms of combined atomic weight of 28.
- Hence the contribution of nitrogen to the total weight of urea in serum is 28/60 that is equal to 0.47. Hence, the serum urea levels can be easily converted to BUN by multiplying it by 0.47. A rise in blood nitrogen level is known as azotemia.

Calcium
- This test measures the amount of calcium in your blood, not the calcium in your bones.
- The body needs it to build and fix bones and teeth, help nerves work, make muscles contraction, help blood clot, and help the heart to work.
- The calcium test screens for problems with the parathyroid glands or kidneys, certain types of cancers and bone problems, inflammation of the pancreas (pancreatitis), and kidney stones.
- **Normal results:** 8.5 to 10.2 mg/dL

Phosphorus
- Phosphorus is a mineral that makes up 1% of a person's total body weight. The body needs phosphorus to build and repair bones and teeth, help nerves function, and make muscles contract.
- The kidneys help control the amount of phosphate in the blood. Extra phosphate is filtered by the kidneys and passes out of the body in the urine.
- It plays an important role in the body's utilization of carbohydrates and fats and in the synthesis of protein for the growth, maintenance, and repair of cells and tissues.
- High levels of phosphorus in blood only occur in people with severe kidney disease or severe dysfunction of their calcium regulation.
- Excessively high levels of phosphorus in the blood, although rare, can combine with calcium to form deposits in soft tissues such as muscle.
- **Normal results:** Standard range not available.

Protein
- Protein in urine is noticeably increased in renal disease of any etiology, except obstruction, and is therefore a very sensitive, general screening test for renal disease, though not specific.
- The extent of proteinuria also provides useful information. The greatest degree of proteinuria is found in the nephrotic syndrome (> 3–4 g/day). In renal disease with the nephritic syndrome, the urinary protein excretion rate is usually about 1–2 g/day.
- In tubulointerstitial disease, urine protein is generally less than 1 g/day. Only in the nephrotic syndrome is the urine protein loss sufficiently great to result in hypoproteinemia.
- Protein in serum can generally be maintained at concentrations above the lower limit of normal by increased hepatic protein synthesis so long as protein loss is less than about 3 g/day.

Serum Creatinine Level
- Creatine is a small tripeptide found in the muscles. It stays in its phosphorylated form and releases energy for any burst of muscular activity.
- It is released from the muscles during regular wear and tear and is converted to creatinine (its internal anhydride).
- It is to be remembered that unlike urea, creatinine is not a toxic waste. It is simply used as a marker of renal function.
- Creatinine is freely filtered at the glomerulus and is also to a very small extent secreted into the tubules. So any problem with gromerular filtrations has a significant effect on the excretion of creatinine resulting in a much substantial rise in serum creatinine level.
- Normal serum creatinine level is 0.6 to 1.5 mg/dL. Serum creatinine is a better indicator of renal function and more specifically glomerular function than urea. For a particular individual the creatinine level is dependent on the muscle mass and muscle wear and tear.
- There may be significant difference in creatinine level of individuals with vastly differing muscle mass. For example, a body builder or athlete will have higher creatinine levels than a sedentary desk worker.
- Similarly creatinine level will also increase in case of any muscle trauma or excessive wear and tear as seems in athletes and people involved in hard physical labor.
- Creatinine is most commonly measured in laboratories calorimetrically by Jaffe's method.

Urea Clearance
- Urea clearance is the hypothetical amount of blood from which kidney clears urea in one minute.

- This is measured by measuring the concentration of urea in blood, concentration of urea in urine and amount of urine excreted over a one hour interval.
- Urea clearance is less than its glomerular filtration as some of the urea that is filtered at the glomerulus is reabsorbed at the tubules.
- To measure urea clearance first the patient is made to void urine and then the made to drink two glasses of water.
- Then the urine is collected after an hour and a blood specimen is also collected at the same time. Then the patient's urine sample is collected after another hour.
- The urea level in the two urine samples and the blood sample is measured. The urine volume is calculated as urine output per minute.
- Maximum urea clearance of an average individual or body surface area of 1.73 sq m is 75 mL/min and a standard urea clearance is 54 mL/min. A urea clearance below 60% of standard is considered impaired.

Creatinine Clearance Rate

- Creatinine is filtered at the glomerulus and its reabsorption at the tubular level is insignificant. Because of this creatinine clearance can be used to measure
- Glomerular filtration rate (GFR). It is measured over a period of 24 hrs.
- For this urine is collected over a 24 hour period and blood sample is also collected. The concentration of creatinine is measured both in the urine as well as the serum sample.
- The normal range of creatinine clearance is—males: 100–120 mL/min, females: 95–105 mL/min this is very close to the glomerular filtration rate.

Inulin Clearance

Inulin is a small polysaccharide of low molecular weight made up of fructose. To measure glomerular filtrate the substance used should have the following qualities:
- It should be non-toxic.
- Should not be metabolized in the body.
- Should be completely filtered at the glomerulus.
- Should neither be secreted or reabsorbed at the tubules. Inulin meets all these criteria and hence makes for a suitable candidate to measure GFR. Inulin clearance hence equals to GFR.
  - GFR is the amount of blood that passes though and is filtered through the glomerulus in a minute.
  - To measure Inulin clearance first Inulin is introduced in the blood by means of a slow continuous infusion to maintain a steady conc. of Inulin in the blood.
  - This is done by first infusing 30 mL of 10% inulin in 250 mL of normal saline infused at a rate of 20 mL/min to achieve desired concentration. Then 70 mL of 10% inulin in 500 mL saline in infused at a rate of 4 mL/min to maintain the desired concentration.
  - The patient is asked to micturate 20 minutes after the second infusion and the urine in discarded and the time noted. After exactly 60 minutes, take another sample of urine and blood is collected.
  - Measure the volume of urine and the conc. of inulin in both the serum and urine. Thereafter, the inulin clearance is measured by the formulae: (Conc. of Inulin in urine volume of Inulin) Conc. of Inulin in serum × Normal inulin clearance is 120 to 130 mL/minute for an average person with a body surface area of 1.73 sqm.
  - This is a close approximation of the GFR. A below normal inulin clearance shows an impaired glomerular function.

Concentration Test

- In case of water shortage in the body the kidney is able to concentrate urine and conserve water.
- This is done by increasing the reabsoption of water from the glomerular filtrate at the tubular level. So in effect the measure of the ability of the kidney to conserve water and concentrate urine is a measure of tubular function.
- For this test the patient is not allowed to take any food or water after the evening meal. The first three urine samples passed in the morning are collected and their specific gravity measured.
- In a normal person the specific gravity of at least one of the samples should be above 1.025 or above. If the specific gravity remains below 1.025 then it is a sign of tubular dysfunction.

Dilution Test

- Like the concentration test the dilution test is also a measure of functioning of the tubules. In cases of fluid overload of our body the tubules reabsorb lesser amounts of water resulting in excretion of diluted urine.
- For this test, the subject is put on overnight fast and then in the morning the subject is made to drink 1200 mL of water over a time period of 30 minutes.
- Then the urine samples are collected every hour for 4 hours.
- The specific gravity of the samples is measured and at least one of the samples should have a specific gravity of 1.003 or less. If none of the samples have the specific gravity of 1.003 or less this is a sign of tubular dysfunction.

Electrolytes

The purpose of the kidney is not just water balance and excretion but also to maintain the electrolyte balance of our body. Kidneys actively reabsorb or excrete electrolytes to maintain the electrolyte balance of the body. Owing to their small size almost all electrolytes are filtered at the glomerulus. After filtration most of the electrolytes are absorbed back at the tubular level but any problem at the tubular level will result in non-absorption and excessive loss of electrolytes in urine. Serum electrolytes that are measured for this purpose are—serum sodium levels (Na+) : 135 to 145 mmols/L
- Serum potassium level (K+) : 3.5 to 5 mmols/L
- Serum chloride level (Cl-) : 95 to 105 mmols/L

LIVER FUNCTION TEST

Liver function tests are a group of tests done to assess the functional capacity of the liver as well as any cellular damage

to the liver cells. To assess all functional capabilities of the liver, such as:
- **Its synthetic ability:** By measuring the various plasma proteins such as albumin and prothrombin that are synthesized by the liver. Also lipids which are also synthesized in the liver.
- **Its secretory/excretory abilities:** By measuring the serum bilirubin level.

Liver function tests are a group of tests done to assess the functional capacity of the liver:
- Synthetic ability of the liver is assessed by measuring the various plasma proteins
- Secretory/excretory ability is assessed by measuring the serum bilirubin level
- The common tests that form part of the liver function test profile are serum bilirubin both conjugated and unconjugated, total serum proteins and albumin globulin ratio, liver enzymes and prothrombin time
- While measuring bilirubin we measure total and conjugated bilirubin (Direct bilirubin) and calculate the indirect bilirubin by substraction the direct from the total.
- The common method of measuring serum bilirubin level is the Diazo method
- The normal total protein level is 5 to 8.5 g/dL. The total serum albumin level is 3.5 to 5 g/dL and the normal range for albumin: globulin ratio is 1.2 to 1.5
- Serum albumin is measured by bromocresol green method and total protein is measured by biuret method
- Prothrombin is a clotting factor (clotting factor II) and it forms an important part of both the intrinsic and extrinsic pathway
- International normalized ratio (INR) is used for measuring the prothrombin time
- The commonly measured enzymes are transaminases: AST (SGOT), ALT (SGPT), and transpeptidases: GGT, phosphatase: ALP.

Common Tests

The common tests that form part of the liver function test profile:
- **Serum bilirubin:** both conjugated and unconjugated.
- Total serum proteins and albumin globulin ratio.
- **Liver enzymes:**
  - *Transaminases:* AST (SGOT), ALT (SGPT)
  - *Others:* ALP, GGT, LDH

Serum Bilirubin

- Bilirubin is one of the end products of heme metabolism and is derived from the heme part of the hemoglobin molecule. It is a yellow colored pigment.
- Liver plays an important role in the metabolism of bilirubin. After the breakdown of heme portion of the hemoglobin molecule 'unconjugated bilirubin' is insoluble in water.
- It is transferred from the site of RBC and heme breakdown such as the spleen to the liver for 'conjugation' bound to albumin.
- At the liver, it is conjugated with glucuronic acid with the help of enzyme glucuronyl transferase.
- This conjugation makes bilirubin water soluble and this conjugated bilirubin is excreted into the bile. While measuring bilirubin we measure total and conjugated bilirubin (Direct bilirubin) and calculate the indirect bilirubin by substracting the direct from the total.

The normal range of bilirubin is:
- **Total bilirubin:** 0.2 to 1 mg/dL
- **Unconjugated bilirubin:** 0.1 to 0.6 mg/dL
- **Conjugated bilirubin:** 0.1 to 0.4 mg/dL

A rise of bilirubin level to that of 2 mg/dL results in the symptoms of jaundice which is marked by deposition of bilirubin in the various mucous membranes. Jaundice is divided into three types depending on its etiology:
- **Pre hepatic jaundice:** In this case, the cause of jaundice is at the level of bilirubin processing before it reaches the liver. Most common cause is over production of bilirubin due to hemolytic disorders. In this case, the rise in the level of unconjugated bilirubin is more than conjugated bilirubin hence there is a rise in total and indirect bilirubin.
- **Hepatic jaundice:** This is caused by cellular dysfunction of the liver hence is also called hepatocellular jaundice. It is caused by the inability of the liver cells to process and excrete the bilirubin in the system. It is seen in hepatitis, cirrhosis of liver, etc. In this jaundice, there is rise in total, direct as well as indirect bilirubin levels.
- **Prehepatic jaundice:** This is also known as obstructive jaundice as it is caused by obstruction to the outflow of bile resulting is reabsoption of conjugated bilirubin and it making an appearance in the serum. It cause by carcinoma of the mouth of gallbladder, stone in the bile duct, etc. In this type of jaundice, we see a rise in total as well as direct (conjugated) bilirubin.

The common method of measuring serum bilirubin level is the Diazo method using Diazotized sufanilic acid to convert bilirubin into a azobilirubin the color intensity of which is measured colorimetrically at a wavelength between 555 nm (550 to 580 nm). The conjugated bilirubin reacts directly with the Diazo sulfanilic acid in an aqueous medium and hence also called direct bilirubin. For unconjugated or free bilirubin which is not water soluble we need to dissolve it into DMSO for the reaction to occur. This method is the 'indirect method' for measuring bilirubin levels and it measures both conjugated and unconjugated bilirubin, i.e., total serum bilirubin.

Test	Normal range	Abnormal range mile-moderate	Abnormal range severe
Liver Enzymes			
Aspartate aminotransferase (AST)	<40 IU/L	40–200 IU/L	>200 IU/IL
Alanine aminotransferase (ALT)	<40 IU/L	40–200 IU/L	>200 IU/L
Gamma-glutamyl transferase (GGT)	<60 IU/L	60–200 IU/L	>200 IU/L
Alkaline phosphatase	< 112 IU/L	112–300 IU/L	>300 IU/L

Contd...

Section 2: Applied Biochemistry

Contd...

Test	Normal range	Abnormal range mile-moderate	Abnormal range severe
Liver function tests			
Bilirubin	<1.2 mg/dL	1.2–2.5 mg/dL	>2.5 mg/dL
Albumin	3.5–4.5 g/dL		
Prothrombin time	<14 seconds	14–17 seconds	>17 seconds
Blood count			
White blood count (WBC)	>6000	3000–6000	<3000
Hematocrit (HCT)	>40	35–40	<35
Platelets	>150,000	100,000–150,000	<100,000
Key			
U = International Unit	L = liter	dL = deciliter	mg = milligrams

Serum Albumin and Albumin Globulin Ratio

❑ Serum albumin is an important serum protein vital for maintaining the plasma oncotic pressure as well as acts as a carrier for various biological substances and drugs. Serum albumin is exclusively synthesized by liver and hence the level of serum albumin gives us a stock of the synthetic ability of the liver.

❑ Another cause of fall of serum albumin maybe protein malnutrition but in that case the fall of all serum proteins including globulins will be seen. The normal total protein level is 5 to 8.5 g/dL.

❑ The total serum albumin level is 3.5 to 5 g/dL. The total plasma globulin level is calculated by subtracting the plasma albumin from the total protein level and is normally in the range of 2 to 2.5 g/dL.

❑ The normal range for albumin: globulin ratio is 1.2 to 1.5. But with hepatic dysfunction this ratio recedes towards 1 as the synthetic function of liver is compromised.

❑ The reversal of the ratio, i.e., if the value recedes below 1, it is an ominous sign and may mark an infective/inflammatory pathology marked by rise in serum globulin level and fall in serum albumin levels.

❑ To measure serum albumin the bromocresol green method is used. Albumin in the presence of bromocresol green at a slightly acidic pH gives a yellow green to blue green color.

❑ The intensity of this color is dependent on the concentration of albumin in the sample.

❑ This intensity is read at a wavelength of 630 nm. To measure the total protein content of the sample the biuret method it used.

❑ In this method, the cupric ions of copper (II) sulfate, present in the biuret reagent, form a violet colored complex with the proteins in a slightly alkaline medium.

❑ The intensity of the color formed is measured at a wavelength of 540 nm (530 to 550 nm).

Figure 22.1 is depicted the summary of liver function tests.

Prothrombin Time

❑ Prothrombin is a clotting factor (clotting factor II) and it forms an important part of both the intrinsic and extrinsic pathway.

❑ Its active form is thrombin (also clotting factor IIa). It is a serine peptidase which converts fibrinogen to fibrin.

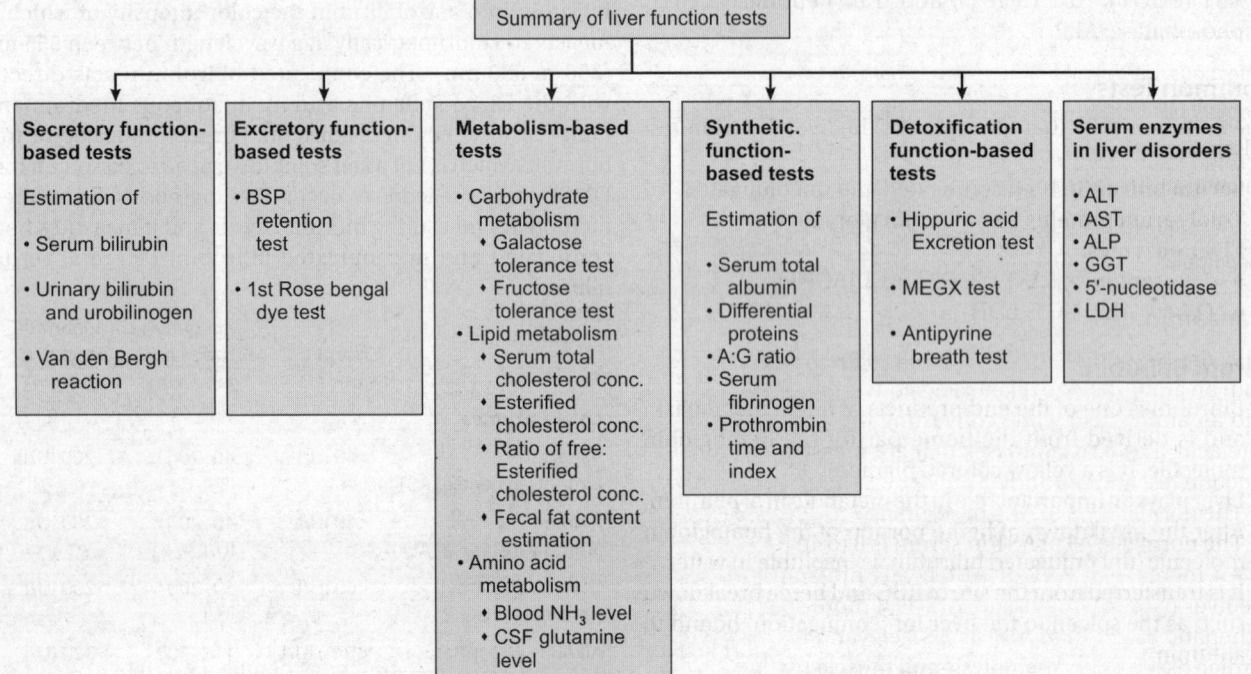

Fig. 22.1: Summary of liver function tests.

- Prothrombin is synthesized in the liver. And hence prothrombin activity in plasma is used to measure the synthetic function of liver.
- Prothrombin time is measured by taking human plasma from blood that has been collected in tube containing citrate as an anticoagulant.
- The plasma in put in an automated machine which adds an excess of calcium to reverse the anticoagulant effects of citrates and measures the time taken for fibrinogen to be converted to fibrin hence measures the activity of thrombin in the plasma.
- The prothrombin time differs in accordance to the analytical method used. Hence to compensate for this International normalized ratio (INR) is used.
- In this, the manufacturers of the kit assign an International sensitivity index (ISI) value. This shows the amount of tissue factor present in the kit as against an internationally accepted standard. The ISI value is generally 1 to 2.

Liver Enzymes

Liver enzymes along with bilirubin are the most commonly measured parameter measured in the liver function test. These enzymes are hepatic in origin and they are leaked into the serum with the destruction of hepatic cells. Liver enzymes are measured to get an idea of the cellular insult on the liver and are increased in a wide variety of conditions such as viral hepatitis, toxic hepatitis, cirrhosis of liver, etc. The commonly measured enzymes are: (a) Transaminases: AST (SGOT), ALT (SGPT) (b) Transpeptidases: GGT (c) Phosphatase: ALP.

Summary of liver function test abnormalities

Disease	ALT	AST	GGT	ALP
Viral hepatitis	+++	+++	++	N/+
Drug-induced hepatitis	++	++	++	N/+
Chronic active hepatitis	++	++	++	++
Infectious mononucleosis hepatitis	++	++	++	N
Primary biliary cirrhosis	++	++	+++	++
Alcoholic cirrhosis	N	++	+++	N/+
Intrahepatic cholestasis	++	++	+++	++
Extrahepatic cholestasis	++	++	+++	+++
Hepatoma	N/+	++	++	++

Transaminases

They are a group of enzymes that transfer the amino group from an amino acid to α keto acid converting the α keto acid into an amino acid while converting the amino acid into a keto acid. The transaminases that are measured in the liver function test are ALT and AST:
- The normal level of ALT in serum is 7 to 40 IU/L.
- The normal level of AST in serum is 8 to 40 IU/L.

An increase in AST or ALT levels hints at an insult to the liver parenchyma tissue. ALT is a more specific marker of hepatic injury than AST as AST elevation is also seen in cardiac tissue injury, hemolysis and muscle tissue.

To measure the level of transaminases the reaction catalyzed by them is coupled to a reaction in which NADH is used up resulting in change in the photometric intensity when read in the UV range at 340 nm. It is a UV kinetic method.

Alkaline Phosphatase

- It is a hydrolase that removes phosphates from all kinds of molecules, such as proteins, nucleotides, etc. It is found in cells lining the billiary system hence a rise in it level is indicative of damage to the billiary tree due to cholestasis.
- It may be due to stone blocking the large ducts or intrahepatic obstruction, inflammation of the biliary channels.
- Alkaline phosphatase is also found in placenta and bones. Hence the level is also increased in growing children in whom bones undergo remodeling and in Paget's disease in adults.
- Normal level of alkaline phosphatase is between 45 to 115 IU/L. The method for measuring the level of alkaline phosphatase is a kinetic method using p-nitrophenyl phosphate as substrate for the enzyme and measuring rate of formation of the colored substrate (p- nitrophenol) formed from the reaction. This measurement of the color intensity is done colorimetrically at a wavelength of 405 nm.

Gamma Glutamyl Transpeptidase

It is another enzyme specific to the biliary tree and a more specific indicator of cholestasis and damage to the biliary tree. It is also a highly specific marker and is raised in even minute and subclinical damage to the biliary tree. Its normal range is in between 0 to 42 IU/L.

THYROID FUNCTION TEST

The thyroid gland is a butterfly-shaped endocrine gland that is normally located in the lower front of the neck. The thyroid's job is to make thyroid hormones, which are secreted into the blood and then carried to every tissue in the body. Thyroid hormones help the body use energy, stay warm and keep the brain, heart, muscles, and other organs working as they should.

Normal thyroid levels

Test	Abbreviation	Typical ranges
Thyroxine serum	T4	4.6–12 ug/dL
Free thyroxine	FT4	0.7–1.9 ng/dL
Triiodothyronine serum	T3	80–180 ng/dL
Free triiodothyronine 1	FT3	230–619 pg/d
Serum thyroglobulin 1	Tg	0–30 ng/m
Thyrotropin serum	TSH	0.5–6 uU/mL

T4 and T3 circulate almost entirely bound to specific transport proteins. If the levels of these transport proteins changes, there can be changes in how much bound T4 and T3 is measured. This frequently happens during pregnancy and with the use of birth control pills. The "free" T4 or T3 is the hormone that is unbound and able to enter and affect the body tissues.

Tests

Blood tests to measure these hormones are readily available and widely used, but not all are useful in all situations. Tests to evaluate thyroid function include the following:

TSH Tests

- The best way to initially test thyroid function is to measure the TSH level in a blood sample. Changes in TSH can serve as an "early warning system"—often occurring before the actual level of thyroid hormones in the body becomes too high or too low.
- A high TSH level indicates that the thyroid gland is not making enough thyroid hormone (primary hypothyroidism). The opposite situation, in which the TSH level is low, usually indicates that the thyroid is producing too much thyroid hormone (hyperthyroidism).

	Value	Normal value
FT4	1.22 ng/dL	0.9–1.8 ng/mL
FT3	3.41 pg/mL	2.4–4.3 pg/mL
TSH	1.46 mU/mL	0.24–3.70 mIU/mL
Tg	540 ng/dL	<30 ng/mL
TgAb	9.4 U/mL	<40 U/mL
TPOAb	0.5 U/mL	<50 U/mL

(FT4: free thyroxine; FT3: free triiodothyronine; TSH: thyroid stimulating hormone; Tg: thyroglobulin; TgAb: anti-thyroglobulin antibody; TPOAb: anti-thyroid peroxidase antibody)

- Occasionally, a low TSH may result from an abnormality in the pituitary gland, which prevents it from making enough TSH to stimulate the thyroid (secondary hypothyroidism). In most healthy individuals, a normal TSH value means that the thyroid is functioning properly.

T4 Tests

- T4 is the main form of thyroid hormone circulating in the blood. A **Total T4** measures the bound and free hormone and can change when binding proteins differ.
- A **Free T4** measures what is not bound and able to enter and affect the body tissues.
- Tests measuring free T4—either a free T4 (FT4) or free T4 index (FTI)—more accurately reflect how the thyroid gland is functioning when checked with a TSH.
- The finding of an elevated TSH and low FT4 or FTI indicates primary hypothyroidism due to disease in the thyroid gland. A low TSH and low FT4 or FTI indicates hypothyroidism due to a problem involving the pituitary gland.
- A low TSH with an elevated FT4 or FTI is found in individuals who have hyperthyroidism.

T3 Tests

- T3 tests are often useful to diagnosis hyperthyroidism or to determine the severity of the hyperthyroidism.
- Patients who are hyperthyroid will have an elevated T3 level. In some individuals with a low TSH, only the T3 is elevated and the FT4 or FTI is normal.
- T3 testing rarely is helpful in the hypothyroid patient, since it is the last test to become abnormal. Patients can be severely hypothyroid with a high TSH and low FT4 or FTI, but have a normal T3.

Free T3

Measurement of free T3 is possible, but is often not reliable and therefore not typically helpful.

Reverse T3

- Reverse T3 is a biologically inactive protein that is structurally very similar to T3, but the iodine atoms are placed in different locations, which make it inactive.
- Some reverse T3 is produced normally in the body, but is then rapidly degraded.
- In healthy, non-hospitalized people, measurement of reverse T3 does not help determine whether hypothyroidism exists or not, and is not clinically useful.

Clinical features of thyroid disease		
Hypothyroidism	Hyperthyroidism	Graves' disease
Lethargy	Tachycardia	Exophthalmos/proptosis
Weight gain	Palpitations (atrial fibrillation)	Chemosis
Cold intolerance	Hyperactivity	Diffuse symmetrical goiter
Constipation	Weight loss with increased appetite	Pretibial myxoedema (rare)
Hair loss	Heat intolerance	Other autoimmune conditions
Dry skin	Sweating	Thyroid bruit
Depression	Diarrhea	
Bradycardia	Fine tremor	
Memory impairment	Hyperreflexia	
Menorrhagia	Goiter	
	Palmar erythema	
	Onycholysis	
	Muscle weakness and wasting	
	Oligomenorrhea/amenorrhea	

Thyroid Antibody Tests

- The immune system of the body normally protects us from foreign invaders, such as bacteria and viruses by destroying these invaders with substances called antibodies produced by blood cells known as lymphocytes.
- In many patients with hypothyroidism or hyperthyroidism, lymphocytes react against the thyroid (thyroid autoimmunity) and make antibodies against thyroid cell proteins.
- Two common antibodies are thyroid peroxidase antibody and thyroglobulin antibody. Measuring levels of thyroid antibodies may help diagnose the cause of the thyroid problem.
- For example, positive anti-thyroid peroxidase and/or anti-thyroglobulin antibodies in a patient with hypothyroidism result in a diagnosis of Hashimoto's thyroiditis.

- While detecting antibodies is helpful in the initial diagnosis of hypothyroidism due to autoimmune thyroiditis, following their levels over time is not helpful in detecting the development of hypothyroidism or response to therapy.
- TSH and FT4 are what tell us about the actual thyroid function or levels. A different antibody that may be positive in a patient with hyperthyroidism is the stimulatory TSH receptor antibody (TSI).
- This antibody causes the thyroid to be overactive in Graves' Disease. If you have Graves' disease, your doctor might also order a thyrotropin receptor antibody test (TSHR or TRAb), which detects both stimulating and blocking antibodies.
- Following antibody levels in Graves' patients may help to assess response to treatment of hyperthyroidism, to determine when it is appropriate to discontinue antithyroid medication, and to assess the risk of passing antibodies to the fetus during pregnancy.

Thyroglobulin

- Thyroglobulin (Tg) is a protein produced by normal thyroid cells and thyroid cancer cells.
- It is not a measure of thyroid function and it does not diagnose thyroid cancer when the thyroid gland is still present. It is used most often in patients who have had surgery for thyroid cancer in order to monitor them after treatment.
- Tg is included in this brochure of thyroid function tests to communicate that, although measured frequently in certain scenarios and individuals, Tg is not a primary measure of thyroid hormone function.

Non-Blood Tests

Radioactive Iodine Uptake

- Because T4 contains iodine, the thyroid gland must pull a large amount of iodine from the bloodstream in order to make an appropriate amount of T4.
- The thyroid has developed a very active mechanism for doing this. Therefore, this activity can be measured by having an individual swallow a small amount of iodine, which is radioactive.
- The radioactivity allows the doctor to track where the iodine goes. By measuring the amount of radioactivity that is taken up by the thyroid gland (radioactive iodine uptake, RAIU), doctors may determine whether the gland is functioning normally.
- A very high RAIU is seen in individuals whose thyroid gland is overactive (hyperthyroidism), while a low RAIU is seen when the thyroid gland is underactive (hypothyroidism).
- In addition to the radioactive iodine uptake, a thyroid scan may be obtained, which shows a picture of the thyroid gland and reveals what parts of the thyroid have taken up the iodine.

Medications that Interfere with Thyroid Function Testing

There are many medications that can affect thyroid function testing. Some common examples include:

- **Estrogens**, such as in birth control pills, or in pregnancy, cause high levels of total T4 and T3. This is because estrogens increase the level of the binding proteins. In these situations, it is better to ask both for TSH and free T4 for thyroid evaluation, which will typically be in the normal range.
- **Biotin**, a commonly taken over-the-counter supplement, can cause the measurement of several thyroid function tests to appear abnormal, when they are in fact normal in the blood. Biotin should not be taken for 2 days before blood is drawn for thyroid function testing to avoid this effect.

CONCLUSION

Organ function tests are the biochemical tests carried out to assess whether particular organ is functioning normally or not. This chapter describes liver function tests, renal function tests and thyroid function tests. Unconjugated hyperbilirubinemia with normal alanine transaminase (ALT) activity indicates the presence of hemolytic jaundice. Conjugated hyperbilirubinemia with raised activity of the ALT indicates hepatic jaundice; however, conjugated hyperbilirubinemia with marked elevation of alkaline phosphatase (ALP) activity suggest obstructive jaundice. The glomerular filtration rate (GFR) is estimated by measuring creatinine clearance. Assessment of concentrating and diluting ability of the kidney provide most sensitive means of detecting early impairment in renal function. Urine analysis reveals the disease anywhere in the urinary tract. The test used to investigate thyroid dysfunction can be performed in vivo or in vitro. Serum T3, T4 and TSH help to assess the severity of thyroid disease.

BIBLIOGRAPHY

1. Bennett WM. Drug Prescribing in Renal Failure. Drugs. 1979;17:111-23.
2. Byrne CJ, Saxton DF, Pelikan PK, Nugent PM. Laboratory Tests: Implications for Nurses and Allied Health Professionals. Menlo Park: Addison-Wesley Publishing Co, 1981.
3. Cockroft DW, Gault MH. Prediction of Creatinine Clearance from Serum Creatinine. Nephron. 1967;16:31-41.
4. Hounkpatin HO, Fraser SDS, Glidewell L, Blakeman T, Lewington A, Roderick PJ. Predicting Risk of Recurrent Acute Kidney Injury: A Systematic Review. Nephron. 2019;142(2):83-90.
5. Kamianowska M, Szczepański M, Wasilewska A. Tubular and Glomerular Biomarkers of Acute Kidney Injury in Newborns. Curr Drug Metab. 2019;20(5):332-49.
6. Koda-Kimble MA, Katcher BS, Young LY (Eds). Applied Therapeutics for Clinical Pharmacists, 2nd edition. San Francisco: Applied Therapeutics Inc, 1975.
7. Okoro RN, Farate VT. The use of nephrotoxic drugs in patients with chronic kidney disease. Int J Clin Pharm. 2019 Jun;41(3):767-75.
8. Ravel R. Clinical Laboratory Medicine: Clinical Application of Laboratory Data, 3rd edition. Chicago: Year Book Medical Publishers Inc, 1978.
9. Ribeiro AJS, Yang X, Patel V, Madabushi R, Strauss DG. Liver Microphysiological Systems for Predicting and Evaluating Drug Effects. Clin Pharmacol Ther. 2019 Jul;106(1):139-47.

10. Sher PP. Drug Interferences with Clinical Laboratory Tests. Drugs. 1982; 24: 24-63.
11. Vagvala SH, O'Connor SD. Imaging of abnormal liver function tests. Clin Liver Dis (Hoboken). 2018 May;11(5):128-34.

REVIEW QUESTIONS

Long Essays
1. Define kidney function test, explain briefly about the components of kidney function test.
2. Explain in detail about liver function test.
3. Describe thyroid function test.

Short Essays
1. Liver enzymes.
2. Serum albumin and albumin globulin ratio.
3. Functional components of a kidney.
4. Thyroid antibody tests.
5. TSH tests.
6. Hepatic jaundice.
7. Radioactive iodine uptake.
8. Medications that interfere with thyroid function testing.

Short Answers
1. Prothrombin time.
2. Thyroglobulin.
3. Alkaline phosphatase.
4. Gamma-glutamyl transpeptidase.
5. Electrolytes.
6. Dilution test.
7. Concentration test.
8. Inulin clearance.
9. Creatinine clearance rate.
10. Urea clearance.
11. Serum creatinine level.
12. Blood urea nitrogen (BUN).
13. Serum urea.
14. Urine examination.

CHAPTER 23

Immunochemistry

CHAPTER OUTLINE
- Structure and Functions of Immunoglobulin
- Investigations and Interpretation—ELISA

TERMINOLOGY

- **Antigens:** Chemical substances which when introduced into the host stimulate the immune system and produce antibodies.
- **Antibodies:** Immunoglobulin (glycoproteins) produced by lymphocytes in response to bacteria, viruses, or other antigenic substances.
- **Cell-mediated immunity:** The mechanism of acquired immunity mediated by T-lymphocytes, which defend from invasion of parasites, fungi, etc.
- **Hormonal immunity:** Immunity that is mediated by circulating antibodies-immunoglobulins.
- **Immunity:** The quality of being insusceptible to a particular disease or condition because of the formation of humoral antibodies or the development of cellular immunity or both.
- **Electrophoresis:** The movement of particles in an electric field. Commonly-used techniques for analysis of mixtures of molecules in solution according to their electrophoretic mobilities.
- **Immune response:** The capacity of a vertebrate to generate antibodies to an antigen, a macromolecule foreign to the organism.
- **Innate immunity:** It is also called natural immunity usually refers to the ability of the body to defend itself against invasion by pathogenic microorganism before the on-set of infection.
- **Autoimmunity:** Usually immune does not react to its own tissues and organs. However, if it does, it results in an immune attack on the host itself leading to autoimmunity.
- **Allergy response:** Allergy represents an inappropriate immune response to antigen. Often these antigens are common, such as pollens, foods, drugs or animal dander.
- **Immunodeficiency:** Immunodeficiency represents an aberration of immune response on a quantitative scale. Due to developmental, physical, chemical or environmental damages, the immune system is not fully developed or functional resulting in inadequate protection.

INTRODUCTION

Immunology is a science that deals with the study of protection of the body from invasion by disease producing micro-organisms. This state of protection of the body is called immunity. It is result of normally functioning immune system which is highly efficient but complex. Our immune system operates at two levels to protect us from these antigens. At the first level, it tries to prevent the attack or entry of the antigen into the body. In this respect, the immune system acts more likely a barrier to block the counter of the body with the antigens. For example, intact normal skin acts as an anatomical barrier preventing the entry of pathogens and antigens. Break or loss of skin, as seen in burn patients, refers the body highly susceptible to infections.

HISTORICAL PERSPECTIVES

Nobel prize winner of immunology

Sl. No.	Year	Contributors	Country	Research work
1.	1901	Emil von Behring	Germany	Serum antitoxin
2.	1905	Robert koch	Germany	Cellular immunity to tuberculosis
3.	1908	Elie Metchnikoff, Paul Ehrlich	• Russia • Germany	• Phagocytosis • Antitoxins
4.	1913	Charles Richet	France	Anaphylasis

Contd...

Contd...

Sl. No.	Year	Contributors	Country	Research work
5.	1919	Jules Bordet	Belgium	Complement-mediated bacteriolysis
6.	1930	Karl Landsteiner	United States	Discovery of human blood groups
7.	1951	Max Theiler	South Africa	Development of yellow fever vaccine
8.	1957	Daniel bovet	Switzerland	Antihistamines
9.	1960	F.Macfarlane Burnet Peter Medawar	• Australia • Great britian	Acquired immunlogical tolerance
10.	1972	• Rodney R Porter • Gerald M Edelman	Great britain	Structure of antibodies
11.	1977	Rosalyn R Yalow	United States	Development of radioimmunoassay
12.	1980	George Snell, Jean Dausset, Baruj Benacerraf	• France • United States	Major histocompatibility complex
13.	1984	Cesar Milstein, George F Kohler, Niels K Jerne	• Great Britian • Germany • Denmark	Monoclonal antibody Immune regulatory theories
14.	1991	E Donnall Thomas, Joseph Murray	• United States • United States	Transplantation immunology
15.	1996	Peter C Doherty Rolf M Zinkernage	• Australia • Switzerland	The specific of the cell-mediated immune response

Structure and Functions of Immune System

The immune system is a lymphoreticular system composed of diverse types of cells distributed widely in organs and tissues. The lymphoreticular system structurally and functionally has different components:

- **Lymphoid system** consisting of lymphoid organs and lymphoid cells.
  The lymphoid system produces humoral and cellular immune response and is responsible for specific immunity.
- **Reticuloendothelial system** consists of phagocytes and is responsible for nonspecific immunity. They have scavenging functions and eliminate microorganisms and other foreign agents from the host.

Lymphoid System

It consists of lymphoid organs and lymphoid cells. Lymphoid organs are classified based on their function into: (1) Central (primary) lymphoid organs, (2) Peripheral (secondary) lymphoid organs.
- **Central lymphoid organs, e.g., thymus:** (a) Bursa of Fabricius in avian species, (b) Bone marrow in mammals
- **Peripheral lymphoid organs:** (a) Lymph nodes, (b) Spleen, (c) Mucosa associated lymphoid tissue (MALT). The lymphoid cells include the lymphocytes and plasma cells.

The central lymphoid organs are responsible for: (a) Development and proliferation of lymphocytes, (b) Development of immunocompetency by lymphocytes.

Cells of Immune System

They are of two types: (1) Structural cells—these include endothelial cells, fibroblasts and reticulum cells, (2) Functional (competent) cells—lymphocytes, plasma cells and macrophages

- **Lymphocyte development:** During embryonic development, blood cell precursors originate mainly in the fetal liver and yolk sac; in postnatal life, the stem cells reside in the bone marrow. Stem cells differentiate into cells of the erythroid, myeloid or lymphoid series. The cells of the lymphoid series evolve into mainly T lymphocytes (T cells) and B lymphocytes (B cells). Thus, in fetus, lymphocytes originate from bone marrow.
- **Processing of lymphocytes:** The cells of the lymphoid series undergo processing in the thymus gland and are therefore called as T lymphocytes. This occurs during the interval just before birth and a few months after birth. The thymus secretes a hormone called thymosin which when released into the circulation accelerates the proliferation and activation of lymphocytes in the thymus. The activity of the lymphocytes in the lymphoid tissue is also increased.
- **Lymphocytes** are of different types in the circulating blood of which 70% are T lymphocytes, 20% B-lymphocytes and 10% null cells. They develop their immunological competence in the central lymphoid organs. They develop the ability to recognize antigens, develop immunological memory and mount an immune response to non-self antigens.

Lymphocytes are classified into 3 main types based on site of development, surface markers and functions into:

1. **T-lymphocytes:** They are thymus derived lymphocytes which carry the T-cell receptor and mediate cell-mediated immune response. After differentiation, they move from the thymus to various lymphoid tissues in lymph nodes, spleen, bone marrow and gastrointestinal tract.

There are two different subsets of T-cells:
a. CD^4 T cells (helper T cells)
b. CD^8 T cells (suppressor/cytotoxic T cells)

a. **CD⁴⁺ T cells:** It recognizes the antigen along with major histocompatibility complex (MHC) class II protein and helps B cell and T cell function. It plays an important role in cell mediated immune response and also in humoral response by influencing antibody production by B cells.
b. **CD⁸¹ T cells:** It recognizes the antigen along with MHC class I protein and can mediate cytotoxic functions (killing of infected cells and malignant cells). These T cells can be activated by cytokines (IFNγ, IL-2) and after activation; they recognize the target cell and destroy it. This is useful against viruses, intracellular bacterial and fungal infections.

2. **B-lymphocytes:** They were first discovered in the bursa of Fabricius in birds and so were named as B-lymphocytes. This bursa is situated near the cloaca in birds but absent in mammals. The processing of these lymphocytes takes place in liver and bone marrow.

The B-cell matures into one of the two types of cells under the influence of antigen presence and interleukins secreted by cells in the environment:
a. Plasma cell—actively secretes large amount of antibody.
b. Memory cell—retains memory of specific antigen exposure

After undergoing transformation, the B cell moves to the blood and the lymphoid tissues in the lymph node, spleen, bone marrow and gastrointestinal tract; it carries immunoglobulin on its surface membrane and is ready to interact with antigen.

Functions:
a. Differentiate into plasma cells and produce antibodies
b. They can present antigen along with MHC class II molecules to CD⁴⁺ T lymphocytes.

3. **Natural killer cells:** It is considered as the third type of lymphocyte and plays an important role in innate host defenses. Approximately 5–10% of peripheral lymphocytes are natural killer cells. They specialize in killing virus infected cells, tumor cells and cancer cells by secreting cytotoxins. They are called so because they kill invading micro organisms or cells without prior exposure. They have no immunological memory and no T-cell receptor and killing does not require recognition of class II MHC proteins. Humans who lack natural killer cells are predisposed to life-threatening infections with Varicella-zoster virus and cytomegalovirus.

MACROPHAGES

They are large phagocytic cells which digest invading microorganisms and release the antigen. They have three main functions:

1. **Phagocytosis:** After ingestion of micro organism, the phagosome containing the microbe fuses with a lysosome to form a phagolysosome. This contains reactive oxygen and nitrogen compounds and lysosomal enzymes which kills the microorganism.
2. **Antigen presentation:** After ingestion and degradation, the antigen fragments are presented along with class II MHC proteins to CD⁴⁺ helper T cells.
3. **Cytokine production:** Interleukin-1 (IL-1) and tumor necrosis factor (TNF) are produced which activate helper T-cells and mediate inflammation. IL-8 is also produced which attracts neutrophils and T-cells by the process of chemotaxis. Macrophages are present as bone marrow histiocytes, Kupffer cells in liver and alveolar macrophages in lungs.

Dendritic cells: They function as antigen presenting cells. They are located in the skin and mucosa (e.g., Langerhans' cell). They express class II MHC proteins and present antigen to CD⁴⁺ T cells. They migrate from their location under skin and mucosa to the local lymph nodes for antigen presentation.

Polymorphonuclear leukocytes: These include neutrophils, eosinophils and basophils.

- **Neutrophils:** They play an important role in innate immunity. They have phagocytic action and contain lysosomal granules which have a bactericidal activity. They have a prominent role to play in acute inflammation.
- **Eosinophils:** They play an important role in hypersensitivity reactions and parasitic diseases. However, they are less phagocytic when compared to neutrophils.
- **Basophils and mast cells:** These cells are present in blood and tissues. They have receptors on their surface for the Fe portion of IgE. When IgE molecules are cross-linked by antigen, degranulation and release of inflammatory mediators occurs. This results in inflammation and hypersensitivity reactions like anaphylaxis.

MAJOR HISTOCOMPATIBILITY (MCH)

It is also known as human leukocyte antigen (HLA) complex. It is a collection of genes arrayed within a long continuous stretch of DNA on chromosome 6 in humans. These HLA antigens which are coded by FILA genes control the success of tissue and organ transplants. These are alloantigens, i.e., they differ among members of the same species. If the HLA proteins on the donor's cells differ from those on the recipient's cell, an immune response occurs in the recipient. The genes which code for the HLA complex fall into three categories:

1. **Class I:** HLA-A, HLA-B and HLA-C code for the class I MHC proteins which are present on the surface of all nucleated cells. They have a role to play in rejection of graft and cell-mediated cytolysis. CD⁸⁺ T cells recognize antigen only when it is presented by antigen presenting cells in association with class I MHC proteins.
2. **Class II:** HLA-DP, HLA-DQ, FILA-DR code for the class II MHC proteins. These are glycoproteins are found on the surface of macrophages, B cells, dendritic cells of the spleen and Langerhans' cells of the skin. These antigens are responsible for the graft-versus-host response.
3. **Class III:** These genes code for the C2 and C4 complement components of the classical pathway and properdin factor B of the alternate pathway.

Immune Response

It is the specific response of the immune system to an antigenic stimulus. The response may be neutral, beneficial

or harmful to the host. The immune response induced can be of two types:
1. Humoral immunity (antibody mediated)
2. Cellular immunity (cell mediated)

Humoral immunity involves the antibodies and B lymphocytes (and plasma cells). It is the first line of defense against most extracellular pathogenic bacteria and defends against viruses causing infection through the respiratory and intestinal tract, It also plays a role in the pathogenesis of hypersensitivity reactions (type I, II and III) and some autoimmune diseases.

Cell mediated immunity involves T lymphocytes (helper T cells and cytotoxic T cells). It defends against infection caused by fungi, viruses and intracellular bacterial pathogens, such as *M. tuberculosis*, and *M. leprae*. It also plays a role in transplantation reactions, such as homograft rejection and graft-versus-host reaction. It also mediates the pathogenesis of delayed hypersensitivity and some autoimmune diseases. It also provides immunity against cancer.

Humoral Immune Response

It is the specific response of the immune system to antigenic stimulus characterized by production of antibodies by B-cells.

The humoral immune response takes place in three stages:
1. **Afferent stage:** It involves the entry and spread of antigens in the body.
2. **Central stage:** This stage is characterized by the uptake of antigen by antigen-presenting cells (APC) mainly miacrophages, and presentation of the antigen by the APC to immunocompetent T cells and B cells.
3. **Efferent stage:** This stage is characterized by recognition of the antigen by the immunocompetent cells and production of lymphokines by T cells which stimulate B cells to produce antibodies and leads to various antibody-mediated actions.

A characteristic pattern is seen in the production of antibodies. They are:
- **Lag phase:** It is the period immediately following an antigenic stimulus during which no antibody is detectable in the circulation.
- **Log phase:** There is a gradual rise in the level of antibodies
- **Plateau phase:** There is equilibrium between the production of antibodies and their catabolism.
- **Phase of decline:** The catabolism of antibodies is more than their production and the antibody level falls.

Primary and Secondary Humoral Response

The primary response is the antibody response following first exposure to antigen where as the secondary response is the antibody response following subsequent exposure to antigen.

The primary response has a long lag phase and a low antibody level that does persist for long whereas in the secondary response, the lag phase is short and the response is fast and effective. The antibody levels are higher and remain for a longer period of time. 1gM is the predominant antibody formed in the primary humoral response whereas IgG is the predominant antibody formed in the secondary humoral response.

Production of antibodies: Immune response to an antigen is brought about it by three types of cells—the antigen processing cells (mainly macrophages and den iritic cells), T cells and B cells. The B cells following activation clonally proliferate and differentiate into antibody secreting plasma cells. B cells carry surface receptors which consist of 1gM or other immunoglobulin classes, Depending on these receptors, plasma cell; secrete 1gM, IgG or any other class of antibodies. However, in the primary response, 1gM is tie antibody initially secreted followed later by secretion of IgG However, a small proportion of of activated B cells, instead of being transformed into plasma cells, develop into memory cells producing a secondary response on subsequent exposure to antigen. T cells regulate the production of antibodies by B cells.

Theories of antibody formation: There are two theories which attempt to explain antibody formation. They are:
1. Instructive theories
2. Selective theories

According to the instructive theory, an immunocompetent cell has the ability to synthesize specific antibodies in response to a specific antigen.

Alternately, the selective theory postulates that the antigen selects the specific immunocompetent cell to synthesize an antibody.

The clonal selection theory is however the most accepted theory. This theory was proposed by Burnet in 1957. It states that during fetal development, clones of immunocompetent cells bearing specific antibody patterns against all possible antigens are produced by a process of somatic mutation of these cells. Those clones which react against self-antigens are eliminated during embryonic development If these clones persist or they appear in later life by somatic mutation, it may lead to autoimmune disease. Each immunocompetent cell can react with one or more antigens. This contact with antigen stimulates cellular proliferation to form clones which can synthesize antibody.

Functions
- Provide passive immunity by neutralizing toxins of diphtheria and tetanus and botulinum toxin by antitoxins.
- Inhibition of rabies and hepatitis A and B viruses.

Monoclonal antibodies: Antibodies produced in response to a single antigen are heterogenous as they are formed from different clones of plasma cells, i.e., polyclonal. If antibodies arise from a single clone of plasma cells, they are monoclonal in nature (e.g., myeloma).

These monoclonal antibodies can also be produced in the laboratory by fusing a myeloma cell with an antibody-producing cell (splenic cells). Such fused cells are called as hybridomas and they have the ability to produce unlimited quantities of monoclonal antibodies. This is because the fused cell has the antibody producing capacity of the splenic cells and the ability to multiply indefinitely as it is a myeloma cell.

Uses

- Treatment of autoimmune disease, cancer prevents or treats allograft rejection and graft-versus-host reaction.
- Detection of bacterial, viral and other antigens
- Production of specific antibodies.

Cellular immune response: It is the response of the immune system to an antigenic stimulus involving T cells, macrophages and their products, such as lymphokines and lymphokine-mediated actions.

This type of immunity is transferable from donor to recipient with intact lymphocytes but cannot be transferred using antisera.

Like humoral immune response, cell mediated immune response also has a primary and a secondary response.

The primary response is when a specific T cell after exposure to an antigen undergoes proliferation to produce a small clone of cells.

The secondary response occurs on subsequent exposure to antigen. The clone of cells further expands to produce more specific T cells.

Induction of cell mediated immune response: It happens when an antigen from micro organisms or other non-microbial cells are presented to T lymphocytes by antigen presenting cells. This presentation of antigens to lymphocytes is an important process in the development of an immune response. This exposure to antigens sensitizes the T cells which undergo blast transformation, clonal proliferation and differentiation into memory cells and effector cells. The activated lymphocytes produce various lymphokines (IL-2 and Gamma interferon) which are responsible for the manifestations of cell mediated immunity.

Cytokines: They are biologically active substances which act as mediators in immune response. They are secreted by macrophages, T lymphocytes, monocytes and other cells. They function as growth and differentiating factors and also exert regulatory influence on other cells.

Chemokines are a group of cytokines which can attract macrophages or neutrophils to the site of infection. They may be secreted by activated mononuclear cells or T cells. For example, of cytokines interleukin-1, interleukin-2, interleukin-6, colony stimulating factor, tumor necrosis factor.

Cell mediated immune response is important in the following situations:
- Immunological defense against infection caused by intracellular pathogens.
- Type IV hypersensitivity reactions
- Immunological surveillance and immunity against cancer
- Pathogenesis of autoimmune conditions, e.g., thyroiditis

Immunological tolerance: It is a state in which an immune response is not produced on exposure to a specific antigen though it produces a response for other antigens. The body usually does not mount an immune response for self antigens but only non-self antigens elicit a response.

Though both B and T cells participate in tolerance, T cell tolerance is more important.

IMMUNITY

Immunity is the resistance of the body against the damage caused by microorganisms and microbial products.

Innate Immunity

It is the inborn resistance of the body against infectious agents. It exists prior to exposure to microbes and is non-specific. It is genetically and physiologically mediated. The functions of innate immunity are to kill or inhibit infectious agents and to activate the acquired immune mechanisms.

Mechanical Barriers

- **Skin:**
  - Intact skin with its keratin layer acts as a mechanical barrier against bacteria and other organisms.
  - Skin secretions, such as sebum and sweat are anti-bacterial and antifungal in nature.
  - Normal flora of skin protects against infection by competing for receptors and nutrients and breakdown of toxins; they also produce toxic metabolites.
- **Respiratory tract:**
  - Anatomy of respiratory tract prevents entry of microorganisms.
  - The mucus lining of the epithelium, the cough reflex and the cilia lining the respiratory tract prevent the entry of microorganisms.
  - Phagocytic cells, such as the alveolar macrophages engulf and destroy the micro organisms that enter the lungs.
- **Gastrointestinal tract:**
  - Gastric pH which is around 1.5 destroys most ingested pathogens.
  - Saliva and other secretions in the oral cavity have an inhibitory effect on many microorganisms; lysozyme in saliva has antibacterial action.
  - Peristaltic movements of the intestine remove infectious agents from the intestinal tract.
  - Normal flora of the intestinal tract competes for receptors and nutrients with potential pathogens and also produces toxic metabolites.
  - Defecation removes infectious agents from intestine.
- **Genitourinary tract:**
  - Flushing action of urine and its acidic pH, vesicoureteric valves prevent the establishment of infection.
  - The acidic pH of the vagina is unfavorable for pathogenic organisms.

Conjunctiva

The flushing action of lachrymal secretions along with lysozyme protects the eye from infectious agents.

Systemic mechanisms

Acquired immunity: It is the resistance that the body develops after exposure to an agent, such as bacteria, viruses or toxins. It improves after repeated exposure to the agent and is specific. It is mediated by antibody and T-lymphocytes (helper and cytotoxic). Acquired immunity is broadly classified into (i) Active immunity (ii) Passive immunity

Active immunity-is of two types
1. Natural—by exposure to infection
2. Artificial—by use of vaccines

Mechanisms of acquired immunity: Development of acquired immunity involves both a humoral and cell-mediated immune response:
1. **Humoral immunity:** It is immunity produced by the activation of B lymphocytes which provide resistance against infectious agents by producing antibodies. It brings about immunity by (i) Neutralization of infectious agents (ii) Opsonization (iii) Complement activation (iv) Antibody dependent cellular cytotoxicity It is important particularly in defense against capsulated and toxic bacterial infections and viral infections.
2. **Cellular immunity:** It is also called as cell mediated immunity. It begins with activation of T-lymphocytes which destroy the infectious agents entering the body of the host. This type of immunity is an important and major defense mechanism of the host against infections caused by viruses, fungi, parasites and certain intracellular bacteria, such as tubercle bacilli. It also has a role to play in delayed hypersensitivity reactions and rejection of foreign tissue transplants.

Types of active immunity:
- **Natural acquired immunity:** It occurs following exposure to infection and may be short lasting (e.g., common cold) or long lasting. (e.g., smallpox)
- **Artificial acquired immunity:** It develops after administration of vaccines which may contain live or killed organisms or toxins.

Vaccines: They are preparations containing non-pathogenic immunogens which when introduced into a host induce protective immunity against a specific infection.

Types of vaccines are:
1. Live attenuated vaccines, e.g., BCG for tuberculosis
2. Killed vaccines, e.g., salk vaccine for poliomyelitis
3. Bacterial products, e.g., tetanus toxoid for tetanus
4. Other vaccines, e.g., subunit vaccines, recombinant DNA vaccines

Passive Immunity

It is immunity acquired by an individual during life in ready form, i.e., antibodies. It is of two types- (a) natural (b) artificial
1. **Natural passive immunity:** It involves passive transfer of antibodies, e.g., maternal IgG antibodies passively transferred to the fetus through the placenta
2. **Artificial passive immunity:** It involves passive transfer of antibodies by parenteral administration. For example, administration of antisera, pooled human gamma globulin

Uses of passive immunization:
- It provides immediate short lasting immunity
- Treatment of severe infections
- To suppress active immunity, e.g., Rh positive baby born to Rh negative mother.

Differences between active and passive immunity:

Active immunity	Passive immunity
It develops actively in the host	Host receives in the form of preformed antibodies
Prior contact not required	Prior contact not required
Immunity usually long lasting	Brief but effective immunity
Immunological memory is present	Immunological memory is absent
Not of use in immunodeficient persons	Useful in immunodeficient persons
Lag period is present	Lag period is absent

Miscellaneous

- **Combined immunization:** It is the simultaneous use of active and passive immunization. Passive immunity provides early protection till active immunity takes effect.
- **Local immunity:** It is the local immunity present on mucosa usually due to secretory IgA. It may be induced by natural infections or oral vaccines. For example, oral polio vaccine.
- **Herd immunity:** It is the overall resistance of individuals in the community against infection. When herd immunity is good, it protects against epidemics of infection. For example, oral polio vaccine gives good herd immunity.

ANTIGEN

Substances capable of inducing a specific immune response are called antigens. Most potent antigens are proteins in nature and include lipoproteins, glycoproteins and nucleoproteins. If antigens are present on the host's own cells, they are called self-antigens or auto-antigens and if those present on non-self cells are called as foreign antigens or non-self antigens.

Examples of non-self antigens include the following:
- Allergens, such as pollen grains, house mite
- Receptors on the cells of microorganisms such as bacteria, viruses and fungi.
- Toxins produced by microbes
- Tissue from transplanted organs or incompatible blood cells.

Based on their ability to induce an immune response, antigens are of two types:
1. **Complete antigen:** It is an antigen which can induce an immune response and also react with its specific antibody.
2. **Hapten:** They are incomplete antigens which cannot induce an immune response on their own. However, when they are linked to carrier molecules, they become complete antigens and can initiate an immune response.

Factors which determine antigenicity are:
- **Foreignness or non-self:** A substance must be foreign or non-self to be able to induce an immune response from the host.
- **Size:** Substances with high molecular weight (above 1,00,000 daltons) are highly antigenic whereas those with

low molecular weight (below 10,000) are weak antigens or non-antigenic.
- **Chemical nature:** Proteins are better antigens than polysaccharides, lipids and nucleic acids.
- **Antigenic determinants (Epitopes):** They are one or more small chemical groups on the antigen (monovalent or multivalent) that react with antibody. This three dimensional structure of antigen determines anti genic specificity.
- **Species specificity:** Organs or tissues in a species possess common antigens called species specific antigens.
- **Isospecificity:** Species may be grouped depending on the presence of isoantigens present in few members of a species. For example, blood grouping
- **Organ specificity:** Some antigens are present in specific organs of different species called as organ specific antigens. For example, some organs, such as brain and lens protein are specific for one species and may induce immune response f transplanted to another species.
- **Autospecificity:** Self antigens are usually not antigenic. Sequestered antigens are those antigens which do not come in contact will the immune system hut when released into circulation, can induce an immune response. For example, eye lens antigen.
- **Heterophile specificity**: They are cross reacting antigens present in different biological specie'. Antibodies produced to such antigens in one species can cross react with antigens (f another biological species.
- **Dosage and route of administration:** Antigen dose varies among antigens and the administration route strongly influences which immune organs and cell populations will be involved in the response.
- **Adjuvants:** They enhance the immune response to an antigen. For example, tetanus toxoid adsorbed vaccine.

ANTIBODIES

They are glycoprotein molecules that are produced by plasma cells in response to an antigen and which function as antibodies. As they migrate with globular proteins when antibody-containing serum is placed in an electrical field, they are also called as immunoglobulins. They are mainly synthesized by plasma cells.

Structure (Fig. 23.1)

The immunoglobulin molecule is made up of four polypeptide chains-two heavy H chains and two light L

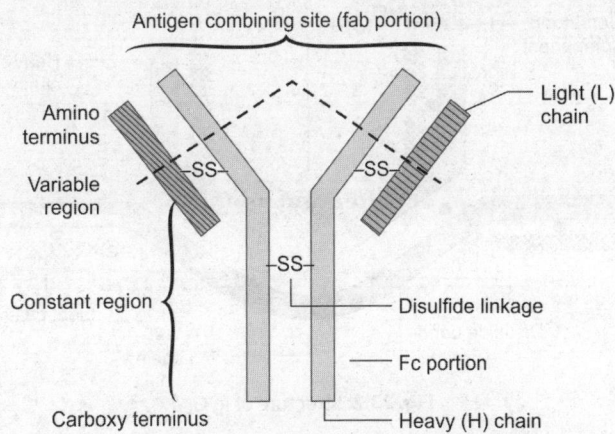

Fig. 23.1: Structure of antibodies.

chains, held together by disulfide bonds and non-covalent interactions.

The heavy chains are structurally and antigenically different in different classes of immunoglobulins. They are composed of five types Ig A, Ig G, Ig E, Ig M, IgD.

The light chains are similar in all classes of immunoglobulins. They are composed of two types (Lambda) and K (Kappa).

Both the light and heavy chains have two regions- a variable (V) region and a constant (C) region. The variable region (amino terminal portion or Fab fragment) of both light and heavy chains is responsible for antigen binding whereas the constant region (F fragment) of the heavy chain is responsible for various biologic functions like complement activation and binding to various cell surface receptors.

Human Immunoglobulin Classes

The immunoglobulins can be divided into five different classes, based on differences in the amino acid sequences in the constant region of the heavy chains.

I. IgG (Fig. 23.2)

IgG is the most abundant (75-80%) class of immunoglobulins. IgG is composed of a single v-shaped unit (monomer). IgG is the only immunoglobulin that can cross the placenta and transfer the mothers immunity to the developing foetus. IgG triggers foreign cell destruction mediated by complement system.
- It is the most abundant immunoglobulin in the serum (>75% of serum immunoglobulin) with a concentration of 8-16 mg/mL.

Type	H-chain	L-chains	Molecular formula	Molecular weight	Percentage carbohydrate	Serum conc. mg/dL	Major functions(s)
IgG	γ	κ or λ	$\gamma_2\kappa_2$ or $\gamma_2\lambda_2$	–150,000	3	800–1,500	Mostly responsible for humoral immunity
IgA	α	κ or λ	$(\alpha_2\kappa_2)_{1-3}$ or $(\alpha_2\kappa_2)_{1-3}$	$-(160,000)_{1-3}$	8	150–400	Protects the body surfaces
IgM	μ	κ or λ	$(\mu_2\kappa_2)_5$ or $(\mu_2\kappa_2)_5$	–900,000	12	50–200	Humoral immunity, serves as first line defense
IgD	δ	κ or λ	$(\delta_2\kappa_2$ or $\delta_2\kappa_2)$	–180,000	13	1–10	B-cell receptor? and histamine release

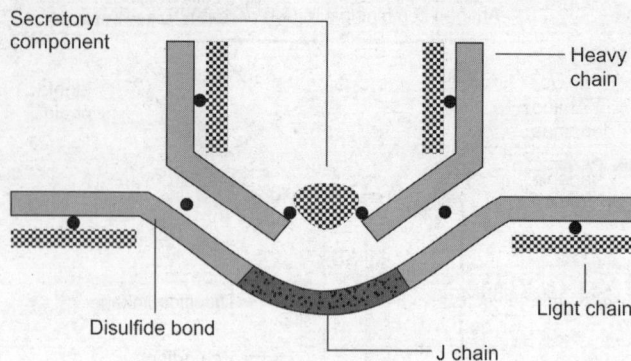

Fig. 23.2: Structure of Ig G.

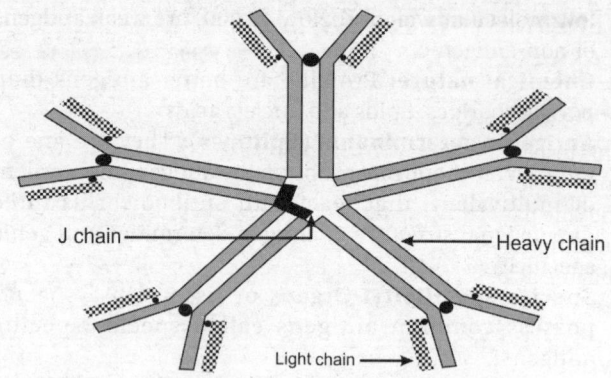

Fig. 23.3: Structure of Ig M.

- IgG has a γ heavy chain.
- Molecular weight is 1,50,000 daltons and has a monomeric structure having a 7S sedimentation coefficient.
- IgG is the major immunoglobulin in extra vascular spaces.
- IgG is the only class of Ig that crosses the placenta and provides passive immunity to the neonate.
- It is important in the secondary immune response and is an important defense against bacterial and viral infections.
- It appears late after the initial IgM response but remains for a longer period.
- It takes part in complement fixation, opsonization and neutralization reactions.

II. IgA

Structure of IgA (secretory IgA): IgA occurs as a single (monomer) or double unit (dimer) held together by J chain. It is mostly found in the body secretions such as saliva, tears, sweat, milk and the walls of intestine. IgA is the most predominant antibody in the colostrum, the initial secretion from the mother's breast after a baby is born. IgA prevents the foreign substances from entering the body cells.

- IgA is the second most common serum immunoglobulin and also exists in secretory form; in dimeric form, the 2 units of the dimer are linked by a J chain.
- Serum concentration is 0.6–4.2 mg/mL.
- IgA is the major class of Ig in secretions—tears, saliva, colostrum, mucus. Since, it is found in secretions, secretory IgA is important in local (mucosal) immunity.
- IgA has an alpha heavy chain.
- Molecular weight is 1,60,000 daltons; it exists as a monomer (7S) in serum and as a dimer (11S) in secretions with the 2 units of the dimer being joined by a J chain.
- IgA provides local immunity by inhibiting adherence, coating microbes and preventing their entry into the tissues, and activating the alternate complement pathway.

III. IgM (Fig. 23.3)

- Largest immunoglobulin in the serum (M stands for Macroglobulin). Accounts for 5–8% of serum immunoglobulin with a concentration of 0.5–2 mg/mL.
- It is a pentamer made up of five immunoglobulin molecules.
- Molecular weight is 9,00,000 to 10,00,000 daltons and sedimentation coefficient is 19S.
- It is the main immunoglobulin produced early in the primary response and is short lived; its presence indicates recent infection.
- It does not cross the placental barrier and is the earliest immunoglobulin synthesized by the foetus; therefore its presence in newborn indicates congenital infection.
- It is useful in the diagnosis of congenital infections like rubella and syphilis (which can be transmitted from mother to fetus).
- It is the most efficient immunoglobulin in agglutination, complement fixation and other antibody reactions and is important in defense against bacteria and viruses.

IV. IgD

- It has no known antibody function and is present in small amounts (3 mg/100 mL) in serum.
- Molecular weight is 1,80,000 daltons and has a monomeric structure (7S).

V. IgE

- It is present in traces in the serum and mostly in the extravascular compartment.
- Molecular weight is 1,90,000 daltons with a sedimentation coefficient of 8S.
- It attaches to surface of basophils and mast cells and acts as a mediator of anaphylaxis.
- It participates in host defenses against parasitic helminthic diseases.

Importance of Immunoglobulins

- It is useful in providing passive immunoprophylaxis (human immunoglobulins to non-immune individuals in conditions, such as diphtheria and tetanus. This provides immediate protection.
- It is useful in the diagnosis of infection. e.g., detection of IgG antibodies in HIV infection by ELISA. Diagnosis of congenital infection (congenital syphilis by detection of IgM antibodies by ELISA).
- Detection of abnormal immunoglobulins in diagnosis. For example, Bence-Jones proteins are abnormal immunoglobulins excreted in patients with multiple myeloma.

ENZYME-LINKED IMMUNOSORBENT ASSAY (ELISA)

Principle
This test is based on covalently linking an enzyme to a known antigen or antibody and reacting the enzyme linked material with the patient's specimen to detect corresponding antibody or antigen. Substrate of the enzyme is then added. The enzyme acts on the substrate to produce a color in a positive test.

Types

I. Antigen Detection Assays

- **Competitive ELISA:** It is called so because there is competition between enzyme labeled antigen and antigen in the patient's serum for binding with limited amount of antibody in the antibody coated wells. Initially, patient's serum is added to the well; if antigens are present, antigen-antibody reaction takes place. This reaction is detected by enzyme labeled antigens. Since the limited amounts of antibodies are already bound by specific antigens in the patient's serum added in the first step, enzyme labeled antigens are unable to bind and remain free. They are washed off during the washing process. Substrate is then added but enzyme is not available (washed off along with labeled antigens in washing process) to act on it. So, no color is produced and indicates a positive result.

  More the color intensity, lesser is the antigen level in the patient's serum.

  The labels used could be the following enzyme systems
  - Alkaline phosphatase as enzyme and p-nitrophenyl phosphate as substrate
  - Horseradish peroxidase as enzyme and O-phenylene-diamine dihydrochloride as substrate

- **Non-competitive ELISA:** In this type of ELISA, there is no competition between labeled and unlabelled reactants.

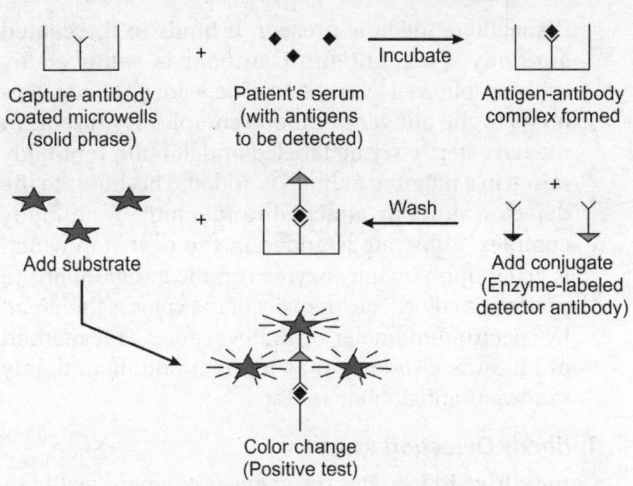

Fig. 23.4: Direct ELISA.

The presence and intensity of color indicates presence of antibodies and the amount of antibodies.

- **Direct ELISA (Fig. 23.4):** The wells of a microtiter plate (solid phase) are coated with specific (capture) antibody to detect antigen in the patient's specimen. If antigen is present, it binds to the specific antibody. After washing to remove free unbound antigen, enzyme labeled detector antibody is added which binds to the antigen-antibody complex in the microtiter plate. Substrate is then added which is acted upon by the enzyme (on the detector antibody) to produce a color. The intensity of the color is then read by spectrophotometer or ELISA reader. This method of ELISA is also known as double antibody sandwich method.

  Applications: Detection of antigens, e.g., ELISA for HBsAg (Hepatitis B surface antigen)

- **Indirect ELISA (Fig. 23.5):** The wells of a microtiter plate (solid phase) are coated with capture antibody to detect specific antigen in the patient's specimen.

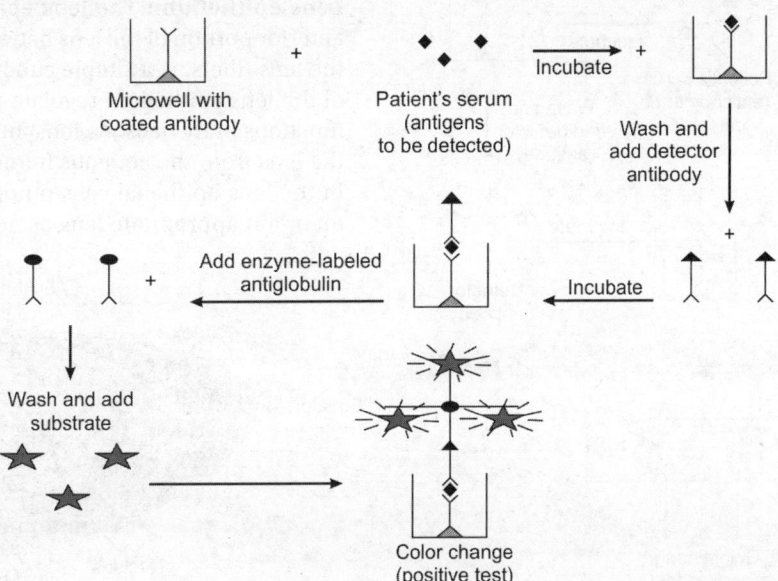

Fig. 23.5: Indirect ELISA.

If specific antigen is present, it binds to the coated antibody. Free unbound antigen is removed by washing followed by addition of detector antibody. This binds to the antigen-antibody complex if present. In the next step, enzyme labeled antiglobulin (antibody raised in a different animal) is added. This binds to the detector antibody attached to the antigen-antibody complex. Substrate is added in the next step which is acted upon by the enzyme (on the antiglobulin) to produce a color. The intensity of the color is then read by spectrophotometer or ELISA reader. This method of ELISA is also known as indirect double antibody sandwich-antiglobulin method.

II. *Antibody Detection Assays*

- **Competitive ELISA:** It is the same as competitive ELISA for detection of antigens, but here limited amount of antigen is coated on the microtiter wells instead of antibody. Also, there is competition between enzyme labeled antibody and unlabeled antibody (in the patient's serum) for limited amount of coated antigen on the microtiter wells.

  No color indicates presence of antibody and hence a positive result but more the color intensity, less is the antibody level in the patient's serum.

- **Non-competitive ELISA (Fig. 23.6):** The wells of a microtiter plate (solid phase) are adsorbed with specific antigen to detect antibody in the patient's serum. If antibody is present, it binds to the adsorbed antigen in the microtiter wells and forms antigen-antibody complex. Enzyme labeled antiglobulin (detector antibody) is added which binds to the antigen-antibody complex in the microtiter plate. Substrate is then added which is acted upon by the enzyme (on the detector antibody) to produce a color. The intensity of the color is then read by spectrophotometer or ELISA reader. The presence and intensity of color indicates presence of antibodies and the amount of antibodies.

Lens Proteins (Fig. 23.7)

The lens is part of the anterior segment of the eye. Anterior to the lens is the iris, which regulates the amount of light entering into the eye. The lens is suspended in place by the suspensory ligament of the lens, a ring of fibrous tissue that attaches to the lens at its equator and connects it to the ciliary body. Posterior to the lens is the vitreous body, which, along with the aqueous humor on the anterior surface, bathes the lens. The lens has an ellipsoid, biconvex shape. The anterior surface is less curved than the posterior. In the adult, the lens is typically circa 10 mm in diameter and has an axial length of about 4 mm, though it is important to note that the size and shape can change due to accommodation and because the lens continues to grow throughout a person's lifetime.

- **Lens structure and functions:** The lens has three main parts—the lens capsule, the lens epithelium, and the lens fibers. The lens capsule forms the outermost layer of the lens and the lens fibers form the bulk of the interior of the lens. The cells of the lens epithelium, located between the lens capsule and the outermost layer of lens fibers, are found only on the anterior side of the lens.

- **Lens capsule:** The lens capsule is a smooth, transparent basement membrane that completely surrounds the lens. The capsule is elastic and is composed of collagen. It is synthesized by the lens epithelium and its main components are Type-IV collagen and sulfated glycosaminoglycans (GAGs) The capsule is very elastic and so causes the lens to assume a more globular shape when not under the tension of the zonular fibers, which connect the lens capsule to the ciliary body. The capsule varies from 2–28 micrometers in thickness, being thickest near the equator and thinnest near the posterior pole. The lens capsule may be involved with the higher anterior curvature than posterior of the lens.

- **Lens epithelium:** The lens epithelium, located in the anterior portion of the lens between the lens capsule and the lens fibers, is a simple cuboidal epithelium the cells of the lens epithelium regulate most of the homeostatic functions of the lens. As ions, nutrients, and liquid enter the lens from the aqueous humor, Na/K ATPase pumps in the lens epithelial cells pump ions out of the lens to maintain appropriate lens osmolarity and volume, with

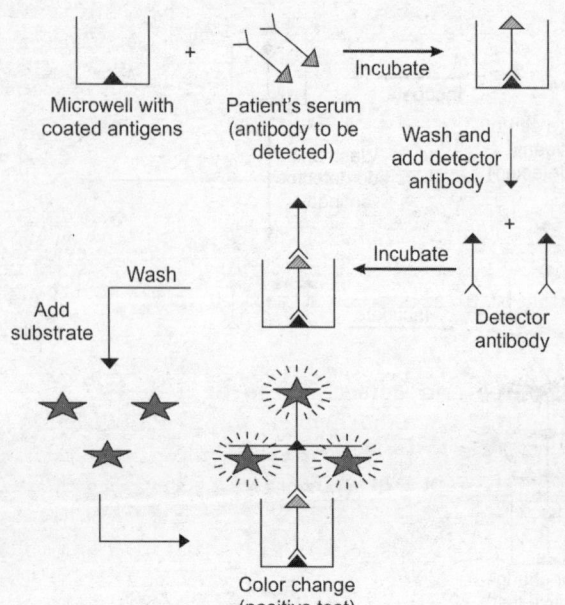

Fig. 23.6: Non-competitive ELISA.

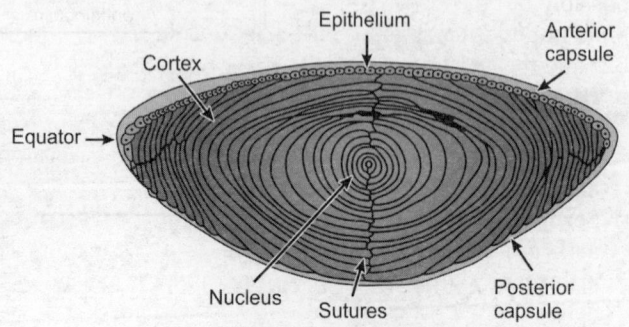

Fig. 23.7: Lens protein.

equatorially positioned lens epithelium cells contributing most to this current. The activity of the Na/K ATPases keeps water and current flowing through the lens from the poles and exiting through the equatorial regions.

The cells of the lens epithelium also serve as the progenitors for new lens fibers. It constantly lays down fibers in the embryo, fetus, infant, and adult, and continues to lay down fibers for lifelong growth

- **Lens fiber:** The lens fibers form the bulk of the lens. They are long, thin, transparent cells, firmly packed, with diameters typically between 4–7 micrometers and lengths of up to 12 mm long. The lens fibers stretch lengthwise from the posterior to the anterior poles and, when cut horizontally, are arranged in concentric layers rather like the layers of an onion. If cut along the equator, it appears as a honeycomb. The middle of each fiber lies on the equator these tightly packed layers of lens fibers are referred to as laminae. The lens fibers are linked together via gap junction and interdigitations of the cells that resemble "ball and socket" forms.

The lens is split into regions depending on the age of the lens fibers of a particular layer. Moving outwards from the central, oldest layer, the lens is split into an embryonic nucleus, the fetal nucleus, the adult nucleus, and the outer cortex. New lens fibers, generated from the lens epithelium, are added to the outer cortex. Mature lens fibers have no organelles or nuclei.

The eyes of older people a diabetics are prone to cataract formation. The normal lens cells possess the usual protein synthesizing machinery. Major lens proteins are alpha, beta and gamma crystallins. The proteins at the center of the lens are as old as the individual. The orderly arrangements of the molecules make the lens protein transparent, when lens proteins change in their three dimensional structure, lens becomes opaque. This leads to increased susceptibility for sulfahydril oxidation and consequent aggregation of proteins resulting in cataract.

HUMAN LEUKOCYTE ANTIGENS (HLA)

These are the main histocompatibility antigens and are responsible for graft rejection. Histocompatibility antigens are now considered important in the regulation of immune response as well as in resistance or susceptibility to a growing list of diseases. The presence of certain HLA antigens is associated with a tendency to develop certain diseases, possibly because the relevant genes occur close together. Most important clinically is the relationship between HLA B27 and rheumatic disease.

- **HLA-B27:** It occurs in 8% of normal Europeans but in 90% of those with ankylosing spondylitis. Its absence makes the diagnosis less likely but not all who have it develop ankylosing spondylitis.
- **Seronegative arthritis:** Ankylosing spondylitis, psoriatic arthropathy, Reiter's syndrome and enteropathic arthropathy come in to this group. The ESR is raised in active disease. The legs, spine and sacroiliac joints are often affected. HLA B27 is present in some patients.

Ankylosing spondylitis is characterized by inflammation at the sites of attachments of ligaments and joint capsules to bone. In cases of doubt the leukocytes should be examined for HLA B27, which is present in 90% of patient. Osteoporosis and periostitis may be seen on X-ray. HLA B27 is positive in two-thirds of patients.

- **Free radicals and antioxidants:** There is a continuous production of H_2O_2 in the living cells which can chemically damage unsaturated lipids, proteins and DNA.

This is however prevented to a large extent through antioxidant reactions involving NADPH. The free radicals are implicated in the development of cancer, heart diseases and also ageing. Vitamin C is a strong biological antioxidant, besides vitamin E and beta-carotene antioxidants prevent the non enzymatic oxidation of various cell components (e.g., unsaturated fatty acids) by molecular oxygen and free radicals such as superoxide (O_2) and hydrogen peroxide (H_2O_2) supplementation of the diet with antioxidants, such as vitamin E, vitamin C and p-carotene has been found to decrease the incidence of chronic diseases, such as cancer and coronary heart diseases. The antioxidants perform a common function to inactivate the toxic free oxygen radicals.

SPECIALIZED PROTEINS

- **Collagen:** Collagen is connective tissue proteins lacking tryptophan. Collagens on boiling with water or dilute acids, yield gelatin which is soluble and digestible.
- **Elastins:** These proteins are found in elastic tissues, such as tendons and arteries.
- **Keratins:** These are present in exoskeletal structures, e.g., hair, nails, horns. Human hair keratin contains as much as 14% cystine.
- **Myosin:** Myosin is a muscle protein. It consists of six polypeptide chains 2 heavy chains and 4 light chains. The two heavy chains are coiled around each other to form double helix; one end of each of these chains is folded in to a globular protein mass called as myosin head. Myosin has a mol. Weight of 4,50,000–5,00,000. Myosin contains ATPase which hydrolyzes ATP to ADP.

CONCLUSION

Immunochemistry is the study of the chemistry of the immune system. This involves the study of the properties, functions, interactions and production of the chemical components (antibodies/immunoglobulins, toxin, epitopes of proteins, such as CD4, antitoxins, cytokines/chemokines, antigens) of the immune system. It also includes immune responses and determination of immune materials/products by immunochemical assays. Immunochemistry is an advanced area of immunology. It deals with the chemical components and chemistry (chemical reactions) of immunological phenomena that is of antibody and antigen. Immunochemical methods are processes utilizing the highly specific affinity of an antibody for its antigen. It detects the distribution of a given protein or antigen in tissues or cells. The methods used for the immunochemical analysis are called

Immunochemical techniques; they are highly important in diagnostic and clinical context, as now even normal cell with many proteins are altered in diseased state (in cancer).

BIBLIOGRAPHY

1. Chandra Sekar. Manipal manual of medical physiology, 1st edition, 2016.
2. Dabbs DJ. Diagnostic immunohistochemistry: theranostic and genomic applications, 4th edition. Philadelphia: Elsevier Saunders; 2014.
3. Kumar V, Abbas AK, Fausto N. Robbins and Cotran pathologic basis of disease, 7th edition. Philadelphia: Elsevier Saunders; 2005.
4. Robinson CH, Marilyn RL, Wanda LC, Anne EG: Normal and Therapeutic Nutrition, 17th edition. Macmillan Publishing Co, New York, USA, 1996.
5. Schacht V, Kern JS. Basics of immunohistochemistry. J Invest Dermatol. 2015;135:e30.
6. Shils MS, Benjamin CA, Catherine R, Robert J. Cousins: Modern Nutrition in Health and Disease, 10th edition. Lippincott, Williams & Wilkins, Baltimore, USA, 2005.
7. Yaziji H, Barry T. Diagnostic Immunohistochemistry: What can go wrong? Adv Anat Pathol. 2006;13:238-46.

REVIEW QUESTIONS

Long Essays

1. Define immunity, explain innate immunity in detail.
2. Define antigen, explain the factors which determine antigenicity.
3. Discuss in detail about human immunoglobulin classes.

Short Essays

1. IgG.
2. Mechanisms of acquired immunity.
3. Theories of antibody formation.
4. Macrophages.
5. Structure and functions of immune system.
6. Major histocompatibility (MCH).
7. Human leukocyte antigens (HLA).
8. Lens proteins.
9. Enzyme-linked immunosorbant assay (ELISA).
10. Importance of immunoglobulins.

Short Answers

1. Humoral immunity.
2. Cellular immunity.
3. Phagocytosis.
4. $CD4^+$ T cells.
5. Cells of immune system.
6. Natural acquired immunity.
7. Lens capsule.
8. Autoimmunity.
9. Allergy response.
10. Immunodeficiency.
11. Innate immunity.
12. Electrophoresis.
13. Antibody detection assays.
14. Hormonal immunity.
15. Cell-mediated immunity.
16. Antibodies.
17. Antigens.

Biochemistry Glossary

A

Absolute configuration: The configuration of four different substituent groups around an asymmetric carbon atom, in relation to D- and L-glyceraldehyde. absolute configuration The configuration of four different substituent groups around an asymmetric carbon atom, in relation to D- and L-glyceraldehyde.

Absolute configuration: The configuration of four different substituent groups around an asymmetric carbon atom, in relation to D- and L-glyceraldehyde.

Absorption: Transport of the products of digestion from the intestinal tract into the blood.

Acceptor control: The regulation of the rate of respiration by the availability of ADP as phosphate group acceptor.

Accessory pigments: Visible light-absorbing pigments (carotenoids, xanthophyll, and phycobilins) in plants and photosynthetic bacteria that complement chlorophylls in trapping energy from sunlight.

Acidosis: A metabolic condition in which the capacity of the body to buffer H^+ is diminished; usually accompanied by decreased blood pH.

Actin: A protein making up the thin filaments of muscle.

Activation energy ($\Delta G^{o\prime}$): The amount of energy (in joules) required to convert all the molecules in 1 mole of a reacting substance from the ground state to the transition state.

Activator: (1) A DNA-binding protein that positively regulates the expression of one or more genes; i.e., transcription rates increase when an activator is bound to the DNA. (2) A positive modulator of an allosteric enzyme.

Active site: The region of an enzyme surface that binds the substrate molecule and catalytically transforms it; also known as the catalytic site.

Active transport: Energy-requiring transport of a solute across a membrane in the direction of increasing concentration.

Activity: The true thermodynamic activity or potential of a substance, as distinct from its molar concentration.

Activity coefficient: The factor by which the numerical value of the concentration of a solute must be multiplied to give its true thermodynamic activity.

Adipocyte: An animal cell specialized for the storage of fats (triacylglycerols).

Adipose tissue: Connective tissue specialized for the storage of large amounts of triacylglycerols.

ADP (adenosine diphosphate): A ribonucleoside 5′-diphosphate serving as phosphate group acceptor in the cell energy cycle.

Aerobe: An organism that lives in air and uses oxygen as the terminal electron acceptor in respiration.

Aerobic: Requiring or occurring in the presence of oxygen.

Alcohol fermentation: The anaerobic conversion of glucose to ethanol via glycolysis. *See* also fermentation.

Aldose: A simple sugar in which the carbonyl carbon atom is an aldehyde; that is, the carbonyl carbon is at one end of the carbon chain.

Alkaloids: Nitrogen-containing organic compounds of plant origin; often basic, and having intense biological activity.

Alkalosis: A metabolic condition in which the capacity of the body to buffer OH^- is diminished; usually accompanied by an increase in blood pH.

Allosteric enzyme: A regulatory enzyme, with catalytic activity modulated by the noncovalent binding of a specific metabolite at a site other than the active site.

Allosteric site: The specific site on the surface of an allosteric enzyme molecule to which the modulator or effector molecule is bound.

α helix: A helical conformation of a polypeptide chain, usually right-handed, with maximal intrachain hydrogen bonding; one of the most common secondary structures in proteins.

Ames test: A simple bacterial test for carcinogens, based on the assumption that carcinogens are mutagens.

Amino acid activation: ATP-dependent enzymatic esterification of the carboxyl group of an amino acid to the 3′-hydroxyl group of its corresponding tRNA.

Amino acids: α-Amino-substituted carboxylic acids, the building blocks of proteins.

Amino-terminal residue: The only amino acid residue in a polypeptide chain with a free a-amino group; defines the amino terminus of the polypeptide.

Aminoacyl-tRNA: An aminoacyl ester of a tRNA.

Aminoacyl-tRNA synthetases: Enzymes that catalyze synthesis of an aminoacylt RNA at the expense of ATP energy.

Aminotransferases: Enzymes that catalyze the transfer of amino groups from α-amino to α-keto acids; also called transaminases.

Ammonotelic: Excreting excess nitrogen in the form of ammonia.

Amphibolic pathway: A metabolic pathway used in both catabolism and anabolism.

Amphipathic: Containing both polar and nonpolar domains.

Amphoteric: Capable of donating and accepting protons, thus able to serve as an acid or a base.

Anabolism: The phase of intermediary metabolism concerned with the energy-requiring biosynthesis of cell components from smaller precursors.

Anaerobe: An organism that lives without oxygen. Obligate anaerobes die when exposed to oxygen.

Anaerobic: Occurring in the absence of air or oxygen.

Anaplerotic reaction: An enzyme-catalyzed reaction that can replenish the supply of intermediates in the citric acid cycle.

Angstrom (Å): A unit of length (10^{-8} cm) used to indicate molecular dimensions.

Anhydride: The product of the condensation of two carboxyl or phosphate groups in which the elements of water are eliminated to form a compound with the general structure R—X(=O)—O—X(=O)—R, where X is either carbon or phosphorus.

Anion-exchange resin: A polymeric resin with fixed cationic groups; used in the chromatographic separation of anions.

Anomers: Two stereoisomers of a given sugar that differ only in the configuration about the carbonyl (anomeric) carbon atom.

Antibiotic: One of many different organic compounds that are formed and secreted by various species of microorganisms and plants, are toxic to other species, and presumably have a defensive function.

Antibody: A defense protein synthesized by the immune system of vertebrates. *See* also immunoglobulin.

Anticodon: A specific sequence of three nucleotides in a tRNA, complementary to a codon for an amino acid in an mRNA.

Antigen: A molecule capable of eliciting the synthesis of a specific antibody in vertebrates.

Antiparallel: Describing two linear polymers that are opposite in polarity or orientation.

Antiport: Cotransport of two solutes across a membrane in opposite directions.

Apoenzyme: The protein portion of an enzyme, exclusive of any organic or inorganic cofactors or prosthetic groups that might be required for catalytic activity.

Apolipoprotein: The protein component of a lipoprotein.

Asymmetric carbon atom: A carbon atom that is covalently bonded to four different groups and thus may exist in two different tetrahedral configurations.

ATP (adenosine triphosphate): A ribonucleoside 5′-triphosphate functioning as a phosphate group donor in the cell energy cycle; carries chemical energy between metabolic pathways by serving as a shared intermediate coupling endergonic and exergonic reactions.

ATP synthase: An enzyme complex that forms ATP from ADP and phosphate during oxidative phosphorylation in the inner mitochondrial membrane or the bacterial plasma membrane, and during photophosphorylation in chloroplasts.

ATPase: An enzyme that hydrolyzes ATP to yield ADP and phosphate; usually coupled to some process requiring energy.

Attenuator: An RNA sequence involved in regulating the expression of certain genes; functions as a transcription terminator.

Autotroph: An organism that can synthesize its own complex molecules from very simple carbon and nitrogen sources, such as carbon dioxide and ammonia.

Auxin: A plant growth hormone.

Auxotrophic mutant (auxotroph): A mutant organism defective in the synthesis of a given biomolecule, which must therefore be supplied for the organism's growth.

Avogadro's number (N): The number of molecules in a gram molecular weight (a mole) of any compound (6.02×10^{23}).

B

Back-mutation: A mutation that causes a mutant gene to regain its wild-type base sequence.

Bacteriophage (phage): A virus capable of replicating in a bacterial cell.

Basal metabolic rate: The rate of oxygen consumption by an animal's body at complete rest, long after a meal.

Base pair: Two nucleotides in nucleic acid chains that are paired by hydrogen bond. ing of their bases; for example, A with T or U, and G with C.

β conformation: An extended, zigzag arrangement of a polypeptide chain; a common secondary structure in proteins.

β oxidation: Oxidative degradation of fatty acids into acetyl-CoA by successive oxidations at the β-carbon atom.

Bilayer: A double layer of oriented amphipathic lipid molecules, forming the basic structure of biological membranes. The hydrocarbon tails face inward to form a continuous nonpolar phase.

Bile salts: Amphipathic steroid derivatives with detergent properties, participating in digestion and absorption of lipids.

Binding energy: The energy derived from noncovalent interactions between enzyme and substrate or receptor and ligand.

Biocytin: The conjugate amino acid residue arising from covalent attachment of biotin, through an amide linkage, to a Lys residue.

Biomolecule: An organic compound normally present as an essential component of living organisms.

Biopterin: An enzymatic cofactor derived from pterin and involved in certain oxidation-reduction reactions.

Biosphere: All the living matter on or in the earth, the seas, and the atmosphere.

Biotin: A vitamin; an enzymatic cofactor involved in carboxylation reactions.

Bond energy: The energy required to break a bond.

Branch migration: Movement of the branch point in branched DNA formed from two DNA molecules with identical sequences. *See also* Holliday intermediate.

Buffer: A system capable of resisting changes in pH, consisting of a conjugate acid-base pair in which the ratio of proton acceptor to proton donor is near unity.

C

Calorie: The amount of heat required to raise the temperature of 1.0 g of water from 14.5 to 15.5°. One calorie (cal) equals 4.18 joules (J).

Calvin cycle: The cyclic pathway used by plants to fix carbon dioxide and produce triose phosphates.

cAMP: *See* cyclic AMP.

CAP: *See* catabolite gene activator protein.

Capsid: The protein coat of a virion or virus particle.

Carbanion: A negatively charged carbon atom.

Carbocation: A positively charged carbon atom; also called a carbonium ion.

Carbon fixation reactions: In photosynthetic cells, the light-independent enzymatic reactions involved in the synthesis of glucose from CO_2, ATP, and NADPH; also known as the dark reactions.

Carboxyl-terminal residue: The only amino acid residue in a polypeptide chain with a free α-carboxyl group; defines the carboxyl terminus of the polypeptide.

Carotenoids: Lipid-soluble photosynthetic pigments made up of isoprene units.

Catabolism: The phase of intermediary metabolism concerned with the energy-yielding degradation of nutrient molecules.

Catabolite gene activator protein (CAP): A specific regulatory protein that controls initiation of transcription of the genes producing the enzymes required for a bacterial cell to use some other nutrient when glucose is lacking.

Catalytic site: *See* active site.

Catecholamines: Hormones, such as epinephrine, that are amino derivatives of catechol.

Cation-exchange resin: An insoluble polymer with fixed negative charges; used in the chromatographic separation of cationic substances.

cDNA: *See* complementary DNA.

Central dogma: The organizing principle of molecular biology: genetic information flows from DNA to RNA to protein.

Centromere: A specialized site within a chromosome, serving as the attachment point for the mitotic or meiotic spindle.

Cerebroside: Sphingolipid containing one sugar residue as a head group.

Channeling: The direct transfer of a reaction product (common intermediate) from the active site of one enzyme to the active site of a different enzyme catalyzing the next step in a sequential pathway.

Chemiosmotic coupling: Coupling of ATP synthesis to electron transfer via an electrochemical H^+ gradient across a membrane.

Chemotaxis: A cell's sensing of and movement toward, or away from, a specific chemical agent.

Chemotroph: An organism that obtains energy by metabolizing organic compounds derived from other organisms.

Chiral compound: A compound that contains an asymmetric center (chiral atom or chiral center) and thus can occur in two nonsuperimposable mirror-image forms (enantiomers).

Chlorophylls: A family of green pigments functioning as receptors of light energy in photosynthesis; magnesium-porphyrin complexes.

Chloroplasts: Chlorophyll-containing photosynthetic organelles in some eukaryotic cells.

Chromatin: A filamentous complex of DNA, histones, and other proteins, constituting the eukaryotic chromosome.

Chromatography: A process in which complex mixtures of molecules are separated by many repeated partitionings between a flowing (mobile) phase and a stationary phase.

Chromosome: A single large DNA molecule and its associated proteins, containing many genes; stores and transmits genetic information.

Chylomicron: A plasma lipoprotein consisting of a large droplet of triacylglycerols stabilized by a coat of protein and phospholipid; carries lipids from the intestine to the tissues.

Cis and trans isomers: *See* geometric isomers.

Cistron: A unit of DNA or RNA corresponding to one gene.

Citric acid cycle: A cyclic system of enzymatic reactions for the oxidation of acetyl residues to carbon dioxide, in which formation of citrate is the first step; also known as the Krebs cycle or tricarboxylic acid cycle.

Clones: The descendants of a single cell.

Cloning: The production of large numbers of identical DNA molecules or cells from a single ancestral DNA molecule or cell.

Closed system: A system that exchanges neither matter nor energy with the surroundings. *See also* system.

Cobalamin: *See* coenzyme B_{12}.

Codon: A sequence of three adjacent nucleotides in a nucleic acid that codes for a specific amino acid.

Coenzyme: An organic cofactor required for the action of certain enzymes; often contains a vitamin as a component.

Coenzyme A: A pantothenic acid-containing coenzyme serving as an acyl group carrier in certain enzymatic reactions.

Coenzyme B_{12}: An enzymatic cofactor derived from the vitamin cobalamin, involved in certain types of carbon skeletal rearrangements.

Cofactor: An inorganic ion or a coenzyme required for enzyme activity.

Cognate: Describing two biomolecules that normally interact; for example, an enzyme and its normal substrate, or a receptor and its normal ligand.

Cohesive ends: *See* sticky ends.

Cointegrate: An intermediate in the migration of certain DNA transposons in which the donor DNA and target DNA are covalently attached.

Colligative properties: Properties of solutions that depend on the number of solute particles per unit volume; for example, freezing-point depression.

Common intermediate: A chemical compound common to two chemical reactions, as a product of one and a reactant in the other.

Competitive inhibition: A type of enzyme inhibition reversed by increasing the substrate concentration; a competitive inhibitor generally competes with the normal substrate or ligand for a protein's binding site.

Complementary: Having a molecular surface with chemical groups arranged to interact specifically with chemical groups on another molecule.

Complementary DNA (cDNA): A DNA used in DNA cloning, usually made by reverse transcriptase; complementary to a given mRNA.

Configuration: The spatial arrangement of an organic molecule that is conferred by the presence of either (1) double bonds, about which there is no freedom of rotation, or (2) chiral centers, around which substituent groups are arranged in a specific sequence. Configurational isomers cannot be interconverted without breaking one or more covalent bonds.

Conformation: The spatial arrangement of substituent groups that are free to assume different positions in space, without breaking any bonds, because of the freedom of bond rotation.

Conformation, β: *See* β conformation.

Conjugate acid-base pair: A proton donor and its corresponding deprotonated species; for example, acetic acid (donor) and acetate (acceptor).

Conjugate redox pair: An electron donor and its corresponding electron acceptor form; for example, Cu^+ (donor) and Cu^{2+} (acceptor), or NADH (donor) and NAD^+ (acceptor).

Conjugated protein: A protein containing one or more prosthetic groups.

Consensus sequence: A DNA or amino acid sequence consisting of the residues that occur most commonly at each position within a set of similar sequences.

Conservative substitution: Replacement of an amino acid residue in a polypeptide by another residue with similar properties; for example, substitution of Glu by Asp.

Constitutive enzymes: Enzymes required at all times by a cell and present at some constant level; for example, many enzymes of the central metabolic pathways. Sometimes called "housekeeping enzymes."

Corticosteroids: Steroid hormones formed by the adrenal cortex.

Cosmid: A cloning vector, used for cloning large DNA fragments; generally contains segments derived from bacteriophages and various plasmids.

e-Transport: The simultaneous transport, by a single transporter, of two solutes across a membrane. *See* antiport, symport.

Coupled reactions: Two chemical reactions that have a common intermediate and thus a means of energy transfer from one to the other.

Covalent bond: A chemical bond that involves sharing of electron pairs.

Cristae: Infoldings of the inner mitochondrial membrane.

Cyclic AMP icAMP): A second messenger within cells; its formation by adenylate cyclase is stimulated by certain hormones or other molecular signals.

Cyclic electron flow: In chloroplasts, the light-induced flow of electrons originating from and returning to photosystem I.

Cyclic photophosphorylation: ATP synthesis driven by cyclic electron flow through photosystem I.

Cytochromes: Heme proteins serving as electron carriers in respiration, photosynthesis, and other oxidation-reduction reactions.

Cytokinesis: The final separation of daughter cells following mitosis.

Cytoplasm: The portion of a cell's contents outside the nucleus but within the plasma membrane; includes organelles such as mitochondria.

Cytoskeleton: The filamentous network providing structure and organization to the cytoplasm; includes actin filaments, microtubules, and intermediate filaments.

Cytosol: The continuous aqueous phase of the cytoplasm, with its dissolved solutes; excludes the organelles such as mitochondria.

D

Dalton: The weight of a single hydrogen atom (1.66×10^{-24} g).

Dark reactions: *See* carbon fixation reactions.

De novo pathway: Pathway for synthesis of a biomolecule, such as a nucleotide, from simple precursors; as distinct from a salvage pathway.

Deamination: The enzymatic removal of amino groups from biomolecules, such as amino acids or nucleotides.

Degenerate code: A code in which a single element in one language is specified by more than one element in a second language.

Dehydrogenases: Enzymes catalyzing the removal of pairs of hydrogen atoms from their substrates.

Deletion mutation: A mutation resulting from the deletion of one or more nucleotides from a gene or chromosome.

Denaturation: Partial or complete unfolding of the specific native conformation of a polypeptide chain, protein, or nucleic acid.

Denatured protein: A protein that has lost its native conformation by exposure to a destabilizing agent such as heat or detergent.

Deoxyribonucleic acid: *See* DNA.

Deoxyribonucleotides: Nucleotides containing 2-deoxy-n-ribose as the pentose component.

Desaturases: Enzymes that catalyze the introduction of double bonds into the hydrocarbon portion of fatty acids.

Desolvation: In aqueous solution, the release of bound water surrounding a solute.

Dextrorotatory isomer: A stereoisomer that rotates the plane of plane-polarized light clockwise.

Diabetes mellitus: A metabolic disease resulting from insulin deficiency; characterized by a failure in glucose transport from the blood into cells at normal glucose concentrations.

Dialysis: Removal of small molecules from a solution of a macromolecule, by allowing them to diffuse through a semipermeable membrane into water.

Differential centrifugation: Separation of cell organelles or other particles of different size by their different rates of sedimentation in a centrifugal field.

Differentiation: Specialization of cell structure and function during embryonic growth and development.

Diffusion: The net movement of molecules in the direction of lower concentration.

Digestion: Enzymatic hydrolysis of major nutrients in the gastrointestinal system to yield their simpler components.

Diploid: Having two sets of genetic information; describing a cell with two chromosomes of each type.

Dipole: A molecule having both positive and negative charges.

Diprotic acid: An acid having two dissociable protons.

Disaccharide: A carbohydrate consisting of two covalently joined monosaccharide units.

Dissociation constant: (1) An equilibrium constant (K_d) for the dissociation of a complex of two or more biomolecules into its components; for example, dissociation of a substrate from an enzyme. (2) The dissociation constant (K_a) of an acid, describing its dissociation into its conjugate base and a proton.

Disulfide bridge: A covalent cross link between two polypeptide chains formed by a cystine residue (two Cys residues).

DNA (deoxyribonucleic acid): A polynucleotide having a specific sequence of deoxyribonucleotide units covalently joined through 3', 5'-phosphodiester bonds; serves as the carrier of genetic information.

DNA chimera: A DNA containing genetic information derived from two different species.

DNA cloning: *See* cloning.

DNA library: A random collection of cloned DNA fragments that includes all or most of the genome of a given organism; also called a genomic library.

DNA ligase: An enzyme that creates a phosphodiester bond between the 3' end of one DNA segment and the 5' end of another.

DNA looping: The interaction of proteins bound at distant sites on a DNA molecule so that the intervening DNA forms a loop.

DNA polymerase: An enzyme that catalyzes template-dependent synthesis of DNA from its deoxyribonucleoside 5'-triphosphate precursors.

DNA replicase system: The entire complex of enzymes and specialized proteins required in biological DNA replication. DNA supercoiling: The coiling of DNA upon itself, generally as a result of bending, underwinding, or overwinding of the DNA helix.

Domain: A distinct structural unit of a polypeptide; domains may have separate functions and may fold as independent, compact units.

Double helix: The natural coiled conformation of two complementary, antiparallel DNA chains.

Double-reciprocal plot: A plot of $1/V_0$ versus $1/[S]$, which allows a more accurate determination of V_{max} and K_m, than a plot of Vo versus [S]; also called the Lineweaver-Burk plot.

E

E_0': *See* standard reduction potential.

E. coli (Escherichia coli): A common bacterium found in the small intestine of vertebrates; the most well-studied organism.

Electrochemical gradient: The sum of the gradients of concentration and of electric charge of an ion across a membrane; the driving force for oxidative phosphorylation and photophosphorylation.

Electrochemical potential: The energy required to maintain a separation of charge and of concentration across a membrane.

Electrogenic: Contributing to an electrical potential across a membrane.

Electron acceptor: A substance that receives electrons in an oxidation-reduction reaction.

Electron carrier: A protein, such as a flavoprotein or a cytochrome, that can reversibly gain and lose electrons; functions in the transfer of electrons from organic nutrients to oxygen or some other terminal acceptor.

Electron donor: A substance that donates electrons in an oxidation-reduction reaction.

Electron transfer: Movement of electrons from substrates to oxygen via the carriers of the respiratory (electron transfer) chain.

Electrophile: An electron-deficient group with a strong tendency to accept electrons from an electron-rich group (nucleophile).

Electrophoresis: Movement of charged solutes in response to an electrical field; often used to separate mixtures of ions, proteins, or nucleic acids.

Elongation factors: Specific proteins required in the elongation of polypeptide chains by ribosomes.

Eluate: The effluent from a chromatographic column.

Enantiomers: Stereoisomers that are nonsuperimposable mirror images of each other.

End-product inhibition: *See* feedback inhibition.

Endergonic reaction: A chemical reaction that consumes energy (that is, for which, ΔG is positive).

Endocrine glands: Groups of cells specialized to synthesize hormones and secrete them into the blood to regulate other types of cells.

Endocytosis: The uptake of extracellular material by its inclusion within a vesicle (endosome) formed by an invagination of the plasma membrane.

Endonuclease: An enzyme that hydrolyzes the interior phosphodiester bonds of a nucleic acid; that is, it acts at points other than the terminal bonds.

Endoplasmic reticulum: An extensive system of double membranes in the cytoplasm of eukaryotic cells; it encloses secretory channels and is often studded with ribosomes (rough endoplasmic reticulum).

Endothermic reaction: A chemical reaction that takes up heat (that is, for which ΔH is positive).

Energy coupling: The transfer of energy from one process to another.

Enhancers: DNA sequences that facilitate the expression of a given gene; may be located a few hundred, or even thousand, base pairs away from the gene.

Enthalpy (H): The heat content of a system.

Enthalpy change (ΔH): For a reaction, is approximately equal to the difference between the energy used to break bonds and the energy gained by the formation of new ones.

Entropy (S): The extent of randomness or disorder in a system.

Enzyme: A biomolecule, either protein or RNA, that catalyzes a specific chemical reaction. It does not affect the equilibrium of the catalyzed reaction; it enhances the rate of a reaction by providing a reaction path with a lower activation energy.

Epimerases: Enzymes that catalyze the reversible interconversion of two epimers.

Epimers: Two stereoisomers differing in configuration at one asymmetric center, in a compound having two or more asymmetric centers.

Epithelial cell: Any cell that forms part of the outer covering of an organism or organ.

Epitope: An antigenic determinant; the particular chemical group or groups within a macromolecule (antigen) to which a given antibody binds.

Equilibrium: The state of a system in which no further net change is occurring; the free energy is at a minimum.

Equilibrium constant (K_{eq}): A constant, characteristic for each chemical reaction; relates the specific concentrations of all reactants and products at equilibrium at a given temperature and pressure.

Erythrocyte: A cell containing large amounts of hemoglobin and specialized for oxygen transport; a red blood cell.

Escherichia coli: *See E. coli.*

Essential amino acids: Amino acids that cannot be synthesized by humans (and other vertebrates) and must be obtained from the diet.

Essential fatty acids: The group of polyunsaturated fatty acids produced by plants, but not by humans; required in the human diet.

Ethanol fermentation: *See* alcohol fermentation.

Eukaryote: A unicellular or multicellular organism with cells having a membranebounded nucleus, multiple chromosomes, and internal organelles.

Excited state: An energy-rich state of an atom or molecule; produced by the absorption of light energy.

Exergonic reaction: A chemical reaction that proceeds with the release of free energy (that is, for which ΔG is negative).

Exocytosis: The fusion of an intracellular vesicle with the plasma membrane, releasing the vesicle contents to the extracellular space.

Exon: The segment of a eukaryotic gene that encodes a portion of the final product of the gene; a portion that remains after post-transcriptional processing and is transcribed into a protein or incorporated into the structure of an RNA. *See* intron.

Exonuclease: An enzyme that hydrolyzes only those phosphodiester bonds that are in the terminal positions of a nucleic acid.

Exothermic reaction: A chemical reaction that releases heat (that is, for which ΔH is negative).

Expression vector: *See* vector.

F

Facilitated diffusion: Diffusion of a polar substance across a biological membrane through a protein transporter; also called passive diffusion or passive transport.

Facultative cells: Cells that can live in the presence or absence of oxygen.

FAD (flavin adenine dinucleotide): The coenzyme of some oxidation-reduction enzymes; it contains riboflavin.

Fatty acid: A long-chain aliphatic carboxylic acid found in natural fats and oils; also a component of membrane phospholipids and glycolipids.

Feedback inhibition: Inhibition of an allosteric enzyme at the beginning of a metabolic sequence by the end product of the sequence; also known as end-product inhibition.

Fermentation: Energy-yielding anaerobic breakdown of a nutrient molecule, such as glucose, without net oxidation; yields lactate, ethanol, or some other simple product.

Fibroblast: A cell of the connective tissue that secretes connective tissue proteins, such as collagen.

Fibrous proteins: Insoluble proteins that serve in a protective or structural role; contain polypeptide chains that generally share a common secondary structure.

Fingerprinting: *See* peptide mapping.

First law of thermodynamics: The law stating that in all processes, the total energy of the universe remains constant.

Fischer projection formulas: *See* projection formulas.

5'-end: The end of a nucleic acid that lacks a nucleotide bound at the 5'-position of the terminal residue.

Flagellum: A cell appendage used in propulsion. Bacterial flagella have a much simpler structure than eukaryotic flagella, which are similar to cilia.

Flavin-linked dehydrogenases: Dehydrogenases requiring one of the riboflavin coenzymes, FMN or FAD.

Flavin nucleotides: Nucleotide coenzymes (FMN and FAD) containing riboflavin.

Flavoprotein: An enzyme containing a flavin nucleotide as a tightly bound prosthetic group.

Fluid mosaic model: A model describing biological membranes as a fluid lipid bilayer with embedded proteins; the bilayer exhibits both structural and functional asymmetry.

Fluorescence: Emission of light by excited molecules as they revert to the ground state.

FMN (flavin mononucleotide): Riboflavin phosphate, a coenzyme of certain oxidation-reduction enzymes.

Footprinting: A technique for identifying the nucleic acid sequence bound by a DNA- or RNA-binding protein.

Frame shift: A mutation caused by insertion or deletion of one or more paired nucleotides, changing the reading frame of codons during protein synthesis; the polypeptide product has a garbled amino acid sequence beginning at the mutated codon.

Free-energy (G): The component of the total energy of a system that can do work at constant temperature and pressure.

Free energy of activation ($\Delta G^{\#}$) *See* activation energy.

Free-energy change (ΔG): The amount of free energy released (negative ΔG) or absorbed (positive ΔG) in a reaction at constant temperature and pressure.

Functional group: The specific atom or group of atoms that confers a particular chemical property on a biomolecule.

Furanose: A simple sugar containing the five-membered furan ring.

Fusion protein: (1) A family of proteins that facilitate membrane fusion. (2) The protein product of a gene created by the fusion of two distinct genes.

Futile cycle: A set of enzyme-catalyzed cyclic reactions that results in release of thermal energy by the hydrolysis of ATP.

$\Delta G°'$: *See* standard free-energy change.

G

Gametes: Reproductive cells with a haploid gene content; sperm or egg cells.

Gangliosides: Sphingolipids, containing complex oligosaccharides as head groups; especially common in nervous tissue.

Gel filtration: A chromatographic procedure for the separation of a mixture of molecules on the basis of size; based on the capacity of porous polymers to exclude solutes above a certain size.

Gene: A chromosomal segment that codes for a single functional polypeptide chain or RNA molecule.

Gene expression: l'inscription and, in the case of proteins, translation to yield the product of a gene; a gene is expressed when its biological product is present and active.

Gene splicing: The enzymatic attachment of one gene, or part of a gene, to another.

General acid-base catalysis: Catalysis involving proton transfer(s) to or from a molecule other than water.

Genetic code: The set of triplet code words in DNA (or mRNA) coding for the amino acids of proteins.

Genetic information: The hereditary information contained in a sequence of nucleotide bases in chromosomal DNA or RNA.

Genetic map: A diagram showing the relative sequence and position of specific genes along a chromosome.

Genome: All the genetic information encoded in a cell or virus.

Genotype: The genetic constitution of an organism, as distinct from its physical characteristics, or phenotype.

Geometric isomers: Isomers related by rotation about a double bond; also called cis and trans isomers.

Germ-line cell: A type of animal cell that is formed early in embryogenesis and may multiply by mitosis or may produce, by meiosis, cells that develop into gametes (egg or sperm cells).

Globular proteins: Soluble proteins with a globular (somewhat rounded) shape.

Glucogenic amino acids: Amino acids with carbon chains that can be metabolically converted into glucose or glycogen via gluconeogenesis.

Gluconeogenesis: The biosynthesis of a carbohydrate from simpler, noncarbohydrate precursors, such as oxaloacetate or pyruvate.

Glycan: Another term for polysaccharide; a polymer of monosaccharide units joined by glycosidic bonds.

Glycerophospholipid: An amphipathic lipid with a glycerol backbone; fatty acids are ester-linked to Gl and C-2 of glycerol, and a polar alcohol is attached through a phosphodiester linkage to C-3.

Glycolipid: A lipid containing a carbohydrate group.

Glycolysis: The catabolic pathway by which a molecule of glucose is broken down into two molecules of pyruvate.

Glycoprotein: A protein containing a carbohydrate group.

Glycosaminoglycan: A heteropolysaccharide of two alternating units: one is either N-acetylglucosamine or N-acetylgalactosamine; the other is a uronic acid (usually glucuronic acid). Formerly called mucopolysaccharide.

Glycosidic bonds: Bonds between a sugar and another molecule (typically an alcohol, purine, pyrimidine, or sugar) through an intervening oxygen or nitrogen atom; the bonds are classified as O-glycosidic or N-glycosidic, respectively.

Glyoxysome: A specialized peroxisome containing the enzymes of the glyoxylate cycle; found in cells of germinating seeds.

Golgi complex: A complex membranous organelle of eukaryotic cells; functions in the post-translational modification of proteins and their secretion from the cell or incorporation into the plasma membrane or organellar membranes.

Gram molecular weight: The weight in grams of a compound that is numerically equal to its molecular weight; the weight of 1 mole.

Grana: Stacks of thylakoids, flattened membranous sacs or discs, in chloroplasts.

Ground state: The normal, stable form of an atom or molecule; as distinct from the excited state.

Group transfer potential: A measure of the ability of a compound to donate an activated group (such as a phosphate or acyl group); generally expressed as the standard free energy of hydrolysis.

H

Half-life: The time required for the disappearance or decay of one-half of a given component in a system.

Haploid: Having a single set of genetic information; describing a cell with one chromosome of each type.

Haworth perspective formulas: A method for representing cyclic chemical structures so as to define the configuration of each substituent group; the method commonly used for representing sugars.

Helicase: An enzyme that catalyzes the separation of strands in a DNA molecule before replication.

Helix, α: See α helix.

Heme: The iron-porphyrin prosthetic group of heme proteins.

Heme protein: A protein containing a heme as a prosthetic group.

Hemoglobin: A heme protein in erythrocytes; functions in oxygen transport.

Henderson-Hasselbalch equation: An equation relating the pH, the pK_a, and the ratio of the concentrations of the protonacceptor (A⁻) and proton-donor (HA) species in a solution.

Hepatocyte: The major cell type of liver tissue.

Heteroduplex DNA: Duplex DNA containing complementary strands derived

Similar sequences, often as a product of genetic recombination. heteropolysaccharide: A polysaccharide containing more than one type of sugar.

Heterotroph: An organism that requires complex nutrient molecules, such as glucose, as a source of energy and carbon.

Heterotropic enzyme: An allosteric enzyme requiring a modulator other than its substrate.

Hexose: A simple sugar with a backbone containing six carbon atoms. high-energy compound: A compound that on hydrolysis undergoes a large decrease in free energy under standard conditions.

High-performance liquid chromatography (HPLC): Chromatographic procedures, often conducted at relatively high pressures, using automated equipment that permits refined and highly reproducible profiles.

Hill reaction: The evolution of oxygen and the photoreduction of an artificial electron acceptor by a chloroplast preparation in the absence of carbon dioxide.

Histones: The family of five basic proteins that associate tightly with DNA in the chromosomes of all eukaryotic cells.

Holliday intermediate: An intermediate in genetic recombination in which two double-stranded DNA molecules are joined by virtue of a reciprocal crossover involving one strand of each molecule.

Holoenzyme: A catalytically active enzyme including all necessary subunits, prosthetic groups, and cofactors.

Homeobox: A conserved DNA sequence of 180 base pairs encoding a protein domain found in many proteins that play a regulatory role in development.

Homeodomain: The protein domain encoded by the homeobox.

Homeostasis: The maintenance of a dynamic steady state by regulatory mechanisms that compensate for changes in external circumstances.

Homeotic genes: Genes that regulate the development of the pattern of segments in the *Drosophila* body plan; similar genes are found in most vertebrates.

Homologous genetic recombination: Recombination between two DNA molecules of similar sequence, occurring in all cells; occurs during meiosis and mitosis in eukaryotes.

Homologous proteins: Proteins having sequences and functions similar in different species; for example, the hemoglobins. made up ride unit.

Homotropic enzyme: An allosteric enzyme that uses its substrate as a modulator.

Hormone: A chemical substance synthesized in small amounts by an endocrine tissue and carried in the blood to another tissue, where it acts as a messenger to regulate the function of the target tissue or organ.

Hormone receptor: A protein in, or on the surface of, target cells that binds a specific hormone and initiates the cellular response.

Hydrogen bond: A weak electrostatic attraction between one electronegative atom (such as oxygen or nitrogen) and a hydrogen atom covalently linked to a second electronegative atom.

Hydrolases: Enzymes (proteases, lipases, phosphatases, nucleases, for example) that catalyze hydrolysis reactions.

Hydrolysis: Cleavage of a bond, such as an anhydride or peptide bond, by the addition of the elements of water, yielding two or more products.

Hydronium ion: The hydrated hydrogen ion (H_2O^+).

Hydropathy index: A scale that expresses the relative hydrophobic and hydrophilic tendencies of a chemical group.

Hydrophilic: Polar or charged; describing molecules or groups that associate with (dissolve easily in) water.

Hydrophobic: Nonpolar; describing molecules or groups that are insoluble in water.

Hydrophobic interactions: The association of nonpolar groups, or compounds, with each other in aqueous systems, driven by the tendency of the surrounding water molecules to seek their most stable (disordered) state.

Hyperchromic effect: The large increase in light absorption at 260 nm occurring as a double-helical DNA is melted (unwound).

I

Immune response: The capacity of a vertebrate to generate antibodies to an antigen, a macromolecule foreign to the organism.

Immunoglobulin: An antibody protein generated against, and capable of binding specifically to, an antigen.

In vitro: "In glass"; that is, in the test tube.

In vivo: "In life"; that is, in the living cell or organism.

Induced fit: A change in the conformation of an enzyme in response to substrate binding that renders the enzyme catalytically active; also used to denote changes in the conformation of any macromolecule in response to ligand binding such that the binding site of the macromolecule better conforms to the shape of the ligand.

Inducer: A signal molecule that, when bound to a regulatory protein, produces an increase in the expression of a given gene.

Induction: An increase in the expression of a gene in response to a change in the activity of a regulatory protein.

Informational macromolecules: Biomolecules containing information in the form of specific sequences of different monomers; for example, many proteins, lipids, polysaccharides, and nucleic acids.

Initiation codon: AUG (sometimes GUG in prokaryotes); codes for the first amino acid in a polypeptide sequence: N-formylmethionine in prokaryotes, and methionine in eukaryotes.

Initiation complex: A complex of a ribosome with an mRNA and the initiating Met-tRNA^{Met} or fMet-tRNA^{fMet}, ready for the elongation steps.

Inorganic pyrophosphatase: An enzyme that hydrolyzes a molecule of inorganic pyrophosphate to yield two molecules of (ortho) phosphate; also known as pyrophosphatase.

Insertion mutation: A mutation caused by insertion of one or more extra bases, or a mutagen, between two successive bases in DNA.

Insertion sequence: Specific base sequences at either end of a transposable segment of DNA.

Integral membrane proteins: Proteins firmly bound to a membrane by hydrophobic interactions; as distinct from peripheral proteins.

Intercalating mutagen: A mutagen that inserts itself between two successive bases in a nucleic acid, causing a frame-shift mutation.

Intercalation: Insertion between two stacked aromatic or planar rings; for example, the insertion of a planar molecule between two successive bases in a nucleic acid.

Interferons: A class of glycoproteins with antiviral activities.

Intermediary metabolism: In cells, the enzyme-catalyzed reactions that extract chemical energy from nutrient molecules and utilize it to synthesize and assemble cell components.

Intron (intervening sequence): A sequence of nucleotides in a gene that is transcribed but excised before the gene is translated.

Ion channel: An integral membrane protein that provides for the regulated transport of a specific ion, or ions, across a membrane.

Ion-exchange resin: A polymeric resin that contains fixed charged groups; used in chromatographic columns to separate ionic compounds.

Ion product of water (K_w): The product of the concentrations of H^+ and OH^- in pure water: $K_W = [H^+][OH^-] = 1 \times 10^{-14}$ at 25 °C.

Ionizing radiation: A type of radiation, such as X-rays, that causes loss of electrons from some organic molecules, thus making them more reactive.

Ionophore: A compound that binds one or more metal ions and is capable of diffusing across a membrane, carrying the bound ion.

Iron-sulfur center: A prosthetic group of certain redox proteins involved in electron transfers; Fe^{2+} or Fe^{3+} is bound to inorganic sulfur and to Cys groups in the protein.

Isoelectric focusing: An electrophoretic method for separating macromolecules on the basis of their isoelectric pH.

Isoelectric pH (isoelectric point): The pH at which a solute has no net electric charge and thus does not move in an electric field.

Isoenzymes: *See* isozymes.

Isomerases: Enzymes that catalyze the transformation of compounds into their positional isomers.

Isomers: Any two molecules with the same molecular formula but a different arrangement of molecular groups.

Isoprene: The hydrocarbon 2-methyl-1,3-butadiene, a recurring structural unit of the terpenoid biomolecules.

Isothermal: Occurring at constant temperature.

Isotopes: Stable or radioactive forms of an element that differ in atomic weight but are otherwise chemically identical to the naturally abundant form of the element; used as tracers.

Isozymes: Multiple forms of an enzyme that catalyze the same reaction but differ from each other in their amino acid sequence, substrate affinity, V_{max}, and/or regulatory properties; also called isoenzymes.

K

Keratins: Insoluble protective or structural proteins consisting of parallel polypeptide chains in α-helical or β conformations.

Ketogenic amino acids: Amino acids with carbon skeletons that can serve as precursors of the ketone bodies.

Ketone bodies: Acetoacetate, D-β-hydroxybutyrate, and acetone; water-soluble fuels normally exported by the liver but overproduced during fasting or in untreated diabetes mellitus.

Ketose: A simple monosaccharide in which the carbonyl group is a ketone.

Ketosis: A condition in which the concentration of ketone bodies in the blood, tissues, and urine is abnormally high.

Kinases: Enzymes that catalyze the phosphorylation of certain molecules by ATP.

Kinetics: The study of reaction rates.

Krebs cycle: *See* citric acid cycle.

L

Lagging strand: The DNA strand that, during replication, must be synthesized in the direction opposite to that in which the replication fork moves.

Law of mass action: The law stating that the rate of any given chemical reaction is proportional to the product of the activities (or concentrations) of the reactants.

Leader: A short sequence near the amino terminus of a protein or the 5'-end of an RNA that has a specialized targeting or regulatory function.

Leading strand: The DNA strand that, during replication, is synthesized in the same direction in which the replication fork moves.

Leaky mutant: A mutant gene that gives rise to a product with a detectable level of biological activity.

Leaving group: The departing or displaced molecular group in a unimolecular elimination or a bimolecular substitution reaction.

Lethal mutation: A mutation that inactivates a biological function essential to the life of the cell or organism.

Leucine zipper: A protein structural motif involved in protein-protein interactions in many eukaryotic regulatory proteins; consists of two interacting α helices in which Leu residues in every seventh position are a prominent feature of the interacting surfaces.

Leukotrienes: A family of molecules derived from arachidonate; muscle contractants that constrict air passages in the lungs and are involved in asthma.

Levorotatory isomer: A stereoisomer that rotates the plane of plane-polarized light counterclockwise.

Ligand: A small molecule that binds specifically to a larger one; for example, a hormone is the ligand for its specific protein receptor.

Light reactions: The reactions of photosynthesis that require light and cannot occur in the dark; also known as the light-dependent reactions.

Lineweaver-Burk equation: An algebraic transform of the Michaelis-Menten equation, allowing determination of V_{max} and K_m by extrapolation of [S] to infinity.

Linking number: The number of times one closed circular DNA strand is wound about another; the number of topological links holding the circles together.

Lipases: Enzymes that catalyze the hydrolysis of triacylglycerols.

Lipid: A small water-insoluble biomolecule generally containing fatty acids, sterols, or isoprenoid compounds.

Lipoate (lipoic acid): A vitamin for some microorganisms; an intermediate carrier of hydrogen atoms and acyl groups in α-keto acid dehydrogenases.

Lipoprotein: A lipid-protein aggregate that serves to carry water-insoluble lipids in the blood. The protein component alone is an apolipoprotein.

Low-energy phosphate compound: A phosphorylated compound with a relatively small standard free energy of hydrolysis.

Lyases: Enzymes that catalyze the removal of a group from a molecule to form a double bond, or the addition of a group to a double bond.

Lymphocytes: A subclass of leukocytes involved in the immune response. B lymphocytes synthesize and secrete antibodies; T lymphocytes either play a regulatory role in immunity or kill foreign and virus-infected cells.

Lysis: Destruction of a cell's plasma membrane or of a bacterial cell wall, releasing the cellular contents and killing the cell.

Lysogeny: One of two outcomes of the infection of a host cell by a temperate phage. It occurs when the phage genome becomes repressed and is replicated as part of the host DNA; infrequently it may be induced, and the phage particles so produced cause the host cell to lyse.

Lysosome: A membrane-bounded organelle in the cytoplasm of eukaryotic cells; it contains many hydrolytic enzymes and serves as a degrading and recycling center for unneeded components.

M

Macromolecule: A molecule having a molecular weight in the range of a few thousand to many millions.

Matrix: The aqueous contents of a cell or organelle (the mitochondrion, for example) with dissolved solutes.

Meiosis: A type of cell division in which diploid cells give rise to haploid cells destined to become gametes.

Membrane transport: Movement of a polar solute across a membrane via a specific membrane protein (a transporter).

Messenger RNA (mRNA): A class of RNA molecules, each of which is complementary to one strand of DNA; carries the genetic message from the chromosome to the ribosomes.

Metabolism: The entire set of enzyme-catalyzed transformations of organic molecules in living cells; the sum of anabolism and catabolism.

Metabolite: A chemical intermediate in the enzyme-catalyzed reactions of metabolism.

Metalloprotein: A protein having a metal ion as its prosthetic group.

Metamerism: Division of the body into segments; in insects, for example.

Micelle: An aggregate of amphipathic molecules in water, with the nonpolar portions in the interior and the polar portions at the exterior surface, exposed to water.

Michaelis-Menten constant (K_m): The substrate concentration at which an enzyme-catalyzed reaction proceeds at onehalf its maximum velocity.

Michaelis-Menten equation: The equation describing the hyperbolic dependence of the initial reaction velocity, V_0, on substrate concentration, [S], in many enzyme-catalyzed reactions: $V_0 = \dfrac{V_{max}[S]}{K_m + [S]}$

Michaelis-Menten kinetics: A kinetic pattern in which the initial rate of an enzyme-catalyzed reaction exhibits a hyperbolic dependence on substrate concentration.

Microbodies: Cytoplasmic, membrane-bounded vesicles containing peroxide forming and peroxide-destroying enzymes; include lysosomes, peroxisomes, and glyoxysomes.

Microfilaments: Thin filaments composed of actin, found in the cytoplasm of eukaryotic cells; serve in structure and movement.

Microsomes: Membranous vesicles formed by fragmentation of the endoplasmic reticulum of eukaryotic cells; recovered by differential centrifugation.

Microtubules: Thin tubules assembled from two types of globular tubulin subunits; present in cilia, flagella, centrosomes, and other contractile or motile structures.

Mitochondrion: Membrane-bounded organelle in the cytoplasm of eukaryotes; contains the enzyme systems required for the citric acid cycle, fatty acid oxidation, electron transfer, and oxidative phosphorylation.

Mitosis: The multistep process in eukaryotic cells that results in the replication of chromosomes and cell division.

Mixed-function oxidases (oxygenases): Enzymes, often flavoproteins, that use molecular oxygen (O_2) to simultaneously oxidize a substrate and a cosubstrate (commonly NADH or NADPH).

Modulator: A metabolite that, when bound to the allosteric site of an enzyme, alters its kinetic characteristics.

Molar solution: One mole of solute dissolved in water to give a total volume of 1,000 mL.

Mole: One gram molecular weight of a compound. *See* Avogadro's number.

Monoclonal antibodies: Antibodies produced by a cloned hybridoma cell, which therefore are identical and directed against the same epitope of the antigen.

Monolayer: A single layer of oriented lipid molecules.

Monoprotic acid: An acid having only one dissociable proton.

Monosaccharide: A carbohydrate consisting of a single sugar unit.

mRNA: *See* messenger RNA.

Mucopolysaccharide: An older name for a glycosaminoglycan.

Multienzyme system: A group of related enzymes participating in a given metabolic pathway.

Mutarotation: The change in specific rotation of a pyranose or furanose sugar or glycoside accompanying the equilibration of its α- and β-anomeric forms.

Mutases: Enzymes that catalyze the transposition of functional groups.

Mutation: An inheritable change in the nucleotide sequence of a chromosome.

Myofibril: A unit of thick and thin filaments of muscle fibers.

Myosin: A contractile protein; the major component of the thick filaments of muscle and other actin-myosin systems.

N

NAD, NADP (nicotinamide adenine dinucleotide, nicotinamide adenine dinucleotide phosphate): Nicotinamide-containing coenzymes functioning as carriers of hydrogen atoms and electrons in some oxidation-reduction reactions.

Native conformation: The biologically active conformation of a macromolecule.

Negative cooperativity: A phenomenon of some multi-subunit enzymes or proteins in which binding of a ligand or substrate to one subunit impairs binding to another subunit.

Negative feedback: Regulation of a biochemical pathway achieved when a reaction product inhibits an earlier step in the pathway.

Neuron: A cell of nervous tissue specialized for transmission of a nerve impulse.

Neurotransmitter: A low molecular weight compound (usually containing nitrogen) secreted from the terminal of a neuron and bound by a specific receptor in the next neuron; serves to transmit a nerve impulse.

Nicotinamide adenine dinucleotide, nicotinamide adenine dinucleotide phosphate: *See* NAD, NADP.

Ninhydrin reaction: A color reaction given by amino acids and peptides on heating with ninhydrin; widely used for their detection and estimation.

Nitrogen cycle: The cycling of various forms of biologically available nitrogen through the plant, animal, and microbial worlds, and through the atmosphere and geosphere.

Nitrogen fixation: Conversion of atmospheric nitrogen (N_2) into a reduced, biologically available form by nitrogen-fixing organisms.

Nitrogenase complex: A system of enzymes capable of reducing atmospheric nitrogen to ammonia in the presence of ATP.

Noncompetitive inhibition: A type of enzyme inhibition not reversed by increasing the substrate concentration.

Noncyclic electron flow: The lightinduced flow of electrons from water to $NADP^+$ in oxygen-evolving photosynthesis; it involves both photosystems I and II.

Nonessential amino acids: Amino acids that can be made by humans and other vertebrates from simpler precursors, and are thus not required in the diet.

Nonheme iron proteins: Proteins, usually acting in oxidation-reduction reactions, containing iron but no porphyrin groups.

Nonpolar: Hydrophobic; describing molecules or groups that are poorly soluble in water.

Nonsense codon: A codon that does not specify an amino acid, but signals the termination of a polypeptide chain.

Nonsense mutation: A mutation that results in the premature termination of a polypeptide chain.

Nonsense suppressor: A mutation, usually in the gene for a tRNA, that causes an amino acid to be inserted into a polypeptide in response to a termination codon.

Nucleases: Enzymes that hydrolyze the internucleotide (phosphodiester) linkages of nucleic acids.

Nucleic acids: Biologically occurring polynucleotides in which the nucleotide residues are linked in a specific sequence by phosphodiester bonds; DNA and RNA.

Nucleoid: In bacteria, the nuclear zone that contains the chromosome but has no surrounding membrane.

Nucleolus: A densely staining structure in the nucleus of eukaryotic cells; involved in rRNA synthesis and ribosome formation.

Nucleophile: An electron-rich group with a strong tendency to donate electrons to an electron-deficient nucleus (electrophile); the entering reactant in a bimolecular substitution reaction.

Nucleoplasm: The portion of a cell's contents enclosed by the nuclear membrane; also called the nuclear matrix.

Nucleoside: A compound consisting of a purine or pyrimidine base covalently linked to a pentose.

Nucleoside diphosphate kinase: An enzyme that catalyzes the transfer of the terminal phosphate of a nucleoside 5'-triphosphate to a nucleoside 5'-diphosphate.

Nucleoside diphosphate sugar: A coenzyme-like carrier of a sugar molecule, functioning in the enzymatic synthesis of polysaccharides and sugar derivatives.

Nucleoside monophosphate kinase: An enzyme that catalyzes the transfer of the terminal phosphate of ATP to a nucleoside 5'-monophosphate.

Nucleosome: Structural unit for packaging chromatin; consists of a DNA strand wound around a histone core.

Nucleotide: A nucleoside phosphorylated at one of its pentose hydroxyl groups.

Nucleus: In eukaryotes, a membranebounded organelle that contains chromosomes.

O

Oligomer: A short polymer, usually of amino acids, sugars, or nucleotides; the definition of "short" is somewhat arbitrary, but usually less than 50 subunits.

Oligomeric protein: A multisubunit protein having two or more identical polypeptide chains.

Oligonucleotide: A short polymer of nucleotides (usually less than 50).

Oligopeptide: A few amino acids joined by peptide bonds.

Oligosaccharide: Several monosaccharide groups joined by glycosidic bonds.

Oncogene: A cancer-causing gene; any af several mutant genes that cause cells to exhibit rapid, uncontrolled proliferation. *See also* proto-oncogene.

Open reading frame: A group of contiguous nonoverlapping nucleotide codons in a DNA or RNA molecule that do not include a termination codon.

Open system: A system that exchanges matter and energy with its surroundings. *See also* system.

Operator: A region of DNA that interacts with a repressor protein to control the expression of a gene or group of genes.

Operon: A unit of genetic expression consisting of one or more related genes and the operator and promoter sequences that regulate their transcription.

Optical activity: The capacity of a substance to rotate the plane of plane-polarized light.

Optimum pH: The characteristic pH at which an enzyme has maximal catalytic activity.

Organelles: Membrane-bounded structures found in eukaryotic cells; contain enzymes and other components required for specialized cell functions.

Origin: The nucleotide sequence or site in DNA where DNA replication is initiated.

Osmosis: Bulk flow of water through a semipermeable membrane into another aqueous compartment containing solute at a higher concentration.

Osmotic pressure: Pressure generated by the osmotic flow of water through a semipermeable membrane into an aqueous compartment containing solute at a higher concentration.

Oxidation: The loss of electrons from a compound.

Oxidation-reduction reaction: A reaction in which electrons are transferred from a donor to an acceptor molecule; also called a redox reaction.

Oxidative phosphorylation: The enzymatic phosphorylation of ADP to ATP coupled to electron transfer from a substrate to molecular oxygen.

Oxidizing agent (oxidant): The acceptor of electrons in an oxidation-reduction reaction.

Oxygen debt: The extra oxygen (above the normal resting level) consumed in the recovery period after strenuous physical exertion.

Oxygenases: Enzymes that catalyze reactions in which oxygen is introduced into an acceptor molecule.

P

Palindrome: A segment of duplex DNA in which the base sequences of the two strands exhibit twofold rotational symmetry about an axis.

Paradigm: In biochemistry, an experimental model or example.

Partition coefficient: A constant that expresses the ratio in which a given solute will be partitioned or distributed between two given immiscible liquids at equilibrium.

Pathogenic: Disease-causing.

Pentose: A simple sugar with a backbone containing five carbon atoms.

Pentose phosphate pathway: A pathway that serves to interconvert hexoses and pentoses and is a source of reducing equivalents and pentoses for biosynthetic processes; present in most organisms. Also called the phosphogluconate pathway.

Peptidase: An enzyme that hydrolyzes a peptide bond.

Peptide: Two or more amino acids covalently joined by peptide bonds.

Peptide bond: A substituted amide linkage between the α-amino group of one amino acid and the α-carboxyl group of another, with the elimination of the elements of water.

Peptide mapping: The characteristic two-dimensional pattern (on paper or gel) formed by the separation of a mixture of peptides resulting from partial hydrolysis of a protein; also known as peptide fingerprinting.

Peptidoglycan: A major component of bacterial cell walls; generally consists of parallel heteropolysaccharides cross-linked by short peptides.

Peripheral proteins: Proteins that are loosely or reversibly bound to a membrane by hydrogen bonds or electrostatic forces; generally water-soluble once released from the membrane.

Permeases: *See* transporters. peroxisome—membrane-bounded organelle in the cytoplasm of eukaryotic cells; contains peroxide-forming and peroxidedestroying enzymes.

pH: The negative logarithm of the hydrogen ion concentration of an aqueous solution.

Phenotype: The observable characteristics of an organism.

Phosphodiester linkage: A chemical grouping that contains two alcohols esterified to one molecule of phosphoric acid, which thus serves as a bridge between them.

Phosphogluconate pathway: An oxidative pathway beginning with glucose-6-phosphate and leading, via 6-phosphogluconate, to pentose phosphates and yielding NADPH. Also called the pentose phosphate pathway.

Phospholipid: A lipid containing one or more phosphate groups.

Phosphorolysis: Cleavage of a compound with phosphate as the attacking group; analogous to hydrolysis.

Phosphorylation potential (ΔG_p): The actual free-energy change of ATP hydrolysis under the nonstandard conditions prevailing within a cell.

Photochemical reaction center: The part of a photosynthetic complex where the energy of an absorbed photon causes charge separation, initiating electron transfer.

Photon: The ultimate unit (a quantum) of light energy.

Photophosphorylation: The enzymatic formation of ATP from ADP coupled to the light-dependent transfer of electrons in photosynthetic cells.

Photoreduction: The light-induced reduction of an electron acceptor in photosynthetic cells.

Photorespiration: Oxygen consumption occurring in illuminated temperate-zone plants, largely due to oxidation of phosphoglycolate.

Photosynthesis: The use of light energy to produce carbohydrates from carbon dioxide and a reducing agent such as water.

Photosynthetic phosphorylation: *See* photophosphorylation.

Photosystem: In photosynthetic cells, a functional set of light-absorbing pigments and its reaction center.

Phototroph: An organism that can use the energy of light to synthesize its own fuels from simple molecules, such as carbon dioxide, oxygen, and water; as distinct from a chemotroph.

pK: The negative logarithm of an equilibrium constant.

Plasma membrane: The exterior membrane surrounding the cytoplasm of a cell.

Plasma proteins: The proteins present in blood plasma.

Plasmalogen: A phospholipid with an alkenyl ether substituent on the C-1 of glycerol.

Plasmid: An extrachromosomal, independently replicating, small circular DNA molecule; commonly employed in genetic engineering.

Plastid: In plants, a self-replicating organelle; may differentiate into a chloroplast.

Platelets: Small, enucleated cells that initiate blood clotting; they arise from cells called megakaryocytes in the bone marrow. Also known as thrombocytes.

Pleated sheet: The side-by-side, hydrogen-bonded arrangement of polypeptide chains in the extended β conformation.

Polar: Hydrophilic, or "water-loving"; describing molecules or groups that are soluble in water.

Polarity: (1) In chemistry, the nonuniform distribution of electrons in a molecule; polar molecules are usually soluble in water. (2) In molecular biology, the distinction between the 5'- and 3'-ends of nucleic acids.

Polyclonal antibodies: A heterogeneous pool of antibodies produced in an animal by a number of different B lymphocytes in response to an antigen. Different antibodies in the pool recognize different parts of the antigen.

Polylinker: A short, often synthetic, fragment of DNA containing recognition sequences for several restriction endonucleases.

Polymerase chain reaction (PCR): A repetitive procedure that results in a geometric amplification of a specific DNA sequence.

Polymorphic: Describing a protein for which amino acid sequence variants exist in a population of organisms, but the variations do not destroy the protein's function.

Polynucleotide: A covalently linked sequence of nucleotides in which the 3'-hydroxyl of the pentose of one nucleotide residue is joined by a phosphodiester bond to the 5'-hydroxyl of the pentose of the next residue.

Polypeptide: A long chain of amino acids linked by peptide bonds; the molecular weight is generally less than 10,000.

Polyribosome: *See* polysome.

Polysaccharide: A linear or branched polymer of monosaccharide units linked by glycosidic bonds.

Polysome (polyribosome): A complex of an mRNA molecule and two or more ribo.

Porphyrin: Complex nitrogenous compound containing four substituted pyrroles covalently joined into a ring; often complexed with a central metal atom.

Positive cooperativity: A phenomenon of some multisubunit enzymes or proteins in which binding of a ligand or substrate to one subunit facilitates binding to another subunit.

Post-transcriptional processing: The enzymatic processing of the primary RNA transcript, producing functional mRNA, tRNA, andJor rRNA molecules.

Post-translational modification: Enzymatic processing of a polypeptide chain after translation from its mRNA.

Primary structure: A description of the covalent backbone of a polymer (macromolecule), including the sequence of monomeric subunits and any interchain and intrachain covalent bonds.

Primary transcript: The immediate RNA product of transcription before any post-transcriptional processing reactions.

Primase: An enzyme that catalyzes the formation of RNA oligonucleotides used as primers by DNA polymerases.

Primer: A short oligomer (of sugars or nucleotides, for example) to which an enzyme adds additional monomeric subunits.

Probe: A labeled fragment of nucleic acid containing a nucleotide sequence complementary to a gene or genomic sequence that one wishes to detect in a hybridization experiment.

Processivity: For any enzyme that catalyzes the synthesis of a biological polymer, the property of adding multiple subunits to the polymer without dissociating from the substrate.

Prochiral molecule: A symmetric molecule that can react asymmetrically with an enzyme having an asymmetric active site, generating a chiral product.

Projection formulas: A method for representing molecules to show the configuration of groups around chiral centers; also known as Fischer projection formulas.

Prokaryote: A bacterium; a unicellular organism with a single chromosome, no nuclear envelope, and no membranebounded organelles.

Promoter: A DNA sequence at which RNA polymerase may bind, leading to initiation of transcription.

Prophage: A bacteriophage in an inactive state in which the genome is either integrated into the chromosome of the host cell or (sometimes) replicated autonomously.

Prostaglandins: A class of lipid-soluble, hormonelike regulatory molecules derived from arachidonate and other polyunsaturated fatty acids.

Prosthetic group: A metal ion or an organic compound (other than an amino acid) that is covalently bound to a protein and is essential to its activity.

Protein: A macromolecule composed of one or more polypeptide chains, each with a characteristic sequence of amino acids linked by peptide bonds.

Protein kinases: Enzymes that phosphorylate certain amino acid residues in specific proteins.

Protein targeting: The process by which newly synthesized proteins are sorted and transported to their proper locations in the cell.

Proteoglycan: A hybrid macromolecule consisting of a heteropolysaccharide joined to a polypeptide; the polysaccharide is the major component.

Proto-oncogene: A cellular gene, usually encoding a regulatory protein, that can be converted into an oncogene by mutation.

Proton acceptor: An anionic compound capable of accepting a proton from a proton donor; that is, a base.

Proton donor: The donor of a proton in an acid-base reaction; that is, an acid.

Proton-motive force: The electrochemical potential inherent in a transmembrane gradient of H^+ concentration; used in oxidative phosphorylation and photophosphorylation to drive ATP synthesis.

Protoplasm: A general term referring to the entire contents of a living cell.

Purine: A nitrogenous heterocyclic base found in nucleotides and nucleic acids; containing fused pyrimidine and imidazole rings.

Puromycin: An antibiotic that inhibits polypeptide synthesis by being incorporated into a growing polypeptide chain, causing its premature termination.

Pyranose: A simple sugar containing the six-membered pyran ring.

Pyridine nucleotide: A nucleotide coenzyme containing the pyridine derivative nicotinamide; NAD or NADP.

Pyridoxal phosphate: A coenzyme containing the vitamin pyridoxine (vitamin B_6); functions in reactions involving amino group transfer.

Pyrimidine: A nitrogenous heterocyclic base found in nucleotides and nucleic acids.

Pyrimidine dimer: A covalently joined dimer of two adjacent pyrimidine residues in DNA, induced by absorption of ITV light; most commonly derived from two adjacent thymines (a thymine dimer).

Pyrophosphatase: *See* inorganic pyrophosphatase.

Q

Quantum: The ultimate unit of energy.

Quaternary structure: The three-dimensional structure of a multisubunit protein; particularly the manner in which the subunits fit together.

R

R groups: (1) Formally, an abbreviation denoting any alkyl group. (2) Occasionally, used in a more general sense to denote virtually any organic substituent tthe R groups of amino acids, for example).

Racemic mixture tracemate): An equimolar mixture of the D and L stereoisomers of an optically active compound.

Radical: An atom or group of atoms possessing an unpaired electron; also called a free radical.

Radioactive isotope: An isotopic form of an element with an unstable nucleus that stabilizes itself by emitting ionizing radiation.

Radioimmunoassay: A sensitive and quantitative method for detecting trace amounts of a biomolecule, based on its capacity to displace a radioactive form of the molecule from combination with its specific antibody.

Rate-limiting step: (1) Generally, the step in an enzymatic reaction with the greatest activation energy or the transition state of highest free energy. (2) The slowest step in a metabolic pathway.

Reaction intermediate: Any chemical species in a reaction pathway that has a finite chemical lifetime.

Reading frame: A contiguous and nonoverlapping set of three-nucleotide codons in DNA or RNA.

Recombinant DNA: DNA formed by the joining of genes into new combinations.

Redox pair: An electron donor and its corresponding oxidized form; for example, NADH and NAD^+.

Redox reaction: See oxidation-reduction reaction.

Reducing agent (reductant): The electron donor in an oxidation-reduction reaction.

Reducing end: The end of a polysaccharide having a terminal sugar with a free anomeric carbon; the terminal residue can act as a reducing sugar.

Reducing equivalent: A general or neutral term for an electron or an electron equivalent in the form of a hydrogen atom or a hydride ion.

Reducing sugar: A sugar in which the carbonyl (anomeric) carbon is not involved in a glycosidic bond and can therefore undergo oxidation.

Reduction: The gain of electrons by a compound or ion.

Regulatory enzyme: An enzyme having a regulatory function through its capacity to undergo a change in catalytic activity by allosteric mechanisms or by covalent modification.

Regulatory gene: A gene that gives rise to a product involved in the regulation of the expression of another gene; for example, a gene coding for a repressor protein.

Regulatory sequence: A DNA sequence involved in regulating the expression of a gene; for example, a promoter or operator.

Regulon: A group of genes or operons that are coordinately regulated even though some, or all, may be spatially distant within the chromosome or genome.

Release factors: See termination factors.

Releasing factors: Hypothalamic hormones that stimulate release of other hormones by the pituitary gland.

Renaturation: Refolding of an unfolded (denatured) globular protein so as to restore native structure and protein function.

Replication: Synthesis of a daughter duplex DNA molecule identical to the parental duplex DNA.

Replisome: The multiprotein complex that promotes DNA synthesis at the replication fork.

Repressible enzyme: In bacteria, an enzyme whose synthesis is inhibited when its reaction product is readily available to the cell.

Repression: A decrease in the expression of a gene in response to a change in the activity of a regulatory protein.

Repressor: The protein that binds to the regulatory sequence or operator for a gene, blocking its transcription.

Residue: A single unit within a polymer; for example, an amino acid within a polypeptide chain. The term reflects the fact that sugars, nucleotides, and amino acids lose a few atoms (generally the elements of water) when incorporated in their respective polymers.

Respiration: The catabolic process in which electrons are removed from nutrient molecules and passed through a chain of carriers to oxygen.

Respiratory chain: The electron transfer chain; a sequence of electron-carrying proteins that transfer electrons from substrates to molecular oxygen in aerobic cells.

Restriction endonucleases: Site-specific endodeoxyribonucleases causing cleavage of both strands of DNA at points within or near the specific site recognized by the enzyme; important tools in genetic engineering.

Restriction fragment: A segment of double-stranded DNA produced by the action of a restriction endonuclease on a larger DNA.

Restriction fragment length polymorphisms (RFLPs): Variations, among individuals in a population, in the length of certain restriction fragments within which certain genomic sequences occur. These variations result from rare sequence changes that create or destroy restriction sites in the genome.

Retrovirus: An RNA virus containing a reverse transcriptase.

Reverse transcriptase: An RNA-directed DNA polymerase in retroviruses; capable of making DNA complementary to an RNA.

Ribonuclease: A nuclease that catalyzes the hydrolysis of certain internucleotide linkages of RNA.

Ribonucleic acid: See RNA.

Ribonucleotide: A nucleotide containing n-ribose as its pentose component.

Ribosomal RNA (rRNA): A class of RNA molecules serving as components of ribosomes.

Ribosome: A supramolecular complex of rRNAs and proteins, approximately 18 to 22 nm in diameter; the site of protein synthesis.

Ribozymes: Ribonucleic acid molecules with catalytic activities; RNA enzymes.

RNA (ribonucleic acid): A polyribonucleotide of a specific sequence linked by successive 3', 5'-phosphodiester bonds.

RNA polymerase: An enzyme that catalyzes the formation of RNA from ribonucleoside 5'-triphosphates, using a strand of DNA or RNA as a template.

RNA splicing: Removal of introns and joining of exons in a primary transcript.

rRNA: See ribosomal RNA.

S

S-adenosylmethionine (adoMet): An enzymatic cofactor involved in methyl group transfers.

Salvage pathway: Synthesis of a biomolecule, such as a nucleotide, from intermediates in the degradative pathway for the biomolecule; a recycling pathway, as distinct from a de novo pathway.

Saponification: Alkaline hydrolysis of triacylglycerols to yield fatty acids as soaps.

Sarcomere: A functional and structural unit of the muscle contractile system.

Satellite DNA: Highly repeated, nontranslated segments of DNA in eukaryotic chromosomes; most often associated with the centromeric region. Its function is not clear.

Saturated fatty acid: A fatty acid containing a fully saturated alkyl chain.

Second law of thermodynamics: The law stating that in any chemical or physical process, the entropy of the universe tends to increase.

Second messenger: An effector molecule synthesized within a cell in response to an external signal (first messenger) such as a hormone.

Secondary metabolism: Pathways that lead to specialized products not found in every living cell.

Secondary structure: The residue-byresidue conformation of the backbone of a polymer.

Sedimentation coefficient: A physical constant specifying the rate of sedimentation of a particle in a centrifugal field under specified conditions.

Shine-Dalgarno sequence: A sequence in an mRNA required for binding prokaryotic ribosomes.

Shuttle vector: A recombinant DNA vector that can be replicated in two or more different host species. *See also* vector.

Sickle-cell anemia: A human disease characterized by defective hemoglobin molecules; caused by a homozygous allele coding for the β chain of hemoglobin.

Sickle-cell trait: A human condition recognized by the sickling of erythrocytes when exposed to low oxygen tension; occurs in individuals heterozygous for the allele responsible for sickle-cell anemia.

Signal sequence: An amino-terminal sequence that signals the cellular fate or destination of a newly synthesized protein.

Signal transduction: The process by which an extracellular signal (chemical, mechanical, or electrical) is amplified and converted to a cellular response.

Silent mutation: A mutation in a gene that causes no detectable change in the biological characteristics of the gene product.

Simple diffusion: The movement of solute molecules across a membrane to a region of lower concentration, unassisted by a protein transporter.

Simple protein: A protein yielding only amino acids on hydrolysis.

Site-directed mutagenesis: A set of methods used to create specific alterations in the sequence of a gene.

Site-specific recombination: A type of genetic recombination that occurs only at specific sequences.

Small nuclear RNA (snRNA): Any of several small RNA molecules in the nucleus; most have a role in the splicing reactions that remove introns from mRNA, tRNA, and rRNA molecules.

Somatic cells: All body cells except the germ-line cells.

SOS response: In bacteria, a coordinated induction of a variety of genes as a response to high levels of DNA damage.

Southern blot: A DNA hybridization procedure in which one or more specific DNA fragments are detected in a larger population by means of hybridization to a complementary, labeled nucleic acid probe.

Specific activity: The number of micromoles (μmol) of a substrate transformed by an enzyme preparation per minute per milligram of protein at 25°C; a measure of enzyme purity.

Specific heat: The amount of energy (in joules or calories) needed to raise the temperature of 1 g of a pure substance by 1°C.

Specific rotation: The rotation, in degrees, of the plane of plane-polarized light (D-line of sodium) by an optically active compound at 25°C, with a specified concentration and light path.

Specificity: The ability of an enzyme or receptor to discriminate among competing substrates or ligands.

Sphingolipid: An amphipathic lipid with a sphingosine backbone to which are attached a long-chain fatty acid and a polar alcohol.

Standard free-energy change ($\Delta G°$): The free-energy change for a reaction occurring under a set of standard conditions—temperature, 298 K; pressure, 1 atm or 101.3 kPa; and all solutes at 1 Ni concentration. $\Delta G°'$ denotes the standard free-energy change at pH 7.0.

Standard reduction potential (E_0'): The electromotive force exhibited at an electrode by 1 M concentrations of a reducing agent and its oxidized form at 25°C and pH 7.0; a measure of the relative tendency of the reducing agent to lose electrons.

Steady state: A nonequilibrium state of a system through which matter is flowing and in which all components remain at a constant concentration.

Stem cells: The common, self-regenerating cells in bone marrow that give rise to differentiated blood cells such as erythrocytes and lymphocytes.

Sterols: A class of lipids containing the steroid nucleus.

Sticky ends: Two DNA ends in the same DNA molecule, or in different molecules, with short overhanging single-stranded segments that are complementary to one another, facilitating ligation of the ends; also known as cohesive ends.

Stroma: The space and aqueous solution enclosed within the inner membrane of a chloroplast, not including the contents within the thylakoid membranes.

Structural gene: A gene coding for a protein or RNA molecule; as distinct from a regulatory gene.

Substitution mutation: A mutation caused by the replacement of one base by another.

Substrate: The specific compound acted upon by an enzyme.

Substrate-level phosphorylation: Phosphorylation of ADP or some other nucleoside 5'-diphosphate coupled to the dehydrogenation of an organic substrate; independent of the electron transfer chain.

Suicide inhibitor: A relatively inert molecule that is transformed by an enzyme, at its active site, into a reactive substance that irreversibly inactivates the enzyme.

Suppressor mutation: A mutation that totally or partially restores a function lost by a primary mutation; located at a site different from the site of the primary mutation.

Svedberg (S): A unit of measure of the rate at which a particle sediments in a centrifugal field.

Symbionts: Two or more organisms that are mutually interdependent; usually living in physical association.

Symport: Cotransport of solutes across a membrane in the same direction.

Synthases: Enzymes that catalyze condensation reactions in which no nucleoside triphosphate is required as an energy source.

Synthetases: Enzymes that catalyze condensation reactions using ATP or another nucleoside triphosphate as an energy source.

System: An isolated collection of matter; all other matter in the universe apart from the system is called the surroundings.

■ T

Telomere: Specialized nucleic acid structure found at the ends of linear eukaryotic chromosomes.

Temperate phage: A phage whose DNA may be incorporated into the host-cell genome without being expressed; as distinct from a virulent phage, which destroys the host cell.

Template: A macromolecular mold or pattern for the synthesis of an informational macromolecule.

Terminal transferase: An enzyme that catalyzes the addition of nucleotide residues of a single kind to the 3'-end of DNA chains.

Termination codons: UAA, UAG, and UGA; in protein synthesis, signal the termination of a polypeptide chain. Also known as stop codons.

Termination factors: Protein factors of the cytosol required in releasing a completed polypeptide chain from a ribosome; also known as release factors.

Termination sequence: A DNA sequence that appears at the end of a transcriptional unit and signals the end of transcription.

Terpenes: Organic hydrocarbons or hydrocarbon derivatives constructed from recurring isoprene units. They produce some of the scents and tastes of plant products; for example, the scents of geranium leaves and pine needles.

Tertiary structure: The three-dimensional conformation of a polymer in its native folded state.

Tetrahydrobiopterin: The reduced coenzyme form of biopterin.

Tetrahydrofolate: The reduced, active coenzyme form of the vitamin folate.

Thiamine pyrophosphate: The active coenzyme form of vitamin B_1; involved in aldehyde transfer reactions.

Thioester: An ester of a carboxylic acid with a thiol or mercaptan.

3'-end: The end of a nucleic acid that lacks a nucleotide bound at the 3'-position of the terminal residue.

Thromboxanes: A class of molecules derived from arachidonate and involved in platelet aggregation during blood clotting.

Thylakoid: Closed cisterna, or disc, formed by the pigment-bearing internal membranes of chloroplasts.

Tissue culture: Method by which cells derived from multicellular organisms are grown in liquid media.

Titration curve: A plot of the pH versus the equivalents of base added during titration of an acid.

Tocopherols: Forms of vitamin E.

Topoisomerases: Enzymes that introduce positive or negative supercoils in closed, circular duplex DNA.

Topoisomers: Different forms of a covalently closed, circular DNA molecule that differs only in their linking number.

Toxins: Proteins produced by some organisms and toxic to certain other species.

Trace element: A chemical element required by an organism in only trace amounts.

Transaminases: *See* aminotransferases.

Transamination: Enzymatic transfer of an amino group from an α-amino acid to an α-keto acid.

Transcription: The enzymatic process whereby the genetic information contained in one strand of DNA is used to specify a complementary sequence of bases in an mRNA chain.

Transcriptional control: The regulation of a protein's synthesis by regulation of the formation of its mRNA.

Transduction: (1) Generally, the conversion of energy or information from one form to another. (2) The transfer of genetic information from one cell to another by means of a viral vector.

Transfer RNA (tRNA): A class of RNA molecules, each of which combines covalently with a specific amino acid as the first step in protein synthesis.

Transformation: Introduction of an exogenous DNA into a cell, causing the cell to acquire a new phenotype.

Transgenic: Describing an organism that has genes from another organism incorporated within its genome as a result of recombinant DNA procedures.

Transition state: An activated form of a molecule in which the molecule has undergone a partial chemical reaction; the highest point on the reaction coordinate.

Translation: The process in which the genetic information present in an mRNA molecule specifies the sequence of amino acids during protein synthesis.

Translational control: The regulation of a protein's synthesis by regulation of the rate of its translation on the ribosome.

Translational repressor: A repressor that binds to an mRNA, blocking translation.

Translocase: (1) An enzyme that catalyzes membrane transport. (2) An enzyme that causes a movement, such as the movement of a ribosome along an mRNA.

Transpiration: Passage of water from the roots of a plant to the atmosphere via the vascular system and the stomata of the leaves.

Transporters: Proteins that span a membrane and transport specific nutrients, metabolites, ions, or proteins across the membrane; sometimes called permeases.

Transposition: The movement of a gene or set of genes from one site in the genome to another.

Transposon (transposable element): A segment of DNA that can move from one position in the genome to another.

Triacylglycerol: An ester of glycerol with three molecules of fatty acid; also called a triglyceride or neutral fat.

Triose: A simple sugar with a backbone containing three carbon atoms.

tRNA: *See* transfer RNA.

Tropic hormone (tropin): A peptide hormone that stimulates a specific target gland to secrete its hormone; for example, thyrotropin produced by the pituitary stimulates secretion of thyroxine by the thyroid.

Turnover number: The number of times an enzyme molecule transforms a substrate molecule per unit time, under conditions giving maximal activity at substrate concentrations that are saturating.

U

Ultraviolet (UV) radiation: Electromagnetic radiation in the region of 200 to 400 nm.

Uncoupling agent: A substance that uncouples phosphorylation of ADP from electron transfer; for example, 2,4-dinitrophenol.

Uniport: A transport system that carries only one solute, as distinct from cotransport.

Unsaturated fatty acid: A fatty acid containing one or more double bonds.

Urea cycle: A metabolic pathway in vertebrates, for the synthesis of urea from amino groups and carbon dioxide; occurs in the liver.

Ureotelic: Excreting excess nitrogen in the form of urea.

Uricotelic: Excreting excess nitrogen in the form of urate (uric acid).

V

Vmax: The maximum velocity of an enzymatic reaction when the binding site is saturated with substrate.

Vector: A DNA molecule known to replicate autonomously in a host cell, to which a segment of DNA may be spliced to allow its replication; for example, a plasmid or a temperate-phage DNA.

Viral vector: A viral DNA altered so that it can act as a vector for recombinant DNA.

Virion: A virus particle.

Virus: A self-replicating, infectious, nucleic acid-protein complex that requires an intact host cell for its replication; its genome is either DNA or RNA.

Vitamin: An organic substance required in small quantities in the diet of some species; generally functions as a component of a coenzyme.

W

Wild type: The normal (unmutated) phenotype.

Wobble: The relatively loose base pairing between the base at the 3'-end of a codon and the complementary base at the 5'-end of the anticodon.

X

X-ray crystallography: The analysis of X-ray diffraction patterns of a crystalline compound, used to determine tha molecule's three-dimensional structure.

Z

Zinc finger: A specialized protein motif involved in DNA recognition by some DNA-binding proteins; characterized by a single atom of zinc coordinated to four Lys residues or to two His and two Lys residues.

Zwitterion: A dipolar ion, with spatially separated positive and negative charges.

Zymogen: An inactive precursor of an enzyme; for example, pepsinogen, the precursor of pepsin.

Index

Page numbers followed by *b* refer to box, *f* refer to figure and *t* refer to table

A

Absorption 8, 12*f*, 71, 83, 109, 111, 137, 155, 226, 471
  fats 72*f*
  site of 82
Accessory pigments 471
Acetyl coenzyme A 375
  formation of 396
Acid phosphatase 422
Acid-base
  balance 424, 433
    maintenance of 58, 424
    renal regulation of 428
    respiratory regulation of 427
  catalysis 477
Acidic amino acid 405
Acidity 110
Acidosis 127, 471
  symptoms of 430*f*
Acquired immunity 463
  mechanisms of 464
Active immunity 464
  types of 464
Adenosine
  diphosphate 471
  triphosphate 472
Adipocyte 471
Adipose tissue 392, 471
Adrenal cortex 392
Adrenal gland 138
Adrenaline 372
Albumin, serum 454
Albuminoids 52
Albumins 52, 402
  bilirubin complex 440
  globulin ratio 454
Alcohol 258, 448
  fermentation 471
  dehydration of 376
Aldolase 420
Aldose 471
Aldosterone secretion 135
Aliphatic side chains 404
Alkaline phosphatase 455
Alkaloids 471
Alkalosis 471
  symptoms of 430*f*
Allergic reaction 3

Allergy response 459
Allosteric site 471
Alpha-helix 401, 471
Alpha-linolenic acid 3
Ames test 471
Amino acid 3, 49, 56, 57, 400, 403, 404, 406, 407, 471
  absorption 408
    mechanism of 408
  activation of 409, 471
  aromatic 50, 406
  basic 405
  carbon skeleton of 410
  catabolism of 410
  chemical structure of 404
  classification of 404, 406
  essential 56, 57, 400, 404, 407, 476
  functions of 407
  general properties of 409
  glucogenic 478
  heterocyclic 50
  ketogenic 480
  non-essential 57, 404, 482
  non-polar 406
  physical classification of 404
  properties of 406
  semi-essential 56
  sources of 57
  symptoms of 410
  transport 99
Aminotransferases 400, 472
Ammonia toxicity 400
Amoxicillin 198
Amphibolic pathway 472
Ampholytes 406
Anabolism 3, 9, 343, 415, 472
Anaerobe 472
Anaplerotic reaction 472
Anderson's disease 385
Anemia 186*f*, 187, 207, 213, 221, 233, 315, 319, 447
  causes of 187
  Control Programme 316
  hemolytic 444
  macrocytic 4
  megaloblastic 79
  microcytic 4
  nutritional 114, 186
  signs 187
  symptoms of 187, 220*f*

Anganwadi worker, selection criteria of 323
Angina pectoris 262
Angstrom 472
Anhydride 472
Animal foods, protein of 57
Anion-exchange resin 472
Anomers 472
Anorexia 206
Anthropometric measurement, steps of 301*f*
Anthropometric methods 301
Antibiotics 196, 472
  use of 277
Antibody 459, 465, 472
  detection assays 468
  formation, theories of 462
  production of 58, 462
  proteins 56
  structure of 465*f*
Anticodon 472
Antigen 459, 464, 472
  complete 464
  detection assays 467
  presentation 461
Antigenic determinants 465
Antioxidant 3, 32, 85, 245, 282, 469
  rich foods 85*t*
Antiport 472
Apoenzyme 472
Apolipoprotein 472
Applied Nutrition Programme, activities of 322
Arginine, formation of 411
Arm 359
Arterial blood gas 428
  measurement of 127
Arterial disease, peripheral 41
Arthritis, seronegative 469
Ascites 256
Ascorbic acid 20, 283
Aspartate aminotransferase 421
Atherosclerosis 262, 397
  dietary management of 77
  sample diet for 77
Atom 106
Autoimmunity 459
Autotroph 472
Auxin 472
Auxotroph 472
Auxotrophic mutant 472
Avogadro's number 472

B

Back-mutation 472
Bacteria 265, 327, 329
Bacterial food poisoning 334
    prevention of 335
    types of 334
Bacteriophage 472
Baking 265, 270, 270f, 274
Balanced diet 3, 155, 156, 156f, 159, 160, 176, 177, 235f
    benefits of 161f
    calculation of 161, 161f
    components of 158, 158f
    elements of 156, 156f
    fundamentals of 164
    health benefits of 160
    long-term effects of 162b
    planning of 176
Balwadi Nutrition Programme 312, 316, 321
Barfoed's test 380
Basal metabolic rate 32, 42, 46, 47t, 472
Basic nutritional assessment 302t
Basophils 461
Behavioral factors 199
Benedict's test 380, 381f
Beriberi 79, 104, 163
    clinical manifestations of 95f
    infantile 211
Beta structure 401
Beta-carotene 3
Beta-oxidation 472
Bicarbonate 127, 134, 427
    buffer system 127
    ions 428
Bifidus factor 3
Bile
    acids 396
    duct
        inflammation of 444
        obstruction of 444
    flow of 202
    production 70
    salts 396, 472
        symptoms of 396
Biliary obstruction 445
Bilirubin 436, 443, 453
    excretion of 440
    serum 453
Binding energy 473
Biochemical
    functions 95b
    methods 303
    processes 426
Biochemistry 343, 345
    concept of 344
    history of 344
Biocytin 473
Biomolecule 343, 473
Biosphere 473
Biotin 457, 473
Bitot's spots 203, 298
Biuret test 403
Blanching 268, 269f, 279
Bland diet 232
Bleeding 207
    ulcer 251
Blood 64, 73
    cholesterol 64
    clotting 111, 246
    count 454
    gases 425
    glucose
        hormonal regulation of 379f
        levels 383
        monitoring 379, 379f
    loss 220
    pH, respiratory regulation of 427f
    plasma 427
    pressure, high 201
    sugar 382
        level 378, 383
        regulation of 39, 378
    test 207, 395, 446
    transfusions 221
    urea nitrogen 450, 451
    vessels 139
B-lymphocytes 461
Body
    building foods 23, 24
    fluids 131f
        consumption of 131
        physiology of 130
        sources of 131
        types of 131
    mass index 3, 32, 42, 45, 75, 298
        classifications 45
    mechanisms 110
    substances, symptoms of 38
    temperature, regulation of 131f
    water intake and output 129f
    weight 168
Boiling 265, 266, 266f
Bond energy 473
Bone
    formation of 110
    growth, maintenance of 85
Boron 218
Bovine spongiform encephalopathy 330
B-oxidation 391
Brain 378
Braising 272f
BRAT diet 226
Breastfeeding 178
Breathing problems 201
Bright's disease, degenerative 259
Bromelain 246
Buffer 473
    systems 426
Bureau of Indian Standards 293

C

Calciferol 85
Calcium 20, 106, 108, 109, 127, 133, 143, 217, 451
    absorption 109
    deficiency 110f, 223, 223f, 224
        causes of 111f, 223
        symptoms of 223
    functions of 109f, 110
    health benefits of 109f
    ions 372
    losses of 133
    regulation of 133
    rich foods 224f
    sources of 110f, 133
Calculi, types of 261
Calibration 327
Calorie 3, 32, 34, 43, 61, 258, 473
    value 35, 66
Calvin cycle 473
Cancer 26, 76
Canning procedure 279
Capsid 473
Carbamoyl phosphate formation 411
Carbanion 473
Carbocation 473
Carbohydrate 10, 14-16, 32, 33, 47, 48, 99, 247, 250, 253, 254, 258, 260, 362
    absorption of 38, 367, 368f
    chemical classification of 33
    classification of 33, 34f, 363f
    composition of 363
    deficiency of 40
    digestion of 38, 39f, 367, 368f
    food sources of 16, 37f
    functions of 17, 38, 38b, 364
    health benefits of 33f
    metabolism 368, 369f
    modified diets 238
    sources of 36t, 37, 37t
    structure of 363
    types of 363
    use of 363
Carbon
    atom, asymmetric 472
    dioxide 127
    fixation reactions 473
Carbonic acid buffer 427
Carboxyl-terminal residue 473
Carboxypeptidases, action of 408
Carcinogen 265
Cardiac diseases 422
Cardiac troponins 421
Cardiovascular disorders 262
Care-digestible diet 248
Carotenoids 473
Catabolism 3, 9, 32, 415, 473
Catabolite gene activator protein 473
Catalysts 58
Catecholamines 473
    formation of 412
Cation-exchange resin 473
Celiac disease 202, 204
Cell 343, 345, 427
    composition of 345, 346
    extensions 357
    functions of 345
    hepatic 377
    mediated immune
        response, induction of 463
    membrane 111, 346, 347, 381
        support 70
    parts of 346f
    protoplasm, symptoms of 407
    structural components of 355f
    structure of 345, 346, 346f
    surface, structure of 348
    wall 357, 358
Cellar storage temperature 278, 278f
Cellobiose 366
Cellular immune response 463
Cellular lipid metabolism 391
Cellulose 32

Index

Central Food Technological Research Institute 295
Central lymphoid organs 460
Central nervous system disorder 213
Centrifugation 475
Centriole 349, 354
Centromere 473
Cephalin 67
Cerebroside 67, 473
Chemical 327, 330
  agents 282
  hazards, types of 290f
  nature 406, 465
  preservative 282f
  properties 407
  toxins 249
  composition 23, 50, 52f
Chemiosmotic coupling 473
Chemistry 83, 86, 90, 98, 99, 102
Chemotaxis 473
Chemotroph 473
Chest circumference 302
Child Survival and Safe Motherhood Programmes 324
Childhood obesity 193, 199, 201f
  causes of 199
  complications of 201f
  consequences of 201f
  health implication of 200
  medical complications 200f
  symptoms of 200
Chloride 106, 124
  deficiency of 124
  functions of 133
  imbalance 124
Chlorine 124
Chlorophylls 473
Chloroplasts 473
Cholelithiasis 255
Cholestasis 256, 444
Cholesterol 3, 64, 67, 392, 395, 396
  biological significance of 70b
  biosynthesis of 396
  content 397
  functions of 70, 395
  health significance of 396
  high 201, 214
  metabolism 396
Chromatin 473
Chromatography 473
Chromium 22, 126, 218
Chromoproteins 52, 403
Chromosome 473
Chylomicron 473
Cilia 349, 355, 356f
Circulatory system 168
Cirrhosis 447
  diet chart 253f
Cis and trans isomers 473
Cistron 473
Citric acid
  cycle 362, 375, 473
    history of 375
    reaction steps 376f
    symptoms of 375
Citrulline formation 411
Clear fluid diet 233
Clear liquid diet 234, 234f

Cloning 473, 474
Cobalamin 474
Cobalt 22, 125
Codon 474
Coenzymes 79, 415, 417, 419, 474
Cofactor 417, 474
Colchicine 395
Cold storage 276, 277f
Collagen 403, 469
Colloidal osmotic pressure 137
Colon 168
Color reaction 402, 403
Colostrum 3
Coma, hepatic 254, 255t
Community 31, 325
  nutrition 314
Complementary feeding 180, 180b, 190
Compound lipids 65, 67
Compound microscope 360
Concentration 110
  test 452
Condenser lens 359
Confocal laser scanning microscope 360
Conjugated bilirubin test 446, 453
Conjugation pili 357
Conjunctiva 463
Constipation 249
  causes of 250
  diet plan 250f
Constitutive enzymes 474
Consumer protection 292
Consumption unit 3
Cooked food
  contamination of 334
  inadequate reheating of 334
Cookery rules 265
Cooking 339
  aims of 266b
  benefits of 266
  methods 266
    combination of 272
  objectives of 266, 266b
  softens connective tissues 266
  sterilizes food 266
Copper 21, 106, 125, 218
Cori cycle 372, 372f
Coronary heart disease 73, 163, 262
Coronavirus disease 2019 (COVID-19) 76
  symptoms, severe 76
Corticosteroids 474
Covalent bond 474
Creatine
  kinase 421
  phosphokinase 420
Creatinine clearance rate 452
Creutzfeldt-Jakob disease 330
Crigler-Najjar syndrome 444
Cristae 474
Critical control point 327
Crohn's disease 202, 204
Crystallization 106
Current nutritional deficiency status 313
Cyanocobalamin 19, 101, 216
Cyclic electron flow 474
Cyclic photophosphorylation 474
Cystic fibrosis 202, 204
Cytochromes 474
Cytokines 463
  production 461

Cytokinesis 474
Cytoplasm 349, 357, 474
  structure of 350f
Cytoskeleton 355f, 357, 474
Cytosol 475

D

Dairy 158, 164
  products 203
Dark reactions 475
De novo pathway 475
Deamination 99, 400, 407, 475
Decarboxylation 99, 376, 410
Decentralization 313
Deep frying 272f
Degenerate code 475
Dehydration 139, 198, 217
  clinical feature of 139f
  effects of 139
  management of 199t
  prevention of 139
  signs of 199t
  types of 198f
Dehydro freezing 279
Dehydrogenases 475
Deletion mutation 475
Dementia 213
Denaturation 475
Dendritic cells 461
Density 106
Dental diseases 26
Dentition 226
Deoxyribonucleic acid 475
  chimera 475
  cloning 475
  library 475
  ligase 475
  looping 475
  polymerase 475
  replicase system 475
Deoxyribonucleotides 475
Dephosphorylation 390
Dermatitis 212
Detergent 51, 327
Detoxification 416
  function 38
Dextrorotatory isomer 475
Dextrose 383
Diabetes mellitus 40, 41, 238, 362, 363, 378, 381, 475
  classification of 381
  complications of 41f
  insulin-dependent 239
  major complications of 42f
  non-insulin-dependent 239
  symptoms of 40f
  type 2 76, 163, 201
Diabetic diet 233
  chart 233f, 239f
Diabetic ketoacidosis 394, 434f
Dialysis 475
Diamino-monocaoxylic acid 50
Diaphragm 359
Diarrhea 198, 212, 249
Diet 26, 77, 185, 228, 230, 233, 245, 247, 257, 393, 448
  management 205

manual 226
modification of 251
order 226
plan 180
principles of 77, 253, 258, 259, 262, 263
roughage of 38
therapy 26, 227, 228b, 229f, 231, 231b, 244, 244f, 247, 249, 251, 259, 262, 263
general objectives of 228
principles of 228, 231, 248
pyramid of 231f
Dietary
assessment 300
considerations 249
counseling 257
energy intake, recommended level of 43
factors 249
fiber 14, 32, 33, 166, 169f
adverse effects of 170
functions of 168
health benefits 169f
intake 170f
recommended dietary allowance of 168
role of 167
sources of 167f
types of 167t
habits 261
history 306, 307
iron 438
management 77, 250, 254, 258-263
modifications 236, 254
protein 110
recommendations 10
restriction 256
sources 68, 100
supplement 32, 226
surveys, types of 306
Dietetics 227
Dietician, responsibilities of 229
Diffusion 136f, 475
Digestion 8, 12f, 32, 38, 70, 155, 368, 416, 475
ease of 247
intestinal 59
mechanism of 369f
Digestive system 9f
Dilution test 452
Dipeptides 408
Diploid 475
Dipole 475
Diprotic acid 475
Direct nutritional
assessment 301f
interventions 199
Direct short-term nutrition intervention 315
Disaccharide 362-365, 475
Discretionary calorie 157
allowance 164
Disulfide bridge 475
Double helix 475
Double-reciprocal plot 475
Doubly labeled water technique 42
Drugs 213, 249
Dry heat methods 269
Dry skin 203f
Drying method 280, 280f
Dubin-Johnson syndrome 444
Dumping syndrome 240
pathophysiology of 240f
Duodenal ulcer diet chart 251f

E

Early warning system 298
Edema 256
Elastin 403, 469
Electrochemical gradient 476
Electrolytes 32, 61, 79, 127, 131, 193, 249, 452
balance, maintenance of 134
imbalance 143
regulation of 132, 138
Electron 106
acceptor 476
carrier 476
donor 476
microscopes 360
transfer 476
Electrophile 476
Electrophoresis 459, 476
Empty calories 3, 226
Emulsification 388
Enantiomers 476
Endergonic reaction 417, 476
Endocrine glands 476
secretion of 47
Endocytosis 347, 348f, 476
Endonuclease 476
Endoplasmic reticulum 349, 350, 476
Endothermic reaction 476
End-product inhibition 476
Energy 32, 41, 244, 247, 250, 252, 254, 255, 259, 260, 262, 263
allowance 36, 55
balance 32
coupling 476
density 191
levels 162
measurement of 45
requirement 42, 43
components of 44
source of 69
units of 42
yielding 16
foods 23, 24
nutrients 226
Entamoeba histolytica 330
Enteral nutrition 79, 226
Entropy 476
Enzymatic functions 56
Enzyme 3, 79, 388, 415, 417, 422, 476, 486
activity, mechanism of 417
allosteric 471
characteristics of 415
classification of 416, 416t
concentration of 418
functions of 416
heterotropic 478
homotropic 479
intracellular 416
linked immunosorbent assay 467
competitive 467, 468
direct 467, 467f
indirect 467, 467f
non-competitive 467, 468, 468f
multiple forms of 419
preparations 285
production of 58
proteins 56
repressible 486

Enzymic proteins 53
Eosinophils 461
Epimerases 476
Epimers 476
Epithelial cell 476
Epithelial tissue, maintenance of 85
Epitope 465, 476
Erectile dysfunction 41
Erythrocyte 476
Erythroid cells 437, 437f
Erythropoietic porphyria 443
Escherichia coli 475, 476
enterohaemorrhagic 329, 330
Essential fatty acid 3, 73, 66, 388, 389, 476
deficiency of 73, 389
functions of 389
Estrogens 457
Ethanol fermentation 476
Ether 388
E-transport 474
Eukaryote 355f, 357, 476
cell
organization 356, 356f
structure of 358f
Excess fluid volume, diagnosis of 141f
Excretion 9, 109, 440
Exercise 382, 393, 448
benefits of 202f
Exergonic reaction 417, 476
Exocytosis 347, 348f, 476
Exon 476
Exonuclease 477
Exothermic reaction 477
Extracellular enzymes 416
Extreme sodium restriction 262
Eye complications 41
Eyepiece lens 359

F

Facultative cells 477
Family food, modified 190
Fasting triglyceride levels 73
Fat 14, 15, 17, 64, 68, 159, 247, 250, 251, 253, 254, 258, 262
absorption of 70, 71f
classification of 65, 65f
controlled diets 241
deficiency of 73
dietary sources of 68
digestion of 70, 71f
functions of 68, 68b
general functions of 69
metabolism 38, 99
modified diets 240
over consumption of 75, 75f
properties of 66
requirements 67, 68
soluble vitamin 79, 81, 82, 82t, 83f
sources of 17
storage of 73
types of 68
Fatty acid 3, 65, 388, 389, 477
activation of 391
biosynthesis of 389, 391
classification of 65f
essential 3, 73, 66, 388, 389, 476
long-chain 66

monounsaturated 4, 65
non-essential 66
oxidation of 391
polyunsaturated 4, 65, 389
saturated 4, 65, 487
short-chain 66, 170
symptoms of 389
syntheses complex, reactions of 389, 390*f*
unsaturated 4, 65, 389, 489
Fatty liver 257
  disease, nonalcoholic 201
Fecal excretion 168
Feeding
  intervals of 247
  requirements 236
Fermentation 265, 477
Ferritin 439
Fertility 203
Fever 247, 394
  diet chart in 247*f*
Fiber 3, 250
  diet, high 262
  mechanism of 166
  role of 169
Fibroblast 477
Fibrous proteins 55, 477
Filtration 137
Fimbriae 357
Fischer projection formulas 477
Five food group plans 23, 24*f*, 24*t*
Five year plan 317, 318
Flagella 349, 355, 357
  structure 356*f*
Flagellum 477
Flaky paint skin 195
Flavin
  adenine dinucleotide 477
  linked dehydrogenases 477
  mononucleotide 477
  nucleotides 477
Flavonoids 3, 33
Flavoprotein 477
Flexibility 313
Fluid 245, 247, 249, 250, 258-262
  balance 131*f*
    maintenance of 58, 134
  control 135*f*
  modified diets 243
  mosaic model 477
  pressure 137
  regulation of 138, 138*f*
  volume deficit 140
    diagnosis of 141*f*
Fluorescence 477
Fluoride 117
  deficiency of 118
  excess of 118
Fluorine 21
  deficiency 118*f*
  sources 118*b*
Folate 81
  rich foods 188
Folic acid 19, 81, 100, 215
  benefits 101*f*
  deficiency 215*f*
  functions of 101*f*
  sources of 216*f*
  supplementation 186

Folin's reaction 403
Folin's test 51
Food 4, 22, 182, 183, 186, 292
  additives 283, 283*f*
    advantages of 285
    agents 284
    disadvantages of 286
    effect 284
    functions of 284*b*
    purpose of 284*f*
    types of 283, 284*f*, 285*f*
  adulteration 286, 286*f*
    Act, prevention of 291, 292
  allergy 163, 226
  and Agricultural Organization 294
    objectives of 294
  and Nutrition Board 294
    activities of 294
  budget 176, 176*f*
  classification of 23, 23*f*
  consumption 266
  contact surfaces 328
  contamination, sources of 333, 334*f*
  diary 307
  digestion 9*f*
  effects of 47
  exchange system 3, 164
  expenditure 176
  fads and fallacies 172
  frequency questionnaire 307
  functions of 24, 25*f*, 69
  groups 23*f*
    basic 24, 24*t*, 157*t*, 164*t*
  handlers
    hygienic practices of 333, 334*f*
    role of 337
  handling of 335
  handling techniques 333
  healthy substances of 29
  hygiene 332
    basic rules of 336
  inadequate cooking of 334
  intake 168
  intolerance 226
  laws 291
  materials 287
  packing materials and techniques 290*f*
  poisoning 328, 333
    bacterial 334
  preparation 328
  preservation 274, 274*f*, 275*f*
    methods of 276
    principles of 275
  processing 69
  purchase of 335
  pyramid and exchange list 164*t*
  record 226
  safety 327, 329*f*, 331, 332, 338
    Act 1990 336
    and Microwave Cooking 338
    concept of 328
    consumer control points for 339
    measures 333*t*
    Regulations 336, 337
  sanitation 332
    principles of 333
  service establishment 328

sources 81, 87, 91, 93, 97, 98, 100, 101, 103, 112-114, 116, 118, 119*f*, 120
  spoilage 275
    causes of 275
  standards 293
  storage of 335
  stuff, types of 287*f*
  thermometer 335*t*
  types of 121, 164
Foodborne
  disease 334, 337
  illness 327
    outbreak 328
  infections 327
  intoxications 328
Foods, functional 33
Foot complications 41
Forbes diseases 384
Fortification 265
Fortified dairy products 205
Fortified soy products 205
Free radicals 3, 469
Free-energy 477
  change 477
Freeze drying 276, 277*f*, 281
Fructose 33, 366
  intolerance, hereditary 386, 386*f*
Frying 265, 271, 271*f*
Full fluid diet 234
Full liquid diet 232
Fumarate, formation of 411
Fundamental unit 42
Furanose 362, 477
Fusion protein 477
Futile cycle 477

G

G proteins 400
Galactose 366
Galactosemia 385
Gallbladder stones diet chart 256*f*
Gametes 477
Gamma-glutamyl transferase 421
Gamma-glutamyl transpeptidase 422, 455
Gangliosides 477
Gastrointestinal disorders 249
Gastrointestinal function 194
Gastrointestinal tract 139, 463
Gastroparesis 41
GCS system 41
Gel filtration 477
Gene 477, 486
  expression 477
  splicing 477
Genetic
  code 477
  disorders 163
  factors 200
  information 478
  map 478
Genitourinary tract 463
Genome 478
Genotype 478
Geometric isomers 478
Germanium 218
Germ-line cell 478
Giardiasis 202

Gilbert's syndrome 444, 448
Globin, fate of 440
Globular proteins 55, 478
Globulins 52, 402
Glomerular filtration rate 457
Glomerulonephritis 259
Glucogenic pathway 410
Gluconeogenesis 362, 369, 478
Glucose 366, 378
   alanine cycle 373, 373f
   formation 39
   maintenance 38
   regulation 379f
   tablets 383
   tolerance test 39, 39f, 379, 380f
   transport of 368
Glutelins 403
Glycans 362, 478
Glycerophosphatides 398
Glycerophospholipid 478
Glycocalyx 357
Glycogen 362
   storage disease 383
      types of 384, 384t
Glycogenesis 362, 368, 371, 372
   pathway of 372
   regulation of 372
Glycogenolysis 362, 368, 377
   pathway 377, 377f
   reaction of 377
Glycolipids 65, 67, 388, 390, 478
Glycolysis 368, 370, 478
   steps of 370, 371f
Glycoprotein 52, 403, 478
Glycosaminoglycan 478
Glycosidic bond 362, 478
Glyoxysome 478
Goiter 298
   endemic 26
   symptoms of 118f
Golgi apparatus 349, 351, 351f
Golgi complex 478
Good quality protein 57
Gout 257, 258, 394, 395
   advanced 395
   recurrent 395
   signs of 394
   symptoms of 394
Grain 156, 159, 164
Gram molecular weight 478
Grilling 265, 269, 270f, 274
Growth 12, 44, 57, 111
   monitoring and promotion 298
Gum disease 41

H

Hair 195
Haploid 478
Hapten 464
Haworth perspective formulas 478
Hazard analysis 328
   critical control point plan 328, 337
Head circumference 302
Health 10b, 11f, 314
   education 325
   status of 47
Hearing loss 41

Heart 139
   attack 420, 421
   beat, irregular 206
   disease 76
   problems 41
   rate monitoring 42
Heat 51
Heavy metals 330
Height-for-age 303
   nutritional index 298
Helicase 478
Heme 436, 478
   catabolism 436, 436f, 440
   degradation 440, 442f
      location of 440
      pathway 441
      significance of 441
   function of 437, 437f
   oxygenase 440
   protein 478
   sources of 440
   synthesis 437, 437f, 438
      steps of 441t
Hemochromatosis 256
   hereditary 441
Hemoglobin 427, 478
   levels 319
   symptoms of 99
Hemosiderin 439
Henderson-Hasselbalch equation 478
Hepatic encephalopathy 256
   diet chart 254f
Hepatitis 447
   A 446
   acute 444
   B 446
   C 446
   infective 252
Hepatocyte 478
Hers disease 385
Heteropolysaccharide 367, 478
Heterotroph 478
Hexose 362, 478
   monophosphate pathway 362
High blood pressure 201
   diet chart 263f
High calorie diets 237
High protein diet 237
   chart 233, 233f, 237f
High triglyceride 214
   levels, treatment of 74
High-performance liquid chromatography 478
Hill reaction 478
Histones 51, 403, 479
Holoenzyme 479
Homeobox 479
Homeodomain 479
Homeostasis 127, 479
Homeostatic mechanism 138
Homeotic genes 479
Homocystinuria 412, 413
Homologous genetic recombination 479
Homopolysaccharides 367
Horizontal nutritional programs 311
Hormone 3, 479, 489
   production of 58, 70
   receptor 479

Human body 129f
Human leukocyte antigens 469
Humoral immune response 462
Hydration 376, 377
Hydrogen bond 479
Hydrolases 416, 479
Hydrolysis 388, 479
Hydronium ion 479
Hydropathy index 479
Hydrophobic interactions 479
Hydrostatic pressure 137
Hydroxy amino acids 405
Hygiene control 335
Hypercalcemia 133, 143, 149
   signs of 148f
   symptoms of 148f
Hypercapnia 428
   signs of 430
   symptoms of 430
Hypercholesterolemia 73
Hyperchromic effect 479
Hyperhydration water intoxication 142b
Hyperkalemia 79, 133, 143, 147
   signs of 147f
   symptoms of 147f
Hyperlipidemia 3
Hypermagnesemia 133, 143, 151, 152f
Hypernatremia 133, 143, 144
   symptoms of 145b
Hyperosmolar hyperglycemic
   nonketotic syndrome 41
Hyperphosphatemia 127, 133, 153, 153f
Hypertension 41, 218, 262
   mild 262
   moderate 262
   risk of 119
   severe 262
Hyperthyroidism 257
   diet chart 257f
Hypervitaminosis 86, 103
Hypocalcemia 133, 143, 148, 148f
   causes of 148b
Hypochloremia 127
Hypoglycemia 382
   causes of 382
   signs of 383f
   symptoms of 383f
   treatment of 383
Hypokalemia 79, 133, 143, 146, 146f, 147
Hypomagnesemia 133, 143, 150, 150f
Hyponatremia 133, 143, 144, 145f
   clinical features 144f
Hypophosphatemia 127, 133, 152, 152f
Hypothalamus 138
Hypothyroidism 257

I

Imino acid 406
Immune response 459, 461, 479
Immune system
   cell of 460
   functions of 460
   response 59
   structure of 460
Immunity 162, 459, 463
   acquired 463
   active 464

artificial
  acquired 464
  passive 464
cell-mediated 459
cellular 464
herd 464
hormonal 459
humoral 464
innate 459, 463
local 464
natural
  acquired 464
  passive 464
passive 464
Immunochemistry 459
Immunoglobulin 466, 479
  A 466
    structure of 466
  D 466
  E 466
  G, structure of 466f
  M 466
    structure of 466f
Induction 479
Infections 41, 203
  bacterial 249
Ingestion 8
Insoluble fiber 33, 166f, 167
Insulin 372
  dose of 382
  long-acting 382
  short-acting 382
  types of 382
Integrated Child Development Services
  objectives of 317, 323
  Scheme 316, 317, 322
    packages of 323
Intercalation 479
International agency, role of 322
Intestinal worms 198
Intrauterine growth retardation 186
Intravenous iron 221
Iodine 21, 106, 115, 125, 218
  deficiency 222
    diagnosis of 223
    disorders 117
    symptoms of 222, 222f
    treatment of 223
  health benefits of 116f
  value 67
Ion
  channel 480
  exchange resin 480
Ionophore 480
Iris 359
Iron 21, 61, 106, 112, 187, 218
  absorption 438, 438f
  abundance 439
  additional sources of 187
  deficiency 117f, 207, 219, 219f, 221, 315, 439
    anemia 114f, 219, 219f, 220, 220f, 221f, 233f, 320, 320t
    test 207
  functions of 113f
  health benefits of 113f
  metabolism 113f
  prophylactic supplements of 222t
  regulation 439, 439f

rich foods 187, 188
sources of 114f, 438
storage 439
supplements 187
transport 438, 438f
Irradiation 277, 277f
Isoelectric pH 480
Isoenzyme 419, 480
Isomerases 416, 480
Isomers 480
Isoprene 480
Isotopes 480
Isozymes 419, 480

J

Jaundice 252, 436, 442-446, 448
  causes of 443
  complications of 446f
  diet chart 253f
  hemolytic 443, 444
  hepatic 444, 453
  hepatocellular 443
  neonatal 443, 444, 448
  obstructive 443
  prehepatic 453
  symptoms of 445, 445f
  types of 444
Joint
  fluid test 395
  pain 201

K

Keratinization 203
Keratins 403, 469, 480
Keratomalacia 203
Ketoacidosis 41, 433
Ketogenesis 393
Ketogenic pathway 411
Ketone bodies 343, 393, 480
  metabolism of 393
Ketose 480
Ketosis 394, 480
Kidney 138, 204
  failure diet chart 260f
  function test 450
    components of 450
  functional components of 450
  stones 395
  stones diet chart 261f
Killer cells, natural 461
Kilocalorie modifications 237
Kinases 480
Kinetics 480
Krebs cycle 362, 480
Kwashiorkor 62, 194, 195, 195t, 196
  clinical features of 61, 195

L

Lactase 33, 39
Lactate dehydrogenase 420
Lactation 44, 55
Lactic acid cycle 372, 372f
Lactoferrin 4
Lactose 33, 110, 366
  intolerance 163, 240

Lead poisoning 443
Lecithin 67
Legislation 336
Lens
  capsule 468
  epithelium 468
  fiber 469
  functions 468
  protein 468, 468f
  structure 468
Lethal mutation 480
Leucine zipper 480
Leukotrienes 480
Levorotatory isomer 480
Ligases 416
Light
  effects of 418
  reactions 480
Lineweaver-Burk equation 481
Linoleic acid 4
Lipase 420, 481
Lipid 4, 14, 17, 73, 388, 481
  biological functions of 389
  blood test 74t
  classification 390
  complex 390
  droplets 392
    functions of 392
    properties of 392
  metabolism 391
    disorders of 392, 393
  properties of 390
Lipoate 481
Lipoic acid 481
Lipoprotein 4, 52, 58, 388, 390, 397, 403, 481
  cholesterol, very low-density 75
  function of 70
  high-density 3, 64, 74, 392
  low-density 4, 64, 74, 392, 393
Liquid diets 232
  chart 232f
Listeria 330
Liver 168, 203, 378, 392, 438
  acute inflammation of 444
  cells 377
  cirrhosis 202, 253, 253f
  diet 252f
  disease 204, 251, 256, 422
    diet chart 252f
    enzyme profile for 422
  enzymes 453, 455
  function test 446, 447f, 452, 454, 454f
    abnormalities 455
Logo of Central Food Technological Research Institute 296f
Logo of Indian Council of Medical Research 295f
Low birth weight 186
Low calorie diet 232, 238t
  chart 232f, 238f
Low energy phosphate compound 481
Low fat diet 241
  chart 232, 232f, 241f
Low protein diet 232, 242f
Low sodium diet chart 232f, 242f
Lungs 139
Lyases 416, 481

Index

Lymphocytes 460, 481
  development 460
  processing of 460
Lymphoid
  organs, peripheral 460
  system 460
Lysis 481
Lysogeny 481
Lysosomes 349, 352, 481
  microscopic identification of 352f

M

Machine drying 276, 276f
Macrominerals 108
Macromolecule 481
Macronutrients 4, 15, 16, 17f, 166
Macrophages 461
Magma 106
Magnesium 21, 106, 121, 133, 143, 217
  deficiency 123f
    symptoms of 123f, 150f
  functions of 122f
  losses of 133
  regulation of 133
  sources of 133
Major histocompatibility 461
Malabsorption 79
Malnutrition 162
  acute 196f
  classification of 62
  clinical features of 198f
  physical signs of 305, 305t
  severe acute 196
  types of 26f
Maltase 39
Maltose 366
Manganese 106, 218
Maple syrup urine disease 412, 413
Marasmic kwashiorkor 61, 62, 193
Marasmus 61, 194, 195, 195t, 196
  clinical features of 61, 195
  nutritional 62
Mass 106
  action, law of 480
Mast cells 461
Matrix 481
McArdle disease 385
Meal planning 170, 171
  goals of 170
  objectives of 170
  steps in 174
Meal replacements 77
Medical nutrition therapy 226
Medium-chain triglycerides, use of 71
Megavitamins 79
Meiosis 481
Melanin, formation of 411
Membrane proteins 56
Menkes' disease 218
Mental health 26, 41
Messenger ribonucleic acid 481
Metabolic acidosis 127, 431f, 432
  mechanism of 433f
Metabolic alkalosis 127, 432
  mechanism of 433f
  symptoms of 434f
Metabolic disorders 257

Metabolism 4, 9, 39, 60, 72, 155, 481
  intermediary 480
  secondary 487
Metabolite 481
Metallic contamination 287
Metalloproteins 52, 403, 481
Metamerism 481
Michaelis-Menten
  constant 481
  kinetics 481
Microbial decomposition 275
Microbody 481
Microfilaments 349, 354, 355, 355f, 481
  structure 356f
Microminerals 108, 125
Micronutrients 4, 15-17, 18f
  deficiencies 198
  types of 18f
Microorganism 265
Microscope 343, 359, 359f
  types of 360
Microsomes 481
Microtubules 349, 354, 355f, 481
Microvilli 349
Microwave 272f, 272
  cooking 272
Mid-day Meal Programme 316, 318
  aims of 318
  concept of 318
  history of 318
Mid-upper arm circumference 196, 298, 302
Milk 30, 157
  hygiene 332
  pasteurization 277f
  products 30
Millon's reactions 403
Minerals 11, 14, 79, 106, 107, 245, 247, 250,
    253, 254, 263
  classification of 107
  deficiency diseases 217
  elements 20
  types of 217t
Ministry of Health and Family Welfare 312
Ministry of Women and Child Welfare 323f
Mission 295, 296
Mitochondria 349, 352
  functions of 354f
  structure of 349f, 353f
Mitosis 481
Mixed-function oxidases 481
MKS system 41
Moist heat methods 266
Molar solution 481
Mole 481
Molybdenum 218
Monoamine monocarboxylic acids 50
Monoamino-dicarboxylic acid 50
Monoclonal antibodies 462, 482
Monoprotic acid 482
Monosaccharide 362-364, 482
Monounsaturated fat 15, 64
Morbidity 12
Mortality 12
Motile proteins 53
Mouth 59, 70
Mucopolysaccharide 482
Mucoprotein 52, 403
Multienzyme system 482

Multi-test systems 379
Muscle
  cells 377
  contraction 111
  diseases 421
  relaxation 111
Mutagenesis, site-directed 487
Mutases 482
Mutation 482
Mycobacterium tuberculosis 263
Myocardial infarction 262
Myofibril 482
Myosin 469, 482

N

Nasogastric tube feeding 235f
National Goitre Control Programme 317, 320
National Institute of Public Cooperation and
    Child Development 296
National Nutritional Anemia Program 319
National Nutritional Policy 27, 315
National Nutritional Programs 311, 315f
  and Role of Nurse 311, 324
Nephropathy 41
Nephrosis 259
Nerve impulse 118
  transmission 111
Neural mechanism 139
Neuron 482
Neuropathy 41
Neurotransmitter 482
Neutral fat 4
Neutron 107
  microscope 360
Neutrophils 461
Niacin 19, 97, 99, 212
  benefits of 98f
  deficiency 104, 213f
  formation of 411
Nicotinamide adenine dinucleotide 482
  phosphate 482
Nicotinic acid 19, 97
Night blindness 86, 86f, 163, 202
Ninhydrin reaction 482
Nitrogen
  cycle 482
  fixation 482
Nitrogenase complex 482
Nitroprusside test 403
Nodules 394
Non-blood tests 457
Noncommunicable disease 11
Noncompetitive inhibition 482
Noncyclic electron flow 482
Nonheme iron proteins 482
Non-protein nitrogenous substances 414
Nonsense mutation 482
Nonsteroidal anti-inflammatory drugs 395
Nuclear envelope, intracellular
    membrane systems of 350
Nucleases 482
Nucleic acids 482
  precursors of 38
Nucleoid 357, 482
Nucleolus 482
Nucleophile 482
Nucleoplasm 482

Index

Nucleoproteins 52, 403
Nucleoside 482
   diphosphate
      kinase 482
      sugar 483
   monophosphate kinase 483
Nucleosome 483
Nucleotide 483
Nucleus 348, 348f, 483
   morphology of 348
   structure of 350f
Nurse
   health promotion role 164
   responsibilities of 309
   role of 30, 30b, 47, 78, 104, 202, 224, 229, 263, 263f
   serving diet 227f
Nursing
   home 30
   intervention 140, 142, 144, 149, 151, 152, 153, 154
   management 382
Nutrients 4, 14, 14f, 32, 53, 165, 193, 266
   caloric values of 34t
   classification of 14, 16f
   elements of 16
   essential 226
   inorganic 14
   malabsorption 249
   modification of 229, 230
   preservation of 265, 273
   proportion of 35f
   recommended dietary allowance of 183t
   review of 16
   source 69
Nutrition 3, 4, 7, 7f, 10b, 11f, 26, 228, 228b, 314
   across life cycle 177
   acute 197f
   assessment 226, 298, 299
      methods 300f
      steps of 308f
   care 243b
      process 226
      protocols 226
   classification of 8f
   concept of 7
   disorders 224
   education 298, 308, 309
      aspects of 308b
      principles of 309
   history of 5, 5b, 6t
   interventions 314
   knowledge 31
   loss 274f
   physiology of 8
   problems 26
   programme 312, 322
   relation of 11
   role of 10, 10f, 227f
   screening 226, 299
   Society of India 294
   status 4
   support 226
   surveillance 299
   survey 298, 299
Nutritional assessment
   methods of 300
   steps 301f
   systems of 299
Nutritional deficiency disorders 162, 163t, 193
Nutritional education 307
   methods of 309
Nutritional index 298
Nutritional status 62, 228, 302
Nutritive foods
   development of 294
   enhancement of 294
Nutritive value 23, 29, 321

O

Obesity 75, 75f, 163, 204
   childhood 193, 199, 201f
   medical complications of 76f
Obstruction 444, 447
Oligomer 483
Oligonucleotide 483
Oligopeptide 483
Oligosaccharides 33, 362, 364, 366, 483
   classification of 34t
Omega-3 fatty acids 64
Oncogene 483
Oncotic pressure 137
Optical microscopes 360
Optimal complementary feeding, benefits of 180f
Optimum
   nutrition 155
   pH 483
Oral contraceptives 213
Oral rehydration
   salt 139
   therapy 139
Organ
   function tests 450
   meat 258
   protection 69
   specificity 465
   systems 426
Organelles 483
Organic compounds 51
Organic nutrients 14
Ornithine 411
Osmolality 137
Osmolarity 137
Osmosis 136, 136f, 281f, 483
Osmotic pressure 137, 483
Osteoarthritis 76
Osteomalacia 89, 90f, 111, 205
   features of 89f
Osteoporosis 90, 90f, 111, 193
Over hydration 139
Over nutrition 162
Oxidation 376, 377, 391, 483
   reduction reaction 483
Oxidative 373f
   deamination 407, 410
   phase 374
   phosphorylation 483
   rancidity 67
Oxidoreductases 416
Oxygen delivery 426
Oxygenases 481, 483

P

Pain, severe 394
Painkillers, natural 246f
Palindrome 483
Pancreas 168, 202, 378, 379f
Pancreatic protease 408
Pantothenic acid 19, 100, 100f, 214
Paradigm 483
Parasites 328, 330
Parathyroid
   gland 139
   hormone 127
Parenteral feeding 236
Parenteral nutrition 79, 226
Partially complete protein 51, 57
Passive immunization, use of 464
Pasteurization 276, 279
Pellagra 79, 104
   symptoms of 213
Pentosans 34
Pentose 362, 483
   phosphate pathway 373, 373f, 374, 374f, 483
Peptic ulcer 250
   diet chart 251f
Peptidase 483
Peptide 400, 403, 483
   bond 400, 483
   mapping 483
Peptidoglycan 483
Peptones 403
Permeases 484
Peroxisomes 352, 353f
Personal hygiene 333, 337
Pest control 336
pH 425, 484
   effects of 418
   function of 426
   scale 424f
Phagocytosis 461
Phenotype 484
Phenylketonuria 412, 415
Phosphate 134
   buffer 427
   functions of 134
Phosphatides 65
Phosphodiester linkage 484
Phosphogluconate pathway 484
Phosphoinositides 398
Phospholipids 65, 67, 388, 390, 398, 484
   biosynthesis of 398
   functions of 69
Phosphoproteins 52, 403
Phosphorolysis 484
Phosphorus 20, 111, 218, 259, 451
Phosphorylation 390
   potential 484
Photochemical reaction center 484
Photon 484
Photophosphorylation 484
Photoreduction 484
Photorespiration 484
Photosynthesis 484
Photosynthetic phosphorylation 484
Photosystem 484
Phototroph 484
Phylloquinone 85
Physical activity 44
   level 42
   ratio 42
Phytochemicals 4

Index

Pickling 282, 282f
Pituitary gland 138
Plant cells 358
Plasma
   membrane 346, 357, 484
      prokaryotic cell structures outside of 357
   proteins 484
Plasmalogen 484
Plasmid 357, 484
Plastids 358, 484
Platelets 484
Poaching 268, 269f
Polar 484
   amino acids 406
Polarity 484
Polyclonal antibodies 484
Polydipsia 381
Polylinker 484
Polymerase chain reaction 484
Polymorphonuclear leukocytes 461
Polynucleotide 484
Polypeptide 49, 400, 408, 484
   chain
      elongation of 409
      initiation of 409
      termination of 409
Polyphagia 382
Polyribosome 484
Polysaccharides 34, 38, 362-364, 366, 484
   complex 34
Polysome 484
Polyunsaturated fat 15, 64
Polyuria 381
Pompe disease 384
Poor diet 220
Porphyria 442
   acute intermittent 443
   cutanea tarda 443
Porphyrin 484
Post-translational modification 484
Potassium 21, 106, 120, 127, 132, 143, 217, 259, 260, 261
   amount of 121
   health benefits of 120f
   losses of 132
   modified diets 242
   sources of 132
Pregnancy 44, 55, 183, 213, 220
   anemia in 186
Pressure
   cooking 268, 268f
   regulation 137f
Primary protein-energy undernutrition 193
Primase 485
Projection formulas 485
Prokaryotes 356, 356f, 485
   genetic material of 357
Prokaryotic cells, structure of 357, 357f
Prolamins 403
Prophage 485
Prostaglandins 485
Prostate specific antigen 422
Prosthetic group 485
Protamines 51, 403
Proteases 403
Protective foods 23, 190

Protein 10, 14, 15, 17, 49, 51-53, 55, 57, 59f, 158, 247, 250, 252, 254, 258-263, 400, 402, 403, 451, 485
   absorption of 60f, 407
   allowances 55
   biological value of 57
   biosynthesis of 408
   buffers 427
   calorie malnutrition 26, 193, 193f, 226
   chemical properties of 51, 51b
   classification of 17, 51, 51f, 52f, 53, 53f, 402
   color reaction of 403
   complementary 226
   complete 51, 52, 57
   conjugated 17, 49, 51, 403, 474
   contractile 53
   deficiency 61
      symptoms of 61
   denatured 475
   digestion of 59, 60f, 407, 408
   energy malnutrition 4, 62, 314
      clinical features of 194
      symptoms of 195
   energy undernutrition
      classification of 193
      clinical manifestations of 194f
      etiology of 193
      pathophysiology of 194
      secondary 194
   excess 61
   foods 251
   functions of 57, 58f
   general characteristics of 50
   good sources of 53
   homologous 479
   incomplete 51, 57
   kinases 400, 485
   metabolism 61f, 99, 409
      disorders 412
   oligomeric 483
   organization, levels of 49f
   over consumption of 62
   peripheral 483
   physical properties of 50
   properties of 50
   quality of 57
   simple 17, 49, 51, 402, 487
   sources of 53
   sparing action 38
   storage of 55, 407
   structural 53, 55
      organization of 401
   structure 50, 426
      types of 50f
   targeting 485
Proteoglycan 485
Prothrombin time 454
Proton 107
   acceptor 485
   donor 485
   motive force 485
Proto-oncogene 485
Protoplasm 485
Pseudojaundice 444
Purines 258, 485
Puromycin 485
Pyranose 485
Pyridine nucleotide 485

Pyridoxal phosphate 485
Pyridoxine 19, 99, 213
   functions 99f
   health benefits of 100f
Pyrimidine 485
   dimer 485
Pyrophosphatase 485
   inorganic 479
Pyruvate metabolism, disorders of 387
Pyruvic acid 368

Q

Quantum 485
Quaternary structure 485
Quetelet's index 45
Quick freezing process 279

R

Racemic mixture tracemate 485
Radiation 283, 283f
   effects of 418
Radioactive iodine uptake 457
Radioactive isotope 485
Radioimmunoassay 485
Raw food, consumption of 335
Reabsorption 137
Redox pair 486
Redox reaction 486
Relax muscles 118
Renal diet chart 259f
Renal diseases 422
Renal failure
   acute 259
   chronic 260
Replication 486
Replisome 486
Repression 486
Reproduction 85
Reproductive and Child Health Programme 324
Resistant starch 33
Respiration 486
Respiratory
   acidosis 127, 429, 431f
   alkalosis 127, 431, 432f
   chain 486
   disorder 263
   system 427f
   tract 463
Restriction endonucleases 486
Restriction fragment 486
   length polymorphisms 486
Reticuloendothelial system 460
Retinol 81, 85
   deficiency 103
Retrovirus 486
Rheumatoid
   arthritis 215, 257
   diet chart 257f
Rhodopsin 79
Riboflavin 19, 96, 211
   deficiency 104, 211, 212f
   use of 96f
   vitamin b2 96f
Ribonuclease 486

Ribonucleic acid 486
  polymerase 486
  splicing 486
Ribonucleotide 486
Ribosomal ribonucleic acid 486
Ribosomes 349, 357, 486
Ribozymes 486
Rickets 79, 88, 89f, 104, 162, 205, 298
Roasting 265, 269, 269f, 274
Rothera's test 393
Rotor's syndrome 444
Rough endoplasmic reticulum 351, 351f

S

S-adenosylmethionine 487
Salmonella enterica 332
Salt
  free diet 232
  high concentration of 281
  inorganic 51
Salvage pathway 487
Sanger's reaction 51
Saponification 487
Sarcomere 487
Saturated fat 15, 64, 66, 68
Scanning
  acoustic microscope 360
  helium ion microscope 360
  probe microscopes 360
Scleroproteins 52, 403
Scurvy 79, 104, 163, 298
Selenium 22, 106, 126, 218
Shine-Dalgarno sequence 487
SI system 42
Sickle cell
  anemia 487
  trait 487
Sickness 230
Silicon 218
Skeletal disease 26
Skeletal muscle 392
Skin 394, 463
  care 214
  complications 41
  irritation 203
Sleep apnea 76
Small intestine 59, 60f, 71, 72f, 168, 392
Smooth endoplasmic reticulum 351, 351f
Sodium 21, 106, 118, 127, 132, 143, 217, 259-262
  balance 134, 135f
  health benefits of 119f
  hypobromide test 414
  imbalance 119
  losses of 132
  regulation of 132
  restricted diets 242, 262
  restriction
    mild 262
    severe 262
  sources of 132
Soft food diet 234
  chart 234f
Soft light diet 232
Solar cooking 265, 272, 273f
Soluble fiber 32, 166f, 167
Somatic cells 487
Sore 207

Southern blot 487
Special feeding methods 235
Special Nutrition Programme 312, 316, 319
Sphingolipids 398, 487
Spray drying 280
Stem cells 487
Stereo microscope 360
Steroids 388, 395
  hormones 396
Sterols 65, 67, 388, 487
  functions of 69
Stewing 265, 267, 267b, 267f
Stomach 59, 71, 168
Stress control 40
Stroke 41, 76
Stroma 488
Substrate 415, 488
  concentration of 418
  level phosphorylation 488
Succinyl coenzyme A, hydrolysis of 376
Sucrase 39
Sucrose 366
Sugar 32, 33
  alcohols 33
  high concentration of 281
Suicide inhibitor 488
Sulfur 106, 218
  containing amino acids 50, 405
Sun drying 280
Supplementary Feeding Programme 316
Suppressor mutation 488
Swollen gums 207
Synergistic activity, convergence of 319
Synthases 488

T

T3 tests 456
T4 tests 456
Taenia solium 330
Tamil Nadu Integrated Nutrition Program 312, 317
Tarui's disease 385
Taste 406
Teeth, maintenance of 110
Telomere 488
Temperature 328
  control 336
  danger zone 338
  effects of 418
  regulation 69
  use of 278
Tetany 111
Tetrahydrobiopterin 488
Tetrahydrofolate 488
Therapeutic diet 226-228, 228f, 231, 263, 263f
  purposes of 229f
Therapeutic feeding interventions 199
Thermodynamics
  first law of 477
  second law of 487
Thiamine 19, 93, 96
  deficiency 104, 208
  pyrophosphate 488
Thioester 488
Thiolester synthesis 376
Three-dimensional endoplasmic reticulum 350f
Thromboxanes 488

Thylakoid 488
Thymus 460
Thyroglobulin 457
Thyroid
  antibody tests 456
  diet chart 257f
  function test 455, 457
  hormone, formation of 412
Tissues 392, 426
  culture 488
T-lymphocytes 460
Toasting 270, 270f
Tocopherols 79, 85, 488
Topoisomerases 488
Topoisomers 488
Toxicity 93, 115, 120-122, 206, 213, 215, 217
  symptoms of 206
Toxins 488
  bacterial 249
Trace elements 21, 124, 124f, 488
Transaminase 421, 455, 488
Transcription 408, 488
Transduction 488
Trans-fatty acids 4, 68
Transferases 416
Transferrin carries iron 439
Translocase 489
Transmethylation 410
Transmission electron microscopy 360
Transport proteins 53, 56
  production of 58
Triacylglycerides 388
Triacylglycerol 489
Triglycerides 4, 64, 65, 393
  functions of 69
Triose 489
Tropin 489
Tryptophan 99
Tube feeding 227, 236
Tuberculosis 263
  diet chart 263f
Twenty-four hour recall method 306
Twenty-Points Programme 323
Typhoid
  diet chart 248f
  fever 247
Tyrosinemia 412, 413

U

Ultraviolet radiation 489
Unconjugated bilirubin test 446, 453
Unit membrane, structure of 347
Unsaturated fats 66, 68
Urea 414
  clearance 451
  cycle 400, 411, 489
  formation of 411
  serum 450
Uric acid 414
  diet chart 258f
  pathway 362
Urinary calculi 261
Urinary disorders 259
Urinary tract, infection of 261
Urine examination 450
Urolithiasis 261
Utensil 328

V

Vaccines 464
Van den Bergh
  reaction 446f
  test 436
Vanadium 218
Vertical nutritional programs 311
Very low calorie diet 238, 238f
Vibrio cholerae 330
Viral vector 489
Viruses 328, 330, 489
Vision 84, 295, 296
Vitamin 10, 14, 17, 79, 81, 85, 94, 163, 245, 247, 250, 253, 254, 263, 303, 489
  A 18, 61, 81-83, 85, 85f, 203
    absorption 84
    deficiency 103, 202, 203, 203f, 315
    health benefits of 83f
    leads, deficiency of 203f
    Prophylaxis Programme 316
    types of 81t
  B1 80
    deficiencies 208, 208f
  B12 19, 81
    benefits of 101f
    deficiency 216f
    rich foods 102f
  B2 80
    deficiency 97f, 212f
  B3 80, 98f
    benefits of 98f
    deficiency 212f
  B5
    deficiency 214f
    rich foods benefits 215f
    sources of 100f
  B6 80, 99f, 100f
    deficiency, symptoms of 213f
    food sources of 214f
  C 81, 102, 246
    deficiency 104, 206, 206f, 207, 208
    food sources of 103f
    functions of 103f
    health benefits of 102f
    prominent food sources of 208f
  classification of 80, 80f
  D 18, 81, 85, 86, 86f, 127
    biological functions of 87f
    deficiency 88f, 104, 203, 204, 204f, 205, 205f, 206, 315, 320
    production 70
  deficiency 26, 103
    disorders 193, 202
  E 18, 81, 85, 90, 91f
    benefits of 91f
    biochemical function of 91, 91b
    deficiency symptoms 92f
    food sources of 93f
  fat-soluble 79, 81, 82, 82t, 83f
  foods 80f
  K 18, 81, 82, 85, 92
    deficiency 93f, 104
    health benefits of 92f
  types of 80t
  water-soluble 79, 82, 82t, 93, 94t, 209t

V

Vomiting 217
Von Gierke's diseases 384

W

Waist circumference 302
Wasting disorders 194
Water 11, 14, 127
  balance 134
  consumption 129
  daily output of 129
  functions of 128b, 129f
  intoxication 139, 142
    symptoms of 142
  ion product of 480
  metabolism 130
  primary functions of 131
  requirement 128
  soluble vitamin 79, 82, 82t, 93, 94t, 209t
Waxes 65, 390
Weaning 189
  foods 4
  problems of 189
Weighed intake method 306
Weight loss 206
  surgeries 204
Weight-for-age 298, 303
Weight-for-height 196, 298, 303
Wheat-based supplementary nutrition programme 312
Wilson disease 218, 256
World Food Programme 321
Wound, healing of 41, 214, 246

X

Xanthoproteic test 51
Xerophthalmia 103, 203
X-ray
  crystallography 489
  microscope 360
  test 207

Y

Yield energy 38
Yolk sac 392

Z

Zinc 22, 106, 115, 125, 218
  deficiency 116f
  finger 489
  role of 115f
Zwitter ions, formation of 407
Zymogen 489